Manual of Dietetic Practice

Manual of Dietetic Practice

Editorial Group
on behalf of the British Dietetic Association

Chairman
Greta Walton
Chairman British Dietetic Association 1983—5
Alison Black
Celia Firmin
Christine Russell
Briony Thomas
Jacki Tredger

Editor
Briony Thomas

The British Dietetic Association was founded in 1936 to advance the science and practice of dietetics and to promote the training and continuing education of dietitians.

Today it is established as the only society to represent the interest of qualified practitioners in the United Kindom and is recognized as such throughout the world.

Manual of Dietetic Practice

Edited for
The British Dietetic Association by

Briony Thomas BSc, PhD, SRD

Formerly Research Nutritionist
Unit for Metabolic Medicine
Department of Medicine
Guy's Hospital
London

Foreword by

R.J.L. Allen

Honorary President
British Dietetic Association

Blackwell Scientific Publications
OXFORD   LONDON   EDINBURGH
BOSTON   PALO ALTO   MELBOURNE

© 1988 by
Blackwell Scientific Publications
Editorial offices:
Osney Mead, Oxford OX2 0EL (*Orders*: Tel. 0865 240201)
8 John Street, London WC1N 2ES
23 Ainslie Place, Edinburgh EH3 6AJ
Three Cambridge Center, Suite 208, Cambridge
Massachusetts 02142, USA
667 Lytton Avenue, Palo Alto, California 94301, USA
107 Barry Street, Carlton, Victoria 3053, Australia

First published 1988

Set by Setrite Typesetters Ltd
Hong Kong
Printed and bound in Great Britain by
Redwood Burn Ltd
Trowbridge, Wilts

DISTRIBUTORS

USA
  Year Book Medical Publishers
  200 North LaSalle Street,
  Chicago, Illinois 60601
  (*Orders*: Tel. 312 726-9733)

Canada
  The C.V. Mosby Company
  5240 Finch Avenue East, Scarborough, Ontario
  (*Orders*: Tel. 416-298-1588)

Australia
  Blackwell Scientific Publications (Australia) Pty Ltd
  107 Barry Street, Carlton, Victoria 3053
  (*Orders*: Tel. (03) 347 0300)

British Library Cataloguing in Publication Data

Manual of dietetic practice.
  1. Diet
  I. British Dietetic Association
  II. Thomas, Briony
  613.2   RA784

ISBN 0-632-01481-4

Contents

SECTION 3
NUTRITIONAL NEEDS OF POPULATION SUB-GROUPS

SECTION 4
THERAPEUTIC DIETETICS FOR DISEASE STATES

A: Metabolic and endocrine disorders

B: Disorders of the mouth and gastrointestinal tract

List of Contributors

RACHEL ABRAHAM BSc, SRD *Senior Metabolic Dietitian, Northwick Park Hospital, Harrow, Middlesex.*

ALISON M ANDERTON BSc, SRD *Senior Renal Dietitian, St Peter's and St Philip's Hospitals, London*

AVRIL DIANE ASLETT-BENTLEY BSc, MSc, SRD *Consultant Nutritionist/Dietitian, Batley*

CAROL BATEMAN SRD *District Dietitian, Royal Free Hospital, London*

SUSAN E BENNETT SRD *Senior Renal Dietitian, Leicester General Hospital*

SHEILA BINGHAM BSc, PhD, SRD *Chief Research Officer, MRC Dunn Clinical Nutrition Centre, Cambridge*

ALISON E BLACK BSc, SRD *Chief Research Officer, MRC Dunn Nutrition Unit, Cambridge*

CAROL BOWYER SRD *Senior Dietitian, St George's Hospital, London*

BRENDA CLARK SRD *Chief Paediatric Dietitian, Royal Hospital for Sick Children, Glasgow*

ISOBEL COLE-HAMILTON BSc, SRD *Project Officer, London Food Commission*

MARY C COOPER SRD *Senior Community Dietitian, St. Mary's Hospital, Leeds*

JENNIFER COUTTS SRD *Chief Dietitian, Royal Manchester Children's Hospital*

PATRICIA E CROOKS SRD *District Dietitian, Walton Hospital, Liverpool*

BARBARA DAVIDSON BSc, SRD *Formerly Senior Dietitian, Royal Free Hospital, London*

NEIL DONNELLY BSc, SRD *District Dietitian, Victoria Hospital, Blackpool*

WENDY DOYLE BA, SRD *Research Dietitian, Institute of Zoology, London*

JANE EATON SRD *District Dietitian, Oxfordshire Health Authority*

LIZ EELEY BSc, SRD *Senior Research Dietitian, Diabetes Research Laboratories, Radcliffe Infirmary, Oxford*

PAULINE M EMMETT BSc, SRD *Senior Research Dietitian, University Department of Medicine, Bristol Royal Infirmary*

STANLEY J EVANS BSc, PhD *Top Grade Biochemist, Northampton General Hospital*

CELIA FIRMIN BSc, SRD *District Dietitian, Staincliffe Hospital, Dewsbury*

MARGARET S N GELLATLY SRD *District Dietitian, Mid Essex Health Authority*

MARGARET HEANEY BSc, SRD *Senior Community Dietitian, Victoria Hospital, Blackpool*

MARGARET D HOLDSWORTH BSc, PhD *Principal Researcher, Gerontology Nutrition Department, Royal Free Hospital School of Medicine, London,*

J P HOWARD SRD *District Dietitian, Bristol Royal Infirmary*

SUSAN M HOWIE SRD *Senior Community Dietitian, North Staffordshire Health Authority*

PATRICIA M HULME BSc, SRD *Chief Research Dietitian, Northwick Park Hospital, Harrow, Middlesex*

MAUREEN HUNTER BSc, SRD *Chief Dietitian, The Royal Marsden Hospital, London*

MONICA B KATAKITY MPhil, SRD *Senior Metabolic Dietitian, Royal National Orthopaedic Hospital, Stanmore, Middlesex*

JENNIFER K KING BSc, SRD *District Dietitian, Stoke Mandeville Hospital, Aylesbury Vale Health Authority*

PETER KING BSc, SRD *Senior Dietitian, St Lawrence Hospital, Chepstow*

CAROL LOGAN BA, SRD *Area Dietitian, Lothian Health Board*

ANNE de LOOY BSc, PhD, SRD *Senior Lecturer in Nutrition and Dietetics, Leeds Polytechnic*

JANET P LOWELL BSc, SRD *Senior Lecturer in Nutritional Science, Robert Gordon's Institute of Technology, Aberdeen*

SUSAN LUPSON BSc, SRD *District Dietitian, Lancaster Health Authority*

ANITA MACDONALD SRD *Senior Paediatric Dietitian, St James University Hospital, Leeds*

JILL METCALFE SRD *Chief Dietitian, British Diabetic Association*

LESLEY A M MICHAEL SRD *Senior Paediatric Dietitian, Alder Hey Children's Hospital, Liverpool*

CHRISTINE MORLEY BSc, SRD *District Dietitian, George Elliot Hospital, Nuneaton*

MARION NOBLE SRD *Senior Paediatric Dietitian, Westminster Children's Hospital, London*

SYLVIA ROBERT-SARGEANT SRD *Consultant Nutritionist, Brentford, Middlesex*

CHRISTINE A RUSSELL SRD *Chief Dietitian, General Hosptial, Northampton*

JENNY SALMON BSc, MSc, SRD *Director, Food Development & Research, KMS Partnership Ltd, Windsor*

DOUGLAS W SCOTT BSc, SRD *District Dietitian, County Hospital, Lincoln*

ROSEMARY SEDDON SRD *Freelance Dietitian, Ruislip, Middlesex*

K E SIMPSON SRD *Consultant Dietitian, Action Research for Multiple Sclerosis, Senior Dietitian, Watford General Hospital*

DIANE SPALDING SRD *District Dietitian, Groby Road Hospital, Leicester*

JOHN STANTON BSc, SRD *Chief Paediatric Dietitian, Booth Hall Children's Hospital, Manchester*

KATE START SRD *Chief Paediatric Dietitian, Evelina Children's Hospital, Guy's Hospital, London*

BRIONY THOMAS BSc, PhD, SRD *Formerly Research Nutritionist, Unit for Metabolic Medicine, Department of Medicine, Guy's Hospital, London*

DENISE THOMAS MPhil, SRD *Senior Dietitian, St. James' Hospital, Portsmouth*

PATRICIA E TORRENS SRD *Formerly Dietetic Adviser, Department of Health and Social Security*

JACKI TREDGER BSc, PhD, SRD *Lecturer in Nutrition, University of Surrey*

E W WALTON MD, FRCPath *Consultant Pathologist, North Tees General Hospital, Stockton-on-Tees*

RAE WARD BSc, SRD *Consultant Dietitian, Henley-on-Thames*

PAMELA WILLIAMS SRD *District Dietitian, Southmead Hospital, Bristol*

RICHARD WILSON BSc, SRD *District Dietitian, King's College Hospital, London*

S A WOOTTON BSc, PhD *Teaching Fellow in Nutrition, Southampton University*

Acknowledgements

Miss Barbara Aitken, *Senior Dietitian, Hammersmith Hospital, London*

Alder Hey Children's Hospital, Liverpool — *Dietetic Department*

Dr CJ Bates, *Member of Scientific Staff, MRC Dunn Nutrition Unit, Cambridge.*

Miss PJ Brereton *District Dietitian, Northwick Park Hospital, Harrow*

Professor Forrester Cockburn *Professor of Child Health, University Department of Child Health, Royal Hospital for Sick Children, Glasgow*

The Coeliac Society

Dr TJ Cole *Member of Scientific Staff, MRC Dunn Nutrition Unit, Cambridge*

Dr CM Colley *Consultant Chemical Pathologist, Princess Margaret Hospital, Swindon*

Professor Michael Crawford *Department of Nutritional Biochemistry, Nuffield Laboratory of Comparative Medicine, Institute of Zoology, London*

Dr TJ David *Senior Lecturer in Child Health, University of Manchester, Hon. Consultant Physician, Booth Hall Children's Hospital, Manchester*

Dr Louise Davies *Head, Gerontology Nutrition Unit, Royal Free Hospital School of Medicine, London*

Miss Sally Day *District Dietitian, St George's Hospital, London*

Miss Dorothy Francis *Chief Dietitian, Great Ormond Street Hospital for Sick Children, London*

Dr DR Fraser *Member of Scientific Staff, MRC Dunn Nutrition Unit, Cambridge*

Mr JG Guest *Consultant Surgeon, Ashington Hospital, Northumberland*

DR WR Hare *Research Fellow, Department of Nutritional Biochemistry, Nuffield Laboratory of Comparative Medicine, Institute of Zoology, London*

Dr George B Haycock *Consultant Paediatric Nephrologist, Evelina Children's Hospital, Guy's Hospital, London*

Dr KW Heaton *Reader in Medicine, University Department of Medicine, Bristol Royal Infirmary*

Mrs Daphne Horder *Community Dietitian, St George's Hospital, London*

Mr DJ Jukes *Lecturer in Food Technology, University of Reading*

Dr ME Knowles *Head, Food Science Section, Ministry of Agriculture, Fisheries and Food*

Dr TML Lang *Director, London Food Commission*

Dr BM Laurance *Formerly Consultant Physician, Queen Elizabeth Hospital for Sick Children, London*

Dr T Lind *MRC Human Reproduction Group, Princess Mary Maternity Hospital, Newcastle-upon-Tyne*

Dr JI Mann *University Lecturer and Hon. Consultant Physician, Department of Community Medicine and General Practice, Radcliffe Infirmary, Oxford*

Dr Martin B Mattock *Principal Biochemist, Unit for Metabolic Medicine, Department of Medicine, Guy's Hospital, London*

Dr JD Maxwell *Senior Lecturer in Medicine, St George's Hospital Medical School, London*

Mental Health Group of the British Dietetic Association

Dr Jane B Morgan *Lecturer in Nutrition, University of Surrey*

National Spinal Injuries Centre, Stoke Mandeville Hospital

Dr M Nelson *Lecturer in Nutrition, Kings College (Kensington), University of London*

Mr AJ Nunn *Principal Pharmacist, Alder Hey Children's Hospital, Liverpool*

Dr Victor Parsons *Director of Renal Medicine, Dulwich Hospital, London*

Miss Alison Paul *Member of Scientific Staff, MRC Dunn Nutrition Unit, Cambridge*

Miss Susan M Pettit *Chief Dietitian, Stoke Mandeville Hospital*

Mrs Marisa Piggott *Secretary, Department of Paediatric Nephrology, Evelina Children's Hospital, Guy's Hospital, London*

Professor TRE Pilkington *Professor of Medicine, St George's Hospital Medical School, London*

Mrs L Puggmur *Secretary, Stockton-on-Tees*

Mrs Pam Quayle *Secretary, Guildford*

Dr Jonathan Reeve *Hon. Consultant Physician, Head of MRC Bone Disease Group, Northwick Park Hospital, London*

Royal National Institute for the Blind

Dr TCB Stamp *Consultant Physician, Royal National Orthopaedic Hospital, Stanmore*

Mrs Diane Talbot *Formerly Chief Dietitian, Addenbrooke's Hospital, Cambridge*

Dr CJ Taylor *Senior Lecturer in Child Health, Alder Hey Children's Hospital, Liverpool*

Dr John Walls *Consultant Nephrologist, Leicester General Hospital*

Ms Joan CE Wells *Senior Nutritionist, Cow and Gate*

Dr AF Winder *Consultant Chemical Pathologist, Leicester Royal Infirmary*

Foreword

The first object of the British Dietetic Association as recited in its original constitution was 'to further the knowledge of dietetics'. It is thus particularly fitting that the golden jubilee of the Association should be closely followed by the publication of a *Manual of Dietetic Practice* that does precisely that. Dr Briony Thomas and the BDA team have put together a source book that will surely become a vade-mecum for dietitians as well as physicians and nutritionists and remain the definitive text in the field for years to come. We have in the *Manual* a comprehensive guide to the role of dietetics in maintaining health and treating disease that to my knowledge is unsurpassed in scope and authority. I know of no other text available here or abroad that deals so fully and in such practical terms with the problems that confront those involved in the application of dietary principles in therapeutic dietetics and to public health issues. It might be claimed fairly that with the publication of the Manual, dietetics in this country has come of age and can assume its due role as a distinct entity among the life sciences and a key sector in medicine and public health.

London, July 1987

R.J.L. Allen
Honorary President
British Dietetic Association

Introduction

Dietetics is, like all scientific disciplines, an ever-expanding and constantly evolving field. It is therefore increasingly difficult for the dietitian to be familiar with all aspects of dietetic practice. This is a particular problem for students, the newly qualified or those who return to the profession after an absence of some years, but even experienced practitioners find that they need to update their knowledge or develop new skills, particularly if they move to a different area of dietetic practice. Yet until now, there has been little dietetic reference material to turn to for guidance. Textbooks of nutrition focus mainly on the theoretical aspects of clinical nutrition and searching for information via journals, symposia and colleagues can be a haphazard and time-consuming process. The *Manual of Dietetic Practice* therefore grew out of a need for a centralized source of up-to-date and essentially practical information.

The Manual is not a collection of diet sheets, indeed the standardized diet sheet has little place in modern dietetic practice; patients and even their disorders, rarely come in a standardized form. A dietitian's skill lies not merely in implementing basic dietetic strategies but in adapting them to suit individual nutritional needs, dietary habits and medical problems. The purpose of this book is to provide the information dietitians need in order to use their skills effectively. Doctors and other health care professionals with a special interest in nutrition will also find the Manual useful.

The Manual is divided into five main sections which complement, and may need to be used in conjunction with, each other:

Section 1, *General Dietetic Principles and Practice*, discusses the basic 'tools of the trade' required by every dietitian. Its three parts cover firstly, aspects of dietary assessment (such as methodology and use of tables of nutrient requirements and food composition) and secondly, anthropometric standards and techniques. The third part deals with basic dietetic practices such as the estimation of nutritional requirements, enteral and parenteral feeding methods and dietary modification techniques.

Section 2, *Foods and Nutrients*, is a compendium of facts about foods, food components and nutrients. It can be used as a reference source by itself but it has also been designed to complement Section 4 (Therapeutic Dietetics) by providing the practical details of how to achieve a required dietary manipulation (such as sodium restriction). This section contains, for example, details of rich or poor sources of certain nutrients, exchange lists, lists of foods free from certain components (such as gluten or caffeine) and the composition of many proprietary dietetic products. Information on food legislation and labelling is also included. Relatively little information is given about the chemistry or metabolism of nutrients because these aspects are well covered in other textbooks.

Section 3, *Nutritional Needs of Population Subgroups*, discusses the nutritional factors which may be relevant when either general or specific advice is required for certain individuals or groups of individuals (such as infants or the elderly, athletes or the physically disabled). The information can also be used to devise educational material either for the general public or for other health care professionals.

Section 4, *Therapeutic Dietetics for Disease States*, details the dietetic management of clinical disorders. As well as familiar topics such as obesity and diabetes, the dietary treatment of a number of rare disorders (such as Prader Willi Syndrome) and some previously poorly documented techniques (such as ketogenic diets) are also discussed in detail. In order to avoid constant repetition of how, for example, to restrict protein intake or increase dietary fibre content, the reader is cross-referred to Section 2 (Foods and Nutrients) for the practical details of these manipulations.

Section 5, *Special Dietetic Procedures and Practice*, covers a number of miscellaneous topics such as the management of burns patients or low birthweight infants or how to conduct metabolic balances or a dietetic research study.

A series of appendices contain information on conversion factors, biochemical reference ranges, abbreviations and useful addresses.

Every effort has been made to ensure that the information given in this Manual is correct. However, its users should be aware that some errors may have inadvertently occurred and that some facts may change in the course of time. The British Dietetic Association cannot accept liability for any such errors or the consequences of them.

Many people have given advice on the content of the Manual and their help is gratefully acknowledged elsewhere. Credit must also be given to Greta Walton who instigated and co-ordinated the whole project, the British Dietetic Association for supporting it and the rest of the editorial team for their hard work. But this book would not have emerged at all without the labours of its contributors, many of whom gave up much of their spare time in order to put their expertise down on paper. To them, and to their long-suffering families who were neglected in the process (including my own), I wish to say a sincere thank you.

Briony Thomas
Editor

Section 1 General Dietetic Principles and Practice

A: Basic Dietetic Principles and Techniques

1.1 Basic Principles of a Healthy Diet

1.1.1 Perspective

Man has been preoccupied since the earliest times with the relationship between food and health. Complex classifications of food according to their 'elemental qualities' survived in orthodox teaching for almost 2000 years. Only over the past 200 years with the development of the science of nutrition has it become possible to make quantitative recommendations about the amount and type of food (the diet) which should be eaten to maintain health.

1.1.2 Essential nutrients

The first principle of healthy eating is that the requirement for the essential nutrients — amino acids, vitamins, inorganic nutrients, essential fatty acids and energy — must be met. Most foods contain a variety of nutrients but, as nearly all are deficient in one or more, requirements for essential nutrients are most likely to be met if a wide variety of foods is eaten in moderation. In general the essential nutrients are found in greater amounts and in more bioavailable forms in animal products such as meat, fish, cheese, eggs and milk. Hence these food groups, together with vegetables and fruit, have traditionally been emphasized in guidelines for healthy eating particularly for those at most risk of classic deficiency disease — the young, the elderly and pregnant or breast feeding women. However, in Westernized countries the occurrence of malnutrition, as judged by poor growth rates or frank clinical symptoms, is now rare and confined to well-defined circumstances — for example certain ethnic minority groups.

1.1.3 Current problems

With the control of undernutrition, and also of infectious diseases in which improved nutrition has played a part, interest in other diseases which may be caused by inappropriate dietary habits in Western populations has increased. Epidemiological studies show clearly that the causes of some of the most common diseases in Western populations (heart disease, stroke and cancer of the breast and bowel) are environmental, since in migrant populations the incidence changes to that of the host country within one or two generations. Diet is one of the environmental factors implicated and comparison of the diets eaten in populations at high risk show that animal protein intake, particularly from meat, is strongly associated with risk from colon cancer; fat intake with cancer of the breast, and salt and animal (saturated) fat intake with stroke and heart disease. The association between sugar consumption and tooth decay is well known, and a substantial proportion of the population in Western countries is overweight. Associations do not prove causation but those who consider all individuals in Western populations to be at risk recommend that salt, fat and sugar in the diet should be reduced, and starch and dietary fibre be increased towards levels found in populations where the occurrence of these diseases is rare.

1.1.4 Practical recommendations

Table 1.1. sets out the recommendations of the COMA Report on Diet and Cardiovascular Disease (DHSS 1984) for changes in the British diet. These entail revisions of traditional guidelines which have emphasized animal protein foods high in fat. Table 1.2 sets out simple guidelines for a prudent and healthy diet incorporating these and other recommendations (NACNE 1983).

However, it must be borne in mind that these recommendations are guidelines and not inflexible rules. Furthermore, they are directed at the general population and are not necessarily appropriate for all individuals within a population. They should not be applied too rigorously in children (who may not be able to eat enough of such a diet to meet energy and nutrient needs) or in the elderly (in whom the disruption to lifestyle may not be justified in terms of health benefit). Some sectors of the population (e.g. adolescents or pregnant women) have special dietary requirements, and the immediate nutritional needs of hospital patients and others with serious illness may be very different from NACNE guidelines.

Even when dietary change is warranted, too much should not be expected too quickly. The entrenched

Table 1.1 Dietary changes recommended in an attempt to reduce the incidence of coronary heart disease

| Dietary component | Current estimated intake | NACNE proposals | | COMA recommendations |
		Long term	Short term	
Energy intake	—	Recommend adjustment of the types of food eaten and an increased exercise programme so that adult body weight is achieved and/or maintained within the optimal limits of weight for height		
Fat intake	42% of total energy	30% of total energy	34% of total energy	35% of total energy
Saturated fatty acid intake	20% of total energy	10% of total energy	15% of total energy	15% of total energy
Polyunsaturated fatty acid intake (Polyunsaturated: Saturated (P/S) ratio)	5% of total energy (0.23)	No specific recommendation		Recommend that the P/S ratio be increased to approximately 0.45
Cholesterol intake	350–450 mg/day	No specific recommendations		
Sucrose intake	38 kg/head/year	20 kg/head/year	34 kg/head/year	The intake of simple sugars should not be increased
Fibre intake	20 g/head/day	30 g/head/day	25 g/head/day	No specific recommendations
Salt intake	8–12 g/head/year	3 g/head/day reduction	1 g/head/day reduction	Salt intake should not be increased. Ways should be sought to decrease the intake. The amount added in and after cooking should be decreased immediately
Alcohol intake	4–9% of total energy	4% of total energy	5% of total energy	An excessive intake should be avoided on general health grounds. No specific recommendation in relation to cardiovascular disease
Protein intake	11% of total energy	No recommendation		No specific recommendation but highlighting that animal protein tends to be associated with saturated fatty acids and vegetable protein with dietary fibre

Table 1.2 General guidelines for a healthy diet

Group	Foods	Daily targets	Principal nutrients provided	Notes
1	Bread, pasta, rice, flour, low salt breakfast cereals, potatoes	Generous amounts at each main meal to satisfy appetite	Energy, protein, B vitamins, fibre, minerals, essential fatty acids	Whole grain cereals are preferable to refined. Fresh potatoes contain vitamin C
2	Fresh vegetables and fruit	Three or more servings including at least one portion of a green or yellow vegetable	Vitamin C, folic acid, vitamin A, minerals, vitamin E, essential fatty acids	Only green and yellow vegetables contain vitamin A
3	Lean meat, poultry, offal, shellfish, fish, peas, beans, lentils, eggs	Two or more servings	Protein, B vitamins, minerals, essential fatty acids	Red meat, offal and soya are good sources of iron. Liver, eggs and fatty fish contain vitamin A
4	Yoghurt, semi-skimmed* or skimmed* milk, low fat cheese	At least $\frac{1}{2}$ pt milk* or 1 small carton yoghurt or 1 serving cheese (reduced fat varieties of cheese & yoghurt)	Calcium	Full cream milk contains vitamin A

GENERAL DIETETIC PRINCIPLES AND PRACTICE

Table 1.2 *contd.*

Group	Foods	Daily targets	Principal nutrients provided	Notes
5	Butter, margarine, oils, cooking fat	Use sparingly. Change to low fat or polyunsaturated varieties	Vitamin A in butter and margarine, vitamin E and essential fatty acids in oils	All fats are high in energy
6	Sugar, sweets, biscuits, sugar-containing soft drinks, cornflour	Use sparingly	Energy	Poor source of all other nutrients
7	Alcoholic drinks	Recommended maximum: Men 3–4 'drinks'/day, Women 2–3 'drinks'/day where one 'drink' is: half a pint of beer or lager, *or* one measure ($\frac{1}{6}$ gill, 24 cm^3) of spirits, *or* one small glass of wine or sherry	Energy	Poor source of all other nutrients

The use of salt in cooking and at the table should be reduced.
*Semi-skimmed or skimmed milk is unsuitable for children under five years of age.

eating habits of a lifetime are unlikely to be transformed overnight. The skill of a dietitian lies in knowing not only which dietary changes are likely to benefit an individual and how these may be accomplished, but also which measures will be acceptable and are therefore likely to be adopted. A healthy diet can only be a healthy diet if it is eaten.

References

DHSS (1984). *Diet and Cardiovascular Disease*, Report on Health and Social Subjects 28. Committee on Medical Aspects of Food Policy. HMSO, London.
National Advisory Committee on Nutrition Education (1983) *Proposals for nutritional guidelines for health education in Britain*. Health Education Council, London.

1.2 Recommended Dietary Allowances

Recommended dietary allowances (RDAs) for the major essential nutrients (protein, energy, vitamins, minerals) are published by most governments and the World Health Organization. Table 1.3 shows the current British RDAs (DHSS 1979) and published WHO and USA recommendations are listed in the references. Except in the case of energy, British RDAs are based on human experimental studies designed to assess the minimum amount of each nutrient necessary to avoid the clinical manifestation of deficiency diseases such as scurvy, beri-beri, anaemia and pellagra. Allowances are made for the bioavailability of nutrients in food and for the range of individual variation in requirements (minimum of 2 standard deviations) in order to arrive at 'safe' or 'recommended' levels for the majority of individuals in a population.

Table 1.3 Recommended daily amounts of food energy and some nutrients for population groups in the United Kingdom (DHSS, 1979)

Age range (year)	Occupational category	Energy (MJ)	(Kcal)	Protein (g)	Thiamin (mg)	Riboflavin (mg)	Nicotinic acid equivalents (mg)	Total* folate (µg)	Ascorbic acid (mg)	Vitamin A retinol equivalents (µg)	Vitamin D cholecalciferol (µg)	Calcium (mg)	Iron (mg)
Boys under 1					0.3	0.4	5	50	20	450	7.5	600	6
1		5.0	1200	30	0.5	0.6	7	100	20	300	10	600	7
2		5.75	1400	35	0.6	0.7	8	100	20	300	10	600	7
3−4		6.5	1560	39	0.6	0.8	9	100	20	300	10	600	8
5−6		7.25	1740	43	0.7	0.9	10	200	20	300		600	10
7−8		8.25	1980	49	0.8	1.0	11	200	20	400		600	10
9−11		9.5	2280	57	0.9	1.2	14	200	25	575		700	12
12−14		11.0	2640	66	1.1	1.4	16	300	25	725		700	12
15−17		12.0	2880	72	1.2	1.7	19	300	30	750		600	12
Girls under 1					0.3	0.4	5	50	20	450	7.5	600	6
1		4.5	1100	27	0.4	0.6	7	100	20	300	10	600	7
2		5.5	1300	32	0.5	0.7	8	100	20	300	10	600	7
3−4		6.25	1500	37	0.6	0.8	9	100	20	300	10	600	8
5−6		7.0	1680	42	0.7	0.9	10	200	20	300		600	10
7−8		8.0	1900	47	0.8	1.0	11	200	20	400		600	10
9−11		8.5	2050	51	0.8	1.2	14	300	25	575		700	12
12−14		9.0	2150	53	0.9	1.4	16	300	25	725		700	12
15−17		9.0	2150	53	0.9	1.7	19	300	30	750		600	12
Men													
18−34	Sedentary	10.5	2510	63	1.0	1.6	18	300	30	750		500	10
	Moderately active	12.0	2900	72	1.2	1.6	18	300	30	750		500	10
	Very active	14.0	3350	84	1.3	1.6	18	300	30	750		500	10
35−64	Sedentary	10.0	2400	60	1.0	1.6	18	300	30	750		500	10
	Moderately active	11.5	2750	69	1.1	1.6	18	300	30	750		500	10
	Very active	14.0	3350	84	1.3	1.6	18	300	30	750		500	10
65−74	Assuming a	10.0	2400	60	1.0	1.6	18	300	30	750		500	10
75+	sedentary life	9.0	2150	54	0.9	1.6	18	300	30	750		500	10
Women													
18−54	Most occupations	9.0	2150	54	0.9	1.3	15	300	30	750		500	12
	Very active	10.5	2500	62	1.0	1.3	15	300	30	750		500	12
55−74	Assuming a	8.0	1900	47	0.8	1.3	15	300	30	750		500	10
75+	sedentary life	7.0	1680	42	0.7	1.3	15	300	30	750		500	10
Pregnancy		10.0	2400	60	1.0	1.6	18	500	60	750	10	1200	13
Lactation		11.5	2750	69	1.1	1.8	21	400	60	1200	10	1200	15

Reproduced, with permission, from DHSS (1979)

*Doubts have been expressed about the validity of the recommended daily amounts for folate and the figures have been withdrawn from the table in the most recent (1985) printing (see p 145).

Whilst RDAs are important in both planning and judging the adequacy of the diet of a particular population (for example, a nation or institution as a whole) they do not cover pathological variations in individual requirements due for example to either inherited or acquired disease. During infection and surgery, requirements may be very much increased. The capacity to excrete excess amounts is markedly reduced in a variety of disorders.

Less than 2% of healthy individuals within a population would, in theory, be at risk of deficiency disease when consuming intakes of protein, vitamins and minerals at or above the RDA. The requirement of the majority of individuals would be lower than this but, nevertheless, it is prudent to give advice about diet (Section 1.1) to an individual whose intakes are shown to be habitually below the RDA. However, a diet containing less than the RDA is not necessarily 'deficient' in a particular nutrient. Dietitians should read the text of RDA booklets carefully before using them.

Recommendations for energy are based on the assumed average requirement for the class of the population concerned, taking into account activity levels, body weight, age and sex. Because it is an average, half the class is expected to require more than the RDA for energy and half less. In practice, a body weight which is in accordance with the ideal (Section 1.8) remains the best indication that requirements for energy expenditure are adequately balanced by energy intake.

References

DHSS (1979) *Recommended daily amounts of food energy and nutrients for groups of people in the United Kingdom.* Report on Health and Social Subjects 15, HMSO, London.
National Research Council (1980) *Recommended Dietary Allowances.* 9th Revised, National Academy of Sciences, National Research Council, Washington DC.
W.H.O. (1985) *Protein and Energy Requirements* Technical Report Series 724, WHO, Geneva.

1.3   Normal Nutrient Intakes

1.3.1   Normal intakes

Knowledge of the expected normal range of nutrient intakes of different age and sex groups is useful

1   to give guidance on whether the intake of a given individual is abnormally high or low.

2   to establish the level which may be regarded as *high* or *low* for research purposes or in planning therapeutic diets (see Section 1.14).

Tables 1.4 and 1.5 show the mean ± s.d., 10th, 50th and 90th centiles* of nutrient intakes in several age/sex groups, as found in studies conducted by the DHSS during 1968 to 1971 (Darke *et al* 1980) and by

*The 10th centile is the value such that 10% of the population studied had lower intakes and 90% had higher intakes.

Table 1.4a–h The mean daily intake, standard deviation, 10th, 50th and 90th centiles for total energy and selected nutrients obtained by seven day weighed dietary studies in 1967 to 1971.

a) Age 12–23 months

	Boys (n = 149)					Girls (n = 154)				
	Mean	SD	10th centile	50th centile	90th centile	Mean	SD	10th centile	50th centile	90th centile
Energy: MJ	5.05	1.22	3.54	4.90	6.49	4.74	1.16	3.42	4.58	6.09
kcal	1207	291	847	1172	1551	1133	277	817	1094	1454
Total protein (g)	37.8	10.4	25.6	36.5	52.2	35.3	9.4	25.0	33.8	44.9
Animal protein (g)	27.4	8.6	16.2	26.7	39.4	26.0	8.7	16.3	25.1	35.1
Fat (g)	51.2	15.2	33.8	49.2	70.6	48.7	13.6	32.5	46.8	65.2
Carbohydrate (g)	157	42	104	154	214	146	42	101	141	197
Calcium (mg)	744	233	459	725	1041	704	272	445	656	958
Iron (mg)	7.0	3.4	3.6	6.3	10.8	6.5	3.1	3.6	5.7	9.9
Retinol equiv. (µg)	821	570	334	616	1641	798	623	287	566	1698
Thiamin (mg)	0.63	0.32	0.40	0.55	0.89	0.57	0.20	0.36	0.52	0.78
Riboflavin (mg)	1.21	0.66	0.71	1.11	1.77	1.10	0.46	0.67	1.01	1.54
Nicotinic acid (mg)	6.56	5.54	3.45	5.53	10.09	5.78	3.01	3.20	4.99	8.17
Pyridoxine (mg)	0.65	0.34	0.41	0.60	0.87	0.60	0.21	0.39	0.57	0.80
Ascorbic acid (mg)	42.6	34.9	13.3	28.4	90.6	41.0	31.3	14.3	32.2	87.8
Cholecalciferol (µg)	3.14	3.85	0.46	1.44	8.14	3.84	4.96	0.42	1.64	10.47

b) Age 24–35 months

	Boys (n = 206)					Girls (n = 201)				
	Mean	SD	10th centile	50th centile	90th centile	Mean	SD	10th centile	50th centile	90th centile
Energy: MJ	5.73	1.49	4.08	5.49	7.50	5.37	1.30	4.11	5.09	6.85
kcal	1370	357	975	1312	1793	1284	310	983	1217	1636
Total protein (g)	39.7	10.9	26.8	38.6	52.0	38.5	10.5	27.6	37.1	50.4
Animal protein (g)	27.4	9.0	17.8	26.3	37.2	27.1	8.7	18.2	25.8	37.7
Fat (g)	57.9	17.8	37.3	56.0	78.8	55.5	16.0	40.0	53.5	73.7
Carbohydrate (g)	182	51	127	174	240	167	42	121	160	211
Calcium (mg)	678	216	425	669	890	660	210	439	620	877
Iron (mg)	6.8	2.4	4.5	6.2	9.2	6.4	2.5	4.0	5.8	9.3
Retinol equiv. (µg)	656	430	300	496	1155	704	635	274	496	1285
Thiamin (mg)	0.65	0.25	0.42	0.60	0.90	0.68	0.51	0.39	0.61	0.91
Riboflavin (mg)	1.06	0.33	0.68	0.99	1.45	1.04	0.39	0.65	0.94	1.66
Nicotinic acid (mg)	7.08	3.15	4.17	6.38	10.94	6.80	3.16	3.97	6.17	10.27
Pyridoxine (mg)	0.70	0.20	0.44	0.67	0.97	0.66	0.20	0.43	0.63	0.88
Ascorbic acid (mg)	36.3	31.0	14.3	25.3	63.7	38.8	37.9	13.1	26.2	80.4
Cholecalciferol (µg)	2.29	3.02	0.45	1.24	5.55	2.63	4.57	0.44	1.21	6.38

GENERAL DIETETIC PRINCIPLES AND PRACTICE

c) Age 36–47 months

	Boys (n = 276)					Girls (n = 262)				
	Mean	SD	10th centile	50th centile	90th centile	Mean	SD	10th centile	50th centile	90th centile
Energy: MJ	6.40	1.58	4.68	6.20	8.44	5.80	1.49	4.40	5.51	7.44
kcal	1529	378	1119	1481	2016	1387	355	1051	1317	1777
Total protein (g)	43.9	12.1	29.9	42.3	59.1	39.2	10.5	28.3	37.6	51.8
Animal protein (g)	29.4	9.6	18.9	28.6	41.0	26.6	11.3	17.2	25.3	36.2
Fat (g)	64.0	20.2	43.6	61.3	86.7	58.6	18.6	40.6	54.1	82.2
Carbohydrate (g)	204	49	149	198	259	186	48	138	180	239
Calcium (mg)	704	225	448	665	964	618	202	397	594	856
Iron (mg)	7.4	2.6	4.8	7.1	10.1	6.7	2.1	4.3	6.3	9.1
Retinol equiv. (µg)	764	630	318	576	1425	636	458	297	491	1185
Thiamin (mg)	0.75	0.27	0.47	0.69	1.08	0.64	0.24	0.43	0.60	0.87
Riboflavin (mg)	1.16	0.39	0.71	1.11	1.62	1.00	0.36	0.61	0.95	1.37
Nicotinic acid (mg)	8.26	3.35	4.88	7.46	12.23	7.29	3.04	4.47	6.90	10.30
Pyridoxine (mg)	0.77	0.23	0.51	0.73	1.03	0.69	0.20	0.48	0.66	0.92
Ascorbic acid (mg)	40.0	34.4	16.0	27.2	84.0	35.8	30.9	14.0	25.3	77.1
Cholecalciferol (µg)	1.94	2.62	0.46	1.16	3.80	1.94	2.59	0.49	1.04	4.34

d) Age 10–11 years

	Boys (n = 163)					Girls (n = 158)				
	Mean	SD	10th centile	50th centile	90th centile	Mean	SD	10th centile	50th centile	90th centile
Energy: MJ	9.08	1.63	6.99	9.13	11.03	8.02	1.56	6.02	7.86	10.20
kcal	2169	390	1670	2181	2634	1916	372	1437	1879	2438
Total protein (g)	62.4	12.5	45.5	62.0	78.8	55.4	11.3	42.3	54.5	70.5
Animal protein (g)	39.1	9.9	25.8	39.0	51.4	35.6	9.2	24.2	35.0	49.2
Fat (g)	90.7	19.6	67.7	90.4	115.3	82.8	19.9	61.1	80.0	106.8
Carbohydrate (g)	292	58	224	292	366.	252	52	183	253	318
Calcium (mg)	899	231	588	904	1172	787	224	495	778	1080
Iron (mg)	10.8	2.6	7.9	10.7	14.3	9.7	2.3	7.0	9.5	12.3
Retinol equiv. (µg)	893	548	409	724	1497	812	453	379	707	1363
Thiamin (mg)	1.03	0.28	0.72	1.00	1.40	0.88	0.21	0.60	0.84	1.14
Riboflavin (mg)	1.43	0.40	0.91	1.42	1.95	1.24	0.36	0.83	1.17	1.76
Nicotinic acid (mg)	11.19	3.13	7.85	10.45	15.94	9.57	2.46	6.62	9.28	12.40
Pyridoxine (mg)	1.16	0.24	0.85	1.16	1.47	1.05	0.23	0.78	1.02	1.35
Ascorbic acid (mg)	48.5	24.4	26.5	42.7	72.0	46.2	23.4	25.6	41.1	68.7
Cholecalciferol (µg)	1.66	1.02	0.82	1.44	2.52	1.44	0.74	0.72	1.30	2.22

e) Age 14–15 years

	Boys (n = 390)					Girls (n = 401)				
	Mean	SD	10th centile	50th centile	90th centile	Mean	SD	10th centile	50th centile	90th centile
Energy: MJ	10.25	2.47	7.28	10.16	13.44	8.00	1.90	5.61	7.98	10.19
kcal	2451	589	1739	2427	3210	1911	454	1340	1907	2435
Total protein (g)	71.2	17.4	48.8	71.0	94.2	57.2	13.9	40.9	56.1	73.6
Animal protein (g)	42.0	13.3	25.2	41.5	58.9	35.1	11.6	22.0	33.1	49.1
Fat (g)	101.8	28.2	66.6	98.7	137.7	84.7	23.0	57.4	83.4	111.3
Carbohydrate (g)	330	87	224	329	445	243	64	160	242	320
Calcium (mg)	870	299	503	841	1261	667	238	393	623	1007
Iron (mg)	12.4	3.5	8.3	12.0	17.1	10.1	2.7	7.0	9.8	13.0
Retinol equiv. (µg)	860	610	382	711	1358	780	574	329	628	1423
Thiamin (mg)	1.17	0.35	0.77	1.14	1.59	0.92	0.50	0.63	0.87	1.19
Riboflavin (mg)	1.48	0.57	0.83	1.40	2.20	1.13	0.71	0.66	1.07	1.63
Nicotinic acid (mg)	13.31	4.22	8.66	12.87	18.04	10.53	5.06	7.17	10.05	13.55
Pyridoxine (mg)	1.40	0.35	0.97	1.38	1.82	1.17	0.53	0.80	1.12	1.49
Ascorbic acid (mg)	53.3	29.2	27.5	49.4	76.6	48.8	27.9	26.0	42.4	77.6
Cholecalciferol (µg)	2.11	1.67	0.70	1.68	3.78	1.81	1.38	0.61	1.43	3.33

f) Age 65–74 years

	Men (n = 213)					Women (n = 225)				
	Mean	SD	10th centile	50th centile	90th centile	Mean	SD	10th centile	50th centile	90th centile
Energy: MJ	9.82	2.44	6.70	9.81	12.58	7.48	1.91	5.11	7.47	9.79
kcal	2347	582	1600	2344	3006	1788	456	1220	1784	2339
Total protein (g)	74.8	17.8	53.8	72.3	96.3	59.2	14.4	42.3	58.4	77.6
Animal protein (g)	50.9	13.9	34.7	48.9	68.1	41.1	11.6	26.3	40.5	53.3
Fat (g)	110.0	32.8	68.5	109.2	150.3	87.4	26.3	55.0	84.6	121.4
Carbohydrate (g)	267	75	175	266	355	200	61	128	195	277
Calcium (mg)	911	282	574	885	1249	796	244	487	790	1063
Iron (mg)	12.2	3.3	8.2	12.1	16.4	9.4	2.6	6.4	9.1	12.9
Retinol equiv. (μg)	1142	686	513	958	2007	1027	676	490	815	1747
Thiamin (mg)	1.05	0.35	0.68	1.01	1.40	0.82	0.23	0.56	0.78	1.11
Riboflavin (mg)	1.55	0.48	0.96	1.46	2.16	1.27	0.42	0.78	1.19	1.78
Nicotinic acid (mg)	16.91	7.42	9.89	14.58	26.97	11.49	4.56	7.12	10.30	17.50
Pyridoxine (mg)	1.37	0.41	0.90	1.31	1.90	1.01	0.28	0.70	0.96	1.38
Ascorbic acid (mg)	42.8	26.0	17.3	38.0	72.2	40.5	27.8	15.9	32.4	74.1
Cholecalciferol (μg)	3.34	3.26	0.93	2.09	6.64	2.32	2.18	0.66	1.60	4.38

g) Age 75+ years

	Men (n = 179)					Women (n = 204)				
	Mean	SD	10th centile	50th centile	90th centile	Mean	SD	10th centile	50th centile	90th centile
Energy: MJ	8.80	2.31	5.94	8.78	11.60	6.81	1.72	4.59	6.78	9.00
kcal	2103	551	419	2098	2771	1627	410	1097	1619	2149
Total protein (g)	67.6	18.4	43.5	67.5	87.5	53.6	13.0	34.9	54.0	69.8
Animal protein (g)	45.9	14.1	28.2	44.7	64.1	37.4	10.4	22.9	37.6	50.1
Fat (g)	97.9	29.2	65.0	95.8	137.4	77.6	22.0	53.8	75.0	105.0
Carbohydrate (g)	244	73	154	240	327	187	59	112	183	255
Calcium (mg)	883	302	503	852	1253	726	253	418	698	1008
Iron (mg)	10.9	3.2	6.5	10.6	14.9	8.5	2.5	5.4	8.4	11.7
Retinol equiv. (μg)	1094	741	512	880	1892	888	588	404	729	1387
Thiamin (mg)	0.93	0.29	0.56	0.90	1.27	0.74	0.23	0.48	0.72	1.02
Riboflavin (mg)	1.40	0.51	0.80	1.34	2.06	1.13	0.39	0.66	1.09	1.71
Nicotinic acid (mg)	13.55	5.04	7.76	12.48	19.51	10.18	3.80	6.18	9.35	14.33
Pyridoxine (mg)	1.18	0.36	0.72	1.17	1.58	0.93	0.27	0.62	0.91	1.27
Ascorbic acid (mg)	37.7	23.1	13.8	33.7	60.8	33.7	20.0	12.3	29.2	58.7
Cholecalciferol (μg)	2.68	2.13	0.75	1.96	5.42	2.09	1.79	0.63	1.48	4.39

h) Pregnant women in the 6th–7th month of pregnancy (n = 435)

	Mean	SD	10th centile	50th centile	90th centile
Energy: MJ	9.01	2.10	6.35	9.04	11.60
kcal	2152	503	1517	2159	2771
Total protein (g)	70.5	16.7	49.6	70.3	92.3
Animal protein (g)	47.8	14.3	31.0	46.8	65.6
Fat (g)	97.9	26.4	65.1	96.6	130.6
Carbohydrate (g)	260	69	172	264	344
Calcium (mg)	959	320	547	946	1363
Iron (mg)	11.7	3.1	8.2	11.5	15.4
Retinol equiv. (μg)	1269	975	516	961	2485
Thiamin (mg)	1.04	0.28	0.70	1.03	1.38
Riboflavin (mg)	1.60	0.67	0.92	1.51	2.30
Nicotinic acid (mg)	14.30	5.30	8.88	13.41	20.34
Pyridoxine (mg)	1.27	0.32	0.88	1.24	1.66
Ascorbic acid (mg)	54.9	24.7	28.0	49.7	89.0
Cholecalciferol (μg)	2.28	2.01	0.76	1.66	4.40

From: Darke *et al* (1980). Reproduced with permission from *Br J Nutr*.

GENERAL DIETETIC PRINCIPLES AND PRACTICE

Table 1.5 The mean daily intake, standard deviation, 10th, 50th and 90th centiles for total energy and selected nutrients obtained by a semi-weighed family dietary record in 1977—8. (From: Nelson 1983; Nelson, Dyson and Paul, 1985 and personal communication)

Age 18—55 years	Men (n = 105)					Women (n = 115)				
	Mean	SD	10th centile	50th centile	90th centile	Mean	SD	10th centile	50th centile	90th centile
Energy: MJ	11.8	2.7	8.9	11.4	14.9	8.2	1.9	5.6	8.2	10.8
kcal	2816	659	2122	2715	3549	1961	452	1419	1943	2575
Protein (g)	89.5	19.5	66.5	87.6	111.0	65.5	14.5	46.7	65.7	84.0
Fat (g)	123.1	31.5	88.5	118.6	166.2	89.9	22.7	60.5	93.4	117.3
Carbohydrate (g)	330	86	231	324	419	226	67	144	222	299
Dietary fibre (g)	20.8	5.9	13.5	21.0	26.7	15.8	4.9	9.2	15.9	21.5
Alcohol (g)	15.4	33.5	0	5.9	33.5	5.5	8.8	0	0	17.4
Calcium (mg)	1131	369	654	1149	1578	901	315	519	885	1283
Iron (mg)	13.86	3.65	9.83	13.01	18.89	10.36	3.06	6.73	10.50	13.74
Retinol equiv (µg)	1639	1869	391	704	4591	1256	1366	304	581	3369
Carotene (µg)	2960	2089	503	2569	5279	2421	1784	518	2077	4831
Thiamin (mg)	1.33	0.35	0.92	1.30	1.75	0.99	0.28	0.66	1.00	1.37
Riboflavin (mg)	2.21	0.75	1.29	2.05	3.30	1.76	0.62	1.00	1.69	2.61
Nicotinic acid (mg)	19.62	5.62	13.71	18.28	26.25	13.69	3.68	9.21	13.66	17.79
Tryptophan/60 (mg)	19.13	4.39	14.05	18.54	24.34	13.84	3.07	10.16	13.99	17.73
Vitamin B6 (mg)	1.409	0.376	1.029	1.388	1.755	1.009	0.230	0.685	1.018	1.279
Vitamin C (mg)	57.5	22.1	31.6	54.9	82.3	54.3	36.7	25.7	46.1	88.4
Vitamin D (µg)	3.261	2.256	1.140	2.828	4.884	2.416	1.608	0.897	2.043	4.111
Sodium (mg)	3481	1073	2227	3466	4747	2383	651	1707	2398	3150
Potassium (mg)	3740	923	2749	3698	4719	2807	629	2038	2803	3511
Magnesium (mg)	331	102	233	314	436	242	64	157	241	326
Phosphorus (mg)	1510	360	1042	1487	1983	1149	304	778	1127	1554
Copper (mg)	1.96	0.84	1.33	1.72	2.89	1.41	0.52	0.88	1.31	2.11
Zinc (mg)	11.29	2.77	8.48	10.73	14.95	8.20	2.10	5.49	8.25	10.73
Chloride (mg)	5499	1655	3508	5492	7614	3735	996	2713	3782	4872
Vitamin E (mg)	5.66	1.88	3.24	5.70	8.02	4.45	1.68	2.53	4.28	5.81
Vitamin B12 (µg)	9.04	8.24	2.98	5.39	20.68	6.25	5.49	2.22	3.94	14.62
Total folate (µg)	196.9	68.4	125.7	184.9	266.6	144.1	54.2	88.2	137.0	223.8
Pantothenic acid (mg)	4.97	1.61	3.24	4.69	6.80	3.64	1.06	2.47	3.63	5.37
Biotin (µg)	29.4	10.3	16.9	28.9	41.2	22.4	9.0	13.8	22.3	34.0

Nelson *et al* during 1978—9 (1984; 1985 and personal communication). Table 1.5 includes a majority of the nutrients listed in McCance and Widdowson's *The Composition of Foods* (Paul and Southgate 1978). Figures for the intake of lesser B vitamins however must be regarded as provisional (Cooke 1983; Black *et al* 1985).

Extremes of nutrient intakes recorded in seven day surveys are probably not *usual* intakes. In any short survey some people will be studied during periods of either lower or higher than average intake. When surveys are conducted for longer periods of time, the range of individual intakes recorded is smaller than the range found in the first few days. This is known as regression to the mean. The 10th and the 90th centiles, and not the full range of intakes, have therefore been given as probably representing the range of *usual* intakes.

Nutrient intake is related to total energy intake. Therefore, to help in assessing the probable ranges of usual intakes for nutrients not shown in the tables,

Figure 1 is included. This shows how the energy intakes of all the age/sex groups in Tables 1.4 and 1.5 relate to each other. Thus, for example, since the range of energy intakes of girls aged 10—11 is only a little less than that of women aged 18—55, then the intakes of other nutrients are likely to have a range similar to that of 18—55 year old women.

1.3.2 Nutrient density

Because total nutrient intake is correlated with total food (energy) consumption the nutrient density of a diet is an important consideration. While it is perfectly possible to choose a diet of high nutrient density such that a good total nutrient intake is obtained for only a small energy intake, the likelihood of a low total nutrient intake is greater for those with small appetites.

Longitudinal studies of dietary intake have shown that individuals tend to be either consistently large or consistently small eaters (Black 1980), and typically for adult women the range of usual energy intakes is

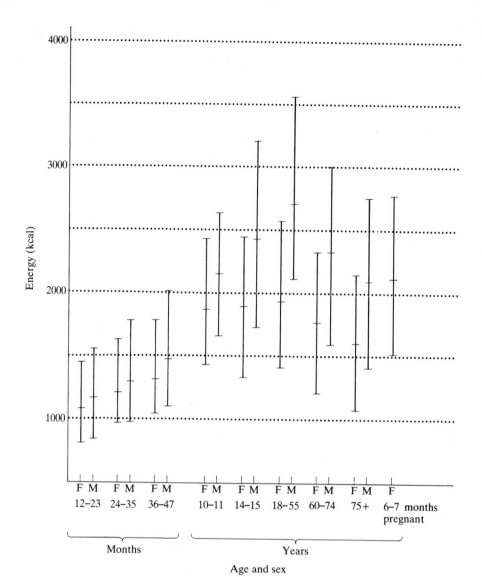

Fig. 1.1 Range (10th, 50th and 90th centiles) of energy intakes in different age and sex groups (Darke *et al* 1980; Nelson and Paul, personal communication).

from 1400−2600 kcal (5.9−10.9 MJ) (see Table 1.5), and some 200 kcal lower in those over 60 years. The distribution of intakes in dietary surveys suggests that possibly 20% of women (aged 20−60 years) have intakes below 1700 kcal, and 10% of them have intakes below 1500 kcal (Black, personal communication).

Table 1.6 shows the required nutrient density (i.e. the quantity/1000 kcal) in diets of 1500, 1600 and 1800 kcal if the RDA for some nutrients for adult women are to be met. This is compared with the actual nutrient densities in diets of women studied by Smithells *et al* (1977). The required nutrient densities for thiamin, iron and pyridoxine are all greater than those found in the actual diets of this population.

While all individuals do not require intakes equal to the RDA, nevertheless if the average intake of a group is low, there is a greater probability of individuals with higher requirements receiving inadequate amounts. The intakes of certain nutrients (e.g. iron, folate) are known to be marginal in UK diets. Other nutrients (e.g. zinc, vitamin B6) may also be marginal (see Sections 2.6 and 2.8). There is possibly a case for routine vitamin/mineral supplementation to hospital patients whose requirements — particularly in infectious or post-traumatic states — are known to be increased and whose appetites are small (Hackett *et al* 1979; Todd *et al* 1984), and also to the elderly in institutional care.

References

Black AE (1980) Pitfalls in dietary assessment. In *Recent advances in clinical nutrition* Howard AN and McLean Baird I (Eds). pp11−18 John Libbey, London.
Black AE, Paul AA and Hall C (1985) Footnotes to food tables 2. The underestimation of intakes of lesser B vitamins by preg-

Table 1.6 Required nutrient density if RDA are to be met at different levels of energy intake, compared with actual nutrient densities for various social groups among pregnant women studied by Smithells *et al* (1977)

Nutrient	Required nutrient density for energy intakes of			Actual nutrient density*				
	1500 kcal	1600 kcal	1800 kcal	I	II	IIINM	IIIM	IV&V
Thiamin	0.6	0.56	0.5	0.58	0.54	0.54	0.53	0.52
Riboflavin	0.87	0.81	0.72	1.1	1.1	0.9	0.9	0.8
Vitamin C	20	18.8	16.7	38	37	32	31	28
Calcium	0.33	0.31	0.28	0.52	0.52	0.51	0.45	0.49
Iron	8.0	7.5	6.7	5.3	5.5	5.2	5.3	4.9
Pyridoxine**	1.3	1.2	1.1	0.6	0.6	0.6	0.6	0.6

*Data presented by social class. NM = Non-Manual; M = Manual.
**USA RDA.

nant and lactating women as calculated using the fourth edition of McCance and Widdowson's *The Composition of Foods. Hum Nutr: Appl Nutr* **39A**, 19–22.

Cooke JR (1983) Food composition tables — analytical problems in the collection of data. *Hum Nutr: Appl Nutr* **37A**, 441–7.

Darke SJ, Disselduff MM and Try GP (1980) Frequency distributions of mean daily intakes of food energy and selected nutrients obtained during nutrition surveys of different groups of people in Great Britain between 1968 and 1971. *Br J Nutr* **44**, 243–52.

Hackett AF, Yeoung CK and Hill GL (1979) Eating patterns in patients recovering from major surgery — a study of voluntary food intake and energy balance. *Br J Surg* **66**, 415–8.

Nelson M (1983) A dietary survey method for measuring family food purchases and individual nutrient intakes concurrently, and its use in dietary surveillance. PhD Thesis; University of London.

Nelson M, Dyson PA and Paul AA (1985) Family food purchases and home food consumption; their nutrient contents compared. *Br J Nutr* **54**, 373–87.

Paul AA and Southgate DAT (1978) McCance and Widdowson's *The Composition of Foods*. HMSO, London.

Smithells RW, Ankers C, Carver ME, Lennon D, Schorah CJ and Sheppard S (1977) Maternal nutrition in early pregnancy. *Br J Nutr* **38**, 497–506.

Todd EA, Hunt P, Crowe PJ and Royle GT (1984) What do patients eat in hospital? *Hum Nutr: Appl Nutr* **38A**, 294–7.

1.4 Dietary Assessment Methodology

1.4.1 General considerations

Methods

There are five basic methods in use for assessing dietary intake in free-living individuals, which were first described 50–60 years ago. Two are records of actual consumption, made at the time of eating food, one with weights of food established by the subjects themselves (Widdowson 1936), and the other with estimated weights of food (Youmans et al 1942). The other three methods attempt to assess diet in the recent past by asking subjects about their food intake the previous day, the 24-hour recall (Wiehl 1942), or over the past few weeks or months, the diet history (Turner 1940). The diet history may be used in an attempt to estimate intake in the distant past. Questionnaires may be used to assess usual diet, either recent or distant past, but are usually devised for completion by the subjects concerned without supervision (Wiehl and Reed 1960) and are rarely used in clinical work.

Accuracy

Accurate results from these methods require a high degree of skill and care on the part of the dietitian. The reason for this is that a number of errors are introduced at each stage of dietary assessment and the net result may be a systematic bias or large random deviations from the true mean. Large random error will entail numerous observations before individuals are classified correctly for their average nutrient intake, and systematic errors invalidate individual comparisons with standards such as, for example, the recommended daily allowance.

Aims

At the outset of a dietary investigation it is essential to establish which nutrients are of interest and how accurate the results are required to be, due to the effect of normal day to day variation in nutrient intake (see below). All results are dependent on (1) the degree of co-operation from the subjects and their ability to give accurate reports or records of their dietary habits, and (2) on adequate food tables (Section 1.6). Food tables cannot be used to measure salt consumption; urine analysis is a preferable method (see subsection 'validity'). Methods for present or recent past dietary assessment, and retrospective dietary investigations are discussed below.

Choice of method

In theory the most accurate method available is the *weighed dietary record* where the weights of all food and beverages consumed are recorded. This requires a robust and convenient set of scales weighing up to 2 kg and accurate to ±1 g which can be given to the subject for use at home. Scales with a taring facility should be avoided because this often causes confusion. People should be given a demonstration of how to weigh a meal on to their normal plates, recording the cumulative weights, and then be asked to repeat the demonstration themselves. Once they have grasped the essence of the technique, a notebook and a set of simple instructions should be provided and the need for adequate details of recipes, brand names and foods consumed away from home explained. Electronic scales with an automatic recording facility can help with illiterate groups. The PETRA scales (available from Cherlyn Electronics, 22 High Street, Histon, Cambs., England) record a spoken description of the item and the weight (undisclosed to the operator) on to a cassette; this is later played back through a special console. The FRED system (available from BC Systems Ltd, 35 Harford Street, Trowbridge, Wilts., England) uses condensed food tables of 95 items, each represented by a separate key on a small desktop computer/scales. The keys can be labelled with pictograms, and weight is recorded automatically, undisclosed to the operator. It must be emphasized to subjects that they must continue with their normal dietary habits, and not change their usual menu or amounts of foods whilst keeping the record. Subjects should be visited at home or asked to return to the clinic to check that they have understood all the instructions and are keeping the record correctly.

If only energy and energy yielding nutrients are to be assessed, a seven day record is sufficient, if an accuracy of ±10% standard error is acceptable (Table

Table 1.7 The effect of day to day variation on the precision of estimates of the average nutrient intake

Item	Average* within person variation %	% standard error [+] of a 7-day record average	Number of days [++] of records necessary to be ±10% of the average
Energy	23	9	5
Carbohydrate	25	9	6
Protein	27	10	7
Fat	31	12	10
Dietary fibre	31	12	10
Calcium	32	12	10
Iron	35	13	12
Thiamin	39	15	15
Riboflavin	44	17	19
Cholesterol	52	20	27
Vitamin C	60	23	36

*Data from up to 19 population samples in Britain, USA, Canada, Israel and others (Bingham 1987).

[+] Calculated from % standard error (se) $= \frac{cv\%}{\sqrt{n}}$ and $n = \frac{cv^2}{\%se^2}$ (Balogh *et al* 1971).
[++]

1.7). This is equivalent to a range of 20 g protein (40 g at $P < 0.05$) assuming an average of 100 g/day. As can be seen from the table, vitamins, minerals and fibre require longer periods of observation, at least 14 days. These do not have to be obtained over a single period of time and four records each of four days duration would be an acceptable compromise. People with stable food habits, and therefore with lower than average within-person coefficients of variation, can be observed for shorter periods, while longer investigations are necessary in those with erratic eating patterns in order to obtain a satisfactory level of precision.

The main disadvantage with the weighed food record is that it is an extremely tedious procedure for the subject and hence requires a considerable amount of co-operation. If this is not forthcoming, the assessor may end up with poorly kept or incomplete records, or even no records at all. In studies of groups of patients (e.g. monitoring dietary compliance or effectiveness) there is always a risk that a high level of non-participation may introduce an element of bias; those who are unable or unwilling to take part may well have different dietary habits from those who do participate. Thus, although the seven or more days weighed food record is the most accurate method, it is not always the most valid or even the most appropriate.

A slightly less invasive, and hence more acceptable, method of assessing dietary intake from a subject's point of view is *the unweighed food record* where the quantity of food is estimated by description using models, standard portions, food replicas and house-hold measures. However, this technique is more demanding for the dietitian who needs to become skilled in interpreting these descriptions and there is a risk that individuals may consistently under- or over-estimate their portion sizes hence introducing systematic errors. Dietary assessments using this method are likely to be less accurate than those derived from weighed records, but may be more readily obtainable from the patients. At least 14 days of records need to be obtained if minerals and vitamins are to be assessed, as detailed above.

The most important, and most commonly used, method in clinical work is the *diet history* which aims to assess the usual nutrient intake by means of dietary questioning. A full dietary history may take as much as $1\frac{1}{2}$ hours to complete properly, although a shortened version is often adequate for the purpose of advising on dietary modification. Practical details have been described in the original publication (Turner 1940). However, because the accuracy of the dietary history is so dependent on the interviewing techniques and method of questioning used to obtain the information, these aspects are discussed in detail at the end of this section (p 16).

Recent studies have shown that intakes assessed by diet history appear to be greater than those obtained from records (Bingham 1987) probably because subjects tend to overestimate how often they consume foods. Nutritionists experienced in taking diet histories can correct for this overestimation with a factor based on the probable numbers of meals eaten during the period of time covered (Calmer, personal communication). Nevertheless, patients are rarely able to recall their food intake with accuracy. Turner (1940) noted that the results from a diet history did not show absolute agreement with those from weighed records, and the dietitian using the diet history should be aware of the approximate amount of error involved. Turner's studies suggested that, for example, protein intakes assessed by the two methods were likely to differ by 32 g on average (standard deviation of difference 16%).

An assessment of the usual diet of a patient based on a single 24-hour recall is not recommended if an accurate estimate of nutrient intake is required; this method tends to be associated with systematic underestimation of food intake and fails to take account of daily variations in dietary habits. At best, it can only give a rough idea of the type of food consumed and approximate meal pattern. Unfortunately, owing to constraints on time, this method of dietary investigation is one on which many dietitians have to rely in clinical practice. If this is unavoidable then dietitians should at least be aware of the limited nature of any information obtained in this way.

Validity

No matter how carefully done, dietary assessments using any of the above methods rely on information given to the dietitian by the patient. Where there is any doubt of the veracity of a report, for example when investigating an obese or anorectic patient, an independent check is needed.

The most practical of these is the 24-hour urinary nitrogen output, which can be compared with the reported nitrogen (protein) intake (Isaksson 1980). Urine nitrogen should not exceed dietary intake and should be within the range of 81 $\pm$5% standard deviation (Bingham and Cummings 1984). In a Swedish study (Warnold et al 1978), the reported dietary intake of obese patients obtained from a diet history was only 46 g protein (7 g nitrogen), whereas their actual intake estimated from 24-hour urinary nitrogen output was 87 g protein, a two-fold difference, or 190% of the supposed dietary intake. Diabetic subjects have been shown to have a tendency to report their prescribed diet rather than their actual food intake as monitored by their 24-hour urine nitrogen output (Steen et al 1977). When 24-hour urine collections are used in this way, or for the assessment of salt consumption, their completeness must be assured by using the para-amino-benzoic acid (PABA) check method. Patients are given an oral dose of PABA and the amount recovered in the urine is an index of the completeness of the urine collection (Bingham and Cummings 1983).

Retrospective dietary assessments

The dietitian may be asked to obtain an assessment of a patient's eating habits in the distant past for diagnostic or research purposes in conditions with a prolonged latent period. In this case, a diet history interview referring patients back to around the time in question may be undertaken. However, a number of recent studies have shown that individuals' reports of past dietary habits are strongly biased towards those of the present (Byers et al 1983; Jensen et al 1984; Rohan and Potter 1984); people cannot remember their dietary habits of several years ago. Estimates of past dietary habits may therefore be misleading.

Dietary survey methodology in research and epidemiology

This is a highly specialized field and dietitians are

advised to consult the following publications (Marr 1971; Black 1982; Black et al 1983; Bingham 1985, 1987) or recommend them to clinicians, before undertaking survey work of either groups or individuals.

1.4.2 Practical guidelines for the assessment of dietary intake in clinical practice

The following guidelines are extracted from 'Guidelines for taking Diet Histories' (British Dietetic Association 1979). Most of the points relate to the dietary history technique itself but some may be relevant to other methods of dietary evaluation used in clinical practice.

Pre-interview information

Is the diet history an individual assessment, or is it part of a series or survey?

In the latter case, it is important that each interview should be conducted in exactly the same way as decided at the start of the series.

What information is required and for what reason?

Defining the specific aims of the evaluation will decide whether a full or a brief diet history is required, which nutrients should be assessed, and therefore which foods should be concentrated on. If for example an estimate of vitamin B12 and folate intake only is required, then less detail may be required on foods such as sugar and fat.

Is any information available about the respondent's background?

Often case notes will give useful information about age, marital status, religion, medical history, nationality and socio-economic background. They may state whether the subject is deaf, or illiterate, or highly intelligent. It is always useful to record what medications are being taken and for how long, because of possible drug nutrient interaction, e.g. contraceptive pills and vitamin B6. Remember that all the information obtained is *confidential*.

Where should the interview be held?

Sometimes there is no choice, but when a choice is available, it pays to consider the alternatives. A hospital ward has many distractions; a quieter side room may be available. Remember the patient's comfort as well as your own, e.g. the chairs, lighting, ventilation and temperature, etc.

When should the interview be held?

Again there may be no choice. However, a diet history is less likely to be reliable if the respondent (or the interviewer) is very hungry; has just had a large meal; is in great pain; is emotionally upset; or is distracted because of a fractious child, a bus to catch, etc.

In hospital wards, try to avoid the time of ward rounds, any time when the patient is undergoing tests or treatment, meal times and visiting times.

Allow sufficient time for the interview

The time required will obviously vary, but if much more than 30 minutes is needed it is usually best to stop and divert the topic for a short while to give the respondent a mental rest, or change the pattern of the interview, e.g. by using cards for the checklist (see pp 20 and 22–26), or even continue on another day.

Interview techniques

There are two main aspects to an interview, the *collection* of information, and the actual *information* to be collected.

General aspects

Thought must be given to the way the interviewer deals with the respondent. Bad techniques can maximize errors and incompleteness and upset people. Good interview technique can get information pleasantly from nearly all respondents. It will enable the interviewer to
1 Keep the respondent at ease throughout the interview.
2 Make the purpose of the interview explicit.
3 Elicit all the required information.
4 Maintain direction of the interview at all times and end it clearly and pleasantly.

Suggested diet history interview model

The interview should be approached systematically as follows (Fieldhouse 1978)
1 Welcome the respondent — seat them comfortably and introduce yourself.
2 Explain the purpose of the interview — reason(s)

for the interview, the time available, and the need for note-taking.
3 Check or collect relevant socio-medical information.
4 Take diet history (see below).
5 Invite questions.
6 Specify future arrangements (if any) — date of next appointment.
7 Terminate the interview — respondent thanked and shown out.
8 Complete records.
9 Attempt evaluation of interview and information.

Essential points to remember in developing good techniques

1 Listen sensitively, information may be volunteered at an earlier stage in the interview than expected.
2 Be interested.
3 Be non-judgemental in words, tone of voice and facial expressions.
4 Tailor question style to the individual respondent.
5 Remember the value of non-verbal encouragement throughout the interview.

Designing questions

Language

The vocabulary and grammatical structure should offer the chance of complete and accurate communication. The language of the questions should approximate to the language of the respondent.

Frame of reference

'Begin where the respondent is' — introduce a topic in a form relevant to the respondent's background.

Open or closed questions

Avoid too many questions requiring 'yes' or 'no' answers. Try to use questions which encourage the respondent to talk, e.g. 'how do you feel about...?' 'what do you think of...?'

Information level

When an interviewer, with the authority given by that role, asks a question, there is the implication that the respondent should be in possession of an adequate answer and if he cannot answer he is somehow discredited; *but* questions need not be limited to those which the respondent can always answer. The interviewer should be cautious in wording a question which may be anticipated as difficult (or embarrassing) to answer. Thus, appropriate introductions are important, e.g. 'many people do...' or 'many people have not...' followed by 'do you happen to...?'

Leading question

A question should be phrased so that it contains no suggestion of the most appropriate response.

Single idea

Questions should be limited to a single idea or reference. Only ask one question at a time.

Question sequence

Arrange the questions so that they make most sense to the respondent. The first few questions are important in showing the respondent what is expected of him.

When changing the subject help the respondent to adjust by making a suitable comment, e.g. 'we have been talking about...now I would like to consider...'

Personal factors

Various personal factors in the respondent may result in the interview taking longer and requiring more effort and ingenuity. Remember that memory and intelligence vary.

Deafness

Speak more slowly, as well as more loudly, enunciate clearly and make sure the respondent can see your mouth. Use your hands to indicate numbers and sizes.

Blindness

This should make little or no difference in taking a diet history. Guide the person to the chair. Do *not* speak more slowly or more loudly. Portion models which the respondent can handle may help in estimating the portion sizes, e.g. cakes, biscuits.

Not fluent in English

Use simple language, speak slowly and enunciate clearly. If no English is spoken, enlist the help of a relative, a member of staff or interpreter who knows the respondent's language. Remember that interpreters may superimpose their own interpretations. In any case, questions need to be very short and clearly phrased. If the interpreter is not acceptable to the respondent, i.e. right age, sex and class, the required information may not be given.

Very young or very old

Greater patience is required. Do not rush. Enlist the help of the person who prepares the food.

Neurotic, aggressive or rude

Maintain a professional approach and do not lose your temper. If necessary terminate the interview and arrange another time.

Limited intelligence

Use simple words and simple grammar. Allow time for respondent's thought processes to work.

Conducting the interview

Introduction — the 'welcome'. It is important to convey a genuine feeling of warmth to the respondent, e.g. standing to greet, handshake, smile, etc. If relevant (e.g. at first meeting) indicate sympathy with possible frustration of being interviewed by another medical specialist at end of a long session. Also be sensitive to the possible state of respondent, e.g. anxiety following diagnosis of an unexpected condition and associated fear of illness concerned.

Introduce self and explain the role played by the dietitian and the purpose and anticipated length of the interview(s). Encourage the respondent to ask questions during interview *and* subsequently make a point of asking at intervals during the interview if there are any questions. During the presentation of questions, remember that communication is both non-verbal and verbal.

Non-verbal communication

The interviewer should be aware of the wide range of possible cues from non-verbal behaviour — by both the interviewer and respondent — a two-way process!
1 Vocal intonation can indicate interest or boredom; vocal stress can be used for emphasis, humour, etc.
2 Gestures can help illustration. Smiling helps to create a relaxed atmosphere!

3 Grunts, mm-mm, eye-gaze, nods, etc. are important cues for sustaining conversation.

4 Posture, pace of speech, pitch of voice and facial expression are possible cues of emotion.

5 Proximity can establish a less formal atmosphere; distance stresses formality.

6 Accent, dialect, clothes, hairstyle, etc. can be possible indications of social group, background, etc.

Verbal communication

During the presentation of questions the following ideas should be considered

1 Your credibility in the eyes of the respondent will increase if you demonstrate expertise and show concern and dedication. Try to be forceful but not overbearing. Rapport is increased if the respondent perceives some similarity with you, e.g. physical similarity — age, sex, race, ethnic features, dress, dialect, etc. However, hidden barriers may be set up by the lack of such similarities, e.g. young dietitian and older respondent, slim dietitian! Rapport is also helped if you begin with an aspect that the respondent would want to hear.

2 Show by your manner that you are interested and that your attention is uninterrupted. Your manner and your words should not indicate shock or surprise at answers and should not imply criticism or impatience towards what is being said. You have the power to reinforce many behaviours of the respondent — to be used judiciously, e.g. attentive listening; eye-contact; addressing the person by name; saying 'good', 'that is interesting', etc. to reinforce specific behaviours.

3 Pause for a few seconds after the respondent has apparently finished and before more questions are asked, in order to give him a chance to speak further. Remember that under normal circumstances there is no time for the respondent to be prepared and there is the inevitable pressure of trying to provide a quick reply when an interviewer is waiting for your answer!

4 Return to topics on which the respondent 'froze' in order to determine if lack of response is significant.

5 Avoid bringing the respondent abruptly back to the point when he digresses. Use appropriate wording for 'probing' questions to maintain a good relationship, e.g. 'I am interested in what you are saying, could you tell me more about that?' You could also adopt a questioning tone when repeating key sentences of the respondent to indicate that you want elaboration.

When clarifying points consider introductory comments, e.g. 'Now let me see if I have understood correctly. You said. . .(and then summarize)!

6 Leave any personal or potentially embarrassing questions as near to the end as possible so that a good rapport has already been established. At the end of the interview thank the respondent and give a positive indication of the usefulness of the interview. Anticipate the next meeting if relevant.

The diet history: the technique of obtaining dietary information

Steps in a diet history

The component parts of a full diet history are described separately here, but an experienced interviewer may be more flexible, combining steps or altering the order to suit their own style. A brief (assessment) diet history consists essentially of the same steps but requires less detailed probing for quantities.

1 24-hour recall. Take the respondent through the previous day noting times of all meals and snacks and what was eaten. This is relatively easy to do, concentrates the respondent's mind on food and gives a guide to meal patterns. If the respondent is an in-patient, establish the pattern of a typical day at home. If the 24-hour recall is difficult, then a diet history is probably impossible!

2 Establish the quantities eaten on the 24-hour recall. This relates to one specific day, and is therefore less hypothetical than 'what quantity might you eat?' Get the respondent to describe quantities, which will give a guide to appetite and a cross-check on reliability of later answers. If possible, use portion models.

3 Establish the weekly pattern. Is the specific 24-hour pattern different in any way from the 'usual' pattern? Take the respondent through the day again. What other dishes might be eaten at each meal? What happens on Saturday and Sunday? What happens if the respondent is working a different shift? How often does he go out? How often does he have visitors? What dishes would be eaten? Probe specifically for sweets, snacks and other items consumed between meals, also alcoholic drinks.

4 Establish likely quantities. Use portion models; it is easier for the respondent to say 'my portion looks like that' than to search for verbal descriptions, particularly if inarticulate. The interviewer's interpretation is also likely to be more accurate. Respondents who do their own shopping can also provide information on quantities bought and for how many people.

5 Establish recipes for composite dishes. This is not always possible with those who do not cook.

6 Cross-check the information already obtained against a list of foods appropriate for the purpose of the study, e.g. to assess vitamin C, only fruit and vegetables (and composite dishes containing them) and squashes, need to be included. The cross-checking can take the form of a set of cards handed to the respondent, rather than the interviewer questioning about each food individually. For each food, ascertain how frequently a 'portion' is eaten on a daily, weekly or monthly basis. Particularly in a full diet history this section demands the best of the interviewer's technique, as it can be lengthy, repetitive and boring.

Essential points to remember

1 Do not *assume* anything about respondent's meal patterns, recipes or portion sizes. It is all too easy to transfer one's own eating patterns on to other people, e.g. 'Fridays we have fried fish'. What does the respondent mean by this? Is it cod coated in batter and deep fried, or plaice lightly tossed in butter, or something else? Do not assume it actually means what *you* think it means; check it. If there is not a full description of the food, you may not be able to select the correct food code or to complete the calculation later.

2 Write everything down. If information is received from the respondent but not recorded, then the interviewer's memory becomes a factor in the accuracy of the diet history. Check that you have not made any obvious mistakes like recording 1000 g instead of 10 g of sugar in tea. Checking that you have recorded the respondent accurately is as important as checking that the respondent has reported fully. It should be possible for someone else to check and calculate a diet history and get the same results as the interviewer. Use a pre-designed form and not scraps of paper (see Table 1.8)

3 Watch for non-verbal clues of boredom or irritation as it is difficult to avoid the inquisitorial aspect. To counteract this, break the flow of questioning by making some comment on how much time is needed to complete the interview or a humorous reference to the number of questions being asked.

Problems of the diet history

1 Holding all the points on which information is needed in one's head is difficult, particularly if inexperienced.

2 Questions may be phrased inappropriately, particularly while thinking of other points to be covered.

3 It is easy to put words into the respondent's mouth. Beware of leading questions.

4 Verbal descriptions of quantity may be very unreliable and may be mistranslated by the interviewer.

Bias is introduced by the respondent's memory and subjective impressions. For instance

(a) A tendency to over-remember 'proper' meals.

(b) A tendency to under-remember snacks.

(c) 'I always have fish on Fridays' may in fact mean two Fridays out of three.

(d) Memory is weighted by the last seven days.

(e) Cross-checking generally overestimates food used infrequently, i.e. if liver is eaten 'once a month', it is probably in fact less frequently. 'Daily', 'weekly' and 'never' frequencies are probably more reliable.

5 The more irregular the eating pattern, the less reliable a diet history tends to be.

6 Respondents may not be entirely truthful.

Analysis and interpretation of information

Assessment of food intake

Depending on the purpose of taking the diet history, the food intake may be assessed or analysed in a variety of ways

1 By relating the food intake to a daily food guide.

2 By using knowledge of food composition to make a judgement about some aspects of the diet, e.g. the adequacy of fibre intake or the likely contribution of the diet to dental caries.

3 By using a table of approximate food values to make a crude calculation of the intake of one or more dietary constituents.

4 By using detailed tables of food composition to calculate the intake of specific nutrients.

Points 1−3 above are relevant to the brief diet history and point 4 to the full diet history.

Assessment of nutrient intake

Nutrient intake = nutrient content of food × portion weight × frequency of consumption. For example, compare the relative contributions of parsley and milk to vitamin C intake

Parsley provides 150 mg/100 g × 1 g portion
                             × once/week = 0.2 mg/day
Milk provides   1.5 mg/100 g × 30 g portion
                             × eight/day = 3.6 mg/day.

Be careful to select from the tables the food which best represents the food described by the respondent. Similarly, care must be taken in translating the respondent's description of portion sizes into weights.

Interpretation

Interpret the results bearing in mind the limitations of the method, your judgement of the quality of information obtained and the variability of individual nutritional requirements. It is meaningless to report results to the nearest mg of calcium or g of protein. It is also more realistic to give results as a range of ±20% on the calculated value.

An *individual's* intake cannot be meaningfully compared directly with RDAs which are standards for *group* intake.

The written interpretation of the results must be expressed *concisely* and clearly. Where appropriate, suggestions should be made for remedying dietary problems.

Evaluation

Examine all aspects of your own work critically (see also Section 1.15). Evaluation of a diet history can be divided into three parts

1 The quality of the personal contact. Was the respondent relaxed and talking at ease? Did the interviewer feel comfortable with the respondent?
2 Validity: Am I measuring what I think I am measuring? Is the answer obtained the correct answer? This is almost impossible to check, but assessing the same respondent by several different methods helps. There is no absolute standard, but a seven day weighed intake is usually assumed to give the most valid results.
3 Reliability: Can I get the same answer as another person? Can I get the same answer on two separate occasions (unless the respondent has changed eating habits)? Standardization of interview technique and of tools used in analysis (and method of use) is essential otherwise different interviews will obtain different results — and how do you decide which is the correct one?

Suggested forms for recording information obtained in the course of taking a diet history (Table 1.8)

The type of form shown here is essentially a blank sheet with some memory-jogging headings. It is the most flexible in application, but its memory-jogging content is minimal and it is up to the interviewer to remember what information must be extracted. This form also gives no guidance on the structure of the interview or on the phrasing of questions. If a series of interviews are to be conducted as part of a research project, it is probably advisable to design a more 'structured' form, so that the phrasing of questions and the shape of the interview are standardized and so that it concentrates on the specific information required.

The first part of the form is for background information. What is included here will obviously vary from department to department and with the purposes of the diet history.

The summary sheet or check list is designed to be used with a set of cards. Each section of the check list is printed on a separate card which can be handed to the patient so that he also has a memory-jogger. The foods which are included on the check list and their order and grouping will depend on the purpose of the diet history, on local eating patterns and the preferences of individual interviewers; the list given here should not be regarded as definitive.

Table 1.8 Suggested forms for use when taking diet history

Background information

Respondent . . . .
Date of history . . . .
Interviewer . . . .

Name.	Registration No. . . . .
Address	Clinic . . . .
. . . .	Physician . . . .
Date of birth	
Place of birth	Sex . . . .
Religion	Height . . . .
Occupation	Weight . . . .

Table 1.8 *contd.*

Working hours . . . .   Standard weight . . . .

Number in household . . . .

Patient's status in household . . . .

Who does the cooking? . . . .

Cooking equipment of relevance . . . .

Storage facilities, e.g. freezer . . . .

Meals taken out . . . .

Food dislikes or intolerances . . . .

Food preferences . . . .

Diet history

Meal pattern

| Respondent . . . . |
| Date of history . . . . |
| Interviewer . . . . |

Meal	Weekdays	Saturday/shift	Sunday/shift
Early morning or Breakfast			
During the morning			
Mid-day			
During the afternoon			
Evening meal			
During the evening			
During the night			

Check list

Food	Cooking method	Handy measure	Weight (g)	Frequency
Beverages				
Coffee				
instant				
ground				
Horlicks, Ovaltine, Bournvita				
Cocoa, Drinking chocolate				
Tea				
Squash				
Fizzy drinks				

Table 1.8 *contd.*

Food	Cooking method	Handy measure	Weight (g)	Frequency
Alcoholic drinks				
beer				
wine				
cider				
spirits				
Fruit juices				
Oxo, Bovril				
Breads, spreads and fats				
Bread (rolls, slices)				
white				
brown				
wholemeal				
wheatgerm				
starch reduced				
Chapattis				
Butter/margarine/low fat spread				
on bread				
on vegetables				
on crispbread				
Dripping				
Jam, marmalade				
Honey				
Lemon curd				
Marmite, Bovril				
Peanut butter				
Meat/fish pastes				
Sandwich fillings				
Brawn				
Other spreads				
Fat for cooking: corn/sunflower/safflower/soya oil				
: vegetable oil				
: lard				
: other				
Breakfast cereals				
Porridge, Ready Brek				
Cold cereals				
Muesli				
Bran				
Dairy products				
Milk (fresh)				
in drinks				
on cereal				
straight				
Other milk				
gold top				
semi-skimmed				
skimmed				
dried, whole				
, skimmed				
evaporated, condensed				
Cream				
single				
double				
whipping				
Cheese				
hard type, full-fat				
, reduced fat				
blue cheese				
cream cheese				
cottage cheese				
cheese spreads				

Table 1.8 *contd.*

Food	Cooking method	Handy measure	Weight (g)	Frequency
processed cheese				
Parmesan				
Yoghurt				
Eggs				
Whole eggs				
Meat and poultry				
Bacon				
back				
middle				
streaky				
gammon				
Cold meats				
ham				
corned beef				
luncheon meat				
haslet				
roast meats				
tongue				
Pork				
roast				
chops				
Beef				
roast				
steaks				
Lamb				
roast				
chops				
Poultry				
Game				
rabbit				
wild fowl				
Offal				
kidney				
liver				
tripe				
other offal				
Meat products				
Sausages				
beef				
pork				
other				
Paté				
Continental sausages, salami				
Sausage rolls				
Meat pies				
Pork pies				
Cornish pasties				
Beefburgers				
Black pudding				
Tinned meat dishes				
Stew, casseroles, hot pots				
Dumplings				
Yorkshire puddings				
Mince				
Curry				
Bolognese sauce				
Chinese dishes				
Pizza				
Pasta dishes				
Egg/cheese flans				

Table 1.8 *contd.*

Food	Cooking method	Handy measure	Weight (g)	Frequency

Fish and fish products
White fish
  cod
  haddock
  plaice
Smoked fish
Oily fish
  mackerel
  herrings
  tuna
  trout
Shellfish
  prawns
  scampi
  crab
  lobster
  cockles
Fish cakes
Fish fingers
Fish pie, kedgeree
Fish roe

Vegetables and meal accompaniments
Potatoes: boiled
       : roast
       : chips
       : jacket
       : mashed
Baked beans
Tinned spaghetti
Salad vegetables
Green vegetables
Root vegetables
Pulse vegetables
Rice white/brown
Spaghetti white/brown

Fruit
Fresh fruit
Tinned fruit
Stewed fruit
Dried fruit

Spices, sauces and soups
Vinegar, mustard
Salt & pepper
Bottled sauces
Salad cream
Mayonnaise
Salad dressings
Gravy
Tomato sauce/ketchup
White sauces; parsley/cheese
Other savoury sauces
Spices; Herbs

Puddings
Custard
  egg
  powder
Instant whip type
Fruit pie, crumble
Steamed sponge puddings

Table 1.8 *contd.*

Food	Cooking method	Handy measure	Weight (g)	Frequency
Christmas pudding				
Jam tarts				
Mince pies				
Cheesecake				
Jelly				
Trifle				
Pancakes				
Ice cream				
Milk puddings				
Sugar and confectionery				
Sugar				
in drinks				
on cereals				
Sweets				
boiled				
mints				
toffees				
gums				
liquorice allsorts				
Chocolate				
plain				
milk				
fancy				
Chocolate bars				
Cakes and biscuits				
Biscuits				
sweet				
semi-sweet				
digestive				
cream crackers				
chocolate digestive				
Cakes				
Victoria sponge (with fat)				
Victoria sponge (fatless)				
Madeira type				
fruit cake				
gateaux				
Meringues				
Doughnuts				
Scones				
Pastries				
Cream buns				
Eclairs				
Yeast buns				
Crumpets				
Gingerbread				
Medications				
Medicines				
Tonics				
Vitamin/mineral supplements				

Table 1.8 *contd.*

Diet history calculation sheet

Respondent	. . . .
Date of history	. . . .
Interviewer	. . . .

Food	Food code	Weight (g)	Fre- quency	Pro- tein	Fat	Carbo- hydrate

Respondent	. . . .
Date of history	. . . .
Interviewer	. . . .

Report: Conclusions and recommendations

References

Balogh M, Kahn HA and Medalie JH (1971) Random repeat 24-hour dietary recalls. *Am J Clin Nutr* **24**, 304–10.

Bingham S and Cummings JH (1983) The use of PABA as a marker to validate the completeness of 24-hour urine collections in man. *Clin Sci* **64**, 629–35.

Bingham S and Cummings JH (1984) Urine 24-hour nitrogen excretion as an independent measure of the habitual dietary protein intake in individuals. *Proc Nutr Soc* **43**, 80A.

Bingham S (1985) Aspects of dietary survey methodology. *BNF Bull* **10**, (44) 90–103.

Bingham S (1987) The dietary assessment of individuals; methods, accuracy, new techniques and recommendations. *Nutr Abstr Rev* (In press).

Black AE (1982) The logistics of dietary surveys. *Hum Nutr: Appl Nutr* **36A** 85–94.

Black AE, Cole TJ, Wiles SJ and White F (1983) Daily variation in food intake of infants from 2–18 months. *Hum Nutr: Appl Nutr* **37A**, 448–58.

British Dietetic Association (1983) *Guidelines for taking dietary histories*. Prepared by a working party for the BDA (unpublished but available from the BDA).

Byers TE, Randall I, Marshall JR, Rzepka TF, Cummings KM and Graham S (1983) Dietary history from the distant past. *Nutr Cancer* **5**, 69–77.

Fieldhouse P (1978) An interview model for use in dietetic training. *J Hum Nutr* **33**, (3), 206–10.

Isaksson B (1980) Urinary nitrogen output as a validity test in dietary surveys. *Am J Clin Nutr* **33**, 4–12.

Jensen OM Wahrendorf J, Rosenquist A and Geser A (1984) The reliability of questionnaire-derived historic dietary information and temporal stability of food habits in individuals. *Am J Epidemiol* **120**, 281–90.

Marr JW (1971) Individual dietary surveys: purposes and methods. *World Rev Nutr Diet* **13**, 105–64.

Rohan TE and Potter JO (1984) Retrospective assessment of dietary intake. *Am J Epidemiol* **120**, 876–7.

Steen B, Isaksson B and Svanborg A (1977) Intake of energy and nutrients in 70 year old males and females in Gothenburg, Sweden. *Acta Med Scand* [Suppl] **611**, 39–86.

Turner D (1940) The estimation of the patient's home dietary intake. *J Am Diet Assoc* **16**, 875–81.

Warnold I, Carlgren G and Krotkiewski M (1978) Energy expenditure and body composition during weight reduction in hyperplastic obese women. *Am J Clin Nutr* **31**, 750–63.

Widdowson EM (1936) A study of English diets by the individual method. Part I. Men. *J Hyg* **36**, 269–92.

Wiehl DG (1942) Diets of a group of aircraft workers in Southern California. *Millbank Memorial Fund Quarterly* **20**, 329–66.

Wiehl DG and Reed R (1960) Development of new or improved methods for epidemiologic investigation. *Am J Public Health* **50**, 824–8.

Youmans JB, Patton EW and Kern R (1942) Surveys of the nutrition of populations. *Am J Public Health* **32** 1371–9.

1.5   Typical Weights and Portion Sizes of Some Common Foods

The information in Tables 1.9 and 1.10 is intended as a guide for students and those inexperienced in assessing food intake. Quantities of foods are expressed either as a typical portion (e.g. a serving of a vegetable) and/or by a convenient unit (e.g. a slice of bread). The average weights of some manufactured foods are also given.

It must be remembered, however, that the term 'typical portion' is a loose one and that there will be considerable variation in the portion sizes consumed by an individual depending on age, sex and appetite.

The values given in Tables 1.9 and 1.10 have been derived from dietary survey data on healthy adults obtained by the Dunn Nutritional Laboratories, Cambridge, the Nuffield Laboratories of Comparative Medicine, London and from information supplied by a number of dietetic departments.

The following spoon sizes have been used

1 level teaspoon (tsp)   = 5 ml
1 level dessertspoon (dsp) = 10 ml
1 level tablespoon (tbs)   = 15 ml

Further weights of food portions are given in Table 2.22 (p 141).

Table 1.9 Typical unit weights/portion sizes of basic foodstuffs

Food	Weight (g)	Food	Weight (g)
Cereal products		Butter/margarine	
Bread		thickly spread on 1 large slice	10
— thin slice, large loaf	25	thinly spread on 1 large slice	7
— medium thick slice, large loaf	33	thinly spread on 1 small slice	5
— thick slice, large loaf	40	Mayonnaise (2 tbs)	30
— medium thick slice, small loaf	20	Cream (single/double)	
Rice, boiled	180	in coffee (1 tbs)	15
Spaghetti. boiled	200	on a dessert (2 tbs)	30
Biscuits		Cheese	
plain or semi-sweet (1)	7	cottage (2 tbs)	60
cream crackers (1)	7	Camembert	40
crispbread (1)	8	Cheddar/Stilton	30
Muffin (1)	40	Cheese spread	20
Croissant (1)	50	Yoghurt	125–150
Crumpet (2)	80	Cooking oil	
Scone (1)	30	1 tbs	18
Roll (1)	40	1 tsp	5
Currant bun (1)	35		
Doughnut (1 medium)	50	*Eggs*	
Fruit cake (1 medium slice)	75	One large (without shell)	54
Gingerbread (1 thick slice)	60	One medium (without shell)	48
Sponge cake	55	One small (without shell)	40
Mince pie (1 medium)	60	Yolk only, medium	17
Yorkshire pudding (1 small)	30	White only, medium	31
Breakfast cereals		Scrambled egg (1)	65
Muesli	60	Fried egg	50
Porridge	180	Omelette (1 egg)	60
Weetabix (2)	35		
Shredded Wheat (2)	50	*Meat and meat products*	
Cornflakes and similar breakfast cereals	30	Bacon	
		back, grilled (2 rashers)	30
Milk, dairy products, oils		streaky, grilled (3 rashers)	30
Milk		Beef	
in tea or coffee (2 tbs)	30	rump steak lean and fat, (small)	120
in tea or coffee (1 tsp)	5	(large)	250
glass	180	roast, (3 slices)	90
Coffeemate (2 tsp)	5	Pork/lamb leg, lean only	90

Table 1.9 *contd*

Food	Weight (g)	Food	Weight (g)
Lamb shoulder, lean only	90	Potatoes, typical portion of	
Pork/lamb chop		baked/chips/boiled/mashed	150
1 large	160	roast	120
1 small	100	Potatoes, per unit	
Chicken/turkey		boiled, the size of an egg	60
roast meat only	100	4 large chips	25
leg and bone	200	1 small roast	40
Corned beef (1 slice)	30	1 heaped tbs mashed	60
Kidney, lamb (2)	60	Sweetcorn, tinned (2 tbs)	60
Liver, lamb, fried	90	Swede	80
Cold meats (2 slices)	50	Tomatoes (1 medium)	60
Salami (2 slices)	30		
Black pudding	50	*Fruit*	
Paté		Apples, baking/eating	
— as starter to a meal	45	— 1 medium	120
— on bread	25	— 1 large	150
Frankfurters (2)	60	Avocado pear, without stone ($\frac{1}{2}$ medium sized)	75
Sausages		Banana	
grilled (2 large)	80	1 small, peeled	70
chipolatas (4)	80	1 medium, peeled	100
Beefburger (1)	60	Dates (2)	15
Savaloy (1)	80	Fruit, tinned/stewed	120
Pizza (7" diameter)	200	Fruit juice (small glass)	100
Pork pies		Grapes (10)	60
large	300	Grapefruit ($\frac{1}{2}$ small)	100
medium	140	Melon (1 slice)	120
small	65	Orange (1 medium, peeled)	120
Beef stew, average portion	200	Strawberries	100
Chilli con carne, average portion	280	Tangerine (1 medium)	60
Lasagne, average portion	300		
Cornish pasty	170	*Miscellaneous items*	
Sausage roll	60	Sugar	
		1 level tsp	5
Fish and fish products		1 rounded tsp	7
Cod/haddock/plaice, fried	130	1 tbs	19
Mackerel, fried ($\frac{1}{2}$)	90	Jam/marmalade/honey (2 level tsp)	15
Herring, edible portion (1 small)	90	Peanut butter (2 tsp)	15
Kipper, baked	120	Syrup (1 tbs)	20
Pilchards/sardines	80	Treacle (1 tbs)	20
Salmon/tuna	60	Cheesecake	150
Anchovies (3 thin fillets)	12	Milk puddings	120
Shrimps, prawns	30	Ice cream (2 scoops)	120–150
Fish fingers (2)	50	Sponge pudding	150
Fish cakes (2)	120	Souffle	120
		Chocolate sauce (2 tbs)	40
Vegetables and salad		Bournvita and malted milk drinks (2 heaped tsp)	15
Beans		Cocoa powder (1 heaped tbs)	6
— runner, boiled	75	White sauce (2 tbs)	33
— haricot, boiled	100	Brown/tomato sauce (1 tbs)	17
— baked in tomato sauce (2 tbs)	40	Oxo cube (1)	6
Beetroot, cooked	40	Instant coffee powder (1 tsp)	2
Brussel sprouts, boiled	80	Soup (1 bowl)	240
Cabbage, boiled	100		
Carrots, boiled	70	*Alcohol*	
Cauliflower, boiled	120	Keg bitter/lager/cider	1 pint (568 ml)
Celery (1 stick)	60		$\frac{1}{2}$ pint (284 ml)
Cucumber (1")	40	Wine, 1 glass (pub measure)	125–150 ml
Leeks, boiled	80	Sherry/vermouth/port	60 ml
Lettuce	25	Spirits (single pub measure)	$\frac{1}{6}$ gill (25 ml)
Peas			
— garden	75		
— chick	75		

Table 1.10 Weights of some manufactured food items

Foods	Weight (g)	Foods	Weight (g)
Biscuits		*Meat and meat products*	
Bandit	20	Harris cottage pie	180
Blue Riband	20	Marks and Spencer minced beef and onion pie	190
Cadbury's Chocolate Wheatmeal biscuit	10	Walls steak and kidney pie	180
Caramel chocolate covered wafer	25	Mattesons spreading pate	113
Chocolate chip cookie	10	St Ivel pan bake pizza	500
McVities			
Chocolate digestive	17	*Fish*	
Digestive	15	John West pink salmon	213 and 440
Sports chocolate biscuits	22	John West tuna	99 and 198
Club (Jacobs)	25	Glenryck pilchards	425
Custard cream	15	Glenryck sardines	120
Gingernut	10		
Harvest crunch	18	*Vegetables*	
Jaffa cake	12	Heinz baked beans	
Penguin	30	large tin	450
Rich tea (2)	15	medium tin	225
Rich tea finger	5	small tin	150
Taxi	18		
Trio chocolate biscuits	25	*Crisps and nuts*	
Wagon wheel	35	*Crisps*	
Yoyo	20	Golden Wonder (small packet)	25
Butter puff	10	KP (small packet)	30
Cornish wafer	10	KP Hula Hoops (small packet)	25
Cream crackers (2)	15	Marks and Spencer (large packet)	75
Tuc	5	Scampi fries (small packet)	25
Water biscuits (2)	15	Walkers (small packet)	28
		(medium packet)	50
Cakes			
Mr Kipling		*Nuts*	
Cherry slice	38	Almonds (6 whole, shelled)	9
Country slice	38	KP almonds (small packet)	30
French fancy	30	KP cashews	25
Fruit pie	53	KP peanuts	50 and 100
Jam tart	40	KP mixed nuts and raisins	50 and 125
Lyons Harvest pie (family size)	300	Golden Wonder mixed nuts and raisins	40 and 78
Harvest pie (individual)	120		
Harvest pie (small)	32	*Sweets and Chocolate*	
Iced tarts (1)	30	*Sweets*	
Caprice	15	Buttered brazil (1)	9
Sainsburys		Chews (1 packet)	30
Chocolate cup cake	40	Chewing gum (1 stick)	4
Fruit pie (1)	55	Jelly babies (1 packet)	113
Eccles cake	42	Maltesers (small packet, 18 sweets)	38
Jam tart	25	Minstrels	
Lemon curd tart	25	— family packet (33 sweets)	90
Mince pie	50	— small packet (15 sweets)	40
Bird's Eye		New Berry fruit (1)	15
Chocolate eclair	35	Smarties (1 tube)	32
		Pastilles	
Yoghurts/desserts		— small packet	33
St Ivel Shape		— medium packet	42
— Natural	150	Polos (1)	1.5
Fruit	125	Rolos (1 packet, 9 sweets)	46
Mr Men	150	Treets (1 packet)	42
Real	125		
Yoplait		*Chocolate*	
Petits Filous	60	Aero	42
Chambourcy		Banjo	47
Nouvelle and Bonjour	125	Bounty (2 small bars)	58
Creme dessert	100	Bournville	50
Black forest dessert	100	Cadburys	
Caramel dessert	92	Milk chocolate bar (small)	60
Eden Vale champagne sundae	125	Fruit and Nut	57
		Whole nut	55
		Creme egg	40

Table 1.10 *contd*

Food	Weight (g)	Food	Weight (g)
Caramac	20 and 38	Mars bar	
Crunchie	35	— Normal size	68
Double decker	50	— King size	100
Drifter	52	Milky Way	32
Flake	35	Marks and Spencer white chocolate bar	30
Fry's chocolate cream	50	Prewetts bars	42
Galaxy bar	70	Star bar	45
Harvest Crunch	18	Toffee crisp	40
Jordans Original Crunchy bar	33	Topic	53
Kit Kat		Twix (2 bars)	50
4 finger	50	Walnut whip	32
2 finger	24	Wispa	35
Lion bar	42	Yorkie bar	60
Marathon	58		

1.6 Food Tables

1.6.1 Available food tables

The standard British food tables are McCance and Widdowson's *The Composition of Foods* (Paul and Southgate 1978). Before using the tables it is essential to read the text (pp 1−34), to be aware of the laboratory and sampling procedures used (pp 313−29), and the recipes adopted (pp 334−45). Paul *et al* (1986) have recently reviewed publications giving the nutritional analysis of UK foods which have been undertaken since the publication of the fourth edition of McCance and Widdowson's *The Composition of Foods*. Twenty-eight publications are quoted. Typographical corrections to the fourth edition, and the weight loss on cooking the recipe dishes are also given. Other food tables which might be of use are listed in Table 1.11, but it should be recognized that the analytical methods used and the factors for converting analytical results into nutrients are not always interconvertible. For example, carbohydrate is measured 'by difference' in American food tables, and directly in British ones. The factors used to convert nitrogen into protein may also vary substantially between tables. It is essential to read the introduction to any set of food tables before using them.

1.6.2 Accuracy of food tables

The values in food tables are averages of representative samples of food or selected values from literature surveys. Like any other biological material, the composition of a particular food will vary considerably from the average. The composition of a diet based on very few foods, a metabolic diet for instance, is therefore likely to differ from that calculated from food tables, and in this instance duplicates of the actual foods concerned must be prepared for direct laboratory analysis.

Provided that the differences from the averages are randomly distributed, then nutrient intake calculated from food tables and from direct analysis will tend to agree more closely if a greater variety of foods is included in the daily diet, or if the length of time individuals are asked to keep records is extended, or if the numbers of individuals chosen to represent a

Table 1.11 A selected list of food tables

Title	Available from
McCance and Widdowson's *The Composition of Foods* 4th edn Paul AA and Southgate DAT (1978) MRC Special Report Series No 297.	HMSO, London, UK.
First supplement to McCance and Widdowson's *The Composition of Foods: Amino acid composition (mg per 100 g food) and fatty acid composition (g per 100 g food)* Paul AA, Southgate DAT and Russell J (1980).	HMSO, London, UK.
Second supplement to McCance and Widdowson's *The Composition of Foods: Immigrant foods* Tan SP, Wenlock RW and Buss DH (1985).	HMSO, London, UK.
McCance and Widdowson's *The Composition of Foods. Supplementary Information and review of new compositional data* Paul AA, Southgate DAT and Buss DH (1986) *Hum Nutr: Appl Nutr* **40A**, 287−99.	
Tables of representative values of foods commonly used in tropical countries Platt BS (1962) MRC Special Report Series No 302.	HMSO, London, UK.
Amino acid content of foods Nutrition Division, FAO: Nutritional Studies No 24. (1970)	HMSO, London, UK.
Composition of Foods Watt BK and Merrill AL (1975) Agricultural Handbook No 8. Revisions of Agricultural Handbook No 8 8−1 Dairy and egg products (1976) 8−2 Spices and herbs (1977) 8−3 Baby foods (1978) 8−4 Fats and oils (1979) 8−5 Poultry products (1979) 8−6 Soups, sauces and gravies (1980) 8−7 Sausages and luncheon meats (1981) 8−8 Breakfast cereals (1982) 8−9 Fruits and fruit juices (1982) 8−10 Pork products (1983) 8−11 Vegetable and vegetable products (1984) 8−12 Nut and seed products (1984) 8−13 Beef products (1986) 8−14 Beverages (1986)	Superintendent of Documents, US Government Printing Office, Washington DC 20402, USA.

population average is increased. For example, with a single day's comparison in individuals consuming their normal mixed diets, the standard deviation of differences between analysed and calculated intakes of protein is 13% on average, meaning that the two can be expected to differ by at least 26 g on any single day (assuming an average intake of 100 g). When the averages from 28 days are compared however, there is complete agreement (standard deviation of difference = 2%).

However, agreement between analysed and calculated values for other nutrients is generally not as good as that for protein. The fat content of meat and cooked dishes is highly variable and micronutrients such as vitamin C and folate are susceptible to destruction by certain cooking practices. Salt consumption is usually underestimated using food tables and is most accurately assessed by analysis of complete 24-hour urine samples (see Section 1.4.1). Paul and Southgate (1978) provide detailed discussions of the accuracy and limitations of values given in food tables.

Certainly nutrient intakes should never be reported with a greater apparent precision than that of the published values.

References

Paul AA and Southgate DAT (1978) McCance and Widdowson's *The Composition of Foods* 4e. MRC Special Report Series No 297. London, HMSO.

Paul AA, Southgate DAT and Buss DH (1986) McCance and Widdowson's *The Composition of Foods*: supplementary information and review of new compositional data. *Hum Nutr: Appl Nutr*, **40A**, 287–99.

1.7 Computers in Dietetics

1.7.1 General considerations

Computers can be used in all aspects of dietetics and are valuable tools in the clinical, educational and management areas of dietetic work (Howard and Hall 1981; Morley 1984). They can store, retrieve and manipulate information which 'the user' provides; they do this using a specially designed set of instructions — the 'program'. Computers vary in size from a hand-held one (Colley *et al* 1985), which can only store a very small amount of information in its memory, to a large mainframe computer which can store a vast amount of information. There are now many good books which explain what computers can do and how they work, and which define some of the computer jargon (BDA 1986). A list of books is given in Appendix 2. For those dietitians needing help initially, the British Dietetic Association runs a 'computer contact' scheme. There are also courses run for dietitians by Regional Training Departments and other outside bodies (Bassham and Fletcher 1986).

The advantages of computers are that they can manipulate data much faster than the human brain; they are more accurate and reliable (provided they are operated and programmed correctly); they can perform complex tasks (e.g. handle many variables and collate different sets of data rapidly); they can cope with increasing volumes of data; and they can store information in a small space. It must be remembered however, that they cannot think for themselves and are only as good as the data which is put into them and the programs (or software) which are used to run them. Disadvantages include the high initial cost, dependence on technology, problems with breakdowns, lack of flexibility and lack of suitable programs.

Computers are being used by dietitians internationally (Youngwirth 1983) and will continue to be used (Williams and Burnet 1984) in all aspects of dietetic work, from data storage to nutrition education (Brook 1971). A summary of the main areas of application is included in Table 1.12.

Although there are many different types of computer on the market, there is at present little software specifically for dietitians. Many of the general business programs can, however, be adapted for dietetic purposes. These programs include *database* (which permits the storage and processing of data in different forms), *spreadsheets* (complex calculation packages) and *authoring* systems (computer assisted learning) (BDA 1986). A list of programs which are of use in dietetics is available from the British Dietetic Association and there is also an American *Journal of Dietetic Software*. The use of computers will become more commonplace within the medical profession over the next few years and there are many plans for future developments that include dietetics.

Table 1.12 Use of computers by dietitians

Use	Details/Program
Computation	
Dietary analysis	Most based on McCance and Widdowson tables. Commercial software available, both specific and linked with catering. Some dietetic departments have developed their own. Smaller programs with limited foods available.
Dietary assessment	Few available, e.g. for assessment of requirements in nutritional support.
Dietary construction	Collation/construction of diets e.g. choosing foods rich in a nutrient, or involving detailed diets, e.g. PKU/ketogenic diets.
Education/training	
Staff/patients	Computer assisted learning packages (CAL) both commercial and tutoring or authoring systems used. Range from 'fun' games to student tutorials.
Interview/counselling	Very few programs available, but other programs could be adapted.
Information storage	Application of database packages for 1 Patient records/lists 2 Manufactured product information 3 Special feeds/regimens 4 Standard recipes/menus
Administration	Using business packages, e.g. word processing, spreadsheets, planners, etc. for 1 Diet sheets/product lists 2 Reports 3 Appointments/records 4 Statistics (Körner information) 5 Budgets/Stock control.
Research	Specific programs written for projects. Statistical packages available, questionnaire analysis.
Links with other systems	Patient administration systems — links with hospital mainframe. Commercial links, e.g. Prestel, Micronet, Food databanks.

Data protection act

The Data Protection Act (1984) came into force in November 1985 and by the middle of 1986 all computers which hold personal data about individuals for practice, private or research purposes will have to be registered with the Registrar (NHSTA 1985). It is important, therefore, that dietitians using computers register under this Act. For those working in the NHS, registration is usually collective at District or Regional level and further information is available from District or Area health boards who have a designated officer. There is also a wealth of material explaining the implications of the Act (National Health Service Computer Policy Committee 1984; The Data Protection Act Guideline No 1 1985; BDA 1986).

1.7.2 Nutrient analysis systems

The process of assessing the nutrient content of any diet involves

1 Establishing the foods eaten and the quantities, either from a pre-determined menu or by dietary assessment (see Section 1.4).
2 Looking up each individual food in the food tables and calculating the amounts of each nutrient provided by the given weight of the food.
3 Totalling the amounts of each nutrient obtained from all the foods.
4 Converting the total intake to amounts per day (or other period of time).

These calculations are simple but laborious and time consuming when done by hand and lend themselves to computerization (Bassham *et al* 1984). Nutrient analysis systems have been developed over the past fifteen years and vary from programs with limited analysis of up to 100 foods, to those which will handle the full McCance and Widdowson food tables (Paul and Southgate 1978; Paul *et al* 1980). The latter are able to analyse at least 950 foods for over 40 nutritional factors, including fatty acids and amino acids. Programs can be used for the analysis of the intake of a single patient on a special diet over a specified period, or the total nutrient content of the hospital menu over a monthly cycle or large numbers of diet records obtained from surveys. A summary of the principle advantages of using computers for detailed diet analysis include

1 It saves time.
2 It gives more reliable results.
3 The intake of many nutrients can be calculated as easily as the intake of one or two. Taking advantage of this facility may therefore enable a better total clinical assessment to be made.
4 Updating information is often easier, and manufactured products can be included in the database.
5 The system can be used in menu planning and could be linked with catering departments for monitoring stores, food uptake and costings.
6 Usage in collation of diet sheets and food lists.

Nutritional analysis programs

Most computerized nutrient analysis programs follow a format similar to that outlined in Fig. 1.2. Any analysis program must have an accurate food and nutrient database. Care must also be taken over the use of the database in any program, especially as many people are inclined to believe that everything produced by a computer must be correct. If McCance and Widdowson food tables are being used, thought must be given as to how to cope with trace values, estimated values and 'no data' values. Consideration must also be given to the handling of composite dishes in programs using food groups. Setting up a food database can be difficult, time consuming and requires expertise (Bassham and Stanton 1984) and only a few dietitians have attempted it. The early programs relied on a paper tape from HMSO containing McCance and Widdowson food data (Russell 1978) and this was used to put together programs for hospital and university mainframe computers (Brereton *et al* 1973). Nutritional analysis programs which use McCance and Widdowson data are now available for microcom-

Table 1.13 Nutritional analysis programs

Programs	Reference
Mainframe computers	
Northwick Park dietary constituents system	Brereton *et al* (1973)
Royal Victoria Hospital, Belfast	McConnell and Wilson (1976)
Recipe	Day (1980)
Diet	Walsh (1976)
	Lowell and Mechie (1983)
Diet 2 and Diet 3	Wise (1986)
Stoke Program (NHS)	
University/Polytechnic/Research unit programs	
Microcomputers	
Microdiet	Bassham *et al* (1984)
Nutricalc	Hall *et al* (1984)
B and W Systems — Dietary Analysis	
XI — Diet	
Superdiet	Gamble *et al* (1980)
Fretwell Downing system	

A full list of dietetic software, including contact names for the different programs, is available from the British Dietetic Association on receipt of an s a e. A list of computer users is also available.

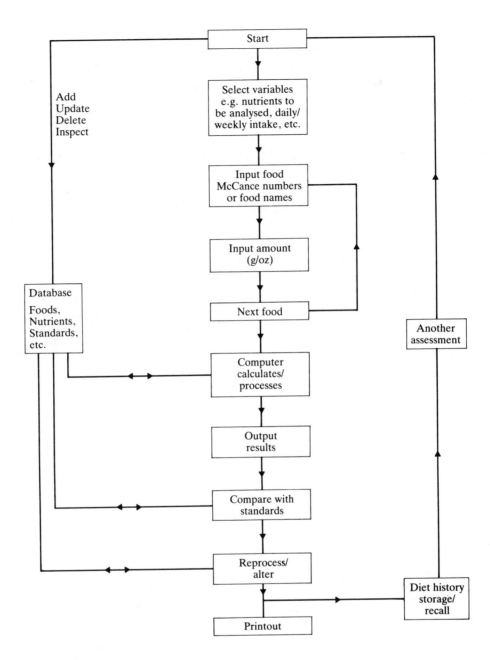

Start

Select variables
e.g. nutrients to
be analysed, daily/
weekly intake, etc.

Add
Update
Delete
Inspect

Input food
McCance numbers
or food names

Input amount
(g/oz)

Database
Foods,
Nutrients,
Standards,
etc.

Next food

Another
assessment

Computer
calculates/
processes

Output
results

Compare with
standards

Reprocess/
alter

Diet history
storage/
recall

Printout

Fig. 1.2 Flowchart of 'typical' diet analysis program.

puters. The Royal Society of Chemistry with the Ministry of Agriculture, Fisheries and Food is in the process of setting up a national food and nutrient database which dietitians should be able to link up with in the future. Nutrient analysis programs presently in use are summarized in Table 1.13. Those which run on mainframe computers may use either on-line analysis or batch analysis.

On-line analysis

On-line analysis is similar to a microcomputer system in that the process is interactive and data/information is fed into the computer using a keyboard and video display unit. This has the advantage of immediate

results, giving a hard copy via a printer, while enabling errors to be checked as the assessment is being processed.

Batch systems

Batch systems on the other hand usually involve recording the data on special forms which are then sent off to a central mainframe computer for processing, the results being returned after a delay in the form of a printout (Brereton *et al* 1973). This method of analysis is being used less often now as it has obvious disadvantages.

Some of the programs listed in Table 1.13 also have facilities additional to straight nutrient analysis such as comparing results with standards which can be specified by the user. Others have additional information in the database, for example the nutrient composites of cooked dishes published as a supplement to McCance and Widdowson (Wiles *et al* 1980) or immigrant food information (Tan *et al* 1985). With any program it is essential to check that it meets the user's specific requirements. It is essential to try out a program before purchasing it. Table 1.14 is a guide to what to look for in a nutritional analysis program.

As well as programs based on the complete McCance and Widdowson food tables, there are some which allow analysis of about 100 foods for five different nutrients and have been designed especially for dietitians using a small hand-held computer. Being portable, this computer has the advantage that it can be taken in a dietitian's pocket to a patient's bedside. Other programs have been written to run on micro-computers for use in schools and some enterprising software firms now produce very simple analysis programs for use on home computers. In the future it may be possible to work out the total nutrient content of a meal whilst it is being cooked in the kitchen!

A word of warning: whether calculated by computer or by hand, the values for the nutrient content of a diet are worth only as much as the method of dietary assessment used to establish the foods and quantities eaten.

Further reading

Davy C and Alcock D (1982) *Illustrating computers.* Pan Information Series, London.
Horton J (19) *Introduction to microcomputing.* Castle House Publications Ltd, Tunbridge Wells.
Corder C. and Reid R. *What is a Computer? How does a computer work? What is a computer program?* Booklets produced by Video Arts to accompany their films and available from: Video Arts, 2nd Floor, Dumbarton House, 68 Oxford Street, London WIN 9LA.
Carrey D (1984) *The computer — how it works?* Ladybird Books, Loughborough.
Smith J (1984) *Microknowledge.* Ladybird Books, Loughborough.
Bradbeer R (1982) *The computer book.* BBC Publications, London.
Bly RW (1984) *The Puffin dictionary of computer words.* Puffin,
Strong BD (1983) *Microcomputer in plain English.* David and Charles (Holdings) Ltd, Newton Abbot.
Maloff C and Zears R (1979) *Computers in nutrition.* Artech.

References

Bassham S, Fletcher LR and Stanton RHJ (1984) Dietary analysis with the aid of a microcomputer. *J Microcomp Applic* **7**, 279−89.
Bassham S and Stanton RHJ (1984) Something to add. *British Dietetic Association ADviser* **12**, 19−20.
Bassham S and Fletcher LR (1986) Computer appreciation training for dietitians. *Hum Nutr: Appl Nutr* **39A**, 400−6.
British Dietetic Association Research Committee (1986) *Computer Guide for Dietitians.* British Dietetic Association.
Brereton P, Healy MJR and Pittaway M (1973) A simple computerized system for dietary calculations. *Nutrition Lond.* **3**, 200−5.
Brook BM (1971) The use of the computer in nutrition education. *Nutrition Lond.* **25**, 24−9.
Colley CM, Fleck A and Howard JP (1985) Pocket computers; a new aid to nutritional support. *Br Med J* **290**, 1403−6.
Data Protection Act (1984) HMSO, London.
Data Protection Act (1985) *Guidelines No. 1* from The Data Protection Registrar, Springfield House, Water Lane, Wilmslow.
Day KC (1980) Recipe — a computer program for calculating the nutrient content of foods. *J Hum Nutr* **34**, 181−7.
Gamble P, Gentry R and Kipps P (1980) The superdiet computer. *Nutr Food Sci* **65**, 17−9.
Hall L, Carter D, Pettit B, Pettit S and Springford J (1984) Chips in the dietetic department. *British Dietetic Association ADviser* **13**, 21−2.
Hoover LW and Perloff BP (1981) *Model for review of nutrient database system capabilities.* University of Missouri.
Howard JP and Hall L (1981) A review of the use of computers in dietetic departments. Unpublished.

Table 1.14 Checklist for assessing a nutrient analysis program (Hoover and Perloff 1981)

General	Can the system be updated/who will do this?
	What back up/support will there be if the system goes wrong?
	Will it work with other systems?
	Check compatability.
Input	How is this done — on-line/batch?
	Are food names or McCance numbers used?
	Can a McCance number be found if needed?
	Are standard portions indicated?
	Can different units, e.g. oz or g, be used?
Analysis	Will it analyse all nutrients including micronutrients?
	How does it cope with values for which there is no information in the database?
	Does it compare with standards?
	Will it do costings?
	Will it work out nutrients in terms of
	Total amount/percentage total?
	Percentage energy intake?
	Percentage of a pre-defined standard?
	Per portion/100 kcal/100 g/kg body weight/unit cost?
	Ratios, e.g. polyunsaturated: saturated fatty acids?
	Will it give exchanges, food groups, or type?
	Does it have conversion factors/averaging factors?
	How accurate is the analysis/What is the error?
Output	What format is used — is this clear?
	Will it give complete analysis per meal/day/week?
	Can you select individual nutrients to be displayed?
	How does it show zero values/estimates/trace amounts on the printout?
	Can you use different output formats, e.g. bar graphs, pie charts, etc.?
Database	Where does the data come from — which food tables have been used?
	Can you add / delete nutrients or foods or add / delete manufactured products?
	Can you list the database?
	Can you set your own standards/recommended daily intakes/dietary goals?
	Does it cope with mixed dishes recipes?
	Can you store/recall information, e.g. diet histories?

Lowell JP and Mechie JR (1983) Computerized dietary calculations: an interactive approach updated. *Hum Nutr: Appl Nutr* **37A**, 36–40.

McConnell FG and Wilson A (1976) Computerized nutritional analysis in the dietetic department of a teaching hospital. *J Hum Nutr* **30**, 405–13.

Morley T (1984) Why compute? *British Dietetic Association ADviser* **13**, 19–20.

National Health Service Computer Policy Committee (1984) *Data protection guidelines for NHS authorities*. Centre for Information Technology, Birmingham.

National Health Service Training Authority (1985) *Data Protection Act — resource pack*, The National Computing Centre Ltd, National Health Service Training Authority, Bristol.

Paul AA and Southgate DAT (1978) McCance and Widdowson's *The Composition of Foods 4ed*. HMSO, London.

Paul AA, Southgate DAT and Russell J (1980) *First Supplement to McCance and Widdowson's The Composition of Foods*. HMSO, London.

Tan SP, Wenlock RW and Buss DH (1985) Immigrant Foods. Second supplement to McCance and Widdowson's *The Composition of Foods*. HMSO, London.

Russell J (1978) The paper tape version of McCance and Widdowsons *The Composition of Foods*. HMSO, London.

Walsh KA (1976) Computerized dietary calculation; an interactive approach. *J Hum Nutr* **30**, 395–403.

Wiles SJ, Nettleton PA, Black AE and Paul AA (1980) The nutrient composition of some cooked dishes eaten in Britain: a supplementary food composition table. *J Hum Nutr* **34**, 189–223.

Williams CS and Burnet LW (1984) Future applications of the microcomputer in dietetics. *Hum Nutr: Appl Nutr* **38A**, 99–109.

Wise A (1986) Interactive computer programs for applied nutrition education. *Hum Nutr: Appl Nutr* **39A**, 407–14.

Youngwirth J (1983) The evolution of computers in dietetics: a review. *J Am Diet Assoc* **82**, 62–7.

B: Anthropometric Standards
and Techniques

1.8 Height and Weight Tables

1.8.1 Infants and children

Weight and height attained

Many height and weight tables have been compiled for children. One well known set were derived from the combined data of Stuart (Boston) and Meredith (Iowa). Published in Nelson's *Textbook of paediatrics* they gained worldwide use and were also the basis for the WHO standards (Jelliffe 1966). These have been superseded for international use by the US National Centre for Health Statistics (NCHS) Standards; these are derived from a very large body of data gathered in the US in the late 1960s and early 1970s. The sample, the construction of the standards, charts and how the data may be used are described by Hamill *et al* (1979), who provide a full list of background references, and NCHS (1977). Tables 1.15 and 1.16 give the recumbent length and weight of children aged 0–3 years, and Tables 1.17 and 1.18 the standing height and weights of children aged 2–18 years.

The British Standards for many years have been those of Tanner *et al* (1966a, b). For ages 0–5 years, these are based on about 80 London children of each sex followed longitudinally and 250 Oxford children of each sex at each age. For ages 5–16 years they are based on approximately 24,000 London schoolchildren and from 16–18, on approximately 30 adolescents followed longitudinally.

A variety of clinical charts for the assessment of growth over different age ranges based on the above data are available from Castlemead Publications, Swain Mill, 4A Crane Mead, Ware, Herts SG12 9PY. They include the Gairdner–Pearson centile charts (1971) for boys and girls from 28 weeks gestation to 2 years of age and the Tanner–Whitehouse charts for boys and girls from 0–5 years.

There is evidence that growth of infants peaked in the 1960s. Australian studies conducted between 1920 and 1980 show similar birth weights, but median weights at 3, 6, 9 and 12 months rising from 1920 and peaking in 1964, with the 1980 values being similar to those found in the 1930s (Hitchcock *et al* 1981; Gracey and Hitchcock 1985.) Studies of breast-fed infants in Western countries in the late 1970s and early 1980s

Table 1.15 Smoothed percentiles of recumbent length (in cm) by sex and age: statistics from NCHS and data from Fels Research Institute, birth to 36 months (NCHS 1977; Hamill *et al* 1979). Reproduced with permission from the National Centre for Health Statistics.

Sex and age	Smoothed percentile						
	5th	10th	25th	50th	75th	90th	95th
Male	Recumbent length (cm)						
Birth	46.4	47.5	49.0	50.5	51.8	53.5	54.4
1 month	50.4	51.3	53.0	54.6	56.2	57.7	58.6
3 months	56.7	57.7	59.4	61.1	63.0	64.5	65.4
6 months	63.4	64.4	66.1	67.8	69.7	71.3	72.3
9 months	68.0	69.1	70.6	72.3	74.0	75.9	77.1
12 months	71.7	72.8	74.3	76.1	77.7	79.8	81.2
18 months	77.5	78.7	80.5	82.4	84.3	86.6	88.1
24 months	82.3	83.5	85.6	87.6	89.9	92.2	93.8
30 months	87.0	88.2	90.1	92.3	94.6	97.0	98.7
36 months	91.6	92.4	94.2	96.5	98.9	101.4	103.1
Female							
Birth	45.4	46.4	48.2	49.9	51.0	52.0	52.9
1 month	49.2	50.2	51.9	53.5	54.9	56.1	56.9
3 months	55.4	56.2	57.8	59.5	61.2	62.7	63.4
6 months	61.8	62.6	64.2	65.9	67.8	69.4	70.2
9 months	66.1	67.0	68.7	70.4	72.4	74.0	75.0
12 months	69.8	70.8	72.4	74.3	76.3	78.0	79.1
18 months	76.0	77.2	78.8	80.9	83.0	85.0	86.1
24 months	81.3	82.5	84.2	86.5	88.7	90.8	92.0
30 months	86.0	87.0	88.9	91.3	93.7	95.6	96.9
36 months	90.0	91.0	93.1	95.6	98.1	100.0	101.5

Table 1.16 Smoothed percentiles of weight (in kg) by sex and age: statistics from NCHS and data from Fels Research Institute, birth to 36 months (NCHS 1977; Hamill *et al* 1979). Reproduced with permission from the National Centre for Health Statistics.

Sex and age	Smoothed percentile						
	5th	10th	25th	50th	75th	90th	95th
Male				Weight (kg)			
Birth	2.54	2.78	3.00	3.27	3.64	3.82	4.15
1 month	3.16	3.43	3.82	4.29	4.75	5.14	5.38
3 months	4.43	4.78	5.32	5.98	6.56	7.14	7.37
6 months	6.20	6.61	7.20	7.85	8.49	9.10	9.46
9 months	7.52	7.95	8.56	9.18	9.88	10.49	10.93
12 months	8.43	8.84	9.49	10.15	10.91	11.54	11.99
18 months	9.59	9.92	10.67	11.47	12.31	13.05	13.44
24 months	10.54	10.85	11.65	12.59	13.44	14.29	14.70
30 months	11.44	11.80	12.63	13.67	14.51	15.47	15.97
36 months	12.26	12.69	13.58	14.69	15.59	16.66	17.28
Female							
Birth	2.36	2.58	2.93	3.23	3.52	3.64	3.81
1 month	2.97	3.22	3.59	3.98	4.36	4.65	4.92
3 months	4.18	4.47	4.88	5.40	5.90	6.39	6.74
6 months	5.79	6.12	6.60	7.21	7.83	8.38	8.73
9 months	7.00	7.34	7.89	8.56	9.24	9.83	10.17
12 months	7.84	8.19	8.81	9.53	10.23	10.87	11.24
18 months	8.92	9.30	10.04	10.82	11.55	12.30	12.76
24 months	9.87	10.26	11.10	11.90	12.74	13.57	14.08
30 months	10.78	11.21	12.11	12.93	13.93	14.81	15.35
36 months	11.60	12.07	12.99	13.93	15.03	15.97	16.54

Table 1.17 Smoothed percentiles of stature (in centimeters), by sex and age: Data and statistics from National Centre for Health Statistics, 2 to 18 years (From NCHS 1977; Hamill *et al* 1979) Reproduced with permission from the National Centre for Health Statistics.

Sex and age	Smoothed percentile						
	5th	10th	25th	50th	75th	90th	95th
Male				Stature (cm)			
2.0 years[1]	82.5	83.5	85.3	86.8	89.2	92.0	94.4
2.5 years	85.4	86.5	88.5	90.4	92.9	95.6	97.8
3.0 years	89.0	90.3	92.6	94.9	97.5	100.1	102.0
3.5 years	92.5	93.9	96.4	99.1	101.7	104.3	106.1
4.0 years	95.8	97.3	100.0	102.9	105.7	108.2	109.9
4.5 years	98.9	100.6	103.4	106.6	109.4	111.9	113.5
5.0 years	102.0	103.7	106.5	109.9	112.8	115.4	117.0
5.5 years	104.9	106.7	109.6	113.1	116.1	118.7	120.3
6.0 years	107.7	109.6	112.5	116.1	119.2	121.9	123.5
6.5 years	110.4	112.3	115.3	119.0	122.2	124.9	126.6
7.0 years	113.0	115.0	118.0	121.7	125.0	127.9	129.7
7.5 years	115.6	117.6	120.6	124.4	127.8	130.8	132.7
8.0 years	118.1	120.2	123.2	127.0	130.5	133.6	135.7
8.5 years	120.5	122.7	125.7	129.6	133.2	136.5	138.8
9.0 years	122.9	125.2	128.2	132.2	136.0	139.4	141.8
9.5 years	125.3	127.6	130.8	134.8	138.8	142.4	144.9
10.0 years	127.7	130.1	133.4	137.5	141.6	145.5	148.1
10.5 years	130.1	132.6	136.0	140.3	144.6	148.7	151.5
11.0 years	132.6	135.1	138.7	143.3	147.8	152.1	154.9
11.5 years	135.0	137.7	141.5	146.4	151.1	155.6	158.5
12.0 years	137.6	140.3	144.4	149.7	154.6	159.4	162.3
12.5 years	140.2	143.0	147.4	153.0	158.2	163.2	166.1
13.0 years	142.9	145.8	150.5	156.5	161.8	167.0	169.8
13.5 years	145.7	148.7	153.6	159.9	165.3	170.5	173.4
14.0 years	148.8	151.8	156.9	163.1	168.5	173.8	176.7
14.5 years	152.0	155.0	160.1	166.2	171.5	176.6	179.5
15.0 years	155.2	158.2	163.3	169.0	174.1	178.9	181.9
15.5 years	158.3	161.2	166.2	171.5	176.3	180.8	183.9
16.0 years	161.1	163.9	168.7	173.5	178.1	182.4	185.4
16.5 years	163.4	166.1	170.6	175.2	179.5	183.6	186.6
17.0 years	164.9	167.7	171.9	176.2	180.5	184.4	187.3
17.5 years	165.6	168.5	172.4	176.7	181.0	185.0	187.6
18.0 years	165.7	168.7	172.3	176.8	181.2	185.3	187.6

GENERAL DIETETIC PRINCIPLES AND PRACTICE

Table 1.17 contd.

Sex and age	Smoothed percentile						
	5th	10th	25th	50th	75th	90th	95th
Female							
2.0 years	81.6	82.1	84.0	86.8	89.3	92.0	93.6
2.5 years	84.6	85.3	87.3	90.0	92.5	95.0	96.6
3.0 years	88.3	89.3	91.4	94.1	96.6	99.0	100.6
3.5 years	91.7	93.0	95.2	97.9	100.5	102.8	104.5
4.0 years	95.0	96.4	98.8	101.6	104.3	106.6	108.3
4.5 years	98.1	99.7	102.2	105.0	107.9	110.2	112.0
5.0 years	101.1	102.7	105.4	108.4	111.4	113.8	115.6
5.5 years	103.9	105.6	108.4	111.6	114.8	117.4	119.2
6.0 years	106.6	108.4	111.3	114.6	118.1	120.8	122.7
6.5 years	109.2	111.0	114.1	117.6	121.3	124.2	126.1
7.0 years	111.8	113.6	116.8	120.6	124.4	127.6	129.5
7.5 years	114.4	116.2	119.5	123.5	127.5	130.9	132.9
8.0 years	116.9	118.7	122.2	126.4	130.6	134.2	136.2
8.5 years	119.5	121.3	124.9	129.3	133.6	137.4	139.6
9.0 years	122.1	123.9	127.7	132.2	136.7	140.7	142.9
9.5 years	124.8	126.6	130.6	135.2	139.8	143.9	146.2
10.0 years	127.5	129.5	133.6	138.3	142.9	147.2	149.5
10.5 years	130.4	132.5	136.7	141.5	146.1	150.4	152.8
11.0 years	133.5	135.6	140.0	144.8	149.3	153.7	156.2
11.5 years	136.6	139.0	143.5	148.2	152.6	156.9	159.5
12.0 years	139.8	142.3	147.0	151.5	155.8	160.0	162.7
12.5 years	142.7	145.4	150.1	154.6	158.8	162.9	165.6
13.0 years	145.2	148.0	152.8	157.1	161.3	165.3	168.1
13.5 years	147.2	150.0	154.7	159.0	163.2	167.3	170.0
14.0 years	148.7	151.5	155.9	160.4	164.6	168.7	171.3
14.5 years	149.7	152.5	156.8	161.2	165.6	169.8	172.2
15.0 years	150.5	153.2	157.2	161.8	166.3	170.5	172.8
15.5 years	151.1	153.6	157.5	162.1	166.7	170.9	173.1
16.0 years	151.6	154.1	157.8	162.4	166.9	171.1	173.3
16.5 years	152.2	154.6	158.2	162.7	167.1	171.2	173.4
17.0 years	152.7	155.1	158.7	163.1	167.3	171.2	173.5
17.5 years	153.2	155.6	159.1	163.4	167.5	171.1	173.5
18.0 years	153.6	156.0	159.6	163.7	167.6	171.0	173.6

[1]Because of a logistic problem the percentiles of stature for children under 2.5 years are not highly reliable. The age interval represented is 2.00–2.25 years.

Table 1.18 Smoothed percentiles of weight (in kilograms), by sex and age: Data and statistics from National Centre for Health Statistics, 1.5 to 18 years (From NCHS 1977; Hamill *et al* 1979) Reproduced with permission from the National Centre for Health Statistics.

Sex and age	Smoothed percentile						
	5th	10th	25th	50th	75th	90th	95th
Male				Weight (kg)			
1.5 years	9.72	10.18	10.51	11.09	12.02	12.95	14.42
2.0 years	10.49	10.96	11.55	12.34	13.36	14.38	15.50
2.5 years	11.27	11.77	12.55	13.52	14.61	15.71	16.61
3.0 years	12.05	12.58	13.52	14.62	15.78	16.95	17.77
3.5 years	12.84	13.41	14.46	15.68	16.90	18.15	18.98
4.0 years	13.64	14.24	15.39	16.69	17.99	19.32	20.27
4.5 years	14.45	15.10	16.30	17.69	19.06	20.50	21.63
5.0 years	15.27	15.96	17.22	18.67	20.14	21.70	23.09
5.5 years	16.09	16.83	18.14	19.67	21.25	22.96	24.66
6.0 years	16.93	17.72	19.07	20.69	22.40	24.31	26.34
6.5 years	17.78	18.62	20.02	21.74	23.62	25.76	28.16
7.0 years	18.64	19.53	21.00	22.85	24.94	27.36	30.12
7.5 years	19.52	20.45	22.02	24.03	26.36	29.11	32.73
8.0 years	20.40	21.39	23.09	25.30	27.91	31.06	34.51
8.5 years	21.31	22.34	24.21	26.66	29.61	33.22	36.96
9.0 years	22.25	23.33	25.40	28.13	31.46	35.57	39.58
9.5 years	23.25	24.38	26.68	29.73	33.46	38.11	42.35
10.0 years	24.33	25.52	28.07	31.44	35.61	40.80	45.27

Table 1.18 *contd.*

Sex and age	Smoothed percentile						
	5th	10th	25th	50th	75th	90th	95th
10.5 years	25.51	26.78	29.59	33.30	37.92	43.63	48.31
11.0 years	26.80	28.17	31.25	35.30	40.38	46.57	51.47
11.5 years	28.24	29.72	33.08	37.46	43.00	49.61	54.73
12.0 years	29.85	31.46	35.09	39.78	45.77	52.73	58.09
12.5 years	31.64	33.41	37.31	42.27	48.70	55.91	61.52
13.0 years	33.64	35.60	39.74	44.95	51.79	59.12	65.02
13.5 years	35.85	38.03	42.40	47.81	55.02	62.35	68.51
14.0 years	38.22	40.64	45.21	50.77	58.31	65.57	72.13
14.5 years	40.66	43.34	48.08	53.76	61.58	68.76	75.66
15.0 years	43.11	46.06	50.92	56.71	64.72	71.91	79.12
15.5 years	45.50	48.69	53.64	59.51	67.64	74.98	82.45
16.0 years	47.74	51.16	56.16	62.10	70.26	77.97	85.62
16.5 years	49.76	53.39	58.38	64.39	72.46	80.84	88.59
17.0 years	51.50	55.28	60.22	66.31	74.17	83.58	91.31
17.5 years	52.89	56.78	61.61	67.78	75.32	86.14	93.73
18.0 years	53.97	57.89	62.61	68.88	76.04	88.41	95.76
Female							
1.5 years	9.02	9.16	9.61	10.38	10.94	11.75	12.36
2.0 years	9.95	10.32	10.96	11.80	12.73	13.58	14.15
2.5 years	10.80	11.35	12.11	13.03	14.23	15.16	15.76
3.0 years	11.61	12.26	13.11	14.10	15.50	16.54	17.22
3.5 years	12.37	13.08	14.00	15.07	16.59	17.77	18.59
4.0 years	13.11	13.84	14.80	15.96	17.56	18.93	19.91
4.5 years	13.83	14.56	15.55	16.81	18.48	20.06	21.24
5.0 years	14.55	15.26	16.29	17.66	19.39	21.23	22.62
5.5 years	15.29	15.97	17.05	18.56	20.36	22.48	24.11
6.0 years	16.05	16.72	17.86	19.52	21.44	23.89	25.75
6.5 years	16.85	17.51	18.76	20.61	22.68	25.50	27.59
7.0 years	17.71	18.39	19.78	21.84	24.16	27.39	29.68
7.5 years	18.62	19.37	20.95	23.26	25.90	29.57	32.07
8.0 years	19.62	20.45	22.26	24.84	27.88	32.04	34.71
8.5 years	20.68	21.64	23.70	26.58	30.08	34.73	37.58
9.0 years	21.82	22.92	25.27	28.46	32.44	37.60	40.64
9.5 years	23.05	24.29	26.94	30.45	34.94	40.61	43.85
10.0 years	24.36	25.76	28.71	32.55	37.53	43.70	47.17
10.5 years	25.75	27.32	30.57	34.72	40.17	46.84	50.57
11.0 years	27.24	28.97	32.49	36.95	42.84	49.96	54.00
11.5 years	28.83	30.71	34.48	39.23	45.48	53.03	57.42
12.0 years	30.52	32.53	36.52	41.53	48.07	55.99	60.81
12.5 years	32.30	34.42	38.59	43.84	50.56	58.81	64.12
13.0 years	34.14	36.35	40.65	46.10	52.91	61.45	67.30
13.5 years	35.98	38.26	42.65	48.26	55.11	63.87	70.30
14.0 years	37.76	40.11	44.54	50.28	57.09	66.04	73.08
14.5 years	39.45	41.83	46.28	52.10	58.84	67.95	75.59
15.0 years	40.99	43.38	47.82	53.68	60.32	69.54	77.78
15.5 years	42.32	44.72	49.10	54.96	61.48	70.79	79.59
16.0 years	43.41	45.78	50.09	55.89	62.29	71.68	80.99
16.5 years	44.20	46.54	50.75	56.44	62.75	72.18	81.93
17.0 years	44.74	47.04	51.14	56.69	62.91	72.38	82.46
17.5 years	45.08	47.33	51.33	56.71	62.89	72.37	82.62
18.0 years	45.26	47.47	51.39	56.62	62.78	72.25	82.47

show mean weights and heights close to the 50th NCHS centile until about six months and then falling close to the 25th centile (Whitehead and Paul 1985). No studies have yet continued beyond two or three years, and more work needs to be done to determine the normal pattern of growth for breast-fed infants and young children. Smoothed centile charts may be disguising the true natural history of growth.

Weight-for-height standards

The NCHS standards include a table of weight-for-height. However it has two disadvantages (a) it only goes up to 11 years and (b) it is unsound for the assessment of weight-for-height in very tall or very short children — just those for whom clinical assessments are most likely to be needed (Cole 1985).

A good measurement of adiposity should be independent of height and highly correlated with weight and with body fat. Cole *et al* (1981) and Rolland-Cachera *et al* (1982, 1984) have argued for the use of W/H^2. However, because the proportions of fat to lean body mass in the individual and the distribution of degrees of adiposity vary with age, the index has to be age standardized. There is a rapid increase in weight for height until about 12 months, a progressive fall to around six years, and a progressive rise to adulthood.

Cole (1979) and Cole *et al* (1981) have devised a hand slide-rule which gives the Tanner height- and weight-for-age standards for boys and girls, and also has a scale which assesses weight-for-height (W/H^2) on an age standardized basis. It is obtainable from Castlemead Publications, Swains Mill, 4A Crane Mead, Ware, Herts SG12 9PY.

Rolland-Cachera and her colleagues (1982, 1984) have produced charts for clinical records which show the distribution of W/H^2 from birth to 21 years. These

Table 1.19 1983 Metropolitan height and weight tables for men and women on metric basis. According to frame, ages 25–59 (Metropolitan Life Insurance Co 1983). Reproduced courtesy of the Statistical Bulletin, Metropolitan Life Insurance Company.

	Men Weight in kg (in indoor clothing)*					Women Weight in kg (in indoor clothing)*			
Height (in shoes)[†] (cm)	Small frame	Medium frame	Mid point	Large frame	Height (in shoes)[†] (cm)	Small frame	Medium frame	Mid point	Large frame
158	58.3–61.0	59.6–64.2	61.9	62.8–68.3	148	46.4–50.6	49.6–55.1	52.4	53.7–59.8
159	58.6–61.3	59.9–64.5	62.2	63.1–68.8	149	46.6–51.0	50.0–55.5	52.3	54.1–60.3
160	59.0–61.7	60.3–64.9	62.6	63.5–69.4	150	46.7–51.3	50.3–55.9	53.1	54.4–60.9
161	59.3–62.0	60.6–65.2	62.9	63.8–69.9	151	46.9–51.7	50.7–56.4	53.6	54.8–61.4
162	59.7–62.4	61.0–65.6	63.3	64.2–70.5	152	47.1–52.1	51.1–57.0	54.1	55.2–61.9
163	60.0–62.7	61.3–66.0	63.7	64.5–71.1	153	47.4–52.5	51.5–57.5	54.5	55.6–62.4
164	60.4–63.1	61.7–66.5	64.1	64.9–71.8	154	47.8–53.0	51.9–58.0	55.0	56.2–63.0
165	60.8–63.5	62.1–67.0	64.6	65.3–72.5	155	48.1–53.6	52.2–58.6	55.4	56.8–63.6
166	61.1–63.8	62.4–67.6	65.0	65.6–73.2	156	48.5–54.1	52.7–59.1	55.9	57.3–64.1
167	61.5–64.2	62.8–68.2	65.5	66.0–74.0	157	48.8–54.6	53.2–59.6	56.4	57.8–64.6
168	61.8–64.6	63.2–68.7	66.0	66.4–74.7	158	49.3–55.2	53.8–60.2	57.0	58.4–65.3
169	62.2–65.2	63.8–69.3	66.6	67.0–75.4	159	49.8–55.7	54.3–60.7	57.5	58.9–66.0
170	62.5–65.7	64.3–69.8	67.1	67.5–76.1	160	50.3–56.2	54.9–61.2	58.1	59.4–66.7
171	62.9–66.2	64.8–70.3	67.6	68.0–76.8	161	50.8–56.7	55.4–61.7	58.6	59.9–67.4
172	63.2–66.7	65.4–70.8	68.1	68.5–77.5	162	51.4–57.3	55.9–62.3	59.1	60.5–68.1
173	63.6–67.3	65.9–71.4	68.7	69.1–78.2	163	51.9–57.8	56.4–62.8	59.6	61.0–68.8
174	63.9–67.8	66.4–71.9	69.2	69.6–78.9	164	52.5–58.4	57.0–63.4	60.2	61.5–69.5
175	64.3–68.3	66.9–72.4	69.7	70.1–79.6	165	53.0–58.9	57.5–63.9	60.7	62.0–70.2
176	64.7–68.9	67.5–73.0	70.3	70.7–80.3	166	53.6–59.5	58.1–64.5	61.3	62.6–70.9
177	65.0–69.5	68.1–73.5	70.8	71.3–81.0	167	54.1–60.0	58.7–65.0	61.9	63.2–71.7
178	65.4–70.0	68.6–74.0	71.3	71.8–81.8	168	54.6–60.5	59.2–65.5	62.4	63.7–72.4
179	65.7–70.5	69.2–74.6	71.9	72.3–82.5	169	55.2–61.1	59.7–66.1	62.9	64.3–73.1
180	66.1–71.0	69.7–75.1	72.4	72.8–83.3	170	55.7–61.6	60.2–66.6	63.4	64.8–73.8
181	66.6–71.6	70.2–75.8	73.0	73.4–84.0	171	56.2–62.1	60.7–67.1	63.9	65.3–74.5
182	67.1–72.1	70.7–76.5	73.6	73.9–84.7	172	56.8–62.6	61.3–67.6	64.5	65.8–75.2
183	67.7–72.7	71.3–77.2	74.3	74.5–85.4	173	57.3–63.2	61.8–68.2	65.0	66.4–75.9
184	68.2–73.4	71.8–77.9	74.9	75.2–86.1	174	57.8–63.7	62.3–68.7	65.5	66.9–76.4
185	68.7–74.1	72.4–78.6	75.5	75.9–86.8	175	58.3–64.2	62.8–69.2	66.0	67.4–76.9
186	69.2–74.8	73.0–79.3	76.2	76.6–87.6	176	58.9–64.8	63.4–69.8	66.6	68.0–77.5
187	69.8–75.5	73.7–80.0	76.9	77.3–88.5	177	59.5–65.4	64.0–70.4	67.2	68.5–78.1
188	70.3–76.2	74.4–80.7	77.6	78.0–89.4	178	60.0–65.9	64.5–70.9	67.7	69.0–78.6
189	70.9–76.9	74.9–81.5	78.2	78.7–90.3	179	60.5–66.4	65.1–71.4	68.3	69.6–79.1
190	71.4–77.6	75.4–82.2	78.8	79.4–91.2	180	61.0–66.9	65.6–71.9	68.8	70.1–79.6
191	72.1–78.4	76.1–83.0	79.6	80.3–92.1	181	61.6–67.5	66.1–72.5	69.3	70.7–80.2
192	72.8–79.1	76.8–83.9	80.4	81.2–93.0	182	62.1–68.0	66.6–73.0	69.8	71.2–80.7
193	73.5–79.8	77.6–84.8	81.2	82.1–93.9	183	62.6–68.5	67.1–73.5	70.3	71.7–81.2

*Indoor clothing weighing 2.3 kilograms for men and 1.4 kilograms for women
[†]Shoes with 2.5 cm heels
Source of basic data *Build Study, 1979*. Society of Actuaries and Association of Life Insurance Medical Directors of America
Copyright 1983 Metropolitan Life Insurance Company

can be obtained from Marie-Francoise Rolland-Cachera, Chargée de Recherches, Section Nutrition, INSERM, 44 chemin de Ronde, 78110 Le Vesinct, France.

1.8.2 Adults

Relative weight

The tables used for many years to judge the weight of adults are those of the Metropolitan Life Insurance Co. of New York (Anon, 1959). These have recently been updated (Anon, 1983) giving slightly higher weights. The tables represent the heights and weights at the time of taking out insurance policies of men and women in apparently good health who subsequently had the best mortality experience, i.e. lived longest. The 1959 tables refer to policies taken out during 1935–54, and 1983 tables to policies of 1954–72. The tables give desirable weights for small, medium and large 'frames'. Table 1.19 gives the 1983 values.

Frame size

Frisancho and Flegal (1983) have suggested that elbow breadth can be used as a measure of frame size, and this concept has been incorporated into the Metropolitan Life Insurance tables. 'The frame designations were developed from elbow breadth measurements taken from the National Health and Nutrition Examination Survey 1971–5 and were devised so that 50%

Table 1.20 Determination of body frame by elbow length. Reproduced courtesy of the Statistical Bulletin, Metropolitan Life Insurance Co. (Metropolitan Life Insurance Co. 1983)

Height (in 1-in heels)	Elbow breadth (in)	Height (in 2.5 cm heels)	Elbow breadth (cm)
Men			
5'2"–5'3"	2½–2⅞"	158–161	6.4–7.2
5'4"–5'7"	2⅝–2⅞"	162–171	6.7–7.4
5'8"–5'11"	2¾–3"	172–181	6.9–7.6
6'0"–6'3"	2¾–3⅛"	182–191	7.1–7.8
6'4"	2⅞–3¼"	192–193	7.4–8.1
Women			
4'10"–4'11"	2¼–2½"	148–151	5.6–6.4
5'0"–5'3"	2¼–2½"	152–161	5.8–6.5
5'4"–5'7"	2⅜–2⅝"	162–171	5.9–6.6
5'8"–5'11"	2⅜–3⅜"	172–181	6.1–6.8
6'0"	2½–3¾"	182–183	6.2–6.9

Source of basic data. Data tape HANES 1–Anthropometry goniometry skeletal age bone density and cortical thickness, ages 1–74. National Health and Nutrition Examination Survey 1971–75. National Center for Health Statistics. Copyright 1983 Metropolitan Life Insurance Company

Table 1.21 The range of the weight-height index (W/H²) calculated from the 'desirable' weights for heights given by the Metropolitan Life Insurance Tables, 1983.

		Small frame	Medium frame	Large frame
Men	158 cm	23.2–24.3	22.7–25.6	25.0–27.4
	193 cm	19.6–21.4	20.7–22.7	22.0–25.2
Women	148 cm	21.3–23.2	22.8–25.4	24.7–27.6
	183 cm	18.8–20.6	20.2–22.1	21.6–24.5

Weights are expressed as kg with an adjustment of 2.3 kg for men and 1.4 kg for women to obtain weight without clothes. Heights are expressed in metres; 2.5 cm were subtracted to obtain height without heels.

of the population falls within the medium frame and 25% each falls within the small and large frames.'

To make a simple approximation of frame size, extend the arm of the subject and bend the forearm upwards at a 90° angle. Keep the fingers straight and turn the inside of the wrist toward the body. With calipers, measure the distance between the two prominent bones on either side of the elbow.

Table 1.20 lists the elbow measurements for men and women of medium frame at various heights. Measurements lower than those listed indicate a small frame while higher measurements indicate a large frame.

Obesity indices

Various indices of obesity have been devised. The most used is the Quetelet index or Body Mass index. It is calculated as

$$\frac{\text{Weight in kilograms}}{\text{Height in metres}^2}$$

Table 1.21 gives the range of W/H^2 expressed in the Metropolitan Life Insurance tables.

Interpretation of these data in relation to obesity are discussed in Section 4.1, Obesity.

References

Anon (1959) Metropolitan Life Insurance Company Statistical Bulletin. **40**, (Nov–Dec).

Anon (1983) Metropolitan Life Insurance Company Statistical Bulletin. **64**, 1–9.

Cole TJ (1979) A method for assessing age standardized weight-for-height in children seen cross-sectionally. *Ann Hum Biol* **6**, 249–68.

Cole TJ (1985) A critique of the NCHS weight for height standard. *Hum Biol* **57**, 183–96.

Cole TJ, Donnet ML and Stanfield JP (1981) Weight-for-height indices to assess nutritional status — a new index on a slide-rule. *Am J Clin Nutr* **34**, 1935—43.

Frisancho AR and Flegel PN (1983) Elbow breadth as a measure of frame size for US males and females. *Am J Clin Nutr* **37**, 311—4.

Gairdner D and Pearson J (1971) A growth chart for premature and other infants. *Arch Dis Childh* **46**, 783—7.

Gracey M and Hitchcock NE (1985) Studies of growth of Australian infants. In *Nutritional needs and assessment of normal growth*. Nestle Nutrition Workshop Series No 7, Gracey M and Falkner F (Eds)., Raven Press, New York.

Hamill PVV, Drizd TA, Johnson CL, Reed RB, Roche AF and Moore WM (1979) Physical growth: National Centre for Health Statistics percentiles. *Am J Clin Nutr* **32**, 607—29.

Hitchcock NE, Owles EN and Gracey M (1981) Breast feeding and growth of healthy infants. *Med J Aust* **2**, 536—7.

Jelliffe DB (1966) *The assessment of the nutritional status of the community*. World Health Organisation, Geneva.

National Centre for Health Statistics (1977): NCHS growth curves for children 0—18 years, United States. *Vital and health statistics* Series 11 No 165, Health Resources Administration. Government Printing Office, Washington DC.

Rolland-Cachera MF, Deheeger M, Bellisle F, Sempé M, Guilloud-Bataille M and Patois E (1984) Adiposity rebound in children: a simple indicator for predicting obesity. *Am J Clin Nutr* **39**, 129—35.

Rolland-Cachera MF, Sempe M, Gilloud-Bataille M, Patois E, Pequignot-Guggenbuhl F and Fautrad V (1982) Adiposity indices in children. *Am J Clin Nutr* **36**, 178—84.

Tanner JM, Whitehouse RH and Takaishi M (1966a) Standards from birth to maturity for height, weight, height velocity and weight velocity: British children 1965, Part I. *Arch Dis Childh* **41**, 454—71.

Tanner JM, Whitehouse RH and Takaishi M (1966b) Standards from birth to maturity for height, weight, height velocity and weight velocity: British children 1965, Part II. *Arch Dis Childh* **41**, 613—35.

Whitehead RG and Paul AA (1985) Human lactation, infant feeding and growth: secular trends. In *Nutritional needs and assessment of normal growth*. Gracey M and Falkner F (Eds). Nestle Nutrition Workshop Series No 7. Raven Press, New York.

1.9   Skinfold Measurements

1.9.1   Uses and techniques

Skinfold measurements are a useful technique both in community studies to assess the prevalence of obesity, and in clinical work for assessing obesity and/or under-nutrition in the individual patient and for monitoring progress. However the technique is a difficult one and subject to large variation both within and between observers.

Variation arises in identifying the location of the skinfold, in the method of picking it up, in the precise placing of the calipers on the fold and in taking a reading. Since a skinfold is compressible when the calipers are placed on, there is a rapid fall in the reading followed by a slow drift downwards, making it difficult to determine the precise moment at which a reading should be taken.

In research studies, one observer only should take all readings. Where more than one observer has to be employed, then it is essential that they frequently take measurements together on the same subject to ensure that their technique is standardized and that they can obtain good agreement. Between and within observer variation has been studied by Womersley and Durnin (1973) and Branson et al (1982).

In clinical work, inevitably many observers are likely to be involved, but, if the measurements are to have any meaning, care should be taken to see that all members of a team standardize their technique together at intervals.

A variety of skinfolds have been measured but the most commonly used are the triceps, biceps, sub-scapular and supra-iliac. All measurements should be repeated three times, normally on the left (or non-dominant) side. Their position is as follows:

Triceps skinfold

With arm bent at right-angles, the length from the tip of the acromion process on the scapula to the olecranon process of the ulna is measured and the mid point marked. With the arm hanging loosely by the side, the skinfold at the mid point level on the back of the arm over the triceps muscle is picked up between the thumb and forefinger of the left hand. The calipers are placed on the skinfold just below the fingers, the fingers removed, and a reading taken.

Biceps

As for the triceps, but over the biceps muscle on the front of the arm.

Subscapular

About 1 inch in and below the angle of the scapula towards the midline and at an angle of approximately 45° to the spine along the natural line of skin cleavage.

Supra-iliac

Midway between the anterior superior iliac spine crest and the lowest point of the ribs, horizontal to the floor, or just above the iliac crest in the mid-axillary line.

A fuller account of the technique can be found in Tanner and Whitehouse (1962), Weiner and Lourie (1969) and Owen (1982).

1.9.2   Skinfold standards

Infancy

Skinfold measurements (like those of adiposity) increase from birth to until they plateau at around 6−9 months of age; they then decrease during early childhood.

The secular trend in infant growth discussed in Section 1.8.1 is also reflected in skinfold measurements. This is illustrated in Table 1.22 which shows the 50th centile values at six and 12 months as reported from studies conducted over the past 25 years.

The three studies conducted in the 1950s and 1960s (Karlberg et al 1968; Hutchinson-Smith 1970; Corbier 1980) gave significantly higher values than the three studies conducted since 1974 (Schlüter et al 1976; Boulton 1981; Whitehead and Paul 1985). It has been suggested that this reflects the changeover from a high incidence of bottle feeding using unmodified formulae, to the much greater frequency of breast feeding and the use of modified formulae for bottle feeding.

Table 1.22 50th centile value for triceps skinfolds in infants aged 6–12 months as measured in different studies (mm)

Author	Place	Year	Sex	Triceps skinfold	
				6 months	12 months
Corbier (1980)	Brussels	1955–8	Boys	10.3	10.4
			Girls	10.6	11.0
Karlberg et al (1968)	Solna, Sweden	1955–8	Boys	9.7	10.4
			Girls	9.8	9.8
Hutchinson-Smith (1970)	Bakewell, Derby, UK	1966–7	Boys	12.0	11.8
			Girls	10.8	11.7
Schluter et al (1976)	W. Berlin	1974–5	Boys + Girls	8.5	8.2
Boulton (1981)	Australia	1976–8	Boys	9.0	8.8
			Girls	8.9	9.0
Whitehead and Paul (1985)	Cambridge	1978–9	Boys	7.8	8.0
			Girls	7.5	8.5

In the UK, Tanner and Whitehouse (1962; 1975) have published two sets of centile charts for triceps and subscapular skinfolds in children. The data for the age-range one month to two years in the 1962 charts are those of Corbier (1980) from the years 1955–58 and in the 1975 charts they are those of Hutchinson-Smith (1970) from the years 1966–67; they are almost certainly no longer appropriate standards. The values from the post 1974 studies tend to cluster round the 10th centile of the Tanner and Whitehouse 1975 charts.

Table 1.23 gives the values from the Australian studies of Boulton (1981). Studies in progress in Cambridge should provide better UK standards in the near future.

Childhood

Information on skinfold measurements in children of 2–18 years is limited. For 2–5 year olds, the Tanner and Whitehouse charts (1962 and 1975) are based on data from the Longitudinal Growth Study of the Institute of Child Health during the 1950s. For 6–16 year olds, the 1962 charts were based on data from a London County Council survey of school children in 1959, and the 1975 charts on an ILEA survey of 1966. Both studies measured approximately 1000 children of each sex at each age. The latter represent children born between 1950 and 1960.

More recent data are those from the USA National Centre of Health Statistics. Preliminary charts of centiles for triceps and subscapular skinfold thicknesses in

Table 1.23a–d Percentile values for skinfold thicknesses. Reproduced with permission from Boulton (1981)

a) Triceps skinfold thickness.

Age group (years)		Percentiles						
		3	10	25	50	75	90	97
0.25	Boys	4.5	5.9	6.9	8.1	9.3	10.5	11.5
	Girls	5.1	5.9	6.7	7.7	8.8	10.3	11.5
0.50	Boys	6.3	6.9	8.1	9.0	10.4	11.5	12.7
	Girls	5.5	5.6	7.6	8.9	10.2	11.4	12.5
1	Boys		6.4	7.5	8.8	10.3	11.5	13.0
	Girls	5.3	6.1	7.4	9.0	10.6	11.8	13.0
2	Boys	5.8	7.2	8.2	9.7	11.2	12.9	14.6
	Girls	5.9	6.9	7.8	9.9	11.9	12.9	14.1
4	Boys	4.0	4.8	6.0	7.7	9.5	11.7	14.0
	Girls	4.5	5.3	6.5	8.6	10.5	12.6	16.0

b) Subscapular skinfold thickness (mm)

Age group (years)		Percentiles						
		3	10	25	50	75	90	97
0.25	Boys	4.5	5.3	6.1	7.1	8.3	10.6	11.0
	Girls	4.7	5.4	6.3	7.2	8.4	9.5	10.5
0.50	Boys		5.3	6.1	7.2	8.5	9.5	11.5
	Girls		5.4	6.3	7.4	8.6	9.7	11.0
1	Boys		5.2	5.9	7.0	8.5	9.8	10.8
	Girls		5.1	6.1	7.5	8.9	11.1	12.5
2	Boys	4.7	5.3	5.9	6.8	8.0	9.0	11.0
	Girls	5.2	5.7	6.2	7.6	8.9	10.1	12.1

c) Biceps skinfold thickness (mm)

Age group (years)		Percentiles						
		3	10	25	50	75	90	97
0.25	Boys		4.3	4.9	5.7	7.8	8.0	9.0
	Girls	3.2	3.9	4.7	5.6	6.7	7.8	8.8
0.50	Boys		4.8	5.5	6.3	8.3	9.5	10.5
	Girls	4.0	4.6	5.4	6.4	7.4	8.7	10.5
1	Boys	4.0	4.4	5.1	5.9	6.9	7.9	10.0
	Girls		4.3	5.1	6.2	7.2	8.5	9.2
2	Boys	3.9	4.8	5.3	5.9	7.0	8.4	10.2
	Girls	4.0	4.7	5.5	6.3	7.3	8.5	9.8

d) Supra-iliac skinfold thickness (mm)

Age group (years)		Percentiles						
		3	10	25	50	75	90	97
0.25	Boys	4.6	5.8	7.3	9.3	11.3	13.8	16.8
	Girls	5.0	6.1	7.3	9.1	11.8	14.7	15.9
0.50	Boys	5.2	6.5	7.8	9.5	11.5	13.5	15.5
	Girls	5.1	6.3	7.8	8.8	11.8	13.8	16.6
1	Boys	4.3	5.3	6.5	8.3	10.7	12.9	16.9
	Girls	4.5	5.6	7.2	9.5	11.6	13.7	15.5
2	Boys	4.0	5.1	5.9	7.7	9.7	11.0	14.8
	Girls	4.9	5.9	7.0	9.1	10.7	13.3	16.0

2–18 year olds have been published (Owen 1982). These are based on measurements of some 20000 children in 1963–74. No secular trend was found in this data over the period of time studied. Owen (1982) describes the sample on which the NCHS charts are based and also discusses the limitations on their use.

The 1975 Tanner & Whitehouse charts and the NCHS charts are similar, both in the median (50th centile) and range of values. The major differences are
1 For the subscapular skinfold in boys, the NCHS chart has lower values at the upper extreme end of the range at all ages.
2 For the subscapular skinfold in girls, the NCHS 50th centile lies on the Tanner and Whitehouse 25th centile.

Adults

Skinfolds and mid upper arm circumference in the clinical assessment of malnutrition (see also Section 1.10)

Jelliffe (1966) published standards for triceps skinfold, the mid upper arm circumference (MUAC) and the mid arm muscle circumference (MAMC), which consisted of a single figure for each measurement for each sex. These figures have been widely used in the assessment of malnutrition. For lack of better data at the time, these standards were derived from a survey of military personnel in Turkey, Greece and Italy in 1960–1 for the design of protective clothing, and a survey among an unspecified sample of American women in 1939–40, to improve garment and pattern construction, and thus are not highly relevant to whole populations in the 1980s.

Burgert and Anderson (1979) and Bishop and Ritchey (1984) have discussed the limitations of these figures and their use in assessing nutritional status. It is recommended that those concerned in the clinical assessment of nutritional status read these papers for the full discussion. A brief summary is given below.
1 The Jelliffe standards were derived from different populations, at different times and by different observers. Neither survey took a random population sample. The precise way in which the standards were derived from the published data is unclear.
2 In 1979 Burgert and Anderson reported an anthropometric study of 77 healthy American adults all within 15% of ideal body weight. The median triceps skinfold thickness, MUAC and MAMC were significantly different from the Jelliffe standards, but not

significantly different from measurements obtained in the USA in the Ten State Nutrition Survey (Frisancho 1974). This suggested that the 'standards' were not appropriate to the US population of the early 1970s.
3 The Jelliffe standards are sex-specific, but not age-specific. However these measurements, particularly in women, increase in middle-age and decline in old age. Thus, if a single figure standard is used at different ages widely varying proportions of the population will be defined as 'malnourished'.
4 Severity of nutritional depletion was defined by Jelliffe as a percentage of the standard without identifying the normal distribution of this measurement in the population. Thus, since the patterns of distribution are not the same for triceps skinfold thickness, MUAC and MAMC, a different proportion of the population will be defined as depleted (say less than 60% of the standard) depending on which measurement is under consideration.

The requirement of a standard is that it should reflect the distribution of that measurement in the population under consideration. Such figures do not exist for the UK, but several sets of age-sex specific centiles for upper arm anthropometry have been published for the USA.

Such centiles are available from the Ten State Nutrition Survey (TSNS) of 1968–70 (Frisancho 1974) and the National Health and Nutrition Examination Survey 1971–4 (NHANES I) (Frisancho 1981; Bishop et al 1981) and also NHANES II (Frisancho 1984). Tables 1.24 and 1.25 give the values published by Bishop, Bowen and Ritchey (1981). These were chosen for several reasons
1 Frisancho (1981) gives data from the TSNS, which was biased towards low income groups, and gives values only to age 44.
2 Frisancho (1984) is based on the largest body of data (NHANES I and II), but gives tables which are over-complicated for routine clinical practice, being broken down into both sexes, two broad age groups, three frame sizes and height in twelve increments of one inch. In addition, while he gives subscapular as well as triceps skinfolds, he does not give MUAC, a direct measurement, but instead gives the derived value 'bone-free arm muscle area'.
3 Bishop et al (1981) give data derived from NHANES I only, but this nevertheless represents 5261 men and 8410 women, and the data are corrected to allow for over-representation among the poor. The authors give the triceps skinfold thickness (TST), MUAC and also

Table 1.24a–c Age- and sex-specific reference values for upper arm anthropometric measurements of American men. (Developed from the data collected during the NHANES Survey of 1971–4.) Bishop, Bowen and Ritchey (1981). Reproduced with permission from the *Am J Clin Nutr*

a) Triceps skinfold thickness (mm)

Age group (years)	Sample size	Mean (mm)	Percentile						
			5th	10th	25th	50th	75th	90th	95th
18–74	5261	12.0	4.5	6.0	8.0	11.0	15.0	20.0	23.0
18–24	773	11.2	4.0	5.0	7.0	9.5	14.0	20.0	23.0
25–34	804	12.6	4.5	5.5	8.0	12.0	16.0	21.5	24.0
35–44	664	12.4	5.0	6.0	8.5	12.0	15.5	20.0	23.0
45–54	765	12.4	5.0	6.0	8.0	11.0	15.0	20.0	25.5
55–64	598	11.6	5.0	6.0	8.0	11.0	14.0	18.0	21.5
65–74	1657	11.8	4.5	5.5	8.0	11.0	15.0	19.0	22.0

b) Mid upper arm circumference (cm)

Age group (years)	Sample size	Mean (mm)	Percentile						
			5th	10th	25th	50th	75th	90th	95th
18–74	5261	31.8	26.4	27.6	29.6	31.7	33.9	36.0	37.3
18–24	773	30.9	25.7	27.1	28.7	30.7	32.9	35.5	37.4
25–34	804	32.3	27.0	28.2	30.0	32.0	34.4	36.5	37.6
35–44	664	32.7	27.8	28.7	30.7	32.7	34.8	36.3	37.1
45–54	765	32.1	26.7	27.8	30.0	32.0	34.2	36.2	37.6
55–64	598	31.5	25.6	27.3	29.6	31.7	33.4	35.2	36.6
65–74	1657	30.5	25.3	26.5	28.5	30.7	32.4	34.4	35.5

c) Mid upper arm muscle circumference (cm)

Age group (years)	Sample size	Mean (mm)	Percentile						
			5th	10th	25th	50th	75th	90th	95th
18–74	5261	28.0	23.8	24.8	26.3	27.9	29.6	31.4	32.5
18–24	773	27.4	23.5	24.4	25.8	27.2	28.9	30.8	32.3
25–34	804	28.3	24.2	25.3	26.5	28.0	30.0	31.7	32.9
35–44	664	28.8	25.0	25.6	27.1	28.7	30.3	32.1	33.0
45–54	765	28.2	24.0	24.9	26.5	28.1	29.8	31.5	32.6
55–64	598	27.8	22.8	24.4	26.2	27.9	29.6	31.0	31.8
65–74	1657	26.8	22.5	23.7	25.3	26.9	28.5	29.9	30.7

Table 1.25a–c Age- and sex-specific reference values for the upper arm anthropometric measurements of American women. (Developed from data collected during the NHANES Survey of 1971–4.) Bishop, Bowen and Ritchey (1981). Reproduced with permission from the *Am J Clin Nutr*

a) Triceps Skinfold Thickness (mm)

Age group (years)	Sample size	Mean (mm)	Percentile						
			5th	10th	25th	50th	75th	90th	95th
18–74	8410	23.0	11.0	13.0	17.0	22.0	28.0	34.0	37.5
18–24	1523	19.4	9.4	11.0	14.0	18.0	24.0	30.0	34.0
25–34	1896	21.9	10.5	12.0	16.0	21.0	26.5	33.5	37.0
35–44	1664	24.0	12.0	14.0	18.0	23.0	29.5	35.5	39.0
45–54	836	25.4	13.0	15.0	20.0	25.0	30.0	36.0	40.0
55–64	669	24.9	11.0	14.0	19.0	25.0	30.5	35.0	39.0
65–74	1822	23.3	11.5	14.0	18.0	23.0	28.0	33.0	36.0

b) Mid upper arm circumference (cm)

Age group (years)	Sample size	Mean (mm)	Percentile						
			5th	10th	25th	50th	75th	90th	95th
18−74	8410	29.4	23.2	24.3	26.2	28.7	31.9	35.2	37.8
18−24	1523	27.0	22.1	23.0	24.5	26.4	28.8	31.7	34.3
25−34	1896	28.6	23.3	24.2	25.7	27.8	30.4	34.1	37.2
35−44	1664	30.0	24.1	25.2	26.8	29.2	32.2	36.2	38.5
45−54	836	30.7	24.3	25.7	27.5	30.3	32.9	36.8	39.3
55−64	669	30.7	23.9	25.1	27.7	30.2	33.3	36.3	38.2
65−74	1822	30.1	23.8	25.2	27.4	29.9	32.5	35.3	37.2

c) Mid upper arm muscle circumference (cm)

Age group (years)	Sample size	Mean (mm)	Percentile						
			5th	10th	25th	50th	75th	90th	95th
18−74	8410	22.2	18.4	19.0	20.2	21.8	23.6	25.8	27.4
18−24	1523	20.9	17.7	18.5	19.4	20.6	22.1	23.6	24.9
25−34	1896	21.7	18.3	18.9	20.0	21.4	22.9	24.9	26.6
35−44	1664	22.5	18.5	19.2	20.6	22.0	24.0	26.1	27.4
45−54	836	22.7	18.8	19.5	20.7	22.2	24.3	26.6	27.8
55−64	669	22.8	18.6	19.5	20.8	22.6	24.4	26.3	28.1
65−74	1822	22.8	18.6	19.5	20.8	22.5	24.4	26.5	28.1

the more simply derived mid arm muscle circumference (MAMC), which is calculated as

$$MAMC = MUAC (cm) - 0.3142 \, TST (mm).$$

In the interpretation of upper arm anthropometry, perhaps the precise value or values used as standards are of minor importance, since each clinical team will develop its own criteria of malnutrition based on their own experience. However, it is useful to have a generally accepted yardstick, if only to facilitate communications between different groups of workers. The figures in Tables 1.24 and 1.25 are put forward as the most appropriate at the time of writing.

Gray and Gray (1979) have suggested that measurements below the 5th percentile be considered as evidence of depletion, and that measurements below the 10th, 15th or other arbitrarily chosen percentile as evidence of marginal depletion.

Skinfold measurements in the assessment of obesity

A number of workers have devised formulae for calculating total body fat from varying combinations of skinfold measurements. This procedure makes the tacit assumption that the quantity of subcutaneous fat stores reflects accurately internal body fat stores. The skinfold values are used to calculate body density: this is used in turn to calculate body fat. The majority of workers have used body density as determined by underwater weighing for deriving their formulae. A useful review of the value of assessing body fat from skinfolds is provided by Schemmel (1980).

One of the best known sets of equations is that developed by Durnin and Womersley using the biceps, triceps, subscapular and supra-iliac skinfolds both individually and in combination. Those interested in estimating body fat from skinfolds are referred to the original paper (Durnin and Womersley 1972).

However, while the estimation of body fat from skinfolds may be useful for research purposes, it is of little value for the day to day clinical management of the obese patient. Garrow (1981) points out that the errors of the method are such that if a man changed body fat content by 5 kg, it is possible but not certain that it would be reflected in skinfold measurements. In contrast, 'it is very unlikely that a change in weight would not correctly indicate a change of 5 kg in fat content, and the measurement of weight is far easier and requires minimal skill in the observer.' Garrow recommends the index W/H^2 as the most convenient and practical measure of obesity.

References

Bishop CW, Bowen PE and Ritchey SJ (1981) Norms for nutritional assessment of American adults by upper arm anthropometry. *Am J Clin Nutr* **34**, 2530−9.

Bishop CW and Ritchey SJ (1984) Evaluating upper arm anthropometric measurements. *J Am Diet Assoc* **84**, 330−5.

Boulton J (1981) Nutrition in childhood and its relationship to early somatic growth, body fat, blood pressure and physical fitness. *Act Paediatr Scand* Suppl 284.

Branson RS, Vaucher YE, Harrison GG, Vargas M and Thies C (1982) Inter and intra-observer reliability of skinfold thickness measurements in newborn infants. *Hum Biol* **54**, 137−43.

Burgert SL and Anderson CF (1979) An evaluation of upper arm measurements used in nutritional assessment. *Am J Clin Nutr* **32**, 2136−42.

Corbier J (1980) L'evolution de l'epaisseur du tissu cellulaire sous-cutane chez l'enfant normal, de la naissance a 3 ans. *Courrier* **30**, 40−53.

Durnin JVGA and Womersley J (1974) Body fat assessed from total body density and its estimation from skinfold thickness measurements on 481 men and women aged from 16 to 72 years. *Br J Nutr* **32**, 77−97.

Frisancho AR (1974) Triceps skinfold and upper arm muscle size norms for assessment of nutritional status. *Am J Clin Nutr* **27**, 1052−8.

Frisancho AR (1981) New norms of upper limb fat and muscle areas for assessment of nutritional status. *Am J Clin Nutr* **34**, 2540−5.

Frisancho AR (1984) New standards of weight and body composition by frame size and height for assessment of nutritional status of adults and the elderly. *Am J Clin Nutr* **40**, 808−19.

Garrow JS (1981) *Treat obesity seriously: a clinical manual.* pp 27−9. Churchill Livingstone, Edinburgh.

Gray GE and Gray LK (1979) Validity of anthropometric norms used in the assessment of hospitalized patients. *J Parent Ent Nutr* **3**, 366.

Hutchinson-Smith B (1970) The relationship between the weight of an infant and lower respiratory infection. *Med Officer* **May 8**, 257−62.

Hutchinson-Smith B (1973) Skinfold thickness in infancy in relation to birth weight. *Dev Med Child Neurol* **15**, 628−34.

Jelliffe DB (1966) *The assessment of the nutritional status of the community.* pp 242. World Health Organisation, Geneva.

Karlberg P, Klackenberg G, Engstrom I, Klackenberg-Larsson I, Lichtenstein H, Stensson J and Svennberg I (1968) The development of children in a Swedish urban community. A prospective longitudinal study. *Acta Paediatr Scand* Suppl, 187.

Owen GM (1982) Measurement, recording and assessment of skinfold thickness in childhood and adolescence: report of a small meeting. *Am J Clin Nutr* **35**, 629−38.

Schemmel R (1980) The assessment of obesity. In *Nutrition, physiology and obesity.* Schemmel R (Ed) pp 1−23. CRC Press, Boca Raton, Florida.

Schluter K, Funfack W, Pachaly J and Weber B (1976) Development of subcutaneous fat in infancy. Standards for tricipital, subscapular and supra-iliac skinfolds in German infants. *Europ J Pediatr* **123**, 255−67.

Tanner JM and Whitehouse RH (1962) Standards for subcutaneous fat in British children. Percentiles for thickness of skinfolds over triceps and below scapula. *Br Med J* **I**, 446−50.

Tanner JM and Whitehouse RH (1975) Revised standards for triceps and subscapular skinfolds in British children. *Arch Dis Childh* **50**, 142−5.

Weiner JS and Lourie JA (1969) *Human biology: A guide to field methods.* IBP Handbook No 9, Blackwell Scientific Publications, Oxford.

Whitehead RG and Paul AA (1985) Human lactation, infant feeding and growth: secular trends. In Nutritional needs and *assessment of normal growth.* Gracey M and Falkner F (Eds). Nestlé Nutrition Workshop Series Vol **7**. Raven Press, New York.

Womersley J and Durnin JVGA (1973) An experimental study on variability of measurement of skinfold thickness in young adults. *Hum Biol* **45**, 281−?2.

C: Basic Dietetic Practice

1.10 The Assessment of Nutritional Status in Clinical Situations

Nutritional status is '...the degree to which the individual's physiological need for nutrients is being met by the foods he/she is eating. It is the state of balance in the individual between the nutrient intake and the nutrient expenditure or need' (Krause and Mahan 1979).

1.10.1 General considerations

Assessment of nutritional status is usually undertaken for three reasons

1   To confirm a diagnosis of undernutrition.
2   To identify the reasons for the presence of undernutrition.
3   To provide a means of monitoring the effectiveness of nutritional support.

Many changes take place in the body in the presence of undernutrition and a multitude of tests have been described which attempt to quantify these changes. Since nutritional assessment can be undertaken in a variety of settings it is important to use indicators which are relatively easy to apply and which do not necessarily need sophisticated resources. This may sometimes mean sacrificing precision for convenience. The following points should always be remembered

1   No test should be considered in isolation — reasons other than undernutrition can cause an abnormal result.
2   Tests should always be applied by the same observer when an element of subjectivity is involved (e.g. anthropometric measurements). Ideally, such tests should be performed three times and an average result taken.
3   In many cases blood levels may reflect recent dietary intake rather than long term nutritional status — fasting samples will give more reliable results in this respect (e.g. glucose, potassium, protein, vitamins).
4   By contrast, homeostatic mechanisms operating in the body can mean that body stores may be nutrient depleted before circulating levels show any measurable decrease (e.g. zinc, calcium).
5   Great care is needed when assessing children — particularly neonates to whom special parameters must be applied. The risk of nutritional deficiencies occurring is increased during times of accelerated growth.

1.10.2 Assessing the nature and extent of nutritional depletion

Nutritional depletion is caused by inadequate nutritional intake or failure to digest, absorb and/or utilize nutrients. All of these can result from illness (Table 1.26).

Table 1.26 Conditions likely to result in nutritional deficiencies. Howard and Herbold (1978). Reproduced with permission

Inadequate intake — quantity	Mechanical feeding problems or undeveloped feeding skills Anorexia (due to emotional problems, disease process, drugs)
Inadequate intake — quality	Lack of education of parents or guardian Institutionalized setting Poor food habits Allergies
Increased metabolism	Fever Infections Malignancy Hyperthyroidism Athetosis Surgery, stress, burns
Increased loss	Vomiting Diarrhoea Decreased food transit time through the gut
Defective utilization	Metabolic diseases (aminoacidopathies, galactosaemia, lipidoses) Disturbed metabolic states (hepatic insufficiency renal tubular acidosis, nephrogenic diabetes insipidus, adrenal cortical hyperplasia with salt loss) Drug interference with nutrients
Defective absorption	Intrinsic disease states (regional enteritis, Hirschsprung's disease) Exogenous states (intestinal parasitosis, coeliac disease, surgical removal of the small bowel) Drugs
Defects in the function of major organ systems	Severe congenital heart disease Severe chest disease Severe liver disease Kidney disease Brain damage
Excessive food or vitamin intake	Obesity Vitamin intoxication — fat-soluble vitamins

The nature and extent of the nutritional depletion can be determined in a number of ways.

Clinical examination

Deficiencies of specific nutrients may result in particular symptoms. Some of the clinical signs associated with undernutrition are summarized in Table 1.27.

Body weight and weight loss

The patient's weight should be measured using *accurate* weighing scales. Actual body weight can then be compared with either the patient's usual body weight or ideal body weight. Percentage weight loss is a useful in-

dicator of nutritional status (Table 1.28) and can be calculated as

$$\% \text{ weight loss} = \frac{\text{Usual weight} - \text{Actual (or ideal) weight}}{\text{Usual weight}} \times 100$$

When recording the patient's weight it is vital to consider the possible presence of

1 Obesity. This can mask significant reductions in lean body mass. One way of detecting obesity is by the Body Mass (or Quetelet) Index (BMI) but this is not infallible and should not be applied in the presence of oedema (see below). The formula and guidance as to its interpretation are given in Table 1.29.

2 Oedema. This will distort weight records. It can be

Table 1.27 Physical signs associated with nutritional depletion. Christakis (1979). Reproduced with permission

Organ system	Physical signs	Nutrient deficiency
Hair	Becomes fine, dull, dry, brittle, stiff, straight; becomes red in Blacks, then lighter in colour; may be 'bleached' in Whites ('flag sign'); is easily and painlessly pluckable; outer one third of eyebrow may be sparse in hypothyroidism (cretinism, iodine deficiency or other causes)	Protein-energy
Nails	Ridging, brittle, easily broken, flattened, spoon shaped, thin, lustreless	Iron
Face	Brown, patchy, pigmentation of cheeks Parotid enlargement 'Moon face'	Protein-energy
Eyes	Photophobia; poor twilight vision; loss of shiny, bright, moist appearance of eyes; xerosis of bulbar conjunctivae; loss of light reflex; decreased lacrimation; keratomalacia (corneal softening), corneal ulceration which may lead to extrusion of lens; Bitot's spot (frothy white or yellow spots under bulbar conjunctivae)	Vitamin A
	Palpebral conjunctivae are pale	Iron or Folate
	Circumcorneal capillary injection with penetration of corneal limbus.	Riboflavin
	Tissue at external angles of both eyes which is red and moist. Angular blepharitis (or palpebritis)	Riboflavin Pyridoxine
	Optic neuritis	B12
Nose	Nasolabial dyssebacea (exfoliation, inflammation, excessive oil production and fissuring of sebaceous glands, which are moist and red). May be found at angles of eyes, ears or other sites	Riboflavin
	Nasolabial seborrhoea	Pyridoxine
Lips	Cheilosis, inflammation of the mucus membranes of the lips and the loss of the clear differentiation between the mucocutaneous border of the lips	Riboflavin
Gums	Interdental gingival hypertrophy	Vitamin C
	Gingivitis	Vitamin A, Niacin Riboflavin
Mouth	Angular stomatitis; cheilosis; angular scars	Riboflavin
	Apthous stomatitis	Folic acid
Tongue	Atrophic lingual papillae, sore, erythematous	Iron
	Glossitis, painful, sore	Folic acid
	Magenta in colour, atrophic lingual papillae; filiform and fungiform papillae hypertrophy	Riboflavin
	Scarlet; raw; atrophic lingual papillae; fissures	Niacin
	Glossitis	Pyridoxine

Table 1.27 *contd.*

Organ system	Physical signs	Nutrient deficiency
Teeth	Caries	Fluoride
	Mottled enamel, fluorosis	Fluoride (excessive)
	Caries	Phosphorus
	Malposition; hypoplastic line across upper primary incisors becomes filled with yellow-brown pigment; caries then occurs and tooth may break off	Protein-energy
Neck	Neck mass (goitre)	Iodine
Skin	Xerosis (dryness of skin)	Vitamin A
	Follicular hyperkeratosis ('goose-flesh,' 'sharkskin,' 'sand-paper skin;' keratotic plugs arising from hypertrophied hair follicles. Acneiform lesions	
	Perifollicular petechiae which produce a 'pink halo' effect around coiled hair follicles intradermal petechiae, purpura, ecchymoses due to capillary fragility. Haemarthroses; cortical hemorrhages of bone visualizable on x-ray	Vitamin C
	Intracutaneous haemorrhages; gastrointestinal haemorrhage	Vitamin K
	Pallor	Iron, folic acid
	Pallor; icterus	B12
	Erythema early, vascularization, crusting, desquamation. Increased pigmentation (even in Blacks), thickened, inelastic, fissured, especially in skin exposed to sun; becoming scaly, dry, atrophic in intertrigenous areas, maceration and abrasion may occur. 'Necklace of Casals' in neckline exposed to sun; Malar and supraorbital pigmentation	Niacin
	Oedema (pitting), 'Flaky paint': dermatosis, Hyperkeratosis or 'Crazy pavement' dermatosis	Protein-energy
	Hyperpigmentation	
	Scrotum dermatitis erythema, hyperpigmentation	Niacin
Vulva	Vulvovaginitis and chronic mucocutaneous candidiasis	Iron
Skeletal	Osteoporosis (in association with low protein intake and fluoride deficiency)	Calcium
	Epiphyseal enlargement, painless.	Vitamin D
	Beading of ribs ('Rachitic Rosary').	
	Delayed fusion of fontaneles, craniotabes. Bowed legs, frontal or parietal bossing of skull. Deformities of thorax (Harrison's Sulcus, pigeon breast).	
	Osteomalacia (adults)	
	Subperiosteal haematoma. Epiphyseal enlargement, painful	Vitamin C
Muscular	Hypotonia	Vitamin D
	Muscle wasting; weakness, fatigue, inactivity; loss of subcutaneous fat	Protein-energy
	Intramuscular haematoma	Vitamin C
	Calf muscle tenderness; weakness	Thiamin
Central Nervous System	Apathy (kwashiorkor); irritability (marasumus); Psychomotor changes.	Protein
	Hyporeflexia; foot and wrist drop. Hypesthesia; parasthesia	Thiamin
	Psychotic behaviour (dementia)	Niacin
	Peripheral neuropathy, symmetrical sensory and motor deficits, especially in lower extremities. Drug resistant convulsions (infants). Dementia, forgetfulness	Pyridoxine
	Areflexia. Extensor plantar responses. Loss of position and vibratory sense. Ataxia, paresthesias	B12
	Tremor, convulsions, behavioural disturbances	Magnesium
Liver	Hepatomegaly (fatty infiltration)	Protein-energy
Gastrointestinal	Anorexia, flatulence, diarrhoea	B12
	Diarrhoea	Niacin, Protein-energy
Cardiovascular	Tachycardia, congestive heart failure (high output type), cardiac englargement, electrocardiographic changes	Thiamin

Reproduced with permission from Christakis G (1979).

Table 1.28 Indicators of nutritional depletion (Jeliffe 1966; Bishop *et al* 1981)

Parameter	Normal range	Depletion Mild	Depletion Moderate	Depletion Severe
Body weight	·100% (i.e. usual weight for height)	95—100%	90—95%	<90%
Mid arm muscle circumference[†]	100% Male = +25.3 cm *or* ++28.7 cm[†] Female = +23.2 cm ++22.0 cm	80—90%	60—80%	<60%
Triceps skinfold thickness[†]	100% Male = +12.5 mm *or* ++12.0 mm[†] Female = +16.5 mm ++23.0 mm	80—90%	60—80%	<60%
Grip strength	100% Male = 40 kg* Female = 27.5 kg*	85%	75—85%	<75%
Creatinine: height index	100%	80—95%	60—80%	<60%
Serum albumin[§]	35—45 g/l	30—35 g/l	25—30 g/l	<25 g/l
Serum transferrin[§]	200—300 mg/100 ml	150—200 mg/100 ml	100—150 mg/100 ml	<100 mg/100 ml
Total lymphocyte[§] count	1500—3500 mm³	1200—1500 mm³	800—1200 mm³	<800 mm³

*This measurement is affected by age.
[†]See page 52 for discussion of the different values given.
+from Jellife (1966).
[§]Remember that these parameters are all more likely to reflect the disease state rather than nutritional status.
++from Bishop *et al* (1981).

Table 1.29 Body mass index

$$\text{Body Mass Index (Quetelet Index)} = \frac{\text{Weight (kg)}}{\text{Height (m)}^2}$$

Interpretation of data obtained
<20 = Long term hazard to health
20—24.9 = Desirable
25—29.9 = Moderate obesity
>30 = Severe obesity

caused by disease, drug therapy or nutritional support (particularly if parenteral regimens are prescribed). It should be remembered that short term weight changes usually reflect alterations in fluid balance.

A record should be made of the patient's usual weight together with the patient's height and the ideal weight for height. These measurements will form the basis of subsequent nutritional support. It is not always easy to obtain a measurement of height but this can be done in the clinical situation by comparing the length of the patient with the length of their hospital bed (a standard King's Fund bed in 7'3" long or 7'14" with raising back-rest including buffers).

Dietary history

The *dietary history* is one of the most important tools in the assessment of nutritional status. Many factors must be considered when recording the dietary intake, particularly in the clinical situation (Section 1.4.2). It is often the dietitian who is able to confirm a diagnosis of undernutrition and, in some cases, a dietary history may reveal previously unsuspected nutritional depletion. A history should therefore provide information about energy and nitrogen intake as well as giving details of related nutrients such as potassium, other minerals and vitamins. Any possible reasons for suspected deficiencies should be highlighted together with appropriate information about the restoration of an adequate nutrition intake (with recommendations for pharmaceutical supplementation if this is considered necessary).

It is also helpful to anticipate possible future depletion which may modify nutritional requirements, for example, planned surgical procedures. Some clinical considerations to take into account are listed in Table 1.30.

Table 1.30 Clinical factors to consider when taking a dietary history

Whether there is an underlying disease state

Whether there is impairment in organic function

Whether undernutrition is present and; if so, its extent and duration

Whether there are likely to be any drug-nutrient interactions

Whether there is an increased requirement for any nutrient and, if so, which and why?

Whether the present situation is likely to change and, if so, will this affect the nutritional status?

Clinical measurement of nutritional status

Many tests have been devised which identify general rather than specific nutrient depletion and provide a guide to the size of the body's fat stores and protein status.

Fat stores

Triceps skinfold thickness. This is a simple reflection of the stores of fat. The measurement obtained is compared with values obtained in normal subjects (see Section 1.9). Any value below this is an indication of depleted nutritional status (Table 1.28).

Total body fat. This can be estimated as a percentage of body weight by taking skinfold measurements at the mid-biceps, mid-triceps, subscapular and supra-iliac sites (see Section 1.9) (Durnin and Womersley 1974). However, it should be noted that the correlations of fat ratios are age and sex dependent.

Note — Always use reliable calipers when making these measurements, and always use the *non*-dominant arm for making measurements. (See Section 1.9 for discussion of anthropometric values.)

Protein stores

The lean body mass is the most important nutritional component in the body. Protein depletion can be masked by both obesity and oedema.

Somatic proteins. These can be measured in several ways.

1 Mid upper arm muscle circumference (MAMC). This is derived from the mid upper arm circumference (MUAC) and triceps skinfold thickness (TSF) (see Section 1.9) using the formula

$$MAMC = MUAC - (TSF \times \pi)$$

2 Dynamometry. Muscle strength has been related to protein status. This can be assessed by measuring hand grip strength using a spring dynamometer. Values are compared with measurements in normal subjects and the extent of depletion can be calculated on a percentage basis (see Table 1.28).

3 Creatinine: height index (CHI). Creatinine is excreted at a constant rate in the presence of normal renal function and an adequate fluid intake unless there is a rapid loss of skeletal muscle mass, e.g. severe sepsis. Creatinine is not affected by normal variations in daily nitrogen intake. It is extremely important to obtain *complete* 24-hour urine collections for analysis. The CHI is calculated using the following procedure

   a) Confirm the patient's height.
   b) Obtain the ideal weight for this height (i.e. the mid-point of medium frame, Metropolitan Life Insurance Tables (Anon 1983); Table 1.19 p 47).
   c) Obtain the ideal creatinine coefficient which is 23 mg creatinine/kg in men and 18 mg creatinine/kg in women (Bistrian *et al* 1975).
   d) Calculate the CHI

$$CHI = \frac{\text{Actual urinary creatinine}}{\text{Ideal urinary creatinine}} \times 100$$

   e) Compare this with standard values (Table 1.28).

Visceral proteins. The visceral protein compartment is responsible for tissue function, protein synthesis and immune competence.

The first two functions can be assessed by monitoring the serum concentrations of transport proteins which are synthesised by the liver. However, *since many factors other than malnutrition affect the levels of these transport proteins, it is important not to place too much reliance on any results.* These factors include stress, trauma, concurrent administration of protein products (such as blood or albumin) and the degree of hydration. Therefore, no single indicator should be considered in isolation either from other indicators of visceral protein status or of general undernutrition.

1 Serum albumin. This indicator is commonly used as a marker for nutritional depletion. However, since it is also affected by stress, renal and hepatic function as well as by posture, it may be more realistic to use it as an indicator of the general clinical condition. The reference range is 35−45 g/l, assuming normal hydration. It may be necessary to correct serum calcium for albumin concentration (Editorial 1979 and see p 605). Some workers have correlated albumin levels with nutritional depletion. These values are given in Table 1.28.

2 Serum transferrin (TF). This has a shorter half life than albumin and is considered to be a more sensitive marker of nutritional status. However, not only is it affected by all the factors listed previously but it is also affected by bleeding episodes. Measurements can be made either directly or by calculation from the total iron binding capacity (TIBC) using the formula

$$\text{Serum TF} = (\text{TIBC} \times 0.8) - 43$$

Note: Several authors recommend that local figures should be used in this derived calculation since a variety of procedures exist for measuring both TIBC and transferrin.

The reference range is 200−300 mg/100 ml.

3 Rapid turnover proteins. These include thyroxin binding prealbumin and retinol binding protein which have a very high turnover rate and are extremely sensitive. They are not usually appropriate indicators of nutritional depletion in the clinical situation.

Immune competence. Impairment of the immune system is one consequence of undernutrition. Immune competence can be measured in two ways

1 Reduced cell mediated immunity. Well nourished subjects respond to an injection of a common recall antigen by showing a weal at the injection site. An anergic response, which is defined as failure to produce a weal of 0.5 cm diameter at 24 hr and 48 hr after injection, may indicate nutritional depletion.

2 Reduced total lymphocyte count (TLC). The lymphocyte count can be *lowered for reasons other than nutritional depletion*, particularly in the clinical situation, such as radiation treatment, surgery, or immunosuppressive drug therapy. It can be calculated using the formula

$$\text{TLC} = \frac{\% \text{ lymphocytes} \times \text{WBC}}{100}$$

The reference range is 1500−3500 mm^3.

Nitrogen balance. An immediate assessment of protein balance can be made by estimating the nitrogen content of a *complete* 24-hour urine collection and relating this to nitrogen intake (Table 1.31). These measurements may need to be modified if the patient has large nitrogen losses from any other sources such as burns or fistulae.

However, nitrogen balance only measures the present state and is more often used when *monitoring* nutritional support. It does not necessarily reflect nutritional status.

Table 1.31 Calculation of nitrogen balance

Nitrogen input	= g protein consumed in 24 hours ÷ 6.25
Nitrogen output	= g urinary urea nitrogen excreted in 24 hours + 2−4 g*
Nitrogen balance	= Nitrogen input − nitrogen output
This should be 0 to +1	

*2−4 g to allow for obligatory nitrogen losses in faeces, sweat, etc.

Summary

The tests which have been described can be considered as general indicators of nutritional status. If a deficiency of a particular nutrient is suspected, e.g. vitamins or minerals, then an appropriate specific test can be used provided any specific constraints which may apply are borne in mind.

The assessment of nutritional status forms a useful basis from which to plan subsequent treatment. No individual indicator is exclusively or uniquely related to nutritional status. A combination of tests should therefore be applied and the results interpreted with caution. It is also important to remember the inherent difficulty of relating general standards to individual patients.

The key to the successful management of the nutritionally vulnerable patient is to be aware of the fact that depletion may exist. This will ensure that the appropriate tests are carried out to confirm the diagnosis and that subsequent therapy is carefully planned to include a suitable level of nutritional support.

Further reading

Blackburn GL, Bistrian BR, Maini BS, Schlamm HT and Smith MF (1977) Nutritional and metabolic assessment of the hospitalized patient. *J Parent Ent Nutr* **1**, 11−12.

Blackburn GL and Bistrian RB (1977) In *Nutritional support in medical practice* Schnieder, Anderson and Coursin Eds pp 139−51. Harpers and Row, Maryland.

Christakis G (1979) How to make a nutritional diagnosis without really trying. *J Flor Med Assoc* **66**, (4), 349−56.

Goode AW (1981) The scientific basis of nutritional assessment. *Br J Anaesth* **53**, (2), 161−7.

Grant JP, Custer PB and Thurlow J (1981) Current techniques of nutritional assessment. *Surg Clin North Am* **61**, (3), 437−63.

Jensen T, Enlert and Dudrick S (1983) *Nutritional assessment — a manual for practitioners.* Appleton Century Crofts.

Krause MV and Mahan LK (1979) Assessment of nutritional status. In *Nutrition and diet therapy* 6e pp 220−41. WB Saunders, Philadelphia.

Shenkin A and Steele LW (1978) Clinical and laboratory assessment of nutritional status. *Proc Nutr Soc* **37**, 95−103.

Shils ME (1981) Indices of the nutritional status of the individual. In *Nutrition in 1980s — constraints on our knowledge* Selvey N and White PL (Eds) pp 71–81. AR Liss Inc, New York.

Solomons NW and Allen LH (1983) The functional assessment of nutritional status: principles, practice and potential. *Nutr Rev* **41**, (2), 33–50.

Woods HF, Newton DJ, Kay R and Clark RG (1981) The nutritional assessment of hospital patients — a critical review. *Proceedings of 2nd European Congress of Parenteral and Enteral Nutrition. Acta Chir Scand* [Suppl] **507**, 171–80.

Wright RA and Heymsfield S (1984) *Nutritional assessment*. Blackwell Scientific Publications, Oxford.

References

Anon (1983) *Metropolitan Life Insurance Company Statistical Bulletin* **64**, 1–9.

Bishop CW, Bowen PE and Ritchley SJ (1981) Norms for nutritional assessment of American adults by upper arm anthropometry. *Am J Clin Nutr* **34**, 2530–9.

Bistrian BR, Blackburn GL and Sherman N (1975) Therapeutic index of nutritional depletion in hospitalized patients. *Surg Gynaecol Obstet* **141**, 512–6.

Christakis G (1979) How to make a nutritional diagnosis without really trying. *J Flor Med Assoc* **66**, (4), 349–56.

Durnin JVGA and Womersley J (1974) Body fat assessed from total density and its estimation from skinfold thickness measurements on 481 men and women aged from 16–72 years. *Br J Nutr* **32**, 77–97.

Editorial (1979) Correcting the calcium. *Br Med J* **1**, 598.

Howard RB and Herbold NH (1978) *Nutrition in clinical care*. McGraw Hill, New York.

Jelliffe DB (1966) *The assessment of the nutritional status of the community* p 242. World Health Organisation, Geneva.

1.11 Estimation of Nutritional Requirements for the Provision of Nutritional Support

1.11.1 General considerations

The aim of nutritional support, whether in a healthy or sick individual, is to provide enough of the essential nutrients to promote and maintain good health. Various sets of tables have been compiled to facilitate these calculations when considering healthy people. However, several factors can influence nutritional requirements — even in the healthy person. These include age, sex and activity as well as the use of various drugs which can modify the need for specific nutrients — especially if they are taken on a long term basis (see Section 5.10).

Disease states modify nutritional requirements further, particularly in respect of energy and nitrogen but also for other nutrients. Much research has been undertaken to identify the precise nutritional needs of sick patients and the results have been widely reported (Bistrian *et al* 1976; Hill *et al* 1977).

It is essential that each patient is considered on an individual basis. In every instance the same procedure should be followed (Fig. 1.3). The aim of nutritional support is to minimize losses by restoring and maintaining the normal homeostatic processes within the body.

Basic objectives

Achieving nitrogen equilibrium or positive nitrogen balance

Positive nitrogen balance must be achieved in order to protect lean body mass and visceral protein status, thus enabling immune competence to be maintained and the functions of the vital organs, particularly the liver, to be preserved.

Prevention or minimization of weight loss

The rate and degree of weight loss are major determining factors in the incidence of post-trauma mortality. It is important to note that patients should *not* be

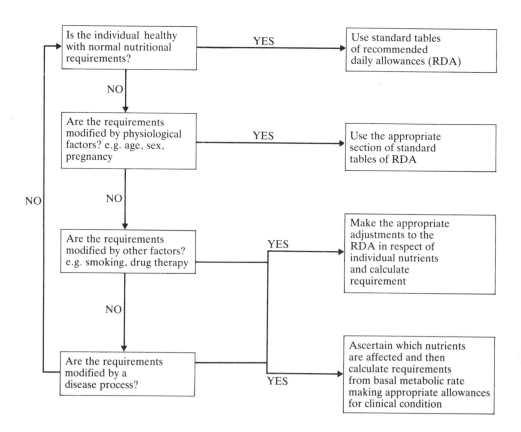

Fig. 1.3 Initial estimation of nutritional requirements.

GENERAL DIETETIC PRINCIPLES AND PRACTICE

prescribed weight reducing regimens while they are acutely ill, even if they are overweight.

Provision of sufficient minerals and vitamins

Adequate provision is required to enable substrate metabolism to take place.

Maintenance of fluid balance

Maintenance of fluid balance is crucial to renal, cardiovascular and respiratory function.

Prevention of overfeeding

Overfeeding could result in metabolic and other clinical problems including obesity. Overfeeding also reduces the cost effectiveness of nutritional support.

There are, of course, many other nutritionally related functions which also have to be considered such as the maintenance of essential systems, e.g. the nervous system. The needs of children merit special consideration; these are outlined in Sections 3.2−3.4 and 5.4. Whatever the category of the patient who is considered for nutritional support, it must not be forgotten that tissue maintenance and/or repletion cannot be achieved if there is a deficiency of any single nutrient. It is also important to remember that there are some patients in whom the nutritional requirement for a particular substrate may exceed their ability to handle it (for example, nitrogen requirements in the critically ill, particularly if there are concurrent extra-renal losses).

Hormonal changes in injury

Hormonal changes affect nutritional requirements and must be considered. The initial metabolic response to injury is an increase in the secretion of catabolic hormones (glucagon, cortisol and the catecholamines) which stimulate glycogenolysis and gluconeogenesis and hence increase the available supply of glucose. Insulin secretion, although initially inhibited by high levels of catecholamines, is also increased during the 'catabolic' phase of injury but, paradoxically, there is often coexistent hyperglycaemia caused by insulin resistance. These changes should not be confused with the changes which occur during starvation (Table 1.32). The hormonal response to injury has been well reviewed by Wilmore (1977) and Woolfson (1978) and is also discussed further in Section 5.1.

Table 1.32 Comparison of the effects of starvation and injury (Woolfson 1978)

	Starvation	Injury
Metabolic rate	Decreased	Increased
Weight	Slow loss	Rapid loss
Energy	Almost all from fat	80% from fat. Remainder from protein
Nitrogen	Losses reduced	Losses increased
Hormones	Early small increases in catecholamines, glucagon, cortisol, hGH, then slow fall.	Increases in catecholamines, glucagon, cortisol, hGH.
	Insulin decreased	Insulin increased but relative insulin deficiency.
Water and Sodium	Initial loss. Later retention	Retention

Assessment of nutritional status

It is necessary to assess the present nutritional status of the patient so that future nutritional requirements can be determined. Particular attention should be paid to clinical appearance, weight loss (particularly if this has occurred during the previous three months) and nitrogen balance (see Section 1.10).

1.11.2 Calculation of nutritional requirements

Energy requirements

One of the two principal nutritional changes which occurs in illness relates to the requirement for energy (the other being the need for nitrogen). The energy requirement is dependent upon the *basal metabolic rate* (BMR). This is the amount of energy which is needed to maintain physiological equilibrium while lying at rest in the fasted state. The BMR may be very difficult to measure in critically ill patients and so the *Resting Metabolic Expenditure (RME)* is often the preferred measurement. This is the BMR with an additional allowance for the energy needed for eating, digestion, respiration and minimal physical activity.

Calculation of the BMR

When constructing a nutritional regimen, it is however possible to calculate the BMR as a basis for treatment. There are several ways of doing this. The two methods most commonly used to data are

1 The standards (BMR per m^2) of Roberston and Reed (1952)
2 Calculation from the Harris−Benedict equation (1919)

However, new equations derived from a compre-

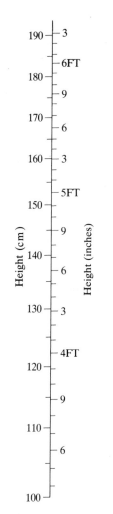

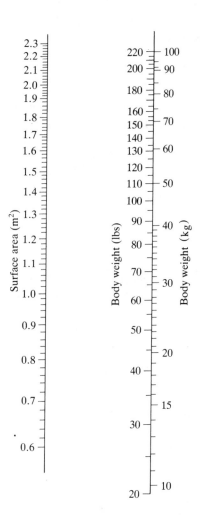

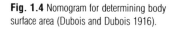

Fig. 1.4 Nomogram for determining body surface area (Dubois and Dubois 1916).

hensive compilation of data from the literature by Schofield (1985) should perhaps now supersede them.

Calculation of BMR from the standards of Robertson and Reed (1952)

1 First, the surface area of the patient is calculated using the formula

$$M^2 = W^{0.425} \times H^{0.725} \times 71.84$$

where M = surface area in m^2; W = weight in kg and H = height in cm.

Alternatively, a nomogram based on the above formula may be used (Fig. 1.4).

2 The surface area is then multiplied by the predicted standard metabolic expenditure for age and sex (Table 1.33).

3 The resulting figure is the basal metabolic requirement.

It is much easier if a small computer can be used for these calculations (Colley *et al* 1985). Alternative, standard tables and forms can be devised.

Calculation of BMR using the Harris-Benedict equation. The following formulae will give an estimate of the BMR for disease-free individuals

1 Males = $66 + (13.7 \times W) + (5 \times H) - (6.8 \times A)$

2 Females = $655 + (9.6 \times W) + (1.7 \times H) - (4.7 \times A)$

3 Infants* = $22.1 + (31.05 \times W) + (1.16 \times H)$

where W = Body weight in kg; H = height/length in cm and A = age in years.

Calculation of BMR from the Schofield equation Schofield (1985) gives twelve equations by age and sex for estimating BMR from weight alone (Table 1.34) and also from height and weight (Table 1.35). For quick reference practical use, he also gives a table of standard BMRs for each sex for weights from 3−85 kg

---

*This formula was derived from studies on infants under the age of two weeks.

Table 1.33 Variation of basal metabolic rate per square metre body surface area for age and sex (Robertson and Reid 1952)**

Standard of ROBERTSON and REID (3–75 years)
Lancet 1, 940 (1952)

| Age | kcal per m² per hour | | Age | kcal per m² per hour | |
	Boys	Girls		Men	Women
3	60.1*	54.5*	17	39.7*	35.3
4	57.9	53.9	18	39.2	34.9
5	56.3	53.0	19	38.8	34.5
6	54.2	51.8	20	38.4	34.3
7	52.1	50.2	25	37.1	34.0
8	50.1	48.4	30	36.4	34.1
9	48.2	46.4	35	35.9	33.5
10	46.6	44.3	40	35.5	32.6
11	45.1	42.4	45	34.1	32.2
12	43.8	40.6	50	33.8	31.9
13	42.7	39.1	55	33.4	31.6
14	41.8	37.8	60	33.1	31.3
15	41.0	36.8	65	32.7	31.0
16	40.3	36.0	70	32.4*	30.7
			75	32.0*	—

*Extrapolated or based on less than 7 subjects.

**Alternative sets of standards have been devised by Fleisch (1951) and Altman and Dittmer (1968).

Table 1.34 Equations for estimating basal metabolic rate from weight (*m*, male, *f* female). (BMR is expressed in MJ/24h; weight in kg; sample size is given as *n*; multiple correlation as R; standard error of the estimate as se) (Schofield 1985). Reproduced with permission

Children:		n	R	s.e.
under 3 years				
m	BMR = 0.249 wt − 0.127	162	0.95	0.2925
f	BMR = 0.244 wt − 0.130	137	0.96	0.2456
3–10 years				
m	BMR = 0.095 wt + 2.110	338	0.83	0.2803
f	BMR = 0.085 wt + 2.033	413	0.81	0.2924
10–18 years				
m	BMR = 0.074 wt + 2.754	734	0.93	0.4404
f	BMR = 0.056 wt + 2.898	575	0.80	0.4661
Adults: 18–30 years				
m	BMR = 0.063 wt + 2.896	2879	0.65	0.6407
f	BMR = 0.062 wt + 2.036	829	0.73	0.4967
30–60 years				
m	BMR = 0.048 wt + 3.653	646	0.60	0.6997
f	BMR = 0.034 wt + 3.538	372	0.68	0.4653
Over 60 years				
m	BMR = 0.049 wt + 2.459	50	0.71	0.6865
f	BMR = 0.038 wt + 2.755	38	0.68	0.4511

(Table 1.36). These however are not applicable to those over 60 years of age.

Estimation of energy requirement from BMR

Several authors have proposed standards to meet the increased energy requirements generated by a variety of disease states. The most commonly used are

Table 1.35 Equations for estimating basal metabolic rate from weight and height (*m*, male, *f*, female). (BMR is given in MJ/24h; weight in kg; height in metres; sample size is given as *n*; multiple correlation as R; standard error of the estimate as se) (Schofield 1985). Reproduced with permission

Children: under 3 years		n	R	s.e.
m	BMR = 0.0007 wt + 6.349 ht − 2.584	162	0.97	0.2425
f	BMR = 0.068 wt + 4.281 ht − 1.730	137	0.97	0.2160
3–10 years				
m	BMR = 0.082 wt + 0.545 ht + 1.736	338	0.83	0.2795
f	BMR = 0.071 wt + 0.677 ht + 1.553	413	0.81	0.2904
10–18 years				
m	BMR = 0.068 wt + 0.574 ht + 2.157	734	0.93	0.4394
f	BMR = 0.035 wt + 1.948 ht + 0.837	575	0.82	0.4525
Adults: 18–30 years				
m	BMR = 0.063 wt − 0.042 ht + 2.953	2879	0.65	0.6408
f	BMR = 0.057 wt + 1.184 ht + 0.411	829	0.73	0.4925
30–60 years				
m	BMR = 0.048 wt − 0.011 ht + 3.670	646	0.60	0.7002
f	BMR = 0.034 wt + 0.006 ht + 3.530	372	0.68	0.4660
Over 60 years				
m	BMR = 0.038 wt + 4.068 ht − 3.491	50	0.74	0.6600
f	BMR = 0.033 wt + 1.917 ht + 0.074	38	0.73	0.4289

Table 1.36 Standard basal metabolic rates for individuals of both sexes (Schofield 1978). Reproduced with permission

| Body weight (kg) | MJ/24 h | | Body weight (kg) | MJ/24 h | | Body weight (kg) | MJ/24 h | |
	m	f		m	f		m	f
3	0.5	0.6	31	5.0	4.6	59	6.7	5.6
4	0.8	0.8	32	5.0	4.6	60	6.8	5.6
5	1.0	1.0	33	5.1	4.7	61	6.8	5.7
6	1.2	1.3	34	5.2	4.7	62	6.9	5.7
7	1.5	1.6	35	5.2	4.8	63	7.0	5.8
8	1.8	1.8	36	5.3	4.8	64	7.0	5.8
9	2.0	2.1	37	5.4	4.8	65	7.0	5.9
10	2.3	2.3	38	5.5	4.9	66	7.1	5.9
11	2.6	2.6	39	5.5	4.9	67	7.1	6.0
12	2.8	2.8	40	5.6	4.9	68	7.2	6.0
13	3.0	3.0	41	5.6	5.0	69	7.2	6.0
14	3.2	3.2	42	5.7	5.0	70	7.3	6.1
15	3.4	3.4	43	5.8	5.0	71	7.3	6.1
16	3.6	3.5	44	5.8	5.1	72	7.3	6.1
17	3.7	3.6	45	5.9	5.1	73	7.4	6.2
18	3.8	3.7	46	6.0	5.1	74	7.4	6.2
19	3.9	3.8	47	6.0	5.2	75	7.5	6.2
20	4.0	3.9	48	6.1	5.2	76	7.5	6.3
21	4.1	3.9	49	6.1	5.2	77	7.6	6.3
22	4.2	4.0	50	6.2	5.3	78	7.6	6.3
23	4.3	4.0	51	6.3	5.3	79	7.7	6.4
24	4.4	4.1	52	6.3	5.3	80	7.7	6.4
25	4.5	4.2	53	6.4	5.4	81	7.7	6.5
26	4.6	4.2	54	6.4	5.4	82	7.8	6.5
27	4.7	4.3	55	6.5	5.4	83	7.8	6.6
28	4.7	4.4	56	6.6	5.5	84	7.8	6.6
29	4.8	4.5	57	6.6	5.5	85	7.9	6.6
30	4.9	4.5	58	6.7	5.5			

Not applicable to the elderly.
For men over 60 years use BMR = 0.049 (wt) + 2.46, or BMR = 0.038 (wt) + 4.07 (ht) − 3.49.
For women over 60 years use BMR = 0.038 (wt) + 2.76, or BMR = 0.033 (wt) + 1.92 (ht) + 0.07.

Table 1.37 Activity and injury factors for estimation of energy requirements (Long 1984)

Basal Energy Expenditure* × activity factor × injury factor

Activity factors
Patients confined to bed × 1.2
Patients out of bed   × 1.3

Injury factors
Minor surgery   × 1.20
Skeletal trauma   × 1.35
Major sepsis   × 1.60
Severe thermal burn** × 2.10

*See p 67 for calculation of basal energy expenditure (or basal metabolic rate).
**See also Section 5.1.3.

Table 1.38 Protein requirements during peak catabolic response in patients following injury or during infection (Wilmore 1977)

Patient Group	Condition	g/kg/day	
		Protein	Nitrogen
Normal	Average level of exercise	0.5−1.0	0.08−0.16
Mildly stressed	Elective operation	0.7−1.1	0.11−0.18
Moderately stressed	Major operations, infections, fractures	1.5−2.0	0.24−0.32
Severely stressed	Multiple injuries, fractures, major burns	2.0−4.0	0.32−0.64

the percentage additions to BMR proposed by Wilmore (1977) or the injury and activity factors devised by Long (1984) (Fig. 1.5 and Table 1.37). Specific formulae have also been devised in respect of thermal injury (see Section 5.1.3).

The daily energy requirement is calculated by making further modifications to the BMR as follows

1 Specific dynamic effect of feeding = BMR + 10%.
2 Activity (if Long's factors are not used)
   a) On ventilator   = BMR − 15%
   b) Unconscious   = BMR
   c) Bedbound and awake = BMR + 10%
   d) Sitting in chair   = BMR + 20%
   e) Walking around ward = BMR + 30%
3 Allowance for weight gain = +300 kcal/day. This will lead to a gain of up to 1 kg/week which is a realistic aim for most patients. Sudden fluctuations in weight usually represent changes in fluid balance.
4 Pyrexia — each 1°C increase in body temperature produces a 10−12% rise in the BMR.

The ambient temperature affects energy requirements. This is only relevant if the patient is nursed in anything other than a thermoneutral environment (23−26°C). Patients nursed in a cooler area have to expend more energy to maintain their body temperature. Conversely, patients nursed in warmer environments such as an intensive care unit need less energy to maintain their temperature.

Another, less precise, method of calculating energy requirements is to allocate an arbitrary allowance of energy based on weight and clinical condition
1 Normal requirement = 30 kcal/kg body weight/day.
2 Moderate stress = 35 kcal/kg body weight/day.
3 Severe stress = 40 kcal/kg body weight/day.

It is interesting to note that the figures for energy requirements which are obtained from these calculations are often significantly lower than those quoted in the standard tables of RDA. The latter are, of course, devised for groups of healthy, active individuals and are not appropriate when considering acutely ill patients in hospital. The calculated figures are also often lower than those used in current clinical practice and some financial savings may be made, particularly when intravenous preparations are being used, if the feeding regimens are based on the calculated individual requirements. There are also many clinical reasons for avoiding overfeeding.

Nitrogen requirements

Patients do not have a requirement for nitrogen *per se*, but for amino acids which are the substrates needed

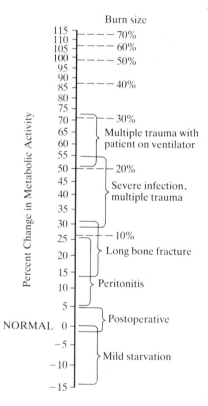

Fig. 1.5 Factors affecting energy requirements in critically ill patients (Wilmore 1977).

for protein synthesis. This may be particularly important if oral or tube feeding regimens are being considered when it may be more difficult to achieve an appropriately balanced intake of amino acids. The aim of nutritional support is to achieve a state of nitrogen balance where the input and output are equal. This should be monitored carefully and can be assessed by measuring the nitrogen input and the total nitrogen output (including urinary, faecal and any other losses). *Nitrogen excretion in g* is approximately equal to

$$\text{g urinary urea excreted in 24 hours} \times \frac{28^*}{60} \times \frac{6^{**}}{5}$$

For practical purposes this formula can be condensed to

$$\text{Nitrogen excretion in g} = \frac{\text{mmol urinary urea excreted in 24 hours}}{30}.$$

Some laboratories may not be able to measure total nitrogen excretion in which case the urinary urea output should be measured and the following formula applied

$$\frac{\text{mmol urinary urea}}{\text{excreted in 24 hours}} \times 0.212 = \frac{\text{g protein lost}}{\text{per 24 hours}}$$

Many factors affect nitrogen requirements including the previous nutritional status of the patient (a nutritionally depleted or stressed patient may only retain 50% of the nitrogen which is given). It is not always either possible or practical to give all the nitrogen which is required especially during the early days following a trauma. All nitrogen losses should be considered carefully including those from faeces and any fistulae or burned areas. The greatest amount of nitrogen is lost 3–5 days after accidental injury or during the peak response to sepsis or burns (Table 1.38). Nutritional support can be based either on these figures or on arbitrary energy — nitrogen ratios (Table 1.39). It is also possible to estimate nitrogen requirements based on 24-hour urinary urea excretions by using a graph. Whichever method is used, it is important to monitor nitrogen balance carefully to ensure optimal nutritional support. Nitrogen input should never be less than 0.16 g/kg body weight.

It is not always possible to measure nitrogen output in patients who have renal failure. The rate of urea nitrogen production can be estimated by referring to

Table 1.39 Commonly used energy:nitrogen ratios

	Total	Non-nitrogen
	Energy:Nitrogen	Energy:Nitrogen
Normal individuals	250–350:1	225–325:1
Convalescence	200 :1	175 :1
Mild catabolism	150 :1	125 :1
Moderate catabolism	125 :1	100 :1
Severe catabolism	100 :1	75 :1

serum urea concentrations. Calculation of nitrogen output in anuric patients with renal failure is as follows

g urea nitrogen produced per day
$$= [(\text{Urea 2} - \text{Urea 1}) \times W \times 0.6 + (W \text{ gain} \times \text{Urea 2})] \times 0.028.$$

Urea 1 = plasma urea at start of period (mmol/l);
Urea 2 = plasma urea at end of period (mmol/l);
0.6 = factor to estimate total body water;
W = weight in kg.

Vitamin requirements

Vitamins are usually administered according to the RDA and customary clinical practice. This may mean that some vitamins need only be given on a weekly or monthly basis (including vitamins A, D B and folic acid). The actual dosage may vary but it is useful to remember that enough should be given to cover not only the RDA but also any expected losses during administration. This is particularly important in parenteral regimens (see Section 1.13, Table 1.13.4).

Certain procedures may modify the requirement for particular vitamins. These include chemotherapy (B vitamins), surgery (vitamin C and vitamin K) and anticoagulant therapy (vitamin K). On the whole it is appropriate to give more rather than less of the water soluble vitamins since they are cheap, particularly in tablet form, and any moderate excess is excreted in the urine.

Fluid requirements

Although not a nutrient as such, the maintenance of fluid balance is often one of the most important aspects of the management of the acutely ill patient. This is particularly critical in the presence of tissue breakdown (e.g. malnutrition or gross sepsis) which may result in an increase in the total body water. It is important to check body weight and serum osmolality regularly (daily if necessary) to monitor any changes in

*The molecular weight of urea is 60 of which 28 parts are nitrogen.
**Approximately 80% of the total urinary nitrogen is urea.

gross fluid balance. Since the fluid requirement is an integral part of the estimation and provision of nutritional support, it must be considered in this context and it will be necessary to know the exact water content of a feeding regimen (see Section 2.9).

Summary

The provision of appropriate nutritional support is an essential part of the management of the patient. The estimate of nutritional requirements must necessarily precede this. Requirements are influenced by many factors, each of which must be considered carefully on an individual basis. Once nutritional therapy has been commenced it is important to monitor the patient regularly and carefully. As the clinical condition changes, so will the requirement for nutritional support and all regimens should be constructed with this in mind.

Further reading

Caldwell MD and Kennedy-Caldwell C (1981) Normal nutritional requirements. *Surg Clin North Am* **61**, (3), 489–507.

Curren PW, Richmond D, Marvin J and Baxter CR (1974) Dietary requirements of patients with major burns. *J Am Diet Assoc* **65**, (4), 415–7.

Elwyn DH (1980) Nutritional requirements of adult surgical patients. *Crit Care Med* **8**, (1), 9–20.

Hill GL and Church J (1984) Energy and protein requirements of general surgical patients requiring intravenous nutrition. *Br J Surg* **71**, 1–9.

Karran SJ and Alberti KGMM (Eds) (1980) *Practical nutritional support*. Pitman Medical Books, Tunbridge Wells.

Kielanowski J (1976) Energy cost of protein deposition. In *Protein metabolism and nutrition* (Cole DJA, Boorman KN, Buttery PJ, Lewis D, Neal RJ and Swan H (Eds) pp 207–15. Butterworths, London.

Kinney JM (1975) Energy requirements of the surgical patient. In *Manual of surgical nutrition* Ballinger WF et al (Eds) pp 223–35. WB Saunders, Philadelphia.

Merritt RJ, Sinatra FR, Smith GA (1983) Nutritional support of the hospitalized child. In *Advances in nutritional research* Vol 5 Draper HH (Ed) pp 77–103. Plenum Press, New York.

Paauw JD, McCarnish MA, Dean RE and Duellette TR (1984) Assessment of caloric needs in stressed patients. *J Am Coll Nutr* **3**, 51–9.

Schofield WN, Schofield C and James WPT (1985) Basal metabolic rate — r. view and prediction, together with an annotated bibliography of source material. *Hum Nutr: Clin Nutr* **39C**, [Suppl 1], 5–96.

Stonor HB (1982) Assessment of energy expenditure. *Proc Nutr Soc* **41**, 349–53.

Sutherland AB (1976) Nitrogen balance and nutritional requirement in the burn patient: a reappraisal. *Burns* **2**, 238–44.

Tweedle DEF (1982) *Metabolic care*. Churchill Livingstone, Edinburgh.

Wilmore DW (1974) Nutrition and metabolism following thermal injury. *Clin Plast Surg* **1**, (4), 603–19.

References

Altman PL and Dittmer DS (1968) *Metabolism* p 345. Federation of American Societies for Experimental Biology, Bethesda.

Bistrian BR, Blackburn GL, Vitale J, Cochran D and Naylor J (1976) Prevalence of malnutrition in general medical patients. *J Am Diet Assoc* **235**, (15), 1567–70.

Colley CM, Fleck A and Howard JP (1985) The pocket computer — a new aid to nutritional support. *Br Med J* **290**, 1403–6.

Dubois D and Dubois EF (1916) Clinical calorimetry — a formula to estimate the approximate surface area if height and weight be known. *Arch Intern Med* **17**, 863–71.

Fleish A (1951) Le metabolisme basal standard et sa determination au moyen du 'metabocalculator'. *Helv Med Acta* **18**, 23.

Harris JA and Benedict FG (1919) *Biometric studies of basal metabolism in man*. Carnegie Institute, Washington.

Hill GL, Blackett RL, Pickford L, Burkinshaw L, Young GA, Warren JV, Schorah CJ and Morgan DB (1977) Malnutrition in surgical patients — an unrecognized problem. *Lancet* **i**, 689–92.

Long CL (1984) The energy and protein requirements of the critically ill patient. In *Nutritional assessment*. Wright RA and Heymsfield S (Eds) pp 157–81. Blackwell Scientific Publications, Boston.

Robertson JD and Reid DD (1952) Standards for the basal metabolism of normal people in Britain. *Lancet* **i**, 940–3.

Schofield WN (1985) Predicting basal metabolic rate, new standards and review of previous work. *Hum Nutr: Clin Nutr* **39C**, [Suppl 1], 5–41.

Wilmore DW (1977) *Metabolic management of the critically ill III*. Plenum Medical Book Company, New York.

Woolfson AMJ (1978) Metabolic considerations in nutritional support. In *Developments in clinical nutrition*. Johnston IDA and Lee HA (Eds) pp 35–47. MSC Consultants, Tunbridge Wells.

1.12   Enteral Feeding

Enteral nutrition can be defined as nutrition provided through or via the gastrointestinal tract. It includes nutrition taken orally or administered via a tube. The term is usually restricted to mean the feeding of patients who are unable or unwilling to feed themselves and/or who require additional or total nutritional support.

The associations between malnutrition and morbidity and mortality have been recognized for some time, but the awareness of the significance of this problem in hospitals increased only relatively recently. Studies have reported that 30–35% of patients (particularly surgical patients) in British and American hospitals show signs of malnutrition (Bistrian *et al* 1974, 1976; Hill *et al* 1977).

Hospitalization presents many fears and anxieties to patients which may result in a reduction of their normal nutritional intake. Uncertainties about their medical or surgical condition, strange surroundings, absence of friends or relatives, different foods served at set meal times, all affect a patient's interest in food. Hospital staff involved in the care of patients and the service of their food can do much to reassure them, help them select suitable meals, ensure that meals are attractively served and identify patients with nutritional problems as early as possible.

Once it is evident that a patient is unable or unwilling to consume an adequate nutritional intake, additional nutritional support should be provided.

When considering nutritional support the following questions should be asked
1   Is the patient malnourished now?
2   Is the patient unable or unwilling to consume a nutritionally adequate diet?
3   Is the patient likely to become malnourished as a consequence of his/her medical/surgical condition?
4   Is the gastrointestinal tract functional?
If the gastrointestinal tract is functional it is by far the most appropriate, natural and the safest route for feeding and considerably less expensive than total parenteral nutrition. The patient's nutritional intake can be improved by one of the following methods
1   Light, appetizing and nourishing foods offered in addition to the normal menu.
2   Soft, semi-solid or liquid meals.
3   Tube feeding.

1.12.1   Additional appetizing and nourishing foods

In a hospital situation it is difficult to cater for patients' individual likes and dislikes. Liaison between the dietitian, nursing and the catering staff should ensure that a limited range of suitable dishes is available for patients who genuinely have difficulty choosing from the normal menus. The advent of cook-freeze or cook-chill catering systems should result in a flexible menu system. Light, nourishing dishes presented attractively will help to tempt the patient to eat and stimulate their appetite. Often patients who have no appetite for meat and two vegetables will manage soup, a sandwich and a milk pudding. Such patients should be encouraged to drink energy-rich fluids (such as milk-based drinks) between meals in preference to water, fruit juice, squash or cups of tea. A daily record of food and fluids taken will help the dietitian assess the approximate energy and protein intake and suggest appropriate improvements.

1.12.2   Soft, semi-solid or liquid diets

A soft, semi-solid or liquid diet is indicated for patients who are physically or psychologically unable to eat a normal diet. Such patients may include those with poor or no teeth; or those with chewing or swallowing difficulties, for example patients recovering from a stroke, those with diseases of the mouth, throat, oesophagus or stomach or those with fractured and wired jaws.

A soft, semi-solid diet may be chopped, minced or pureed depending on individual needs. Meals should be served with plenty of sauce or gravy to facilitate feeding and swallowing.

Liquidized hospital meals are unattractive and additional liquid is usually required to achieve the correct consistency. The nutrient content of the meal may therefore be reduced if the patient cannot consume the volume produced. However, many patients enjoy liquidized meals because of the familiar taste of the foods in them. Soups and milk puddings fortified with protein supplements (e.g. skimmed milk powder

Table 1.40 Proprietary protein and energy supplements*

Protein and energy sources	Protein sources	Carbohydrate sources	Fat sources
Build Up (Carnation)	Casilan (Farley Health Products)	Calonutrin (Geistlich)	Calogen / Liquigen } (Scientific Hospital Supplies)
Complan (Farley Health Products) Fresubin (Fresenius)	Forceval (Unigreg)	Caloreen (Roussel)	
Fortimel Fortisip Fortify } (Cow and Gate)	Maxipro HBV (Scientific Hospital Supplies)	Fortical (Cow and Gate)	Medium chain triglyceride oil (Cow and Gate, Mead Johnson)
Supplement (Wyeth Laboratories)	Protifar (Cow and Gate) Promod (Abbott Laboratories)	Hycal (Beecham)	
		Maxijul (Scientific Hospital Supplies)	Duocal (Scientific Hospital Supplies)
		Polycal (Cow and Gate)	
		Polycose (Abbott Laboratories)	
		Duocal (Scientific Hospital Supplies)	

*Compositional details of these products are given in Section 2.12

or Maxipro) and energy supplements (e.g. Maxijul, Polycal, Polycose or Caloreen), may be included to increase the protein and energy intake.

Excellent commercially available preparations (Table 1.40) are available which may be offered to the patient either between meals to supplement their protein and energy intake or as a meal replacement.

Palatability, acceptability and variety are important factors and many patients prefer to have a selection of suitable meals and nourishing fluids throughout the day, rather than to rely on an individual product as the sole source of nutrition.

Sip feeding

This is the term used when a patient's nutritional intake is provided by nourishing fluids taken at frequent intervals. Fluids may be taken from a cup, glass, feeding beaker or via a straw. Liquidized meals are not usually very suitable and commercially produced preparations of known nutritional content tend to be preferred, e.g. Build-Up, Complan, Fortimel, or any of the enteral feeding preparations (see Tables 1.40 and 1.43). Patients will tire of a monotonous flavour, so a range of flavours, both sweet and savoury, should be offered. If patients are unable or unwilling to consume an adequate nutritional intake by this method, tube feeding should be considered.

Clear fluids

These are indicated post-operatively in acute inflam-

matory conditions of the gastrointestinal tract and acute stages of many illnesses. Suitable fluids include water, fruit juices, fruit cordials, plain jelly, clear soups (e.g. consomme), black tea and coffee, soda water and lemonade. The diet is nutritionally inadequate and should be used only for a brief period of time. Additional energy may be provided by sugar, glucose polymers and glucose drinks (e.g. Hycal, Fortical).

1.12.3 Tube feeding

It is important to re-emphasize the fact that most patients requiring nutritional support have a functional gastrointestinal tract and can therefore be fed enterally. Administration of nutrients via the enteral route is more natural, safer and less expensive than parenteral feeding. A wide range of enteral feeds can be administered via nasogastric, nasoduodenal or nasojejunal tubes as well as via oesophagostomy, gastrostomy or jejunostomy tubes (see Fig. 1.6).

Formulating a tube feed

Patients with normal gastrointestinal function are capable of digesting and absorbing whole protein and unhydrolysed triglycerides. The composition of an ideal standard enteral feed is shown in Table 1.41.

Patients with impaired gastrointestinal function due to digestive insufficiency or reduced absorptive capacity may benefit from a pre-digested enteral feed. The term 'elemental' diets has been used to describe the early, free amino-acid and glucose-containing feeds

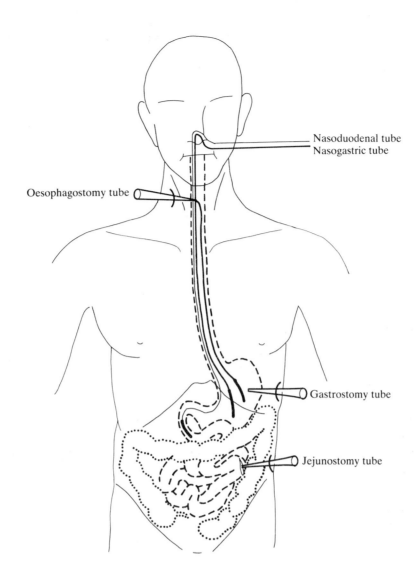

Fig. 1.6 Routes of enteral feeding.

Table 1.41 Composition of an ideal standard enteral feed. (After Silk 1983)

Nitrogen source	Whole protein
Energy source	Carbohydrate (65%) high molecular weight glucose polymers
	Fat (35%) triglycerides
Non-protein energy: nitrogen ratio (kcal/g)	150–200 : 1
Electrolytes	
Minerals	
Vitamins	
Osmolality	285–300 mosmol/kg

Table 1.42 Indications for use of predigested 'elemental' diets. (After Silk 1983)

1	Impaired luminal nutrient digestion	Total pancreatectomy
	Severe exocrine pancreatic insufficiency	Carcinoma of pancreas
		Severe chronic pancreatitis
	Short bowel syndrome	Intestinal resections
		Intestinal fistulae
2	Reduced functional absorptive capacity	Intestinal resections
		Intestinal fistulae
		Severe untreated coeliac disease
		Severe active Crohn's disease

and also the amino-acid and short chain peptide-containing feeds which have been developed recently.

Short chain peptides are absorbed more rapidly by the mucosa than free amino acids (Silk 1974) and the use of 'elemental' diets has been advocated in a variety of gastrointestinal conditions (Russell 1975). However, there seems to be little justification for their general use (Koretz and Meyer 1980; Jones *et al* 1980) and they should be restricted to conditions of maldigestion and malabsorption (see Table 1.42).

Choice of feed

Hospital-made tube feeds

Over recent years the range of commercially available feeds has increased and attitudes towards tube feeding have changed. In the past, tube feeds were prepared in hospital kitchens under the supervision of the dietetic department and indeed this still continues in some hospitals. The most frequently prepared hospital feed was based on a mixture of Complan, Caloreen, Prosparol and milk with vitamin, and occasionally mineral and electrolyte, supplementation (Tredger *et al* 1981).

Although the actual cost of the ingredients of such feeds is low, their preparation may place a considerable burden on the dietetic department and catering staff. It is doubtful whether the patient's trace elements, electrolyte and vitamin requirements are adequately met and many formulations result in a hyperosmolar feed. The ingredients of these feeds are an ideal medium for bacterial contamination (Casewell 1979) and care should be taken to ensure that they are prepared under very 'clean' conditions and do *not* contain raw eggs. Aseptic conditions in hospital kitchens are seldom possible. Many hospitals have now changed to using sterile commercially prepared, ready to use feeds.

Commercially prepared tube feeds

A wide range of commercially prepared nutritionally complete enteral feeds are available (see Table 1.43). They are produced as liquids or powders and packed in bottles, cans or sachets. They fall into two main groups.

'Whole protein' or 'polymeric' feeds — containing whole protein as the nitrogen source, hydrolysed fat and carbohydrate. They have a relatively low osmolality, require normal digestion and the majority are low residue. Their palatability varies but they can be administered either orally, flavoured as required, or via a tube. The non-protein energy to nitrogen ratio of the different feeds varies, the majority falling between 130:1 to 170:1 with Clinifeed Iso providing 200:1.

Chemically defined 'elemental' feeds — containing free amino acids as the nitrogen source, e.g. Vivonex, Vivonex HN, Elemental 028 or a mixture of amino acids and short chain peptides, e.g. Nutranel, Peptisorbon, Pepdite. The triglyceride content is low but they may contain medium chain triglycerides. The main source of energy is provided by oligosaccharides and monosaccharides. They are hyperosmolar (and therefore require slow introduction), unpalatable and more expensive than whole protein feeds. They require minimal digestion, are readily absorbed in the upper small intestine and are low residue.

Nutritional considerations

When selecting a suitable feed or range of feeds the following points should be considered
1 Non-protein energy: nitrogen ratio.
2 Osmolality.
3 Lactose content.
4 Residue.
5 Vitamin, mineral and trace element content.
6 Cost.

Non-protein energy: nitrogen ratio

The estimation of nitrogen and energy requirements is discussed in Section 1.11.

The variety of commercially available enteral feeds offers a choice of preparations with non-protein energy: nitrogen ratios ranging from 100:1 to 200:1 (see Table 1.43). The approximate energy and nitrogen requirements in different groups of patients is outlined in Table 1.44 (Woolfson 1978). The energy content of ready prepared feeds can be increased by the addition of glucose polymers, e.g. Caloreen, Maxijul (glucose polymer solutions such as Polycose or Maxijul are particularly convenient) or a mixture of fat and glucose, e.g. Duocal.

Osmolality

The molar concentration of a solute in a solution is expressed either in terms of osmolality (mosmol per kg solvent) or osmolarity (mosmol per litre of solution). Osmolality is greater than osmolarity (see p 605).

A high osmotic load in the duodenum draws fluid into the gut and is likely to cause diarrhoea. Ideally, a feed should be isotonic with plasma and have an osmolality of 280–300 mosmol/kg. Feeds providing 1 kcal per ml will have a relatively low osmolality.

The lower the osmolality, the more quickly the feed can be introduced. If the osmolality is high, the feed must be introduced more slowly and may need to be diluted. This will result in a reduced nitrogen and energy intake over the first few days until full strength feeding is tolerated. It is possible to administer hyperosmolar

Table 1.43 Proprietary enteral feeds — composition per standard pack (Table prepared April 1987)

Manufacturer	Product	Presentation	Pack size	Dilution to full strength feed	Energy (kcal)	Protein (g)	Nitrogen (g)	Non-protein energy:nitrogen ratio (kcal/gN)	Osmolality (mosmol/kg)
Whole protein preparations									
Abbott Laboratories	Enrich (+ fibre)	Liquid	250 ml		260	9.4	1.5	148	484
	Ensure	Liquid (or powder)	250 ml* 400 g		250	8.8	1.4	154	450
	Ensure Plus	Liquid	250 ml		375	15.6	2.5	125	600
	Two Cal HN	Liquid	237 ml		475	19.8	3.2	124	747
	Osmolite	Liquid	250 ml*		250	10.5	1.7	124	310
	Pulmocare	Liquid	237 ml		355	14.8	2.4	125	490
Bristol Myers	Isocal	Liquid	250 ml		250	8.0	1.3	170	300
Cow and Gate	Fortison								
	Standard	Liquid	500 ml		500	20.0	3.2	131	300
	Energy Plus	Liquid	500 ml		750	25.0	3.9	166	410
	Soya	Liquid	500 ml		500	20.0	3.2	131	300
	Pre-Fortison	Liquid	500 ml		250	10.0	1.6	131	150
Fresenius Dylade	Fresubin	Liquid	500 ml		500	19.0	3.0	140	360 (vanilla)
Kabivitrum	Nutrauxil	Liquid	500 ml		500	19.0	3.0	140	350
Merck	Triosorbon	Powder	85 g	+ 400 ml	400	16.1	2.6	130	250
	Liquisorb	Liquid	500 ml		500	20.0	3.2	131	320 (neutral)
	Liquisorbon MCT	Liquid	500 ml		500	25.0	4.0	100	270 (neutral)
MCP Pharmaceuticals	Salvimulsin MCT	Liquid	500 ml		500	24.0	3.8	106	285**
Oxford Nutrition	Hipernutril MCT	Powder	90 g	+ 500 ml	400	19.0	3.0	108	424
	Stressnutril	Powder	91 g	+ 330 ml	400	18.0	2.5	131	770
Roussel	Clinifeed								
	Iso	Liquid	375 ml		375	10.5	1.7	200	338
	400	Liquid	375 ml	+ 125 ml	400	15	2.4	142	414 undiluted 293 diluted
	Favour	Liquid	375 ml		375	14.1	2.25	145	388
	Protein rich	Liquid	375 ml	+ 125 ml	500	30.0	4.8	79	700 undiluted 486 diluted
Scientific Hospital Supplies	Enteral 400	Powder	86 g	+ 330 ml	400	11.5	1.8	193	300
Peptide preparations									
Bristol Myers	Flexical	Powder	454 g	As per instructions	2002	44.9	7.2	256	580
MCP Pharmaceuticals	Salvipeptid	Powder	129 g	+ 400 ml	500	16.7	2.7	160	430**
Merck	Peptisorbon	Powder	83 g	+ 400 ml	333	15.0	2.4	114	400
	Petisorb	Liquid	500 ml		500	18.75	3.0	142	400
Roussel	Nutranel	Powder	101 g	+ 350 ml	400	16.0	2.6	137	480
	Reabilan	Liquid	375 ml		375	11.5	1.9	175	360
Scientific Hospital Supplies	Pepdite 2+	Powder	100 g	+ 400 ml	450	13.9	2.2	178	288
	MCT Pepdite 2+	Powder	100 g	+ 400 ml	460	13.9	2.2	182	360
Elemental preparations									
Norwich Eaton	Vivonex								
	Standard	Powder	80 g	+ 300 ml	300	6.2	1.0	275	550 (USA figs)
	HN	Powder	80 g	+ 300 ml	300	13.3	2.0	123	810
Scientific Hospital Supplies	Elemental 028	Powder	100 g	+ 650 ml + 400 ml	400	10.0	1.9	189	520 (flavoured) 720 (flavoured) 450 (unflavoured)

*Also available in 1 litre cans.
**Measured in hospital laboratory.

feeds without inducing osmotic diarrhoea provided that they are administered slowly. The rate of administration should be controlled by an enteral feeding pump if possible. It is more important to control the number of osmoles administered per unit time than the number of osmoles administered per unit volume (Bastow *et al* 1985).

In theory, isotonic feeds may be introduced at full strength as it has been shown that the use of starter regimens for hypertonic feeds does not reduce the gas-

Table 1.44 Approximate requirements for energy and nitrogen in different patients. Normal men are included for comparison. (After Woolfson 1978)

	Normal active men*	Catabolic	Intermediate	Non-catabolic
Energy requirements				
MJ/24 hours	11−14	15−18	11−14	7−9
(kcal/24 hours)	(~3000)	(~4000)	(~3000)	(~2000)
Optimal Ratio (kJ/g)	1365	630	840	1050
Non-protein energy/nitrogen/(kcal/g)	(325)	(135)	(200)	(250)
Nitrogen requirement for equilibrium (g/24 hours)	8.5	25	14	7.5

*From Calloway and Spector (1954)

trointestinal side effects (Keohane *et al* 1984). However, in practice, feeds are often introduced at a dilute strength for one to two days.

A commercially produced, half strength preparation is available (Pre-Fortison) which offers a convenient way of introducing enteral feeding. The need for dilution is overcome and the risk of microbial contamination is reduced.

Lactose and milk intolerance

Many enteral feeds contain milk or milk-based solids. For patients who are milk intolerant a range of soya based feeds is available. The lactose in milk-based feeds has a bad reputation for causing diarrhoea, although this is probably over-emphasized. There are some patients for whom a lactose-free feed would be advisable (McMichael 1978)
1 Cases of known lactase deficiency.
2 Asian or African patients (Simoons 1969).
3 Patients with a mildly damaged gut, e.g. due to malnutrition or intestinal inflammation.

Lactose-free or 'clinically lactose-free' feeds are available to help overcome this problem.

Residue

All enteral feeds may be described as low residue. Provided there is normal gastrointestinal digestion and absorption there is no benefit from using 'elemental' enteral feeds in preference to whole protein enteral feeds. (Jones *et al* 1980; Russell and Evans 1984.) Nursing staff and patients should be assured that a normal bowel action is not always to be expected during tube feeding and the unnecessary use of suppositories should be discouraged. A fibre-rich feed (Enrich) is available which may be of benefit in producing a more normal bowel action in patients receiving enteral nutrition for a long period of time. As well as resolving constipation, it may also relieve the problem of diarrhoea. This feed *will not* pass through a fine bore tube without the use of an enteral feeding pump.

Vitamins, minerals and trace elements

Proprietary enteral feeds are of known vitamin, mineral and trace element content. Additional vitamins and electrolytes and minerals can be given according to individual requirements based on biochemical and haematological measurements. The high vitamin K content of some enteral feeds may have serious consequences with patients taking oral anticoagulants (Watson *et al* 1984).

Cost

Proprietary enteral feeds are more expensive than hospital-made feeds and the price varies quite considerably. The chemical composition of many of the preparations is fairly similar and it is not practical for hospitals to stock a wide range of feeds. The cost of the feed is therefore an important consideration when selecting a suitable preparation for use for the majority of patients requiring tube feeding. Which feed is selected should ideally be a joint decision made between dietitian and pharmacist or by the hospital nutritional team. It is often preferable, more convenient and efficient for the pharmacy department to be responsible for ordering, stock control and issuing of the feed to the wards.

Administration of tube feeds

Routes of administration

Tube feeds may be provided via the following routes
1 Nasogastric tube feeding by fine or narrow bore tube. Fine bore tubes are more comfortable than wide bore tubes and less likely to cause oesophageal erosions, oesophagitis or strictures. Occasionally, wider

bore tubes may be preferable in patients who require gastric aspiration during intermittent feeding.

2 Nasoduodenal or nasojejunal feeding — via a weighted narrow bore tube.

3 Oesophagostomy, gastrostomy or jejunostomy feeding (Fig. 1.6).

Choice of tube

There are several feeding tubes available differing in material, length, bore, luer fitting and price. There are two main types

1 Simple unweighted or open-ended tubes (1–2 mm internal diameter, e.g. Clinifeed (Roussel)) which are introduced with the aid of a guide wire or nylon stylette.

2 Tubes with a tungsten weighted tip, e.g. Dobhoff tube, Entriflex tube. Mercury used to be used in these tubes but tungsten is now recommended. These tubes may also have a wire introducer to aid intubation if necessary. They are more expensive than the open-ended tubes.

A simple, open-ended tube is suitable for most patients but a weighted tube may be preferable in patients with oesophageal strictures or when nasoduodenal or nasojejunal feeding is indicated.

Specifications for fine bore enteric tubes are detailed by the British Standards Institution (Ref BS 6314, (1983).) It should be noted that most tubes produced in the United States of America are made with a luer fitting which is not compatible with most British administration sets. Care must always be taken to ensure that they are not inadvertently connected to any intravenous infusion administration sets.

Passing fine bore tubes

An internal guide wire or nylon stylette will stiffen a fine bore tube and facilitate nasogastric intubation. Fine bore tubes can also be placed endoscopically into the stomach or duodenum. Tubes should be radio-opaque and the position of the feeding tube checked by aspiration of gastric acid, by injecting air down the tube and listening with a stethoscope over the stomach, or by chest X-ray. Most hospitals have a standard nursing procedure for the passing of fine bore tubes and the frequency of tube replacement.

Administration reservoirs and sets

A range of bags and bottles of varying sizes and shapes are available with compatible giving sets, with or without a pump insert. The luer fitting on the giving sets should be 'female' to avoid the risk of connection to intravenous lines. The choice of administration sets is largely one of cost, convenience and nurse preference.

Control of infusion rate

Many patients can be fed successfully when the feed is administered by gravity drip infusion, using the giving set clamp to control the infusion rate. Enteral feeding pumps are available to control the rate of infusion but are expensive. However, some methods of feeding (e.g. jejunostomy) and the more viscous feeds, should be administered using an enteral feeding pump.

Preparation of feeds

The preparation of enteral feeds, whether hospital-made or commercially prepared, necessitates careful attention to aseptic technique. Pre-sterilized enteral feeds should be used where possible (Bastow et al 1982) and should be administered via sterile giving sets using sterile water to dilute the feed if required. Any additives required should be added aseptically. Hospital-made or powdered enteral feeds should be mixed, preferably with sterile equipment under aseptic conditions (Anderton 1983). The pharmacy department may be able to assist in the preparation of proprietary products. Guidelines for the control of microbial contamination of enteral feeds are given by Anderton et al (in press).

Prescribing the regimen

Estimation of nutritional requirements should be made following the guidelines outlined in Section 1.11. It is not necessarily correct to assume that all patients fit a standard regimen. Gastric emptying should be established, especially in unconscious patients before fine bore feeding is commenced. Continuous drip feeding over 20–24 hours eliminates many of the problems associated with bolus feeding (such as diarrhoea, abdominal distension, regurgitation or nausea) although some patients prefer to be fed intermittently (e.g. feeding over two hours, resting for two hours). This method of feeding is possibly more 'normal' physiologically, and provides time between feeds to encourage patient mobilization whenever possible. Intermittent feeding may be preferable in unconscious patients who have an increased risk of developing aspiration pneumonia, as the stomach can be aspirated before each feed thereby preventing regurgitation and aspiration of the feed into the lungs. In restless or uncontrollable patients bolus feeding may be more practical.

If full strength feeds are introduced too quickly, abdominal distension, discomfort, colic and diarrhoea may occur (Silk 1980). Feeds introduced at half strength increasing to full strength over 1–2 days are usually well tolerated. If gastrointestinal function is impaired or slow to return post-operatively, it may be advisable to even start the feed at quarter strength and at a reduced volume. The feeds should be increased slowly over 5–6 days increasing first the volume and then the density of the feed until full strength feeding is tolerated.

When prescribing enteral feeding regimens it is important to consider the nursing staff who will be responsible for· their administration. The regimen should be as simple as possible and follow a standard method of administration to which the nursing staff are accustomed. Complicated or unusual regimens often result in confusing the nursing staff and the feed may be incorrectly or inadequately administered.

Gastrostomy feeding

The feeding gastrostomy has been a classical method of post-operative long term feeding, particularly in patients with upper gastrointestinal lesions. Liquidized meals may be given but proprietary enteral feeds are more appropriate. They should be administered at room temperature and each feed should be given by slow, continuous drip rather than as a bolus. The tube should be flushed with sterile water after each feed.

Jejunostomy feeding

Jejunostomy feeding also offers a means of providing enteral nutrition in patients following upper gastrointestinal surgery. Large bore catheters have been used for jejunostomy feeding for some years. More recently fine bore catheters have been inserted and 'jejunostomy kits' comprising a fine bore polyurethane catheter with introducer wire and needles are now available. The catheter jejunostomy provides a safe, cost-effective means of providing nutritional support. (Page *et al* 1979).

Chemically defined 'elemental' feeds or whole protein feeds may be administered via a catheter jejunostomy. Unless there is pancreatic or biliary insufficiency, or a reduced absorptive capacity, whole protein feeds should be used in preference to chemically defined 'elemental' preparations.

Jejunostomy feeding can commence in the early post-operative period. The feed should be administered by continuous drip over 24 hours and introduced at half strength and at a slow rate of administration (e.g. 30–50 ml per hour). The volume and then the density of the feed should be increased slowly to full volume and full strength over at least 4–5 days. The rate of infusion should be controlled using an enteral feeding pump. Flushing the catheter every 4–6 hours with 10–20 ml of sterile water will help to prevent blockage. Abdominal distension may occur which can be relieved by reducing the rate or the density of the feed. Diarrhoea can be controlled by the use of anti-diarrhoeal agents.

Complications of tube feeding

Gastrointestinal side effects

Nausea, diarrhoea, abdominal distension and discomfort are the most common side effects of enteral feeding. Diarrhoea is the major problem and can be provoked by any of the following
1 Rapid introduction of full strength feed into a previously rested gut.
2 The administration of hyperosmolar feeds.
3 Inadequate control of rate of infusion.
4 Bolus administration.
5 Antibiotic therapy (Editorial 1975). This is often the most common cause of diarrhoea during enteral feeding.
6 Lactose intolerance.
7 Bacterial contamination of the feed.
8 Rapid gastric emptying.

Diarrhoea should be treated as soon as it begins using an anti-diarrhoeal agent, e.g. codeine phosphate or Imodium, rather than the feed halted.

Tube related problems are associated more often with the use of wide bore tubes, e.g. Ryles tubes when used for feeding or gastric aspiration. Oesophageal erosions and haemorrhages can occur and may give rise to oesophageal strictures. Nasal necrosis can occur, particularly if wide bore tubes are *in situ* for some time.

Blockage of fine bore tubes occurs occasionally but can be prevented by· flushing the tube regularly with 10–20 ml of sterile water.

Regurgitation and aspiration

Regurgitation followed by pulmonary aspiration may occur. Unconscious patients or those with neurological disease are at risk of regurgitation of enteral feeds or possible pulmonary aspiration. It can be prevented by feeding intermittently via a wider bore tube and aspirating 4-hourly or by instigating nasoduodenal feeding.

Metabolic complications

Hyperglycaemia may occur and routine urinalysis should be undertaken as well as routine serum biochemistry to monitor the blood glucose level. Electrolyte abnormalities are more likely to be due to the patient's medical or surgical condition, but adjustments to the feed may be necessary. Abnormal liver function tests have been reported (Tweedle *et al* 1979) but the cause of this is not certain.

Monitoring

A complete nutritional assessment based on clinical, biochemical, anthropometric, haematological and immunological (if possible) investigations should be performed before enteral feeding is commenced (see Section 1.10) and repeated at regular intervals throughout of the period of feeding (Table 1.45). Changes in these measurements during the period of feeding are best observed by recording them on suitably designed forms which can be completed by nursing, medical or dietetic staff. The value of simply looking at the patient and observing changes in clinical appearance must not be forgotten. More detailed patient monitoring is described in the textbooks listed under Further reading.

It is also advisable to make random checks on the microbiological quality of the feed both during and at the end of administration.

Table 1.45 Patient monitoring during enteral feeding

Body weight	Daily, twice weekly or weekly, according to nursing time
Urinalysis	4—6 hourly
Blood glucose	4—6 hourly if glycosuria is present
24-hour urine for urinary urea	Twice weekly (daily if required for nitrogen balance studies)
Full serum profile and electrolytes	Twice weekly
Accurate fluid balance	Daily

Home tube feeding

With careful instruction and supervision, patients can tube feed themselves successfully at home either during the day or overnight. The majority of commercially prepared feeds are available on prescription and feeding reservoirs and administration sets can be provided by the hospital or community nursing departments.

The development of portable feeding systems (Viomedex carry pack) has made home feeding more convenient and the patient is free to move about the home and garden as desired.

Discontinuing tube feeding

Where possible, any method of nutritional support should be phased out gradually as normal eating is resumed or improved. Close dietetic supervision should be given to patients who are resuming their oral diet to ensure that their energy and nitrogen intake is maintained. Patients in whom tube feeding is discontinued will benefit from sip feeding in addition to their normal diet until an adequate diet is taken.

Many patients leaving hospital are still not eating very well and regular follow-up at out-patient clinics or in the community is advisable whenever possible.

Further reading

Grant AM and Todd E (1982) *Enteral and parenteral nutrition: a clinical handbook*. Blackwell Scientific Publications, Oxford.

Johnston IDA and Lee HA (1978) *Developments in clinical nutrition*. Proceedings of a symposium held at the Royal College of Physicians, London. MCS Consultants, London.

Moghissi K and Boore J (1984) *Parenteral and enteral nutrition for nurses*. Heinemann, London.

Ryan JA and Page CP (1984) Intrajejunal feeding: development and current status. *J Parent Ent Nutr* **8**, 187—8.

Silk DBA (1983) *Nutritional support in hospital practice*. Blackwell Scientific Publications, Oxford.

References

Anderton A Howard JP and Scott DW (1986) *Microbial control in enteral feeding — a guidance document*. The Parenteral and Enteral Nutrition Group of the British Dietetic Association.

Anderton A (1983) Microbiological aspects of the preparation and administration of nasogastric and nasoenteric tube feeds in hospitals: a review. *Hum Nutr: Appl Nutr* **37A**, 426—40.

Bastow MD, Greaves P and Allison SP (1982) Microbial contamination of enteral feeds. *Hum Nutr: Appl Nutr* **36A**, 213—7.

Bastow MD, Rawlings J and Allison SP (1985) Overnight nasogastric tube feeding. *Clin Nutr* **4**, 7—11.

Bistrian BR, Blackburn GL, Vitale J, Cochran D and Naylor J (1976) Prevalence of malnutrition in general medical patients. *J Am Med Assoc* **235**, 1567—70.

Bistrian BR, Blackburn GL, Hallowell E and Heddle R (1974) Protein status of general surgical patients. *J Am Med Assoc* **230**, 858—60.

Calloway DH and Spector H (1954) Nitrogen balance as related to calorie and protein intake in active young men. *Am J Clin Nutr* **2**, 405—12.

Casewell MW (1979) Nasogastric feeds as a source of klebsiella infection for intensive care patients. *Res Clin Forums* **1**, (1), 101−5.

Editorial (1975) Antibiotic diarrhoea. *Br Med J* **4**, 243−4.

Hill GL, Blacket RL, Pickford L, Burkinshaw L, Young GA, Warren JV, Schorah CJ and Morgan DB (1977) Malnutrition in surgical patients. *Lancet* **i**, 689−92.

Jones BJM, Lees R, Andrews J, Frost P and Silk DBA (1980) Elemental and polymeric tube feeding in patients with normal gastrointestinal function: a controlled trial. *Gut* **21**, A905.

Keohane PP, Attrill H, Love M, Frost P and Silk DBA (1984) Relation between osmolality of diet and gastrointestinal side effects in enteral nutrition. *Br Med J* **288**, 678−80.

Koretz RL and Meyer JH (1980) Elemental diets — facts and fantasies. *Gastroenterology* **78**.393−410.

McMichael HB (1978) Physiology of carbohydrate, electrolyte and water absorption. In *Developments in clinical nutrition*. Proceedings of a symposium held at the Royal College of Physicians, London, pp 25−8. MCS Consultants, London.

Page CP, Carlton PK, Andrassy RJ, Feldtman RW and Shield CF (1979) Safe, cost-effective post-operative nutrition: defined formula diet via·needle catheter jejunostomy. *Am J Surg* **138**, 939−45.

Russell CA and Evans SJ (1984) A comparison of the absorption from 'chemically defined elemental' and 'whole protein' enteral feeds by the human small bowel. *Proc Nutr Soc* **43**, 123A.

Russell CA (1984) Fine needle catheter jejunostomy in patients with upper gastrointestinal carcinoma. *Appl Nutr* **11**, 1−7.

Russell RI (1975) Elemental diets. *Gut* **16**, 68−79.

Silk DBA (1974) Peptide absorption in man. *Gut* **15**, 494−501.

Silk DBA (1980) Enteral nutrition. *Hosp Update* **8**, 761−76.

Silk DBA (1983) *Nutritional support in hospital practice*, pp 68−101. Blackwell Scientific Publications, Oxford.

Simoons FJ (1969) Primary adult lactose intolerance and the milking habit: a problem in biological and cultural inter-relations. 1: Review of the medical research. *Am J Dig Dis* **14**, 819−36.

Tredger J, Bazin C and Dickerson JWT (1981) Nasogastric tube feeding: a survey to investigate current practices and attitudes of dietitians. *Hum Nutr* **35**, 118−22.

Tweedle DE, Skidmore FD, Gleave EN, Gowland E and Knass DA (1979) Nutritional support for patients undergoing surgery for cancer of the head and neck. *Res Clin Forums* **1**, (1), 59−69.

Watson AJM, Pegg M and Green JRB (1984) Enteral feeds may antagonize Warfarin. *Br Med J* **288**, 557.

Woolfson AMJ (1978) Metabolic considerations in nutritional support. In *Development in clinical nutrition*. Proceedings of a symposium held at the Royal College of Physicians, London, pp 35−47. MCS Consultants, London.

1.13 Parenteral Feeding

Total parenteral nutrition (TPN) is the aseptic delivery of nutritional substrates directly into the circulatory system. This route may be necessary when

1 The gastrointestinal tract is inaccessible (e.g. oesophageal stricture).

2 Complete rest of gastrointestinal tract is indicated (e.g. gastrointestinal fistula and exacerbation of inflammatory bowel disease).

3 The gastrointestinal tract, although accessible, cannot be used for enteral feeding because of a functional derangement (e.g. post-operative ileus).

4 The total requirements cannot be met because the gastrointestinal tract has limited function (e.g. in premature infants or patients with severe burns).

Although a potentially life-saving therapy, parenteral nutrition is expensive and may expose an already debilitated patient to serious complications, notably catheter related sepsis and metabolic disorders. Furthermore, the gastrointestinal tract has, in addition to the absorption of nutrients, important metabolic and hormonal functions which may be bypassed in the patient on total parenteral nutrition. Wherever possible, patients should be fed enterally rather than parentally.

1.13.1 Management of the nutritional support system

There are four essential elements to the management of any parenteral nutritional support system

1 Establishing and maintaining access.

2 A method of administering the nutrition to the patient.

3 Selecting the quantity and type of substrate.

4 Observation, monitoring and assessment.

Access

Establishing and maintaining suitable access to the circulation is essential for the successful management of a parenteral nutrition regimen. This aspect is not the immediate concern of dietitians and is not discussed in detail here, but they should be familiar with principles and problems involved (Grant and Todd

1982; Tweedle 1982; Silk 1983).

The hyperosmotic nature of solutions usually used necessitates access to a central vein. Typically, a catheter is inserted via the subclavian vein into the superior vena cava (Fig. 1.7) under strict aseptic conditions. To reduce the risk of infection, it may then be tunnelled a few inches under the skin. It is possible, or even preferable, to use a peripheral vein in certain circumstances, for example

1 In neonates.

2 In short term (up to ten days) feeding in adults where 10 g nitrogen, 1500 non-protein kcal will meet requirement.

3 In 'protein sparing' therapy using amino acids alone in the post-operative period (see p 91).

In the first two situations, the regimen will include lipid emulsion; this may have a protective effect on the vein.

The feeding line into a central or peripheral vein should be regarded as the patient's nutritional life line and ideally only parenteral nutrition should be given via this line. Separate venous access is then required for blood, plasma protein fraction, saline, drugs and measurement of central venous pressure.

Administration

Maintenance of flow rate

This is essential in parenteral nutrition in order to control blood glucose and avoid hyperglycaemia and rebound hypoglycaemia, to avoid occlusion of the venous line and to optimize the utilization of infused nutrients. Various methods are used to maintain flow rate

1 Mechanical controllers, e.g. clamps and other types of variable resistance devices.

2 Electro-mechanical devices, e.g. peristaltic pumps; flow controllers and volumetric pumps.

With the exception of the volumetric pumps, control of flow rate relies on counting the rate of drop flow. Because of the complex composition of parenteral nutrition solutions, the drop size differs from that of simple intravenous fluids on which the devices are calibrated (Allwood 1984a).

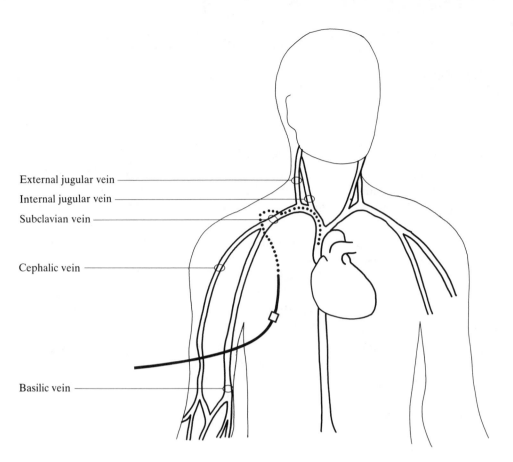

External jugular vein

Internal jugular vein

Subclavian vein

Cephalic vein

Basilic vein

Fig. 1.7 Illustration of a feeding catheter inserted via the subclavian vein into the superior vena cava and tunnelled under the skin (dotted line). Other entry sites may be used as indicated.

Method of administration

Unlike enteral feeds, parenteral nutrition fluids cannot be purchased easily in a complete form because there are problems with stability. Usually, therefore, several fluids have to be given. Three different methods of administration can be used.

Sequential single bottle regimen. The disadvantage of this method is that if different solutions are being given sequentially (e.g. amino acids, then dextrose, then lipid) the nutrients may not be used optimally by the body.

Multiple bottle regimen. This uses 'Y' or 'W' lead connectors to run energy and nitrogen sources simultaneously. Although nutritionally and metabolically superior to single bottle regimens, it increases the nursing workload considerably and problems occur with refluxing of solutions of different densities between bottles.

The following rules may be helpful in planning a multiple bottle regimen

1   Keep it simple with minimal additions.
2   Give nitrogen and energy simultaneously.
3   Consult nursing staff and pharmacists regarding administration.
4   Where possible give glucose continuously over 24 hours.
5   In order to avoid breakdown of the fat emulsion, never add anything to Intralipid other than Vitlipid, Solvito and Heparin.
6   To minimize nutrient losses due to precipitation or degradation. (see p 92) avoid adding phosphate to preparations containing calcium or magnesium, and avoid mixing vitamins with trace elements or amino acids.

Big bag regimen. Pharmacy sterile production units will prepare, under strict aseptic conditions, a complete feeding regimen (including lipid) in a 2–3 litre bag. This has many advantages; it saves nursing time, greatly reduces infection risk, improves metabolic tolerance of substrates (i.e. lipid, glucose and amino acids) and optimizes utilization of substrate over 24 hours. However, it requires facilities to prepare the bags and there are problems with stability and nutrient availability in compounding such a complex mixture (see p 91). Standard regimens are frequently used but care should be taken not to compromise the individual needs of the patient. It is possible to purchase prepared big bags with a shelf life of 90 days which only require the addition of lipid and vitamins. These are useful for long term and home TPN patients.

Nutritional aspects

Nutritional requirements

Requirements during parenteral nutrition for energy, nitrogen, fluid, sodium and potassium are quantitatively the same as those for enteral nutrition (see Section 1.11). There are however, notable differences with respect to the *qualitative* requirements for energy and nitrogen intake and these are discussed later.

Quantitative differences do exist in the requirements for certain mineral, trace element and vitamin requirements because there is, firstly, no loss from the gastrointestinal tract and secondly, a greater risk of overdosage. Table 1.46 gives suggested recommended daily intravenous intakes. They should only be used for guidance in selecting the most appropriate preparations from those available. Actual requirements vary between individuals and there are variable losses during mixing and administration of solutions (Table 1.51). Providing reasonable precautions are taken, the recommendations given in Table 1.46 will be adequate. However, meeting recommended intakes is no substitute for the regular assessment of patients for early signs of nutritional deficiencies or excesses (see p 92).

It is desirable to keep the number of additives in parenteral nutrition regimens to a minimum. The question inevitably arises of when to add micronutrients. Several factors need to be taken into account

1 The patients concerned are generally nutritionally depleted before starting nutritional support, this may have occurred over a period of several weeks or months.

2 The disease process itself may increase turnover and losses of micronutrients or may impair their metabolism (e.g. folate).

3 The availability of certain micronutrients may be impaired by the administration process (see p 93).

Whenever possible, complete nutritional support should be given from the start of parenteral feeding. However, it is not always necessary to give the nutrient daily in order to achieve the desired intake.

Sources of nutrients

The types of products used to provide a parenteral feeding regimen are summarized in Table 1.47. Tables 1.48−1.50 give the composition of commercially available products for parenteral nutrition.

Energy

The sources of energy in a parenteral nutrition regimen are carbohydrate and/or lipid. (It is assumed, perhaps optimistically on occasions, that the amino acid content of a parenteral regimen makes no contribution to its energy yield.) There are important qualitative considerations to be taken into account when deciding which source of energy to use.

Table 1.46 Suggested micronutrient requirements* in parenteral nutrition

Nutrient	Infants 0−1 year (per kg body weight per day)		Children 1−15 years[1] (per kg body weight per day)	Adults[2] (per day)
	pre-term	full term		
Ca (mmol)	1.5	1.0 − 1.5	0.5 − 1.0	7.7 − 14.0
Mg (mmol)	0.3	0.15− 0.3	0.1 − 0.15	2.8 − 28.0[3]
P (mmol)	0.5 − 1.5	0.5 − 1.5	0.12− 0.4	10 − 50
Fe (μmol)	2.0 − 3.0	2.0 − 3.0	1.0 − 2.0	19.5 − 70
Mn (μmol)	0.3 − 1.0	0.3 − 1.0	0.3	2.7 − 14.4[4]
Zn (μmol)	2.0 − 6.0	0.6 − 2.3	0.3 − 0.6 (1.5 for 1−5 years)	37.5 −100[3]
Cu (μmol)	0.4 − 0.85	0.3 − 0.4	0.1 − 0.3	7.5 − 22.5[4]
Cr (μmol)	0.01− 0.02	0.01− 0.02	0.01	0.19− 2.9
Se (μmol)	0.04	0.04	0.4	0.4
Mo (μmol)	0.12	0.12		0.2
F (μmol)	1.3	1.3	0.7 − 1.5	49 −105
I (μmol)	0.04	0.04	0.02−. 0.04	1.0

Table 1.46 contd.

Nutrient	Infants 0–1 year (per kg body weight per day)		Children 1–15 years[1] (per kg body weight per day)	Adults[2] (per day)	
	pre-term	full term			
Thiamin (mg)	0.05– 2.0	0.05– 2.0	0.02– 2.0	3.0	
Riboflavin (mg)	0.1 – 0.4	0.1 – 0.4	0.03– 0.4	3.6	
Nicotinic acid (mg)	1.0 – 4.0	1.0 – 4.0	1.0 – 4.0	40	
Pyridoxine (mg)	0.1 – 0.6	0.1 – 0.6	0.03– 0.6	4.0	
Folic acid (µg)	20 –100	20 – 50	3.0 – 50.0	500[5]	
Vitamin B12 (µg)	0.2 – 5.0	0.2 – 5.0	0.3 – 5.0	5.0[5]	
Vitamin B5 (mg)	1.0 – 2.0	1.0 – 2.0	0.2 – 2.0	15.0	
Biotin (µg)	30 – 60	30 – 60	5 – 60	60 –200	
Vitamin C (mg)	30 – 20	30 – 20	0.5 – 25.0	100 –500	
Vitamin A (µg)	100 –150	100 –150	10 –150	1000	
Vitamin D (µg)	2.5	2.5	2.5	5	
	(max 10 µg/day)	(max 10 µg/day)	(max 10 µg/day)		
Vitamin E (mg)	0.7 – 1.0	0.7 – 1.0	0.4 – 1.0	7	
Vitamin K (µg)	50 –150	50 –150	2.0 –150	20 –140[5]	
Linoleic acid (µg)	0.5 – 1.0	0.5 – 1.0	0.3 – 0.7	10 – 50	

[1]The wide variations in quoted requirements for children (1–15 years) are due to the variations caused by age differences and disease effects on requirements (see Grotte *et al* 1982).

[2]The higher requirements for adults indicate requirements for more catabolic patients.

[3]For increased gastrointestinal losses (adults): Additional zinc: 256 µmol/l, stool and ileostomy losses. 183 µmol/l, small bowel fistula losses. Additional chromium: 0.38 µmol/day. Total magnesium at least 10 mmol/day.

[4]Avoid high Cu and Mn intakes if there is biliary obstruction.

[5]Can be given as 15 mg folic acid, 1000 µg vitamin B12 and 10 mg vitamin K intramuscularly initially and weekly thereafter (Bradley *et al* 1978). This vitamin B12 and vitamin K dose may be adequate given monthly, but patients with prolonged prothrombin time (e.g. if also receiving antibiotics) may require more vitamin K; up to 10 mg/day (Hands *et al* 1985).

*Requirements devised from the following sources: Adamkin (1982); AMA (1979); Bradley *et al* (1978); Freund *et al* (1979); Friel *et al* (1984); Grotte *et al* (1982); Hands *et al* (1985); Innis and Allardyce (1983); Kien and Ganther (1983); Jeejeebhoy *et al* (1973); Kingsnorth (1984); Lockitch *et al* (1983); Mock *et al* (1985); Quercia *et al* (1984); Ruberg and Mirtallo (1981); Russell (1985); Shike *et al* (1981); Shenkin and Wretlind (1978); Tovey *et al* (1977); Strelling *et al* (1979); Wolfram *et al* (1978); Wolman *et al* (1979); Zlotkin and Buchanan (1983).

Table 1.47 Types of products used in parenteral nutrition

Nutrient	Sources
Energy	Glucose solutions in concentrations from 5% to 50%. Glucose/electrolyte solutions. Fructose solutions (rarely used now). Some amino acid solutions also contain glucose, fructose, sorbitol and/or ethanol. Lipid emulsions of 10% or 20%
Nitrogen	Crystalline amino acid solutions ranging in nitrogen concentrations from 5 g/l to 24 g/l. Specialist amino acid solutions, e.g. branched chain amino acids, essential amino acids, paediatric formulations, isotonic solutions
Electrolytes and trace elements	Glucose/electrolyte/trace element solutions, e.g. Glucoplex, Nutracel Amino acid solutions may contain electrolytes and some trace elements. Sodium chloride and acetate solutions. Potassium, phosphate, calcium and magnesium additives. The phospholipid emulsifier in lipid emulsions provides phosphate but usually in insufficient quantities for requirements. Composite trace element additives, e.g. Addamel, Ped–el, TEC for local preparations Single trace element additives
Vitamins	Composite additives, e.g. Solivito, Vitlipid adult/infant, Multibionta, Parentrovite, Multiple Vitamin Solution. Individual vitamin preparations. Intralipid provides some vitamin E and essential fatty acids
Albumin/plasma protein fraction	These may be given to compensate severe hypoproteinaemia and can comprise albumin, plasma protein fraction, or blood. They should not be regarded as sources of nitrogen or trace elements when calculating intakes.

GENERAL DIETETIC PRINCIPLES AND PRACTICE

Table 1.48 Composition of commercially available amino acid solutions (prepared April 1987)

	Aminofusin forte	Aminoplasmal L3	Aminoplasmal L5	Aminoplasmal L10	Aminoplasmal PED	Aminoplex 5	Aminoplex 12	Aminoplex 14	Aminoplex 24	Freamine III
Manufacturer	M	BB	BB	BB	BB	G	G	G	G	B
Packaging 100 ml					Yes					
250 ml					Yes					
500 ml	Yes	Yes	Yes	Yes			Yes	Yes	Yes	Yes
1000 ml						Yes				
Nitrogen (total) (g/l)	15.2	3.5	5.8	11.6	5.7	5.0	12.4	13.4	24.9	13.0
Energy (Non-N) (kcal/l)	—	400	400	400	—	850	—	—	—	—
Glucose (g/l)	—	—	—	—	—	—	—	—	—	—
Fructose (g/l)	—	—	—	—	—	—	—	—	—	—
Sorbitol (g/l)	—	100	100	100	—	125	—	—	—	—
Ethanol (g/l)	—	—	—	—	—	50	—	—	—	—
Sodium (mmol/l)	40	48	48	48	50	35	35	35	35	10
Potassium (mmol/l)	30	25	25	25	25	28	30	30	30	—
Magnesium (mmol/l)	5	2.5	2.5	2.5	2.5	4	2.5	—	2.5	—
Acetate (mmol/l)	10	59	59	59	27	28	5.0	—	5	72
Chloride (mmol/l)	28	18	31	62	15	43	67	79	67	3
Phosphate (mmol/l)	—	9	9	9	—	—	—	—	—	20
Calcium (mmol/l)	—	—	—	—	—	—	—	—	—	—
Valine (mg/g N)	197	418	415	415	281	360	360	388	360	431
Leucine (mg/g N)	289	734	770	770	439	466	466	328	466	592
Isoleucine (mg/g N)	204	447	441	441	246	306	305	239	305	454
Methionine (mg/g N)	276	331	329	329	140	386	386	478	386	346
Tryptophan (mg/g N)	59	58	156	156	105	112	113	119	112	100
Threonine (mg/g N)	132	360	355	355	526	258	257	239	257	262
Phenylalanine (mg/g N)	289	447	441	441	333	554	547	328	553	369
Lysine (mg/g N)	329	605	606	606	789	548	547	634	692	669
Histidine (mg/g N)	132	447	450	450	526	178	177	209	177	185
Alanine (mg/g N)	789	1182	1185	1185	1018	806	804	110	803	462
Arginine (mg/g N)	526	793	796	796	386	740	740	687	739	623
Aspartate/Ornithine (mg/g N)	—	389	389	389	533	160	161	149	—	—
Cyst(e)ine (mg/g N)	—	63	62	63	256	—	—	—	—	<15
Glutamic acid (mg/g N)	1184	403	398	398	1719	160	161	—	161	—
Glycine (mg/g N)	1316	677	683	683	860	354	354	896	353	915
Proline (mg/g N)	921	764	770	770	474	966	965	299	964	731
Serine (mg/g N)	—	202	208	208	175	194	193	—	193	385
Tyrosine (mg/g N)	—	121	126	132	204	—	—	—	—	—

Carbohydrate

1 Glucose is the preferred carbohydrate source; it is well utilized by all tissues, has an established nitrogen sparing effect and serum levels can easily be measured. Disadvantages of glucose include hyperglycaemia, particularly in the glucose intolerant stressed patient; glucose solutions over 5% concentration are hyperosmotic and thrombophlebitic particularly when given via peripheral veins; excessive glucose infusion may lead to increased CO_2 production delaying the weaning of patients off ventilators; and excessive glucose infusion may lead to fatty infiltration of the liver and hepatic dysfunction.

2 Fructose, sorbitol, xylitol and ethanol all have established nitrogen sparing abilities, are less thrombophlebitic than glucose and do not readily result in hyperglycaemia. However, fructose and sorbitol may cause lactic acidosis, serum levels cannot be monitored easily and they require metabolism by the liver to glucose before being utilized by other tissues for energy. More detailed discussion on the utilization of these energy substrates is given by Silk (1983) and Tweedle (1982). Glucose remains the carbohydrate-energy source of choice.

Lipid emulsions. The only lipid emulsion currently available in the UK is Intralipid (Kabi Vitrum UK Ltd) which is available as either a 10% or 20% emulsion. These are soya bean oil emulsions with egg

Table 1.48 contd.

	Perifusin	Synthamin 9	Synthamin 14	Synthamin 14 w/e	Synthamin 17	Vamin 9 glucose	Vamin 9	Vamin 14	Vamin 14 w/e	Vamin 18 w/e	4% Branched chain amino acid solution
Manufacturer	M	T	T	T	T	K	K	K	K	K	T
Packaging 100 ml						Yes					
250 ml											
500 ml		Yes	Yes	Yes	Yes	Yes	Yes	Yes	Yes	Yes	Yes
1000 ml	Yes	Yes	Yes	Yes	Yes	Yes	Yes	Yes	Yes	Yes	
Nitrogen (total) (g/l)	5.0	9.1	14.0	14.0	16.5	9.4	9.4	13.5	13.5	18.0	4.4
Energy (Non-N) (kcal/l)	—	—	—	—	—	400	—	—	—	—	—
Glucose (g/l)	—	—	—	—	—	100	—	—	—	—	—
Fructose (g/l)	—	—	—	—	—	—	—	—	—	—	—
Sorbitol (g/l)	—	—	—	—	—	—	—	—	—	—	—
Ethanol (g/l)	—	—	—	—	—	—	—	—	—	—	—
Sodium (mmol/l)	40	73	73	—	73	50	50	100	—	—	—
Potassium (mmol/l)	30	60	60	—	60	20	20	50	—	—	—
Magnesium (mmol/l)	5	5	5	—	5	1.5	1.5	8	—	—	—
Acetate (mmol/l)	10	100	130	68	150	—	—	135	—	—	—
Chloride (mmol/l)	9	70	70	34	70	55	55	100	—	—	—
Phosphate (mmol/l)	—	30	30	—	30	—	—	—	—	—	—
Calcium (mmol/l)	—	—	—	—	—	2.5	2.5	5.0	—	—	—
Valine (mg/g N)	198	351	352	352	352	457	457	407	407	406	2818
Leucine (mg/g N)	290	441	443	443	442	564	564	437	437	439	3136
Isoleucine (mg/g N)	212	363	364	364	364	415	415	311	311	311	3136
Methionine (mg/g N)	278	242	243	243	242	202	202	311	311	311	—
Tryptophan (mg/g N)	66	109	109	109	109	106	106	104	104	106	—
Threonine (mg/g N)	132	254	255	255	255	319	319	311	311	311	—
Phenylalanine (mg/g N)	290	338	340	340	339	585	585	437	437	439	—
Lysine (mg/g N)	330	351	352	352	352	415	415	504	504	500	—
Histidine (mg/g N)	132	290	291	291	291	255	255	378	378	378	—
Alanine (mg/g N)	792	1251	1257	1257	1255	319	319	889	889	889	—
Arginine (mg/g N)	528	695	699	699	697	351	351	622	622	628	—
Aspartate/Ornithine (mg/g N)	—	—	—	—	—	436	436	185	185	189	—
Cyst(e)ine (mg/g N)	—	—	—	—	—	149	149	31	31	31	—
Glutamic acid (mg/g N)	—	—	—	—	—	957	957	378	378	311	—
Glycine (mg/g N)	1320	622	626	626	624	223	223	437	437	439	—
Proline (mg/g N)	924	411	413	413	412	862	862	378	378	378	—
Serine (mg/g N)	—	302	304	304	303	798	798	252	252	250	—
Tyrosine (mg/g N)	—	24	24	24	24	53	53	13	13	13	—

Key: w/e: Without electrolytes

Manufacturers: B = Boots PLC; BB = B. Braun Ltd; G = Geistlich Ltd; K = Kabi Vitrum UK Ltd; M = E Merck; T = Travenol Laboratories Ltd.

lecithin emulsifiers and they have a proven record as safe intravenous energy sources. Early experiences with certain cottonseed oil emulsions in the USA revealed toxic effects for some patients and as a result the use of lipid was discontinued there for several years.

However, lipid emulsions do have some advantages over glucose solutions

1 They provide essential fatty acids (efa). In sick neonates, biochemical evidence of efa deficiency can be seen in the first week of life on lipid-free regimens (Friedman et al 1976) although clinical signs may take three weeks to three months to develop. Stressed adults may also develop efa deficiency within 30 days.

Stable patients on long term parenteral nutrition may also develop the symptoms after several months. Estimated requirements vary and it is possible that a high carbohydrate load and high insulin level may suppress the outflow of linoleic acid from adipose tissue to plasma (Wolfram et al 1978). A requirement of 10 g linoleic acid daily, increasing to 50 g daily or more for the critically ill, has been suggested by Wolfram et al (1978). Others have suggested 2−7 g daily (Collins et al 1971) and 25 g daily (Jeejeebhoy et al 1973). The lipid fraction of Intralipid contains 46−48% linoleic acid and 8% linolenic acid so that 500 ml of 10% Intralipid or 250 ml 20% Intralipid daily should cover most adult requirements.

Table 1.49 Some commercial composite vitamin sources used in parenteral nutrition (prepared April 1987)

	Multibionta	Parentrovite 1	Parentrovite 2	Solivito	Vitlipid adult	Vitlipid infant*
Manufacturer	M	Ben	Ben	K	K	K
Packaging (ml)	10	5	5	1 Vial	10	10
Thiamin (mg/unit)	50	250	—	1.2	—	—
Riboflavin (mg/unit)	10	4.0	—	1.8	—	—
Nicotinic acid (mg/unit)	100	—	160	10	—	—
Pyridoxine (mg/unit)	15.0	50	—	2	—	—
Folic acid (μg/unit)	—	—	—	0.2	—	—
Vitamin B12 (μg/unit)	—	—	—	2.0	—	—
Vitamin B5 (mg/unit)	25	—	—	10	—	—
Biotin (μg/unit)	—	—	—	0.3	—	—
Vitamin C (mg/unit)	500	—	500	30	—	—
Vitamin A (μg/unit)	3000	—	—	—	753	102.5
Vitamin D (μg/unit)	—	—	—	—	3	2.5
Vitamin E (mg/unit)	5	—	—	—	—	—
Vitamin K (μg/unit)	—	—	—	—	15	50
Linoleic acid (g/unit)	—	—	—	—	—	—

Key. Manufacturers: Ben = Bencard; K = Kabi Vitrum UK Ltd; M = E. Merck Ltd.
*Composition of Vitlipid infant given is per ml.

When fat is not given intravenously or orally, Press *et al* (1974) found, perhaps surprisingly, that as little as 230 ml sunflower oil rubbed into the flexor muscle of the forearm could provide sufficient linoleic acid to prevent deficiency symptoms. If lipid is included in the parenteral feeding regimen it is important to include adequate vitamin E (see Table 1.46) Soya bean oil emulsions provide 4–10 mg vitamin E per litre depending upon the soya bean crop.

2 Lipid emulsions, being approximately isotonic, may be given via a peripheral vein. This advantage has been used for many years with multiple bottle systems. More recently lipid has been added to big bags to produce regimens suitable for administration via a peripheral vein. However, it should be noted that no more than 1600 non-nitrogen kcal and 10 g nitrogen should be provided per 3 litres and the osmolarity should be kept below 600 mosmol/kg (Gazitua *et al* 1979). Such a regimen is not a substitute for central vein feeding in those patients with moderate to high nutritional requirements unless it is being used to complement limited enteral nutrition.

3 The partial substitution of glucose with lipid decreases the respiratory quotient (RQ) to below 1.0 and reduces CO_2 production. This may be a significant advantage for the patient with respiratory failure (Askanazi *et al* 1981).

4 Lipid may be beneficial in the prevention of fatty liver and hepatic dysfunction in long term feeding.

Lipid emulsions may also have some disadvantages compared with glucose solutions

1 Lipid emulsions have been reported to have a poorer nitrogen sparing ability when compared with glucose. However, this finding was derived from studies which were carried out over short periods, 3 days in the study of Long *et al* (1977). Measured

Table 1.50 Some commercial composite electrolyte and trace element sources used in parenteral nutrition (prepared April 1987)

	Addamel (adults)	Addiphos	Glucoplex 1000	Glucoplex 1600	TEC	Nutracel 400	Nutracel 800	Ped-El (instants)
Manufacturer	K	K	G	G	T	T	T	K
Packaging (ml)	10	10	500/1000	500/1000	3	500	1000	20
Energy (glucose) (kcal/unit)	—	—	1000	1600	—	400	800	—
Sodium (mmol)	<1	30	50	50	—	—	—	—
Potassium (mmol)	<1	30	30	30	—	—	—	—
Magnesium (mmol)	1.5	—	2.5	2.5	—	9.0	9.0	0.025
Acetate (mmol)	—	—	—	—	—	80	80	—
Chloride (mmol)	13.3	—	67	67	—	33	33	0.35
Calcium (mmol)	5	—	—	—	—	7.5	7.5	0.15
Phosphate (mmol)	—	40	18	18	—	—	—	0.075
Iron (μmol)	50	—	—	—	—	—	—	0.5
Manganese (μmol)	40	—	—	—	5.4	40	40	0.25
Zinc (μmol)	20	—	45.6	45.6	45	40	40	0.15
Copper (μmol)	5	—	—	—	18	—	—	0.075
Chromium (μmol)	—	—	—	—	0.23	—	—	—
Selenium (μmol)	—	—	—	—	—	—	—	—
Molybdenum (μmol)	—	—	—	—	—	—	—	—
Fluorine (μmol)	50	—	—	—	—	—	—	0.75
Iodine (μmol)	1	—	—	—	—	—	—	0.01

Key. Manufacturers: G = Geistlich Sons Ltd; K = Kabi Vitrum UK Ltd; T = Travenol Laboratories.
Composition of Ped-El given is per 1 ml and composition of Glucoplex solutions is per 1000 ml.

nitrogen retention/excretion will be influenced by a flux in the amino acid pool on changing from glucose to lipid energy; this does not in itself indicate a better nitrogen sparing ability. Rogaly *et al* (1982) showed that a glucose calorie and a lipid calorie were equally nitrogen sparing provided that the obligatory glucose requirement of approx 150 g per day in adults was met first. Stoner *et al* (1983) studying oxidative metabolism of glucose and fat in 27 patients with sepsis, found a reduction in glucose oxidation but a continued oxidation of fat as the principal metabolic fuel. There is now a large body of evidence which supports the view that there is an increased rate of lipid clearance from serum after trauma. It is pertinent to note however that the removal of lipid from plasma cannot be used as a measure of fat utilization (Nordenstrom 1982).

2 The presence of some nutrients in certain concentrations may cause a breakdown in the fat emulsion. The inclusion of lipid emulsions in big bags may therefore limit the flexibility of the regimen.

3 Some lipid emulsions have been found to block the reticulo-endothelial system and to interfere with the coagulation system. These complications are not found with the soya bean oil emulsion, Intralipid (Shenkin and Wretlind 1978).

4 Lipid emulsions may increase the risk of bilirubin encephalopathy (kernicterus) in icteric neonates. Free fatty acids released into the plasma following lipid infusion may compete with bilirubin for binding sites on plasma albumin thus reducing bilirubin binding capacity. From *in vitro* and *in vivo* studies, Whittington and Burckart (1982) considered there to be insufficient evidence to withhold intravenous lipid from jaundiced neonates where proper monitoring techniques are available and when energy supplementation is crucial.

5 Pulmonary impairment has been reported as a temporary phenomenon following Intralipid infusion. The significance of this when compared with the advantage in reducing the CO_2 load through reducing glucose intake must be considered. Any pulmonary impairment is of greater concern in neonates, particularly in the light of reports of lipid deposition in the lung capillaries of low birth weight infants (Hertel 1982) and pre-term infants (Levene 1980). For infants there may be an advantage in using 10% Intralipid over 20% Intralipid because of a smaller particle size in the former.

6 Blood samples should not be taken within two hours of lipid infusions as lipaemic blood samples may give inaccurate biochemical results. Thought is therefore required when timing bottle changes in multiple bottle regimens. However, lipaemia does not appear to be a problem when lipid is added to 24-hour big bag regimens.

7 As a source of energy, lipid emulsions are considerably more expensive than glucose infusions.

The use of MCT emulsions as an energy substrate is still under clinical evaluation.

Choosing glucose or lipid: a summary. For most patients there is no inherent metabolic problem in giving either lipid or glucose as an energy substrate, only in knowing how much of either to give. Unless lipid is contraindicated, a rule of thumb is to limit glucose to between 30 and 70% of non-amino acid energy, and provide the remainder as lipid emulsion.

Nitrogen

The choice of amino acid solution depends upon several issues, not all of which are nutritional

1 The concentration of nitrogen per litre of the amino acid solution.

2 The energy, electrolyte and mineral content of the amino acid solution.

3 An amino acid profile for optimum utilization.

4 Factors relevant to the safe and simple compounding of big bags by pharmacy especially if lipid is to be included. These include the nitrogen concentration, amino acid profile, pH, content of calcium and magnesium and total electrolyte concentration.

5 Cost.

All nitrogen sources currently sold in the UK for parenteral nutrition are crystalline amino acid solutions. The wide range of amino acid solutions available bears testimony to the unresolved debate on the optimum amino acid profile for parenteral nutrition. It is generally advised that the E:T ratio (essential amino acid (g) to total nitrogen (g)) should be about 1:3 and the majority of solutions currently available meet this criterion. However in the sick patient and in the infant the concept of essential and non-essential amino acids must be questioned. Certain amino acids may not be essential in the strict sense but they may significantly improve the utilization of other amino acids.

Glycine has been much criticized as a cheap 'filler' amino acid. However, Kingsnorth *et al* (1980) found the half-life of glycine to be considerably shorter than that of alanine which is recognized as a most efficacious source of nitrogen (glutamate had an even shorter half-life). Nevertheless, large amounts of glycine or glutamic acid should not be given. The inclusion of arginine will prevent hyperammonaemia occurring when glycine is given.

Cyst(e)ine is reported to be essential for infants (Sturman *et al* 1970) and for patients with cirrhosis (Rudman *et al* 1981; Chawla *et al* 1984). There can be technical problems in measuring cyst(e)ine levels (Malloy *et al* 1983) and there are difficulties in maintaining a stable form of cyst(e)ine in amino acid solutions particularly in higher nitrogen concentrations. The cyst(e)ine argument remains unresolved, but any solution should contain either cyst(e)ine or an enhanced level of methionine as a precursor of cyst(e)ine. Additional methionine may increase folate requirements (Connor *et al* 1978).

Tyrosine. The ability of infants and the very ill to synthesize tyrosine is questionable, but if it is not included in the mixture then additional phenylalanine should be given.

Histidine is essential in infants as well as the very ill and patients with renal failure.

Carnitine is an important trimethylamine normally synthesized in the liver from lysine, methionine and glycine in the presence of ascorbic acid and pyridoxine. It has an important role in the oxidation of fatty acids by facilitating their transport across the mitochondrial membrane. No parenteral nutrition solution yet contains carnitine but its synthesis may be impaired in sick patients (Tao and Yoshimura 1980) and in premature infants (Schmidt-Sommerfield *et al* 1983) thus prejudicing fat utilization.

Safety however must come before optimum profile and all amino acids are individually toxic if administered in large enough dosages. There are two schools of thought

1 To supply all amino acids since the conversion of 'essential' amino acids to 'non-essential' amino acids is in doubt in these patients.

2 To supply adequate amounts of important precursors (e.g. alanine) and avoid giving amino acids which may accumulate to toxic levels (e.g. glutamic acid and aspartic acid) or which may be unstable in solution (e.g. cyst(e)ine and tyrosine).

The amino acid profile is also of significance when the amino acid solution is to be mixed with lipid emulsions. Aspartic and glutamic acids may accelerate the coalescence of lipid particles, whereas arginine, lysine and histidine may help to maintain emulsion stability (Hardy *et al* 1982).

Amino acid solutions for special situations

1 Essential amino acids. These have been advocated for patients in acute renal failure (Wilmore and Dudrick 1969). However, such patients have the same nutritional needs as others with similar medical or surgical problems. They do not require special amino acid formulations but they do require dialysis to allow full nutritional requirements to be met. Amino acid solutions without electrolytes may be useful in such situations (see Section 4.16.2).

2 Branched chain amino acids (BCAA) i.e. Valine, Leucine and Isoleucine. Patients with hepatic precoma or severe hepatic damage may benefit from a higher proportion of BCAA. These amino acids, which are not metabolized by the liver directly but by the peripheral tissues, may also be of benefit to patients with severe burns or sepsis and possibly also severely traumatized patients. Currently, a 4% w/v BCAA solution is available for use in conjunction with other amino acid solutions. Unfortunately, it is too dilute to be useful for the latter groups of patient.

3 Isotonic amino acid solutions. These, when administered peripherally without additional energy, have been advocated as a means of achieving a positive nitrogen balance in the post-operative patient (Blackburn *et al* 1973). However, when healthy subjects are given intravenous amino acids alone, the level of ketones in the blood is less than that found in prolonged starvation, showing that gluconeogenesis of amino acids takes place in order to provide energy for cerebral tissues.

A second important observation which weakens Blackburn's hypothesis is that the administration of amino acids alone stimulates rather than suppresses the secretion of insulin and thus will inhibit lipogenesis. The clinical benefit of this method of nutritional support remains to be proven (Collins *et al* 1978).

Stability of solutions and availability of nutrients

Having overcome the hurdles of aseptic administration and selection of appropriate nutritional substrate in the correct quantities, it may be found that the compatibility of preparations will restrict what can be given to the patient. Much research has been done and remains to be done in this field and the subject has been reviewed recently by Allwood (1984b). With present knowledge it should be possible to meet the needs of all patients. Problems occur when big bags are prepared, especially if lipid emulsion is to be included. Care is also required when using additives in multiple bottle regimens. Pharmacy departments will have access to the necessary data but it is important that dietitians understand the problems involved as they affect nutrient availability. Table 1.52 shows many of the common problems, the possible causes and the courses of preventative action. Big bag formulations are very complex chemical mixtures and many as yet unknown reactions and losses may occur. The main reasons for loss of nutrient availability or stability are

1 Precipitation, particularly of calcium phosphate. Folic acid may also precipitate.
2 Photodegradation can affect many nutrients to varying degrees (see Table 1.51). Artificial light is not of concern but daylight even from a nearby window can cause significant losses of vitamin A and riboflavin. The solution must also be protected from the intense ultra-violet light used in neonatal phototherapy.
3 Oxidation, principally of vitamin C (see Table 1.51).
4 Degradation.
5 Adsorption on to plastic bags and administration sets.
6 Breakdown of fat emulsion. This may result in irreversible lipid/water phase separation and can be caused by a high concentration of total electrolytes, in particular of divalent and trivalent cations. There are many other factors which may affect emulsion stability (Table 1.51).

Complications and monitoring

Monitoring is necessary to detect and minimize complications of the feeding regimen. Some metabolic complications and suggested parameters for monitoring are given in Table 1.52. The frequency with which they should be monitored initially is suggested, but in practice this depends upon the clinical condition of the patient, the nature of the feeding regimen and the results of previous measurements. A monitoring protocol should be prepared for each hospital in consultation with all concerned (including the laboratory staff) and adapted for each patient. The most common non-metabolic complication in parenteral nutrition is catheter related sepsis which can be minimized by good nursing practices and by using big bag regimens in preference to multiple bottle regimens.

Long term or home TPN patients are generally more stable, and may be fed at home using cyclical (interrupted) feeding, but various metabolic complications can occur.

Hepatic dysfunction

This may be seen after four weeks or longer on parenteral nutrition (see Table 1.52). There tends to be a characteristic pattern of an initial increase in the serum aspartate and alanine amino transferases followed by a mild progressive rise in alkaline phosphatase and eventually a rise in serum bilirubin. Clinically the patient is seen to become jaundiced due to cholestasis. The phenomenon is generally reversible on cessation of feeding and is also seen occasionally in enteral feeding (Tweedle et al 1978). The cause is unclear but several possibilities have been suggested

1 Excessive glucose intake leading to fatty liver.
2 Deficiency of essential fatty acids.
3 Insufficient nitrogen intake, possibly in relation to energy intake.
4 Continuous 24-hour feeding.
5 Suppression of trophic and/or secretion stimulant gut hormones.
6 Lithocholate toxicity.
7 Toxic breakdown products of tryptophan.
8 Choline deficiency.
9 Methionine deficiency.

In several reports lipid has been withdrawn from the feeding regimen and an improvement in cholestasis has occurred (although it has not always been made clear whether the lipid was substituted with equicaloric quantities of glucose or whether the total energy intake was reduced). The type of energy substrate given is undoubtedly important in avoiding this complication (Buzby et al 1981). In a few infants developing cholestatic jaundice on long term TPN the problem has developed into a progressive disease leading to cirrhosis.

If hepatic changes are sufficient to give rise to clinical concern the following procedure is suggested

1 consider whether there is a non-nutritional cause (e.g. sepsis).
2 If glucose alone is being used for energy, then substitute 30—50% of calories with lipid.
3 If practical (i.e. in a stable long term patient) cyclical feeding (e.g. 12 hours in 24 hours) can be tried.
4 Reduce the total energy intake by reducing lipid or glucose, maintain nitrogen intake and monitor.
5 If jaundice worsens, consider stopping feeding for 3—4 days and observe.

Table 1.51 Losses of nutrient availability in parenteral nutrition solutions

Nutrient	Nature of loss(es)	Possible causes of loss(es)	Preventative action(s)
Dextrose	None	None	None
Lipid	Flocculation (reversible) ↓ Coalescence (irreversible) ↓ Lipid/water phase separation	High total electrolyte concentration particularly divalent and trivalent cations. Calcium affecting phospholipid emulsifier. Low pH from dextrose and amino acid content Over-dilution of emulsifier	Careful control over electrolyte content in bags. Correct procedure in preparing bags. Inclusion of certain amino acids in big bag regimens may aid stability (see p 000) Limit storage time of bags containing lipid. Add only Vitlipid and Solivito to Intralipid bottles
	Photodegradation of essential fatty acids	Exposure to intense phototherapy in neonatal units	
Amino acids	Photodegradation of glycine, leucine, tryptophan, methionine and tyrosine	Long term exposure to daylight Exposure to intense phototherapy in neonatal units	Cover in storage
Trace elements	Precipitation of iron Other trace elements appear stable	Precipitation of iron phosphate when iron compounds are added to certain amino acid solutions (e.g. Synthamin)	Include 500 mg vitamin C in big bags Add trace element/iron additive to dextrose rather than to amino acid solution in multiple bottle regimen.
Electrolytes	Precipitation of calcium phosphate	Excessive calcium and phosphate concentrations Increasing pH. Sudden change of temperature (removing from refrigerator). Mixing of lipid emulsion in line with calcium/phosphate mixtures as may occur in infant feeding	Calcium (mmol/l) × Phosphate (mmol/l) not to exceed 185 Do not mix calcium with phosphate in multiple bottle regimens
Vitamin A	Photodegradation	Short term exposure to daylight	Give sufficient Vitamin A for unavoidable loss. Cover during storage and infusion. Give in lipid containing bottle/bag. Do not hang near a window.
	Loss from solution	Acetate vitamin A ester absorbed on to plastic bag	Use palmitate vitamin A ester
Thiamin	Degraded	Metabisulphite in undiluted amino acid solutions Low pH	Give sufficient thiamin for unavoidable losses. Use big bag or add to another component of regimen or add to amino acid solution not containing metabisulphite.
Riboflavin	Photodegradation (up to 57%)	Exposure to daylight, Phototherapy	Add sufficient to cover unavoidable losses.
Pyridoxine	Photodegradation (small)	Exposure to direct sunlight	Protect from daylight
Vitamin K	Photodegradation	Exposure to daylight	Protect from daylight or give intramuscularly
Folic acid	Loss from solution	Absorption to plastic bags	Add sufficient folic acid for unavoidable losses.
	Precipitation	High calcium concentrations Increased risk if added to certain amino acid solutions pH less than 5.0	Watch calcium content in bag. Give intramuscular folate weekly Avoid storing bags containing folate
Vitamin C	Oxidation	Dissolved oxygen introduced when filling big bags or absorbed through plastic bag. Copper if added acts as a catalyst in vitamin C oxidation	Add sufficient vitamin C for unavoidable losses. Give vitamin C and copper in separate bags, e.g. alternate days or use a cystine/cysteine containing amino acid solution (inhibits catalytic action of copper) or add excess vitamin C (see also trace elements — preventing iron precipitation)
		Low pH	

Table 1.52 Some metabolic complications of parenteral nutrition

Complication	Possible causes(s)	Treatment(s)	Suggested monitoring	Suggested initial monitoring frequency
Hyperglycaemia	Excessive glucose Glucose intolerance in stress	Decrease glucose Increase lipid: carbohydrate ratio Give insulin	Urinalysis for glycosuria Serum glucose	Six hourly
Hypoglycaemia	Rebound hypoglycaemia on ending glucose infusion	Revise regimen	Serum glucose	As required
Osmotic diuresis	Uncorrected hyperglycaemia	Control serum glucose as above Rehydrate with 5% dextrose and hypotonic saline rather than TPN	Serum glucose, sodium and potassium. Fluid balance Serum and urine osmolarity in critically ill	Daily Daily Twice weekly
Hypokalaemia	Large glucose infusion Insulin/glucose infusion Excessive gastrointestinal or urinary potassium loss	Increase potassium based on patients requirements	Serum potassium	Daily
Hypophosphataemia	Inadequate inorganic phosphate especially with high glucose infusions and in very stressed patients	Add phosphate	Serum phosphate and corrected calcium	Twice weekly
Elevated serum urea	Dehydration Excessive nitrogen intake Renal impairment	Rehydrate with 5% dextrose or hypotonic saline rather than TPN Revise TPN regimen for individual patient Appropriate treatment for renal failure	Serum urea, creatinine and potassium	Daily
Metabolic acidosis	Excessive gastrointestinal (or renal) loss of base Excessive chloride intake Excessive carbohydrate intake Infusion of excessive amounts of fructose, sorbitol or ethanol Excessive amino acid intake	Careful monitoring of serum biochemistry and losses Increase acetate in regimen Use glucose and fat for energy Avoid amino acid solutions with large quantities of any single amino acid	Serum bicarbonate chloride and potassium	Daily
Hypomagnesaemia	Insufficient intake of magnesium Excessive gastrointestinal or renal losses	Increase magnesium in regimen	Serum magnesium	Weekly
Hepatic dysfunction	Excessive glucose and/or deficiency of essential fatty acids, leading to fatty infiltration of liver. Overfeeding of energy and amino acids. In prolonged TPN (over two weeks) aberrations of liver function can occur occasionally leading to cholestasis. The aetiology is probably multifactorial and it is usually mild and reversible.	Reduce glucose intake Temporarily reduce glucose and lipid and observe. If condition permits try cyclic TPN, e.g. 12-hour feeding in 24 hours. If severe cholestasis stop feeding 2—4 days if condition permits.	Serum SGOT, SGPT, alkaline phosphatase and bilirubin	Weekly
Acute folate deficiency	In trauma patient there is an increased requirement for folate and an impaired metabolism of folate Infusion of ethanol Infusion of amino acid especially methionine Loss of folate in bag (Table 1.52)	Give additional folate 0.5—1 mg daily or 15 mg weekly Before commencing TPN give loading doses of 15 mg folate and 1000 μg Vitamin B12 intramuscularly	Serum folate and vitamin B12	Weekly

Cholelithiasis

Cholelithiasis may be found in both adults and children receiving long term TPN. Prolonged TPN (over one year), ileal resection and no oral intake are all major contributions to the formation of gallstones.

Polymyopathy

Polymyopathy with muscular pain and high serum creatinine phosphate has been reported in long term 'fat free' TPN and is probably due to deficiency of essential fatty acids.

Metabolic bone disease

A metabolic bone disease characterized by skeletal pain and hypercalcuria has been reported in long term parenteral nutrition (Klein *et al* 1980; Shike *et al* 1980). This syndrome is seen after at least three months of parenteral nutrition. A number of causes have been suggested in conflicting reports namely

1 Excess vitamin D intake (Shike *et al* 1980).
2 Excess aluminium in solutions, especially casein hydrolysates (Klein *et al* 1980).
3 High nitrogen intake particularly as part of a cyclic PN regimen (Vernejoul *et al* 1985).

A transient hypercalcuria occuring after one week PN and persisting for 1–4 weeks was reported by Gordon *et al* (1984). This was not found to be related to calcium intake and was not considered to represent a major mineral metabolic problem.

Hypercholesterolaemia and hypertriglyceridaemia

Elevated serum levels of cholesterol and triglycerides have been reported in patients receiving TPN, but should be minimized by careful control of energy intake, lipid, carbohydrate balance and weight.

Deficiency of trace elements

Deficiencies of trace elements including zinc, copper, chromium and selenium have been reported.

Deficiencies of vitamins

Deficiencies of vitamin A, vitamin E and biotin have been reported.

1.13.2 Parenteral nutrition for infants

When properly managed, parenteral nutrition is a safe and effective method of nutritional support for infants, comparable in efficacy to enteral nutrition (Yu *et al* 1979). It may be crucial to the infant's survival.

Typical indications for parenteral nutrition for infants include

1 Major gastrointestinal surgery.
2 Supplemental or total parenteral nutrition in premature and low birth weight infants, and infants of less than 30 weeks gestation.
3 Necrotising enterocolitis.
4 Protracted diarrhoea.
5 Crohn's disease.
6 Extensive burns.

Administration is usually via a peripheral vein.

Parenteral nutrition for infants has been well reviewed (Grotte *et al* 1982; Booth and Harries 1982; Cockburn 1985). The quantitative requirements for energy and nitrogen are the same as those for enteral nutrition. The limited fluid handling capacity of the low birth weight infant can present difficulties in achieving these requirements; a 1 kg infant for example has a plasma volume of about 45 ml.

Energy requirements vary from 90–110 kcal/kg for a basal requirement to 150 kcal/kg in catabolic states. Energy should be provided as glucose alone or as glucose with lipid. It is desirable, even when a central vein is used, to keep osmolarity low. Lipid emulsions (being approximately isotonic) appear to have a clear advantage, but, as discussed previously, lipid may present problems for the infant with respiratory distress or jaundice. Grotte *et al* (1982) suggest that for premature and small-for-date infants, Intralipid should be started at 1.5–3 g lipid/kg and plasma turbidity checked daily. Once the infant is able to clear lipid from the circulation, a dosage of up to 4 g lipid/kg may be given. It is advisable to give less than this to jaundiced neonates.

Nitrogen requirements vary from 0.3 g/kg basal requirements to 0.63 g/kg in catabolic states. Care must be exercised to avoid excessive nitrogen intakes particularly as an excessive intake of glutamic acid may cause brain damage. Nitrogen retention in low birth weight infants depends not only on adequate energy provision but also on the amino acid composition of the formulation (Chessex *et al* 1985). The optimum amino acid requirement for infants is unknown but in addition to the eight 'essential' amino acids, histidine, cysteine and tyrosine are also regarded as essential. To achieve optimum utilization of the amino acids given, alanine, glutamic acid and proline are required. Glycine is required to maintain normal levels of serum glycine and serine and sufficient arginine is required to prevent hyperammonaemia arising from glycine infusion. Carnitine is also considered necessary for the infant (Schmidt-Sommerfield *et al* 1983) but as yet it is not included in any commercially available amino acid solution.

Simultaneous administration of nitrogen, glucose and lipid is metabolically desirable (Whitfield *et al* 1983).

It is important to ensure that the nutritional support given is adequate in all respects, including vitamins and trace elements, so that in addition to daily maintenance requirements, sufficient substrates are available to sustain brain growth (especially in first year of life) and to establish adequate body stores in the premature infant.

Several problems may influence the nutritional regimen

1 Limited glucose tolerance.

2 Limited fluid volume tolerance.

3 Limitations on lipid metabolism.

4 Care is required over calcium and phosphate intakes.

5 Certain requirements (e.g. carnitine) may not be met using products available at present.

6 Increased losses with phototherapy and radiant heaters.

7 The optimum amino acid requirement must be met.

8 Immaturity of organ function including skin, kidney, endocrine system, gastrointestinal tract, liver, pancreas, respiratory system, cardiovascular system and central nervous system.

9 Body stores of certain nutrients (e.g. fat soluble vitamins) are low and these are compromised by increased utilization rates of these nutrients.

If any enteral nutrition can be tolerated safely, this should be encouraged no matter how small the nutritional contribution. This will minimize atrophy of the gut and pancreas during the period on parenteral nutrition.

References

Adamkin DH (1982) Intravenous fat emulsions: a neonatologist's point of view. In *Current perspectives in the use of lipid emulsion*, Johnston IDA Ed pp1−10 MTP Press, Lancaster.

Allwood MC (1984a) Drop size of infusions containing fat emulsion. *Br J Parent Ther* **5**, 113−6.

Allwood MC (1984b) Compatibility and stability of TPN mixtures in big bags. *J Clin Hosp Pharm* **9**, 181−98.

American Medical Association (1979) Multi vitamin preparations for parenteral use — a statement by the Nutrition Advisory Group. *J Parent Ent Nutr* **3**, 258−67.

American Medical Association (1979b) Guidelines for essential trace element preparations for parenteral use — a statement by the Nutrition Advisory Group. *J Parent Ent Nutr* **3**, 258−67.

Askanazi J, Nordenstrom J, Rosenbaum SH, Elwyn DH, Hyman AI, Carpentier YA and Kinney JM (1981) Nutrition for the patient with respiratory failure: glucose vs fat. *Anesthesiology* **54**, 373−7.

Blackburn GL, Flatt JP, Clowes GHA and O'Donnell TE (1973) Peripheral intravenous feeding with isotonic amino acid solutions. *Am J Surg* **125**, 447−54.

Booth IW and Harries JT (1982) Parenteral nutrition in young children. *Br J Intrav Ther* **3**, 31−40.

Bradley JA, King RFJG, Schorah CJ and Hill GL (1978) Vitamins in intravenous feeding: a study of water soluble vitamins in critically ill patients receiving intravenous nutrition. *Br J Surg* **65**, 492−4.

Buzby GP, Mullen JL, Stein P and Rosato EF (1981) Manipulation of TPN caloric substrate and fatty infiltration of the liver. *J Surg Res* **31**, 46−54.

Chawla RK, Lewis FW, Kutner MH, Bate DM, Roy RGB and Rudman D (1984) Plasma cysteine, cystine and glutathione in cirrhosis. *Gastroenterology* **87**, 770−6.

Chessex P, Zebiche H, Pineault M, Lepage D and Dallaine L (1985) Effect of amino acid composition of parenteral solutions on nitrogen retention and metabolic response in very low birth weight infants. *J Paediatr* **105**, 111−7.

Cockburn F (1985) Parenteral nutrition in low birth weight infants. *Br J Parent Ther* **6**, 68−74.

Collins FD, Sinclair AJ, Royle JP, Coats DA, Maynard AT and Leonard RF (1971) Plasma lipids in human linoleic acid deficiency. *Nutr Metab* **13**, 150−67.

Collins JP, Oxby CB and Hill GL (1978) Intravenous amino acids and intravenous hyperalimentation as protein sparing therapy after major surgery: a controlled clinical trial. *Lancet* i, 788−91.

Connor H, Newton DJ, Preston FE and Woods HF (1978) Oral methionine as a cause of acute serum folate deficiency: its relevance to parenteral nutrition. *Postgrad Med J* **54**, 318−20.

Freund H, Atamain S and Fisher JE (1979) Chromium deficiency during total parenteral nutrition. *J Am Med Assoc* **241**, 496−8.

Friedman A, Donon A, Stahlman MT and Oates JA (1976) Rapid onset of essential fatty acid deficiency in the newborn. *Paediatrics* **58**, 640.

Friel JK, Gibson RS, Peliowski A and Watts J (1984) Serum zinc, copper and selenium concentrations in preterm infants receiving enteral nutrition or parenteral nutrition supplemented with zinc and copper. *J Paediatr* **104**, 763−8.

Gazitua R, Wilson KN, Bistrian BR and Blackburn GL (1979) Factors determining peripheral vein tolerance to amino acid infusions. *Arch Surg* **114**, 897−900.

Gordon D, Allan A, Sim AJW and Shenkin A (1984); Transient hypercalciuria after commencing total intravenous nutrition. *Clin Nutr* **3**, 215−9.

Grant A and Todd E (1982) *Enteral and parenteral nutrition — a clinical handbook.* Blackwell Scientific Publications, Oxford.

Grotte G, Meurling S and Wretlind A (1982) Parenteral nutrition. In *A textbook of paediatric nutrition* 2e McLaren DS and Burman D Eds pp 228−54. Churchill Livingstone, London.

Hands LJ, Royle GT and Kettlewell MGW (1985) Vitamin K requirements in patients receiving total parenteral nutrition. *Br J Surg* **72**, 665−7.

Hardy G, Cotter R and Dawe R (1982) The stability and comparative clearance of TPN mixtures with lipid. In *Current perspectives in the use of lipid emulsion* Johnston IDA Ed pp 63−82. MTP Press Ltd, Lancaster.

Hertel J, Tygstrup I and Anderson GE (1982) Intravascular fat accumulation after Intralipid infusion in the very low birth weight infant. *J. Paediatr* **100**, 975−6.

Innis SM and Allardyce DB (1983) Possible biotin deficiency in adults recieving long term total parenteral nutrition. *Am J Clin Nutr* **37**, 185−7.

Jeejeebhoy KN, Zohrab WJ, Langer B, Phillips MJ, Kuksis A and Anderson GH (1973) Total parenteral nutrition at home for 23 months without complications and with good rehabilitation. *Gastroenterology* **65**, 811−20.

Kien CL and Ganther HE (1983) Manifestations of chronic selenium deficiency in a child receiving total parenteral nutrition. *Am J Clin Nutr* **37**, 319−28.

Kingsnorth AN, Ross BD and Kettlewell M (1980) Cost effective parenteral feeding. *Lancet* ii, 1371.

Kingsnorth AN (1984) Trace elements in adult total parenteral nutrition. *Br J Parent Ther* **5**, 8−22.

Klein GL, Targoff CM, Ament ME, Sherrard DJ, Bluestone R, Young JH, Norman AW and Coburn JW (1980) Bone disease associated with total parenteral nutrition. *Lancet* ii, 1041−4.

Levene MI, Wigglesworth JS and Desai R (1980) Pulmonary fat accumulation after Intralipid infusion in the preterm infant. *Lancet* ii, 815−8.

Lockitch G, Godolphin W, Pendray MR, Riddell D and Quigley G (1983) Serum zinc, copper, retinol binding protein, pre-albumin and ceruloplasmin concentrations in infants recieving intravenous zinc and copper supplementations. *J Paediatr* **102**, 304–8.

Long JM III, Wilmore DW, Mason AD and Pruitt BA (1977) Effect of carbohydrate and fat intake on nitrogen excretion during total intravenous feeding. *Ann Surg* **185**, 417–22.

Malloy MH, Russin DK and Richardson CJ (1983) Cyst(e)ine measurements during total parenteral nutrition. *Am J Clin Nutr* **37**, 188–91.

Mock DM, Baswell DL, Baker H, Holman RT and Sweetman L (1985) Biotin deficiency complicating parenteral alimentation: diagnosis, metabolic repercussions and treatment. *J Paediatr* **106**, 762–9.

Nordenstrom J (Ed) (1982) Utilization of exogenous and endogenous lipids for energy production during parenteral nutrition. *Acta Chir Scand* [Suppl] **510**, 1–79.

Press M, Hartop PJ and Prottey C (1974) Correction of essential fatty acid deficiency in man by the cutaneous application of sunflower seed oil. *Lancet* **i**, 597–9.

Quercia RA, Korn S, O'Neill D, Doughty JE, Ludwig M, Schweizer R and Sigman R (1984) Selenium deficiency and fatal cardiomyopathy in a patient receiving long term home parenteral nutrition. *Clin Pharm* **3**, 531–5.

Rogaly E, Clague MB, Carmichael MJ, Wright PD and Johnston IDA (1982) Comparison of body protein metabolism during total parenteral nutrition using glucose or glucose and fat as the energy source. *Clin Nutr* **1**, 80–90.

Ruberg RL and Mirtallo J (1981) Vitamin and trace element requirements in parenteral nutrition: an update *Ohio State Med J* **12**, 725–9.

Rudman D, Kutner M, Ansley J, Jansen R, Chippani J and Bain RP (1981) Hypotyrosinaemia, hypocystinaemia and failure to retain nitrogen during total parenteral nutrition of cirrhotic patients. *Gastroenterology* **81**, 1025–35.

Russell RI (1985) Magnesium requirements in patients with chronic inflammatory bowel disease receiving intravenous nutrition. *Br J Parent Ther* **6**, 86–94.

Schmidt-Sommerfield E, Penn D and Wolf H (1983) Carnitine deficiency in premature infants receiving total parenteral nutrition: effect of L-carnitine supplementation *J Paediatr* **102**, 931–4.

Shenkin A and Wretlind A (1978) Parenteral nutrition. *World Rev Nutr Diet* **28**, 1–111.

Shike M, Harrison JE, Sturtridge WC, Tam CS, Bobecko PE, Jones G, Murray TM and Jeejeebhoy KN (1980) Metabolic bone disease in patients receiving long term total parenteral nutrition. *Ann Int Med* **92**, 343–50.

Shike M, Rouet M, Kurain R, Whitewell J, Stewart S and Jeejeebhoy KN (1981) Copper metabolism and requirements in total parenteral nutrition. *Gastroenterology* **81**, 290–7.

Silk DBA (1983) *Nutritional support in hospital practice.* Blackwell Scientific Publications, Oxford.

Stoner HB, Little RA, Frayn KN, Elebute AE, Tresaden J and Gross E (1983) The effect of sepsis on the oxidation of carbohydrate and fat. *Br J Surg* **70**, 32–5.

Strelling MK, Blackledge DG and Goodall HB (1979) Diagnosis and management of folate deficiency in low birth weight infants. *Arch Dis Childh* **54**, 271–7.

Sturman JA, Gaull G and Raiha NCR (1970) Absence of cystathionase in human fetal liver: is cystine essential? *Science* **169**, 74–6.

Tao RC and Yoshimura NN (1980) Carnitine metabolism and its application in parenteral nutrition *J Parent Ent Nutr* **4**, 469–86.

Tovey SJ, Benton KGF and Lee HA (1977) Hypophosphataemia and phosphorus requirements during intravenous nutrition. *Postgrad Med J* **53**, 289–97.

Tweedle DEF, Skidmore FD, Gleave EN and Knass DA (1978) Nutritional support for patients undergoing surgery for cancer of the head and neck. In *Developments in clinical nutrition* Johnston IDA and Lee HA Eds pp 59–69. MCS Consultants, Tunbridge Wells.

Tweedle DEF (1982) *Metabolic care.* Churchill Livingstone, Edinburgh.

Vernejoul MC de, Messing B, Modrowski D, Bielakoff J, Buisine A and Miravet L (1985) Multifactorial low remodelling bone disease during cyclic total parenteral nutrition. *J Clin Endocrinol Metab* **60**, 109–13.

Whitfield MF, Spitz L and Milner RDG (1983) Clinical and metabolic consequences of two regimens of total parenteral nutrition in the newborn. *Arch Dis Child* **58**, 168–75.

Whittington PF and Burckart GT (1982) Changes in binding of bilirubin due to intravenous lipid emulsion. In *Current perspectives in the use of lipid emulsion* Johnston IDA Ed pp 15–28. MTP Press, Lancaster.

Wilmore DW and Dudrick SJ (1969) Treatment of acute renal failure with intravenous essential L-amino acids. *Arch Surg* **99**, 669–73.

Wolfram G, Eckart J, Walther B and Zollner N (1978) Factors influencing essential fatty acid requirement in total parenteral nutrition. *J Parent Ent Nutr* **2**, 634–9.

Wolman SL, Anderson GH, Marliss EB and Jeejeebhoy KN (1979) Zinc in total parenteral nutrition and metabolic effects. *Gastroenterology* **76**, 458–67.

Yu VYH, James B, Hendry P and MacMahon RA (1979) Total parenteral nutrition in very low birth weight infants: a controlled trial. *Arch Dis Childh* **54**, 653–61.

Zlotkin SH and Buchanan BE (1983) Meeting zinc and copper requirements in the parenterally fed preterm and full term infant. *J Paediatr* **103**, 441–6.

1.14 Dietary Modification and the Giving of Dietary Advice

1.14.1 Dietary modification in clinical practice — essential factors to consider

Purpose

A modified diet is more likely to be adhered to if the patient and relatives are given clear and simple instructions as to why the diet has to be changed.

Dietary composition

Quantitative requirements must be discussed with the clinician. A change in one nutrient will usually lead to changes in other directions and these must also be considered with the clinician. For example, a low carbohydrate diet will inevitably be a high fat diet and a low fat regimen may result in diets containing less than the recommended allowance of vitamin A. A low calcium diet, unless supplemented, is a low riboflavin diet since milk is the major source of both. Water soluble vitamin losses may be hastened in homogenized foods kept hot for long periods. The overall adequacy of therapeutic diets must always be checked and the diet supplemented if necessary.

'Low' and 'high' diets

The absolute level of a nutrient in a therapeutic diet is established ideally by reference to the desired biochemical/physiological/clinical effect. Thus a low protein diet for a patient in renal failure contains a level of protein only as low as is necessary to keep blood urea at acceptable levels while maintaining nitrogen balance.

Alternatively, a statistical definition can be made. Thus an intake which is more than two standard deviations away from the average is likely to occur in less than 5% of a given population, and can be classified as *low* if below and *high* if above the average intake. For example, Bingham (1979) defines low-fibre diets as follows. 'The standard deviation of fibre intakes in a random British population aged 20–80 years was 5.2 g/day with a mean of 20 g/day. A low dietary fibre diet would therefore contain 10 g of dietary fibre or less on this basis'. Similar reasoning may be applied to the average nutrient intakes in UK populations shown

in Section 1.3. Where there is no biochemical or other yardstick, then *low X diet* usually implies a level which is as low as is practicable and acceptable in terms of usual eating patterns. The generally accepted nutrient levels in *low* or *high* therapeutic diets will be found in the relevant clinical sections.

'Low' and 'high' foods

There are two basic methods of constructing therapeutic diets

1   The desired level of intake is specified and the diet is constructed from an exchange list, i.e. the size of the portion of each food containing a given amount of the nutrient is defined and the patient is allowed a specified number of these portions. Thus a 40 g protein diet may be constructed from 5×6 g protein exchanges and 5×2 g protein exchanges plus unlimited quantities of foods virtually free from protein. This method is used typically for carbohydrate and protein controlled diets.

2   The diet is constructed from normal sized portions of foods but those foods which have the highest nutrient content *per portion* are excluded from the diet. However, *frequency* of consumption must also be taken into account, and it may be necessary to limit the number of portions of foods of moderate content of the given nutrient if they are eaten very frequently, e.g. bread, milk and butter. The amount of the given nutrient in the diet is thus allowed to achieve an unspecified, but lower-than-habitual intake. This method is typically used for low fat and low calcium diets.

In-patients

The diet must be of a suitable and palatable form and may differ in several respects from that prescribed on leaving hospital, for example in energy content or texture. It is essential that the therapeutic diet service within the hospital is efficient and this requires well-informed catering and ward staff. Diet cooks must be trained regularly and supervised in the techniques of diet cookery and all members of the ward staff must be made aware of the dietary requirements of patients by use of diet sheets and nutritional intake charts. Ward staff can also help to check that the patient receives the prescribed diet but the dietitian should also make occasional spot checks at meal times.

The amount of dietary information given to the in-patient will vary with the length of time the patient is to remain on a diet. If the patient is to leave hospital on the same diet then some of the time spent as an in-patient can be used to teach them about their dietary modifications. Information should also be given to relatives about foods which can be brought in for the patient, for example boiled sweets for those on a low sodium diet or low energy drinks for those trying to lose weight.

Out-patients

Diets must be tailored to fit individual patients' habits and needs. Factors such as shift work, income and lifestyle must be considered and are discussed in detail in the following section.

Ideally, more than one interview should be arranged and should, wherever possible, include the person who prepares most of the patient's meals. Relevant advice concerning modification of usual recipes and suitable cookery books and/or food lists should be given.

In certain very specialized diets, where culinary skills need to be developed, verbal information may be insufficient and demonstrations will be necessary, e.g. coeliac or renal disease.

Follow-up

Patients will require considerable encouragement and interest from the dietitian if a permanent change in food habits is to be achieved. Frequent out-patient appointments and referral to a community dietitian for domiciliary visits may be necessary. Patients can be given a record book for recording their menus in the intervening time between returning home and the first out-patient attendance. Following this, patients should be asked to keep records of, for example, the week preceding an out-patient visit. Where there is doubt about compliance, it is sometimes possible to check dietary adherence by independent measures, such as subcutaneous fat biopsy for determination of P:S ratio, the measurement of glycosylated haemoglobin (HbA1) as a reflector of diabetic control and assessment of the 24-hour urinary output of sodium or nitrogen/urea for sodium and protein restriction respectively (see Sections 1.4 and 1.15).

1.14.2 Giving nutritional and dietetic advice

For nutrition education and therapeutic dietetic advice to have a chance of being effective, many considerations must be taken into account by the dietitian. These fall into two main categories (1) the context in which the information is received and (2) the way in which it is given. Some guidelines which may be of use to dietitians involved in both therapeutic and preventive nutrition are outlined below.

Factors affecting food choice

The context in which nutritional or dietetic advice is received will be different for each individual and will differ between people on therapeutic diets and those with no immediate health problem. There are many factors which have a bearing on individual food choice and the relative importance of these to each individual person must be assessed by the dietitian so that specific dietary advice is realistic. These factors should also be considered when general nutrition advice is given to groups of people rather than to individuals.

The availability of food

People can only eat regularly the foods they can buy in the shops they can get to. Many small shops stock a limited range of foods and it is often impossible for people without cars to shop in large supermarkets situated away from main shopping centres. Dietitians should be familiar with the type of shops in the areas their patients live and the products available in them.

The cost of food

The cost of food is important in determining people's food choice. People can only eat regularly the foods they can afford. A 25% difference between the price of a white and a wholemeal loaf of bread is likely to be a deciding factor for a household on a low income. The price of an individual food is often more influential than the cost of the diet as a whole. For example, for a person advised to eat lean meat, fish and fruit instead of steak pies, sausages and biscuits the increased cost of the individual types of food would seem to be prohibitive. They may at the same time be being advised to cut down on other expensive foods such as alcoholic drinks, cream, chocolate and cheese, but it is more difficult to look at overall costs.

The actual use of the food also affects people's

perceptions of price. For example, a person on a reducing diet may be advised to eat fruit instead of chocolate bars. Piece for piece the chocolate is probably more expensive. However, chocolate is bought one piece at a time by the individual and consumed in that way. Fruit is bought in quantity and left in a bowl to be eaten when required by all members of the household. It is not rationed in the same way as chocolate and so, used in this way, *is* more expensive. Dietitians need to be sensitive to the needs of people on low incomes and their perceptions of price as well as actual food costs.

Even if a sufficient choice of suitable foods is easily accessible at a price the consumer can regularly afford, there are still many other factors involved in determining what is actually eaten.

Cultural influences

Among the strongest determinants of food choice are cultural factors. These include peer group pressures, social conventions, religious practices, the status value afforded to different foods, the influence of other members of the household and individual lifestyles.

Every dietitian is familiar with instances of, for example, the child who is ridiculed or feels ostracized for taking wholemeal bread to school or for not buying an ice cream on the way home; the business executive who 'has' to eat rich meals when entertaining clients; the Muslim child who cannot get suitable school meals; the demeaning associations of eating large amounts of bread and potatoes as an indication of poverty; the woman who always cooks chips for the whole household because that is all 'he' will eat and the teenagers who 'do not have time' to eat a sit down meal because they are far too busy. These and many other cultural factors are also compounded by economic considerations.

Economic influences

Lack of money is rarely the only problem in households on a low income. Health problems and depressive illness, poor housing and deprivation generally, are highest among the unemployed and low paid. It is very easy for well-meaning professional workers, such as dietitians, to give advice on, for example, 'budgeting', 'careful shopping' and 'planning meals and menus' but this advice is often totally unrealistic. It is often based on the cultural background from which

the professional comes and the concepts may be totally alien to many of the people to whom it is given. Priorities for different individuals and groups of people vary widely and dietitians or other professionals should not impose their own priorities on others. Sensitivity to a particular person's *own* perceived needs and priorities is essential and advice must be structured around those needs.

Advice about saving money by buying cheaper foods, if it is information requested by the client, must also be realistic. Cheaper foods (e.g. cheap cuts of meat or beans and pulses) often use considerably more fuel during cooking than more expensive foods and in terms of overall expenditure may well make the meal more expensive. Fuel saving equipment such as slow-cookers and pressure cookers are expensive pieces of equipment and for many households on low incomes it is inconceivable to pay out that amount of money all at once.

The other important economic influence on eating habits is time. Women are still the main providers of food in the home. However, more and more women are now going out to work and are effectively doing two full-time jobs — running the home and bringing in a significant proportion of the income. For many women time is at a premium and shopping for and cooking the meals takes enough time without having to spend extra time planning, budgeting and finding out about and looking round for nutritionally suitable foods.

There is a real need for nutritionally sound, cheap, convenience foods and until these exist dietitians must accept the limitations of the advice they are giving. (For more information on advising people on low incomes see Section 3.7.)

Psychological influences

For many people the strongest influence over their eating behaviour is psychological. Food, especially sweet food, is often used as an important form of reward or punishment for children and some may be given sweets by their parents as a means of dealing with their own feelings of guilt, caused, perhaps, by the conflict between the necessity for many mothers to go out to work and the condemnation from society in general for so doing. Compulsive eating is, for many adults, a way of finding comfort during depression, loneliness and boredom. Anorexia nervosa can be a way of coping with hate or anger towards a parent or fear of maturity. Whatever the cause, the problem is unlikely to be resolved by dietary advice — although in some cases it can be part of the solution.

Individual choices and preferences

Every individual has personal food preferences and tastes. These may change from time to time but will affect what is eaten at a given time. Taste preferences are based primarily on the flavour, colour, texture and smell of food, but may also be based on association of a certain food with an unpleasant incident. On the whole, tastes are acquired early in life but are subject to many other influences. Dietitians need to take personal preferences into account whenever advice is being given.

Moral and political convictions may also influence the foods people buy and eat. The most common examples of this are vegetarianism, veganism, or not eating products from countries with particular political regimes. There is no point in telling someone to eat an orange every day, or fruit tinned in water if the only types available in their area come from a country whose goods they personally boycott.

Information and knowledge

In order for people to have more control over what they eat, they must be informed. Information on its own, however, is not sufficient. People also need to know how to evaluate that information and to act upon it.

Information about food and nutrition comes from a wide variety of sources including friends, relatives, teachers, health professionals, advertisements, magazine and newspaper articles, promotions and food manufacturers. It is wide-ranging and can be inconsistent, confusing, often inaccurate and open to misinterpretation. Dietitians should be aware of the diversity of information that the general public receives and the impact some of it, particularly television advertisements, can have.

Outlined above are some of the factors which will influence the way in which dietetic advice is acted upon. This, however, is just one aspect of the issue. The way in which the information is given is also crucial.

Communication

Most dietetic advice is given in a one-to-one interview, although with the increasing emphasis on preventive nutrition, group work and the production of information for mass markets is developing rapidly. The basic principles which should be followed in such circumstances are outlined below.

Basic principles of communication

Expertise. When a dietitian is giving advice she is indeed an expert in her own field. However, it is easy to forget that in most situations that expertise is extremely limited. The dietitian will know what is best for a person's nutritional health but probably has little knowledge of the problems and other things of importance to a particular individual. The client is the expert on many of the issues which will be under discussion. How many dietitians, when talking with a group of pensioners, have first-hand experience of being a pensioner? Nutrition and dietetic interviews are two-way discussions with each participant being able to learn as much from the other.

Know the 'audience'. It is impossible to give realistic advice unless something is known and understood about the client or audience. What is their socio-economic and cultural background? Where do they live? What sort of household and peer group pressures are they subjected to? What problems might they have in effecting the advice? What level of knowledge do they already have? What do they want to know about? What is their degree of literacy in the language of any written material? The best way to find out this information is to ask the person or audience. However, the dietitian needs to put people at ease and help them to relax in the early stages of an interview or meeting so careful, sensitive discussion is more appropriate than straight, point blank questions. With groups, informal quizzes are often helpful to assess current knowledge and act as a basis for discussion.

Building on what already exists. Once the level of knowledge which already exists, and exactly what the person or audience wants to know more about, has been established, it is possible to build on that knowledge, correct misconceptions and give requested information. Starting with what the client is already interested in, it is possible to widen the discussion and interest to include points the dietitian feels to be important.

Style of advice. The style of the dietitian will depend

to a certain extent on her own personality but should also reflect the needs of the person or audience. It is easy to be dogmatic and prescriptive and for a few people this may be appropriate. That is for the dietitian to assess. It is often more appropriate to give people information — the pros and cons if they exist — and then help them to make their own decisions. Fear is a very short-term motivating factor. The dietitian's role is to give information, advice and support as required and as appropriate.

Language. The level and type of language used varies as much with different individuals or groups of people as does the type of information being given. However, in general, language must be simple and accessible, without the use of long and technical words.

Feedback and assessment of understanding. During a session it is crucial that the dietitian obtains feedback on whether or not the advice is being understood. This can be aided by

1 Giving the person or audience frequent opportunities to ask questions.
2 Asking simple questions on what has already been said and relating to the needs of the person or group.

It is important to respond to this type of feedback by further discussions on the points which have been misunderstood or missed.

Amount of information. The number of important points the dietitian wants to put over should be kept to a minimum. Learning capacity and memory is surprisingly low, especially when the recipient of the information is feeling anxious or under stress. Two or three major points are enough for any session. These can of course be illustrated by examples and anecdotes to help their clarity.

Most people's concentration span is about 5−8 minutes. The dietitian should be sensitive to the concentration level of the recipient(s) and respond accordingly. The amount of repetition necessary in one session will depend on the feedback the dietitian is receiving.

Follow-up. People should always go away with the feeling that they can approach the dietitian at any time for more information. It should be made clear that at follow-up sessions there will be a chance for the person to discuss any problems which have been encountered and to have any questions which have arisen in the intervening time answered.

Information to take away. Leaflets or diet sheets giving clear information which reinforces what has been said and provides more detail as appropriate should be available at the end of the session.

Teaching methods

Information can be passed from one person to another in a number of ways. Those most commonly used by dietitians are one-to-one interviews, lectures and discussion groups. Perhaps the most fundamental rule is that a dietitian is talking *with* people and not *to* them. This may seem a small point but it is crucial. Any teaching method used in therapeutic dietetics or nutrition education must involve two-way communication between the giver and the receiver of information and conventional 'lectures' are, therefore, inappropriate. It is often easier for a dietitian who is nervous or not very self-confident to prepare a 'talk' or 'lecture' and give it. In most dietetic settings this is unsuitable as it allows for virtually no feedback or assessment of how much the audience is understanding or interested in.

One-to-one interviews. These must be as relaxed as possible and always give time for both people involved to put their own points across. The dietitian is often a counsellor as well as a teacher in these sessions and must assess the needs of the person and respond to them appropriately. A dietitian will get nowhere with her advice if she is not prepared to discuss the problems or misunderstandings of her patients.

Group sessions. Group sessions may be used for therapeutic purposes or for nutrition education of people who do not currently have health problems. Ideally, everyone in the group should have a chance to participate but this will depend on the size of the group. The optimum size for participation and exchange of ideas is between seven and ten people. Larger groups can always be divided for discussions with report-back sessions to the whole group. The major advantage of group discussions is that the information and ideas people put to each other spark off new ideas which may not otherwise have emerged. People learn more if they are able to take part, think ideas through for themselves and build on their own experiences.

Dietitians talking with community groups can use, for example, quizzes and question and answer techniques to involve people in the 'talks' and encourage exchange of ideas and expertise between participants.

Audio-visual aids

Most people remember things better if they have something visual as well as verbal to recall. For example, saying that a plate of chips is high in fat is less effective than showing them exactly how much fat is present. Visual aids can be of great help to dietitians in giving information. There are numerous types, many of which can be used with individuals as well as groups:

Writing boards, flip charts, flannel boards, magnetic boards and overhead projectors can be used to illustrate and clarify points while the dietitian is speaking, in response to questions or for recording the main points of discussions. The writing and pictures must be clear and legible for the person furthest away and must complement the teaching.

Food models, actual foods and food packets make the best teaching aids. People can recognize them immediately and relate to them in a personal way. *Posters, slides and photographs* are also useful but have limitations. When using slides in particular it is easy to lose some contact with the audience because of the need for dimmed lights.

Tape slides, videos and films can be useful but care is needed to ensure that they do not replace the teaching but complement it. Videos are particularly useful because they can be stopped and repeated, picking up on specific points of interest to the group.

Leaflets and quizzes are also often useful as they can help focus the audience's attention and expand on ideas picked up during the session. All written information must be thought out carefully and the language clear and simple. Each sentence should contain only one idea and the words kept short and simple. It is always worth working out the 'readability' level of leaflets and other written information. Leaflets also should complement, not replace, teaching and on their own are often of relatively limited value.

Exhibitions and displays

Dietitians involved in nutrition education will frequently find the need for exhibitions and displays designed for large groups of people. They may or may not be serviced by the dietitians while they are *in situ*.

The same basic principles apply with exhibitions and displays as with any other form of communication

1 Know the audience.
2 Keep the information clear, concise and simple.
3 Give information and be careful about dogma.
4 Have leaflets and more detailed information for those interested to take away.

Exhibitions and displays should be as visual as possible with a minimum of text. They are there to attract people's attention, provoke their thoughts and tempt them to delve deeper into the subject by taking away leaflets and information sheets or by talking to the dietitians servicing the display. They cannot be comprehensive tools of education on their own and should not be expected to be.

The mass media

The widest audiences are reached by dietitians via the mass media. Once again, the same basic principles of communication apply. For most dietitians the mass media they will have ready access to are local newspapers, although local radio and television are becoming increasingly interested in health issues.

Writing press releases. Press releases are one of the most useful ways for dietitians to communicate with the media. Press rooms receive dozens of press releases everyday and many of the articles in any newspaper are taken from them.

There are no hard and fast rules about writing press releases, but there are a few basic principles which can be applied.

All press releases must be typed, preferably with wide margins and double spaced. They must give information about what is happening and why, who is doing it, and where and when it is happening.

The first two sentences are the most important and should contain all the main points. The rest of the press release should concentrate on giving facts and information. Quotes from people involved in the event are also useful.

All press releases must give the name and telephone number of a contact person who is available and able to give more details to interested journalists. They should also have a simple title, designed to help the news editor spot the interest of the story.

Responding to the press. If a dietitian is contacted unexpectedly by the press great care should be taken over what is said via the telephone. Authors and people who comment on issues have very little control over what is finally published. However, on the whole, the media are sympathetic towards issues raised by or involving dietitians and do not deliberately try to denigrate the profession or misrepresent the issues.

Television and radio interviews. Media interviews may be live or recorded; either way it is essential to be well prepared.

If invited to an interview, the dietitian will have some idea of the issues to be discussed. It is useful to have a few well prepared main points to put across — the number will depend on the amount of time — and to stick to these as far as possible. The whole experience can be very nerve-racking but when in the situation very few people are unable to contribute. It is worth remembering that, when listening to the interview later, it always sounds better than it seemed at the time!

Further reading

Curzon LB (1976) *Teaching in further education.* Cassell, London.
Gowers E (1984) *The complete plain words.* Penguin Books, London.
Hopson B and Scally M (1981) *Life skills teaching.* McGraw-Hill, London.
Inner London Education Authority (1985) *Nutrition guidelines.* Heinemann Educational Books, London.
MacShane D (1979) *Using the media.* Pluto Press, London.
Rodwell-Williams S (1978) *Essentials of nutrition and diet therapy* 2e. The C V Mosby Company, St Louis.
TACADE (1981) *Informal methods in health and social education.* TACADE, 2 Mount Street, Manchester, M2 5NG.

Reference

Bingham SA (1979) Low residue diets: a reappraisal of their meaning and content. *J Hum Nutr* **33**, 516.

1.15 Evaluation of Dietetic Practice

'The dietitian would seem to be faced with a wide range of topics to proselytize, frequently in adverse surroundings. Her audience is likely to be up to 15 in number, female and under 45 years of age, but there is no certainty in predicting any of these and she has to use her own initiative in devising aids and supplying examples. She cannot guarantee that her audience really wishes to be involved and she is likely to be left in severe doubt about whether her information has been absorbed or the attitudes of the audience altered' (Earl 1984).

Section 1.14.2 describes in detail the conditions which must exist if dietetic practice is to be, in any way, successful. However, very little research into the effectiveness of dietetic advice or nutrition education in the UK has ever been undertaken. If dietitians are to increase their professionalism and to continue to improve their service to the public and National Health Service, evaluation of dietetic practice is essential.

Evaluation of dietetic practice can be divided into three broad categories

1 Self assessment by the dietitian to ensure she is giving the best advice in the best way possible.

2 Evaluation of patient compliance with the advice they are given.

3 Evaluation of the effectiveness of the advice or treatment.

1.15.1 Self-assessment by dietitians

Earl (1984) recognized the need for self-assessment by dietitians. In evaluating a self-assessment sheet, she found that talks given by 21 dietitians ranged from ten minutes to one hour in length; audience numbers ranged from one to eighty; locations varied 'from the living rooms of houses and the waiting rooms of doctors' surgeries, through hospital kitchens and corridors, to meeting rooms in health clinics and official lecture theatres.' Generally, the venue for the talk was considered unsatisfactory by the dietitian 'seating and interruptions being the most common problems.'

Whatever the preconceived ideas the dietitian has about how a talk ought to be, this is how it is. Dietitians need to be very flexible and learn to assess their own performance in the context of each talk, and to remember that people will learn more if they are relaxed and in familiar surroundings. It is the dietitian's responsibility to adapt to those surroundings.

Self-assessment is never easy and it is hard to be objective about one's own work. Using a routine assessment form after each talk or session can help systematize the assessment, aid consistency and chart growth and development in the dietitian's work.

Table 1.53 is the self-assessment sheet developed at Robert Gordon's Institute of Technology by Earl and her colleagues (Earl 1984). It is a useful guide and can be adapted and supplemented by dietitians keen to evaluate their own work.

Table 1.54 gives some additional questions which dietitians could include in their own self-assessment forms.

To answer all the questions in these tables after every talk could be very time consuming and it may be that after a little practice most of the points become automatic. However, never forget that there is *always* room for improvement, imagination and new ideas.

Table 1.53 Professional talk — self-assessment sheet

This sheet should take only four minutes to complete. Nevertheless, it should encourage critical self-appraisal. For the purposes of definition 'talk' includes any time spent on the topic in the presence of the audience, e.g. screening of film, actual talk and question time would all be incorporated.

Name . . . .   Date . . . .

Subject of talk (be precise) . . . .

Duration (minutes) Anticipated . . . . Actual . . . .

Location   e.g. Church Hall, 20 m × 10 m . . . .

Unfavourable factors (underline as appropriate)
External noise   Interruption   Seating   Ventilation
Other (please specify): . . . .

Table 1.53 *contd.*

Audience (circle as appropriate, more than one circle allowed in each column):

SEX/RACE	AGE	NO. OF PEOPLE	LEVEL OF EDUCATION
Male	Under 18 years	One person	Primary
Female	18–45 years	2–15 people	Secondary
Multi-racial	46–65 years	16–30 people	Further
(Describe	Over 65 years	Over 30 people	Graduate
. . . .)			

Aids used (circle as appropriate, more than one circle allowed):

Blackboard	Tape	Handout
Chart	Slides	Questionnaire
Flip board	Photographs	Pamphlet
Overhead projector	Film/video	Other (please specify) . . . .
Poster	3-D model	. . . .

Delivery (Please tick appropriate boxes):
Did *you* —

	Yes	No
Introduce yourself?	☐	☐
Establish a rapport?	☐	☐
Introduce the subject clearly?	☐	☐
Develop material in a logical manner?	☐	☐
Summarize at the end?	☐	☐
Allow time for questions/discussion?	☐	☐
Recapitulate after the discussion?	☐	☐

Audience response. Now consider the audience and estimate the strength of their response

	Strong	Considerable	Slight	Weak
Attention	☐	☐	☐	☐
Interest	☐	☐	☐	☐
Questioning/participation in discussion	☐	☐	☐	☐
Extension of knowledge	☐	☐	☐	☐
Change of attitude	☐	☐	☐	☐

Think about your response to the section on delivery and think about giving the talk again. With a similar group *next time* would you:

	Yes	No
Shorten the talk?	☐	☐
Lengthen the talk?	☐	☐
Simplify the language?	☐	☐
Modify sections of the talk?	☐	☐

State which and how . . . .

	Yes	No
Increase your vocal volume?	☐	☐
Alter the aids?	☐	☐
Improve the summary?	☐	☐
Give greater opportunity for audience participation?	☐	☐
Give more examples related to the audience's experience?	☐	☐
Allow more time for discussion?	☐	☐
Make any other adjustment?	☐	☐

Give details . . . .

Table 1.54 Questions which could be included in a self-assessment questionnaire

Did I know enough about the audience beforehand?

	Yes	No
Size	☐	☐
Living environment	☐	☐
Social circumstances	☐	☐
Age	☐	☐
Previous knowledge	☐	☐
Main areas of interest	☐	☐

Other (specify) . . . .

Did I know enough about the venue beforehand?

	Yes	No
Size	☐	☐
Seating arrangements	☐	☐
Acoustics	☐	☐
Presence of other people e.g. children	☐	☐
Position of electrical points	☐	☐
Visual aid facilities	☐	☐

Other (specify) . . . .

Did I arrive early enough to arrange the room as I wanted it?

Yes ☐   No ☐

Did I manage to set the group at ease and make sure they felt able to participate?

Yes ☐   No ☐

Can I improve on this ? . . . .

Did I find out the level of knowledge and the areas of interest from the group during the session?

Yes ☐   No ☐

What techniques can I use to improve this? (e.g. quizzes, questions and answers, etc.). . . . .

Did I allow verbal feedback and questions during the session?

Yes ☐   No ☐

Can I improve on this?-. . . . .

Was I aware of any non-verbal feedback? (e.g. people laughing, smiling, nodding in understanding, looking puzzled, mentally wandering off, staring blankly, falling asleep).

Yes ☐   No ☐

Did I respond to verbal and non-verbal feedback?

Yes ☐   No ☐

How can I improve on this? . . . .

Did I build on existing knowledge among the group?

Yes ☐   No ☐

Did I actively involve the audience in the session?

Yes ☐   No ☐

How can I do so in future? . . . .

Did I allow exchange of ideas and experience between members of the group?

Yes ☐   No ☐

Table 1.54 contd.

How can I improve on this? . . . .

How many main points did I try to put across? Was it more than three?

	Yes	No
	☐	☐

If yes — was that alright? Did I succeed?

	Yes	No
	☐	☐

Was my language level suitable?

	Yes	No
	☐	☐

Did I use jargon words?

	Yes	No
	☐	☐

Did I explain complicated terms and ideas?

	Yes	No
	☐	☐

Did my visual aids complement what I was saying effectively?

	Yes	No
	☐	☐

Did I provide or arrange any follow-up? (e.g. leaflets, further sessions)

	Yes	No
	☐	☐

Should I have done?

	Yes	No
	☐	☐

Being aware of all the possible pitfalls and generally being well prepared helps the dietitian to teach with relaxed confidence. She always has something to offer the audience and always something to learn from them.

Tables 1.53 and 1.54 are designed mainly for critical self-assessment for dietitians working with groups of individuals rather than for one-to-one counselling and interviews. Nevertheless, many of the issues still apply to the counselling of individuals and it should not be difficult to design departmental assessment forms for both one-to-one and group situations. The same basic principles of communication as outlined in Section 1.14.2 are applicable in both instances.

1.15.2 Evaluating patient compliance

However effective the dietitian thinks she has been in communicating her message it is still crucial to find out whether or not that advice has been acted upon.

Patient compliance may need to be assessed for research purposes (e.g. to ensure that an experimental or control diet is being followed) or for improving the effectiveness of the care of specific individuals. The methods used will to some extent depend on the

reason for the study. In research programmes accurate measurements of compliance may be essential (see Section 5.11) whereas in individual care the sensitivity and specificity requirements can be less stringent (Gordis 1976). A detailed description of dietetic research procedures is given in Section 5.11.

On a day to day basis it is important for dietitians to be able to assess the value of their time spent with patients. Patient non-compliance shows itself in a number of ways. These may include failure of the dietary treatment to improve the condition, failure to keep follow-up appointments and disregard for the dietitian's advice. More specific parameters which can be examined include:

Symptom relief

If a special diet is well established and accepted as the means of treatment for a specific illness then dietary compliance will result in the relief of visible symptoms. For example

1 In coeliac disease, the presence or absence of symptoms depends on dietary compliance.
2 In obesity, weight loss depends on reduced food energy intake.

3 In food allergies, non-compliance results in a return of the symptoms.

4 In dietary iron, vitamin B12 or folate deficiency anaemias, a cure will only be maintained if the diet is altered.

5 Constipation caused by insufficient dietary fibre is relieved by dietary compliance.

Biochemical or histological changes

In some conditions where diet is the key form of treatment, biochemical or histological tests may be useful in assessing compliance. For example

1 The measurement of glycosylated haemoglobin (HbA1) in diabetics is a good indication of diabetic control and compliance with treatment.

2 In coeliac disease, jejunal biopsies reveal whether gluten has been included in the diet.

3 Serum lipid levels may indicate if a modified fat diet has been consumed.

Assessment of dietary understanding

Quizzes and questionnaires can be used to assess various aspects of compliance but such methods are less objective and may be less reliable. They can be useful to examine patients' knowledge and understanding of their dietary regimen which is the first step towards compliance; however, they do not necessarily give any indication of the degree of behaviour change. Without knowledge and understanding, dietary compliance is impossible. With it, it is far from assured.

Dietary records

These may also be a useful too and can be in a number of forms. For example by questions such as 'What was eaten yesterday?', 'What is a typical day's food', 'Which of the following types of foods do you normally eat?'. Alternatively, written records in the form of diaries or more precise weighed intakes can be kept for various periods of time (depending on which nutrients or dietary parameters are the focus of study). The choice of technique also depends on the dietitian's access to the patient, i.e. whether contact will be via a one-to-one interview, a group discussion or by post.

Dietary investigations can give valuable information about a patient's actual eating habits but dietitians must be aware that some people will be tempted to give an account of what they understand they *should have* been eating rather than what they have actually eaten. This possibility must always be borne in mind.

If the patient is not complying with the dietary advice then the reasons for this should be examined and acted upon. If a patient does not believe the diet to be important, he will not bother to follow it. If he has not fully understood the advice, he cannot follow it. If the advice is too general and not geared specifically to the needs, lifestyle, income, cooking and storing facilities, tastes and eating habits of the individual then it will fail. If maintaining the diet causes more strain, trouble or social rejection than the condition itself it will be soon abandoned. Dietitians must never underestimate how difficult it is for some people to change the eating habits of a lifetime.

1.15.3 Evaluating the effectiveness of the dietary treatment

It is also important that dietitians evaluate the effectiveness of the treatment itself. If the patient genuinely appears to be complying with the advice given but the condition is not improving or the symptoms are not disappearing then the treatment, as it has been offered, is wrong for that person. There may be a number of reasons for this:

A wrong diagnosis. If the condition has been diagnosed incorrectly the dietary advice will be inappropriate. This possibility should always be considered.

Inappropriate dietary parameters. Prescribing nutrient intake based on average needs (i.e. from standard RDA tables) may seriously over or underestimate the actual requirement for a particular individual. If the diet is inappropriate in terms of content, it will not be beneficial however carefully it is followed.

Only the symptoms of the condition are being treated, not the cause. This often happens in the case of chronic obesity. Very few dietitians, when advising patients, try and find out the cause of the obesity. Superficially it is overeating but in reality that is a symptom of a much more complicated problem. Ultimately, unless the real cause is tackled, the treatment or dietary advice will be ineffective.

The treatment does not work. The rational on which a treatment is based may be faulty.

If a person has a health problem for which they are being given a programme of treatment, whether it be diet, drugs, exercise or another, it is in their interest to follow that treatment. If the patient is not noticing any change in the condition despite the treatment, the incentive to continue is very small. People want to get better and feel fit and well; they do not disregard advice out of cussedness. If a patient is not responding to treatment, for whatever reason, the treatment needs to be reviewed and discussed with them. If necessary, an alternative form of treatment needs to be found. It is all too easy to blame the patient for failing whilst more often than not it is the practitioner who is to blame. It is irresponsible and damaging to continue offering a treatment which is not working.

In the UK very little research into dietary compliance and the effectiveness of dietetic practice has been published. The few studies which have appeared in the last five years have looked at nutrition education and its effect on infant feeding practices (Kirk 1980) and on the behaviour of primary school children (Murray et al 1984); and at dietary compliance among diabetics (Henry et al 1981; Westgarth et al 1981; McCullock et al 1983; Sheard 1984), among coronary patients (Reid et al 1984) and at out-patient attendance (Gallagher 1984).

A discussion of dietary compliance, with particular reference to diabetics, was published in 1981 (Thomas 1981) and the problems of compliance with therapeutic regimens generally has been discussed in detail elsewhere (Kelly 1973; Sackett 1976; Karvetti 1981; Schwartz and Clampett 1983).

References

Earl SE (1984) Self-appraisal: a formalized tool for improving dietitians' communication. *Hum Nutr: Appl Nutr* **38A**, (2), 119–25.

Gallagher C (1984) Next please: a review of dietetic out-patient attendance. *Hum Nutr: Appl Nutr* **38A**, (3), 181–6.

Gordis L (1976) Methodologic issues in the measurement of patient compliance. In *Compliance with therapeutic regimens*. Sackett DL and Haynes RB (Eds). The John Hopkins University Press, Baltimore and London.

Henry CL, Heaton KW, Manhire A and Hartog M (1981) Diet and the diabetic: the fallacy of a controlled carbohydrate intake. *Hum Nutr* **35**, (2), 102–5.

Karvetti RL (1981) Change in the diet of myocardial infarction patients. Effects of nutrition education. *J Am Diet Assoc* **79**, (6), 660–7.

Kelly MW (1973) Diet therapy of diabetes: an analysis of failure. *Ann Intern Med* **79**, 425–34.

Kirk TW (1980) Appraisal of the effectiveness of nutrition education in the context of infant feeding. *J Hum Nutr* **34**, (6), 425–38.

McCulloch DK, Young RJ, Steel JM, Wilson EM, Prescott RJ and Duncan LJP (1983) Effect of dietary compliance on metabolic control in insulin dependent diabetics. *Hum Nutr: Appl Nutr* **37A**, (4), 287–92.

Murray M, Rona RJ, Morris RW and Tait N (1984) The smoking and dietary behaviour of Lambeth school children. *Public Health* **98**, (3), 163–72.

Reid V, Graham I, Hickey N and Mulcahy R. (1984) Factors affecting dietary compliance in coronary patients included in a secondary prevention programme. *Hum Nutr: Appl Nutr* **38A**, (4), 279–87.

Sackett DL (1976) The magnitude of compliance and non-compliance. In *Compliance with therapeutic regimens*. Sackett DL and Haynes RB (Eds). The John Hopkins University Press, Baltimore and London.

Schwartz NE and Clampett DM (1983) Evaluation of a nutrition innovation in secondary school home economics education. *Hum Nutr: Appl Nutr* **37A**, (3), 180–8.

Sheard CM (1984) How effective is our advice to diabetics? A preliminary evaluation. *Hum Nutr: Appl Nutr* **38A**, (2), 138–41.

Thomas BJ (1981) How successful are we at persuading diabetics to follow their diet — and why do we sometimes fail? In *Nutrition and diabetes*. Turner M and Thomas B (Eds) pp 57–66. John Libbey, London.

Westgarth SA, De Looy AE and Buckler JMH (1981) An investigation into the dietary habits of some diabetic children. In *Applied nutrition 1*. Bateman EC (Ed). John Libbey, London.

Section 2   **Foods and Nutrients**

2.1   Dietary Energy

2.1.1   Energy requirements

The energy requirements of individuals vary widely, even between people who are apparently similar in terms of age, sex and activity level. The standard deviation observed for energy in population intake studies is about 25% (Darke *et al* 1980). Energy intakes also vary widely from day to day for a given individual. Caution therefore needs to be exercised when using tables of average energy requirements for groups of people e.g. Recommended Daily Amounts (see Sections 1.2 (RDAs) and 4.1 (Obesity)).

2.1.2   Dietary sources of energy

Principal dietary sources in the average British diet

Figure 2.1 shows the contributions made by different food groups to energy intakes in the UK excluding the contribution from alcohol and chocolate and sugar

confectionery (MAFF 1985). The national average energy intake for 1983 was 2140 kcal (9.0 mJ) per person per day. In addition, the national supplies of alcoholic drinks provided 151 kcal (0.63 MJ) and those of chocolate and sugar confectionery 137 kcal (0.57 MJ) per person per day on average.

Factors affecting the contribution of a food to total energy intake

Energy content per 100 g

Energy content per 100 g is just one of the factors which are important when considering the contribution which a particular food makes to energy intake. Also of relevance are:

The portion size typically consumed. Foods with a relatively high energy content per 100 g may not neces-

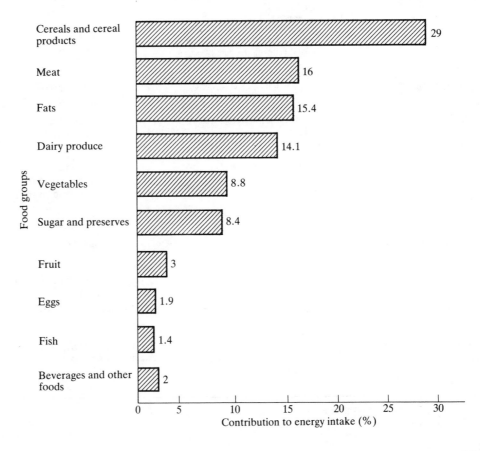

Fig. 2.1 Sources of energy in the British diet. Contribution made by groups of foods to energy intake of the average British household (MAFF 1985).

sarily be high energy providers if only consumed in 5 or 10 g portions (e.g. jam or marmalade).

The frequency of consumption. Milk, for instance, contains less energy than cream but because milk is usually consumed more often, (as well as in larger quantities) it makes a more significant contribution to energy intake.

Other considerations

Nutrient density. As a general rule, foods in their natural state tend to have a high nutrient density for their energy value, e.g. fruit, vegetables and wholemeal cereals. In contrast, foods which have been fried or have added sugar tend to have a low nutrient density for energy, e.g. jam compared with fresh fruit.

Energy density. Fat and alcohol provide approximately twice as much energy per gram as protein or carbohydrate. It is therefore not surprising that food and drinks containing significant amounts of either fat or alcohol have a high energy content. However, most foods are complex and contain a mixture of the energy-providing nutrients. Protein, for instance, rarely occurs in isolation from fat in its natural state (white fish

Table 2.1 Energy contribution of different foods taking typical portion size** into account

Food group	High energy (>150 kcal/portion)	Medium energy (75–150 kcal/portion)	Low energy (<75 kcal/portion)
Cereal and cereal products	Pastry*, pies*, puddings* cakes*, scones*, doughnuts* pancakes*, sweetened breakfast cereals, chocolate and sweet biscuits*, pizza, quiches	Bread, flour, pasta, rice, semi-sweet and water biscuits*, unsweetened breakfast cereals	Crispbreads
Milk and milk products	Channel Island and full-fat milk, cream*, milk puddings, full and medium fat cheeses	Semi-skimmed milk, reduced fat cheeses, sweetened yoghurts	Low fat cheeses, natural yoghurt
Eggs	Egg yolk	Whole eggs	Egg white
Fats and oils	Butter*, margarine*, cooking and vegetable oils*, lard* suet*, dripping*, all fried foods*	Low fat spreads*	—
Meat and meat products	Fat on meat*, fatty meats* poultry skin*, sausages*, meat pies*, pasties, cold cuts e.g. luncheon meat*, salami*, spam, mortadella*, tongue, samosas*	Lean meat, poultry without skin	—
Fish and fish products	Oily fish, fish tinned in oil/tomato sauce, taramasalata	White fish, shellfish, fish tinned in brine, fish fingers	—
Vegetables	Fried and roast vegetables*, potato crisps*	Potatoes, pulses, baked beans, parsnips, sweetcorn, beetroot, yams, sweet potatoes, plantain	Green leafy vegetables, onions, leeks, swede, turnips runner/French beans, beansprouts, peppers, salad vegetables
Fruit	Avocado pears, dried fruit	Bananas, grapes, cherries mangoes, stewed dried fruit, fruit cooked with sugar, tinned fruit in syrup*, olives	All other fresh fruit, fresh fruit stewed without sugar
Nuts and seeds	All nuts except chestnuts, all seeds, peanut butter	Chestnuts	—
Sugar, preserves and confectionery	Sugar*, sweets*, chocolates*	Jam*, marmalade*	Reduced sugar jams
Beverages	Chocolate and malted drinks made with whole milk	Sugar-containing fizzy drinks*, fruit squash*, fruit juice (sweetened)* fruit juice (unsweetened)	Tea, coffee, Bovril, tomato juice, low calorie drinks*
Alcoholic beverages (per measure or ½ pint)	—	Spirits*, wine*, beer*, lager*, low alcohol beers and lager*	—
Sauces, soups and miscellaneous	Mayonnaise, salad cream*, French dressing*, crisps* and savoury snacks*, oily pickles and chutneys*	Proprietary sauce mixes*, gravy mixes*, sweetened pickles*, thickened soups	Oxo, Bovril, Marmite, low calorie and thin soups, low calorie salad dressings made without oil*, herbs and condiments, pickles in vinegar, Worcester sauce

*Foods with a relatively low nutrient density.
**See Section 1.5

excepted) and so foods containing protein tend to be energy dense. Foods naturally rich in carbohydrate are not linked with fat in the same way as protein. Moreover, fibre is not utilized by humans, so foods high in complex carbohydrates generally have a low energy content. However, it should be borne in mind that this relationship does not necessarily apply to manufactured or created foods such as cakes or biscuits.

The water content of foods. This influences the energy value of a food. For instance, 90% of broccoli is water and it provides only 18 kcal/100 g; a refined source of carbohydrate such as sugar contains only a trace of water and provides 394 kcal/100 g.

Satiety value. It can be argued that the bulk of low energy foods will provide a higher sense of satiety than energy dense foods, e.g. 285 g of apple has the same energy value as 25 g of cheddar cheese (100 kcal).

2.1.3 Altering the energy content of the diet

The energy contribution of different foods, taking typical portion size (see p 29) into account, is given in. Table 2.1.

Energy reduction

The diet should be composed of foods relatively low in energy with high nutrient density and high satiety value (see Table 2.1).

Energy supplementation

Emphasis should be on the use of energy dense foods which also have a high nutrient density. Proprietary energy supplements (see Section 2.12) can be used to modify recipes and supplement meals.

References

Darke SJ, Disselduff MM and Try GP (1980) Frequency distributions of mean daily intakes of food energy and selected nutrients obtained during nutrition surveys of different groups of people in Great Britain between 1968 and 1971. *Br J Nutr* **44**, 243–52.

Ministry of Agriculture, Fisheries and Food (1985) Household food consumption and expenditure: 1983. *Annual Report of the National Food Survey Committee.* HMSO, London.

2.2   Dietary Protein and Amino Acids

2.2.1   Sources of protein in the average British diet

The average British diet (as estimated from the survey of Household Food Consumption, MAFF 1985) provides approximately 70 g protein/person/day, about two-thirds of which is obtained from animal sources and one-third from vegetable sources (Fig. 2.2).

Most proteins contain about 16% nitrogen so the concentration of protein in a particular food can be obtained by multiplying its nitrogen content by 6.25. The approximate protein density (g protein/100 g food) of some common foods is listed in Table 2.2. However, as with all foods, the nutrient density alone does not necessarily reflect the importance of a food as a contributor to the daily protein intake; the likely portion size and the frequency of consumption must also be taken into account. For example, skimmed milk is one of the most concentrated sources of protein yet usually makes a minimal contribution to dietary protein content; in contrast, cereal foods contain a lower percentage of protein yet provide about one-quarter of the average person's daily protein intake.

It is important to remember that, unlike fat and carbohydrate, protein consumed in excess of immediate requirement cannot be stored by the body. In essence, only the energy component of any surplus will be retained and the excess nitrogen will be excreted.

2.2.2   Protein quality

In addition to considerations of quantity, the quality of the protein consumed is of vital importance. The quality of a particular dietary protein depends on the following factors.

Bioavailability

Usually over 90% of the amino acids in animal proteins are absorbed. The availability of those in vegetable proteins may be 80% or less.

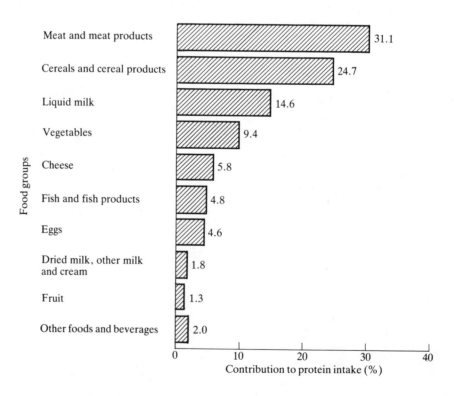

Fig. 2.2 Sources of protein in the average British diet. Percentage contribution made by groups of foods to the protein intake of the average British household (MAFF 1985).

Table 2.2 Typical protein content of some foods

Food	Protein content (g/100 g)
Dairy produce	
Dried skimmed milk	36.4
Liquid milk	3.3
Cheese (cheddar)	26.0
Yoghurt	5.0
Meat, fish and eggs	
Beef, lamb, pork, chicken (lean, raw)	20.5
Liver (raw)	20.1
Kidney (raw)	16.5
White fish (raw)	17.5
Mackerel (raw)	19.0
Pilchards (in tomato sauce)	18.8
Prawns (boiled)	22.6
Eggs	12.3
Cereals and cereal products	
Bread	
wholemeal	8.8
white	7.8
Flour	
wholemeal	13.2
white	9.5
Cornflakes	8.6
Muesli	12.9
All-bran	15.1
Rice (boiled)	2.2
Pasta (boiled)	4.2
Vegetables	
Beans	
baked (canned)	5.1
broad (boiled)	4.1
butter (boiled)	7.1
haricot (boiled)	6.6
runner (boiled)	1.9
Brussels sprouts (boiled)	2.8
Cabbage (boiled)	1.7
Carrots (boiled)	0.6
Lentils (boiled)	7.6
Peas (boiled)	5.0
Potatoes (boiled)	1.4

Table 2.3 Amino acids

Essential amino acids	Leucine
	Isoleucine
	Valine
	Lysine
	Threonine
	Methionine
	Phenylalanine
	Tryptophan
	Histidine
Semi-essential	Cystine (can be synthesized from methionine)
	Tyrosine (can be synthesized from phenylalanine)
Non-essential	Glycine
	Arginine
	Proline
	Glutamic acid
	Aspartic acid
	Serine
	Alanine

Amino acid content (see Table 2.3)

Amino acids can be classified as follows
1 Essential, i.e. they cannot be synthesized by the body.
2 Semi-essential, i.e. they can be supplied by the metabolism of certain amino acids provided that these are consumed in adequate amounts.
3 Non-essential, i.e. they can be synthesized from carbon and nitrogen precursors.

Proteins which contain all the essential amino acids in sufficient amounts to support growth or maintain nutritional status are termed high biological value (HBV) protein. Proteins with a relatively low concentration of one or more essential amino acids are of low biological value (LBV).

Animal foods generally contain HBV protein while plant foods supply LBV protein. The major limiting essential amino acids in vegetable proteins are
1 Lysine (cereals).
2 Tryptophan (maize).
3 Sulphur-containing amino acids i.e. methionine and cystine (peas, beans and pulses).

However, by combining plant proteins limited in certain essential amino acids with others which contain relatively high amounts of those amino acids, a plant protein mixture which is of high biological value can be produced. This is a cardinal principle of vegan diets (see Section 3.9) where pulse dishes must be eaten with rice, bread or other cereal foods.

2.2.3 Altering the protein content of the diet

Protein supplementation

For those able to eat a normal diet, an increase in protein intake is usually achieved by eating foods which are relatively protein-dense and of high biological value (e.g. meat, fish, milk, cheese and eggs).

For those with poor appetites, the addition of skimmed milk to milk-based drinks and to some cooked foods is a useful way of boosting protein intake.

There are also a number of proprietary supplements high in protein which can be used as sip feeds, or as meal or between-meal supplements. These products are listed on p 74.

Protein restriction

A protein restriction is frequently indicated in the

Table 2.4a, b 6g and 7g protein exchanges **a)** High biological value (HBV) protein exchanges

Food	Quantity for a 7 g protein exchange	Quantity for a 6 g protein exchange	Also high (√) in		
			Na[1]	K[1]	P[1]
Dairy produce					
Milk					
cows'/goats'	$\frac{1}{3}$ pt	180 ml		√	√
evaporated	3 fl.oz	70 ml		√	√
breast, modified baby milk	$\frac{3}{4}$ pt	400 ml			
Cheese (cheddar)	1 oz	25 g	√	√	√
Cottage cheese[2]	$1\frac{3}{4}$ oz	45 g			
Cheese curd[2]	$1\frac{1}{4}$ oz	30 g			√
Yoghurt	5 oz	120 g		√	√
Eggs					
Hen's egg	One large	One small			
Meat					
Bacon (lean, cooked)	$\frac{3}{4}$ oz	20 g	√		
Meat (lean, cooked)	1 oz	25 g			
Poultry (cooked)	1 oz	25 g			
Liver/kidney	1 oz	25 g			√
Fish					
White fish (e.g. cod)	$1\frac{1}{2}$ oz	35 g			
Smoked fish (steamed)	1 oz	25 g	√		
Sardines	1 oz	25 g	√		
Fish fingers[2]	2	$1\frac{1}{2}$			
Shrimps/prawns (with shells)	1 oz	25 g	√		√
Mussels	$1\frac{1}{2}$ oz	35 g	√		√

b) Low biological value (LBV) protein exchanges

Food	Quantity for a 7 g protein exchange	Quantity for a 6 g protein exchange	Also high (√) in		
			Na[1]	K[1]	P[1]
Meat products					
Sausage (cooked)	$1\frac{1}{2}$ oz	45 g	√		
Haggis	$2\frac{1}{4}$ oz	55 g	√		
Peas and beans					
Baked beans	5 oz	120 g		√	√
Haricot beans					
raw	1 oz	25 g		√	√
cooked	$3\frac{1}{2}$ oz	90 g		√	√
Peas (fresh, frozen)	4 oz	100 g		√	√
Mung beans (raw)	1 oz	25 g		√	√
Lentils					
raw	1 oz	25 g		√	√
cooked	$3\frac{1}{4}$ oz	80 g		√	√
Nuts					
Almonds	$1\frac{1}{2}$ oz	35 g		√	√
Brazil nuts	2 oz	40 g		√	√
Chestnuts	11 oz	250 g		√	√
Hazel nuts	3 oz	75 g		√	√
Peanuts (unsalted)	1 oz	25 g		√	√

[1]Na = sodium; K = potassium; P = phosphorus.
[2]Contains some sodium; usually allowed on a 'No added salt' diet.

Table 2.4c. 2 g protein exchanges. (All are low biological value (LBV) unless marked with an asterisk.)

Food	Imperial	Metric	Na[1]	K[1]	P[1]
Cereal products					
Bread (1 large thin slice)	1oz	25 g			
Flour (wheat, plain)	½ oz	15 g			
Pastry	1 oz	25 g	✓		
Pasta					
raw	½ oz	15 g			
boiled	1¾ oz	50 g			
Oatmeal	½ oz	15 g			
Rice					
raw*	1 oz	30 g			
cooked*	3½ oz	100 g			
Breakfast cereals					
Cornflakes	1 oz	25 g			
Puffed Wheat	½ oz	15 g			✓
Rice Krispies*[2]	1 oz	25 g			✓
Shredded Wheat	1	1 g			✓
Sugar Puffs	1 oz	25 g			
Weetabix	1	1 g		✓	✓
Biscuits and cakes					
Cream crackers[2]	3	3			
Digestive biscuits[2]	2	2			
Semi-sweet biscuits	4 small	4 small			
Sponge cake (without fat)	1 oz	25 g			
Dairy produce					
Cream cheese*	2 oz	60 g	✓		
Double cream*	4½ oz	125 g			
Malted drink[2]	3 tsp	3 tsp	✓		
Vegetables					
Green vegetables	2½ oz	75 g		✓	
Carrots/celery/cucumber/lettuce	11 oz	300 g		✓	
Sweetcorn (boiled)	1¾ oz	50 g		✓	
Potatoes (boiled)*	5 oz	140 g		✓	
Yam (raw)	3½ oz	100 g		✓	
Miscellaneous					
Chocolate					
milk	1 oz	25 g		✓	✓
plain	1¾ oz	50 g		✓	✓
Crisps*	1 small pkt	30 g	✓	✓	
Chappati	1 small	1 small			
Yorkshire pudding*	1 oz	25 g			✓

[1]Na = sodium; K = potassium; P = phosphorus.
[2]contain some sodium — usually permitted on 'No added salt' diets.
*High biological value protein.

management of disorders associated with liver and renal dysfunction (see Sections 4.13 and 4.16).

The degree of protein restriction required will depend on the severity of the disease state and will be a compromise between the body's requirement for protein and the clinical indications. Because protein intake is limited, the biological value of the protein which is consumed is a vital consideration.

In some instances, the intake of other nutrients such as sodium, potassium or phosphorus may also have to be controlled and this further limits the choice, as well as the amount, of protein foods which can be consumed. In such cases protein-containing foods high in sodium, potassium and phosphorus must also be identified and excluded from or limited in the patient's diet.

These potentially complicated dietary manipulations are usually achieved by means of protein exchange lists. These give the quantity of food which provides a certain amount of protein of either high or low biological value.

Table 2.5 Composition of low protein diets

	Protein intake				
	20 g	30 g	40 g	50 g	60 g
Daily allowance of					
Milk	150 ml	150 ml	200 ml	200 ml	200 ml
Protein exchange[1]	1 × 6 g protein exchange divided between two meals	2 × 6 g protein exchanges divided between two meals	3 × 6 g protein exchanges divided between three meals	5 × 6 g protein exchanges divided between three meals	7 × 6 g protein exchanges divided between three meals
Breakfast cereal[2]	—	—	1 × 2 g protein exchange	1 × 2 g protein exchange	1 × 2 g protein exchange
Bread[3]	2 × 2 g protein exchanges	2 × 2 g protein exchanges	3 × 2 g protein exchanges	3−4 × 2 g protein exchanges	3−4 × 2 g protein exchanges
Potatoes, rice or pasta[4]	2 × 2 g protein exchanges	2 × 2 g protein exchanges	2 × 2 g protein exchanges	2 × 2 g protein exchanges	2 × 2 g protein exchanges
Average portions of	Low protein vegetables or salad[6], fruit[6], sugar and butter or polyunsaturated margarine[5]				
	Extra energy from glucose polymers and/or fat emulsions if necessary. An allowance of double cream can be given.				

[1]6 g Protein exchanges: 1 exchange = 25 g cooked meat/35 g fresh cooked fish 1 egg. (80 g cooked lentils — not suitable in renal disease)
[2]Type of cereal not specified unless soldium intake is restricted. Muesli should be avoided due to variability of composition and protein content.
[3]Standard thin slice from large loaf.
[4]Potatoes should be limited or avoided if potassium restriction is necessary.
[5]Salt free butter should be used if there is need for a strict sodium restriction.
[6]Fruit and vegetables will need to be limited if a potassium restriction is indicated.
Low protein products (Table 2.7) may be required to add variety and increase energy intake.

Table 2.6 Foods not allowed on a low protein diet. Meat, fish, eggs and cheese should be eaten only in the quantities specified in the diet plan

Dairy products
Extra milk (see exchange list)
Milk powders*
Instant creams
Single cream
Yoghurt (can be exchanged for milk allowance)
Tinned milk
Sour cream
Skimmed milk
Buttermilk

Cereal products
Extra bread (see exchange list)
High protein breads and cereals
Biscuits (see exchange list)
Bought cakes (see exchange list)
Bought pastry (see exchange list)
Semolina
Macaroni
Barley
Breakfast cereals (see exchange list)
Muesli
Extra porridge oats (see exchange list)

Sweet foods
Lemon curd
Fruit pastilles and gums
Fancy chocolates
Extra chocolate (see exchange list)
Drinking chocolate
Cocoa
Malted drinks (see exchange list)

Marzipan
Extra nuts (see exchange list)
Dried fruit and prunes
Ice cream (see exchange list)
Ice cream mixes
Mousse
Jelly, (agar jelly allowed)
Whips and instant puddings
Virol
Advocaat

Vegetables
Extra butter beans
Baked beans
Broad beans — see
Haricot beans — exchange
Peas — list
Lentils
Spinach
Mushrooms (except as a garnish)

Savoury foods
Salad cream
Mayonnaise
Tinned and packet soups
Sauce mixes
Batter mixes
Packet stuffings
Meat pastes
Fish pastes
Bemax
Bovril

*Coffeemate and similar whiteners not made from milk can be used to extend the milk allowance.

Table 2.7 Proprietary low protein foods

Food	Manufacturer/distributor**
Bread	
Juvela low protein loaf	GF Dietary Supplies Ltd
Rite Diet gluten-free low protein bread	
Rite Diet gluten-free low protein bread with soya bran	Welfare Foods Ltd
*Rite Diet low protein white bread with added fibre	
*Rite Diet low protein bread with no added salt	
Flour and bread mixes	
Juvela low protein mix	GF Dietary Supplies Ltd
*Rite Diet low protein flour mix	Welfare Foods Ltd
Aproten flour	Ultrapharm
Tritamyl PK PF flour	Procea
Rite Diet gluten-free baking powder (NP)	Welfare Foods Ltd
Biscuits	
Aproten low protein biscuits	Ultrapharm
*Aglutella cream-filled wafers	GF Dietary Supplies Ltd
dP cookies	
*Rite Diet low protein vanilla cream wafers	
*Rite Diet low protein chocolate flavoured cream wafers	Welfare Foods Ltd
*Rite Diet low protein sweet biscuits	
*Rite Diet low protein cream-filled biscuits — chocolate flavour	
Crackers/crispbread	
Aproten crispbread	Ultrapharm
Rite Diet low protein, gluten-free crackers	Welfare Foods Ltd
Pasta	
*Aglutella pasta and semolina	GF Dietary Supplies Ltd
*Aproten pasta	Ultrapharm
*Rite Diet low protein pasta	Welfare Foods Ltd

*Low sodium content
**Addresses of manufacturers/distributors are given on p 617
NP = Not prescribable

The dietary plan should specify the number of exchanges to be eaten at each meal but the patient, if well enough, is free to choose the food. The patient will also require guidance as to which foods may be eaten freely and which are contraindicated.

The most commonly used protein exchanges are 6 g or 7 g of HBV protein and 2 g of LBV protein. 7 g protein exchanges lend themselves to imperial measures whilst 6 g exchanges are more appropriate for metric quantities. Most adults prefer to use imperial measures but there are an increasing number of adolescents who are more familiar with metric quantities.

Tables 2.4, 2.5 and 2.6 provide details of protein exchanges and the construction of low protein regimens. However, it should be noted that these tables are for use by dietitians and are not presented in a format which is suitable to be given directly to the patient.

Proprietary low protein foods

Some proprietary low protein foods are prescribable for some disorders (e.g. liver or renal failure). A list of low protein foods currently available is given in Table 2.7. Up-to-date information regarding the availability and prescribability of these products can be found in the Monthly Index of Medical Specialities (MIMS) or the British National Formulary.

It should be noted that while most proprietary low protein foods can be used on a gluten-free diet (see p 188), only some proprietary gluten-free products can be used on a low protein diet.

Reference

Ministry of Agriculture, Fisheries and Food (1985) Household food consumption and expenditure; 1983. *Annual report of the National Food Survey Committee.* HMSO, London.

2.3 Dietary Fats

2.3.1 Composition of food fats

Fats in food differ widely in both amount and type. This makes it very difficult to estimate the nutritional value of foods which contain fat. However, it is possible to get some idea of the quantity and nutritional quality of the different fats which occur in food if one understands something of the properties of fats, their biological functions and the effects of refining or other processing.

About 21 different fatty acids are found in significant quantities in the fats of an average diet (Table 2.8). The contrasts in the properties and nutritional values of different fats are due to variation in the amounts and types of fatty acids they contain. Both the common and the systematic names are frequently used for many fatty acids. For others, the common name is more frequently used because it is equally precise and more convenient. Some fatty acids do not have a common name.

Fatty acids are composed of a chain of carbon atoms with an acid (carboxyl) group at one end. They are described according to two characteristics: chain length and the degree of saturation with hydrogen. Saturated fatty acids are hard at room temperature, and often referred to as 'storage' fats. They are chemically stable if stored in the body and have long shelf lives if used in food. Their use minimizes the formation of rancid flavours in food during storage and hence are of obvious value to food manufacturers. However, they are not 'essential' in the diet and may well have harmful effects if they predominate in the dietary fat intake.

Increased fluidity is achieved in animal tissues by the addition of unsaturated bonds to the carbon chain. One to six unsaturated bonds are common. These more unsaturated fatty acids (called mono- or poly-unsaturated fatty acids) are used for cell structures and prostaglandin synthesis and are important in all tissues. Muscles in particular require a high fluidity in order to allow the tissue to expand and contract. Fish fats are the most unsaturated, reflecting their need for flexibility at low temperatures. Polyunsaturated fatty acids (PUFA) readily oxidize, which is one cause of the rapid deterioration of fish once caught.

2.3.2 Metabolism of fatty acids in humans

Animals, including humans, can synthesize saturated fatty acids from carbohydrate and from some amino acids when there is excess energy in the diet. They can also add one double bond to a saturated fat, and thus synthesize a monounsaturated fatty acid. However, almost all of the fatty acids containing more than one double bond i.e. the polyunsaturated fatty acids, cannot be synthesized and must be obtained from the diet. These polyunsaturated fatty acids are thus called 'essential fatty acids' (efa).

There are two families of efa — the omega-6 and the omega-3 families (Fig. 2.3). The most common efa in the diet is linoleic acid.

2.3.3 P/S ratio

The P/S ratio refers to the balance of the essential polyunsaturated fatty acids to the non-essential, saturated fatty acids. The P/S ratio is a useful concept owing to the fact that saturated fats compete with the utilization of the essential fatty acids. A high intake of saturated fat increases the requirement for efa. The FAO/WHO (1980) recommended a dietary P/S ratio of 1.0, The National Advisory Committee on Nutrition Education (1983) also suggested that a value of about 1.0 is likely to be beneficial while the COMA report (1984) recommended a ratio of 0.45. The British Medical Association (1986) suggested a ratio of 0.48. They also pointed out that present evidence suggests that a P/S ratio of two or more is not conducive to a reduction in total mortality rates even though the incidence of coronary heart disease may decline.

2.3.4 Cis and trans fatty acids

Double bonds in mono and poly-unsaturated fatty acids can occur in one of two shapes, cis or trans. Most naturally occurring fatty acids contain cis double bonds although significant proportions of fatty acids

Table 2.8 Nomenclature of fatty acids commonly found in food

Carbon: double bonds	Common name	Systematic name	Common natural sources
Saturated			
4:0	Butyric	Tetranoic	
6:0	Caproic	Hexanoic	
8:0	Caprylic	Octanoic	
10:0	Capric	Decanoic	Coconut oil and dairy products.
12:0	Lauric	Dodecanoic	
14:0	Myristic	Tetradecanoic	
16:0	Palmitic	Hexadecanoic	Palm oil, cottonseed oil, butter, meat fat.
18:0	Stearic	Octadecanoic	Meat fat, butter, chocolate.
20:0	Arachidic	Eicosanoic	Nut and seed oils.
22:0	Behenic	Docosanoic	Peanut oil, peanuts.
Monounsaturated			
16:1n7	Palmitoleic	9 cis-hexadecenoic	Cod liver oil, meat fat, fish.
18:1n9	Oleic	9 cis-octadecenoic	Olive oil, nut and seed oils, meat fat, butter, eggs, avocado.
18:1n9	Elaidic	9 trans-octadecenoic	Hydrogenated oils, fats from ruminants.
20:1n9	—	11 cis-eicosenoic	Fish, peanut oil.
22:1n9	Erucic	13 cis-dodecenoic	Rapeseed if not a low erucic variety.
Polyunsaturated			
18:2n6	Linoleic	—	Vegetable oils, nuts, lean meat and eggs.
18:3n3	Alpha-linolenic	—	Soyabean and rapeseed oils.
18:3n6	Gamma-linolenic	—	Evening Primrose oil
20:4n6	Arachidonic	—	Offal, game, lean meat, egg.
20:5n3	—	Eicosapentaenoic(EPA)	Fish.
22:6n3	—	Docosahexanoic	Fish, liver, egg yolk.

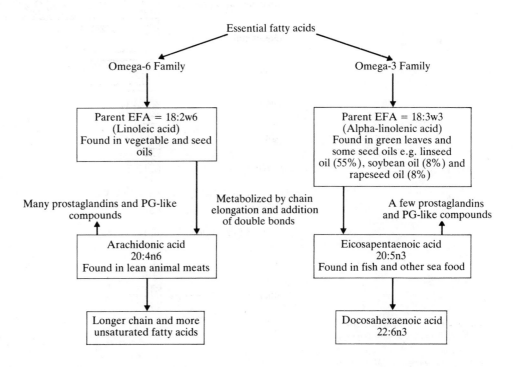

Fig. 2.3 Essential fatty acids.

with trans double bonds are found in partially hydrogenated vegetable oils, margarines made from them and in fat from ruminant meats, milk and milk products. Trans isomers of efa are of no use to the body and therefore are no longer 'essential'. Since they can affect the metabolism of cis essential fatty acids they may also be undesirable. Because they are metabolized similarly to saturated fats, some expert committees (COMA 1984; BMA 1986) recommend that they should be regarded as equivalent to saturated fats for the purpose of recommendations.

2.3.5 Reduction of dietary fat intake

The total amount of fat consumed may need to be reduced either as a general health measure of for a specific therapeutic purpose. In order to do this the principal sources of fat in the diet must be identified and the intake of these foods reduced and/or the food replaced with a low fat alternative. For most people, this will mean alteration in the intake of spreading fats and cooking oils, meat and meat products and milk

(Fig. 2.4). In addition, the consumption of other foods high in fat (such as cheese, double cream and pastry) may also need to be adjusted. However, it must be remembered that the fat density (g/100 g) of a food is not necessarily a good reflector of that food's importance to the daily fat consumption. The frequency of consumption and quantity consumed must also be taken into account. For example, on a g/100 g basis, full fat milk is a relatively low fat food yet is usually one of the major contributors to total fat intake. Substituting full fat milk with a skimmed or semi-skimmed alternative is therefore an important therapeutic measure. Similarly, a food such as a roast potato also contains a relatively low percentage of fat compared to some foods, but patients should still be advised to cook potatoes by an alternative method which avoids the use of fat. The data in Table 2.9, which stratifies foods according to their fat density and lists the amount of each which will provide 10 g fat, therefore needs to be used with caution. However, some patients, particularly those requiring severe fat restriction, may find a 'fat exchange' list compiled from this information helpful.

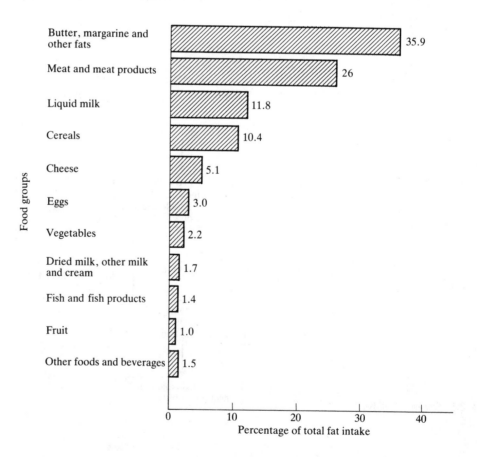

Fig. 2.4 Sources of fat in the average British diet. Percentage contribution made by groups of foods to the fat intake of the average British household. (MAFF 1985).

Table 2.9 Food portions which contain 10 g fat

Food group	High fat foods Fat density ≥ 20 g/100 g	Portion containing 10 g fat	Medium fat foods Fat density 10–20 g/100 g	Portion containing 10 g fat	Low fat foods Fat density 5–10 g/100 g	Portion containing 10 g fat	Very low fat foods Very low fat density or fat free	Portion containing 10 g fat
Milk, cream	Butter	12 g	Full fat yoghurt	300 g	Evaporated, condensed milk	100 g	Gold top milk[a]	⅓ pt
	Double cream	20 g					Silver top milk[a]	½ pt
	Whipping cream	30 g					Semi-skimmed[a]	1 pt
	Milk powder	40 g					Skimmed milk, fresh	
	Single or soured cream	50 g					or dried, low fat yoghurt	
Oils, fats, spreads	Vegetable oils, lard, dripping	10 g	Low fat spread	25 g			Bottled sauces and pickles, marmite,	
			Salad cream,	35 g			jams, honey, bovril,	
	Margarine, butter	12 g					tomatoes etc,	
	Mayonnaise	12 g					onions, herbs, spices	
Eggs	Scrambled eggs	45 g	Boiled eggs (2)	100 g			Egg white	
	Fried eggs	50 g						
	Scotch egg	50 g						
Cheese	Stilton	25 g	Feta	50 g			Cottage cheese	
	Cream cheese	20 g	Tendale	70 g				
	Cheddar, Cheshire	30 g	Curd cheese	90 g				
	Danish blue, Parmesan,	35 g						
	Edam, cheese spread (e.g. dairylea)	45 g						
Cheese dishes	Quiche	35 g	Cheese souffle	55 g	Macaroni cheese	100 g		
	Welsh rarebit	40 g	Pizza	90 g	Cauliflower cheese	125 g		
			Cheese pudding	95 g				
Meats	Fried streaky bacon	20 g	Grilled lean back bacon	50 g	Home cooked lean ham	100 g	Turkey breast, White fish	
	Boiled brisket	40 g	Fried rump steak, (with fat)	70 g	Lean grilled rump steak	170 g		
			Stewed mince	70 g	Lean roast beef	110 g		
	Lamb chop (with fat)	30 g	Lean lamb chop	85 g	Lean roast leg lamb	120 g		
	Pork chop (with fat)	40 g	Lean pork chop	95 g	Lean roast leg pork	150 g		
	Roast duck, (with fat)	25 g	Roast chicken, (with skin)	70 g	Roast chicken (no skin)	185 g		
	Liver paté	40 g	Fried lamb's liver	70 g	Grilled lamb's kidney	100 g		
	Luncheon meat	40 g	Corned beef	80 g	Canned lean ham	195 g		
	Pork sausages	40 g	Steaklets, beefburgers, hamburgers	60 g				
	Sausage roll	25 g	Moussaka	75 g	Lean meat in stew, hot pot, shepherd's pie, curry	150–200 g		
	Pork pie	35 g	Bolognese sauce	100 g				
	Pastie, meat pie,	50 g						
Fish	Taramosalata	20 g	Fried cod in batter	100 g	Pichards in tomato sauce	185 g	All poached or steamed white fish and shellfish	
	Fried whitebait	20 g	Canned salmon	120 g				
	Fried scampi	55 g	Sardines	85 g				
			Fish fingers	100 g				
Vegetables and nuts and soups	Crisps	30 g	Thick chips	100 g	Roast potatoes	200 g	All potatoes cooked without fat. All	
	Low fat crisps	50 g	Olives	90 g	Oven ready chips	140 g	vegetables, salad,	
	Frozen fried chips	50 g	Cream and thick soups (e.g tomato, lentil, oxtail)	250g			peas, beans, lentils (except soya) with no added fat	
	Soya beans	45 g						
	Avocado pears	45 g						
	Nuts and nut butters	20 g						
Sweets and chocolates	Milk chocolate	35 g	Mars bar	50 g			All plain sweets	
			Toffees	60 g				

Table 2.9 *contd.*

Food group	High fat foods Fat density ≥ 20 g/100 g	Portion containing 10 g fat	Medium fat foods Fat density 10–20 g/100 g	Portion containing 10 g fat	Low fat foods Fat density 5–10 g/100 g	Portion containing 10 g fat	Very low fat foods Very low fat density or fat free	Portion containing 10 g fat
Breads, breakfast cereals	Fried bread	25 g	Chapatis	80 g	Muesli Ready brek Soft rolls	133 g 115 g 150 g	All other bread, pasta, rice, cereals, breakfast cereals	
Biscuits	Chocolate (orange creams, Penguins, etc.) Filled wafers Custard creams Chocolate digestive Shortbread Home made Easter Lincoln, crunch biscuits	35 g 35 g 40 g 40 g 40 g 45 g 45 g	Cream crackers Rich tea Oatcakes Ginger nuts Water biscuits	60 g 60 g 55 g 65 g 80 g	Starch reduced	130 g	Matzo, rye crispbread	
Cakes	Flaky pastry Short pastry Victoria sponge Chocolate eclairs Mince pies	25 g 30 g 40 g 40 g 50 g	Madeira, rock cakes Doughnuts, jam tarts Scones Plain iced cakes Fruit cake	60 g 65 g 70 g 70 g 85 g	Currant bun Sponge with no fat, (e.g. Swiss roll)	130 g 150 g	Meringues	
Puddings	Cheesecake	30 g	Custard tart Pancakes Sponge pudding Fruit pie (two crust) Lemon meringue pie, Treacle tart	60 g 60 g 60 g 65 g 70 g	Trifle Fruit tart Bread and butter pudding Ice cream Apple crumble Egg custard	165 g 130 g 130 g 140 g 150 g 170 g	Jelly, low fat yoghurt, fresh, canned or frozen fruit, custard or other milk pudding made with skimmed milk (fresh or powdered)	

[a]Milk contains the following fat per 100 g: gold top (Jersey) 4.8 g; silver top (Fresian) and red top (homogenized) 3.8 g; silver and red top (semi-skimmed) 2.0 g; blue top (skimmed) 0.1 g.

Reproduced (with permission) from Bingham (1987).

2.3.6 Low fat substitutes

This is a relatively new market area and one which is being expanded steadily. Dietitians should therefore alert themselves to new products as they appear. At the time of writing, statutory regulations apply only to claims on fat in foods relating to the PUFA and cholesterol content. There are no regulations on 'low fat' claims as such, so any such product must be evaluated individually on the grounds of total fat content in relation to the parent food. 'Low fat' foods currently available include

1 Low fat and semi-skimmed milks. These are often identified by blue (or striped blue and silver) and striped red and silver tops respectively.
2 Low fat yoghurts.
3 Low fat spreads. Outline and St. Ivel Gold are popular brands and many supermarket chains provide similar products under their own label.
4 Low fat cheeses. These include St. Ivel Shape, Tendale and similar supermarket own brands. They

are an acceptable and lower fat alternative to full or medium fat cheeses but none of these are as low in fat as cottage cheese.

Other products such as low fat sausages, low fat pies and low fat salad dressings are also available from some food outlets.

2.3.7 Fat labelling

Currently the only food labelling requirements regarding fat relate to polyunsaturates and cholesterol. By law (Food Labelling Regulations SI No 1305, 1984) those foods which contain a minimum of 35 g per 100 g food, e.g. margarines, which are claimed by their manufacturers to be high in PUFA must contain a minimum of 45% by weight as polyunsaturated and no more than 25% saturated fat. In this instance, saturated fat is not required to include trans fatty acids. Margarines claiming to be low in cholesterol must contain no more than 0.005% cholesterol by weight. In the absence of such claims by the manufacturer, it is not possible to determine the degree of saturation or cholesterol level in a product.

Food labelling is currently under review (see Section 2.18). The Ministry of Agriculture, Fisheries and Food have issued proposals (1986) on labelling. They have suggested that almost all foods should be labelled with their fat and saturated fat (including trans fatty acids) content. Foods to be exempted are currently suggested to be those containing less than 0.5 g fat/100 g food (for example fresh fruit, vegetables, spices and herbs and alcohol) and bread and flour (as defined by bread and flour regulations). Foods sold for immediate consumption (e.g. in restaurants) will probably also be exempt.

2.3.8 Fatty acid content of principle fat sources

An overwhelming variety of oils and margarines is available for human consumption. The fatty acid composition of margarines, blended vegetable oils and foods to which fat is added (such as biscuits, cakes and pastry products) will vary from one manufacturer to another. Individual manufacturers may also change the fat used according to the market price of oils and fats. For many foods, the fatty acids have been derived predominantly from the manufacturing or cooking process rather than from the food itself. This means that differences in the fats used will alter the contents of saturated, polyunsaturated and trans fatty acids.

The result is a wide variation between foods of the same type (Table 2.10). Therefore, it is important, when assessing fatty acid intakes, to obtain not only the make of fats used for spreading and cooking but also the name of the manufacturer of foods in which fat is an ingredient.

A breakdown of fatty acid contents of the principle fats and oils is given in Table 2.11 and of the principle food fat sources in Table 2.12.

2.3.9 Dietary cholesterol

A 'cholesterol-lowering diet' is not the same as a 'low cholesterol diet'. The former might incorporate high linoleic acid foods, e.g. sunflower oil which has the effect of lowering blood cholesterol; the latter simply

Table 2.10 Range of total saturates, linoleic, alpha-linolenic and trans fatty acids in some manufactured foods of different makes

Fatty acids	Potato crisps Range (g/100 g) ($n = 11$)	Cheesecakes Range (g/100 g) ($n = 6$)	Gateaux Range (g/100 g) ($n = 7$)	Solid cooking fats Range (g/100 g) ($n = 15$)
Saturates	5.8−14.3	3.7−10.5	4.4−11.3	19.2−48.9
18:2n6	4.5−18.1	0.5− 0.8	0.4− 4.7	0.4−43.0
18:3n3	0.1− 2.1	0.1− 0.2	0.1− 1.1	0.02− 4.6
Trans	0.3− 5.0	0.7− 1.1	0.4− 1.2	0.7−39.8

Table 2.11 Fatty acid content and P/S ratios of the principle edible fats and oils in order of PUFA content

Oils/fats	Total fat (g/100 g)	Saturates (excl. trans) (g/100 g)	Monoenes (g/100 g)	PUFA (g/100 g)	P/S ratio
Grapeseed oil	99.9	13.9	16.8	64.6	4.7
Safflower oil	99.9	15.6	16.7	64.5	4.1
Corn oil	99.9	11.3	24.5	59.5	5.3
Soya oil	99.9	14.0	24.3	56.7	4.0
Sunflower oil	99.9	13.1	31.8	49.9	3.8
Sesame seed oil	99.9	14.2	35.7	45.0	3.2
Margarine (good quality)	81.0	14.2	12.6	43.5	3.1
Peanut/groundnut/arachis oil	99.9	18.8	47.8	28.5	1.5
Blended oil (good quality)	99.9	6.5	60.2	28.4	4.4
Blended oil (poor quality)	99.9	13.8	53.5	23.1	1.7
Lard (pork fat)	99.0	36.2	44.4	10.3	0.3
Palm oil	99.0	49.3	37.0	9.3	0.2
Olive oil	99.9	13.5	73.7	8.4	0.8
Margarine (poor quality)	81.0	34.7	32.0	3.8	0.1
Dripping	99.0	58.8	44.2	3.6	0.06
Butter	82.0	48.8	27.2	2.4	0.05
Coconut oil	99.0	85.2	6.6	1.7	0.02
Coconut cream	82.0	87.2	6.3	1.0	0.01

Analysed by Nuffield Laboratory of Comparative Medicine.

Table 2.12 Fatty acid content of the principle fat sources in food

		Total fat (g/100 g)	Saturates (g/100 g)	Monoenes (g/100 g)	PUFA (g/100 g)	Trans (g/100 g)
Dairy foods						
(mean of summer and winter)						
Cheese						
cottage	*	4.0	2.6	0.9	0.1	0.2
cheddar	*	33.5	21.3	7.8	0.5	1.9
cream	*	47.4	30.1	11.1	0.7	2.8
Egg						
whole raw	*	10.5	3.5	5.4	1.3	Tr
fried in dripping	*	19.5	6.8	7.4	1.4	0.3
fried in corn oil	*	19.5	4.6	6.6	5.1	Tr
Milk						
skimmed, fresh	*	0.1	0.05	0.02	0.0	Tr
whole, fresh	*	3.8	2.4	0.9	0.1	0.2
Channel Island	*	4.8	3.1	1.1	0.1	0.3
Cream						
single	*	21.2	13.5	4.9	0.3	1.2
whipping	*	35.0	22.2	8.2	0.5	2.1
double	*	48.2	30.6	11.3	0.7	2.8
Meat						
Chicken (roast)						
no skin	§	5.4	1.8	2.4	0.8	—
with skin	§	14.0	4.6	6.3	2.1	—
Beef topside (roast)						
lean	*	4.4	1.9	1.4	0.7	0.1
lean and fat	*	12.0	1.9	4.5	1.0	0.4
Lamb, leg (roast)						
lean	*	8.1	4.0	2.4	0.7	0.5
lean and fat	*	17.9	9.2	5.3	0.9	1.3
Pork, leg (roast)						
lean	*	6.9	2.6	2.3	1.7	0.02
lean and fat	*	19.8	7.9	7.3	3.7	0.08
Corned Beef	*	12.1	5.6	4.9	0.3	0.6
Sausages (grilled)						
pork	*	24.6	9.9	9.4	4.0	0.1
beef	*	17.3	8.0	7.0	0.4	0.8
Pork pie	*	27.0	10.5	13.0	2.8	—
Cornish pastie	*	20.4	8.9	8.7	2.2	—
Fish						
Oily fish						
Herring (grilled)	§	13.0	2.6	6.5	2.3	0.9
Kipper (baked, net weight)	§	11.4	2.3	5.7	2.0	0.9
Mackerel (raw)	§	16.3	3.9	6.3	4.1	1.0
Pilchards in tomato sauce	§	5.4	1.7	1.2	1.8	1.0
Salmon (tinned)	§	8.2	2.0	3.1	2.1	1.0
Sardines (fish only)	§	13.6	2.7	7.4	2.7	1.0
White fish						
Haddock (steamed)		0.8	0.11	0.14	0.26	2.4

Note. The fat content of fish will vary with maturity of fish and time of year. Oily fish caught in British waters, e.g. herring and mackerel, are highest in fat content in the winter months.

Nuts and seeds (net weights)						
Almonds	§	53.5	4.2	36.6	10.0	0.0
Brazil nuts	§	61.5	15.7	20.2	22.9	0.0
Cashew (dry roasted)	†	46.4	9.2	27.3	7.8	0.0
Coconut (fresh)	§	36.0	30.9	2.4	0.6	0.0
Hazel nuts	§	36.0	2.6	27.9	3.7	0.0
Peanuts	§	49.0	9.2	23.5	13.9	0.0
Peanut butter	§	53.7	10.6	27.2	13.4	0.0
Sesame seeds (dried)	†	49.7	7.0	18.8	21.8	0.0
Walnuts	§	51.5	5.6	8.0	35.1	0.0
Plant foods (net weights)						
Avocado[1]	§	22.2	2.6	16.7	1.9	0.0

Table 2.12 *contd.*

		Total fat (g/100 g)	Saturates (g/100 g)	Monoenes (g/100 g)	PUFA (g/100 g)	Trans (g/100 g)
Olives (in brine)	§	11.0	1.5	7.7	1.2	0.0
Potato crisps (mean of 7 brands)	*	·36.8	11.0	12.5	9.4	1.5
Cakes and Biscuits						
Biscuits						
Cream crackers	*	16.3	8.8	6.8	0.6	—
Digestives	*	20.5	8.3	10.3	1.8	—
Semi-sweet	*	16.6	7.8	7.5	1.1	—
Cakes (shop bought, mean of *n* samples)						
Cheesecake (*n* = 6)	*	13.6	6.4	5.2	0.9	0.8
Gateau (*n* = 7)	*	17.1	8.7	5.9	1.1	0.8
Fruit cake (*n* = 4	*	16.8	8.7	5.9	1.0	0.7
Chocolate						
Mars bar	*	18.9	10.4	5.9	1.2	0.5
Chocolate (milk)	*	30.3	18.2	8.9	1.1	0.3
Chocolate (plain)	*	29.2	17.8	8.2	1.5	0.2

Analysed by: *Nuffield Laboratories; †USA Agricultural Handbook; §McCance and Widdowson, First Supplement.
[1]Fat content of avocados varies according to season.

aims to reduce the intake of foods containing cholesterol. It must be pointed out that the amount of cholesterol synthesized and metabolized by the body itself is far greater than the amount usually consumed in the diet, of which only 50% may be absorbed. It is also worth noting that in healthy people, little correlation has been found between the intake of cholesterol and blood cholesterol levels. However, the level of cholesterol in the blood is increased with high intakes of dietary saturated fat and it can be lowered by increasing the intake of linoleic acid. A high intake of fibre, particularly gel-forming fibres (found for example in beans and other pulses), also leads to a reduction in cholesterol absorption from the intestine and increased faecal excretion of dietary cholesterol (Kritchevsky and Story 1974). A list of high, medium and low sources of cholesterol is given in Table 2.13.

Table 2.13 Sources of dietary cholesterol

Rich sources	All offal including paté, egg yolk, fish roes, mayonnaise, shell fish and dishes made with these ingredients.
Moderately rich sources	Fat on meat, duck, goose and cold cuts (e.g. salami) whole milk, tinned milks, cream, ice cream, cheese, butter, most commercially made cakes, biscuits and pastries, homemade dishes containing any of the above ingredients. Crisps and all shop bought foods made with unspecified fat/oil.
Poor sources	All fish (white and oily) and fish tinned in vegetable oil, very lean meats, poultry (no skin), skimmed milk, low fat yoghurt, cottage cheese, bread, margarines claiming to be low in cholesterol (i.e. <0.005% cholesterol).
Cholesterol-free	All vegetables and vegetable oils, fruit including avocado and olives, nuts, cereals, pasta (without added eggs), rice, popcorn (unbuttered), egg white, meringue, sugar.

References

Bingham SA (1987) *Everyman companion to food and nutrition.* LM Dent and Sons, London.

British Medical Association (1986) Diet, nutrition and health. Report of the Board of Science and Education. BMA, London.

FAO/WHO (1980) *Dietary fats and oils in human nutrition.* FAO Food and Nutrition Series No 20 Rome.

Computer fatty acid analysis of foods by modem. Nuffield Laboratories of Comparative Medicine, Institute of Zoology, London NW1 4RY.

Committee on Medical Aspects of Food Policy (1984) *Diet and cardiovascular disease. Report on Health and Social Subjects No 28.* HMSO, London.

Kritchevsky D and Story JA (1974) Binding of bile salts *in vitro* by non-nutritive fibre. *J Nutr* **104**, 458.

Ministry of Agriculture, Fisheries and Food (1984) *The food labelling regulation.* SI No 1305 Schedule 6, Part 2. HMSO, London.

Ministry of Agriculture, Fisheries and Food (1985) *Household food consumption and expenditure 1983.* Annual report of the National Food Survey Committee. HMSO, London.

National Advisory Committee on Nutrition Education (1983) *Proposals for nutrition guidelines for health education in Britain.* Health Education Council, London.

Paul AA, Southgate DAT and Russell J (1980) *First Supplement to McCance and Widdowson's The Composition of Foods.* HMSO, London.

2.4   Dietary carbohydrate

2.4.1   Composition

Dietary carbohydrate which is available to the human body is comprised of
1   Monosaccharides — glucose, fructose and galactose.
2   Disaccharides — sucrose (glucose + fructose), lactose (glucose + galactose) and maltose (glucose + glucose).
3   Polysaccharides — starch (a polymer of glucose synthesized by plants).

2.4.2   Sources of carbohydrate in the average British diet

In the UK, carbohydrate consumption has declined in recent years both in absolute terms and as a proportion of total energy intake. In the average British diet, carbohydrate comprises about 47% of the total energy intake or approximately 250 g per person per day (MAFF 1985). Of this, about one third is comprised of sucrose, approximately 7% is lactose and most of the remainder is starch.

The sources of carbohydrate in the average British diet (MAFF 1985) are shown in Fig. 2.5.

2.4.3   Alteration of carbohydrate intake

Carbohydrate supplementation

An increase in carbohydrate intake may be required in order to help meet the body's requirement for energy. This may be necessary as a result of energy requirements being increased (e.g. during catabolic states) or because the existing requirement for energy is not being met (e.g. due to loss of appetite or a therapeutic diet which curtails the intake of other energy-providing nutrients). In some patients, carbohydrate supplementation is relatively easy because there are so many foods which are concentrated sources of sucrose or starch. However, when appetite is poor or solid foods cannot be eaten, proprietary drinks or supplements based on glucose or liquid glucose polymers may be required. These provide a concentrated source of readily assimilable energy and in a form which is less sweet, and hence more palatable, than an equivalent

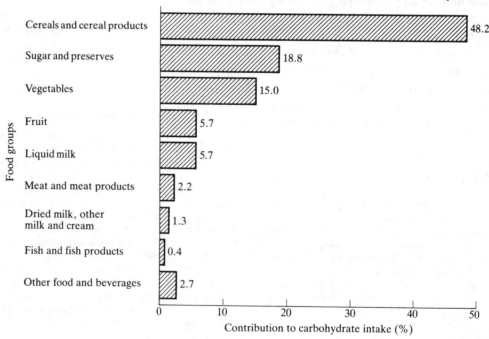

Fig. 2.5   Sources of carbohydrate in the average British diet. Percentage contribution made by groups of foods to the carbohydrate intake of the average British household (MAFF 1985).

GENERAL DIETETIC PRINCIPLES AND PRACTICE

amount of sucrose. Proprietary carbohydrate supplements are listed on p 74.

Carbohydrate restriction or regulation

There are two types of dietary carbohydrate restriction, general and specific

1 General. The total amount of carbohydrate consumed per day, and possibly per meal, has to be either restricted (e.g. Type IV hyperlipidaemia) or regulated (e.g. diabetes). In addition, the presence or absence of other nutrients in a particular carbohydrate food (e.g. in diabetes, its fibre content; in liver disease, its sodium content) may limit its suitability.

2 Specific. The intake of one or more types of carbohydrate (e.g. sucrose or lactose) must be either severely restricted or eliminated from the diet as a result of a specific intolerance.

General regulation or restriction of carbohydrate intake

If careful regulation of carbohydrate intake is required, this may necessitate the use of a carbohydrate exchange list. Such patients will usually be diabetics on insulin or some of those on oral hypoglycaemic therapy. Most diabetics treated mainly or solely by diet alone will not need to use a carbohydrate exchange list, although some may find one helpful. Table 2.14 provides a carbohydrate exchange list primarily designed for use in the treatment of diabetes. Each of the foods in the

list contains about 10 carbohydrate when eaten in the amount stated. The energy content of each serving is given in kcal. The most suitable forms of carbohydrate for the diabetic (i.e. fibre-rich sources) are marked with an asterisk. Not all patients will need to weigh their food portions although many may prefer to do so initially. Those who use household measures should use standard kitchen measuring spoons obtainable from the British Diabetic Association. In the exchange list, 1 tablespoon (tbs) = 1 level 15 ml spoon and 1 teaspoon (tsp) = 1 level 5 ml spoon.

Table 2.15 lists some low sodium 10 g carbohydrate exchanges and may be useful in the management of some cases of liver disease.

It should be noted that the information in Tables 2.14 and 2.15 is intended as a reference source for dietitians and is not necessarily in a format which is suitable to be handed to a patient. Some diabetics, particularly those who are elderly, will only be able to cope with simple information, e.g. a short list of the most common foods, with quantities expressed only in household measures. Asian or West Indian diabetics may require information about foods not usually included in a standard exchange list.

Much of the information in Table 2.14 has been derived from the *Food values list of diabetics* produced by the British Diabetic Association. Details of the carbohydrate content of many manufactured foods can be obtained from *Countdown*, also produced by the Association.

Table 2.14 10 g carbohydrate exchange list	Food item	Household measure	Weight (g)	Energy content (kcal)
	Bread[1]			
	*Wholemeal bread	Thin slice small loaf	25	55
		$\frac{3}{4}$ large slice (medium thickness)		
	White bread	1 small slice (medium thickness)		
		$\frac{2}{3}$ large slice (medium thickness)	17	44
		$\frac{1}{2}$ large thick slice		
	Breakfast cereals			
	*All Bran	5 tbs	20	50
	*Bran buds	4 tbs	20	50
	Cornflakes	5 tbs	10	40
	*Muesli (unsweetened)	2 tbs	15	50
	Puffed Wheat	15 tbs	15	50
	Rice Krispies	6 tbs	10	40
	*Shredded Wheat	$\frac{2}{3}$ of one	10	50
	Special K	8 tbs	15	50
	*Spoonsize Cubs	12—14	—	45
	*Weetabix	1 biscuit	15	60
	*Weetaflakes	4 tbs	15	50
	Porridge (made with water)	4 tbs	120	55
	Biscuits[2]			
	Plain or semi-sweet	2	15	60

Table 2.14 *contd.*

Food item	Household measure	Weight (g)	Energy content (kcal)
*Oatcake	1	15	55
*Digestive or wholemeal	1	15	70
Crackers (plain)	2	15	70
Crispbread	2	15	50
Flours and grains			
Flour			
white, plain or self-raising	1½ tbs	10	40
*wholemeal	2 tbs	15	50
Arrowroot, custard powder, cornflour	1 tbs	10	35
Barley (raw)	1 tbs	10	40
*Oats (uncooked)	3 tbs	15	60
Rice			
*brown (uncooked)	1 tbs	10	40
white (uncooked)	1 tbs	10	45
Spaghetti			
*wholewheat	20 10″ strands	15	50
white	6 long (19″) strands	10	45
Sago, tapioca, semolina, uncooked	2 tsp	10	35
Vegetables[3]			
*Beans			
*baked (canned)	4 tbs	75	55
*broad (boiled)	10 tbs	150	75
*dried (all types, raw)	2 tbs	20	55
*Beetroot (cooked whole)	2 small	100	45
*Lentils dry (raw)	2 tbs	20	60
Onions (raw)	1 large	200	45
Parsnips (raw)	1 small	90	45
*Peas (marrowfat or processed)	7 tbs	75	60
*Peas (dried, all types, raw)	2 tbs	20	60
Plantain, green (raw, peeled)	Small slice	35	40
Potatoes —			
raw	1 egg sized	50	45
boiled	1 egg sized	50	40
chips (cooked weight)	4–5 average chips	25	65
*jacket (weighed with skin)	1 small	50	45
mashed	1 small scoop	50	80
roast	1 egg sized	40	65
*Sweetcorn			
canned or frozen	5 tbs	60	45
on the cob	medium cob	75	60
*Sweet potato (raw peeled)	1 small slice	50	45
Fruits[4]			
Apples —			
eating (whole)	1 medium	110	50
cooking (whole)	1 medium	125	55
stewed without sugar	6 tbs	125	40
Apricots			
fresh (whole)	3 medium	160	40
dried (raw)	4 small	25	45
Bananas with skin	5″ in length	90	40
Blackberries (raw)	10 tbs	150	45
Blackcurrants (raw)	10 tbs	150	45
Cherries (fresh, whole)	12	100	40
Currants (raisins, dried)	2 tbs	15	35
Damsons (raw, whole)	7	120	40
Dates			
fresh, whole	3 medium	50	40
dried, without stones	3 small	15	40
Figs			
fresh whole	1	100	40
dried	1	20	40
Grapes (whole)	10 large	75	40
Grapefruit (whole)	1 very large	400	45
Greengages (fresh, whole)	5	90	40

Table 2.14 *contd.*

Food item	Household measure	Weight (g)	Energy content (kcal)
Guavas (fresh, flesh only)	1	70	45
Mango (fresh whole)	$\frac{1}{3}$ of a large one	100	40
Melon (all types, weighed with skin)	large slice	300	40
Nectarine (fresh, whole)	1	90	40
Orange (fresh whole)	1 large	150	40
Paw-paw (fresh, whole)	$\frac{1}{6}$ of a large one	80	50
Peach (fresh, whole)	1 large	125	40
Pear (fresh, whole)	1 large	130	40
Pineapple (fresh, no skin or core)	1 thick slice	90	40
Plums			
cooking (fresh, whole)	4 medium	180	40
dessert (fresh, whole)	2 large	110	40
Pomegranate (fresh, whole)	1 small	110	40
Prunes (dried, without stones)	2 large	25	40
Raisins (dried)	2 tbs	15	35
Strawberries (fresh)	15 medium	160	40
Sultanas (dried)	2 tbs	15	40
Tangerines (fresh, whole)	2 large	175	40
Fruit juices (unsweetened)			
Apple juice	6 tbs	85	40
Blackcurrant juice	7 tbs	100	40
Grapefruit juice	8 tbs	125	45
Orange juice	7 tbs	100	40
Pineapple juice	6 tbs	85	40
Tomato juice	1 large glass	275	50
Milk and milk products			
Milk —			
fresh, whole	$\frac{1}{3}$ pint	200 ml	130
fresh, semi-skimmed	$\frac{1}{3}$ pint	200 ml	90
fresh skimmed	$\frac{1}{3}$ pint	200 ml	70
dried, whole	8 tsp	25	125
dried, skimmed	10 tsp	20	70
evaporated	6 tbs	90 ml	145
Yoghurt (plain)	1 small carton	150 ml	80
Manufactured foods[5]			
Beefburgers (frozen)	3 small	—	450
Fish fingers	2	—	110
Ice cream	1 scoop	—	90
Sausages	2 thick	110	400
Soup (thickened)	1 cup	200	115
Beer (draught)	$\frac{1}{2}$ pint	275	100
Lager (draught)	$\frac{3}{4}$ pint	425	135
Sugar-rich foods[6]			
Glucose	2 tsp	10	40
Dextrosol	3 tablets	—	40
Sugar	2 tsp	10	40
Golden syrup	1 tbs	15	40
Marmalade/jam/honey	2 tsp	15	40
Lucozade	3–4 tbs	50 ml	36
Cola	8 tbs	100 ml	40

[1]Figures for carbohydrate and energy are contained on the packaging of many sliced breads. Details are also given in *Countdown*.

[2]Details of many individual brands are given in *Countdown*.

[3]A portion of the following will not add more than 5 g of carbohydrate and 20–25 kcal to the diet and need not be counted as an exchange:

Artichokes, asparagus, aubergine, beans (runner), beansprouts, broccoli, brussels sprouts, cabbage, carrots, cauliflower, celery, courgettes, cucumber, leeks, lettuce, marrow, mushrooms, mustard and cress, okra (raw), peas (fresh or frozen), peppers, pumpkin, radishes, spinach, spring onions, swede, tomatoes (raw and canned), turnip, watercress.

[4]Cranberries, gooseberries, lemons, loganberries and rhubarb need not be counted into the diet.

[5]Different brands of the same product vary considerably in nutrient composition. Precise figures can be obtained from *Countdown*. The figures in the table are given for guidance only.

[6]For use at times of illness or hypoglycaemia by the insulin dependent diabetic.

Table 2.15 Low sodium, 10 g carbohydrate exchange list

Food item	Household measure
Salt-free bread	1 small, thin slice
	$\frac{1}{2}$ large, thick slice
Tea Matzos	2 biscuits
Matzos (large)	$\frac{1}{2}$
Salt-free crackers	2
Pasta (macaroni, noodles, spaghetti)	
raw cooked	1 heaped tbs
cooked	3 heaped tbs
Rice (boiled)	2 heaped tbs
Sago, semolina, rice, tapioca (raw)	1 level tbs
Puffed Wheat	5 heaped tbs
Shredded Wheat	$\frac{2}{3}$ biscuit
Porridge (cooked)	4 tbs
Flour, cornflour, custard powder (raw)	1 rounded tbs
Potato	
boiled, roast	1 egg sized
mashed	1 heaped tbs
chips	6 large chips
Unsalted crisps (Salt'n shake)	1 small packet

Specific restriction or avoidance of carbohydrate

Sucrose avoidance. Sucrose intolerance may be either primary (congenital sucrase deficiency) or secondary to some other malabsorption state (see Section 4.12.1).

Many sources of dietary sucrose are readily apparent i.e. table sugar and obviously sweetened foods. How-ever, most fruits, many vegetables and many manu-factured (especially canned) products contain sucrose and must also be eliminated from the diet.

Sucrose intolerant infants will require a milk formula in which the sucrose is replaced by glucose. Weaning presents less of a problem than it used to as many manufactured baby foods are free from added sucrose; however, fruit and some vegetable-based weaning foods will still contain sucrose of natural origin and must be avoided. Vitamin supplementation (especially of vitamin C) is vital.

Secondary sucrose intolerance is commonly ac-companied by lactose intolerance and if this is the case, products containing milk, milk solids, and lactose must also be excluded (see lactose-free foods).

Table 2.16 provides broad guidelines for a sucrose-free diet (and associated lactose intolerance). The presence or absence of *added* sucrose in a manufactured food can be determined from its label. However, 'sucrose' will not appear on the list of ingredients if it originated naturally, e.g. fruit canned in natural juice.

Lactose avoidance. Lactose intolerance may be primary (and is common in certain racial groups) or secondary as a result of acute diarrhoeal illness. In the former instance, complete avoidance of lactose is usually unnecessary; there is usually a threshold for

Table 2.16 Guidelines for a sucrose-free diet (with or without associated lactose intolerance)

Food group	Permitted foods	Excluded foods
Cereals and cereal products	Porridge oats Sugar-free breakfast cereals* Bread* Sucrose-free biscuits* Some crispbreads* Flour, cornflour Rice, tapioca and sago* Pasta	Sugar-containing breakfast cereals Sweetened bread, biscuits, cakes, pastries and pies Manufactured desserts and puddings Canned pasta
Milk and milk products	Milk* Evaporated milk (unsweetened)* Most coffee whiteners* Unsweetened yoghurt* Cheese* Cream*	Condensed milk Sweetened yoghurt
Eggs	Egg yolk, egg white and whole egg	Meringues (unless made with a sucrose substitute)
Fats and oils	All types*	
Meat and meat products	Beef, lamb and pork Poultry Ham and bacon (unless sweet cured)	Most canned meats Meat paste Some meat products Casseroles with unsuitable vegetables (see below)

Table 2.16 contd.

Food group	Permitted foods	Excluded foods
Fish and fish products	Fresh and frozen fish Most tinned fish	
Vegetables	Green leafy vegetables — broccoli, cabbage, spinach, brussels sprouts and cauliflower Salad vegetables — lettuce, cucumber, chicory, cress, celery and tomato Asparagus Marrow Mushrooms Potatoes Runner beans	Pulses — peas, beans and lentils Root vegetables — carrots, parsnips, turnips and swede Beetroot Leeks Sweetcorn Many canned vegetables Some varieties of baked beans
Fruit	Cherries Grapes Figs	All other fruit (fresh, canned or dried) Glace cherries Fruit juice (except unsweetened tomato juice)
Nuts		All
Sugars, preserves, confectionery	Glucose, fructose Saccharine, aspartame and other sucrose-free artificial sweeteners Sugarless drinks Some brands of honey	Sugar Sugar-containing drinks and baked products Jam, marmalade Syrup, treacle Ice-cream, jelly Confectionery Drinking chocolate, Bournvita and malted milk drinks
Alcoholic drinks	Spirits Sugar-free mixers	Wines, sherries and ports Beer, lager Liqueurs
Miscellaneous	Gelatine Marmite, Bovril Oxo, stock cubes Salt, pepper, herbs and spices	Gravy browning Canned or packet soups Pickles, chutneys Salad cream Syrup-based medicines
Baby foods	Baby milks* without added sugar Sugar-free weaning foods Baby rice	Sugar-containing milks or foods Fruit-based weaning foods

*Items which contain milk, milk products or lactose and will need to be excluded if there is associated lactose intolerance.

lactose (in the region of around 10 g/day) below which no symptoms of intolerance will occur. However, some individuals and some cases of secondary lactose intolerance will have a very low lactose tolerance.

Lactose is contained in human, cows', sheep's and goats' milk, in milk products and manufactured foods containing milk. It is also present in some medicines and artificial sweeteners.

Lactose intolerant infants will require a low lactose milk based on soya. Lactose intolerant children may require extra protein from meat, fish and eggs. Calcium supplements may also be needed.

For practical purposes, no differentiation is generally made between cows' milk protein intolerance and lactose intolerance. The construction of milk-free diets is discussed in detail in Section 2.11 on p 193. However, guidelines for a low lactose diet are summarized in Table 2.17.

Manufactured foods free from lactose are included in the list of foods free from milk and milk products printed by the British Dietetic Association (but see p 615). Proprietary products which are prescribable in cases of lactose intolerance with associated gluten intolerance are listed on p 192.

Table 2.17 Principle sources of dietary lactose (and suggested alternatives)

Food group	Foods containing lactose	Lactose-free alternative
Milk and milk products	Human, cows' and goats' milk Yoghurt Cream and cheese	Low lactose milk substitute (see p 195)
Fats and oils	Butter Most margarines	Tomor margarine Some low fat spreads Lard Vegetable oil
Manufactured and baked products	Cakes, biscuits, bread and pastry containing milk Milk puddings Ice cream	Milk-free products (see p 194)
Miscellaneous	Lactose-containing sweeteners Tablets with a lactose filler Many manufactured products	

Note: Milk-free diets are discussed in detail in Section 2.11, p 193.

Galactose avoidance. Galactosaemia, an inborn error of metabolism (see Section 4.7.7), requires a galactose-free diet. Since galactose is a constituent of lactose, this entails *severe* restriction of lactose-containing foods as well as other sources of galactose and galactosides.

It is usually possible to replace milk with a low lactose milk substitute, but in young infants a feed based on comminuted chicken, milk-free cereal, egg and glucose may be required.

Guidelines for a galactose-free diet are given in Table 2.18. These should be used in conjunction with an up-to-date list of manufactured foods free from milk and milk derivatives printed by the British Dietetic Association (but see p 615). The construction of milk-free regimens is also discussed in detail on p 193.

Table 2.18 Guidelines for a galactose-free diet

Food group	Permitted foods	Excluded foods
Milk and milk products	Lactose-free or low lactose milk substitute (e.g. Formula S (Cow and Gate), Prosobee (Mead Johnson) or Wysoy (Wyeth)** Some coffee whiteners	Human, cows' and goats' milk, cheese, cheese spread, yoghurt and cream Any manufactured food containing milk, milk solids, lactose, galactose, whey, casein or caseinate
Cereals	Breakfast cereals without added milk solids Flour, cornflour Milk-free bread, biscuits, cakes and puddings Baby rice Rice, sago, tapioca and semolina (made without milk) Pasta	Some baby cereals
Eggs	Egg yolk, egg white, whole egg	Scrambled egg made with milk
Fats and oils	Tomor margarine Some low fat spreads Lard Vegetable oils	Butter Margarine
Meat and meat products	Cooked without milk	Meat products containing milk solids or lactose Offal*
Fish and fish products	Cooked without milk	Fish products containing milk solids or lactose
Vegetables	All except those listed opposite	Peas*, beans*, lentils*, soya*, legumes* and pulses
Fruits	All	
Nuts	All	
Sugar and preserves	Boiled sweets Water ices Sugar	Milk-containing confectionery (chocolate, fudge and toffees)

Table 2.18 *contd.*

Food group	Permitted foods	Excluded foods
	Jam, honey, marmalade Syrup, treacle Jelly	Ice cream Milk-based desserts
Beverages	Milk or lactose-free tea, coffee, fruit juice, squash and fizzy drinks	Malted milk or chocolate drinks
Miscellaneous	Marmite, Bovril Oxo, stock cubes, salt, pepper, herbs and spices	Soups made with milk or cream Tablets with lactose filler Some artificial sweeteners Many canned or manufactured foods

*Contain galactosides
**Details of products suitable for use in milk-free diets are given on p 194.

Starch avoidance. Primary starch intolerance is due to isomaltase deficiency and is usually associated with primary sucrose intolerance. This will require exclusion of the sucrose-containing foods listed in Table 2.16 as well as foods which contain the following

1 Flour and foods containing flour (i.e. bread, cakes and biscuits).
2 Breakfast cereals.
3 Cornflour (and most manufactured desserts).
4 Rice.
5 Pasta.
6 Food coated in breadcrumbs or batter.
7 Potatoes.
8 Many manufactured meat products (e.g. sausages,

beefburgers, rissoles and meat and fish pastes).

It may be possible to use a soya-based flour as an alternative for baking.

Further reading

Francis D (1986) *Diets for sick children* 2e. Blackwell Scientific Publications Ltd, Oxford.

Reference

Ministry of Agriculture, Fisheries and Food (1985) *Household food consumption and expenditure: 1983.* Annual Report of the National Food Survey committee. HMSO, London.

2.5 Dietary Fibre (non-starch polysaccharides)

2.5.1 Definition and principal fibre components

Dietary fibre is a class of carbohydrate; it is defined chemically as non-starch polysaccharides (NSP). The average UK diet for example contains approximately 280 g total carbohydrate, of which 110 g is composed of sugars such as glucose, fructose, and sucrose. Approximately 155 g is starch, and the remainder, 13−14 g, is NSP.

NSP are complexes of cellulose, a polysaccharide of glucose, which comprises about 20% of total NSP in the average UK diet, and of various other polysaccharides (the non-cellulosic polysaccharides). These contain the pentose sugars, xylose and arabinose (36% of the total NSP), the hexose sugars, glucose and arabinose (27% of the total) and the uronic acids found particularly in pectin (15% of the total). Small amounts of mannose may also be found. Lignin is sometimes included in the definition of dietary fibre but it is extremely difficult to measure. Current analytical methods which attempt to measure it in human foods actually isolate various inert substances which are better referred to as 'substances analysing as lignin'. These amount in total to less than 1 g in human diets.

The term 'hemicellulose' is sometimes used together with 'pectin' to mean non-cellulosic polysaccharides, but this nomenclature is now rarely used.

2.5.2 Analysis

Dietary fibre is extremely difficult to measure, particularly in starch-rich foods such as potatoes and cereals. In these, starch may be inadequately removed and contaminate the analyses, giving erroneously high results. Conversely, some of the polysaccharides, particularly water soluble ones, may be lost and dietary fibre values will be underestimated. As a result of these and other problems, the several different methods of analysis give different results (Table 2.19). The Southgate method used in the current set of British food tables (see Section 1.6) gives higher results for cereals and potatoes than others. To establish the most accurate technique for reference purposes, a

Table 2.19 Total dietary fibre (g/100 g fresh weight) as assessed by different methods

Method	White rice	White bread	Cabbage
Hellendoorn *et al* (1975)	1.4	2.4	2.1
Southgate *et al* (1978)	2.4	2.7	3.4
Holloway *et al* (1977)	—	2.4	2.1
NDF (Van Soest 1978)	—	1.5	1.1
Angus *et al* (1981)	1.7	2.0	1.0
Englyst *et al* (1983)	0.7	1.6	3.3

number of collaborative trials are in progress and it is probable that the Englyst technique (Englyst *et al* 1982, 1983; Englyst and Cummings 1984) will be chosen for the standard, and the values shown in Table 2.20 are based on the few food analyses currently available using this technique. Analyses of fruits and vegetables are in progress and dietitians should keep a look-out for new information until the dietary fibre values in the food tables are updated. Meanwhile the present food table values will of necessity continue to be used in clinical work.

2.5.3 Low/high fibre foods

In human diets, NSP is derived mainly from the cell walls of plants. Gums and mucilages used as food additives and sometimes fibre supplements, are also NSP. Ispaghula, for example, consists mainly of soluble pentose sugar-containing polysaccharides, and the polysaccharides of guar gum contain mainly the hexose sugars, galactose and mannose.

In general, unrefined cereals are the best source of fibre and the outer husk or bran contains the most (see Table 2.20). Of the fruits and vegetables, pulses and nuts are probably the best sources of dietary fibre but only limited analytical values are available.

Fresh fruits and vegetables in general tend to have a high water content and usually less than 5% of their weight is dietary fibre. When attempting to increase the fibre content of diets therefore, emphasis must be given to unrefined cereal products, such as wholemeal bread, wholemeal pasta and wholewheat breakfast cereals. To achieve an intake of 30 g dietary fibre for example, six slices or equivalent of wholemeal bread must be eaten per day. Large quantities of unprocessed

Table 2.20 Non-starch polysaccharide (i.e. 'fibre') content of some foods (Englyst *et al* 1982, 1983; Englyst and Cummings 1984)

Foods	g/100 g fresh weight
Good sources	
Cereals	
Wheat Bran	41.9
All Bran	22.9
Weetabix	9.8
Shredded Wheat	9.8
Oats	6.6
Wholemeal bread	5.8
Brown bread	4.3
Wholewheat spaghetti (cooked value)	3.0
Vegetables	
Dried peas (cooked value)	5.6
Dried haricot beans (cooked value)	5.0
Cabbage	3.3
Runner beans	3.1
Brussel sprouts	1.8
Tomato	1.1
Hazelnuts	2.8
Potato	1.0[†]
Poor sources	
Brown rice (cooked value)	1.7
White bread	1.6[†]
Cornflakes	0.6
Rice Krispies	0.8
White rice (cooked value)	0.5
Sago	0.5
Cornflour	0.1
Tapioca	0.4
Arrowroot	0.1

[†]On cooling or storing, retrograded or resistant starch is formed (see text).

bran should be avoided because of its high phytic acid content; the enzyme phytase is present in yeast so leavened bread contains smaller amounts of phytic acid than bran.

Low fibre foods are shown in Table 2.20. When devising diets low in residue however, it is probably important to limit starch in addition, since if this escapes digestion in the small bowel it will act in a similar manner to NSP by acting as an energy source for bacterial growth in the large bowel, and faecal weight will be increased. Potatoes for example contain little NSP and the starch in these is readily digested if they are eaten freshly cooked. On cooling, the starch retrogrades or becomes 'resistant' and in cooked cooled potatoes (for instance eaten as potato salad) a significant quantity of the starch will enter the large

bowel. In practice, low residue diets are difficult to achieve if they contain cereals, even highly refined cereals. In some cases, specially designed diets may be necessary for research purposes, consisting entirely of meat, cheese, eggs, fish and sugar; alternatively, a liquid formula diet may be necessary.

2.5.4 Sources of different fibre constituents

Different fibre constituents are identified in the analytical method, for example pentose sugars, uronic acids, soluble fibre, but the physiological significance of these constituents is not always clear. In general, fruit and vegetables contain more of their NSP as cellulose and uronic acids (pectin). The presence of soluble fibre (for example, gums or pectins) may be particularly important in the control of plasma glucose and cholesterol levels. Oat fibre, which is higher in soluble fibre than other cereal fibres, can also reduce elevated blood cholesterol levels. NSP from other cereals, particularly wheat, which contain a greater proportion of pentose sugars and insoluble dietary fibre, may be particularly important in increasing faecal weight and therefore valuable in the treatment of constipation and diverticular disease. Some soluble NSP such as guar and pectin, however, do not bring about an increase in faecal weight.

References

Angus R, Sutherland TM and Farrell DJ (1981) Insoluble dietary fibre contents of some local foods. *Proc Nutr Soc Aust* **6**, 161.

Englyst HN, Anderson V and Cummings JH (1983) Starch and NSP in some cereal foods. *J Sci Food Agric* **34**, 1434–40.

Englyst HN and Cummings JH (1984) Simplified method for the measurement of total NSP by GLC. *Analyst* **109**, 937–42.

Englyst H, Wiggins HS and Cummings JH (1982) Determination of NSP in plant foods by GLC of constituent sugars as alditol acetates. *Analyst* **107**, 307–18.

Hellendoorn EW, Noordhoff MG and Slagman J (1975) Enzymatic determination of the indigestible residue content of human food. *J Sci Food Agric* **26**, 1461.

Holloway WD, Tasman-Jones C and Maher D (1977) Towards an accurate measurement of dietary fibre. *N Z Med J* **85**, 420.

Southgate DAT, Bailey B, Collinson E and Walker AF (1976) A guide to calculating intakes of dietary fibre. *J Hum Nutr* **30**, 303.

Van Soest PJ (1978) Fibre analysis tables. *Am J Clin Nutr* [Suppl] **31**, S284.

2.6 Vitamins

2.6.1 Dietary sources of vitamins

Figure 2.6 shows the contributions of various food groups to the intake of vitamins in the UK. These figures are taken from data derived from the National Food Survey (Spring *et al* 1979; Bull and Buss 1982; MAFF 1984). For comparative purposes, the intakes from the food groups are expressed as a percentage of the total intake. It is thus possible to see at a glance

which foods make the most important contribution to the intake of each vitamin.

While Fig. 2.6 indicates the relative importance of certain food groups in providing vitamins it does not indicate which individual foods are most valuable in boosting intake. The contribution which an individual food makes to nutrient intake depends on three factors: the vitamin content/100 g; the size of the portion eaten, and the frequency of consumption.

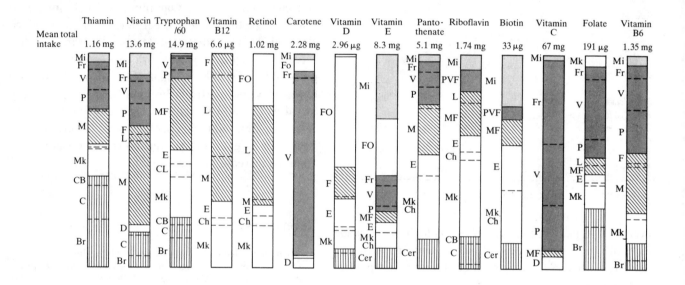

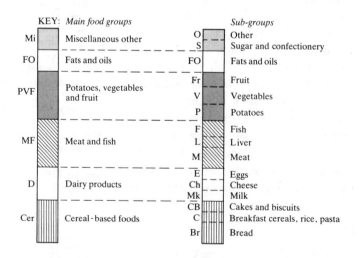

Fig. 2.6 Mean intakes of vitamins in British household diets and the proportion derived from different food groups. Drawn from Spring *et al* 1979; Bull and Buss 1982; MAFF 1984.

Therefore, it is not sufficient, when identifying foods to increase or reduce intake, to simply run the eye down the tables of content/100 g. The other two factors also have to be considered. This is illustrated in Table 2.21. Parsley contains almost three times as much vitamin C as oranges, but makes a negligible contribution to total intake, while milk, containing 1/33rd as much makes a significant contribution.

Table 2.21 The contribution of three foods to vitamin C intake

	Parsley	Milk	Oranges
Portion weight (g)	1	30	80
× frequency	1/month	8/day	2/week
× content/100 g (mg)	130	1.5	50
= Intake per day (mg)	0.04	3.6 mg	11.4 mg

Table 2.22 lists some 130 commonly eaten foods (as the cooked form if usually eaten cooked) and their nutrient content *per portion*. It is left to the dietitian to consider how frequently the food might be eaten by the group or individual under consideration.

The portion weights in Table 2.22 are derived from dietary studies of families in Cambridge (Nelson, personal communication); 105 families provided 805 days of records from adult women, and 735 days from adult men. The portions eaten by women were cross-checked with those eaten by Cambridge mothers (73 mothers, 3185 days; Black, personal communication) and found to be similar. The portions eaten by women have been used to calculate the nutrient contents per portion; portions eaten by men are given in brackets for comparison. For many foods they were similar, but the men did eat larger portions of meat and also many cereal foods. Where too few portions of specific food items (codes) had been recorded to provide a reliable average portion weight, similar foods were grouped together, e.g. three kinds of liver. For fresh fruit, it

Table 2.22 Vitamin contents of foods in portions eaten by adult women in Cambridge, UK. (Portions eaten by men are given in brackets for comparison). (Derived from the data of M Nelson, personal communications). Tr = trace − = No data ( ) = Estimated value

Food code[1]	Food	Women's portion[2]	Men's portion[3]	Retinol μg	Carotene (μg)	Vitamin D (μg)	Thiamin (mg)	Riboflavin (mg)	Nicotinic acid (mg)	Tryptophan/60 (mg)	Vitamin C (mg)	Vitamin E (mg)	Vitamin B6 (mg)	Vitamin B12 (μg)	Total folate (μg)	Pantothenic acid (mg)	Biotin (μg)
4	Bemax	10		0	0	0.000	0.15	0.06	0.58	0.53	0.0	1.10	0.095	0.00	(33.0)	(0.17)	0.0
5	Bran (wheat)	8		0	0	0.000	0.07	0.03	2.37	0.24	0.0	0.13	0.110	0.00	20.8	0.19	1.1
18	Porridge	190	(240)	0	0	0.000	0.09	0.02	0.19	0.57	0.0	(0.00)	0.019	0.00	11.4	0.19	(3.8)
20	Rice, polished (boiled)	140	(160)	0	0	0.000	0.01	0.01	0.42	0.70	0.0	(0.14)	(0.070)	0.00	(8.4)	(0.28)	(1.4)
27	Spaghetti (boiled)	190	(240)	0	0	0.000	0.02	0.02	0.57	1.71	0.0	—	(0.019)	0.00	(3.8)	(Tr)	(Tr)
30	Bread (wholemeal)	60	(65)	0	0	0.000	0.16	0.04	2.34	1.02	0.0	(0.12)	0.084	0.00	23.4	0.36	3.6
31	Bread (brown)	55	(75)	0	0	0.000	0.13	0.03	1.60	0.99	0.0	(Tr)	0.044	0.00	19.8	0.16	1.7
32	Bread (Hovis)	55	(70)	0	0	0.000	0.29	0.05	2.14	1.10	0.0	—	0.049	0.00	11.0	0.16	1.1
33	Bread (white)	55	(85)	0	0	0.000	0.10	0.02	0.77	0.88	0.0	Tr	0.022	0.00	14.9	0.16	0.5
47	All Bran	30	(20)	0	0	0.000	0.22	0.84	14.70	0.96	0.0	0.60	0.249	0.00	30.0	—	—
48	Cornflakes	30	(40)	0	0	0.000	0.54	0.48	6.30	0.27	0.0	0.12	0.009	0.00	2.1	—	—
50	Muesli	60	(50)	0	0	0.000	0.20	0.16	1.62	1.80	Tr	1.92	0.084	0.00	28.8	—	—
53	Rice Krispies	30	(35)	0	0	0.000	0.69	0.51	7.20	0.39	0.0	0.18	0.057	0.00	4.2	—	—
57	Weetabix	35	(35)	0	0	0.000	0.35	0.52	4.20	0.80	0.0	0.63	0.084	0.00	17.5	—	—
60	Crispbread (rye)	20	(20)	0	0	0.000	0.06	0.03	0.22	0.36	0.0	0.10	0.058	0.00	(8.0)	(0.22)	(1.4)
62	Biscuits (digestive, plain)	30	(30)	0	0	0.000	(0.04)	(0.02)	(0.45)	0.60	0.0	—	(0.018)	0.00	(3.0)	—	—
70	Biscuits (short sweet)	25	(25)	0	0	0.000	0.04	0.01	0.22	0.32	0.0	0.32	0.012	0.00	(2.5)	—	—
75	Fruitcake (rich)	70	(100)	84	7	0.798	0.86	0.06	0.35	0.56	0.0	0.98	0.091	Tr	2.8	0.14	2.8
81	Spongecake (with fat)	50	(60)	150	0	1.380	(Tr)	0.06	0.30	0.80	0.0	1.35	0.030	Tr	3.5	0.25	4.0
124	Milk, cows, fresh, whole (summer)	30		11	7	0.009	0.01	0.06	0.02	0.23	0.4	0.03	0.012	0.09	1.5	0.11	0.6
125	Milk, cows, fresh, whole (winter)	30		8	4	0.004	0.01	0.06	0.02	0.23	0.4	0.02	0.012	0.09	1.5	0.11	0.6
131	Milk, fresh (skimmed)	30		0	0	0.000	0.01	0.06	0.02	0.24	0.5	0.00	0.012	0.09	1.5	0.11	0.6
124	Milk, cows, fresh, whole (summer)	200		70	44	0.060	0.08	0.38	0.16	1.56	3.0	0.20	0.080	0.60	10.0	0.70	4.0
125	Milk, cows, fresh, whole (winter)	200		52	26	0.026	0.08	0.38	0.16	1.56	3.0	0.14	0.080	0.60	10.0	0.70	4.0
131	Milk, fresh (skimmed)	200		0	0	0.000	0.08	0.40	0.16	1.60	3.2	0.00	0.080	0.60	10.0	0.72	4.0
140	Butter (salted)	12	(16)	90	56	0.091	Tr	Tr	Tr	0.01	Tr	0.24	Tr	Tr	Tr	Tr	Tr
142	Cream, single (summer)	30	(45)	60	38	0.050	0.01	0.04	0.02	0.17	0.4	0.15	0.009	0.06	1.2	0.09	0.4
143	Cream, single (winter)	30	(45)	44	21	0.024	0.01	0.04	0.02	0.17	0.4	0.12	0.009	0.06	1.2	0.09	0.4
151	Camembert type cheese	35		75	47	0.063	0.02	0.21	0.28	1.88	0.0	(0.21)	0.070	0.42	21.0	0.49	2.1
152	Cheddar type cheese	35	(45)	109	72	0.091	0.01	0.18	0.04	2.14	0.0	0.28	0.028	0.52	7.0	0.11	0.6
154	Edam type cheese	40	(30)	86	54	0.072	0.02	0.16	0.02	2.29	0.0	(0.32)	0.032	0.56	8.0	0.12	0.6

Table 2.22 *contd.*

Food code[1]	Food	Women's portion[2]	Men's portion[3]	Retinol μg	Carotene (μg)	Vitamin D (μg)	Thiamin (mg)	Riboflavin (mg)	Nicotinic acid (mg)	Tryptophan/60 (mg)	Vitamin C (mg)	Vitamin E (mg)	Vitamin B6 (mg)	Vitamin B12 (μg)	Total folate (μg)	Panthothenic acid (mg)	Biotin (μg)
156	Stilton cheese	30	(40)	111	69	0.094	0.02	0.09	—	1.81	0.0	(0.30)	—	—	—	—	—
157	Cottage cheese	70		22	13	0.016	0.01	0.13	0.06	2.25	0.0	—	0.007	(0.35)	6.3	—	—
160	Cheese spread	20		36	21	0.027	0.00	0.05	0.01	0.86	0.0	—	—	—	—	—	—
161	Yoghurt (low fat natural)	140	(140)	11	7	Tr	0.07	0.36	0.17	1.46	0.6	0.04	0.056	Tr	2.8	—	—
169	Egg (boiled)	60	(60)	84	Tr	1.050	0.05	0.27	0.04	2.17	0.0	0.96	0.060	1.02	13.2	0.96	15.0
140	Butter (salted)	12	(16)	90	56	0.091	Tr	Tr	Tr	0.01	Tr	0.24	Tr	Tr	Tr	Tr	Tr
187	Margarine (all kinds)	12	(16)	108	0	0.953	Tr	Tr	Tr	Tr	0.0	0.96	Tr	Tr	Tr	Tr	Tr
220	Bacon, gammon rashers, grilled (lean only)	80		Tr	Tr	Tr	0.80	0.22	5.68	4.72	0.0	(0.03)	(0.296)	Tr	(1.6)	(0.56)	(2.4)
227	Bacon, rashers, fried middle, (lean and fat)	35		Tr	Tr	Tr	0.14	0.07	1.75	1.58	0.0	0.07	0.102	Tr	0.4	0.11	0.7
230	Bacon, rashers, grilled, average (lean only)	35		Tr	Tr	Tr	0.21	0.08	2.17	1.99	0.0	0.01	0.130	Tr	0.7	0.25	1.0
232	Bacon, rashers, grilled middle (lean and fat)	35		Tr	Tr	Tr	0.14	0.06	1.54	1.61	0.0	0.04	0.091	Tr	0.4	0.18	0.7
250	Beef, rump steak, fried (lean and fat)	90	(100)	Tr	Tr	Tr	0.07	0.31	4.95	5.49	0.0	0.30	0.261	1.80	13.5	0.72	Tr
258	Beef, sirloin, roast (lean only)	90	(100)	Tr	Tr	Tr	0.06	0.28	5.40	5.31	0.0	0.26	0.297	1.80	15.3	0.81	Tr
286	Lamb, leg, roast (lean only)	80	(100)	Tr	Tr	Tr	0.11	0.30	5.28	5.04	0.0	0.08	0.176	1.60	3.2	0.56	1.6
292	Lamb, shoulder, roast (lean and fat)	80	(100)	Tr	Tr	Tr	0.06	0.16	2.48	3.36	0.0	0.10	0.128	1.60	2.4	0.40	0.8
304	Pork chops, grilled (lean and fat)	85	(125)	Tr	Tr	Tr	0.56	0.17	4.85	4.51	0.0	0.03	0.263	0.85	5.1	0.85	1.7
310	Pork, leg, roast (lean only)	85	(125)	Tr	Tr	Tr	0.72	0.30	5.61	4.85	0.0	0.00	0.349	1.70	5.9	1.11	2.6
321	Chicken, roast (meat only)	80	(130)	Tr	Tr	Tr	0.06	0.15	6.56	3.68	0.0	0.09	0.208	0.00	8.0	0.96	2.4
322	Chicken, roast (meat and skin)	85	(135)	Tr	Tr	Tr	(0.05)	(0.14)	(5.35)	3.57	0.0	—	—	Tr	—	—	—
323	Chicken, roast (light meat)	80	(130)	Tr	Tr	Tr	0.06	0.11	8.24	4.00	0.0	0.06	0.280	Tr	5.6	0.88	1.6
324	Chicken, roast (dark meat)	80	(130)	Tr	Tr	Tr	0.07	0.19	4.88	3.44	0.0	0.12	0.128	0.80	10.4	1.04	2.4
344	Turkey, roast (meat only)	100		Tr	Tr	Tr	0.07	0.21	8.50	5.40	0.0	Tr	0.320	2.00	15.0	0.80	2.0
365	Kidney, lamb (fried)	60		96	—	—	0.34	1.38	5.76	3.18	5.4	0.25	0.180	47.40	47.4	3.06	25.2
367	Kidney, ox (stewed)	60		150	—	—	0.15	1.26	2.88	3.30	6.0	0.25	0.180	18.60	45.0	1.80	29.4
369	Kidney, pig (stewed)	60		84	0	—	0.11	1.26	3.66	3.12	6.6	0.22	0.168	9.00	25.8	1.44	31.8
376	Liver, lamb (fried)	90	(135)	18540	54	0.450	0.23	3.96	13.68	4.41	10.8	0.29	0.441	72.90	216.0	6.84	36.9
378	Liver, ox (stewed)	90	(135)	18090	1386	1.017	0.16	3.24	9.27	4.77	13.5	0.40	0.468	99.00	261.0	5.13	45.0
380	Liver, pig (stewed)	90	(135)	10440	0	1.017	0.19	2.79	10.35	4.95	8.1	0.14	0.576	23.40	99.0	4.14	30.6
393	Beef, corned (canned)	50	(65)	Tr	Tr	Tr	Tr	0.11	1.25	3.25	0.0	0.39	0.030	1.00	1.0	0.20	1.0
394	Ham (canned)	40	(40)	Tr	Tr	Tr	0.21	0.10	1.56	1.20	0.0	0.03	0.088	Tr	Tr	0.24	0.4
395	Ham and pork chopped (canned)	40	(65)	Tr	Tr	Tr	0.08	0.08	1.28	1.08	0.0	0.04	0.020	0.40	0.4	0.16	0.8
396	Luncheon meat (canned)	40	(65)	Tr	Tr	Tr	0.03	0.05	0.72	1.08	0.0	0.04	0.008	0.40	0.4	0.20	Tr
398	Tongue (canned)	60		Tr	Tr	Tr	0.02	0.23	1.50	2.28	0.0	0.16	0.024	3.00	1.2	0.24	1.2
401	Black pudding (fried)	45	(75)	Tr	Tr	Tr	0.04	0.03	0.45	1.26	0.0	0.11	0.018	0.45	2.3	0.27	0.9
404	Liver sausage	35	(45)	(2905)	Tr	(0.210)	0.06	0.55	1.51	0.84	Tr	0.04	0.049	2.80	6.6	0.52	2.4
405	Frankfurters	55		Tr	Tr	Tr	0.04	0.07	0.83	0.83	0.0	0.14	0.016	0.55	0.5	0.22	1.1
407	Salami	30		Tr	Tr	Tr	0.06	0.14	1.38	1.08	0.0	0.08	0.045	0.30	0.9	0.24	0.9
413	Sausages, pork (grilled)	70	(90)	Tr	Tr	Tr	0.01	0.11	2.80	1.96	0.0	0.15	0.042	0.70	2.1	0.42	2.1
442	Cod (fried in batter)	125	(135)	Tr	Tr	Tr	(0.09)	(0.09)	(2.13)	4.63	Tr	—	(0.475)	(2.50)	(15.0)	(0.25)	(3.8)
446	Cod (steamed)	100	(150)	Tr	Tr	Tr	(0.09)	(0.09)	(2.10)	3.50	Tr	(0.54)	(0.370)	(3.00)	(12.0)	(0.20)	(3.0)
489	Kipper (baked)	105	(145)	(51)	Tr	(26.250)	Tr	(0.19)	(4.20)	5.04	Tr	(0.31)	(0.599)	(11.55)	(10.5)	(0.92)	(10.5)
492	Mackerel (fried)	95	(49)	Tr		(20.045)	(0.09)	(0.36)	(8.26)	3.80	Tr	—	(0.798)	(11.40)	—	(0.91)	(7.6)
494	Pilchards (canned in tomato sauce)	75		Tr	Tr	6.000	0.02	0.22	5.70	2.63	Tr	0.52	—	9.00	—	—	—
498	Salmon (canned)	30	(45)	27	Tr	3.750	0.01	0.05	2.10	1.14	Tr	0.45	0.135	1.20	3.6	0.15	(1.5)
500	Sardines, canned in oil (fish only)	70	(85)	Tr	Tr	5.250	0.03	0.25	5.74	3.08	Tr	0.21	0.336	19.60	5.6	0.35	3.5
508	Tuna (canned in oil)	70	(85)	Tr	Tr	4.060	0.03	0.08	9.03	3.01	Tr	4.41	0.308	3.50	10.5	0.29	2.1
523	Prawns (boiled)	40	(40)	Tr	Tr	Tr	—	—	—	1.68	Tr	—	—	—	—	—	—
563	Beans, runner (boiled)	75	(75)	0	300	0.000	0.02	0.05	0.38	0.22	3.8	0.15	0.030	0.00	21.0	0.03	0.4
568	Beans, haricot (boiled)	90	(115)	0	Tr	0.000	—	—	—	0.99	0.0	—	—	0.00	—	—	—
569	Beans baked (canned in tomato sauce)	115	(160)	0	—	0.000	0.08	0.06	0.58	0.92	Tr	0.69	0.138	0.00	33.3	—	—
575	Beetroot (boiled)	40	(40)	0	Tr	0.000	0.01	0.02	0.04	0.12	2.0	0.00	0.012	0.00	(20.0)	0.04	Tr
579	Brussels sprouts (boiled)	85	(100)	0	340	0.000	0.05	(0.08)	0.34	0.43	34.0	0.76	0.144	0.00	73.9	0.24	0.3
583	Cabbage, spring (boiled)	90	(135)	0	450	0.000	0.03	0.03	0.18	0.18	22.5	0.18	0.090	0.00	(45.0)	0.13	Tr
586	Cabbage, winter (boiled)	90	(115)	0	270	0.000	0.03	0.03	0.18	0.27	18.0	0.18	0.090	0.00	31.5	0.13	Tr
588	Carrots, old (boiled)	60	(80)	0	7200	0.000	0.03	0.02	0.24	0.06	2.4	0.30	0.054	0.00	4.8	0.11	0.2
592	Cauliflower (boiled)	120	(115)	0	36	0.000	0.07	0.07	0.48	0.48	24.0	0.12	0.144	0.00	58.8	0.50	1.2
594	Celery (raw)	45	(50)	0	Tr	0.000	0.01	0.01	0.13	0.09	3.2	0.09	0.045	0.00	5.4	0.18	0.0

Table 2.22 *contd.*

Food code[1]	Food	Women's portion[2]	Men's portion[3]	Retinol μg	Carotene (μg)	Vitamin D (μg)	Thiamin (mg)	Riboflavin (mg)	Nicotinic acid (mg)	Tryptophan/60 (mg)	Vitamin C (mg)	Vitamin E (mg)	Vitamin B6 (mg)	Vitamin B12 (μg)	Total folate (μg)	Panthothenic acid (mg)	Biotin (μg)
597	Cucumber (raw)	30	(40)	0	Tr	0.000	0.01	0.01	0.06	0.03	2.4	Tr	0.012	0.00	4.8	0.09	(0.1)
602	Leeks (boiled)	80	(80)	0	32	0.000	0.06	0.02	0.32	0.24	12.0	0.64	0.120	0.00	—	0.08	0.8
606	Lettuce (raw)	25	(30)	0	250	0.000	0.02	0.02	0.08	0.02	3.8	0.13	0.017	0.00	8.5	0.05	0.2
623	Peas, frozen (boiled)	60	(70)	0	180	0.000	0.14	0.04	0.90	0.54	7.8	Tr	0.042	0.00	46.8	(0.19)	0.2
624	Peas, canned (garden)	60	(70)	0	180	0.000	0.08	0.06	1.26	0.42	4.8	Tr	0.036	0.00	31.2	0.09	(0.2)
625	Peas, canned (processed)	85	(90)	0	255	0.000	0.08	0.03	0.43	0.85	Tr	Tr	0.025	0.00	2.6	(0.07)	(5.1)
632	Peas, chick (cooked)	75		0	—	—	0.06	0.02	0.30	0.53	Tr	—	—	0.00	22.3	—	—
640	Potatoes, old (boiled)	140	(235)	0	Tr	0.000	0.11	0.04	1.12	0.42	12.6	0.14	0.252	0.00	14.0	0.28	Tr
641	Potatoes, old (mashed)	140	(235)	Tr	Tr	Tr	0.11	0.06	1.12	0.56	11.2	0.14	0.252	0.00	(14.0)	0.28	Tr
642	Potatoes, old (baked)	140	(235)	0	Tr	0.000	0.14	0.06	1.68	0.84	14.0	0.14	0.252	0.00	14.0	0.28	Tr
644	Potatoes, old (roast)	110	(170)	0	Tr	0.000	0.11	0.04	1.32	0.77	11.0	0.11	0.198	0.00	7.7	0.22	Tr
645	Potatoes, old (chips)	130	(170)	0	Tr	0.000	0.13	0.05	1.56	0.17	13.0	0.13	0.234	0.00	(13.0)	0.26	Tr
648	Potatoes, new (boiled)	140	(235)	0	Tr	0.000	0.15	0.04	1.68	0.56	25.2	0.14	0.280	0.00	14.0	0.28	Tr
660	Swedes (boiled)	80	(125)	0	Tr	0.000	0.03	0.02	0.64	0.16	13.6	0.00	0.096	0.00	16.8	0.06	Tr
666	Tomatoes (raw)	50	(55)	0	300	0.000	0.03	0.02	0.35	0.05	10.0	0.60	0.055	0.00	14.0	0.16	Tr
675	Apples (eating)	80	(80)	0	24	0.000	0.03	0.02	0.08	Tr	2.4	0.16	0.024	0.00	4.0	0.08	0.2
691	Apricots (canned)	100		0	1000	0.000	0.02	0.01	0.30	0.10	2.0	—	0.050	0.00	(5.0)	0.10	—
692	Avocado pears	75		0	75	—	0.08	0.08	0.75	0.60	11.3	2.40	0.315	0.00	49.5	0.80	2.4
693	Bannanas (raw)	70	(70)	0	140	0.000	0.03	0.05	0.42	0.14	7.0	0.14	0.357	0.00	15.4	0.18	0.0
710	Currants, black (stewed with sugar)	25		0	40	0.000	0.00	0.01	0.05	0.02	35.0	0.20	0.012	0.00	—	0.07	0.5
724	Dates (dried)	25		0	13	0.000	0.02	0.01	0.50	0.22	0.0	—	0.038	0.00	5.3	0.20	—
734	Gooseberries, green (stewed with sugar)	100		0	140	0.000	0.03	0.02	0.20	0.10	28.0	0.30	0.020	0.00	—	0.11	0.4
736	Grapes, black (raw)	55		0	(Tr)	0.000	0.02	0.01	0.16	Tr	2.2	—	0.055	0.00	3.3	0.03	0.2
740	Grapefruit (raw)	85		0	Tr	0.000	0.04	0.02	0.17	0.08	34.0	0.25	0.025	0.00	10.2	0.24	(0.9)
758	Mandarin oranges (canned)	100		0	50	0.000	0.07	0.02	0.20	0.10	14.0	Tr	0.030	0.00	8.0	(0.15)	(0.8)
762	Melons, canteloupe (raw)	105		0	2100	0.000	0.05	0.03	0.52	Tr	26.3	0.11	0.074	0.00	31.5	0.24	—
764	Melons, yellow, honeydew (raw)	105		0	105	0.000	0.05	0.03	0.52	Tr	26.3	0.11	0.074	0.00	(31.5)	0.24	—
773	Oranges (raw)	105	(90)	0	53	0.000	0.11	0.03	0.21	0.11	52.5	0.21	0.063	0.00	38.8	0.26	1.0
784	Peaches (canned)	100		0	250	0.000	0.01	0.02	0.60	Tr	4.0	—	0.020	0.00	(3.0)	0.05	0.2
790	Pears (canned)	100		0	10	0.000	0.01	0.01	0.20	0.10	1.0	Tr	0.010	0.00	(5.0)	0.02	Tr
792	Pineapple (canned)	100		0	40	0.000	0.05	0.02	0.20	Tr	12.0	—	0.070	0.00	—	0.10	Tr
806	Prunes (stewed with sugar)	100		0	470	0.000	0.04	0.09	0.70	0.20	Tr	—	0.100	0.00	Tr	0.20	(Tr)
813	Raspberries (canned)	100		0	(75)	0.000	0.01	0.03	0.30	0.10	7.0	—	0.040	0.00	—	0.17	—
817	Strawberries (raw)	90	(80)	0	27	0.000	0.02	0.03	0.36	0.09	54.0	0.18	0.054	0.00	18.0	0.31	1.0
820	Tangerines (raw)	45	(30)	0	45	0.000	0.03	0.01	0.09	0.05	13.5	—	0.031	0.00	9.5	0.09	—
848	Honey (in jars)	15		0	0	0.000	Tr	0.01	0.03	Tr	Tr	—	—	0.00	—	—	—
849	Jam (fruit with edible seeds)	25		0	Tr	0.000	Tr	Tr	Tr	Tr	2.5	Tr	Tr	0.00	Tr	Tr	Tr
853	Marmalade	20		0	10	0.000	Tr	Tr	Tr	Tr	2.0	Tr	Tr	Tr	1.0	Tr	Tr
857	Chocolate (milk)	25	(35)	0	(10)	Tr	0.02	0.06	0.05	0.35	0.0	0.13	(0.005)	Tr	(2.5)	(0.15)	(0.8)
867	Bournvita	7		0	0	0.000	—	—	—	0.13	0.0	—	—	0.00	—	—	—
868	Cocoa powder	4		0	(2)	0.000	0.01	0.00	0.07	0.22	0.0	0.02	0.003	0.00	1.5	—	—
873	Drinking chocolate	7		0	—	0.000	0.00	0.00	0.03	0.11	0.0	0.01	0.001	0.00	0.7	—	—
874	Horlicks malted milk	10		47	—	0.155	0.08	0.11	1.12	0.29	0.0	—	—	—	—	—	—
875	Ovaltine	7		—	—	(2.142)	(0.12)	—	—	0.15	—	—	—	—	—	—	—
895	Keg bitter beer[4]	283	(334 868)	0	Tr	0.000	Tr	0.08	0.91	0.37	0.0	—	0.054	0.42	13.0	(0.28)	(1.4)
896	Lager (bottled beer)[4]	283	(331 669)	0	Tr	0.000	Tr	0.06	0.93	0.59	0.0	—	0.059	0.40	12.2	(0.28)	(1.4)
898	Stout (bottled)[4]	283	(307 567)	0	Tr	0.000	Tr	0.08	0.74	0.48	0.0	—	0.040	0.31	12.5	(0.28)	(1.4)
902	Cider (sweet)[4]	283	(252 —)	0	Tr	0.000	Tr	Tr	0.03	Tr	0.0	—	0.014	Tr	—	0.08	1.7
904	Wine (red)[4]	116	(163 256)	0	Tr	0.000	Tr	0.02	0.10	Tr	0.0	—	0.017	Tr	0.2	(0.05)	—
907	Wine white (medium)[4]	116	(163 256)	0	Tr	0.000	Tr	0.01	0.09	Tr	0.0	—	0.016	Tr	0.2	(0.03)	—
912	Sherry (medium)[4]	60	(71 182)	0	Tr	0.000	Tr	0.01	0.05	Tr	0.0	0.00	0.005	Tr	0.1	—	—
914	Vermouth (dry)[4]	60	(68 122)	0	0	0.000	Tr	Tr	0.02	0.00	0.0	0.00	0.005	Tr	Tr	—	—
915	Vermouth (sweet)[4]	60	(68 122)	0	0	0.000	Tr	Tr	0.02	0.00	0.0	0.00	0.002	Tr	Tr	—	—

[1]Food code = the number of the food in McCance and Widdowson's *The Composition of Foods* (Paul and Southgate, 1978).
[2]Womens' portion: see text for definition.
[3]Mens' portion: see text for definition. Where no weight is given, either men did not eat this food or data for both sexes was combined.
[4]For alcoholic beverages, the nutrient content is given per typical glass. The actual average portion weights for each sex are given in brackets.

was necessary to combine data from both sexes. Lack of space makes it impossible to provide lists of foods ranked for content per portion for each separate nutrient. However, it is relatively easy to run the eye down this table and pick out the foods of high or low content.

2.6.2 Vitamin requirements

For information on the biochemistry of the vitamins and for accounts of the classical deficiency diseases the reader is referred to the standard textbooks of nutrition (e.g. Passmore and Eastwood 1986).

For summaries of the body of work on which the Recommended Dietary Allowances (RDAs) are based, the relevant reports should be studied (DHSS 1979; NRC 1980; NRC 1985; Palmer et al 1982, 1984). This section notes some of the most recent work with implications for the vitamin requirements of normal populations.

Vitamin A

Deficiency of vitamin A is unknown in the UK and dietary surveys show intakes well above the RDA. However, there is currently much interest in the possible role of vitamin A in protecting against the development of certain cancers. Two studies (Wald et al 1980; Kark et al 1981) have shown that subjects with a higher plasma retinol concentration had a reduced risk of developing cancer; however, three other studies have found no such association (Haines et al 1982; Stähelin et al 1982; Willett et al 1984). Recent reviews (Wolf 1982; Anon 1982a; Anon 1984) regard the case as 'not proven'. 'It would be appealing if a...policy that prescribes carotene-rich foods rather than proscribing cigarettes would have a substantial effect on...lung cancer. It would be equally appalling if such a proclamation were made...on the present evidence' (Avon 1982a).

Vitamin D

Dietary vitamin D is listed in the both UK food tables and UK RDAs, and nutritionists still continue to measure dietary intake. However, it is clearly established that in people regularly exposed to sunlight, dietary vitamin D (about 2.5 µg; 100 iu/day) makes an insignificant contribution to plasma 25(OH)D levels. In only a minority of the population does it play a significant role in maintaining vitamin D status. Fraser (1983) provides an important review of recent advances.

Elderly people

In people deprived of sunshine, dietary vitamin D does make a valuable contribution to vitamin D status even though it has been calculated that an intake of about 12.5 µg (500 iu) is necessary to maintain plasma 25(OH)D at satisfactory levels. For the elderly therefore, particularly the housebound and those in institutions, supplements of 10 µg (400 iu) are to be recommended (Fraser 1983; Holdsworth et al 1984; Dattani et al 1984; Sheltawy et al 1984).

Infants

It has been shown in animals (Clements and Fraser 1984) that there is active transport of vitamin D from the mother to the foetus; the newborn therefore, even in the absence of sunlight and dietary vitamin D, do not develop rickets if maternal vitamin D status is adequate. Therefore, the vitamin D status of the infant is best determined by ensuring an adequate prenatal status in the mother rather than by giving oral vitamin D2 supplements to the infant. There is also a suspicion from experience with animals that giving oral vitamin D to infants promotes arteriosclerosis, and may therefore be harmful. (Peng et al 1978).

Milk, it must be noted, contains very little vitamin D. The suggestion by Lakdawala and Widdowson (1977) that it contains considerable amounts of water soluble vitamin D sulphate has not been confirmed by other workers (Leerbeck and Sondergaard 1980; Hollis et al 1981; Reeve et al 1982).

Asians

Asian mothers have a low vitamin D status and many Asian infants show signs of vitamin D deficiency e.g. neonatal tetany. Attempts to get Asians to increase dietary vitamin D have not been very successful and concerned people would like to see fortification of chapatti flour. However, this action has been rejected by the Committee on Medical Aspects of Food Policy (COMA). Arguments for and against fortification are set out in DHSS (1980) and Sheiham and Quick (1982).

The incidence of neonatal tetany has a seasonal variation, indicating that sunlight does make an important contribution to vitamin D status, and that it is not a total absence of exposure to sunlight which causes low vitamin D status in Asian women. Recent work (Clements and Fraser in preparation) suggests that deficiency is precipitated by the low Ca:P ratio and the low availability of calcium in the Asian diet. It is thought that this leads to enhanced destruction of vitamin D in the liver. Thus strategies for preventing vitamin D deficiency other than supplementation with pills or fortification of foods with vitamin D may emerge.

Welfare foods scheme supplements

COMA (DHSS 1980) recommended that vitamin tablets (vitamins A and D) continue to be made available to expectant and nursing mothers up to 30 weeks after parturition, and children's vitamin drops (vitamins A, D and C) for children up to the age of 5 years. They are probably unnecessary except among the Asian community.

Some 'lesser' vitamins

The RDAs are sometimes used rather uncritically to assess the dietary adequacy in population groups. When diets of healthy populations are apparently very deficient, this conclusion must be questioned. In a group of Cambridge mothers, Black *et al* (1986) found intakes of the 'lesser' vitamins to be much below the USA RDA or Estimated safe and adequate daily intake (ESADI) (NRC 1980), even though the diets were of above average nutrient density (see Table 2.23).

Table 2.23 Mean vitamin intakes of non-pregnant, non-lactating Cambridge women in Social Classes I, II and IIIA (Black *et al* 1986)

Vitamin	Intake	RDA or ESADI* (NRC 1980)	Intake as percentage of RDA or ESADI
Vitamin B6 (mg)	1.2 ± 0.2	2.0	60
Total folate (μg)	170 ± 45	400	43
Pantothenic acid (mg)	4.2 ± 0.9	4−7*	105−60
Biotin (mg)	25 ± 7	100−200*	25−13
Vitamin E (mg)	5.3 ± 1.7	8	66

The authors reviewed the bases of the RDA and concluded that folate is probably a marginal nutrient, so that people with high requirements and low intakes have a high probability of being deficient; that vitamin B6 may be marginal; and that the RDA/ESADIs for pantothenate, biotin and vitamin E were based on limited data with a generous safety allowance added and that these nutrients are unlikely to be deficient in the UK diet. The evidence is summarized below.

Vitamin B6

The various forms of pyridoxine, pyridoxal, pyridoxamine and their phosphates and some other conjugated forms all contribute to the vitamin B6 activity in foods. Bioavailability has been found to vary widely (Gregory and Kirk 1981), and uncertainty exists over how well this is reflected by the current forms of assay. The figures given in food tables must be regarded as tentative (Paul and Southgate 1978; Cooke 1983).

The RDA (NRC 1980) are based primarily on depletion−repletion experiments. Semi-synthetic diets containing around 0.5 mg vitamin B6 were given until biochemical indications of deficiency appeared, when subjects were repleted with supplements of varying magnitude. Supplements >2 mg/day reversed signs of deficiency, while supplements >0.5 mg/day and <2 mg/day had variable effects. (For a more recent comprehensive summary and bibliography see Rutishauser (1982).)

Vitamin B6 requirements are related to protein intake. The Australian RDA (Rutishauser 1982) propose a *minimum* intake of 0.015 mg/g protein/day and an RDA of 0.02 mg/g protein from a mixed diet providing 10−15% energy from protein, i.e. 1.2 mg for a 2000 kcal diet containing 12% energy from protein. Intakes in the UK range from 1.0−1.8 mg/day (adult men) 0.7−1.3 mg/day (adult women) — see Table 2.23.

Vitamin B6 may be a marginal nutrient among groups taking low energy diets of low nutrient density (see Section 1.3.2). There have been some reports of vitamin B6 deficiencies in the elderly (Vir and Love 1977), in patients on poor diets (Spies *et al* 1939) and in infants on a formula containing only 60 μg of vitamin B6 (Coursin 1955). However, it has proved remarkably difficult to obtain real evidence of biochemical deficiency in human populations. A wide variety of biochemical indices exist, e.g. plasma vitamin B6 levels, urinary excretion of trypotophan metabolites after tryptophan loading, and several enzyme activation tests, but they tend to give conflicting evidence about the existence of deficiency. More research is needed to determine the biological availability and the true dietary intake, and to assess the vitamin B6 status of normal populations on known intakes of vitamin B6.

Folate

On the one hand recorded total folate intakes generally range between 120−300 μg/day although some intakes as low as 30 µg/day have been recorded; on the other hand, the US (NRC 1980) and other countries' RDAs are 400 µg total folate/day for adults rising to 800 µg/day in pregnancy. Yet the population does not suffer from widespread folate deficiency. The reasons for this discrepancy between intakes and RDAs have been reviewed by Bates *et al* (1982) and Truswell (1984). In brief

1 There are several sources of error in the methods currently used for assaying folate in foods, and food table values are likely to be revised upwards in the future.

2 The availability of folates in foods is poorly understood, but the poor absorption of polyglutamates from the gut may have been exaggerated. Rodriguez (1978) summarized work on the availability from different foods; the average is 52.5% which is well above the 37.5% assumed in the US RDA report (NRC 1980). The distinction between free folate and conjugated folate is now considered inappropriate.

3 Evidence on which the RDA is based is limited and the NRC (1980) added very large safety factors.

In the UK, an RDA for folate was initially included in the 1979 COMA report (DHSS 1979) but it was withdrawn from subsequent reprints However, other countries continue to make recommendations regarding folate intake. The most recent RDAs are those of Australia (Truswell 1984). They are expressed as total folate and recommend an intake of 200 µg/day for adult men and women. This figure is based on three principles

1 The amount of absorbed folate required to treat or fully prevent deficiency disease in non-pregnant adults is 100 µg/day.

2 The average absorption of folates from foods is around 50%.

3 The average total folate consumption in Britain and North America is about 200 µg/day.

In pregnancy, folate needs are increased by the demand from increased cell turnover. That these needs cannot always be met from an individual's normal diet is shown by the significant number of women who developed megaloblastic anaemia of pregnancy before antenatal supplementation became routine (Chanarin 1973). The amount necessary to prevent a fall in red cell folate is an additional 100 µg/day in women who start pregnancy with adequate stores, but this cannot be assumed and an additional 200 µg/day is generally accepted as necessary. The Australian RDA for pregnancy is 400 µg/day. For lactation they recommend 300–350 µg/day, and for infants and young children 4 µg/kg/day.

For discussion of folates in preconceptional nutrition see Section 3.1.

Pantothenic acid

Food table values are derived from microbiological assays after enzyme treatment to release bound forms. Data is lacking for many foods. Calculated intakes must be regarded as tentative. Deficiency has been produced only by use of semi-synthetic diets (Fry *et al* 1976) or by giving an antagonist (Hodges *et al* 1959). Indications of deficiency take several weeks to appear, and studies of intake and excretion (Fry *et al* 1976) suggest the body has considerable stores. It is probable that the lower limit of the ESADI (4 mg) is sufficient to maintain health.

Biotin

Biotin occurs in bound and unbound forms and the biological availability in foods varies enormously. Food table values are based on 'values obtained by microbiological assay...after acid hydrolysis to release the bound form. Recent improvements have resulted in lower amounts...and these are believed to be more correct than the older ones' (Paul and Southgate 1978). Data is lacking for many foods. Calculated food intakes must be regarded as tentative. Biochemical evidence on which to assess the daily requirement is virtually non-existent. Deficiency syndromes are rare except in individuals who have consumed large amounts of egg white, although lowered urinary excretion, or lowered blood levels are said to have been reported in infants with seborrhoeic dermatitis, pregnant women, the elderly and athletes (Bonjour 1977), and deficiency has been reported as a complication of total parenteral nutrition (Mock *et al* 1981; Gillis *et al* 1982). It is thought that synthesis by intestinal microorganisms may contribute significantly to intake. All in all, it seems unnecessary, and even inappropriate, to attempt to estimate 'safe and adequate intake' for the general population.

Vitamin E

The RDA of 8 mg for adult females (NRC 1980) was based on the assumption that US diets are adequate and the statement that they contain 7–13 mg/day. However, the studies quoted in support of this statement have calculated intakes from selected meals, and not from total diets (Bunnell *et al* 1965; Bieri and Evarts 1973). Studies of total diets (Thompson *et al*

1973; Witting and Lee 1975; Bull and Buss 1982; Black *et al* 1986) find intakes of 2.3−3.0 mg/1000 kcal, (or 4−9 mg in diets of 1800−3000 kcal). Since deficiency is unknown except in premature infants and malabsorption syndromes, it is probable that the RDA is higher than necessary.

Lipids and lipid vitamins are poorly absorbed by neonates weighing less than 1500 g at birth. Low serum levels of vitamin E are commonly seen and are associated with haemolytic anaemia, bronchopulmonary dysplasia and retrolental fibroplasia.

Vitamin E deficiency also occurs in patients with malabsorption syndromes such as cystic fibrosis, massive ileal resection, blind loop syndrome and congenital cholestatic jaundice. It is associated with neuropathological syndromes (Anon 1986). In these cases, pharmacological doses of vitamin E are required for treatment.

Megadoses of vitamins

The use of vitamins in doses far exceeding the RDA has grown in recent years. They are claimed to cure or prevent a variety of conditions including the common cold, schizophrenia, cancer, hyperactivity, to increase ability to deal with stress and to delay ageing. Megadosing is promoted primarily by food faddists and 'orthomolecular' physicians. It can also arise through injudicious medical prescribing or by unwitting self-administration of high content vitamin preparations from health food shops. The best controlled studies have found no benefits from megadosing and significant toxic effects have emerged.

The toxic effects of the fat soluble vitamins are well recognized, but the water soluble vitamins are generally regarded as safe on the grounds that excess is eliminated in the urine. This is not so. All biologically active substances have a toxic level. The toxic effects of water soluble vitamins have been reviewed by Alhadeff *et al* (1984) and the toxic effects of all vitamins by Miller and Hayes (1982). Adverse effects are of four kinds

1 Direct toxicity.
2 Induced dependency.
3 The masking of other diseases.
4 Interactions with other drugs.

The reported adverse effects are summarized in Table 2.24, together with an indication of the doses at which adverse effects have been reported. Toxic effects of thiamin, riboflavin, pantothenic acid, biotin, folic acid and vitamin K have been rarely or never reported. Vitamin E is also of low toxicity, although an excess

could cause problems in patients on anticoagulant therapy.

References

Alhadeff L, Gualtieri CT and Lipton M (1984) Toxic effects of water soluble vitamins. *Nutr Rev* **42**, 33−40.

Anon (1982a) Dietary carotene and the risk of lung cancer. *Nutr Rev* **40**, 265−8.

Anon (1982b) The pathophysiological basis of vitamin A toxicity. *Nutr Rev* **40**, 272−4.

Anon (1983) Megavitamin E supplementation and vitamin K dependent carboxylation. *Nutr Rev* **41**, 268−70.

Anon (1984) Serum vitamin and provitamin A levels and the risk of cancer. *Nutr Rev* **42**, 214−5.

Anon (1986) Vitamin E deficiency. *Lancet* **i**, 423−4.

Bates CJ, Black AE, Phillips DR, Wright AJA and Southgate DAT (1982) The discrepancy between normal folate intakes and the folate RDA. *Hum Nutr: Appl Nutr* **36A**, 422−9.

Bieri JG and Evarts RP (1973) Tocopherols and fatty acids in American diets. *J Am Diet Assoc* **62**, 147−51.

Black AE, Wiles SJ and Paul AA (1986) The nutrient intakes of pregnant and lactating mothers of good socioeconomic status in Cambridge, UK: some implications for recommended daily allowances of minor nutrients. *Br J Nutr* **56**, 59−72.

Bonjour JP (1977) Biotin in man's nutrition and therapy — a review. *Int J Vitam Nutr Res* **47**, 107−18.

Bull NL and Buss DH (1982) Biotin, pantothenic acid and vitamin E in the British household food supply. *Hum Nutr: Appl Nutr* **36A**, 190−6.

Bunnell RH, Keating J, Quaresimo A and Parman GK (1965) Alphatocopherol content of foods. *Am J Clin Nutr* **17**, 1−10.

Chanarin I (1973) Dietary deficiency of vitamin B12 and folic acid. In *Nutritional deficiencies in modern society* Howard AN and McLean Baird I (Eds) Newman Books, London.

Clements MR and Fraser DR (1984) Quantitative aspects of vitamin D supply to the rat foetus and neonate. *Calcif Tissue Int* **36**, [Suppl 2] S31.

Clements MR, Johnson L and Fraser DR (1987) A new mechanism for induced vitamin D deficiency in calcium deprivation. *Nature* **324**, 62−5.

Cooke JR (1983) Food composition tables — analytical problems in the collection of data. *Hum Nutr: Appl Nutr* **37A**, 441−7.

Coursin DB (1955) Vitamin B6 (pyridoxine) in milk. *Q Rev Pediatr* **10**, 2.

Dattani JT, Exton-Smith AN and Stephen JML (1984) Vitamin D status of the elderly in relation to age and exposure to sunlight. *Hum Nutr: Clin Nutr* **38C**, 131−8.

Department of Health and Social Security (1979) *Recommended daily amounts of food energy and nutrients for groups of people in the United Kingdom*. Report on Health and Social Subject No 15. HMSO, London.

Department of Health and Social Security (1980) *Rickets and osteomalacia*. Report on Health and Social Subjects No 19. HMSO, London.

Fraser DR (1983) The physiological economy of vitamin D. *Lancet* **i**, 969−72.

Fry PC, Fox HM and Tas HG (1976) Metabolic response to a pantothenic acid deficient diet in humans. *J Nutr Sci Vitaminol* **22**, 339−46.

Gillis J, Murphy FR, Boxall LBHG and Pencharz PB (1982) Biotin deficiency in a child on long term TPN. *J Parent Ent Nutr* **6**, 308−10.

Gregory JF and Kirk JR (1981) The bioavailability of vitamin B6 in foods. *Nutr Rev* **39**, 1−8.

Table 2.24 Toxicity of vitamins (compiled from Alhadeff *et al* 1984 except where otherwise stated)

Vitamin	Reported effects/mechanisms of megadosis	RDA	Reported toxic intakes (per day)
Nicotinic acid	Histamine release; flushing, aggravation of asthma Hyperglycaemia; aggravation of diabetes, aggravation of peptic ulcer (by histamine release and acidity), hepatotoxicity, cholestatic jaundice, gouty arthritis from raised serum uric acid, cardiac arrhythmias and dermatological problems	18 mg	Flushing may occur at doses as low as 100 mg 750 mg for 3 months 1—3 g for 5—6 months 3—3.75 g for 96 weeks 3 g for 5 years
Vitamin B6	Peripheral neuropathy; destruction of dorsal roots (effect can be permanent) Antagonizes levodopa used to treat Parkinson's disease, penicillamine in treatment of Wilson's disease and the anticonvulsant phenytoin Dependency in adults, and in infants of mothers taking large doses in pregnancy	2.2 mg (USA)	2 g for 4 months 5 g for 2 months 10—25 mg 200 mg 5—300 mg
Vitamin C	Kidney stones due to acidification of urine and increased excretion of urate and oxalate, increased lysis of red blood cells, impaired bactericidal activity of white blood cells, diarrhoea Decreased absorption of vitamin B12, increased absorption of iron and aggravation of idiopathic haemochromatosis, thalassaemia major or siberoblastic anaemia Dependency in adults, and infants of mothers taking large doses in pregnancy	30 mg	5 g for 2 days or 2 g for 15 days can cause early biochemical changes 0.5—1 g 200 mg
Folic acid	Insomnia and irritability, masking of vitamin B12 deficiency, reduction of serum phenytoin levels (phenytoin itself reduces serum folate levels)	0.4 mg	5—15 mg
Vitamin A (Anon 1982b)	Skin changes: dryness, rash, fissures, depigmentation, pruritus. Hair loss Anorexia, weight loss, muscle soreness Headaches: raised intracranial pressure Chronic liver disease	750 µg	6000—12000 µg for years 30000—60000 µg for months 5400 µg in children
Vitamin D (DHSS 1980)	Hypercalcaemia in infants Hypercalcaemia and metastatic calcification Renal caluriosis; urolithiosis, hypercholesterolaemia, hypertension	10 µg	25—100 µg in infants 1000—3000 µg in adults
Vitamin E (Anon 1983)	Prolongs clotting time by antagonizing Vitamin K Increases the anticoagulant action of warfarin	8 mg	

Haines AP, Thompson SG, Basu TK and Hunt R (1982) Cancer, retinol binding protein, zinc and copper. *Lancet* i, 52—3.

Hodges RE, Bean WB, Ohlson MA and Bleiler B (1959) Human pantothenic acid deficiency produced by omega-methyl panthothenic acid. *J Clin Invest* **38**, 1421—5.

Holdsworth MD, Dattani JT, Davies L and Macfarlane D (1984) Factors contributing to vitamin D status near retirement age. *Hum Nutr: Clin Nutr* **38C**, 139—50.

Hollis BW, Roos BA, Draper HH and Lambert PW (1981) Occurrence of vitamin D in human milk whey. *J Nutr* **109**, 384—90.

Kark JD, Smith AH, Switzer BR and Hames CG (1981) Serum vitamin A (retinol) and cancer incidence in Evans County, Georgia. *J Nat Cancer Inst* **66**, 7—16.

Lakdawala DR and Widdowson EM (1977) Vitamin D in human milk, *Lancet* i, 167—8.

Leerbeck E and Sondergaard H (1980) The total content of vitamin D in human milk and cows' milk. *Br J Nutr* **44**, 7—12.

Miller DR and Hayes KC (1982) Vitamin excess and toxicity. In *Nutritional toxicology* Vol 1 Darby WJ (Ed) pp 81—133. Academic Press, New York.

Ministry of Agriculture, Fisheries and Food (1984) *Household food consumption and expenditure: 1982.* Annual report of the National Food Survey Committee. HMSO, London.

Mock DM De Lorimer AA, Liebman W, Sweetman L and Baker H (1981) Biotin deficiency: an unusual complication of parenteral alimentation. *New Engl J Med* **304**, 820—3.

National Research Council (1980) *Recommended dietary allowances*, 9e. National Academy of Sciences, Washington DC.

National Research Council (1985) *Recommended dietary allowances*, 10e. National Academy of Sciences, Washington DC. In preparation.

Palmer N *et al* (1982) Recommended dietary intakes for use in Australia. *J Food Nutr* **39**, 157−93.

Palmer N *et al* (1984) Recommended dietary intakes for use in Australia. *J Food Nutr* **41**, 109−54.

Passmore R and Eastwood M (1986) *Human nutrition and dietetics*. 8e. Churchill Livingstone, Edinburgh.

Paul AA and Southgate DAT (1978) McCance and Widdowson's *The Composition of Foods*. HMSO, London.

Peng SK, Taylor CB, Tham P and Mikkelson B (1978) Role of mild excesses of vitamin D3 in arteriosclerosis. A study in squirrel monkeys. *Paroi Arterielle* **4**, 229−43.

Reeve LE, Jorgensen NA and DeLuca HF (1982) Vitamin D compounds in cows' milk. *J Nutr* **112**, 667−72.

Rodriguez MS (1978) A conspectus of research on folacin requirements of man. *J Nutr* **108**, 1983−2103.

Rutishauser IHE (1982) Vitamin B6. *J Food Nutr* **39**, 158−67.

Sheiham H and Quick A (1982) *The rickets report. 'Why do British Asians get rickets?* Haringey Community Health Council, London.

Sheltawy M, Newton H, Hay A, Morgan DB and Hullin RP (1984) The contribution of dietary vitamin D and sunlight to the plasma 25-hydroxyvitamin D in the elderly. *Hum Nutr: Clin Nutr* **38C**, 191−4.

Spies TD, Bean WB and Ashe WF (1939) A note on the use of vitamin B6 in human nutrition. *J Am Med Assoc* **112**, 2414.

Spring JA, Robertson J and Buss DH (1979) Trace nutrients 3. Magnesium, copper, zinc, vitamin B6, vitamin B12 and folic acid in the British household food supply. *Br J Nutr* **41**, 487−93.

Stähelin HB, Buess E, Rösel F, Widmer LK and Brubacher G (1982) Vitamin A, Cardiovascular risk factors and mortality. *Lancet* **i**, 394−5.

Thompson JN, Beare-Rogers JL, Erdödy P and Smith DC (1973) Appraisal of human vitamin E requirements based on an examination of individual meals and a composite Canadian diet. *Am J Clin Nutr* **26**, 1349−54.

Truswell AS (1984) Folate. *J Food Nutr* **41**, 143−54.

Vir SC and Love AHG (1977) Nutritional evaluation of B groups of vitamins in institutionalized aged. *Int J Vitam Nutr Res* **47**, 211−8.

Wald N, Idle M, Boreham J and Bailey A (1980) Low serum vitamin A and subsequent risk of cancer. *Lancet* **ii**, 813−5.

Willett WC, Polk BF, Underwood BA, Stampfer MA, Pressel S, Rosner B, Taylor JO, Schneider K and Hames CG (1984) Relation of serum vitamins A and E and carotenoids to the risk of cancer. *New Engl J Med* **310**, 430−4.

Witting LA and Lee L (1975) Dietary levels of vitamin E and polyunsaturated fatty acids and plasma vitamin E. *Am J Clin Nutr* **28**, 571−6.

Wolf G (1982) Is dietary beta-carotene an anti-cancer agent? *Nutr Rev* **40**, 257−61.

2.7 Minerals

2.7.1 Sodium and potassium

Requirements

Sodium and potassium are of major importance in the body as they maintain fluid volume and pressure both intracellularly and extracellularly. They are both essential minerals and it is possible to find signs of deficiency if the dietary intake is reduced. (Whitney and Boyle 1984).

The body normally has a good homeostatic mechanism for control of the body content of these two minerals. The major excretory route is urine. Losses in the stools amount to only 2% of ingested sodium (Sanchez-Castillo and James 1984) and about 11% of potassium (Caggiula et al 1985). Loss of sodium in sweat is very small (2%/day) and individuals can become acclimatized, thereby reducing the loss. This does not appear to be the case with potassium and large losses can occur with profuse sweating (Lane and Cerda 1978, cited by Whitney and Boyle 1984).

The requirements for sodium and potassium are not easy to establish but 500 mg (22 mmol)/day has been quoted for sodium (BNF 1981) and 1560 mg (40 mmol)/day for potassium (Lee 1974) in adults. The requirement for potassium is higher because there is an obligatory loss of potassium in the urine and stools which amounts to about 590 mg (15 mmol)/day.

Sodium

Dietary sources and intake

The dietary intake of sodium may be divided into discretionary, (i.e. added to the food by the individual) and non-discretionary (the sodium which is added to food during manufacture or present naturally in foods.)

It has been estimated, that 84–88% of sodium intake in the UK is non-discretionary (Shepherd et al 1984; Sanchez-Castillo et al 1984). Bull and Buss (1980b) estimated from National Food Survey data that the intake of sodium in the British diet was between 2.9 and 3.7 g/day from non-discretionary sources, 86% being from processed foods.

Foods which make a significant contribution to the non-discretionary intake are the staples in the diet such as cereal products (bread and breakfast cereals in particular) and margarine or butter. A study in Australia (Greenfield et al 1984b) demonstrated that this group of staples provided 36% of the total sodium intake and that if cakes were also added, nearly 50% of sodium intake came from this group which would not be classified as 'highly salted foods'. In fact, 'highly salted foods' were shown to contribute 33% to the total. The remaining 17% of the total came from milk, beer and meat. Similar percentages have been shown for British diets although cereals provided 40% of the total (Bull and Buss 1980b). A diet relying heavily on processed foods could supply up to 6.5 g of sodium/day (282 mmol sodium or 16.6 g of salt) while one relying on take-away foods could contain about 5.1 of sodium (Greenfield et al 1984b). The same authors estimated that a diet which included very few processed foods and no take-away foods may supply as little as 1.6 g of sodium (70 mmol sodium or 4.1 g of salt).

Discretionary addition of sodium includes salting of food at the table and during cooking, although Sanchez-Castillo et al (1984) estimated that 29% of the sodium added when cooking was discarded with the cooking water. In a large observational study of over 2000 people, 64% were observed to add salt to their food, 16% of them without prior tasting (Greenfield et al 1984a). The amount added to the meal was largely dependent on the total diameter of the holes in the shaker but could be as much as 1.2 g of salt or 20.4 mmol (469 mg) of sodium. The use of a single-holed shaker of hole area 3 mm resulted in smallest addition of salt. The amount added to foods has been shown to correlate with preference for salty foods (Shepherd et al 1984) but not with total sodium intake nor sensitivity to the salt taste (Pangborn and Pecore 1982). However, it was of interest to find that in a controlled experiment, those men and women who added salt to their food did so in an amount proportional to the energy content of the diet, 0.4–0.6 g/1000 kcal (Kumanyika and Jones 1983). The amount added per day by individuals showed little intraindividual variability.

Clearly there is much more that needs to be done to establish just how individuals perceive the need for adding salt to food and to estimate the real contribution that this discretionary addition of sodium makes to total intake. What, perhaps, is clear is that the processed/ manufactured foods in the diet make a larger contribution to sodium intake than does individual salting. Therefore, salt taken in processed foods needs to be reduced in order to reduce the sodium intake of the population. Furthermore, if sodium intake is reduced then the preference for salty foods also decreases (Bertino *et al* 1982), i.e. the sensitivity to salt taste increases. Since a preference for salt in food and sensitivity to salty taste has been recognized in infants of only two years of age (British Nutrition Foundation 1981), the sodium content of food offered to this age group could conceivably affect their preference for salt in later life.

Estimation of sodium consumption is notoriously difficult (Pangborn and Pecore 1982). The 24-hour excretion of sodium provides a more realistic estimate of sodium intake. Caggiula *et al* (1985) found the urinary excretion of sodium in salt users to be 157 mmol (estimated intake was 119 mmol) and 119 mmol excretion in non-salt users (estimated intake was 104 mmol). This study demonstrates that the error in estimating sodium intake is likely to increase where the individual adds salt to his food; the percentage underestimate of sodium intake (as judged from excretion) was 24% for salt users and 13% for non-salt users.

One other source of sodium which must be considered when estimating intake of sodium, especially where the individual has been advised to reduce sodium, is in laxative and other drug usage (British Nutrition Foundation 1981).

Sodium restriction

Three categories of sodium restriction are used in clinical practice, depending on the degree of restriction required

1   No added salt — 80–100 mmol sodium/day (1.8–2.3 g sodium/day).
2   Low salt — 40 mmol sodium/day (1 g sodium/day).
3   Low sodium — 22 mmol sodium/day (0.5 g sodium/day).

A 'no added salt' (NAS) diet requires that the patient does not use salt in cooking or at the table. In addition, the consumption of salt-rich foods (Table 2.25) may need to be limited if the usual intake of these is particularly frequent or excessive.

Guidance for the construction of low salt or low sodium regimens is given in Tables 2.26 a and b. In some disorders, additional constraints on protein or fluid intake may have to be taken into account. Rite Diet low sodium bread (Welfare Foods Ltd) is prescribable for some patients on a low sodium regimen.

Because sodium restricted diets tend to be bland in flavour, alternative ways of flavouring foods using freely allowed herbs and spices should be suggested to patients. Some suggestions are given in Table 2.27. The formulation of a low sodium baking powder is given in Table 2.28. Retail pharmacists are often unwilling to make this up in small quantities and patients may

Table 2.25 Foods high in sodium

Food group	High sodium foods
Meat and meat products	All meat and poultry which is either tinned, smoked, cured or pickled, e.g. bacon, ham, sausages, salt beef, salt tongue, corned beef, luncheon meat and haslet. Meat paste and paté. Made-up, frozen, ready prepared meat stews, casseroles and other dishes.
Fish and fish products	Smoked or tinned fish, shellfish, kippers, sardines, etc. Fish paste and paté, made-up fish dishes.
Dairy products	Cheese (cottage cheese is lower in sodium)
Vegetables	All tinned vegetables
Miscellaneous	Dehydrated prepacked meals. Tinned, packet and bottled sauces and soups. Marmite, Oxo, Bovril, yeast extracts, stock cubes and gravy powders. Crisps and other snacks. Instant puddings and cake mixes.

Table 2.26 a and b Sodium restricted regimens

a) Daily allowances

Food	22 mmol sodium (Low sodium)	40 mmol sodium (Low salt)
Milk	200 ml	300 ml
Ordinary bread	None*	2 thin slices

NO SALT to be used in cooking or added to food at the table.
*Rite-Diet low sodium bread (Welfare Foods Ltd) is prescribable as a substitute in certain disorders (especially liver and renal disease).

b)

Foods allowed	Foods to avoid
[†]Meat	
Fresh or frozen meat, poultry, game, sweet-breads, tripe or liver	Bacon, ham, sausages, kidney, tongue tinned meat, meat pastes, and spreads; any salted and/or smoked meats or smoked meats or sausages. Manufactured meat products, e.g. meat pies and beefburgers
[†]Fish	
Fresh or frozen fish or fish roe	Tinned or smoked fish, shell-fish molluscs, fish pastes and spreads.

Table 2.26b *contd.*

Foods allowed	Foods to avoid
	Manufactured fish products, e.g. fish fingers and fish in sauce.
Dairy products Milk and eggs as an allowance. Unsalted butter, double cream and unsalted cream cheese. Yoghurt may be used in exchange for milk (but has a slightly higher sodium content)	Milk in excess of allowance. Cheese, evaporated or condensed milk and single cream.
Cereals Plain flour, wholemeal flour, salt-free bread, salt-free cakes and salt-free biscuits. Matzos and kosher crackers. Shredded Wheat, Puffed Wheat, Sugar Puffs and porridge. Rice, spaghetti, macaroni, semolina, tapioca, arrowroot and sago.	Self-raising flour, ordinary bread, cakes and biscuits (unless otherwise directed). Breakfast cereals other than those listed opposite.
Vegetables All fresh or frozen vegetables except those listed opposite. Unsalted potato crisps.	Baked beans, instant mashed potato and tinned vegetables. Salted potato crisps. *Use sparingly* carrots, spinach, celery and beetroot.
Fruit and nuts All fresh, tinned or stewed fruit, fruit juices, dates and unsalted nuts.	Dried fruit (except dates) Pickled olives, salted nuts and peanut butter.
Sugar products All sugars, glucose, jam, marmalade, honey, jelly, plain chocolate, boiled sweets, peppermints, marshmallows and marzipan.	Toffee, fudge, milk chocolate and filled chocolates. *Use sparingly* golden syrup and treacle.
Soups, sauces and gravies Home made salt-free soups and sauces. Salt-free meat or vegetable stock. Salt-free stock cubes, salt-free gravy browning (made from pure caramel). Salt-free tomato puree (check label).	Tinned and packet soups, gravy mixes and brownings. Stock cubes (unless salt-free). Salted yeast and meat extracts (e.g. Marmite, Bovril and Oxo). Commercial sauces, ketchups, salad creams, pickles, chutneys and tomato puree, unless labelled unsalted.
Beverages Tea, coffee and fresh fruit juices. Suitable low sodium fruit squashes, minerals and fizzy drinks, (manufacturers will usually provide information).	Soda water, mineral waters (unless permitted brand). Lucozade, tomato juice, cocoa powder, drinking chocolate, Bournvita, Horlicks and rosehip syrup.
Miscellaneous Herbs (see Table 2.27) Spices e.g. turmeric, ginger, nutmeg, curry powder, cloves, chilli, pepper, paprika, garlic and powdered mustard. Lemon juice, vinegar (check label for salt). Cooking oils, lard, suet and yeast. Salt substitute (based on potassium chloride[§]). Salt-free baking powder, custard powder and blancmange powder (check label).	Salt, celery salt or other flavoured salt. Bicarbonate of soda, baking powder, ready-mixed mustard and any products containing salt, soda or sodium.

*In cases of renal and liver disease, a sodium restriction may need to be accompanied by a fluid restriction.
[†]In cases of renal and liver disease, a protein restriction may also be indicated.
[§]Not allowed in renal disease.

Table 2.27 Flavouring food on low sodium diets

Food	Suggested flavourings
Fish	Allspice, bay leaf, dill, red cayenne pepper.
Roast meat	Allspice. Pork — cloves, apples. Lamb — marjoram, rosemary, apricot. Veal — tarragon. Chicken — tarragon, dill, grapes. Liver — oranges.
Grills and roasts	Fresh lemon juice.
Stews	Basil, bay leaf, dill, garlic, bouquet garni, marjoram, oregano, chilli, sage, thyme, orange or lemon peel, red cayenne pepper.
Tomatoes	Basil, marjoram, oregano.
Potatoes	Bay leaf, nutmeg, dill, garlic, mint.
Rice	Bay leaf, nutmeg, coriander, cardamom, peppercorns, turmeric.
Scrambled egg	Chilli, chives, red paprika pepper.
Omelette	Chives, chervil, tarragon, garlic, red paprika pepper.
Courgettes	Coriander, garlic.
Carrots	Thyme
Cauliflower, cabbage	Dill, caraway.
All dishes	Freshly ground black and white pepper.

Table 2.28 Low sodium baking powder (makes 100 g)

21 g starch

30 g potassium bicarbonate

6 g tartaric acid

43 g potassium acid tartrate

The powder should be stored in a cool, dry place.

experience difficulty in getting the baking powder for this reason. If a number of patients at any centre are going to need this baking powder the hospital pharmacist should be asked to prepare it. The powder can then be used within the hospital for low sodium diets, and patients be given a supply when they leave and on subsequent visits.

Potassium

Dietary sources and intake

Potassium is found widely distributed in foods. Bull and Buss (1980c) have calculated the contributions which various food groups made to the supply of potassium in the UK diet. Out of a total intake of 2.99 g (76.6 mmol/day), root vegetables supplied the greatest percentage (27%), and significant amounts were also provided by milk (19%), meats and eggs (13%), cereal products (11%) and other vegetables (10%). From

Table 2.29 Foods high in potassium

Food group	Foods high in potassium
Wholegrain cereals*	These may be incorporated into the diet. The absorption of K^+ varies between subjects and therefore blood biochemistry needs careful monitoring.
Meat and meat products	All meat*
Fish and fish products	All fish*
Dairy products	Milk*, eggs* and yoghurt*.
Fruit	All fruit, especially dried and crystallized fruit, bananas, apricots, rhubarb and blackcurrants. Fruit juices, tomato juice.
Nuts	All nuts
Vegetables	Dried pulses, baked beans, beetroot, sweetcorn, mushrooms, spinach. Instant potatoes*, chips*, jacket potatoes*, potato waffles*, crisps and other manufactured potato snacks. Vegetable juice.
Beverages	Build Up, drinking chocolate, Horlicks, Ovaltine, other malted milk drinks. Coffee and cocoa. Wine and sherry.
Sugar and confectionery	Chocolate and all foods containing it, toffees, liquorice. Molasses, black treacle, syrup, mincemeat and dried fruit.
Miscellaneous	Marmite and all yeast extracts, Oxo, Bovril, gravy powders, stock cubes, bottled sauces and ketchups, pastes, pickles and chutneys. Packet sauces, tinned and packet soups. Instant puddings, Gram flour, Cream of Tartar.
Herbs and spices	Salt substitutes, e.g. Ruthmol, Selera. Reduced sodium salts. Curry powder, chilli and ginger.

*these foods may be incorporated into the diet using an exchange list.
Note that some foods may be unsuitable in renal or liver failure due to their high sodium and/or protein content.

Table 2.30 Low potassium foods

Food group	Low potassium foods
Bread and cereals	Arrowroot, cornflour, custard powder, flour, oatmeal porridge, rice, sago, tapioca, white bread.
Fats and oils	Butter, dripping, margarine, oils, suet, fats.
Sugar and confectionery	Boiled sweets, barley sugars, glucose, honey, glacé cherries, jam, marshmallows, Opal fruits, Opal mints, pastilles, peppermints, marmalade
Beverages	Tea, weak ground coffee, spirits e.g. whisky, ginger ale, lemonade, orangeade, Lucozade, soda water, Hycal, lime juice cordial, Tizer, Pepsi-cola, water. Schweppes: American sweet ginger, bitter lemon, dry ginger, sparkling grapefruit, lemonade, sparkling golden orange, sugar-free tonic and tonic water.

Note that some items will not be suitable if a sodium and/or protein restriction is necessary.

analysis of diet samples, Bull and Buss (1980c) found the total intake of potassium to be slightly less at 2.51 g/day and the proportion supplied by cereals higher (16%) and that from root vegetables lower (23%).

Dietary potassium is not completely absorbed and 24-hour urinary potassium excretion is a more accurate way of measuring potassium intake (Caggiula *et al* 1985).

Potassium restriction

Potassium is present in nearly all foods. Foods which are particularly high in potassium are summarized in

Table 2.31 *Potassium exchange list.* Each exchange provides approximately 4 mmol potassium

Food group	Foods	Exchange	Food group	Foods	Exchange
High biological value protein foods	Milk	100 ml	Cereals *contd*	Millet flour	40 g
	Soya milk	300 ml		Poppadums	15 g
	Yoghurt	60 g	Fruit	Apple	
	Cheddar cheese	130 g		Bilberries	
	Eggs, hens	2 eggs		Pineapple, canned (with syrup)	
	Meat, average, lean (cooked)	50 g		Strawberries, canned (with syrup)	125 g
	Fish (cooked)	50 g		Cranberries	
	Tofu	200 g		Pear	
Cereals	White wheat flour	120 g		Tangerine (weighed with skin)	
	Wholemeal flour	45 g		Watermelon (weighed with skin)	
	Wheat bran	13 g		Peaches, canned (with syrup)	
	Wholemeal bread	70 g		Strawberries, fresh	
	White bread	160 g		Lemon (whole or juice)	
	Rye crispbread	30 g		Orange (weighed with skin)	100 g
	Digestive biscuits	100 g		Passion fruit (weighed with skin)	
	All Bran	15 g		Tangerine (weighed without skin)	
	Cornflakes	160 g		Blackberries	
	Rice Krispies	100 g		Gooseberries	
	Weetabix	3 biscuits		Lychees	
	Noodles (raw)	60 g		Mango	75 g
	Spaghetti (raw)	60 g		Melon (weighed with skin)	
	Rice, brown (raw)	60 g		Plums	

Table 2.31 *contd.*

Food group	Foods	Exchange	Food group	Foods	Exchange
Fruit *contd*	Quince		Vegetables *contd*	Tomato	
	Raspberries	}		Ginger root	}
	Apricots (fresh)			Beans	
	Cherries			mung	
	Damsons			haricot	
	Figs, fresh (raw)			Cassava	
	Grapes			Gourd (dried)	
	Loganberries			Lentils (dried)	
	Melon (weighed without skin)			Mushrooms	
	Mulberries	50 g		Peas	<25 g
	Nectarines			chick	
	Orange (weighed without skin)			dried	
	Peach			Pigeon peas (dried)	
	Pineapple			Plantain	
	Pomegranate			Potato	
	Redcurrants			jacket	
	Whitecurrants			chips	
	Apricots (dried)			roast	
	Avocado pear			crisps	
	Banana			Spinach	
	Blackcurrants			Yam	
	Currants (dried)		Beverages*	Milk	100 ml
	Figs (dried)	<25 g		Soya milk	300 ml
	Prunes (dried)			Pure orange juice	
	Raisins (dried)			canned	120 ml
	Rhubarb			fresh	90 ml
	Sultanas (dried)			Pure grapefruit juice (canned)	140 ml
Vegetables	Carrots, old (boiled)			Pineapple juice	110 ml
	Chayote			Tomato juice	60 ml
	Marrow (boiled)	125 g		Coffee	
	Onions			instant	4 g
	Swede (boiled)			ground, infusion	240 ml
	Cabbage			Tea (infusion)	920 ml
	Cucumber			Bournvita	40 g
	Runner beans (boiled)	100 g		Cocoa	10 g
	Turnip (boiled)			Drinking chocolate	40 g
	Water chestnuts			Horlicks	20 g
	Cauliflower			Ovaltine	20 g
	Chicory (raw)			Beer	
	Courgettes			keg bitter	1 pint
	Green pepper	75 g		pale ale	350 ml
	Marrow (raw)			stout	350 ml
	Okra			stout extra	180 ml
	Radish			strong ale	140 ml
	Ackee			Cider	200 ml
	Artichokes, globe (edible portion)			Wine	
	Aubergine			red	120 ml
	Beans			white, average	200 ml
	broad (boiled)			Sherry	
	baked			dry	175 ml
	Beetroot (raw)			sweet	140 ml
	Broccoli (boiled)			Vermouth	400 ml
	Brussels sprouts (boiled)		Miscellaneous	Golden syrup	60 g
	Cabbage (raw)			Black treacle	10 g
	Carrots (raw)			Jam (not low sugar)	150 g
	Leeks	50 g		Marmalade (not low sugar)	350 g
	Lettuce			Chocolate	
	Cress			plain	50 g
	Parsnips			milk	35 g
	Peas			Toffee	75 g
	Potato (boiled)			Marzipan	40 g
	Pumpkin			Indian sweets (average)	25 g
	Sweetcorn				
	Sweet potato				

Table 2.31 *contd.*

Food group	Foods	Exchange
Spices[†]	Anise seeds	10 g
	Allspice	1 g
	Caraway seeds	10 g
	Cardamom powder	10 g
	Chilli powder	5 g
	Cinnamon powder	30 g
	Coriander seeds	10 g
	Cumin seeds	5 g
	Dill seeds	10 g
	Fennel seeds	5 g
	Fenugreek seeds	20 g
	Ginger (ground)	15 g
	Mustard powder	15 g
	Nutmeg	40 g
	Paprika	5 g
	Saffron	5 g
	Sesame seeds	35 g
	Turmeric	5 g

*Spirits, carbonated drinks, fruit-flavour drinks and fruit squashes contain negligible amounts of potassium.
[†]White pepper has a negligible potassium content.

Table 2.29. Low potassium foods are listed in Table 2.30. In some instances (for example, certain renal disorders), dietary potassium intake may need to be regulated by means of a system of potassium exchanges. A 4 mmol potassium exchange list is given in Table 2.31.

2.7.2 Calcium, phosphorus and magnesium

Requirements

These minerals can be considered together as they have several features in common. They are meta-bolically and physiologically linked so that altering the status with respect to one mineral has an effect on the other two

1 Calcium and phosphorus are known to be vitamin D responsive (DeLuca 1982; Weiser 1984) while magnesium may well be too (Bengoa and Wood 1984).
2 All three can moderate the levels of parathyroid hormone (Aikawa 1978; DeLuca 1982).
3 Symptoms and signs of deficiency for all three minerals include neuromuscular abnormalities indi-cating a key role in nerve transmission and muscle physiology.
4 A major route of excretion is through the kidneys and this represents the major homeostatic control mechanism for phosphorus and magnesium (Marshall *et al* 1976).

Table 2.32 shows the estimates for dietary intake of the three minerals, together with the observed intakes in the UK for adults. Tables 2.33, 2.34, 2.35 and 2.36 show some of the factors which can affect body status of calcium and magnesium in health and disease. (Aikawa 1978; Allen 1982; Weiser 1984; Bengoa and Wood 1984).

Dietary sources of calcium

The principal sources of calcium in a typical British diet (MAFF 1985) are milk, cheese, bread, flour (if fortified) and vegetables (Table 2.37). The average calcium content of some common foods is given in Table 2.38; more complete data can be obtained from McCance and Widdowson's *The Composition of Foods* (Paul and Southgate 1978).

Table 2.32 Intake, requirement and absorption of calcium, magnesium and phosphorus

Mineral	Absorption (%)	Estimated daily requirement	Recommended daily intake	Actual daily intake (adult)
Calcium	Range: 24–75% Normally:[a,b] 30–40%	Obligatory losses:[a,b,c] 100–190 mg (GI) 110–130 mg (urine) 15 mg (sweat) Total: 235 mg	500 mg (Men and women[d]) 1200 mg Pregnant and lactating women[d]	800 mg[e]
Magnesium	Range:[f,g] 24–76% Normally: 45%	Approximately[c] 100 mg (to induce a deficiency, a level of 10–20 mg is needed).	300–350 mg[h]	249 mg[i]
Phosphorus	Approximately 60%[c]	Approximately 400 mg[c]	800 mg[h]	1223–1300 mg[j]

[a]Allen (1982); [b]Weiser (1984); [c]Marshall *et al* (1976); [d]DHSS (1979); [e]MAFF (1985); [f]Bengoa and Wood (1984); [g]Aikawa (1978); [h]Whitney and Boyle (1984); [i]Spring *et al* (1979) and [j]Gilbert *et al* (1985).

Table 2.33 Dietary factors affecting the availability of calcium and magnesium for absorption

	Calcium	Magnesium
Factors causing increased availability	Bile salts, Solubility greatest in the presence of gastric juice and where pH is <6.0. Congeners in wine?	
Factors causing decreased availability	Abnormally high levels of saturated fats (e.g. in steatorrhoea and when bile salts are reduced). Phytic acid,* oxalates* and phosphates* (very little effect[c]). Fibre (especially the uronic acid group found in fruit and vegetables). However, degradation of complexes may occur in the large bowel, releasing Ca^{2+}	As for calcium

*Probably only important when dietary calcium levels are low and over short periods.
[c]Spencer et al (1984).

Table 2.34 Factors affecting the absorption of calcium and magnesium

	Calcium	Magnesium
Factors causing increased absorption	Physiological status — growth, pregnancy and lactation (oestrogens). Increase of simple dietary sugars — lactose, glucose, galactose. Increased dietary protein? Occurs in postmenopausal women[e] but not in young men[f]. The amount of mineral available to the mucosa and the length of contact time, particularly on the unsaturated absorption in the distal bowel (ileum and colon). Increased vitamin D intake.	Slow transit time may enhance absorption. Concentration of Mg in the lumen — low = 76% absorption; high = 24% absorption. But independent of Mg status? Increase in simple sugars. Vitamin D may enhance absorption. High levels of sodium
Factors causing decreased absorption	Increasing age. Increased alcohol consumption. Low vitamin D status. High zinc intake.	High levels of calcium or phosphorus. High levels of zinc.

[e]Lutz and Linkswiler (1981); [f]Allen et al (1977).

Details of proprietary mineral supplements are given on p 205. The composition of other calcium supplements can be found in a current edition of the *Monthly Index of Medical Specialities* (MIMS) or the *British National Formulary*.

Table 2.35 Factors causing excretion and body losses of calcium and magnesium

Calcium	Magnesium
Low physical activity Increased dietary phosphate Increased dietary protein Increased dietary sodium Oxalates	Renal — increased intake causes increased urinary losses. Gut — diarrhoea and vomiting incur losses as secretions contain large amounts of Mg. Sweat — profuse sweating may result in high losses since acclimatization does not take place. Sweat accounts for 10–15% of total Mg losses per day, up to 25%.

Dietary sources of phosphorus

Foods which are high in protein and calcium are also, in general, high in phosphorus. Therefore if the phosphorus content of the diet needs to be limited, this entails restriction of all foods of animal origin, and in particular: milk, yoghurt, hard cheese, eggs, offal, shellfish and meat extracts.

In addition, the intake of nuts, dried pulses and wholegrain cereals should be limited (although the extent to which phosphorus is available for absorption in the latter remains uncertain).

The phosphorus content of some foods is listed in Table 2.39.

Table 2.36 Clinical conditions which can affect mineral status

Area of clinical interest	Calcium	Magnesium	Phosphorus
Intestinal and hepato-biliary tracts	In Crohn's disease, losses occur proportional to enteric protein losses[a]. Jejuno-ileal bypass (resection) results in reduced absorption,[d] proportional to the amount of ileum (colon) removed. Cholestatic liver disease and reduction in bile salts result in impaired absorption.[d,e]	Increased losses in Crohn's disease[b] and ulcerative colitis Pancreatic insufficiency Pancreatitis,[b,c] Reduced absorption (also greater deposition in fat leads to hypomagnesaemia). Jejuno-ileal bypass, diarrhoea and/or accelerated transit times lead to reduced absorption[b]. As for calcium	Prolonged treatment with antacids ($Mg(OH)_2$ and $Al(OH)_3$) reduces serum phosphate levels[a]
Renal	Hypocalcaemia can result from altered vitamin D metabolism in the kidney[a]; hypercalcaemia can result from reduced clearance in uraemia[f].	Hypermagnesaemia may result from high levels of magnesium in dialysate[b], possibly causing neuropathy/uraemic pruritis[g].	Hyperphosphataemia may develop as phosphates are not excreted due to nephron destruction in renal disease[h].
Diabetes	(In the rat the absorption of calcium is altered, perhaps because of altered vitamin D metabolism)[a].	Hypomagnesaemia in insulin dependent diabetes[c] is suggested to influence insulin sensitivity of tissues[j] inverse relationship between magnesium levels and blood glucose in young women has been reported[k].	
Cancer	Hypercalcaemia has been described in later stages. (Low sodium diet is used to enhance calcium loss[l].)		
Hypertension	Calcium excretion has been found to be greater in hypertensives, with a lower dietary intake.[m,n,o] A supplement of 2 g calcium reduced blood pressure in the third trimester of pregnancy.		Depressed serum phosphorus levels enhanced renal clearance in hypertensives.
Drugs	Glucocorticoids reduce intestinal absorption and inhibit bone resorption.[d,p] Anticonvulsants influence body status through their effect on vitamin D[d].	Aminoglycoside antibiotics,[q] thiazide and loop diuretics and laxatives enhance magnesium losses.[r]	

Dietary sources of magnesium

Magnesium is widespread in foods, especially those of vegetable origin (Table 2.40). Dietary deficiency is rare and magnesium deficiency is usually a result of gastrointestinal losses, for example, due to diarrhoea.

2.7.3 Iron

Although not usually regarded as such, iron can be classified as a 'trace element' because the body's requirement for it, although vital, is very low compared with other minerals such as calcium. Some general

Table 2.36 contd.

Area of clinical interest	Calcium	Magnesium	Phosphorus
Altered dietary patterns	Osteoporosis has been described[s] in starvation as in anorexia nervosa. During long term parenteral feeding mineral status needs careful monitoring;[d] hypercalcaemia has been reported with TPN and oliguria.[f]	Starvation but with chronic laxative or diuretic abuse enhanced losses (e.g. anorexia nervosa)[t] As for calcium	
Miscellaneous	Hypocalcaemia has been described with pernicious anaemia. Hypercalcuria has been described with a high protein diet[v]. Lactose intolerance may reduce calcium absorption[w].		Hypophosphataemia has been described after a fun run, and may be due to an increase in catecholamines[x].

[a]Allen (1982); [b]Bengoa and Wood (1984); [c]Aikawa (1978); [d]Weiser (1984); [e]Epstein *et al* (1982); [f]Crookes and Graham (1984); [g]Graf *et al* (1979); [h]DeLuca (1982); [i]Yajnik *et al* (1984); [j]Mather *et al* (1979); [k]Poston (1982); [l]Heller and Hosking (1986); [m]McCarron and Morris (1982); [n]Belizan *et al* (1983); [o]Henry *et al* (1985); [p]Jibani and Hodge (1985); [q]Wilkinson *et al* (1986); [r]Swales (1982); [s]Szmukler *et al* (1985); [t]Fonseca and Havard (1985); [u]Fairris *et al* (1984); [v]Allen *et al* (1977); [w]Finkenstedt *et al* (1986); [x]Bushe (1986).

Table 2.37 Sources of calcium in the typical British diet (MAFF 1985)

Food group	% of daily calcium intake
Milk and cream	42%
Cereals	26%
Cheese	14%
Vegetables	7%
Meat and meat products	3%
Fish and fish products	2%
Eggs	2%
Fruit	2%
Miscellaneous	2%

aspects of iron requirement, absorption and excretion are therefore included in the following section on trace elements. However, more specific considerations of iron can be found in the following sections of this Manual in relation to the following

1   Iron deficiency anaemia (Section 4.18; p 473.)

2   Iron requirements during pregnancy (Section 3.1; p 247.)

Further reading

Wright M (1984) *The salt counter, a quick and easy checklist of the salt content of natural and packaged foods.* Pan, London.

References

Aikawa JK (1978) Biochemistry and physiology of magnesium. *World Rev Nutr Diet* **28**, 112−142.

Allen LH (1982) Calcium bioavailability and absorption: a review. *Am J Clin Nutr* **35**, 783−808.

Allen LH, Oddoye EA and Margen S (1977) The calcium metabolism of young men fed high protein diets. *Proc Nutr Soc* **36**, 101A.

Belizan JM, Villar J, Pineda O, Gonzalez AE, Sainz E, Garrera G and Sibrain R (1983) Reduction of blood pressure with calcium supplementation in young adults. *J Am Med Assoc* **249**, 1161−5.

Bengoa J and Wood R (1984) Magnesium In *Absorption and malabsorption of mineral nutrients* pp 69−88. A R Liss Inc, New York.

Bertino M, Beauchamp GK and Engleman K (1982) Long term reduction in dietary sodium alters taste of salt. *Am J Clin Nutr* **36**, 1134−44.

British Nutrition Foundation (1981) *Salt in the diet.* British Nutrition Foundation Briefing Paper (2). British Nutrition Foundation, London.

Bull NL and Buss DH (1980b) Contributions of foods to sodium intakes. *Proc Nutr Soc* **39**, 30A.

Bull NL and Buss DH (1980c) Contributions of foods to potassium intakes. *Proc Nutr Soc* **39**, 31A.

Bushe CJ (1986) Profound hypophosphataemia in patients collapsing after a 'fun run'. *Br Med J* **292**, 898−9.

Caggiula AW, Wing RR, Nowalk MP, Milas NC, Lee S and Langford H (1985) The measurement of sodium and potassium intake. *Am J Clin Nutr* **42**, 391−8.

Crookes PF and Graham HK (1984) Hypercalcaemia precipitated by oliguria during total parenteral nutrition. *Br Med J* **289**, 561.

De Luca HF (1982) Vitamin D. In *Human nutrition: current issues and controversies.* Neuberger A and Jukes TH (Eds). MTP Press Ltd, Lancaster.

Department of Health and Social Security (1979) *Recommended daily amounts of food energy and nutrients for groups of people in the United Kingdom.* Report on Health and Social Subjects No 15. HMSO, London.

Fairris GM, Mason PD and Fairris N (1984) Hypocalcaemia in pernicious anaemia. *Br Med J* **288**, 607.

Table 2.38 Calcium content of foods

Food group	Calcium content (mg/100 g)
Dairy products	
Milk	
liquid	120
dried skimmed	1190
Cheese	
cheddar	800
cottage	60
Yoghurt, natural	180
Cream, single	79
Cereal products	
Bread	
white	100
wholemeal	23
Flour	
white (fortified)	150
wholemeal	35
Cornflakes	3
Muesli	200
All Bran	74
Puffed wheat	26
Pasta (cooked)	8
Rice	1
Biscuits (digestive)	110
Pastry (cooked)	92
Scone	620
Meat, fish and eggs	
Beef, lamb, pork (lean, raw)	8
Cod, haddock (raw)	17
Herring (raw)	33
Pilchards (in tomato sauce)	300
Sardines (in tomato sauce)	460
Eggs (whole)	52
Vegetables	
Broccoli (boiled)	76
Cabbage (boiled)	40
Carrots (boiled)	37
Cauliflower	18
Peas	31
Potatoes (old, boiled)	4
Fruit (raw, edible portion)	
Apple (eating)	4
Banana	7
Blackberries	63
Melon	19
Orange	41
Rhubarb	100
Sultanas	52

Table 2.39 Phosphorus content of foods

Food group	Phosphorus content (mg/100 g)
Dairy produce	
Milk	95
Cheese (cheddar)	520
Yogurt	140
Meat, fish and eggs	
Beef, lamb, pork, chicken (lean, raw)	190
Liver (raw)	370
Kidney (raw)	270
White fish (raw)	170
Pilchards (canned in tomato sauce)	350
Prawns	350
Eggs (whole)	220
Pulses	
Beans	
butter (boiled)	87
baked (canned)	91
haricot (boiled)	120
broad (boiled)	99
Peas (boiled)	85
Lentils (boiled)	77
Nuts (edible portion)	
Almond	440
Brazil	590
Coconut	94
Peanuts	370
Cereal products	
Bread	
white	97
wholemeal	230
Bran	1200
Flour	
white	110
wholemeal	340
All Bran	900
Cornflakes	47
Muesli	380
Rice Krispies	150
Miscellaneous	
Marzipan	220
Chocolate	
milk	240
plain	140
Cocoa powder	660
Baking powder	8430
Yeast extract (Marmite)	1700

Finkenstedt G, Skrabal F, Gasser RW and Braunsteiner H (1986) Lactose absorption, milk consumption and fasting blood glucose concentrations in women with idiopathic osteoporosis. *Br Med J* **292**, 161–2.

Fonesca V and Havard CWH (1985) Electrolyte disturbances and cardiac failure with hypomagnesaemia in anorexia nervosa. *Br Med J* **291**, 1680–2.

Gilbert L, Wenlock RW and Buss DH (1985) Phosphorus in the British household food supply. *Hum Nutr: Appl Nutr* **39A**, 208–12.

Graf H, Kovarik J, Stummvoll HK and Wolf A (1979) Diappear-ance of uraemic pruritis after lowering dialysate magnesium concentration. *Br Med J* **279**, 1478–9.

Greenfield H, Smith AM, Maples J and Wills RBH (1984b) Contributions of foods to sodium in the Australian food supply. *Hum Nutr: Appl Nutr* **38A**, 203–10.

Heller SR and Hosking DJ (1986) Renal handling of calcium and sodium in metastatic and non-metastatic malignancy. *Br Med J* **292**, 583–6.

Henry HJ, McCarron DA, Morris CD and Parrott-Garcia M (1985) Increasing calcium intake lowers blood pressure: the literature reviewed. *J Am Diet Assoc* **85**, 182–5.

Table 2.40 Magnesiium content of foods

Food group	Magnesium content (mg/100 g)	Food group	Magnesium content (mg/100 g)
Dairy produce		Potatoes (boiled)	15
Milk	12	Beans	
Cheese (cheddar)	25	runner (boiled)	17
Yoghurt	17	baked	31
Meat, fish and eggs		*Fruit* (edible portion)	
Beef, lamb, pork (lean, raw)	18	Apple (eating)	5
White fish	23	Banana	42
Sardines (in tomato sauce)	51	Orange	13
Shrimps (boiled)	110		
Eggs	12	*Nuts* (edible portion)	
		Almonds	260
Cereal products		Brazil	410
Bread		Chestnuts	33
white	26	Peanuts	180
wholemeal	93		
Flour		*Miscellaneous*	
white	20	Cocoa powder	520
wholemeal	140	Chocolate (plain)	100
All Bran	370	Treacle	140
Cornflakes	14	Marzipan	120
		Yeast extract (Marmite)	180
Vegetables			
Cabbage (boiled)	8		

Jibani M and Hodge H (1985) Prolonged hypercalcaemia after industrial exposure to vitamin D. *Br Med J* **290**, 748−9.

Kuminyika SK and Jones DY (1983) Patterns of week to week table salt use by men and women consuming constant diets. *Hum Nutr: Appl Nutr* **37A**, 348−56.

Lee HA (1974) Normal fluid and electrolyte requirements. In *Parenteral nutrition in acute metabolic illness* pp 97−112. Academic Press, London and New York.

Lutz J and Linkswiller HM (1981) Calcium metabolism in post-menopausal women consuming two levels of dietary protein. *Am J Clin Nutr* **34**, 2178−86.

McCarron DA and Morris CD (1982) Calcium consumption and human hypertension: report of a national survey. *Clin Res* **30**, 338A.

Marshall DH, Nordin BEC and Speed R (1976) Calcium, phosphorus and magnesium requirement. *Proc Nutr Soc* **35**, 163−73.

Mather HM, Nisbet JA, Burton GH, Poston GT, Bland JM, Bailey PA and Pilkington TRE (1979) Hypomagnesaemia in diabetes. *Clinica Chimica Acta* **95**, 235−42.

Ministry of Agriculture, Fisheries and Food (1985) *Household Food Consumption Survey: 1983.* HMSO, London.

Pangborn RM and Pecore SD (1982) Taste perception of sodium chloride in relation to dietary intake of salt. *Am J Clin Nutr* **35**, 510−20.

Paul AA and Southgate DA (1978) McCance and Widdowson's *The Composition of Foods.* 4e MRC Special Report Series No 297.

Poston GJ (1982) Insulin resistance and hypomagnesaemia. *Br Med J* **255**, 575−6.

Sanchez-Castillo CP and James WPT (1984) Estimating dietary sources of sodium with lithium tagged salt. *Proc Nutr Soc* **43**, 154A.

Sanchez-Castillo CP, Warrender S, Whitehead T and James WP (1984) Epidemiological assessment of sodium sources in the diet by the use of the lithium-marker technique. *Proc Nutr Soc* **43**, 153A.

Shepherd RE, Farleigh CA and Land DG (1984) Effects of taste sensitivity and preference on salt intake. *Proc Nutr Soc* **43**, 87A.

Solomons NW (1982) Mineral interactions in the diet. *ASDC J Dent Child* **49**, (6), 445−8.

Spencer H, Kramer L and Osis D (1984) Effect of calcium on phosphorus metabolism in man. *Am J Clin Nutr* **40**, 219−25.

Spring JA, Robertson J and Buss DH (1979) Trace nutrients 3: Magnesium, copper, zinc, vitamin B6, vitamin B12 and folic acid in the British Household Food Supply. *Br J Nutr* **41**, 487−92.

Swales JD (1982) Magnesium deficiency and diuretics. *Br Med J* **285**, 1377−8.

Szmukler GI, Brown SW, Parsons V and Darby A (1985) Premature loss of bone in chronic anorexia nervosa. *Br Med J* **290**, 26−7.

Weiser MM (1984) Calcium. In *Absorption and Malabsorption of mineral elements* Solomons NW and Rosenberg IH (Eds). pp 15−68. AR Liss Inc, New York.

Whitney EN and Boyle MA (1984) *Understanding nutrition* 3e. West Publishing Co.

Wilkinson R, Lucas GL, Heath DA, Franklin IM and Boughton BJ (1986) Hypomagnesaemia tetany associated with prolonged treatment with aminoglycosides. *Br Med J* **292**, 818−9.

Yajnik CS, Smith RF, Hockaday TDR and Ward NI (1984) Fasting plasma magnesium concentrations and glucose disposal in diabetes. *Br Med J* **288**, 1032−4.

2.8 Trace Elements

2.8.1 General considerations

Tremendous advances in our understanding of trace element nutrition have been made in the past 30 years. Newer analytical techniques and the ability to produce environments and diets free of individual trace elements have made the study of the metabolism of such elements possible. A deficiency of trace elements which are ubiquitous in the environment can now be produced in animals.

However, the question then arises, if such stringent experimental conditions need to be imposed, how could such elements ever be deficient in a normal diet and therefore be worthy of consideration by dietitians? Frank deficiencies of trace metals are rare, but sub-optimal levels of the element in the body can arise and may be responsible for conditions of clinical importance. A frank deficiency of chromium (Jeejeebhoy *et al* 1977) only occurred after inadvertent omission of chromium from a TPN regime for five years. However, sub-optimal deficiency of chromium has been suggested to occur in certain cases of diabetes mellitus where chromium supplementation has improved glucose tolerance (Guthrie 1982). A relative silicon deficiency has been suggested in atherosclerosis (Nielsen 1984). Both chromium and silicon are present in food and it would seem impossible for low tissue levels to arise and impair metabolic function. Yet this can happen for any trace element. Even on apparently adequate dietary intakes of a trace element, overall status can be compromised through several mechanisms

1 Interactions between trace elements. A marginal deficiency or excess of an element can influence the utilization and function of another (Kirchgessner *et al* 1982).

2 Interactions between trace elements and other dietary components. For example, between fibre and silicon (Kelsey *et al* 1979) or iron and tannin (Cook *et al* 1981).

3 The form in which the element appears in the food. Organically complexed selenium is much more readily absorbed than the simple inorganic form (Combs and Combs 1984).

4 Drugs. These can affect absorption, tissue distribution and excretion of trace elements (Section 2.8.4).

Chelating agents such as EDTA enhance loss of zinc (Shah 1981), vitamin D enhances uptake of lead (Moore 1979) and oral contraceptives affect blood levels of many trace elements (Smith and Brown 1976).

5 Clinical conditions. These can affect tissue levels of trace elements. Where there is impaired absorption and possible dietary restriction, selenium levels have been found to be low (Hinks *et al* 1984). Zinc excretion is enhanced in alcoholism (Prasad 1982).

Table 2.41 Trace elements in the human diet

Essential	Possibly essential	Non-essential (toxic)
Chromium	Arsenic	Aluminium
Cobalt (as vitamin B12)	Fluorine	Cadmium
Copper	Nickel	Lead
Iodine	Silicon	Mercury
Iron	Tin	
Manganese	Vanadium	
Molybdenum		
Selenium		
Zinc		

Other elements found in human tissue include beryllium, boron, bromine, gold, lithium, silver and rubidium.

Dietitians should also consider the dietary factors which may affect trace element toxicity. Trace elements which are toxic to humans behave in the same way as elements which are essential. This means it may be possible to manipulate the dietary intake to minimize absorption or enhance excretion of toxic elements.

2.8.2 Trace element requirements

Some trace elements have been identified as being essential to humans, some as possibly essential and others as non-essential, or toxic (Table 2.41).

To establish a level of consumption which will ensure a nutritional adequacy is difficult. In animal models this is relatively easy, although as different species often display different signs and symptoms of deficiency, requirements may well vary between species and at different times of the life cycle. In humans who eat a great variety of foods, live in complex environments and for longer periods of time than experimental

Table 2.42 Trace element composition per kg wet weight[a]

Food	Chromium (µg)	Cobalt (µg)	Fluorine (mg)	Manganese (mg)	Molybdenum (mg)	Nickel (mg)	Selenium (µg)	Vanadium (µg)[f]	Aluminium (mg)	Cadmium (µg)	Mercury (µg)	Lead (µg)
Cereals and grain products												
Wheat germ (Bemax)	<20*	20	1.4	180	0.3	0.8	30		11	150	<4	<50
Wheat bran	50	70	1.7	150	0.2	1.2	20		26	100	7	<50
Whole wheat	20*	20	0.6	36	0.2	0.4	10, 530d		8	50	<4	<50
Wheat flour (white)	20	20	<0.5	8	<0.2	0.1	10, 40d		7	30	<4	<50
Rolled oats (porridge) (raw)	<20	80	0.8	58	<0.2	0.7	10, 30d		<5	60	6	<50
Rice, whole grain (raw)	30	30	0.4	24	0.2	0.2	20		28	6	9	70
Rice, polished (raw)	20	<20	<0.5	9	0.2	0.1	20, 100d		5	<10	4	<50
Spaghetti (raw)	40	<20	N	6.0	N	0.1	10		<5	40	<4	110
Bread (wholemeal)	20*	40	0.9	17.0	<0.2	0.1	<10		<5	30	<4	80
Bread (white)	30	20	0.5	6.0	<0.2	0.1	<10		<5	20	<4	<50
Cornflakes	70*	30	0.5	110	<0.2	0.4	20, 20d		16	<10	<4	50
Puffed rice (Rice Krispies)	50	20	0.6	10	0.2	0.1	20		<5	50	4	<50
Crispbread (rye)	80	60	1.0	36	0.2	0.2	30		20	20	<4	90
Biscuits/cookies	60	30	<0.5	3.5	<0.2	0.05	<10		<5	20	<4	90
Sponge cake	60	20	<0.5	3.1	<0.2	<0.05	20		5	10	<4	50
Swiss roll	80	<20	<0.5	2.4	<0.2	<0.05	20		<5	10	<4	70
Milk and dairy												
Milk, cows', fresh (whole)	10	<5	0.1	0.09	0.05	0.01	3,<10d	0.09	<1	<2	<1	10
Milk, fresh (skimmed)	5*	<5	0.8	0.08	<0.05	<0.01	2		<1	<2	<1	10
Milk, dried (skimmed)	20	<20	N	0.8	N	<0.05	20	0.2	<5	5	<4	100
Butter	60	10	N	0.11	N	0.1	5,<10d		<3	5	2	40
Cream (whipping)	40	5	0.2	0.04	0.2	0.03	2		1	4	<1	70
Cheddar type/full fat[b] cheese	10	10	0.5	0.48	0.06	<0.03	40, 120d		3	60	<2	70
Edam type cheese (40% Fat)	20	10	0.7	0.59	0.06	0.1	40		2	<5	<2	40
Cottage cheese	20	5	0.3	0.26	0.05	0.02	20		1	<2	1	20
Cheese (processed) (45% Fat)	60*	10	0.3	0.41	0.06	0.03	10		4	10	<2	100
Yoghurt, low fat, (Natural)	5	<5	0.1	0.1	<0.05	0.01	3		<1	<2	<1	20
Egg (whole)	5	5	0.3	0.46	<0.05	0.01	110		1	4	7	10
Egg (white)												
Egg (yolk)[b]	200	<20	2	0.97	N	<0.05	300, 200d		<10	10	<4	<50
Margarine[b]	<20	40	N	0.12	N	0.1	<10,<10d		<5	20	<4	<50
Meat												
Beef	20	10	0.2	0.1	<0.1	<0.02	10, 30d		5	5	<2	30
Pork	40	<10	0.2	0.1	<0.1	<0.02	70, 140d		4	<5	3	30
Mutton	40	10	0.2	0.1	<0.1	0.02	20,<10d		4	5	<2	30
Liver (mean of beef, pig and sheep)	10*	50	<0.2	3.6	1.5	<0.02	180, 130d	6.0	13	70	10	20
Kidney (mean of beef, pig and sheep)	20	50	<0.2	1.3	0.7	<0.02	1020		9	170	5	70
Gelatin												
Chicken	40*	10	<0.2	0.2	<0.1	<0.02	110		4	<5	2	40
Fish												
Cod (raw)	10	<10	1.6	0.25	<0.1	<0.02	270, 100d		<2	<5	170	30
Sardines (in oil)	40	20	1.3	1.5	<0.1	0.03	350		3	30	19	770
Salmon (canned)	10	10	6.8	0.48	0.1	0.06	420		4	5	82	250
Tuna (in oil)	90	10	0.9	0.55	<0.1	0.02	420		9	20	420	290
Oysters												
Lobster								430				
Fruit and vegetables (all raw, unless stated[g])												
Beans, green	5	10	0.1	2.5	0.2	0.5	<2		2	2	<1	10
(frozen)	20e	20e				0.35e						
Beetroot	10, 82e	10, 30e	0.1	6.0	<0.1	0.1 ,0.17e	<2		3	30	1	20
Broccoli	10, 190e	50, 20e	0.1	5.8	<0.1	0.5 ,0.11e	<2		2	10	6	40

Table 2.42 *contd.*

Food	Chromium (µg)	Cobalt (µg)	Fluorine (mg)	Manganese (mg)	Molybdenum (mg)	Nickel (mg)	Selenium (µg)	Vanadium (µg)[f]	Aluminium (mg)	Cadmium (µg)	Mercury (µg)	Lead (µg)
Cabbage (winter)	5, 150[e]	5, 30[e]	<0.1	2.4	<0.1	0.1, 0.2[e]	<2,<10[d]		<1	5	<1	10
Carrots	10, 80[e]	<5, 20[e]	0.1	3.6	<0.1	0.04,0.03[e]	<2,<10[d]		3	30	2	20
Cauliflower	5	<5	0.1	2.3	<0.1	0.3	<2	0.08	5	10	1	<10
Cucumber	<5, 170[e]	<5, 10[e]	<0.1	0.98	<0.1	0.02,0.08[e]	<2	2.1	1	5	<1	10
Leeks	30, 80[e]	<5,<10[e]	0.1	1.9	0.1	0.1, 0.13[e]	<2		16	10	2	10
Lettuce	10, 170[e]	5, 10[e]	0.2	5.2	<0.1	0.1, 0.05[e]	<2	21	3	50	1	70
Onion	10, 190[e]	5,<10[e]	<0.1	2.3	<0.1	0.05,0.09[e]	<2		2	30	<1	20
Parsnips	10	<5	0.1	4.0	0.1	0.2	<2		3	50	1	20
Peas (green)	20	5	<0.1	3.8	0.2	0.5	2		1	30	1	30
Peas (frozen)	10, 380[e]	30, 20[e]	0.2	3.7	0.2	0.6, 0.35[e]	3		0.9	10	<1	20
Peas (dried)	40	100	0.7	12.0	0.7	1.8	<10		12	20	4	80
Potatoes (old)	5, 150[e]	10, 20[e]	0.1	2.2	<0.1	0.1, 0.16[e]	<2,<10[d]	0.82	3	10	2	20
Potatoes (new)	10	20	<0.1	2.5	N	0.2	<2		1	30	1	10
Spinach	20, 200[e]	10, 50[e]	0.4	17.0	<0.1	0.2, 0.4[e]	<2		13	150	4	110
(frozen)	(60[e])	(20[e])				(0.02[e])						
Swedes	5, 90[e]	5, 10[e]	<0.1	1.4	<0.1	0.05, 0.06[e]	<2		1	5	<1	20
Tomatoes	5, 240[e]	<5, 10[e]	0.1	1.1	N	0.05, 0.09[e]	<2	0.03	1	10	<1	10
(tinned)	(30[e])	(<10[e])				(0.49[e])						
Apples (eating)	5, 110[e]	<5, 10[e]	0.2	0.47	<0.1	0.01, 0.01[e]	<2,<10[d]	1.1	1	<2	2	40
Apple juice	40	10	0.1	0.56	<0.1	0.05	<2		2	<2	<1	60
Apricots (canned)	120, 40[e]	10, 10[e]	0.2	0.43	<0.1	0.1, 0.2[e]	2		7	<2	1	600
Bananas	30	<5	0.1	2.4	<0.1	0.02	5		5	<2	1	30
Currants (black)	30	<5	0.2	3.1	0.1	0.1	<2		9	2	1	60
(tinned)	(30[e])	(10[e])				(0.13[e])						
Dates	60	10	<0.3	4.0	<0.1	0.1	30		3	4	3	100
Gooseberries	10	<5	<0.1	1.7	<0.1	0.03	<2		2	2	<1	20
Grapes	10	<5	0.1	0.85	<0.1	0.02	<2		2	<2	<1	670
Grapefruit	10	<5	0.1	0.36	<0.1	0.1	2		<1	<2	<1	20
Mandarin oranges	10	<5	0.1	0.55	<0.1	0.03	<2,<10[d]		1	<2	<1	30
Oranges	10	5	0.1	0.42	<0.1	0.03	<2,<10[d]		1	<2	<1	40
Orange juice	10	<5	0.3	0.29	<0.1	0.01	<2		<1	<2	<1	40
Peaches	20	<5	0.1	0.7	<0.1	0.4	<2		4	4	1	40
(tinned)	(50[e])	(10[e])				(0.09[e])						
Pears	20, 440[e]	<5, 20[e]	<0.1	0.5	<0.1	0.1, 0.2[e]	<2		<1	10	1	30
Pineapple (canned)	110, 90[e]	5, 10[e]	<0.1	15	<0.1	0.5, 0.85[e]	<2		2	3	<1	220
Plums	20,<10[e]	<5,<10[e]	0.1	1.0	<0.1	0.05, 0.2[e]	<2		2	<2	<1	40
Prunes (dried)	190	10	0.7	3.8	<0.1	0.6	5		7	4	3	230
Raisins	100	10	1.0	3.1	<0.1	0.03	5		29	4	3	620
Raspberries (frozen)	20	30	0.2	12	<0.1	0.9	<2		10	20	<1	40
Strawberries	10	10	0.1	4.3	<0.1	0.04	<2		5	10	<1	20
Mushrooms[b]	10, 25[e]	<5, 30[e]	N	0.83	N	0.02, 0.08[e]	30, 80[d]		14	10	220[c]	10
(tinned)	(330[e])	(20[e])				(0.2[e])	100[d]					
Almonds	120	140	N	25	N	1.3	20, 40[d]		7	10	<4	90
Peanuts[b]	80	<20	N	8.6	N	3.9	20, 30[d]		14	30	<4	70
Hazelnuts	140	210	1.0	14.0	<0.2	1.8	30,<10[d]		<5	20	<4	200
Preserves and sweets												
Honey	50	<20	0.8	3.7	<0.2	0.2	<10		<5	<10	<4	100
Jam, fruit (with edible seeds)[b]	30	10	N	2.5	N	0.2	3		4	10	<2	110
Marmalade[b]	20	10	N	1.4	N	0.1	3		<3	5	<2	40
Chocolate (milk)	60	60	1.0	2.6	<0.2	0.7	20		<5	30	<4	260
Toffee and fudge	170	50	1.0	0.83	<0.2	0.2	<10		<5	10	<4	50
Beverages												
Tea (as drunk)	5	<2	0.49	1.6	<0.02	0.07	<1		3	<1	<0.4	2
Coffee, drip grind (as drunk)	<2	<2	0.05	1.1	<0.02	0.01	<1		0.7	<1	<0.4	<5
Coffee (instant)	<20	<20	4.0	18.0	<0.2	0.9	30		7	10	<4	170
Cocoa beverage (as drinking chocolate)	140	140	N	7.7	N	2.0	15		15	20	<4	240

Table 2.42 contd.

Food	Chromium (µg)	Cobalt (µg)	Fluorine (mg)	Manganese (mg)	Molybdenum (mg)	Nickel (mg)	Selenium (µg)	Vanadium (µg)[f]	Aluminium (mg)	Cadmium (µg)	Mercury (µg)	Lead (µg)
Carbonated cola drink	8	2	0.2	0.02	<0.02	<0.01	1		1	<1	<0.4	7
Carbonated lemonade	3	<2	0.05	<0.01	<0.02	<0.01	<1		<0.5	<1	<0.4	<5
Beer (3–3.7% alcohol by weight)	9	<2	<0.05	0.27	<0.02	0.01	<1,<10[d]		<0.5	<1	<0.4	9
Red wine[b] (Spanish)	10	1.5	0.08	1.1	0.02	0.05	0.25		2.3	2	<1	15
White wine (medium)[b] (French)	120	<2	0.08	0.22	0.02	<0.01	0.8		10	<2	<1	340

*High biological Chromium (GTF) Toepfer et al (1973). [a]Unless stated otherwise, annotated values taken from Koivistoinen (1980). [b]Only one sample analysed. [c]High compared to other varieties — range 5–94 µg/kg. [d]Taken from Thorn et al (1978) values for UK foods. [e]Taken from Thomas et al (1974) values for UK foods. [f]Taken from Soremark (1967) worldwide values. [g]Tinned concentrations will vary with storage. (Henriksen et al 1985). N, No data available.

or farm animals, it is very much more difficult to define a minimum intake or even optimal intake. It would seem that the following criteria would need to be met in order to begin to make some recommendations

1 Identify the signs and symptoms of a sub-optimal intake (manifestations may take many years to develop).
2 Record the level of trace element intake.
3 Assess the absorption of the trace element (this may be difficult due to many factors which can influence absorption).
4 Monitor body levels of trace elements.
5 Assess changing needs for trace elements at different stages of the life cycle, physiological status and periods of environmental stress.

Dietitians and human nutritionists need to consider trace element status so that our understanding of dietary requirements can be advanced. A clear understanding of those factors which influence the assessment of dietary intake, absorption and excretion is needed before predictions about requirements can be made.

2.8.3 Assessment of trace element intake

Trace element composition of food

In order to estimate the trace element content of the diet, food composition tables are needed. The only large study undertaken recently in this area was in Finland. Table 2.42 is based largely on data from this survey (Koivistoinen 1980) but only those foods in common use in the UK have been selected. The reader is referred to the original for more analyses. Where analysis has been undertaken in the UK or elsewhere, these values are also given. It is of interest that in many cases the UK and Finnish values are in close agreement. The table can be used to give an estimate of the trace element intake.

However, the following points should be borne in mind when using there and other publishing values of the trace element content of food

1 Analytical techniques need to be sensitive, often

Table 2.43 Factors affecting trace element concentrations in food

Factor	Example of effect on trace element concentration
Geographical location of production	Iodine in potatoes[1] (µg/kg dry weight) Scotland = 89 Somerset = 163. Zinc in apples[2] (mg/kg wet weight) Finnish = 1.2 Imported = 0.23.
Annual variation	Chromium in winter wheat[2] (µg/kg wet weight) In 1973 = 31 In 1975 = 9.
Seasonal variation	Iodine in milk[1,6] (µg/litre) Summer = 8 Winter = 32.
Maturity	The trace element content of cereal grains decreases during maturation. The trace element content of animal tissues may also decrease — eggs from young hens have 34% more copper than those from older hens.
Processing 1 Milling	Zinc in rice[4] (mg/100 g wet wt) Unpolished = 0.65 Polished = 0.16.
2 Fractionating	Molybdenum in milk (mg/100 g wet wt) Whole milk = 0.02 Skimmed milk = 0.002.
3 Cooking	Copper in spinach[3] On boiling = 29% loss On pressure cooking = 16% loss On steaming = 9% loss Lead in potatoes[5] (µg/kg wet wt) Uncooked = 400 Boiled = 250.
4 Grinding/ homogenizing	Iron in meat[2] (mg/kg wet wt) Homogenized in liquidizer = 7.4 Ground in meat grinder = 8.9.

[1]Chilean Iodine Educational Bureau (1952); [2]Koivistoinen (1980); [3]Pennington and Calloway (1973); [4]Schroeder (1971); [5]Zoetman and Brinkman (1976); [6]Wenlock et al (1982).

to parts per billion, and selective in order to provide data about trace element concentrations in food and biological material. Wolf (1982) considers present procedures to be reliable for only the following elements: copper, manganese, cadmium, mercury, iron, selenium, lead and zinc.

2 If data has been produced for only one or two samples of a food it may not be applicable to the foodstuff as eaten by any one individual. Table 2.43 shows the factors which can influence the trace element content of food.

3 The presence of a trace element in a food does not necessarily mean it is biologically available.

Trace elements in water

Tap water probably supplies about 60% of our water intake (Zoeteman and Brinkmann 1976), so that where dietary intakes are marginal, trace elements in water could be important. Hardness of the water supply, and the piping through which it flows, can influence the trace element concentration (Masironi 1978). There is also the consideration of whether tap water reflects

adequately the trace element intake where it is used to make other beverages, such as tea and coffee, as elements may be lost or added (Gillies and Paulin 1982). Zoeteman and Brinkman (1976) report that manganese, nickel and zinc were particularly increased in tea and coffee by 10–100 fold, 3–6 fold, and 7 fold respectively.

Bottled mineral waters may have a higher concentration of trace elements than tap water. In one study (Zoeteman and Brinkman 1976) levels of arsenic, beryllium, boron, chromium, lithium, manganese and nickel were all higher in mineral water (lithium by a factor of 700). The levels of cadmium (a hardener in plastic piping), cobalt, copper, lead, mercury and zinc were higher in some tap waters in the same study.

2.8.4 Absorption and excretion of trace elements

Information on the absorption of trace elements for men is limited and for women and children even more so. The reasons for this are

1 Traditional balance studies are difficult to interpret

Table 2.44 Estimated intake, body content, absorption and requirements of trace elements in adults (not pregnant, not lactating)[4]

Trace element	Estimated intake	Body content[3]	Percentage absorption	Estimated daily requirement
Essential				
Chromium (μg)	30 –200[a]	1000– 5000[b] ↓	1– 25[a]	50 –200[a,b]
Cobalt (mg)	0.2 – 0.6[c]	1.1[b]	73– 97[b,c]	Only as B12
Copper (mg)	2 – 5[e]	80[e]	30[e]	2 – 3[f,d]
Iodine (μg)	100 –400[g]	10000–20000[c] (50000)[b]	100[b]	100 –200[c]
			6♂[i]	10♂[m]
Iron (mg)	7 – 20[i,j] (9 – 12% haem[o])	1000[j]	15♀[i]	12♀[m]
Manganese (mg)	2.4 – 7.0	10– 20[e]	3– 4[f]	2.5– 5.0[f]
Molybdenum (μg)	100[c]	9000–16000[b]	40–100[b]	150 –500[f]
Selenium (μg)	60 –216[j,e]	14000–21000[b,e]	35– 85[b]	30 –200[e,h]
Zinc (mg)	5 – 22[c]	1400– 2300[c]	10– 40[e]	15[f]
Possibly essential				
Arsenic (mg)	0.07– 0.4[c]	8– 20[b]	[1](5[b])> 90[c]	?
Fluorine (mg)	0.6 – 1.8[n]	2600– 4000[c,d] ↑	50– 90[c]	1.5– 4[f,d]
Nickel (μg)	600[g]	5000–10000[b]	3– 6[b]	50 – 80[2]
Silicon (mg)	21 – 46[e]	1100[b]	1– 4[b]	?
Tin (mg)	1.5 – 3.5[e](17[k])	42[b,c]	<3[e]	?
Vanadium (μg)	22[e]	10000[b] ↑	≤1[b,e]	10– 25[e]
Non essential				
Aluminium (mg)	3.8 – 51.6	50– 150[b] ↑	0.1[b]	None
Cadmium (μg)	13 – 24[e]	15000–30000[b] ↑	5[e,l]	None
Lead (μg)	140 –400[k]	122000[b] ↑	≃10[l]	None
Mercury (μg)	4 – 20[k]	13000[b]	*5– 10[b](90[e])	None

[1]Depends on form, as the organic complex is very easily absorbed. [2] Estimated on the basis of 50–80 ng per g of diet. [3]Arrows indicate increasing (↑) or decreasing (↓) with age. [4]Northern hemisphere.
[a]Guthrie (1982); [b]Linder (1978); [c]Underwood (1971); [d]Nordstrom (1982); [e]Prasad (1982); [f]Whitney and Boyle (1984); [g]Abdulla *et al* (1979); [h]Golden (1982); [i]Barber *et al* (1985); [j]Barber *et al* (1985); [k]Lynch and Morck (1983); [k]Prasad (1976); [l]Waldron (1982); [m]DHSS (1979); [n]WHO (1970); [o]Bull and Buss (1980).

as endogenous excretion of trace elements (mainly in the bile) are indistinguishable from exogenous sources.

2 *In vivo* tracer techniques, to identify exogenous and endogenous sources, have relied on radioisotopes which are potentially hazardous for children and women of child-bearing years.

3 Newer tracer techniques, which are safer, use stable isotopes. However, these are expensive and not all trace elements have a suitable isotope for study in this way.

Nevertheless, some factors which can influence trace element absorption have been identified. The absorption of some elements, such as chromium, decrease with age (Guthrie 1982). Low zinc status may enhance zinc absorption and this homeostatic mechanism may well exist for other trace elements (Solomons and Rosenberg 1984). Periods of rapid growth also affect the absorption of both essential and non-essential elements, it is thought that about 10% of lead is absorbed in adults and possibly as much as 50% is absorbed in young animals and children (Smith 1976). Estimates of the absorption and requirements for trace elements are shown in Table 2.44.

The principal routes of excretion are summarized in Table 2.45. Body losses may well be enhanced

1 During periods of malabsorption.

2 During catabolic periods (note sweat losses).

Table 2.45 Excretion of trace elements (values in *italics* indicate part of homeostatic mechanism)

Trace element	Faecal Percent of dietary intake (actual amount/day)	Urine (per day)	Sweat (per 100 ml)	Menses (per day)	Breast milk (μg/l)
Essential					
Chromium (μg)	95– 99[a]	0.3– 0.6[a]			39[c], 20[b]
Cobalt (μg)	15[d], 80[e](40–60)	140 –190[d]			<5[b]
Copper (μg)	(100–300)[d]	60♂[f] 12♀[f]	55♂[f] 148♀[f]	20[d]	50, 330[b]
Iodine (μg)	(5–20)[d]	40[d]	Significant		9– 43[g]
Iron (mg)	*Variable*[2](0.6)[h]	0.1[h]		0.45[h]	300–600[i]
Manganese (μg)	*95[d]*	11 – 23[f]			14[e], 25[b]
Molybdenum (μg)	40[d]	*11 – 58[f]*			10[b]
Selenium (μg)	40– 70[d]	*50 – 60% of dietary intake[j]*			10– 20[k]
Zinc (mg)	70[d]	0.6♂[f] 0.3♀[f]	0.05♂[f] 0.125♀[f]		2000[f]
Possibly essential					
Arsenic (mg)	*Variable[2]*	Variable[p] *(0.23[3,e])*			<0.010[b]
Fluorine (μg)	10[m]	(80% dietary intake)			0.1[m], 100[b]
Nickel (μg)	95[d](258)	15 – 47[3,d]	4.9[n]		10[b]
Silicon (mg)	60– 97[f]	12 – 16[f]			<2[b]
Tin (μg)	99[d]	8 – 16[d]			(2–3 ng/g[a] dry weight)
Vanadium (μg)	95[d]	*0 – 8[f]*			
Non essential					
Aluminium (μg)	95[d]	15[o]			<100[b]
Cadmium (μg)	95[e]	1 – 2(1.5[3,e])* (0.9[3,e])[t]			<2[b]
Lead (μg)	90[f]	10 – 80[f]	5.0[f] 11.8[f]		5–12, 10[b]
Mercury (μg)	*Variable[2]*	1.5–200[3,t]			Readily transferred <1[b]

[1]Mature milk
[2]See Table ?
[3]Estimated on basis 1.5 litres/day
*Smokers
[t]Non-smokers

[a]Byrne and Kosta (1979); [b]Koivistoinen (1980); [c]Kumpulainen and Vuori (1980); [d]Underwood (1971); [e]Waldron (1982); [f]Prasad (1982); [g]Chilean Iodine Educational Bureau (1952); [h]Lynch and Morck (1983); [i]Linder (1978); [j]Levander and Morris (1984); [k]Thorn *et al* (1978); [l]Digest (1982); [m]Prasad (1976); [n]Horak and Sunderman (1973); [o]Boegman and Bates (1984); [p]Solomons and Rosenberg (1984).

GENERAL DIETETIC PRINCIPLES AND PRACTICE

Table 2.46 Trace elements — dietetic and clinical significance in adults

Trace element	Major manifestation of deficiency and (toxicity)	Instances when trace element status may be compromised	Reported daily consumption (country of study)	Dietary sources Good	Poor
Copper	Anaemia, neutropenia, bone demineralization[a] (50 mg dose, nausea[f])	Prolonged TPN,[b] protein-energy malnutrition[d], impaired intestinal absorption (coeliac)[e,a,f], nephrotic syndrome[e], chelating drugs. Diets low in energy or fat (<25%)[c] Diets low in protein Supplementary zinc[f]	1.74 – 12.51 mg (USA)[c]	Offal, pulses, nuts, shellfish. (Food cooked in copper pots)	Dairy produce
Chromium	Impaired glucose tolerance[g], possibly impaired fat metabolism[h] (3 g as a single dose[h])	Diabetes, multiparous women, protein-energy malnutrition[h], prolonged periods of exercise, diets high in refined carbohydrate[1], the elderly[2].	0.005 – 0.115 mg (USA)[m] 0.033 – 0.126 mg (USA)[h] 0.014 – 0.045 mg (Fin)[h] 0.014 – 0.048 mg (UK)[3]	Brewers yeast, meat, cheese, vegetables, unrefined carbohydrate, wine, beer.	Fruit, seafood, refined carbohydrate.
Iron	Anaemia[i] (100 mg per day for at least 20 years)	Malabsorption, low energy diets, pregnancy, diets with a high phytate and/or tannin content[i], (Iron overload may occur in cirrhosis, renal failure (when transfused often) and chronic iron ingestion/supplementation)[i]	6.75 – 26.0 mg (USA)[j] 3.5 – 9.4 mg (♀UK)[k]	Red meat, offal, potatoes, dark green vegetables.	Dairy produce, fruit, unsupplemented cereals.
Manganese	Possibly (but poor evidence) causes reduction in blood clotting factors and haemoglobin level. Also possibly causes hypocholesterolaemia[n]. (High manganese intake severely compromises iron)[f]	May be a need in prolonged TPN with poor Mn (high levels reported in liver of cirrhotic patients and rats given alcohol)[n].	0.7 – 10.8 mg (Can)[o] 1.6 – 11.2 mg (Can)[p] 2.4 – 5.0 mg (USA)[c] 1.4 – 5.2 mg (FRG)[q] Average 4.6 mg (UK)[r]	Tea, cereals, nuts, fruit and vegetables.	Meat and dairy produce.
Molybdenum	Probably only through effect on copper balance[f] i.e. excess molybdenum causes copper deficiency[3]	Increased catabolism; high protein diets[i].	75 – 100 μg (USA)[i] 5 – 1010 μg (FRG)[q]	Legumes, offal, leaf vegetables, cereals.	Fruit, roots, meat, dairy produce.
Selenium	Cardiac myopathy[t] (Keshans disease); possible role in malignancy[s] and cardiovascular disease[t]. (2400 – 3000 μg/day)	Chronic malabsorption/disease of the gastrointestinal tract, coeliac disease[t,u].	8 – 96 μg (Swe)[v] 6 – 103 μg (Fin)[4] 113 – 220 μg (USA)[w] Average 60 μg (UK)[x]	Meat, fish, eggs, cereals (but depends on source).	Fruit, dairy produce vegetables.
Zinc	Skin rash, hair loss, anorexia, diarrhoea[d], possibly growth retardation, anaemia[y]. (>150 – 5000 mg/day)[f]	Catabolic states, especially with TPN[d], proteinuria, chelation therapy[f], alcoholism[f], low energy diets[z], low protein diets[z], general chronic malabsorption[f]. Iron therapy where iron:zinc ratio >2:1[f].	4.9 – 8.6 mg (USA)[z] (low protein) 6.4 – 16.1 mg (USA)[c] 3.5 – 16.2 mg (USA)[m]	Red meat egg, offal, whole grain, shellfish, cheese.	Fruit, refined cereals.

[a]Prasad (1982); [b]Fleming et al (1976); [c]Walker and Page (1977); [d]Kay (1981); [e]Nordstrom (1982); [f]Solomons and Rosenberg (1984); [g]Jeejeebhoy et al (1977); [h]Guthrie (1982); [i]Underwood (1971); [j]Prasad (1976); [k]Barber et al (1985); [l]Lynch and Morck (1983); [m]Murthy et al (1971); [n]Waldron (1982); [o]Gibson and Scythes (1982); [p]Gibson et al (1985); [q]Schelenz (1977); [r]Wenlock et al (1979); [s]Combs and Combs (1984); [t]Fell et al (1981); [u]Hinks et al (1984); [v]Abdulla et al (1979b); [w]Thompson et al (1975); [x]Thorn et al (1978); [y]Fell (1980); [z]Brown et al (1976); [1]Anderson et al (1982); [2]Bunker et al (1984); [3]Agarawal (1975); [4]Mutanen (1984).

Table 2.47 Toxic elements — dietetic and clinical significance in adults

Toxic element	Major manifestations of toxicity	Major routes into the body	Factors affecting concentration of element in the body	
			Enhance	Reduce
Aluminium	Encephalopathy in dialysis therapy, possible bone disease[a], memory loss, pre-senile dementia[b,c].	Air (dust) Drugs (antacids) Food Drinking water Deodorants[a]	Deficiency of calcium or magnesium[a], zinc or manganese[c].	Supplementary zinc, manganese or magnesium[c].
Cadmium	Chronically, itai-itai disease, (proteinuria, glycosuria, decalcification) but may interfere with renal or hepatic function as these are the main deposition sites[e].	Air (especially cigarette smoke, may increase exposure 12x that of air alone) Drinking water Food, especially cereals and fruit[e]	Iron or zinc deficiency[d].	Possibly supplementary zinc and/or vitamin C, iron [e,d].
Lead	At blood levels up to 40 µg%* there is equivocal evidence of mental dysfunction. At blood levels 40−60 µg%, there may be neurological (e.g. insomnia) and abdominal (e.g. nausea) symptoms or neuropathy (e.g. muscle weakness). At blood levels ≃80 µg%, anaemia. At blood levels 130−>150 µg%, renal function deterioration and encephalopathy[e].	Air, estimated 10−20% intake[f] (especially people who work with lead, paint stripping, stained glass window workers or gasoline (petrol) sniffing)[g,h]. Dust, this will contaminate food (in adults 30% of air-borne lead is deposited in the lungs, 40−50% is absorbed)[e]; Food, an estimated 45−90% of the intake is via this route; Fluids, an estimated 0−45% in water[f] and alcoholic drinks[i] may also contribute.	low dietary calcium or calcium deficiency,[i] low dietary iron,[e] high fat diets.	

*(1 µmol/l = 21 µg%)

[a]Boegman and Bates (1984); [b]Sohler *et al* (1981); [c]Howard (1984); [d]Underwood (1981); [e]Waldron (1982); [f]Gloag (1981); [g]Waldron (1985); [h]Ross (1982); [i]Prasad (1976); [j]Shaper *et al* (1982).

---

3 During lactation.
4 During heavy menstrual blood loss.
5 When treatment compromises absorption, e.g. vitamin and mineral supplementation.

2.8.5 Clinical/dietetic implications of trace elements

The foregoing discussion has outlined the difficulties involved when studying trace elements. Trace element balances on humans in clinical situations are scarce, so it is difficult to say with any certainty which trace element may be compromised and when.

Table 2.46 attempts to summarize, for major trace elements, areas when the dietitian should consider trace element status. The table only relates to adults. Also, such is the dearth of information that only caucasian, non-pregnant adults are considered. Different ethnic groups may have other needs when consideration of dietary intake is made.

Table 2.47 is concerned with information about non-essential or toxic elements. It cannot be over-emphasized that essential trace element status can affect the absorption and possibly the retention of toxic elements. Dietitians can minimize the risk of toxic element intoxication by not only monitoring intake from food and other sources, but also by promoting a more-than adequate intake of essential elements, especially to those patients known to be at risk.

References

Abdulla M, Jagerstand M, Melander A, Norden A, Svenson S and Wahlin E (1979) Iodine. *Scand J Gastroenterol* **14**, 185.

Abdulla M, Kolar K, and Svenson S (1979b) Selenium. *Scand J Gastroenterol* **14**, 181.

Anderson AA, Polansky MM, Bryden NA, Roginski EE, Patterson KY and Ramer DC (1982) Effect of exercise (running) on serum glucose, insulin and chromium excretion. *Diabetes* **31**, 212−16.

Barber SA, Bull NL and Buss DH (1985) Low iron intakes among young women in Britain. *Br Med J* **290**, 743−4.

Boegman RJ and Bates LA (1984) Neurotoxicity of aluminium. *Can J Physiol Pharmacol* **62**, 1010−4.

Bull NL and Buss DH (1980) Haem and non-haem iron in British household diets. *J Hum Nutr* **34**, 141−5.

Bunker VW, Lawson MS, Delves HT and Clayton BE (1984) The uptake and excretion of chromium by the elderly. *Am J Clin Nutr* **39**, 797−802.

Brown ED, McGluckin MA, Wilson M and Smith JC (1976) Zinc in selected hospital diets. *J Am Diet Assoc* **69**, 632–5.

Byrne AR and Kosta L (1979) On the vanadium and tin contents of diet and human blood. *Sci Total Environ* **13**, 87–90.

Chilean Iodine Educational Bureau (1952) *Iodine contents of foods.* Chilean Iodine Educational Bureau, London.

Combs GF and Combs SB (1984) The nutritional biochemistry of selenium. *Ann Rev Nutr* **4**, 257–80.

Cook JD, Morck TA, Silkine BS and Lynch SR (1981) Biochemical determinants of iron absorption. In *Symposia from XII International Congress in Nutrition.* Eds Harper AE and Davis GK, pp 323–32. AR Liss Inc, New York.

Department of Health and Social Security (1979) *Recommended daily amounts of food energy and nutrients for groups of people in the United Kingdom.* Report on Health and Social Subjects No 15. HMSO, London.

Fell GS, Stromberg P, Main A, Spooner R, Campbell R, Russell R, Brown A and Ottaway JM (1981) Biochemical signs of human selenium deficiency. *Proc Nutr Soc* **40**, 76A.

Fleming CR, Hodges RE and Hurley LS (1976) Serum copper and zinc levels of patients receiving TPN. *Am J Clin Nutr* **29**, 70–7.

Gibson RS, MacDonald AC and Martinez OB (1985) Dietary chromium and manganese intakes of a selected sample of Canadian elderly women. *Hum Nutr: Appl Nutr* **39A**, 43–52.

Gibson RS and Scythes CA (1982) Trace element intakes of women. *Br J Nutr* **48**, 241–8.

Gillies ME and Paulin HV (1982) Estimations of daily mineral intakes from drinking water. *Hum Nutr: Appl Nutr* **36A**, 287–92.

Gloag D (1981) Sources of lead pollution. *Br Med J* **284**, 41–4.

Golden MHN (1982) Trace elements in human nutrition. *Hum Nutr: Appl Nutr* **36C**, 185–202.

Guthrie BE (1982) *Biological and environmental aspects of chromium.* Langard S (Ed) pp 118–48. Elsevier Medical Press,

Henriksen LK, Mahalko JR and Johnson LK (1985) Canned foods: appropriate in trace element studies. *J Am Diet Assoc* **85**, 563–8.

Heinz Baby Foods Advisory Service (1982) *Digest: Zinc and Nutrition.*

Hinks LJ, Inwards KD, Lloyd B and Clayton BE (1984) Body content of selenium in coeliac disease. *Br Med J* **288**, 1862–3.

Horak E and Sunderman EW (1973) Faecal nickel excretion by healthy adults. *Clin Chem* **19**, 429–30.

Howard JMH (1984) Clinical importance of small increases in serum aluminium. *Clin Chem* **30**, 1722–3.

Jeejeebhoy KN, Chu RC, Marliss EB, Greenberg GR and Bruce-Robertson A (1977) Chromium deficiency, glucose intolerance and neuropathy reversed by chromium supplementation, in a patient receiving long term total parenteral nutrition. *Am J Clin Nutr* **30**, 532–8.

Kay RG (1981) Zinc and copper in human nutrition. *J Hum Nutr* **35**, 25–36.

Kelsay JK, Behall KM and Prather ES (1979) The effect of fibre from fruits and vegetables in metabolic response of human subjects II. Calcium, magnesium, iron and silicon. *Am J Clin Nutr* **32**, 1876–8.

Kirchgessner M, Schwartz FJ and Schnegg A (1982) Interactions of essential metals. In *Clinical, biochemical and nutritional aspects of trace elements* Prasad AS (Ed) p 476. AR Liss Inc, New York.

Koivistoinen P (Ed) (1980) Mineral composition of Finnish food. N, K, Ca, P, S, Fe, Cu, Mn, Zn, Mo, Co, Ni, Cr, F, Se, Si, Rb, Al, B, Br, Hg, As, Cd, Pb and ash. *Acta Agric Scand* [Suppl] **22**,

Kumpulainen J and Vuori E (1980) Longitudinal study of chromium in human milk. *Am J Clin Nutr* **33**, 2299–302.

Levander OA and Morris VC (1984) Dietary selenium levels needed to maintain balance in North American adults consuming self-selected diets. *Am J Diet Assoc* **39**, 809–15.

Linder MC (1978) Functions and metabolism of trace elements. In *Perinatal physiology* Stave U (Ed; pp 425–54. Plenum Medical Book Co, London.

Lynch SR and Morck TA (1983) Iron deficiency anaemia. In *Nutrition and haematology* Lindenbaum J (Ed) pp 143–65. Churchill Livingstone, New York.

Masironi R (1978) How trace elements in water contribute to health. *WHO Chronicle* **32**, 382–5.

Moore MR (1979) Diet and lead toxicity. *Proc Nutr Soc* **38**, 243–50.

Murthy BK, Rhea U and Peeler JT (1971) Levels of antimony, cadmium, chromium, cobalt, manganese and zinc in institutional diets. *Environment Sci Tech* **5**, 436–42.

Mutanen M (1984) Dietary intake and sources of selenium in young Finnish women. *Hum Nutr: Appl Nutr* **38A**, 265–9.

Nielsen FH (1984) Ultra trace elements. *Ann Rev Nutr* **4**, 21–41.

Nordstrom JW (1982) Trace mineral nutrition in the elderly. *Am J Clin Nutr* **36**, 788–95.

Pennington JT and Calloway DH (1973) Copper contents of foods. *J Am Diet Assoc* **63**, 143–53.

Prasad AS (1976) *Trace elements in human health and disease* Vol II. Essential and toxic elements. Academic Press, New York.

Prasad AS (1982) *Clinical, biochemical and nutritional aspects of trace elements.* AR Liss Inc, New York.

Ross CA (1982) Gasoline sniffing and lead encephalopathy. *Can Med J* **127**, 1195–7.

Schelenz R (1977) Dietary intake of 25 elements by man, estimated by neutron activation analysis. *J Radio Anal Chem* **37**, 539–48.

Schroeder HA (1971) Losses of vitamins and trace minerals resulting from processing and preservation of foods. *Am J Clin Nutr* **24**, 563–73.

Shah BG (1981) Bioavailability of trace elements in human nutrition. In Symposia from XII International Congress in Nutrition. Harper AE and Davis GK (Eds) pp 199–208. AR Liss Inc, New York.

Shaper AG, Pocock SJ, Walker M, Wale CJ, Clayton B, Delves HT and Hinks L (1982) Effects of alcohol and smoking on blood lead levels in middle-aged British men. *Br Med J* **284**, 299–302.

Smith JL (1976) Metabolism and toxicity of lead. In *Trace elements in human health and disease* Vol II Prasad AS (Ed) pp 443–52. Academic Press Inc, New York.

Sohler A, Pfeiffer CC and Papaioannou R (1981) Blood aluminium levels in a psychiatric out-patient population. *J Orthomol Psychiatry* **10**, 54–60.

Solomons NW and Rosenberg IH (1984) Absorption and malabsorption of mineral nutrients. In *Current topics in nutrition and disease* Vol 12. AR Liss Inc, New York.

Soremark R (1967) Vanadium in some biological speciments. *J Nutr* **92**, 183–90.

Thomas B, Roughan JA and Watters ED (1974) Cobalt, chromium and nickel content of some vegetable foodstuffs. *J Sci Food Agric* **25**, 771–6.

Thompson JN, Erdody P and Smith DC (1975) Selenium content of food consumed by Canadians. *J Nutr* **105**, 274–7.

Thorn J, Robertson J and Buss DH (1978) Trace nutrients: selenium in British food. *Br J Nutr* **39**, 391–6.

Toepfer EW, Mertz W, Roginski EE and Polansky MM (1973) Chromium in foods in relation to biological activity. *J Agric Food Chem* **21**, 69–73.

Underwood EJ (1971) *Trace elements in human and animal nutrition* 3e. Academic Press, London.

Underwood EJ (1981) Trace elements in human and animal health. *J Hum Nutr* **35**, 37–48.

Waldron HA (Ed) (1982) *Metals in the environment.* Academic Press, London.

Walker MA and Page L (1977) Nutritive value of college meals. *J Am Diet Assoc* **70**, 260−6.

Wenlock RW, Buss DH and Dixon EJ (1979) Trace elements 2: manganese in British foods. *Br J Nutr* **41**, 253−5.

Wenlock RW, Buss DH, Moxon RE and Bunton NG (1982) Trace elements 4: iodine in British foods. *Br J Nutr* **7**, 381−90.

Whitney EN and Boyle MA (1984) *Understanding nutrition* 3e. West Publishing Co,

Wolf WR (1982) Trace element analysis in food. In *Clinical, biochemical and nutritional aspects of trace elements* Prasad AS (Ed) pp 427−46. AR Liss Inc, New York.

Zoetman BCJ and Brinkman FJJ (1976) Hardness of drinking water and public health. In *Proc Eur Sci Coll Luxembourg.* Pergamon Press, Oxford.

2.9 Fluid

Fluid forms 50–70% of total body weight in adults. This percentage varies according to age (it is higher in infants than in adults) and sex (women have larger stores of adipose tissue and therefore less body water than men). Body water is divided between the intracellular and extracellular compartments, the latter being composed of the interstitial fluid and the plasma volume (Table 2.48). The compartments are separated by semi-permeable barriers which permit the free passage of salt and water but only limited movement of other solutes such as proteins. All three compartments are interdependent and movement of fluid between them is regulated largely by pressure gradients and osmosis. It is difficult to gain access to the intracellular fluid compartment so extracellular fluid volume is considered when providing clinical care for a patient.

2.9.1 Regulation of body fluid

Regulation of the body fluid is called homeostasis. This is a dynamic function governed by biochemical and physiological processes. Normally the total fluid volume fluctuates by less than 1%/day, despite variations in intake. Changes of as little as 1–2% can lead to illness and sometimes death. An understanding of the functions of fluid within the body helps to clarify the factors affecting its regulation. Fluid is needed

1 To act as a solvent for ions and molecules.
2 To act as a transport medium especially for the excretion of osmotically active solutes such as urea and salts.
3 As a lubricant.
4 To regulate body temperature.

Fluid requirement and fluid balance

Fluid intake

Fluid intake is normally controlled by the sensation of thirst which is regulated by the hypothalamus. Fluid is present in food as well as in oral liquids. Small quantities of water are also produced by the metabolic processes of the body.

Fluid output

Fluid output is governed by the kidneys, although there are also insensible losses via the skin, lungs and gastrointestinal tract. These insensible (obligatory) losses can vary significantly depending on factors such as climate, activity, state of health and dietary intake.

Management of the patient should always be influenced by the need to maintain a state of balance between fluid intake and output (Table 2.49). Assessment of current fluid status requires meticulous completion of daily fluid balance charts and careful monitoring of blood results including sodium and serum osmolality.

Individual requirements for additional fluids vary considerably. The *minimum* intake should be sufficient to replace losses from all sources and provide adequate dilution for the excretion of solutes via the kidney. The *maximum* intake from oral liquids (or enteral or parenteral fluids) should be that which the kidney can excrete. In normal circumstances this is approximately 30 ml/kg body weight *or* 1 ml/kcal in adults and 1.5 ml/kcal in children.

Table 2.48 Body fluids — location, percentage and composition

Compartment	Location	% Body weight	Principal cation	Principal anion
Extracellular				
Interstitial	Fluid surrounding the cells	16%	Na^+	Cl^-
Vascular	Fluids within the blood vessels (6.5% solids-mainly protein)	4%		
Intracellular	Fluids within the cells (Protein content higher than plasma)	30–40%	K^+	PO_4^- (+ protein)

The only common feature between these three compartments is the osmolality which is 290 mosmol/kg water.

Table 2.49 Fluid balance

Input		Output	
Source	Typical volume (ml)	Source	Typical volume (ml)
Oral liquids	1500	Urine	1500
Water contained in food*	1000	Faeces	150
Metabolism†	300	Lungs	400
		Insensible losses	750
Total	2800	Total	2800

*The water content of food can be ascertained by looking up the appropriate item in McCance and Widdowson's *The Composition of Foods*. It may not always be necessary to calculate this figure accurately, but an estimate of the fluid derived from food should be included in the daily input. If the patient is not eating, the fluid usually derived from food should be replaced by another source.
†Metabolism of 1 g starch yields 0.6 g water; 1 g protein yields 0.4 g water and 1 g fat yields 1.1 g water.

Factors affecting fluid movement

Movement of water

Water movement between the three fluid compartments is controlled by a variety of sensitive and highly complex mechanisms including osmosis and the effects of hydrostatic pressure gradients. Particles within the body fluid are electrically charged; the main extracellular cation is sodium and the main intracellular cation is potassium (Table 2.48). In normal circumstances the osmolality (see p 605) of the plasma and interstitial fluid are equal. Plasma osmolality usually reflects the serum sodium which, in turn, reflects the total extracellular volume. It may be useful to note that, provided water is distributed normally between the three compartments, a high serum sodium level may indicate dehydration while a low level could point to overhydration.

Plasma osmolality

This is a key factor in the determination of fluid movement and slight alterations in plasma osmolality are usually corrected by the movement of fluid between the interstitial compartment and the plasma. This may be accompanied by variations in oral intake. If the plasma osmolality increases then the hypothalamus is stimulated by a sensation of thirst and increased amounts of antidiuretic hormone (ADH) are released. This leads to the reabsorption of water from the distal renal tubules and correction of the plasma osmolality. Decreased plasma volume can also lead to a raised osmolality; aldosterone is then released which results in increased sodium and water retention.

Renal function is therefore an important factor in the regulation of fluid balance and any impairment is often characterized by oedema.

'Pitting oedema'

This is the commonest clinical symptom of an expanded interstitial volume. Fluid balance is normally maintained within the extracellular compartment but can be upset for a number of reasons. It is important to remember that the location of pitting oedema is affected by gravity and that a bedridden patient may show signs of sacral oedema in the absence of ankle oedema. Correction of oedema should never be attempted without a precise knowledge of its cause. It is also important to remember that severe cases of disturbed osmolality or volume depletion can lead to the movement of water between the intracellular and extracellular compartments; this is more difficult to diagnose and can have fatal consequences if not treated promptly.

Hydrostatic pressure

Plasma volume is also maintained by the effects of hydrostatic pressure. Essentially, a higher pressure is exerted within the arterial end of the capillary. At the same time there is the lesser effect of osmotic pressure exerted by the plasma proteins (oncotic pressure) resulting in the movement of fluid into the interstitial space. The process is reversed at the venous end of the capillary with a consequent movement of fluid back into the plasma (Starling's hypothesis, summarized in Fig. 2.7). The plasma proteins therefore play an important role in the movement of fluid between the vascular and interstitial compartments.

Correction of fluid balance

This is sometimes effected by the administration of Plasma Protein Fraction (PPF) or additional nutritional support. The fluid level in the intracellular compartment is maintained by a shift of water from the extracellular space. Administration of extra protein as PPF will lead to the retention of water and consequent expansion of the plasma volume.

It is important to note however, that serum albumin levels are maintained by a balance between albumin synthesis, breakdown and redistribution. Giving a bolus of additional protein may help to restore fluid balance but it is unlikely to confer any long term benefit on the serum albumin level. Approximately

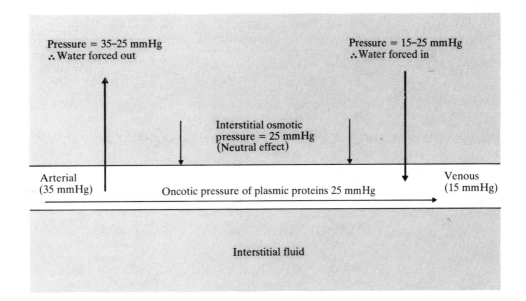

Pressure = 35–25 mmHg
∴ Water forced out

Pressure = 15–25 mmHg
∴ Water forced in

Interstitial osmotic
pressure = 25 mmHg
(Neutral effect)

Arterial
(35 mmHg)

Oncotic pressure of plasmic proteins 25 mmHg

Venous
(15 mmHg)

Interstitial fluid

Fig. 2.7 Starling's hypothesis.

one-third of the albumin pool is in the plasma and the remaining two-thirds are distributed throughout the extracellular compartment. The plasma pool is maintained by the movement of albumin from the extracellular space. PPF administration will result in albumin diffusing back to the extracellular compartment rather than remaining in the plasma pool and thus the serum albumin level should not be used as an isolated clinical indicator when considering the nutritional status of patients. It is also the reason why longer term nutritional support should be initiated as soon as possible in order to maintain protein levels.

Intestinal control of fluid balance

This is chiefly related to any losses incurred during bouts of diarrhoea and/or vomiting. Normally the large quantities of digestive juices which are secreted into the gastrointestinal tract are reabsorbed. If there is abnormal gastrointestinal function leading to excessive fluid losses this is replaced by extracellular fluid which crosses the mucosa into the gut. This may be caused by a variety of conditions including short bowel syndrome and ileostomy losses. The average composition of various intestinal fluids is shown in Table 2.50.

Insensible losses

The *respiratory system* is involved to a lesser degree in the maintenance of fluid volume. Normally a constant amount of water (approximately 400 ml) is lost daily from the lungs. This loss can increase dramatically in hyperventilation, whatever the cause.

Fluid is also lost by evaporation from the *skin*. Losses amount to approximately 500–750 ml daily, but will increase as a result of a hot climate, fever, burns or any other situation which increases the metabolic rate.

Summary

Fluid is essential to life and, although man can survive for remarkably long periods without food, he cannot

Table 2.50 Volume and composition of gastrointestinal secretions and sweat (Adapted from Harper 1971; Caldwell and Kennedy-Caldwell 1981)

Fluid	Average adult volume (ml/24 hours)	Electrolyte concentration (mEq/l)			
		Na$^+$	K$^+$	Cl$^-$	HCO$_3^-$
Gastric juice	2500	31– 90	4.3–12	52–124	0
Bile	700–1000	134–156	3.9– 6.3	83–110	38
Pancreatic juice	700–1000	113–153	2.6– 7.4	54–95	110
Small bowel (Miller-Abbott Section)	3000	72–120	3.5–.6.8	69–127	30
Ileostomy					
Recent	100–4000	112–142	4.5–14	93–122	30
Adapted	100– 500	50	3	20	15–30
Caecostomy	100–3000	48–116	11.1–28.3	35– 70	15
Faeces	100	<10	<10	<15	<15
Sweat	500–1000	30– 70	0 – 5	30– 70	0

Table 2.51 Patients at particular risk of inadequate fluid intake and consequent depletion

Increased requirements for fluid	Patients with tracheostomies or on ventilators; diarrhoea and/or vomiting; increased fluid losses e.g. sepsis, any other conditions associated with pyrexia, diabetes insipidus.
	Patients receiving high protein/high osmolar diets (e.g. tube feeding regimens; patients with nephrotic syndrome)
	Infants — particularly with any of the above conditions.
Lack of awareness of, or inability to express, the need for fluid	Patients who are unable to communicate — those who are unconscious; those who have suffered a stroke.
	Patients who are unable to eat normally — those with dysphagia (e.g. cancer of the oesophagus); those with diminished food intake (e.g. anorexia nervosa); those with a poor appetite (e.g. the elderly or chronically ill); those on 'nil by mouth' regimens who are receiving inadequate fluids intravenously.

Patients on long term diuretic therapy should have their fluid balance monitored closely to avoid any risk of dehydration.

Some patients may require a *reduced* fluid intake. These could include patients in various stages of renal failure; congestive cardiac failure; respiratory failure; or post-operative recovery — especially chest surgery.

withstand a prolonged deprivation of fluid. It is unlikely that the majority of patients will suffer from severe fluid imbalance. However, there are certain groups of patients in whom the possibility of fluid imbalance should be considered carefully and these are listed in Table 2.51. Awareness of the problems created by fluid imbalance is the key to the successful management of these patients.

Further reading

Bunton GL (1976) *Fluid balance without tears.* Lloyd-Luke Medical Books, London.
Martin DW (1983) Water and minerals. In *Harpers review of biochemistry.* 17e. Martin DW, Mays PA and Rodwell VW (Eds). Lange, Los Altos.
Moghissi K and Boore J (1983) *Parenteral and enteral nutrition for nurses* p 18. Heinemann Medical Books, London.
Richards P and Truniger B (1983) *Understanding water, electrolyte and acid-base balance.* Heinemann Medical Books, London.
Smith, Kinsey (1980) *Fluids and electrolytes — a conceptual approach.* Churchill Livingstone, Edinburgh.
Tweedle DEF (1982) *Metabolic care.* Churchill Livingstone, Edinburgh.
Willatts M (1982) *Lecture notes on fluid and electrolyte balance.* Blackwell Scientific Publications, London.

References

Caldwell MD and Kennedy-Caldwell C (1981) Normal nutritional requirements. *Surg Clin North Am* **61**, (3), 489—507.
Harper HA (197) *Physiological chemistry* 13e. Large Medical Publications, Los Altos.

2.10   Miscellaneous Substances

2.10.1   Caffeine, theophylline and theobromine

Caffeine, theophylline and theobromine are all methyl derivatives of xanthine. They are pharmacologically active substances. Caffeine is the most potent and acts as a stimulant to the heart and central nervous system. It also increases gastric acid secretion and is known to cause vasodilatation. Effects are most likely when excessive quantities are taken or in highly sensitive individuals.

Caffeine is added as a flavour to foods and may only be listed on the label as 'flavouring' with no E number.

The principal sources of dietary caffeine are summarized in Table 2.52.

2.10.2   Monoamines

Monoamine oxidase inhibitors (MAOI) are drugs used in the treatment of depression. Current MAOI drugs in use include

Generic name	Trade name
Tranylcypromine	Parnate
Phenelzine	Nardil
Isocarboxazid	Marplan
Iproniazid	Marsilid

Monoamine oxidase is required for the metabolism of catecholamines. There are biologically active amines (e.g. tyramine, histamine and dopamine) in certain foods which, if taken during a course of MAOI, can result in unpleasant and even life threatening reactions. The most commonly reported reactions are headaches, but substantial rises in blood pressure leading to sub-arachnoid haemorrhage and death have also been documented.

Massey Stewart (1976) reviewed this area of food and drug interaction and concluded that some dangers of MAOI drugs and food have been exaggerated. The main problem is the presence of tyramine (produced by the decarboxylation of tyrosine). There is a wide variation in the tyramine content of different samples of the same type of food and there is also a variation in patient tolerance to tyramine.

Eating fresh foods, including freshly prepared meals from tinned and frozen ingredients, reduces the risk of consuming protein which has undergone degradation and possibly resulted in the production of tyramine.

Foods to be avoided when MAOI drugs are taken are listed in Table 2.53.

Foods where evidence of the need for avoidance on MAOI drugs is poor include chocolate, soy sauce, yoghurt, tea, coffee and cola beverages.

2.10.3   Oxalates

Oxalates are found mainly in foods of plant origin. The actual content varies considerably with season, species, variety, age, maturity and part of the plant.

Table 2.52 Principal food sources of caffeine (Nagy 1974; Bunker and McWilliams 1979)

Food	Caffeine content
Coffee (mg/cup)	
instant	61– 70
percolated ground	97–125
Tea (mg/cup) loose/teabags	15– 75
Cocoa (mg/cup)	10– 17[a]
Chocolate bar	60– 70[a]
Chocolate beverages	—[b]
Carbonated cola drinks (mg/12 oz can) e.g. Pepsi Cola, Tab, Diet Coke, Coca Cola	43– 65
Lucozade (mg/100 g)	18

[a]Main stimulant is theobromine.
[b]Figure not available.

Table 2.53 Foods to be avoided on MAOI drugs and for 14 days after the end of treatment (Massey Stewart 1976; BMA 1984)

Red wine (especially chianti) and real ale. Other forms of alcohol can be consumed in moderation.

Broad bean pods

Cheese, fermented (e.g. blue cheeses) matured, processed and cheese spreads

Game

Meat extracts and yeast extracts (e.g. Oxo, stock cubes, Marmite and Bovril). These extracts are also added to manufactured foods (check food labels).

Pickled herrings

Any food which has been kept for a long time

Any food which has previously produced unpleasant symptoms

All patients placed on MAOI drugs should be given a card by the pharmacist which lists the foods to be avoided.

The oxalate content of the diet may need to be modified as part of the treatment of some renal stones (see Section 4.17).

A typical UK diet contains approximately 70–150 mg oxalic acid per day (Zarembski and Hodgkinson 1962). A low oxalate diet should provide 60–70 mg oxalic acid daily. Sources of dietary oxalate are summarized in Table 2.54.

2.10.4 Purines

Drug therapy has largely replaced dietary restriction of purines in the treatment of gout (hyperuricacidaemia). However, it is still reasonable to advise patients with recurrent gout to eliminate the principal sources of purines from their diet because this is not difficult and dietary nucleoproteins contribute about 5% of urate present in blood. Purine restriction is not effective in treating uric acid stones (see p 467).

Principal sources of uric acid are summarized in Table 2.55.

2.10.5 Salicylates, benzoates and glutamates

Salicylates, benzoates and glutamates occur naturally in a wide range of foods. All have been implicated in the causation of certain food intolerances. Salicylates in particular may cause or exacerbate urticaria or asthma in certain individuals (see Section 5.9). Such people may also be sensitive to aspirin or similar analgesics such as sodium salicylate.

Salicylates are stable to food processing, occur in a wide range of foods and may be used as a synthetic flavouring in certain types of food without being specifically recorded on the food label. Data on the salicylate content of foods has therefore been difficult to obtain and is scarce. Until recently, most of the available figures have been derived from the work of Lockey (1971) but further information is now available from Swain et al (1985a; 1985b) (see below).

Foods thought to contain significant quantities of salicylates are summarized in Table 2.56. For further guidance, the values for the salicylate content of some foods as determined by Swain et al (1985b) are also reproduced in Table 2.57. The availability of other salicylate values in the literature is indicated in the two right hand columns.

Tables 2.58 and 2.59 give some values determined for the natural benzoate and free glutamate content of certain foods. These may also be used as a guide to naturally occurring levels. It should be noted however, that actual levels will vary according to variety, soil and growing conditions. It addition, the number of samples that have been analysed is small and few, if any, are likely to have originated from the British Isles.

2.10.6 Yeast

Yeast has been implicated in certain food allergy conditions. Yeast can be an ingredient in foods or occur as a microbiological contaminant. Possible sources of yeast in the diet are listed in Table 2.60.

Table 2.54 Principal sources of oxalate to be avoided on a low oxalate diet (Kasidas 1980)

Food	Oxalic acid content (mg/100 g)
Beetroot	500
Chocolate (and all other products containing cocoa)	117
Parsley	100
Peanuts	187
Rhubarb	600
Spinach	600
Tea infusion (mg/100 ml)	55–78

Moderate sources of oxalate to be taken in controlled amounts on a low oxalate diet include strawberries; celery; coffee (instant) and malted milk drinks.

Table 2.55 Principal sources of purines (Clifford et al 1976; Wyngaarden and Kelly 1976)

Meat sources	Fish sources
Liver	Anchovies
Heart	Crab
Kidney	Fish roes
Sweetbreads	Herring
Meat extracts (e.g. Oxo)	Mackerel
	Sardines
	Shrimps
	Sprats
	Whitebait

Table 2.56 Foods thought to contain salicylates (Lockey 1971; Swain et al 1985a, b)

Food group	Foods
Fruit	Apples, apricots, blackberries, blueberries, cherries, gooseberries, grapes and dried fruit, melon, nectarines, oranges, pineapple, plums, prunes, raspberries, rhubarb. Jam prepared from any of these fruits.
Vegetables	Carrots, cucumber, onion, peas and tomatoes.
Nuts	All nuts, especially peanuts and almonds.
Cereals	Maize
Beverages	Tea, coffee, wine, sherry, beer and cider.
Miscellaneous	Yeasts. Many manufactured foods especially ice cream, sweets, liquorice, soft drinks and cake mixes.

Table 2.57 Salicylates in 333 foods* (Swain *et al* 1985b Reproduced with permission)

Food	Type	State	Salicylate (mg/100 g)[1]	Reported in literature	References
Fruit					
Apple	Golden Delicious	Fresh	0.08 ⎱		
	Red Delicious	Fresh	0.19		
	Granny Smith	Fresh	0.59 ⎰	yes	33
	Jonathan	Fresh	0.38		
	Ardmona	Canned	0.55‡		
	Mountain Maid	Juice	0.19‡	yes	36
Apricot		Fresh	2.58	yes	33, 34
	Ardmona	Canned	1.42‡		
	Letona	Nectar	0.14‡	yes	34
Avocado		Fresh	0.60‡		
Banana		Fresh	0‡	yes	33
Blackberry	John West	Canned	1.86	yes	8, 16
Blueberry	Socomin	Canned	2.76		
Boysenberry	John West	Canned	2.04		
Canteloupe	Australian rockmelon	Fresh	1.50‡		
Cherry	sweet	Fresh	0.85	yes	8, 10, 34
	John West	Canned	2.78		
	Morello Sour	Canned	0.30	yes	6
Cranberry	S. & W.	Canned	1.64	yes	11, 12
		Sauce	1.44		
Currants	Black currant	Frozen	3.06	yes	8, 33
	Red currant	Frozen	5.06		
Custard apple	(from Queensland)	Fresh	0.21		
Dates		Fresh	3.73		
	Cal-Date	Dried	4.50‡		
Figs		Fresh	0.18	yes	34
	S. & W. Kadota	Canned	0.25		
	Calamata string	Dried	0.64		
Guava	Gold Reef	Canned	2.02		
Grapes	Red Malaita	Fresh	0.94 ⎱		
	Sultana	Fresh	1.88	yes	8
	S. & W. light seedless	Canned	0.16 ⎰		
	Berri Dark	Juice	0.88		
	Sanitarium Light	Juice	0.18		
	Currants I.P.C.	Dried	5.80	yes	8, 36
	Raisins A.D.F.A.	Dried	6.62‡	yes	34
	Sultana	Dried	7.80		
Grapefruit		Fresh	0.68‡	yes	1, 33
	Berri	Juice	0.42		
Kiwi fruit		Fresh	0.32	yes	33
Lemon		Fresh	0.18‡	yes	1
Loganberry	John West	Canned	4.40		
Loquat		Fresh	0.26		
Lychee		Canned	0.36		
Mandarin		Fresh	0.56‡	yes	34
Mango		Fresh	0.11		
Mulberry		Fresh	0.76		
Nectarine		Fresh	0.49	yes	33
Orange		Fresh	2.39‡	yes	1, 33, 35
	Berri	Juice	0.18‡	yes	34, 35
Passion fruit		Fresh	0.14‡	yes	9, 13
Pawpaw		Fresh	0.08‡		
Peach		Fresh	0.58‡	yes	33, 34
	Letona	Canned	0.68‡	yes	14, 15, 33
	Letona	Nectar	0.10‡	yes	34
Pear	Packham (with skin)	Fresh	0.27‡		
	Packham (no skin)	Fresh	0‡		
	William (with skin)	Fresh	0.31‡		
	Letona Bartlett	Canned	0‡		
Persimmon		Fresh	0.18‡		
Pineapple		Fresh	2.10‡	yes	33, 34, 35

Table 2.57 *contd.*

Food	Type	State	Salicylate (mg/100 g)[1]	Reported in literature	References
	Golden Circle	Canned	1.36		
	Golden Circle	Juice	0.16‡	yes	34
Plum	Blood (red)	Fresh	0.21		
	Kelsey (green)	Fresh	0.095	yes	33
	Wilson (red)	Fresh	0.11		
	S.P.C. dark red	Canned	1.16		
	Letona prunes	Canned	6.87	yes	33, 34
Pomegranate		Fresh	0.07		
Raspberries		Fresh	5.14	yes	8, 16, 33
		Frozen	3.88		
Rhubarb		Fresh	0.13	yes	33
Strawberry		Fresh	1.36‡	yes	8, 16, 33, 36
Tamarillo		Fresh	0.10	yes	33
Tangelo		Fresh	0.72	no	7#
Watermelon		Fresh	0.48‡	yes	3, 33
Youngberry		Canned	3.06		
Vegetables					
Alfalfa		Fresh	0.70		
Asparagus		Fresh	0.14‡	yes	33
	Triangle Spears	Canned	0.32‡		
Bamboo shoots	Sunshine	Canned	0		
Beans	Blackeye	Dried	0		
	Borlotti	Dried	0.08		
	Broad, "vicia faba"	Fresh	0.73		
	Brown	Dried	0.002		
	Green French	Fresh	0.11‡	yes	3, 33, 34
	Lima	Dried	0	yes	34
	Mung	Dried	0		
	Soya	Dried	0	yes	22
	Soya grits	Dried	0		
Bean sprouts		Fresh	0.06		
Beetroot		Fresh	0.18‡	yes	4, 33
	Golden Circle	Canned	0.32‡		
Broccoli		Fresh	0.65‡		
Brussels sprouts		Fresh	0.07		
Cabbage	Green	Fresh	0‡	yes	33
	Red	Fresh	0.08‡	yes	2
Carrot		Fresh	0.23‡	yes	4, 34
Cauliflower		Fresh	0.16‡	yes	33
Celery		Fresh	0‡		
Chicory		Fresh	1.02	no	5
Chives		Fresh	0.03	no	5
Choko	(Chayote)	Fresh	0.01‡		
Cucumber	(no peel)	Fresh	0.78‡	yes	3
	Aristocrat gherkin	Canned	6.14‡	yes	3
Eggplant	(with peel)	Fresh	0.88‡	yes	3
	(no peel)	Fresh	0.30‡		
Endive		Fresh	1.9	no	5
Horseradish	Eskal	Canned	0.18	yes	2
Leek		Fresh	0.08		
Lentil	Brown	Dried	0		
	Red	Dried	0		
Lettuce		Fresh	0‡	no	3
Marrow	(Cucurbita pepo)	Fresh	0.17		
Mushroom		Fresh	0.24		
	Champignon	Canned	1.26		
Okra	Zanae	Canned	0.59		
Olive	Black Kraft	Canned	0.34‡		
	Green Kraft	Canned	1.29‡	yes	24
Onion		Fresh	0.16‡	no	3

Table 2.57 *contd.*

Food	Type	State	Salicylate (mg/100 g)[1]	Reported in literature	References
Parsnip		Fresh	0.45		
Peas	Chick-pea	Dried	0		
	Green	Fresh	0.04‡	yes	3, 33, 34
	Green split pea	Dried	0		
	Yellow split pea	Dried	0.02		
Peppers	Green chili	Fresh	0.64‡		
	Red chili	Fresh	1.20‡		
	Yellow-green chili	Fresh	0.62‡		
	Sweet, green (Capsicum)	Fresh	1.20‡	yes	3, 33
Pimentos	Arson sweet red	Canned	0.15		
Potato	White (with peel)	Fresh	0.12‡	yes	17, 33
	White (no peel)	Fresh	0‡		
Pumpkin		Fresh	0.12‡	yes	3, 34
Radish	Red, small	Fresh	1.24‡	yes	4
Shallots		Fresh	0.03		
Spinach		Fresh	0.58	yes	5, 34
		Frozen	0.16‡		
Squash	Baby	Fresh	0.63		
Swede		Fresh	0		
Sweet corn		Fresh	0.13‡	yes	33
	Mountain Maid niblets	Canned	0.26‡	yes	33
	Mountain Maid creamed	Canned	0.39‡	yes	33, 34
Sweet potato	White	Fresh	0.50‡		
	Yellow	Fresh	0.48‡	yes	33
Tomato		Fresh	0.13‡	yes	3, 18, 19, 20, 33, 34
	Letona	Canned	0.53‡	yes	34
	Goulburn Valley	Juice	0.10‡		
	Heinz	Juice	0.12‡		
	Letona	Juice	0.18‡		
	Campbell	Paste	0.57‡ ⎫		
	Leggo	Paste	1.44‡ ⎬	yes	33
	Tom Piper	Paste	0.43‡ ⎭		
	Heinz	Soup	0.54‡ ⎫		
	Kiaora	Soup	0.54‡ ⎬	yes	33, 34
	P.M.U.	Soup	0.32‡ ⎭		
	Fountain	Sauce	0.94‡ ⎫		
	Heinz	Sauce	2.48‡ ⎪		
	I.X.L.	Sauce	1.06‡ ⎬	yes	32, 33, 34, 35
	P.M.U.	Sauce	0.98‡ ⎪		
	Rosella	Sauce	2.15‡ ⎭		
Turnip		Fresh	0.16‡		
Watercress		Fresh	0.84‡		
Zucchini		Fresh	1.04‡	no	3
Condiments					
Allspice	Powder	Dry	5.2		
Aniseed	Powder	Dry	22.8	yes	38
Bay leaf	Leaves	Dry	2.52		
Basil	Powder	Dry	3.4		
"Bonox"		Liquid	0.28		
Canella	Powder	Dry	42.6		
Cardamom	Powder	Dry	7.7		
Caraway	Powder	Dry	2.82		
Cayenne	Powder	Dry	17.6		
Celery	Powder	Dry	10.1		
Chili	Flakes	Dry	1.38		
	Powder	Dry	1.30		
Cinnamon	Powder	Dry	15.2‡	yes	39, 40, 41
Cloves	Whole	Dry	5.74	yes	37
Coriander	Leaves	Fresh	0.20		
Cumin	Powder	Dry	45.0		

Table 2.57 *contd.*

Food	Type	State	Salicylate (mg/100 g)¹	Reported in literature	References
Curry	Powder	Dry	218		
Dill		Fresh	6.9		
	Powder	Dry	94.4		
Fennel	Powder	Dry	0.8	no	5
Fenugreek	Powder	Dry	12.2		
Five spice	Powder	Dry	30.8		
Garam masala	Powder	Dry	66.8		
Garlic	Bulbs	Fresh	0.10‡	yes	5
Ginger	Root	Fresh	4.5		
Mace	Powder	Dry	32.2		
Marmite	Sanitarium	Paste	0.71‡		
Mint	Common garden	Fresh	9.4‡		
Mixed herbs	Leaves	Dry	55.6		
Mustard	Powder	Dry	26		
Nutmeg	Powder	Dry	2.4‡		
Oregano	Powder	Dry	66		
Paprika	Hot powder	Dry	203		
	Sweet powder	Dry	5.7		
Parsley	Leaves	Fresh	0.08‡	yes	4, 5
Pepper	Black powder	Dry	6.2‡		
	White powder	Dry	1.1‡		
Pimento	Powder	Dry	4.9		
Rosemary	Powder	Dry	68		
Saffron	Powder	Dry	0		
Sage	Leaves	Dry	21.7		
Soy Sauce		Liquid	0		
Tabasco Pepper	McIlhenny	Sauce	0.45	yes	21, 23
Tandori	Powder	Dry	0		
Tarragon	Powder	Dry	34.8		
Turmeric	Powder	Dry	76.4		
Thyme	Leaves	Dry	183		
Vanilla	Essence	Liquid	1.44		
Vinegar	Malt	Liquid	0		
	White	Liquid	1.33		
Worcestershire Sauce		Liquid	64.3		
Vegemite	Kraft	Paste	0.81‡		
Drinks					
Aktavite		Powder	0		
Cereal coffee¶	Bambu	Powder	0.15		
	Dandelion	Powder	0.08		
	Ecco	Powder	0		
	Nature's Cuppa	Powder	2.26		
	Reform	Powder	0.38		
Coca-Cola		Liquid	0.25		
Coffee¶	Andronicus Instant	Powder	0		
	Bushells Instant	Powder	0.21		
	Bushells Turkish Style	Powder	0.19		
	Gibsons Instant	Powder	0.12		
	Harris Mocha Kenya	Beans	0.45		
	Harris Instant I	Powder	0		
	Harris Instant II	Powder	0.10		
	International Roast	Powder	0.96	yes	28
	Maxwell House Instant	Powder	0.84		
	Moccona Instant	Granules	0.64		
	Moccona Decaffeinated	Powder	0		
	Nescafé Instant	Granules	0.59		
	Nescafé Decaffeinated	Powder	0		
	Robert Timms Instant	Powder	0.16		
Herbal tea‖	Camomile	Bag	0.06		
	Fruit	Bag	0.36		
	Peppermint	Bag	1.10		
	Rose hip	Bag	0.40		

Table 2.57 contd.

Food	Type	State	Salicylate (mg/100 g)[l]	Reported in literature	References
Milo		Powder	0.01		
Ovaltine		Powder	0		
Rose hip tea‖	Delrosa	Syrup	1.17		
Tea‖	Asco	Bag	6.4		
	Billy	Leaves	2.48		
	Burmese Green	Leaves	2.97		
	Bushells	Bag	4.78		
	Golden Days Decaffeinated	Bag	0.37		
	Harris	Bag	4.0		
	Indian Green	Leaves	2.97		
	Peony Jasmine	Leaves	1.9		
	Old Chinese	Leaves	1.9	yes	29, 30, 31
	Tetley	Bag	5.57		
	Twinings:				
	Earl Grey	Bag	3.0		
	English Breakfast	Bag	3.0		
	Darjeeling	Leaves	4.24		
	Irish Breakfast	Bag	3.89		
	Lapsang Souchong	Bag	2.40		
	Lemon Scented	Bag	7.34		
	Orange Pekoe	Leaves	2.75		
	Prince of Wales	Bag	2.97		
Cereals					
Arrowroot	Powder	Dry	0		
Barley	Unpearled	Dry	0		
Buckwheat	Grains	Dry	0		
Maize	Meal	Dry	0.43		
Millet	Grains	Dry	0		
	Hulled grains	Dry	0		
Oats	Meal	Dry	0		
Rice	Brown grains	Dry	0‡		
	White Grains	Dry	0‡		
Rye	Rolled	Dry	0		
Wheat	Grains	Dry	0		
Nuts and seeds					
Almonds		Fresh	3.0		
Brazil nuts		Fresh	0.46		
Cashew nuts		Fresh	0.07		
Coconut	Dessicated	Dry	0.26		
Hazelnuts		Fresh	0.14		
Macadamia nuts		Fresh	0.52		
Peanuts	Unshelled	Fresh	1.12		
	Sanitarium butter	Paste	0.23		
Pecan nuts		Fresh	0.12		
Pine nuts		Fresh	0.51		
Pistachio nuts		Fresh	0.55		
Poppyseed		Dry	0		
Sesame seed		Dry	0.23		
Sunflower seed		Dry	0.12		
Walnuts		Fresh	0.30		
Water chestnut	Socomin	Canned	2.92		
Sugars					
Carob	Powder	Dry	0‡		
Cocoa	Powder	Dry	0‡		
Honey	Allowrie	Liquid	2.5		
	Aristocrat	Liquid	3.7		
	Capillano	Liquid	10.14		
	Mudgee	Liquid	3.9		
	"No Frills"	Liquid	11.24		
Golden syrup	C.S.R.	Liquid	0.10‡		
Maple syrup	Camp	Liquid	0		

Table 2.57 *contd.*

Food	Type	State	Salicylate (mg/100 g)[1]	Reported in literature	References
Sugar	White granulated	Dry	0		
Molasses	C.S.R.	Liquid	0.22		
Confectionery					
Caramel	Pascall Cream	Dry	0.12		
Liquorice	Barratts	Dry	9.78		
	Giant	Dry	7.96		
Peppermints	Allens Strong Mint	Dry	0.77		
	Allens "Koolmint"	Dry	7.58		
	Lifesavers	Dry	0.86		
	"Minties"	Dry	1.78		
	Allens "Steamrollers"	Dry	2.92		
Dairy					
Cheese	Blue Vein	Fresh	0.05		
	Camembert	Fresh	0.01		
	Cheddar	Fresh	0		
	Cottage	Fresh	0		
	Mozarella	Fresh	0.02		
	Tasty Cheddar	Fresh	0		
Milk	Fresh full cream	Liquid	0‡		
Yoghurt	Full cream	Fresh	0		
Meat, fish and eggs					
Beef		Fresh	0‡		
Chicken		Fresh	0‡		
Egg	White	Fresh	0		
	Yolk	Fresh	0		
Kidney		Fresh	0		
Lamb		Fresh	0‡		
Liver		Fresh	0.05		
Oyster		Fresh	0		
Pork		Fresh	0		
Prawn		Fresh	0.04		
Salmon	Lunchtime Pink	Canned	0		
Scallop		Fresh	0.02		
Tripe		Fresh	0		
Tuna	Seakist	Canned	0		
Alcoholic drinks					
Beer	Reschs Dinner Ale		0.35 ⎫		
	Tooheys Draught		0.23 ⎬	no	26
	Tooths Sheaf Stout		0.32 ⎭		
Cider	Bulmer's Dry		0.17		
	Bulmer's Sweet		0.19		
	Lilydale Dry		0.17		
	Mercury Dry		0.16		
Liqueurs	Benedictine		9.04		
	Cointreau		0.66		
	Drambui		1.68		
	Tia Maria		0.83		
Port	McWilliams Royal Reserve		1.4		
	Stonyfell Mellow		4.2		
Sherry	Lindemans Royal Reserve Sweet		0.56		
	Mildara Supreme Dry		0.46		
	Penfolds Royal Reserve Sweet		0.49		
Spirits	Brandy — Hennessy		0.4		
	Gin — Gilbey's		0		
	Rum — Bundaberg		0.76 ⎫		
	Rum — Captain Morgan		1.28 ⎬	yes	25
	Vodka — Smirnoff		0		
	Whisky — Johnnie Walker		0	no	26
Wines	Buton Dry Vermouth		0.46 ⎫		
	Kaiser Stuhl Rosé		0.37		
	Lindemans Riesling		0.81		
	McWilliams Dry White Wine		0.10		
	McWilliams Cabernet Sauvignon		0.86		
	McWilliams Private Bin Claret		0.90 ⎭	yes	26, 27

Table 2.57 *contd.*

Food	Type	State	Salicylate (mg/100 g)[1]	Reported in literature	References
	McWilliams Reserve Claret		0.35		
	Penfolds Traminer Riesling Bin 202		0.81		
	Seaview Rhine Riesling		0.89		
	Stonyfell Ma Chére		0.69		
	Yalumba Champagne		1.02		

*Most trade names are those of products of various Australian companies. Some varieties of foods also are Australian.

†Edible portion.

‡Multiple extractions.

#Ashoor found no detectable salicylate in grapefruit, lemon, orange, strawberry and tangelo.

¶For coffee, mg salicylate per 100 ml made from 2 g powder in 100 ml water.

‖For tea, mg salicylate per 100 ml infusion made from two standard tea bags (4 g dry leaves).

[1]Stöhr and Herrmann (1975a); [2]Schmidtlein and Hermann (1975a); [3]Schmidtlein and Herrmann (1975b); [4]Stöhr and Herrmann (1975b); [5]Schmidtlein and Herrmann (1975c); [6]Stöhr *et al* (1975); [7]Ashoor and Chu (Unpublished); [8]Nursten and Williams (1967); [9]Winter and Klöti (1972); [10]Gierschner and Baumann (1968); [11]Anjou and Von Sydow (1967); [12]Anjou and Von Sydow (1969); [13]Murray (1973); [14]Do *et al* (1969); [15]Kemp *et al* (1971); [16]McGlumphy (1951); [17]Buttery *et al* (1970); [18]Johnson *et al* (1971); [19]Pyne and Wick (1965); [20]Buttery *et al* (1971); [21]Haymon and Aurand (1971); [22]Arai *et al* (1966); [23]Buttery *et al* (1969); [24]Fedeli and Jacini (1970); [25]Liebich *et al* (1970); [26]Kahn (1969); [27]Christensen and Caputi (1968); [28]Stoffelsma *et al* (1968); [29]Saijo and Kuwabara (1967); [30]Yamanishi (1978); [31]Stahl (1962); [32]Daenens and Larvelle (1973); [33]Robertson and Kermode (1981); [34]Thornberg (1976); [35]Guppy *et al* (1977); [36]Bellanca (1971); [37]Deyama and Horiguchi (1971); [38]Porsch *et al* (1965); [39]Heide (1972); [40]Dodge (1918); [41]Onishi and Yamamoto (1956).

Table 2.58 Natural benzoic acid content of foods

	Benzoic acid (mg/kg)	Range	Reference		Benzoic acid (mg/kg)	Range	Reference
Milk and milk products				*Fruit juices*			
Milk	0.3	(0.2– 0.3)		Apple	1.0		
Processed cheese	23.6	(22.0–25.1)	1	Grape	0.2		3
Whey	3.8	(2.9– 5.5)		Grapefruit	3.8		
Yoghurt				Orange	2.3		
Full-fat	26.0	(18 –37)					
Low fat	25.0	(13 –34)		*Wine*			
Apricot	31	(22 –39)		Average all types	0.4		
Bilberry	25.0	(22 –32)	4				
Blackberry	21.0	(18 –25)		*Dried fruit*			
Pineapple	16.0			Apple	0.6		
Raspberry	26.0	(22 –31)		Apricot	30.4		
Strawberry	20.0	(15 –28)		Banana	1.2		4
				Grape (raisin/sultana)	0.4		
Fruit				Peach	4.2		
Apple	Tr, 0.2*			Pineapple	0.5		
Avocado	1.7			Plum (prune)	12.1		
Banana	0.2						
Cherry	1.1			*Peel*			
Fig (fresh)	0.2, 0.8*			Candied lemon	0.7		4
Grapefruit	0.7, 6.1*			Candied valencia orange	0.5		
Grapes	Tr						
Kiwi fruit	Tr			*Jam*			
Kumquat	0.5, 2.7*			Apple	0.7		
Lemon	0.7, 2.7*			Apricot	16.4		
Melon	Tr, 1.2†			Blackberry	0.4		
Orange Valencia	0.6, 5.0*			Blueberry	3.5		4
Orange Mandarin	0.5, 4.3*			Cherry	Tr		
Orange Navel	2.3		3	Cranberry	140.0		
Nectarine	1.3			Strawberry	2.5		
Papaya	1.5, 4.0*, 18.1†						
Peach	2.7			*Marmalade*			
Persimmon	Tr			Grapefruit	3.0		
Pineapple	0.1			Lemon	0.7		4
Plum	0.4, 0.6*			Valencia Orange	1.9		
Pomegranate	0.3						
Quince	0.7, 1.1*, 25.5†			*Honey*			
Strawberry	13.9			Acacia	0.8		
Watermelon	0.3			Clover	13.2 (2.7–46.9)		
				Forest	3.5 (1.7– 5.1)		2
				French Heather	143.0		
				German Heather	11.3		
				Scottish Heather	215.8		

*Content in peel of fruit. †Content in seeds of fruit. [1]Drawert and Leupold (1978); [2]Speer and Montag (1984); [3]Nagayama *et al* (1983); [4]Stivje and Hischenhuber (1984).

MISCELLANEOUS SUBSTANCES

Table 2.59 Free glutamate content of various animal-based foods (Maga 1983 Reproduced with permission)

Food	Free glutamate (%)	Reference
Meat products		
Beef	0.042	1
Beef, tenderloin	0.042	4, 8
Beef, shank	0.014	4, 8
Beef, standing rib, medium rare	0.057	7
Beef, standing rib, medium rare, juice from slicing	0.088	7
Beef, standing rib, well done	0.013	7
Bologna	0.004	7
Chicken	0.055	1
Chicken	0.056	4, 8
Chicken bone	0.051	4, 8
Chicken	0.051	7
Duck	0.064	4
Eggs	0.029	1
Frankfurters, boiled	0.001	7
Lamb	0.003	7
Mutton	0.008	4, 8
Pork	0.029	1
Pork, loin	0.029	4, 8
Pork, loin	0.012	7
Sausage, fried, grease removed	0.003	7
Milk products		
Milk, cows'	0.003	1
Milk, cows' 2 months after giving birth	0.0008	2
Milk human	0.024	1
Milk, human, second day after giving birth	0.015	2
Milk, human 3 weeks after giving birth	0.008	2
Milk, human, 2 months after giving birth	0.005	2
Cheese, Camembert	0.760	1
Cheese, Camembert	0.495	2
Cheese, Danish blue	0.850	2
Cheese, Emmental	1.155	9
Cheese, Gouda	0.584	2
Cheese, Gouda	1.244	9
Cheese, Gruyere	1.333	2
Parmesan	0.762	1
Parmesan	1.524	2
Parmesan	2.755	9
Roquefort	1.605	2
Saint Paulin	0.266	2
Stilton	1.041	2
Fish products		
Albacore	0.007	4, 8
Abalone	0.138	4, 8
Carp	0.009−0.022	4, 8
Clam, hard	0.316	4, 8
Clam, Surf	0.192	4, 8
Clam, Little Neck	0.296	4, 8
Clam, minced, canned	0.121	7
Clam chowder, canned	0.031	7
Cod	0.011	4, 8
Corbicula	0.029	4, 8
Crab, King, canned	0.072	7
Crab, deviled, canned	0.032	7
Croaker, white	0.016	4, 8
Eel	0.013	4, 8
Fishing frog	0.065	4, 8
Halibut	0.012−0.013	4, 8
Herring	0.009	4, 8
Loach	0.028	4, 8
Lobster	0.009	4, 8
Mackerel	0.025	4, 8
Mackerel, frigate	0.047−0.075	4, 8
Mackerel, horse	0.024	4, 8
Mackerel, pike	0.046	4, 8
Octopus	0.037	4, 8
Oyster	0.335	4, 8
Pilchard	0.356	4, 8
Prawn	0.065	4, 8
Salmon, canned	0.025	7
Scallop	0.191	4, 8
Sea bream	0.012−0.024	4, 8
Sea urchin	0.381−0.508	4, 8
Squid	0.004−0.056	4, 8
Tuna, yellow fin	0.005−0.011	4, 8
Tuna, canned	0.025	7
Trunk fish	0.009	4, 8
Yellowtail	0.023	4, 8
Animal proteins		
Albumin (egg white)	20.9	2
α-Casein	28.5	2
β-Lactoglobulin (milk)	25.4	2
Actin (muscle)	18.8	2
Myosin (muscle)	26.6	2
Fruits		
Apple	0.005	4, 8
Grape	0.044	4, 8
Grape, red malaga	0.228	2
Grape juice	0.330	2
Grapefruit, white meat	0.146	2
Grapefruit juice	0.236	2
Kumquat	0.019	4, 8
Lemon	0.009	4, 8
Nectarine	1.219	2
Orange	0.015	4, 8
Orange juice	0.026	2
Peach juice	0.041	2
Pear	0.020	4, 8
Persimmon	trace	4, 8
Plum, Yellow	0.100	2
Prunes, fresh	0.017	2
Prunes, dry	0.022	2
Strawberry	0.055	2
Vegetables		
Asparagus, fresh, cooked	0.051	7
Asparagus, canned	0.076	7
Beans, garbonzo, canned	0.012	7
Beans, green, canned	0.012	7
Beans, fresh, cooked	0.025	7
Beans, lima, canned	0.025	7
Beans, yellow wax, canned	0.005	7
Beets, canned	0.038	7
Broccoli	0.213	2
Burdock	0.001	4, 8
Carrot	0.004	4, 8
Corn	0.165	1
Corn, canned	0.051	7
Corn, very young, cooked fresh	0.146	7
Corn, medium, cooked fresh	0.063	7
Corn, mature, cooked fresh	0.076	7
Corn, raw, young	0.165	7
Corn, raw, medium	0.102	7
Corn, raw, mature	0.078	7
Corn, young, cooked after 24 hr refrig.	0.101	7
Corn, young, cooked after 48 hr refrig.	0.088	7
Corn, young, cooked after 72 hr refrig.	0.101	7
Corn, medium, cooked after 24 hr refrig.	0.051	7
Corn, medium, cooked after 48 hr refrig.	0.051	7
Corn, medium cooked after 72 hr refrig.	0.051	7
Corn, mature, cooked after 24 hr refrig.	0.051	7
Corn, mature, cooked after 48 hr refrig.	0.038	7
Corn, mature, cooked after 72 hr refrig.	0.051	7

Corn, young, cooked and refrig. 24 hr	0.152	7
Corn, young, cooked and refrig. 48 hr	0.152	7
Corn, young, cooked and refrig. 72 hr	0.139	7
Corn, medium, cooked and refrig. 24 hr	0.076	7
Corn, medium, cooked and refrig. 48 hr	0.076	7
Corn, medium, cooked and refrig. 72 hr	0.076	7
Corn, mature, cooked and refrig. 24 hr	0.063	7
Corn, mature, cooked and refrig. 48 hr	0.051	7
Corn, mature, cooked and refrig. 72 hr	0.063	7
Corn, medium, cooked on cob	0.114	7
Corn, medium, cooked after removal from cob	0.101	7
Cucumber	0.001	4, 8
Egg plant	0.001	4, 8
Garlic	0.002	4, 8
Ginger	0.001	4, 8
Lotus root	0.001	4, 8
Melon, pickling	0.0005	4, 8
Mushroom, canned	0.285	7
Mushroom, wild, cooked fresh	0.171	7
Mushroom, Shiitake, dried	0.177−0.635	5
Mushroom, *Agaricus bisporus*	0.175	6
Mushroom, *Coprinus comatus*	0.457	10
Mushroom, *Agaricus bisporus*, fresh	0.685	3
Mushroom, *Agaricus bisporus*, dried	0.571	3
Mushroom, *Agaricus bisporus*, sterilized	0.850	3
Mushroom, *Agaricus bisporus*, fresh	0.787	3
Mushroom, *Boletus edulis*, canned	0.076	3
Mushroom, *Boletus edulis*, dried	0.025	3
Mushroom, *Calvatia gigantea*, fresh	0.596	3
Mushroom, *Cantharellus cibarius*, canned	0.063	3
Mushroom, *Coprinus comatus*, fresh	0.444	3
Mushroom, *Gyromitra esculenta*, dried	0.279	3
Mushroom, *Lactarius sanguefluus*, fresh	0.444	3
Mushroom, *Lentinus edodes*, dried	0.266	3
Mushroom, *Marajmius scorodonius*, dried	0.127	3
Mushroom, *Pholiota squarrosa*, fresh	0.177	3
Mushroom, *Pleurotus ostreatus*, fresh	0.368	3
Mushroom, *Tricholoma nudum*, fresh	0.393	3
Mushroom, *Tricholoma protentosum*, canned	0.535	3
Okra, canned	0.038	7
Onion	0.001	4, 8
Peas	0.254	1
Peas, canned	0.152	7
Peas, small, raw	0.254	7
Peas, medium, raw	0.228	7
Peas, large, raw	0.203	7
Peas, medium, cooked after 24 hr refrig.	0.152	7
Peas, medium, cooked after 48 hr refrig.	0.165	7
Peas, medium, cooked after 72 hr refrig.	0.165	7
Peas, medium, raw after 72 hr refrig.	0.165	7
Peas, medium, cooked and refrig. 24 hr	0.209	7
Peas, medium, cooked and refrig. 48 hr	0.216	7
Peas, medium, cooked and refrig. 72 hr	0.196	7
Peas, small, cooked fresh	0.241	7
Peas, medium, cooked fresh	0.209	7
Peas, large cooked fresh	0.196	7
Peas, pods	0.051	7
Potato, fresh	0.254	3
Potato	0.129	2
Potato, whole, canned	0.051	7
Potato, small, cooked fresh	0.053	7
Potato, boiled, variety Bintje	0.092	11, 12
Potato, boiled, variety Ostara	0.045	11, 12
Potato, sweet, canned	0.051	7
Pepper, red	0.002	4, 8
Pork and beans, canned	0.012	7
Pumpkin	0.004	4, 8
Radish	0.002	4, 8
Spinach	0.005	4, 8
Spinach	0.049	1

Spinach, canned	0.031	7
Tomato	0.005	4, 8
Tomato, fresh	0.724	7
Tomato	0.177	1, 2
Plant proteins		
Barley	48.7	2
Coconut	26.6	2
Cottonseed	29.9	2
Flax	26.2	2
Lupine	34.5	2
Maize	34.1	2
Peanut	26.4	2
Soybean	26.0	2
Wheat	58.0	2
Miscellaneous products		
Tea, green	0.264−0.640	4, 8
Tangle, dried	2.26 −5.36	4, 8

Data originally reported as free-glumatic acid were converted to MSG equivalents by using a conversion factor of 1.27.[2]

[1]Anon (1980); [2]Giocometti (1979); [3]Dijkstra (1976); [4] Technical Bulletin; [5]Sugahara *et al* (1975); [6]Dijkstra and Wiken (1976); [7]Hac *et al* (1949); [8]Maeda *et al* (1960); [9]Muller (1970); [10]Dijkstra and Wiken (1976b); [11]Solms and Wyler (1979); [12]Solms (1971).

Table 2.60 Possible sources of yeast in the diet (Warin 1976; Workman *et al* 1984)

Bread	Bread made with yeast or yoghurt (soda breads are yeast-free)
	Buns and cakes made with yeast (e.g. crumpets, doughnuts, teacakes, bath buns)
	Foods made with bread (e.g. bread sauce, stuffing, bread and butter pudding, apple charlotte, summer pudding)
	Foods containing bread as a 'filler' (e.g. sausages, beefburgers, rissoles, meat loaf,)
	Foods coated in breadcrumbs (e.g. fish fingers, fish cakes, breaded fish, potato cakes, scotch eggs)
	Pizza
Fermented foods	Cheese, yoghurt, buttermilk, soured cream, some synthetic creams
	Wine, fortified wines (e.g. vermouth), beer, cider.
	Fruit juices (unless freshly prepared and consumed)
	Grapes, plums and any over-ripe fruit
	Dried fruit such as sultanas, raisins, currants, dates, figs or prunes and foods containing dried fruit (e.g. fruit cake, mincemeat, muesli, eccles cakes)
	Soy sauce
	Pickles (e.g. pickled onions, pickled beetroot)
	Vinegar and vinegar-containing products (e.g. tomato sauce, salad dressing, mayonnaise)
Yeast and meat extracts	Marmite, Bovril
	Oxo and similar beef, chicken or vegetable stock cubes
	Gravy mixes
	Many tinned and packet savoury foods (e.g. soups, sauces)
Vitamin tablets	Brewers yeast tablets
	B vitamins, either as multivitamin or single preparations, are often produced from yeast
Miscellaneous	Malted milk drinks
	Cream crackers
	Twiglets
	Any manufactured food with yeast as an ingredient on the label.

References

Anjou K and Von Sydow E (1967) Aroma of cranberries I. Vaccinium vitisidaea. *Acta Chem Scand* **21**, 945.

Anjou K and Von Sydow E (1969) Aroma of cranberries III. Juice of vaccinium vitisidaea. *Acta Chem Scand* **23**, 109.

Anon (1980) Monososium glutamate (MSG). *Food Technol* **34**, (10), 49.

Arai S, Suzuki H, Fujimaki M and Sakurai Y (1966) Flavour components in soybean III. Volatile fatty acids and volatile amines. *Agric Biolog Chem (Tokyo)* **30**, 363.

Ashoor S and Chu FS. Analysis of salicylic acid and methyl salicylate in fruits and almonds. Food Research Institute, University of Wisconsin, Madison. Unpublished typescript.

Bellanca N (1971) In *Fenaroli's handbook of flavour ingredients* Furia TE and Bellanca N (Eds). Cleveland Chemical Rubber Co, Cleveland.

BMA (1984) and The Pharmaceutical Society of Great Britain. *British National Formularly* No 7.

Bunker ML and McWilliams M (1979) Caffeine content of common beverages. *J Am Diet Assoc* **74**, 28.

Buttery RG, Siefert RM, Gaudagni DG and Ling LC (1969) Characterization of some volatile constituents of bell peppers. *J Agric Food Chem* **17**, 1322.

Buttery RG, Siefert RM and Ling LC (1970) Characterization of some volatile potato components. *J Agric Food Chem* **18**, 538.

Buttery RG, Siefert RM, Gaudagni DG and Ling LC (1971) Characterization of additional volatile components of tomato. *J Agric Food Chem* **19**, 524.

Christensen EN and Caputi A (1968) The quantitative analysis of flavonoids and related compounds in wine by gas-liquid chromatography. *Enology Viticulture* 238.

Clifford AJ, Riumullo JA, Young VR and Scrimshaw NS (1976) Effect of oral purines on serum and urinary uric acid of normal and gouty humans. *J Nutr* **106**, 428.

Daenens P and Larvelle L (1973) Column chromatographic clean up and gas-liquid determination of hydroxybenzoic esters in food. *J Assoc Off Anal Chem* **56**, 1515.

Deyama T and Horiguchi T (1971) Studies of the components of essential oil of clove. *Yakugaku Zasshi* **91**, 1383.

Dijkstra FY (1976) Studies on mushroom flavours 3. Some flavour compounds in fresh, canned and dried edible mushrooms. *Z Lebensm Unters Forsch* **160**, 401.

Dijkstra FY and Wiken TO (1976a) Studies on mushroom flavours 1. Organoleptic significance of constituents of the cultivated mushroom, *Aquaricus bisporus*. *Z Lebensm Unters Forsch* **160**, 255.

Dijkstra FY and Wiken TO (1976b) Studies on mushroom flavours 2. Flavour compounds in *Coprinus cornatus*. *Z Lebensm Unters Forsch* **160**, 263.

Do JE, Salunkhe DK and Olson LE (1969) Isolation, identification and comparison of volatiles of peach fruit as related to harvest maturity and artificial ripening. *J Food Sci* **34**, 618.

Dodge FD (1918) Constituents of oil of cassia. *J Indus Engineer Chem* **10**, 1005.

Drawert F and Leupold G (1978) Über das vorkommen von benzoesäure in milch und milcherzeugnissen. *Lebensmittelchemie u. gerichtl. Chemie* **32**, 77–8.

Fedeli 'E and Jacini G (1970) Odorous components of olive oil. *Chim Indust (Milan)* **52**, (2), 161.

Gierschner K and Baumann G (1968) Aromatic substances in fruit. *Reichstoffe Aromen Koerperflegemittel* **18**, (1), 3.

Giocometti T (1979) Free and bound glutamate in natural products, glutamic acid. In *Advances in biochemistry and physiology* Filer *et al* (Eds). Raven Press, New York.

Guppy H, Whitfield FB and Woodhill JB. Salicylic acid in fruit and vegetables. Report of Research 1977–8. CSIRO Division of Food Research, Sydney, Australia.

Hac LR, Long ML and Blish MJ (1949) The occurrence of free L-glutamic acid in various foods. *Food Technol* **3**, 351.

Haymon LW and Aurand LW (1971) Characterization of volatile constituents of Tabasco peppers. *J Agric Food Chem* **19**, 1131.

Heide R (1972) Qualitative analysis of the essential oil of cassia (cinnamomum cassia blume). *J Agric Food Chem* **20**, 747.

Johnson AE, Nursten HE and Williams AA (1971) Vegetable volatiles. Survey of components identified. *Chem Indust* July, 1212.

Kahn JH (1969) Compounds identified in whisky, wine, beer. A tabulation. *J Assoc Off Anal Chem* **52**, 1166.

Kasidas GP (1980) Oxalate content of some common foods: Determination by an enzymic method. *J Hum Nutr* **34**, 255–66.

Kemp TR, Knavel DE and Stoltz LP (1971) Characterization of some volatile components of muskmelon fruit. *Phytochemistry* **10**, 478.

Liebich HM, Koenig WA and Bayer E (1970) Analysis of the flavour of rum by gas-liquid chromatography and mass spectrometry. *J Chromatogr Sci* **8**, 527.

Lockey SD (1971) Reactions to hidden agents in foods, beverages and drugs. *Annals of Allergy* **29**, 461–6.

Maeda S, Eguchi S and Sasaki H (1960) Distribution of free glutamic acid in various foods. *Microbioassay* **2**, 23.

Maga JA (1983) *Critical Reviews in Food Science and Nutrition* **18**, 266–70.

Massey Stewart M (1976) MAOIs and food — fact and fiction. *J Hum Nutr* **30**, 415–9.

McGlumphy JH (1951) Fruit flavours. *Food Technol* **5**, 351.

Muller H (1970) Occurrence of free glutamic acid in foods. *Z Ernährungswissenschaft* **10**, 83.

Murray KE (1973) The flavour of purple passionfruit. *Food Technol Aust* **25**, 446.

Nagayama T, Nishijima M, Yasuda K, Saito K, Kamimura H, Ibe A, Ushiyama H, Nagayama M and Naoi Y (1983) Benzoic acid in fruits and fruit products. *J Food Hyg Soc* **24**, 416–22.

Nagy M (1974) Caffeine content of beverages and chocolate. *J Am Med Assoc* **229**, 337.

Nursten HE and Williams AA (1967) Fruit aromas: A survey of components identified. *Chem Indust* March, 468.

Onishi I and Yamamoto K (1956) Essential oils of tobacco leaves. *Chem Abstr* **50**, 15028.

Porsch F, Farnow H and Winkler H (1965) The constituents of star aniseed oil. *Dragoco Rep* **12**, 123.

Pyne AW and Wick EL (1965) Volatile components of tomatoes. *J Food Sci* **30**, 192.

Robertson GL and Kermode WJ (1981) Salicylic acid in fresh and canned fruit and vegetables. *J Sci Food Agric* **32**, 883.

Saijo R and Kuwabara U (1967) Volatile flavour of black tea. *Agric Biolog Chem (Tokyo)* **31**, 389.

Schmidtlein H and Herrmann K (1975a) Über die phenolsäuren des gemüses I. Hydroxyzimtsäuren und hydroxybenzoesäuren der kohlartern und anderer cruciferen-blatter. *Z Lebensm Unters Forsch* **159**, 139.

Schmidtlein H and Herrmann K (1975b) Über die phenolsäuren des gemüses II. Hydrozyzimtsäuren und hydroxybenzoesäuren der frucht und samengemüsearten. *Z Lebensm Unters Forsch* **159**, 213.

Schmidtlein H and Herrmann K (1975c) Über die phenolsäuren des gemuses IV. Hydroxyzimtsäuren und hydroxybenzoesäuren weiterer gemüsearten und der kartoffeln. *Z Lebensm Unters Forsch* **159**, 255.

Solms J (1971) Non-volatile compounds and the flavour of foods. In *Gustation and Olfaction* Ohloff, G and Thomas AF (Eds.), p. 92. Academic Press, New York.

Solms J and Wyler R (1979) Taste components of potatoes. In *Food Taste Chemistry* Boudreau JC (Ed), p. 175. American Chemical Society, Washington D.C. Series No 115.

Speer VK and Montag A (1984) Beitrag zum Verkommen von Ben-

GENERAL DIETETIC PRINCIPLES AND PRACTICE

zoesäure und Phenylessigsäure in Honig. *Deutsche Lebensmittel-Rundschau* **80**, 103–5.

Stahl WH (1962) The chemistry of tea and tea manufacturing. *Adv Food Res* **11**, 201.

Stivje T and Hischenhuber C (1984) High performance liquid chromatographic determination of levels of benzoic acid and sorbic acid in yoghurts. *Deutsche Lebensmittel-Rundschau* **80**, 81–5.

Stoffelsma J, Sipma G, Kettenes DK and Pypker J (1968) New volatile components of roasted coffee. *J Agric Food Chem* **16**, 1000.

Stöhr H and Herrmann K (1975a) Über das vorkommen von verbindungen der hydroxyzimtsäuren, hydroxybenzoesäuren und hydroxycumarine in citrusfrüchten. *Z Lebensm Unters Forsch* **159**, 305.

Stöhr H and Herrmann K (1975b) Über die phenolsäuren des gemüses III. Hydroxyzimtsäuren und hydroxybenzoesäuren des wurzelgemüses. *Z Lebensm Unters Forsch* **159**, 219.

Stöhr H, Mosel H and Herrmann K (1975) The phenolics of fruits VII. The phenolics of cherries and plums and the changes in catechins and hydroxycinnamic acid derivatives during the development of fruits. *Z Lebensm Unters Forsch* **159**, (11), 85.

Sugahara T, Aral S, Aoyagi Y and Kunisaki N (1975) Contents of 5'-nucleotides and free amino acids in different varieties of dried shiitake mushroom. *Eiyo to Shokuryo* **28**, 477.

Swain AR, Soutter V, Loblay R and Truswell AS (1985a) Salicylates, oligoantigenic diets and behaviour. *Lancet* **ii**, 41–2.

Swain AR, Dutton SP and Truswell AS (1985b) Salicylates in foods. *J Am Med Assoc* **85**, 950–60.

Technical Bulletin of Ajinomoto Co. Nucleotides Part I. Savoury substances. Ajinomoto Co, Inc., Tokyo, Japan.

Thornberg W (1976) Salicylic acid and methyl salicylate in canned Delmonte products. Delmonte Foods, Unpublished typescript.

Warin RP (1976) Food factors in urticaria. *J Hum Nutr* **30**, (3), 181–2.

Winter M and Kloti R (1972) Über das aroma der gelben passionsfrucht. *Helv Chim Acta* **55**, 181.

Workman E, Hunter J and Alun Jones V (1984) *The allergy diet* (Positive Health Guide) Martin Dunitz Ltd, London.

Wyngaarden JB and Kelly WN (1976) *Gout and hyperuricaemia* pp 453–5. Grune and Stratton, New York.

Yamanishi T (1978) The aroma of various teas. In *Flavour of foods and beverages: Chemistry and technology* Charalambous G and Inglett GE (Eds). Academic Press, New York.

Zarembski PM and Hodgkinson A (1962) The oxalic acid content of English diets. *Br J Nutr* **16**, 627–34.

2.11 Specific Food Avoidance

2.11.1 Gluten/gluten and soya/gluten and lactose avoidance

Gluten-free foods

Gluten-free foods are required by those with coeliac disease (Section 4.12.2) and dermatitis herpetiformis (Section 4.33). It is generally accepted that a gluten-free diet involves the complete avoidance of all foods made from, or containing, wheat, rye, barley and usually oats (Table 2.61). Oats may be permitted, this will be decided by the consultant, however the Coeliac Society advise *against* their inclusion in the gluten-free diet.

Some manufactured products bear the gluten-free symbol on their label

indicating their suitability for inclusion in gluten-free diets. However, not all manufacturers have adopted this policy and it is not satisfactory to attempt to deduce suitability of a given product by looking at the ingredients listed on the label.

The Coeliac Society publishes a list of gluten-free manufactured products in booklet form which is updated every year. Where the column of permitted foods states 'certain brands', these should be sought in the Coeliac Society's list. Where necessary, categories of products are prefaced by an informative, explanatory paragraph.

It is essential that the *current* edition of the list should be referred to in order to complement the basic diet sheet. Patients should be strongly recommended to enrol as members of the Coeliac Society, not only in order that they be in receipt of the list but also for the other benefits which membership affords.

The address of the Society is The Coeliac Society, PO Box 220, High Wycombe, Bucks HP11 2HY, Tel: 0494-37278.

Communion wafers

Ordinary Communion wafers do contain gluten, however gluten-free wafers can be obtained at a small cost from The Monastery of Poor Colettines, Mossley Hill, Liverpool, L18 3ES.

The Coeliac Society's list of gluten-free manufactured products may list alternative sources.

Prescribable items

A wide range of specially manufactured gluten-free items, e.g. biscuits, bread, bread mix, cakes, crispbread, flour, flour mix, pastas and rusks are prescribable under the National Health Service for gluten-sensitive enteropathies.

Full use of these products should be encouraged. Their inclusion in the diet not only adds variety, palatability and bulk but also aids compliance. Dietary indiscretions are much more likely to occur in a hungry patient.

Table 2.61 Gluten-free and gluten-containing foods

Food group	Gluten-free foods	Gluten-containing foods
Cereals and flours	Arrowroot, buckwheat, corn or maize, cornflour or maize flour, gluten-free flour, potato flour (or fecule or farina), rice and rice flour, sago, soya, soya flour, tapioca. Oats* (if permitted).	Wheat, wholemeal, wholewheat and wheatmeal flours, bran, barley, rye, rye flour, pasta (macaroni, noodles, spaghetti, etc.), semolina.
Prepared cereals	Made from corn or rice e.g. Cornflakes, Rice Krispies, baby rice. Porridge oats* (if permitted).	Cereals made from wheat, barley or rye, e.g. muesli, Shredded Wheat, Sugar Puffs, Weetabix.
Baked goods	*Gluten-free* biscuits, bread, bread mix, cakes, crispbread, flour, flour mix, pasta, rusks. *Certain brands* of oatcakes* (if permitted).	*All ordinary baked goods* made from wheat, barley, rye flour, suet and semolina. Crispbreads and starch reduced bread and rolls. Ice cream wafers and cones. Communion wafers (see above)

Table 2.61 *contd.*

Food group	Gluten-free foods	Gluten-containing foods
Milk	Fresh, condensed, dried, evaporated, skimmed, sterilized. Fresh or tinned cream. Most brands of yoghurt. Coffee creamers and whiteners.	Artificial cream containing flour. Yoghurt containing muesli.
Cheese	Plain, e.g. Cheddar, cottage cheese, cream cheese, curd cheese. *Certain brands* of cheese spreads.	Cheese spreads containing flour.
Eggs	Prepared and cooked without flour and breadcrumbs.	Prepared and cooked with flour or breadcrumbs e.g. 'Scotch' eggs.
Fats and oils	Butter, margarine, oil, lard, dripping.	Suet.
Meat and fish	All varieties prepared and cooked without flour and breadcrumbs. *Certain brands* of canned meat and canned fish in sauce. *Certain brands* of meat and fish pastes. *Certain brands* of continental sausages. *Certain brands* of burgers.	Savoury pies and puddings containing flour, breadcrumbs, stuffing and suet. Sausages and burgers containing breadcrumbs. Battered or crumbed fish, fish fingers, fish cakes.
Vegetables	Fresh, cooked, canned, dried, frozen, pulses, soya. *Certain brands* of baked beans. *Certain brands* of potato crisps.	Vegetables canned in sauce e.g. creamed mushrooms. Potato croquettes. Textured vegetable protein containing wheat.
Fruit	Fresh, cooked, canned, dried, frozen.	
Nuts	Fresh and plain, salted.	
Preserves and confectionery	Sugar, glucose, jam, honey, malt, malt extract, marmalade, molasses, treacle, *certain brands* of mincemeat. *Certain brands* of sweets and chocolate. Plain ice lollies.	Sweets containing or rolled in flour, e.g. liquorice, unwrapped sweets, Smarties, Twix.
Puddings and desserts	Jelly, milk puddings made from permitted cereals **NOT** semolina. Home-made puddings using gluten-free ingredients. *Certain brands* of instant desserts. *Certain brands* of ice cream.	Puddings and desserts containing flour, breadcrumbs and suet. Ice cream cones and wafers.
Beverages	Tea, pure instant or fresh ground coffee, cocoa, fizzy drinks, squashes and cordials, fresh fruit juices, wines, spirits, keg beers.	Barley-based instant coffee, barley flavoured fruit drinks. Bengers, malted drinks e.g. Horlicks. Home brewed beer, cloudy real ale, hot drinks from vending machines.
Soups, sauces and gravies	Soup, sauce and gravy if thickened with suitable cereal. *Certain brands* of tinned and dried soups. *Certain brands* of stock concentrates, gravy brownings and gravy salts.	Soup, sauce and gravy thickened with or containing wheat, barley, rye or pasta. Bisto.
Seasonings	Salt, fresh ground or pure pepper. Herbs, pure spices, vinegar. *Certain brands* of ready-to-eat mustard. *Certain brands* of ready mixed spices, seasonings and curry powders. Monosodium glutamate.	Pepper compound, ready-mixed spices, seasonings and curry powders containing flour as a 'filler'.
Miscellaneous	Bicarbonate of soda, cream of tartar, tartaric acid. *Certain brands* of baking powder, fresh and dried yeast, colourings and essences, gelatine.	Medication containing gluten.

The foregoing lists are intended only as a basic guide to the suitability of 'everyday' foods.

Gluten-free bread is now available vacuum-packed in sealed plastic/polythene packs for longer shelf life, as well as in tins. Bread can also be made easily from a variety of mixes. Gluten-free bread can be frozen and will keep for a long time in a freezer — it can even be sliced prior to freezing to allow economical use of small amounts.

Gluten-free flours and flour mixes are available to make cakes, biscuits and other baked goods and now give results which look and taste exactly like items cooked with ordinary flour. To obtain the best results, the recipes given by individual manufacturers for their own products *must* be followed; it is no longer satisfactory to substitute gluten-free flour for ordinary flour in ordinary recipes, or to interchange one gluten-free flour for another.

A list of prescribable items appears in the current editions of *Monthly Index of Medical Specialities* (MIMS) and the *British National Formulary* under the Borderline Substances Appendix, and in Appendix 1 of the current Coeliac Society food list. Prescriptions should be marked 'ACBS' (Advisory Committee for Borderline Substances). Prescribable items (at the time of going to press) are listed in Table 2.62.

Children under 16 years, pregnant women, men aged 65 years or over and women aged 60 years or over are exempt from prescription charges. Other adults may find it economical to buy a 'season ticket', (prepayment of charges) for their prescriptions. Form FP 95 (EC 95 in Scotland) is available from Post Offices, local social security offices and chemists. Further information may be found in leaflet P11 — '*NHS prescriptions, how to get them free*'.

Certain other gluten-free products are considered non-essential luxuries rather than staple items, and therefore must be purchased — they *are not* available on prescription. These products can be ordered from a chemist. Alternatively, certain products may be available by mail order direct from the manufacturers or distributors. Non-prescribable gluten-free foods available at the time of going to press are listed in Table 2.63.

Gluten-free, soya-free foods

Reference should be made to the foregoing section covering 'everyday' gluten-free foods. In addition to the forbidden foods listed, the following should also be avoided

1 Soya beans
2 Soya grits
3 Soya flour

Table 2.62 Gluten-free foods available on prescription

Product	Manufacturer/distributor*
Bread	
Juvela gluten-free loaf	
Juvela gluten-free fibre loaf	GF Dietary Group Ltd
Juvela low protein loaf	
Rite-Diet gluten-free white bread	
Rite-Diet gluten-free, high fibre bread (with soya bran)	
Rite-Diet gluten-free and low protein bread	Welfare Foods (Stockport) Ltd
Rite-Diet gluten-free low protein bread with added soya bran (brown)	
Rite-Diet low protein white bread with added fibre	
Ener-G Brown Rice bread	General Designs Ltd
Flour and bread mixes	
Aproten flour	Farmitalia Carlo Erba Ltd
Juvela gluten-free mix	
Juvela gluten-free fibre mix	GF Dietary Group Ltd
Juvela low protein mix	
Rite-Diet gluten-free white bread mix	
Rite-Diet gluten-free brown bread mix	
Rite-Diet gluten-free flour mix	Welfare Foods (Stockport) Ltd
Rite-Diet low protein flour mix	
Tritamyl gluten-free flour	
Trufree or Jubilee	
No 1 flour	
No 2 flour (with rice bran)	
No 3 flour for Cantabread	
No 4 white flour	The Cantassium Company
No 5 brown flour	
No 6 flour (plain)	
No 7 flour (self raising)	
Biscuits	
Aproten low protein biscuits	Farmitalia Carlo Erba Ltd
Bi-Aglut gluten-free biscuits	
Glutenex	Cow and Gate Ltd (Distrib)
Farley's gluten-free biscuits	Farley Health Products Ltd
Verkade gluten-free biscuits	GF Dietary Group Ltd
Rite-Diet gluten-free digestive biscuits	
Rite-Diet gluten-free savoury biscuits	Welfare Foods (Stockport) Ltd
Rite-Diet gluten-free sweet biscuits	
Crackers/crispbread	
Aproten crispbread	Farmitalia Carlo Erba Ltd
Bi-Aglut gluten-free cracker toast	
GF brand gluten-free crackers	GF Dietary Group Ltd
Rite-Diet low protein, gluten-free crackers	Welfare Foods (Stockport) Ltd
Rite-Diet gluten-free high fibre crackers	
Pasta	
Aproten Anellini (small pasta rings)	
Aproten Ditalini (small macaroni)	Farmitalia Carlo Erba Ltd
Aproten Rigatini (ribbed macaroni)	
Aproten Tagliatelle (flat noodles)	
Aglutella Gentili spaghetti	
Aglutella Gentili spaghetti rings	GF Dietary Group Ltd
Aglutella Gentili macaroni	
Aglutella Gentili semolina	
Rite-Diet low protein pasta (macaroni, spaghetti, spaghetti rings)	Welfare Foods (Stockport) Ltd

*Addresses of manufacturers/distributors can be found on p 617.

Table 2.63 Non-prescribable gluten-free foods

Product	Manufacturer/distributor*
Bread	
GF Dietary thin wafer bread	GF Dietary Group Ltd
Mixes, brans and flours	
Ener-G rice bran	
GF Dietary pastry mix	GF Dietary Group Ltd
Juvela gluten-free corn mix	
Rite-diet processed soya bran (gluten-free)	Welfare Foods (Stockport) Ltd
Tritamyl gluten-free bread mix	Procea
Biscuits	
Aglutella low protein gluten-free cream filled wafers	
GF Dietary maize biscuits with chocolate	
GF Dietary maize biscuits with hazelnuts	
GF Dietary fruit bran biscuits	GF Dietary Group Ltd
GF Dietary muesli fruit biscuits	
GF Dietary coconut cookies	
GF Dietary ginger cookies	
GF Dietary fibre cookies	
Rite-Diet gluten-free half-covered milk chocolate biscuits	
Rite-Diet gluten-free sultana biscuits	
Rite-Diet gluten-free custard creams	
Rite-Diet gluten-free sweet biscuits (Shortcake/Lincoln)	
Rite-Diet gluten-free chocolate chip cookies	Welfare Food (Stockport) Ltd
Rite-Diet low protein vanilla cream wafers	
Rite-Diet low protein chocolate flavoured cream wafers	
Rite-Diet low protein sweet biscuits	
Rite-Diet low protein cream filled biscuits (chocolate flavour)	
Cakes	
Country Basket carob rice cakes	
Country Basket rice cakes (salted and unsalted)	Newform Foods
Rite-Diet gluten-free rich fruit cake (canned)	Welfare Foods (Stockport) Ltd
GF Dietary banana cake	
GF Dietary date and walnut cake	GF Dietary Group Ltd
GF gluten-free rich fruit cake	
Miscellaneous	
GF Dietary muesli (without added sugar)	GF Dietary Group Ltd
GF Dietary hot breakfast cereal	
Rite-Diet gluten-free baking powder	Welfare Foods (Stockport) Ltd
GF Dietary baking powder	GF Dietary Group Ltd

4 Hydrolysed, 'spun' or 'textured' vegetable protein of soya origin
5 Soya milk
6 Soya-based flavouring
7 Soya oil
8 Soya protein isolate.

Using the Coeliac Society food list, the ingredients of those foods listed should be checked for the presence or absence of soya.

Up to 2% soya (usually as soya isolate) fulfils such purposes as water binding emulsification and whippability in a wide range of foods including baby foods,

hams, sausages, pastes and other meat products, fish products, dessert toppings, yoghurt, coffee whiteners, dairy products and ice cream, snack foods and sugar confectionery.

Soya products may be the major component of products intended for use as meat 'extenders' usually in textured forms such as extruded defatted soya flour or spun soya isolate. These textured products may be present in some meat products in addition to the legally required minimum meat content. Soya flour is often present in sausages as a binder at levels of 2−3%.

Prescribable items

Many gluten-free prescribable items contain soya to improve protein content, palatability and texture, and are therefore contraindicated. Prescribable and non-prescribable foods which are both gluten-free and soya-free are listed in Tables 2.64 and 2.65.

Table 2.64 Prescribable gluten-free, soya-free foods

Product	Manufacturer/distributor*
Bread	
Juvela gluten-free loaf	
Juvela gluten-free fibre loaf	GF Dietary Group Ltd
Juvela low protein loaf	
Rite-Diet gluten-free white bread	
Rite-Diet gluten-free and low protein bread (canned)	Welfare Foods (Stockport) Ltd
Rite-Diet low protein white bread (with added fibre)	
Ener-G Brown Rice bread	General Designs Ltd
Flour and bread mixes	
Aproten flour	Farmitalia Carlo Erba Ltd
Juvela gluten-free mix	
Juvela gluten-free fibre mix	GF Dietary Group Ltd
Juvela low protein mix	
Rite-Diet low protein flour mix	Welfare Foods (Stockport) Ltd
Biscuits	
Bi-Aglut gluten-free biscuits	
Aproten low protein biscuits	Farmitalia Carlo Erba Ltd
Verkade gluten-free biscuits	GF Dietary Group Ltd
Crackers/crispbread	
Aproten crispbread	Farmitalia Carlo Erba Ltd
Rite-Diet low protein, gluten-free crackers	Welfare Foods (Stockport) Ltd
Pasta	
Aproten Anellini (small pasta rings)	
Aproten Ditalini (small macaroni)	Farmitalia Carlo Erba Ltd
Aproten Rigatini (ribbed macaroni)	
Aproten Tagliatelle (flat noodles)	
Aglutella Gentili spaghetti	
Aglutella Gentili spaghetti rings	GF Dietary Group Ltd
Aglutella Gentili macaroni	
Aglutella Gentili semolina	
Rite-Diet low protein pasta (macaroni, spaghetti, spaghetti rings)	Welfare Foods (Stockport) Ltd

*Addresses of manufacturers/distributors are given on p 617.

Table 2.65 Non-prescribable gluten-free, soya-free foods

Product	Manufacturer/distributor*
Brans and mixes	
Ener-G rice bran	GF Dietary Group Ltd
Juvela gluten-free corn mix	
Biscuits	
Rite-Diet low protein sweet biscuits	Welfare Foods (Stockport) Ltd
Rite-Diet low protein vanilla cream wafers	
Rite-Diet low protein chocolate flavoured cream wafers	
Rite-Diet low protein cream filled biscuits (chocolate flavour)	
GF Dietary coconut cookies	GF Dietary Group Ltd
GF Dietary ginger cookies	
GF Dietary fibre cookies	
Cakes	
Country Basket carob rice cakes	Newform Foods
Country Basket rice cakes (salted and unsalted)	
Rite-Diet gluten-free rich fruit cake (canned)	Welfare Foods (Stockport) Ltd
GF Dietary banana cake	GF Dietary Group Ltd
GF Dietary date and walnut cake	
Miscellaneous	
GF Dietary muesli (without added sugar)	GF Dietary Group Ltd
GF Dietary hot breakfast cereal	
Rite-Diet gluten-free baking powder	Welfare Foods (Stockport) Ltd

*Addresses of manufacturers/distributors are given on p 617.

Gluten-free low lactose foods

A gluten-free, low lactose diet involves the complete avoidance of several cereals (See 'gluten-free foods'; Table 2.61) and of milk, most milk products and milk derivatives (See 'milk-free foods'; Table 2.68).

Combining these two sections will provide comprehensive lists of everyday foods which are permitted and forbidden on a gluten-free, milk-free diet.

However, the percentage of lactose in butter is so small (approximately 0.4−1% maximum) as to render it suitable for use in most cases of simple lactose intolerance. Similarly, most types of pure cheese contain only traces of lactose. Norwegian Mysost does contain significant quantities of lactose, as does cottage cheese and processed cheeses such as cheese spreads and cheese portions. Hence apart from allowing butter and pure cheese, the permitted and forbidden foods are the same for a low lactose regimen as for a milk-free regimen.

A list of 'wheat-free, milk-free manufactured foods' is available to dietitians at a small cost from The British Dietetic Association (but see p 615). This may be used as a basis for ascertaining suitable gluten-free, low lactose proprietary items.

Prescribable items

At the time of going to press items which may be prescribed for gluten sensitive enteropathies with associated lactose intolerance are listed in Table 2.66. Non-prescribable items are listed in Table 2.67.

Table 2.66 Foods prescribable for gluten sensitive enteropathies with associated lactose intolerance

Product	Manufacturer/distributor*
Milk/milk substitutes	
Formula S Soya Food	Cow and Gate Ltd
Nutramigen	Mead Johnson
Pregestimil	
Prosobee	
Wysoy	Wyeth Laboratories
Isomil	Abbott Laboratories
Bread	
Juvela low protein loaf	GF Dietary Group Ltd
Rite-Diet gluten-free low protein bread (canned)	Welfare Foods (Stockport) Ltd
Rite-Diet low protein bread with added soya bran	
Riet-Diet low protein white bread with added fibre	
Flour and mixes	
Aproten flour	Farmitalia Carlo Erba Ltd
Juvela low protein mix	GF Dietary Group Ltd
Tritamyl gluten-free flour	Procea
Tritamyl PK protein-free flour	
Rite-Diet low protein flour mix	Welfare Foods (Stockport) Ltd
Biscuits	
+Aproten low protein biscuits	Farmitalia Carlo Erba Ltd
+Bi-Aglut gluten-free biscuits	
++Farley's gluten-free biscuits	Farley Health Products Ltd
Glutenex (a gluten-free biscuit)	Cow and Gate Ltd
Rite-Diet gluten-free sweet biscuits	Welfare Foods (Stockport) Ltd
Rite-Diet gluten-free savoury biscuits	
Rite-Diet gluten-free digestives	
Crispbread/crackers	
+Aproten crispbread	Farmitalia Carlo Erba Ltd
GF brand gluten-free crackers	GF Dietary Group Ltd
Rite-Diet low protein gluten-free crackers	Welfare Foods (Stockport) Ltd
Rite-Diet gluten-free high fibre crackers	
Pasta	
Aproten Anellini (small pasta rings)	Farmitalia Carlo Erba Ltd
Aproten Rigatini (ribbed macaroni)	
Aproten Tagliatelle (flat noodles)	
Aproten Ditalini (small macaroni)	
Aglutella Gentili spaghetti	GF Dietary Group Ltd
Aglutella Gentili spaghetti rings	
Aglutella Gentili macaroni	
Aglutella Gentili semolina	
Rite-Diet low protein pasta (macaroni, spaghetti, spaghetti rings)	Welfare Foods (Stockport) Ltd

*Addresses of manufacturers/distributors are given on p 617.
+contains negligible lactose but is contraindicated in cases of milk protein intolerance.
++contains 0.6% lactose which may be tolerated in cases of lactose intolerance, but is contraindicated in cases of milk protein intolerance.

Table 2.67 Non-prescribable foods suitable for gluten sensitive enteropathies with associated lactose intolerance

Product	Manufacturer/distributor*
Bread	
GF Dietary thin wafer bread	GF Dietary Group Ltd
Brans, flour and mixes	
Ener-G rice bran	GF Dietary Group Ltd
Juvela gluten-free corn mix	
Rite-Diet processed soya bran (gluten-free)	Welfare Foods (Stockport) Ltd
Biscuits	
Aglutella low protein gluten-free cream filled wafers	
GF Dietary fruit bran biscuits	GF Dietary Group Ltd
GF Dietary coconut cookies	
GF Dietary ginger cookies	
GF Dietary fibre cookies	
Rite-Diet gluten-free custard creams	
Rite-Diet gluten-free sweet biscuits (Shortcake, Lincoln)	
Rite-Diet gluten-free chocolate chip cookies	
Rite-Diet low protein vanilla cream wafers	
Rite-Diet low protein chocolate flavoured cream wafers	Welfare Foods (Stockport) Ltd
Rite-Diet low protein sweet biscuits	
Rite-Diet low protein cream filled biscuits (chocolate flavour)	
Rite-Diet low protein sultana biscuits	
Cakes	
Country Basket rice cakes (salted and unsalted)	Newform Foods
GF Dietary banana cake	
GF Dietary date and walnut cake	GF Dietary Group Ltd
GF gluten free rich fruit cake	
Miscellaneous	
GF Dietary muesli (without added sugar)	GF Dietary Group Ltd
GF Dietary hot breakfast cereal	
Rite-Diet gluten-free baking powder	Welfare Foods (Stockport) Ltd
GF Dietary Baking Powder	GF Dietary Group Ltd

*Addresses of manufacturers/distributors are given on p 617.

2.11.2 Wheat avoidance

Wheat is present in a wide variety of foods, including flour, pasta, many breakfast cereals, cakes, biscuits and in many manufactured foods in the form of, for example, gluten, wheat starch, rusk and hydrolysed vegetable protein of wheat origin. It is important that all sources of wheat (including wheat protein and starch) are excluded from a patient's diet. Many gluten-free special products, e.g. bread and biscuits, contain wheat starch and are not suitable for use in wheat intolerance. This, in fact, reduces the variety of special foods available, which ultimately increases the difficulties of adhering to the diet. In practice, many patients react not only to wheat but also to rye and this should be excluded on a wheat free diet initially and reintroduced at a later stage. A list of wheat-free manufactured foods is available to dietitians from the British Dietetic Association (but see p 615).

2.11.3 Egg avoidance

Egg intolerance is very common. An egg-free diet involves the complete avoidance of eggs and foods containing whole egg, dried egg, egg yolk, egg albumin or egg lecithin. Such foods include egg pasta, most biscuits and cakes, meringues and mayonnaise. The British Dietetic Association produces a list of manufactured egg-free foods (but see p 615).

Substitutes for egg

GF Dietary egg replacer

This is a low protein, low phenylalanine, low fat and cholesterol-free product which can be used as a substitute for egg. It is composed of potato starch, modified maize starch, thickener, cellulose gum, calcium polyphosphate, carotene and potassium carbonate. It may be used to replace eggs using one teaspoon of egg replacer to two tablespoons of water. GF Dietary egg replacer is available in 250 g tubs (equivalent to approximately 50 eggs) from GF Dietary Supplies Ltd, 494−496 Honeypot Lane, Stanmore, Middlesex HA7 1JH.

Edifas A

This composed of purified methyl ethyl cellulose which, when made up into a 5% solution, provides the basis for producing an excellent meringue substitute. Edifas A is distributed for ICI by Bow Produce Ltd, 15 Ashurst Close, Northwood, Middlesex HA6 IEL.

2.11.4 Milk avoidance

Milk is particularly difficult to exclude from a patient's diet. In addition to the fact that milk and products based on milk are important components of the average diet, many popular manufactured foods contain milk or milk derivatives. A dietitian's help is essential if a patient (or parent) is to remove milk completely from a diet without adverse nutritional consequences.

A milk-free diet involves the complete avoidance of cows' (and sometimes goats' and sheep's milk), milk products such as butter, cheese, cream and yoghurt and milk derivatives such as casein, whey, skimmed milk, non-fat milk solids and hydrolysed whey. Lactose is also found in many foods and in retail brands of monosodium glutamate (MSG), certain low calorie sweeteners and as a constituent of some crisps, stock cubes and dried soups. Lactose is also used by the pharmaceutical industry as a filler in some tablets.

For practical purposes, no differentiation is usually made between cows' milk protein intolerance and lactose intolerance. However, goats' and sheep's milk may be permissible in the diet of some cases of cows' milk protein intolerance but, since these milks contain lactose, are unsuitable for those with lactose intolerance.

Foods which are either suitable or unsuitable for inclusion in a milk-free diet are listed in Table 2.68. However, these are only guidelines and it must be stressed to patients that the ingredient list of manufactured brands of items should be checked for the presence of milk or a milk derivative. The British Dietetic Association regularly prints a list of milk-free manufactured foods for use by dietitians (see p 615) but it must be remembered that this rapidly becomes out of date owing to changes in the formulation of foods or the introduction of new products.

Fortunately, many recipes can be adapted by using milk-free margarines to replace butter or ordinary

Table 2.68 Foods suitable or unsuitable for a milk-free diet

Milk-free foods	Foods containing milk or milk products
Complete milk substitutes Formula S Soya Food — Cow and Gate Nutramigen Pregestimil } Mead Johnson Prosobee Isomil Abbots Wysoy Wyeth Laboratories	*All milk* Fresh, condensed, dried, evaporated, skimmed.
Milk-free margarines Rakusens, Telma, Tomor, Vitaquell. *Certain brands* of low fat spread, e.g. Weight Watchers, Co-op Slimmers Spread. Lard, suet, dripping, vegetable oil.	Milk products Butter, all types of cheese. Fresh and tinned cream. Margarines and spreads containing milk. Yoghurt, ice cream, dairy desserts, mousse.
Prepared Cereals *Certain brands* of baby cereals, e.g. pure baby rice — Robinsons, Boots. *Certain brands* of rusks, e.g. Farley's Original rusks. *Certain brands* of breakfast cereals, e.g. Cornflakes, Rice Krispies.	Baby cereals containing milk, e.g. Farley's baby rice. Rusks containing milk, e.g. Farley's low sugar rusks, Cow and Gate Liga rusks. Breakfast cereals containing milk, e.g Special K, some brands of muesli.
Cereals and Flours Cornflour, all varieties of flour *Certain brands* of blancmange powder,	Instant desserts. Instant porridge, milk puddings.

Table 2.68 *contd.*

Milk-free foods	Foods containing milk or milk products
oats, rice, sago, semolina, tapioca, spaghetti, macaroni, etc.	
Baked goods and puddings Bread (standard white, brown and wholemeal). Home-made cakes, biscuits and puddings using milk-free ingredients. *Certain brands* of cakes, biscuits and puddings.	Milk loaf, 'toasting' loaf, fancy bread and buns. Cakes, biscuits and puddings made with milk or milk products.
Meat and Fish All varieties prepared and cooked without milk and milk products. *Certain brands* of sausages, fish fingers, etc.	Meat products containing milk derivatives. Fish in batter or crumbs or sauce made with milk or milk products.
Eggs	
Vegetables Fresh, cooked, canned, dried, frozen, pulses, soya beans. *Certain brands* of baked beans. *Certain brands* of instant potato. *Certain brands* of potato crisps.	Vegetables canned in sauce containing milk or milk products. Instant potato containing milk or milk products.
Fruit Fresh, cooked, canned, dried, frozen, fruit pie fillings. Fresh fruit juice.	
Nuts Fresh and plain salted. Peanut butter.	Dry roasted nuts with a lactose-containing flavouring.
Preserves and confectionery Sugar, glucose, jam, honey, syrup, marmalade, molasses, treacle, mincemeat, *certain brands* of lemon curd. *Certain brands* of sweets and plain chocolate. Plain ice lollies. Sorbet, jelly.	Toffee, fudge, caramels, butterscotch, milk chocolate.
Beverages Soya milks, e.g. Granogen, Granose Soya Milk, Plamil, Itona Soya Bean Milk. Tea, coffee, cocoa. *Certain brands* of 'drinking' chocolate, Bovril, Marmite. Squashes and cordials, fizzy drinks, wines, spirits, beers, etc.	Malted milks, e.g. Bournvita, Horlicks, Ovaltine.
Soups, sauces, gravies and salad cream Home-made using milk-free ingredients. *Certain brands* of convenience soups, sauces and gravies. *Certain brands* of mayonnaise and salad cream, seasonings. Salt, pepper, herbs, spices, vinegar, mustard.	Soups, sauces, gravies and salad cream containing milk products or milk derivatives. Monosodium glutamate with a lactose filler.
Miscellaneous Bicarbonate of soda, cream of tartar, tartaric acid, baking powder, fresh and dried yeast, colourings and essences, gelatine.	Tablets containing a lactose filler. Low calorie sweeteners containing lactose, e.g. Sweet 'n' Low, Canderel.

When the column of milk-free foods states 'certain brands' these should be sought in the 'Milk-free manufactured foods products list'. This list is available to dietitians at a small cost from the British Dietetic Association (but see p 615).

margarine and by using a milk substitute to replace milk. Since milk normally provides a major source of protein, energy, calcium, riboflavin and vitamin A in the diet of infants and young children, it is vitally important that a nutritionally complete milk substitute is given to those who are milk intolerant. Nutritionally complete milk substitutes are prescribable in cases of milk or lactose intolerance and galactosaemia. A list of prescribable milk substitutes can be found in the *Monthly Index of Medical Specialities* (MIMS) or the *British National Formulary* and those currently available (October 1987) are listed in Table 2.69. Casein hydrolysate milk (i.e. Nutramigen and Pregestimil) show virtually no antigenic cross-reactivity with cows' milk (McLaughlan *et al* 1981) and because of their low allergenic properties they are preferable to soya, goats' and sheep's milks, especially for children under one year. However, the choice of milk substitute will depend on the age of the patient, the range of foods included in the diet and the quantity consumed. Casein hydrolysate

Table 2.69 Milk substitutes available for children

Type of milk	Recommended dilution	Protein source	Fat source	Carbohydrate source	Comments
Hydrolysed casein milks					
Pregestimil* (Mead Johnson)	1 scoop + 1 oz water	Enzymatically hydrolysed casein (charcoal treated)	Corn oil MCT oil Lecithin	Glucose syrup solids Tapioca starch	Nutritionally adequate infant formula. Has added vitamins and minerals
Nutramigen* (Mead Johnson)	1 scoop + 1 oz water	Enzymatically hydrolysed casein (charcoal treated)	Corn oil	Glucose polymers Tapioca starch	Nutritionally adequate infant formula. Has added vitamins and minerals.
Soya milks					
Formula S* (Cow and Gate)	1 scoop + 1 oz water	Soya protein isolate + L-methionine	Palm oil Coconut oil Maize oil Safflower oil	Glucose syrup	Nutritionally adequate infant formula. Has added vitamins and minerals
Prosobee powder* (Mead Johnson)	1 scoop + 1 oz water	Soya protein isolate + L-methionine	Coconut oil Corn oil	Glucose syrup	Nutritionally adequate infant formula. Has added vitamins and minerals
Prosobee liquid* (Mead Johnson)	50% solution	Soya protein isolate + L-methionine	Soya oil Coconut oil	Glucose syrup	
Wysoy* (Wyeth)	1 scoop + 1 oz water	Soya protein isolate + L-methionine	Oleo oil (destearinated beef fat) Oleic oil Soya oil Coconut oil	Sucrose Corn syrup solids	Nutritionally adequate infant formula. Has added vitamins and minerals
Isomil* (Abbott)	1 scoop + 1 oz water	Soya protein isolate + L-methionine	Corn oil Coconut oil	Sucrose Corn syrup solids	Nutritionally adequate infant formula. Has added vitamins and minerals
Miscellaneous					
Pepdite 0–2 (SHS) Pepdite 0–2 MCT (SHS)	15% solution	Hydrolysed meat and soya. Peptides and amino acids	Vegetable and animal fats Vegetable oils + MCT oil	Maltodextrin	Nutritionally adequate infant formula. Has added vitamins and minerals
Comminuted chicken* (Cow and Gate)	See data sheet or p 200	Finely ground chicken meat dispersed in water	Chicken fat	None	This is only a source of protein and fat. It needs diluting with an additional fat source, carbohydrate, vitamins and minerals. Refer to data sheet for use
Other animal milks					
Goats milk	—	Goats' milk protein		Lactose	This is high in protein and minerals and low in carbohydrate, vitamins A, D, C, folic acid and B12. It should be boiled before use
Sheep milk	—	Sheep's milk protein		Lactose	This milk is high in protein, fat, energy and minerals. It is low in carbohydrate. It should not be used for infants under one year

*May currently (1986) be prescribed in the UK (ACBS) for cows' milk intolerance on a FP 10 prescription.

milks, for example, have a strong taste and smell and may be unacceptable to a young child drinking from an open feeding cup. Nutritionally adequate soya protein-isolate formuale such as Formula S, Wysoy, Isomil and Prosobee may be more agreeable to a child over the age of one year. Many other available soya preparations, containing soya and sugar only, are nutritionally incomplete and therefore unsuitable for infants and young children.

If a child refuses to drink a milk substitute, a daily calcium supplement should be prescribed to supply approximately 300−400 mg of elemental calcium (e.g. Sandocal, 1 tablet = 400 mg elemental calcium or Calcium Sandoz, 15 ml = 325 mg elemental calcium). It may also be necessary to recommend an appropriate vitamin supplement.

Nutritionally incomplete milk replacements are available from health food shops and some supermarkets. These do not provide the same nutrients as cows' milk and should never be regarded as an adequate nutritional substitute. Such 'social' milk replacements may be a useful adjunct to the diet of older children and adults.

2.11.5 Low allergen foods

The use of low allergen foods and diets is discussed in detail in Section 5.9 (Food allergy and food intolerance).

There still is considerable disagreement as to what constitutes a 'low allergenic' diet and consequently considerable variation in the advice given. The most common food allergens are thought to be: milk; eggs; wheat; some meats (especially pork); some fish (especially shellfish); some vegetables (including legumes, mushrooms, cucumber and brassicas); some fruit (including citrus fruits); soya; azo dyes; and some preservatives.

The following foods are usually considered to have a *low allergenic potential*: Lamb, rabbit; *rice, sago, arrowroot, buckwheat, carrots, *potatoes (fresh, not powdered), pears, rhubarb, *apricots, *peaches, Tomor margarine, Vitaquel margarine, olive oil, bottled 'spring waters', soda water, *tap water, *sugar, *golden syrup, sea salt, herbal teas.

*Indicates that some authorities exclude this item. This usually will depend on what condition a food intolerance is suspected of causing.

Reference

McLaughlan P, Anderson KJ and Coombs RRA (1981) An oral screening procedure to determine the sensitizing capacity of infant feeding formulae. *Clin Allergy* **11**, 311−8.

2.12 Proprietary Energy and Nutrient Supplements

Tables 2.70–2.82 give the current (1986) composition of the following proprietary energy and nutrient supplements

1 Table 2.70. Products containing carbohydrate.

2 Table 2.71. Products containing fat or fat and carbohydrate.

3 Table 2.72. Products containing protein, with or without fat, carbohydrate, vitamins and minerals.

4 Table 2.73. Amino acid supplements.

5 Table 2.74. Multivitamin supplements.

6 Table 2.75. Single vitamin preparations.

7 Table 2.76. Mixed mineral supplements.

8 Table 2.77. Iron preparations.

9 Table 2.78. Potassium, sodium, calcium, phosphorus and zinc supplements.

10 Table 2.79. Vitamins with minerals for general use.

11 Table 2.80. Over-the-counter vitamin and mineral preparations.

12 Table 2.81. Substances used in vitamin preparations.

13 Table 2.82. Some mineral salts used in pharmaceutical preparations.

These tables indicate whether or not a specific product is currently prescribable. Prescriptions should be marked 'ACBS' (Advisory Committee for Borderline Substances). Up-to-date information regarding their prescribability and composition can be found in the *Monthly Index of Medical Specialities (MIMS)* or the *British National Formulary*.

Details of the following proprietary products can be found elsewhere in the Manual:

1 Enteral feeds (Section 1.12) Whole protein preparations (p 77); Peptide preparations (p 77) and Elemental preparations (p 77).

2 Parenteral regimens (Section 1.13) Amino acid solutions (p 87); Vitamin sources (p 89) and Electrolyte and trace element sources (p 89).

3 Milk substitutes (Section 2.11) Hydrolysed casein milks (p 195) and Soya milks (p 195).

4 Proprietary low protein foods (Section 2.2) (p 121).

5 Proprietary gluten-free foods (Section 2.11) Gluten-free foods (p 190); Gluten-free, soya free foods (p 191) and gluten-free, low lactose foods (p 192).

The tables of vitamin and mineral preparations have been compiled from *MIMS* (February 1986) and *The Extra Pharmacopoeia* (Martindale 1982).

Tables 2.74–2.79 list preparations that are primarily intended for supply against prescriptions written by medical practitioners. Table 2.80 lists proprietary medicines licensed in Great Britain (excluding herbal preparations) and advertised for over the counter sale to the public. No sharp distinction can be drawn between preparations in Tables 2.74–2.79 and those in Table 2.80, since some of those in Tables 2.74–2.79 may be lawfully supplied to the public without prescription.

A number of differing forms of vitamins are available for inclusion in pharmaceutical products. These are listed in Table 2.81. In Tables 2.74, 2.75 and 2.79, the vitamins are described as fully as in the publications consulted. However, in Table 2.80 generic alphabetic names have been used, since the precise form of the vitamin used is frequently not specified. Martindale states 'the contents of those preparations are as described by the manufacturers'.

Information on mineral preparations is given sometimes in terms of the mineral of interest e.g. zinc, and sometimes in terms of the whole salt/compound, e.g. zinc sulphate. A list of mineral salts used in pharmaceutical preparations, their chemical formulae and molecular weight is given in Table 2.82 to enable appropriate calculations.

Vitamin and mineral preparations designed specifically for parenteral nutrition are excluded from the Tables. They can be found in Section 1.13 (p 89).

Product (manufacturer)	Description	Protein (g)	Fat (g)	CHO (g)	Energy (kJ)	Energy (kcal)	Sodium (mg)	Sodium (mmol)	Potassium (mg)	Potassium (mmol)	Intended use	Prescribable for
Calonutrin (Geistlich)	Polysaccharides, maltose, glucose. Unflavoured powder	Nil	Nil	108.0	1720	410	<92.0	<4.0	<12.0	<0.3	To increase oral energy consumption by adding to foods, drinks and tube feeding regimens	Amino acid abnormalities, disaccharide intolerances (without isomaltase intolerance), high energy, low fluid diets; hypoglycaemia; liver cirrhosis; protein intolerances; renal failure
Caloreen (Cassenne)	Low osmolar glucose polymer. Unflavoured powder	Nil	Nil	96.0	1674	400	<41.0	<1.8	<12.0	<0.3		
Polycal (Cow and Gate)	Low osmolar glucose polymer. Unflavoured powder	Nil	Nil	94.5	1610	380	50.0	2.2	50.0	1.3		
Maxijul (SHS)	Low osmolar glucose polymer. Unflavoured powder	Nil	Nil	96.0	1536	360	46.0	2.0	4.0	0.1		As for Calonutrin plus malabsorptive states
Polycose (Abbott)	Low osmolar glucose polymer. Unflavoured powder	Nil	Nil	94.0	1596	380	110.0	4.8	10.0	0.3		Not prescribable
Liquid Maxijul (SHS)	Glucose polymers. Natural and three flavours	Nil	Nil	50.0	800	188	<23.0	<1.0	<4.0	<0.1		Not prescribable
Maxijul LE (SHS)	Low osmolar, low electrolyte glucose polymer. Unflavoured powder	Nil	Nil	96.0	1536	360	0.23	0.1	0.4	0.01	Energy supplement, very low electrolyte diets	As for Maxijul plus high energy, low fluid, low electrolyte diets
Fortical (Cow and Gate)	Low osmolar, low electrolyte glucose polymer liquid. Neutral and five flavours	Nil	Nil	61.5	1045	246	7.0	<0.3	1.0	0.03	Energy supplement, low electrolyte, low fluid diets	High energy, low fluid, low electrolyte diets; liver cirrhosis; renal failure
Hycal (Beechams)	Low osmolar, low electrolyte glucose polymer liquid. Natural and four flavours.	Nil	Nil	49.5	845	198	13.8	0.6	0.6	0.02		As for Fortical

*All products are lactose-free.

Table 2.71 Products containing fat or fat and carbohydrate.* Composition per 100 g or 100 ml product

Product (manufacturer)	Description	Protein (g)	Fat (g)	CHO (g)	Energy (kJ)	Energy (kcal)	Sodium (mg)	Sodium (mmol)	Potassium (mg)	Potassium (mmol)	Intended use	Prescribable for
Calogen (SHS)	Peanut oil/water emulsion	Nil	50.0 (56%C18:1 26%C18:2)	Nil	1880	450	21.0	0.9	19.5	0.5	As an energy source in low protein diets, with or without electrolyte restriction; inborn errors of amino acid metabolism; carbohydrate intolerance tube feeds and ketogenic diets	Amino acid abnormalities; ketogenic diets in epilepsy; high energy, low fluid, low electrolyte diets; renal failure
MCT oil (Mead Johnson)	Fractionated coconut oil containing medium chain triglycerides	Nil	93.0 (Approx 70%C8:0 25%C10:0)	Nil	3250	775	—	—	—	—	Energy source in malabsorptive states; ketogenic diets	Ketogenic diets in epilepsy; hyperlipoproteinaemia (Type I); intestinal lymphangectasia; liver cirrhosis; steatorrhoea (associated with cystic fibrosis); intestinal surgery
MCT oil (Cow and Gate)	Fractionated coconut oil containing medium chain triglycerides	Nil	100 g (Approx 56% C8:0 40% C10:0)	Nil	3469	830	—	—	—	—	As MCT oil	
Alembicol D (Alembic)	Coconut oil (MCT)	Nil	100.0 (50–60%C8:0 35–40%C10:0)	Nil	3500	837	—	—	—	—	As MCT oil	As MCT oil (not hyperlipoproteinaemia, Type I)
Liquigen (SHS)	Coconut oil (MCT)/water emulsion	Nil	50:0 (81%C8:0 16%C10:0)	Nil	1700	400	39.0	1.7	27.0	0.7	As MCT oil	As MCT oil and malabsorptive states
Duocal (SHS)	Mixture of glucose polymers, peanut oil and coconut oil. Powder	Nil	22.3 (34% MCT)	72.7	1960	470	28.0	1.22	3.5	0.09	Increase energy	Renal failure; liver cirrhosis; disaccharide intolerance; amino acid metabolism disorders and/or whole protein intolerance. Malabsorption states and other conditions requiring a high energy, low fluid intake
Duocal liquid (SHS)	Mixture of glucose polymers, peanut oil and coconut oil. 50% solution	Nil	7.1	23.4	627	150	20.0	0.9	30.0	0.8	As Duocal	As Duocal
MCT Duocal (SHS)	Glucose polymers and coconut oil. Powder	Nil	23.2 (83%C8:0 + C10:0 12%C18:2)	74.0	1960	470	175.0	7.6	6.0	0.15	Energy source in malabsorptive states	Not prescribable

*All products are lactose-free.

Table 2.72 Products containing protein, with or without fat, carbohydrate, vitamins and minerals. Composition per 100 g or 100 ml product

Product (manufacturer)	Description	Protein (g)	Fat (g)	CHO (g)	Lactose (g)	Energy (kJ)	Energy (kcal)	Sodium (mg)	Sodium (mmol)	Potassium (mg)	Potassium (mmol)	Intended use	Prescribable for	Notes
Build-Up (Carnation)	Skimmed milk powder with a complete range of vitamins and minerals added. Six flavours	22.4	0.5¹	67.0¹	36.0	1442	345	350	15.0	950¹	24.0¹	Meal supplement when reconstituted with milk	Not prescribable	¹Chocolate flavour — 2.65 g fat, 62.0 g CHO, 1010 mg (26.0 mmol) potassium
Casilan (Farley)	Calcium caseinate powder	90.0	1.8	<0.5	<0.5	1600	376	7.0	0.3	7.0	0.2	Hyperproteinaemia; hypercatabolic states; nephrotic syndrome. Oral and nasogastric feeding	Hypoproteinaemia	
Comminuted chicken meat (Cow and Gate)	Suspension of chicken meat and water	7.5*	3.0*	Nil	Nil	239*	57*	10*	0.4*	50*	1.3*	As a source of protein in infants who are intolerant to milk	Cows' milk protein or glucose, galactose or lactose intolerance	Figures for protein, fat and energy are approximate
Complan (Farley)	Skimmed milk powder, maltodextrins and hydrolysed vegetable fat with a complete range of vitamins and minerals added. Natural + four flavours	20.0²	16.0	55.0²	28.0²	1870²	444²	340²	15.0²	850²	22.0²	Total oral fluid feed (not savoury), tube feeding (natural only). Meal supplement	Not prescribable	²Savoury varieties — 22.5 g protein, 51.0 g CHO, 7.0 g lactose, 1830 kJ (436 kcal) 2000 mg (87.0 mmol) sodium, 620 mg (16.0 mmol) potassium
Forcival protein (Unigreg)	Calcium caseinate powder with added vitamins and minerals	55.0	<1.0	30.0	30.0	1530	366	<120	<5.2	50	1.3	Supplement for protein, vitamin and mineral deficiencies	Not prescribable	
Fortify (Cow and Gate)	Skimmed milk powder	18.8	18.3	57.3	<0.1	1914	455	375	16.3	630	16.2	Meal supplement	Not prescribable	Flavours: savoury — chicken, tomato vegetable; sweet — banana, strawberry, chocolate, natural
Fortimel (Cow and Gate)	Protein-enriched modified skimmed milk drink with sucrose, corn oil, vitamins and minerals. Four flavours	9.7	2.1	10.4	4.4	420	100	50.0	2.2	200	5.1	Meal supplement	As for Fortisip	
Fortisip (Cow and Gate)	Sodium caseinate maltodextrin, oils, vitamins and minerals	Standard 4.0 / Energy plus 5.0	4.0 / 6.5	12.0 / 17.9	<0.025 / <0.025	420 / 630	100 / 150	80 / 80	3.5 / 3.5	150 / 150	3.8 / 3.8	Meal supplement / Meal supplement	Short bowel syndrome; intractable malabsorption; inflammatory bowel syndrome; preoperatively with undernourished patient; total gastrectomy; dysphagia, bowel fistulae and anorexia nervosa	³Minerals (see below)
Liquisorb (Merck)	Skimmed milk protein, casein, soya oil, mono-, di-, oligo- and polysaccharides	4.0	4.0	11.8	Tr	420	100	103	4.5³	176	4.5³	Complete diet or supplement pre- and postoperatively	Short bowel syndrome, intractable malabsorption, pre-operative undernourished patients, total gastrectomy, dysphagia, bowel fistulae, anorexia nervosa	
Maxipro HBV (SHS)	Supplemented whey protein powder	88.0	4.0	Tr	Tr	1640	390	230.0	10.0	450	11.5	Hypoproteinaemia, as a supplement in short bowel syndrome and related conditions requiring tube feeds and minimal oral nutrition.		
Maxisorb (SHS)	Soya and milk protein-based soups and desserts	Soups 40.0 / Desserts 40.0	1.3 / 20.0	43.0 / 30.0	? / ?	1400 / 1880	333 / 450	2000.0 / 138.0	87.0 / 6.0	550 / 529	14.0 / 13.7	High protein supplement for those with a poor appetite	Not prescribable	Figures represent typical composition. Soups — vegetable and chicken; desserts — vanilla, strawberry and chocolate flavours
Nutribisk (Oxford Nutrition)	Biscuit containing wheat flour, soya oil, skimmed milk powder and sucrose	9.4	29.7	52.6	?	2092	500	117	5.0	—	—	High energy supplement	Not prescribable	
Promod (Abbott)	Whey protein powder	75.8	9.1	10.2	<6.0	1788	426	198	8.6	987	25.3	Protein supplement	Not prescribable	
Protifar (Cow and Gate)	Skimmed milk powder	88.5	1.6	0.5	0	1575	370	30	1.3	50	1.3	Increased protein requirement, compensation for negative nitrogen balance. Protein supplement	Biochemically proven hypoproteinaemia	
Vitadrink (Oxford Nutrition)	Soya protein drink with maltodextrin, sucrose, sunflower oil, vitamins and minerals. three flavours	3.9	2.9	12.0	Nil	385	92	50.0	2.2	150	3.8	Supplement for lactose intolerance; milk protein intolerance/allergy	Not prescribable	

³Minerals:

	Na mg	Na mmol	K mg	K mmol
Chocolate	115	5	235	6
Banana	115	5	72	1.8

*Average figures

Table 2.73 Amino acid supplements. Composition per 100 g product

Product (manufacturer)	Description	Amino acids (g)	Fat (g)	CHO (g)	Energy (kJ)	Energy (kcal)	Sodium (mg)	Sodium (mmol)	Potassium (mg)	Potassium (mmol)	Intended use	Prescribable for
Albumaid complete (SHS)	Mixture of amino acids with vitamins and trace elements	89.4	0	0	1246	298	800	34.8	160	4.1	Malabsorption states	Malabsorption states with failure to hydrolyse or absorb protein
Amin-Aid (Boots)	Mixture of essential amino acids, maltodextrins sucrose and soyabean oil. Powder, four flavours.	4.5	10.7	85.4	1885	457	<115	<5	Neg	Neg	Chronic renal failure	Not prescribable
Dialamine (SHS)	Mixture of essential amino acids, maltodextrins and sucrose with some trace elements, minerals and vitamin C. Orange flavoured powder.	30.0	Nil	62.0	1500	360	168	7.3	9.2	0.2	Hypoproteinaemia; chronic renal failure	Renal failure; hypoproteinaenia; wound leakage with protein loss; controlled nitrogen intake
Hepatamine (SHS)	Mixture of amino acids, maltodextrins and sucrose. Reduced aromatic amino acids and methionine, raised branched chain amino acids (BCAA) and arginine. Yellow, flavoured powder.	30.0 (40% BCAA)	Nil	65.0	1443	345	138	6.0	24.0	0.6	Hepatic failure	Not prescribable
Hepatic-Aid (Boots)	Mixture of amino acids, aspartame maltodextrin, sucrose and hydrogenated soya bean oil. Reduced aromatic amino acids (no phenylalanine) and methionine, raised BCAA	11.5 (46% BCAA)	9.8	77.9	1835	444	<115	<5.0	Neg	Neg	Hepatic failure	Not prescribable

Table 2.74 Multivitamin supplements

(Compiled from MIMS, February 1986)

	Abidec (Warner-Lambert)	Allbee with C (Robins)	BC 500 (Ayerst)	Becozyme (Roche)	Becozyme Forte (Roche)	Benerva compound (Roche)	Bravit (Galen)	Ce-cobalin (Paines and Byrne)	Concavit capsules (Wallace)	Concavit Drops	Concavit syrup	Dalivit drops (Paines and Byrne)	Dayovite [effervescent] (Cox)	Forceval capsules (Unigreg)	Forceval Junior	Gevral (Lederle)
Dosing unit	per 0.6 ml	per capsule	per capsule	per tablet	per tablet or 5 ml	per tablet	per tablet	per tablet	per ml	per capsule	per ml	per 5 ml	per 0.6 ml	per 4 g sachet		
		X	X	X	G	X	G	X	X	X	X		X	X	X	X
Vitamin A (i.u.)	4000	4000							5000	10 000	5000	5000				
Vitamin D (i.u.) Ergocalciferol (D$_2$)	400	400							500	1000	500	400				
Vitamin E (i.u.) Tocopheryl acetate (mg)									2							
Vitamin K Acetomenaphthone (mg)																
Ascorbic acid (mg)	50	25	300				100	2	40	100	50	50	500			
Na ascorbate (mg)				500												
Thiamin hydrochloride (mg)	1	1					1	25								
Thiamin mononitrate (mg)			15	25												
Thiamin (mg)					5	15			2.5	4	2	1	25			
Riboflavin (mg)	0.4	1	10	12.5	2	15	1	5	2.5	2	1	0.4	12.5			
Riboflavin sodium phosphate (mg)																
Pyridoxine hydrochloride (mg)	0.5	0.5	5	10				5					10			
Pyridoxine (mg)					2	10			1	2	1	0.5				
Nicotinamide (mg)	5	10	50	100	20	50	15	200	20	25	12.5	5	20			
Nicotinic acid (mg)																
Pantothenic acid																
Ca pantothenate (mg)			10	20					5	4	2		20			
Pantothenyl alcohol (mg)																
Cyancobalamin (μg)				5				6	5	10	5		5			

GENERAL DIETETIC PRINCIPLES AND PRACTICE

Table 2.74 *contd.*

(Compiled from MIMS, February 1986)

	Halycitrol (LAB)	Hemoplex (Paines and Byrne)	Hepacon-B Forte (Consolidated)	Hepacon-Plex (Consolidated)	Juvel (Tablets and syrup) (Bencard)	Ketovite tablets	Ketovite liquid (Paines and Byrne)	Lance B + C (Kirby-Warrick)	Lederplex (Lederle)	Lipotriad (Lewis)	Multibionta (Merck)	Multivite (Duncan Flockhart)	Orovite (Bencard)	Orovite-7 (Bencard)	Pabrinex (Paines and Byrne)	Intravenous high potency (IVHP)	Intramuscular high potency (IMHP)	Intramuscular maintenance (IMM)
Dosing unit	per 5 ml	per 10 ml vial	per 2 ml ampoule	per 2 ml ampoule	per tablet or 6.25 ml	per tablet	per 5 ml	per tablet	per 5 ml	per capsule or 1.67 ml	per 10 ml ampoule	per tablet	per tablet or 12.5 ml syrup	per 5 g sachet	per pair ampoules			
	X	PX	PX	PX	X	P		X	X	X	P	X	X	X	P			
Vitamin A (i.u.)	4600				5000		2500				10 000	2500		2500				
Vitamin D (i.u.)	460						400											
Ergocalciferol/calciferol (D$_2$) (i.u.)					500							250		100				
Vitamin E (i.u.) / Tocopheryl acetate (mg)						5					5							
Vitamin K / Acetomenaphthone (mg)						0.5												
Ascorbic acid (mg) / Na ascorbate (mg)					50	16.6		100			500	12.5	100	60	500			
Thiamin HCl (mg)		100			2.5	1		50	2	0.33			50		250			
Thiamin mononitrate (mg)														1.4				
Thiamin (mg)			50	100							50	0.5						
Riboflavin (mg)		5		2	2.5	1		5	2	0.33	10		5		4			
Riboflavin sodium phosphate (mg)														1.7				
Pyridoxine HCl (mg)		25			2.5	0.33		5	0.2	0.33	15		5	2	50			
Pyridoxine (mg)				5														
Nicotinamide (mg) / Nicotinic acid (mg)		100		150	50	3.3		200	10	3.33	100		200	18	160			
Pantothenic acid (mg)										2								
Ca pantothenate (mg)				10		1.16												
Pantothenyl alcohol (mg)										0.33	25							
Cyancobalamin (μg)			15	8				12.5	5									
Hydroxocobalamin (μg)										1.66								
Folic acid (μg)			2500			250												
Choline chloride (mg)							150		20									
Choline bitartrate (mg)										233								
Inositol (mg)							50		10	111								
Biotin (mg)						0.17												
Pro-lintane hydrochloride (mg)																		
dl-Methionine (mg)										28					1000			
Dextrose (mg)																		
Liver extract			√	√						√								

Notes (right-hand columns):
- IMHP: As for IVHP but without 1000 mg dextrose and with 140 mg benzyl alcohol.
- IMM: As for IMHP but with 100 mg thiamin hydrochloride and 80 mg benzyl alcohol.

Table 2.74 *contd.*

(Compiled from MIMS, February 1986)

Dosing unit	Parentrovite (Bencard) Intravenous high potency (IVHP) Intramuscular high potency (IMHP) Intramuscular maintenance (IMM) per pair ampoules	Polyvite (Medo) per capsule	Surbex-T (Abbott) per tablet	Tonivitan (Medo) per capsule	Vi-Daylin (Abbott) per 5 ml syrup	Vitavel (Bencard) per 5 ml	Villescon (Boehringer) per tablet	Villescon liquid (Boehringer) per 5 ml
	P	PX	X	PX	X	X	PX	PX
Vitamin A (i.u.)		4500		4500	3000	500		
Vitamin D (i.u.)					400			
Ergocalciferol/calciferol (D_2) (i.u.)		440		600		200		
Vitamin E (i.u.)								
Tocopheryl acetate (mg)								
Vitamin K (Phytomenadione)								
Acetomenaphthone (mg)								
Ascorbic acid (mg)	500	30		15	50	10	50	
Na ascorbate (mg)			500					
Thiamin HCl (mg)	250	2.5		1	1.5			1.67
Thiamin mononitrate (mg)			15			0.3	5	
Thiamin (mg)								
Riboflavin (mg)	4	1.5	10		1.2	0.4	3	
Riboflavin sodium phosphate (mg)								1.36
Pyridoxine HCl (mg)	50	1.5	5		1		1.5	0.5
Pyridoxine (mg)								
Nicotinamide (mg)	160	15	100		10	4.5	15	5
Nicotinic acid (mg)				15				
Pantothenic acid (mg)								
Ca pantothenate (mg)		2						
Pantothenyl alcohol (mg)								
Cyancobalamin (μg)								
Folic acid (mg)								
Choline chloride (mg)								
Inositol (mg)								
Biotin (mg)								
Prolintane hydrochloride (mg)							10	2.5
dl-Methionine (mg)								
Dextrose (mg)	1000							
Yeast, dried (mg)					50			
Liver extract								

Notes (Parentrovite column): As IVHP but without 1000 mg dextrose and with 140 mg benzyl alcohol. As IMHP but with 100 mg thiamin HCl and 80 mg benzyl alcohol.

P = prescription only; X = not available on NHS; G = only generic equivalents available at NHS expense. FP10 prescriptions must be written in generic name.

Table 2.75 Single vitamin preparations. Compiled from MIMS, February 1986

Preparation (manufacturer)	Availability[†]	Vitamin	Dose
AT10 (Sterling Research Laboratories)		Dihydrotachysterol	0.25 mg per ml oily solution
Benerva (Roche)	G	Thiamin HCl	3, 10, 25, 50, 100 or 300 mg per tablet
Cobalin-H (Paines and Byrne)	PG	Hydroxocobalamin	1000 μg per 1 ml ampoule
Complement Continus (Napp)	X	Pyridoxine HCl	100 mg per tablet
Cytacon (Duncan Flockhart)	X	Cyancobalamin	50 μg per tablet, 35 μg per 5 ml
Cytamen (Duncan Flockhart)	PG	Cyancobalamin	250 or 1000 μg per 1 ml ampoule
Ephynal (Roche)		Tocopheryl acetate	3, 10, 50 or 200 mg per tablet
Hepacon-B$_{12}$ (Consolidated)	PX	Cyancobalamin	1000 μg per 1 ml ampoule
Lexpec (RP Drugs)	P	Folic acid	2500 μg per 5 ml
Neocytamen (Duncan Flockhart)	PG	Hydroxocobalamin	250 or 1000 μg per 1 ml ampoule
One-alpha (Leo)	P	Alfacalcidol (I α OHD$_3$)	0.25 or 1.0 μg per tablet
Redoxon (Roche)	G	Ascorbic acid	25, 50, 200, 500 or 1000 mg per tablet
Refolinon (Farmitalia C E)	P	Ca folinate	15 mg per tablet
Ro-A-Vit (Roche)	P	Vitamin A acetate	50 000 i.u. per tablet
Rocaltrol (Roche)	P	Calcitrol (1,25(OH)$_2$D$_3$)	0.25 or 0.5 μg per capsule
Sterogyl-15 (Roussel)	G	Ergocalciferol	600 000 i.u. per 1.5 ml
Tachyrol (Duphar)		Dihydrotachysterol	0.2 mg per tablet

(See also Table 2.79) Over the counter preparations include Boots effervesent vitamin C, Delrosa syrups, Boots vitamin E tablets, Effer-C, Hip-C, Redoxon, Sanatogen vitamin E. [†]See footnote Table 2.74.

Table 2.76 Composition of mixed mineral supplements (per 100 g)

Mineral	Metabolic Mineral Mix (SHS)	Calcium-free Mineral Mix (SHS)	Aminogran Mineral Mix (Allen and Hanbury)
Sodium (g)	3.96	9.73	4.0
(mmol)	172.2	423.0	170.0
Potassium (g)	8.3	20.4	8.3
(mmol)	212.3	522.0	210.0
Chloride (g)	1.8	—	—
(mmol)	50.8	—	—
Calcium (g)	8.2	—	8.1
(mmol)	204.6	—	200.0
Phosphorus (g)	5.96	14.64	6.0
(mmol)	192.4	473.0	190.0
Magnesium (g)	0.97	2.38	0.97
(mmol)	39.9	98.0	40.0
Iron (mg)	63.0	155.0	63.0
Zinc (mg)	48.0	118.0	48.0
Iodine (mg)	0.76	1.87	Tr
Manganese (mg)	5.7	14.0	4.0
Copper (mg)	13.0	32.0	13.0
Aluminium (μg)	20.0	50.0	Tr
Molybdeum (μg)	150.0	370.0	Tr
Chromium (μg)	—	—	—
Dose	1.5 g/kg/day (up to 5.5 kg), then 8 g/day	0.7 g/kg/day (up to 5.5 kg), then 4 g/day	1.5 g/kg/day (up to 5.5 kg), then 8 g/day

Table 2.77 Iron preparations. (Compiled from MIMS, February, 1986.)

Preparations (manufacturer — unit — availability):

- BC 500 with iron (Ayerst) — per tablet — X
- Feac (Robins) — per tablet — X
- Fe-Cap (MCP) — per capsule
- Fe-Cap C (MCP) — per capsule — X
- Fe-Cap Folic (MCP) — per capsule — P
- Fefol Spansule (SK and F) — per capsule — P
- Fefol Vit Spansule (SK and F) — per capsule — PX
- Fefol Z Spansule (SK and F) — per capsule — P
- Feospan Spansule (SK and F) — per capsule
- Feospan Z Spansule (SK and F) — per capsule
- Fergon (Winthrop) — per tablet
- Ferrocap (Consolidated) — per capsule
- Ferrocap F-350 (Consolidated) — per capsule — P
- Ferrocontin Continus (Napp) — per tablet
- Ferrocontin Folic Continus (Napp) — per tablet — P
- Ferrograd (Abbott) — per capsule — P
- Ferrograd C (Abbott) — per tablet — X
- Ferrograd Folic (Abbott) — per tablet — P
- Ferromyn (Calmic) — per tablet
- Ferromyn Elix (Calmic) — per 5 ml
- Ferromyn B (Calmic) — per tablet or 5 ml — XX
- Ferromyn B Elix (Calmic) — per tablet or 5 ml — XX
- Feraday (Duncan Flockhart) — per tablet
- Fersamal (Duncan Flockhart) — per tablet
- Fersamal syrup (Duncan Flockhart) — per 5 ml
- Fesovit Spansule (SK and F) — per capsule — X
- Fesovit Z Spansule (SK and F) — per capsule — X
- Folex-350 (Rybar) — per tablet — P
- Folicin (Paines and Byrne) — per tablet — P
- Galfer (Galen) — per capsule — P
- Galfer FA (Galen) — per capsule — P
- Galfervit (Galen) — per capsule — X
- Gastrovite (MCP) — per tablet — X

	BC 500	Feac	Fe-Cap	Fe-Cap C	Fe-Cap Folic	Fefol	Fefol Vit	Fefol Z	Feospan	Feospan Z	Fergon	Ferrocap	Ferrocap F-350	Ferrocontin	Ferrocontin Folic	Ferrograd	Ferrograd C	Ferrograd Folic	Ferromyn	Ferromyn Elix	Ferromyn B	Ferromyn B Elix	Feraday	Fersamal	Fersamal syrup	Fesovit	Fesovit Z	Folex-350	Folicin	Galfer	Galfer FA	Galfervit	Gastrovite
Ferrous sulphate (mg)						150	150	150	150	150						325	325	325								150	150	308	200				
Ferrous fumarate (mg)	200	150										330	330											✓	140					290	290	305	
Ferrous gluconate (mg)											300																						
Ferrous succinate (mg)																			100	106	106	–											
Ferrous glycine sulphate (mg)			565	565	450									✓	✓								✓										225
Iron dextran complex (mg)																																	
[Fe equivalent (mg)]			[100]	[100]		[47]	[47]	[47]	[47]	[47]	[35]	[110]	[110]	[100]	[100]	[105]	[105]	[105]	[37]	[37]	[37]	[37]	[100]	[65]	[45]	[47]	[47]	[100]	[60]	[100]	[100]		[40]
Thiamin mononitrate (mg)	25	7.5					2														1	1				2	2					2	
Riboflavin (mg)	12.5	5					2														1	1				2	2					2	
Nicotinamide (mg)	100	25					10														10	10				10	10					10	
Folic acid (μg)					350	500	500	500					350		500			350										350	2500		350		
Pyridoxine hydrochloride (mg)	10	2.5					1																			1	1						
Ascorbic acid (mg)		150		300			50																			50	50					56	
Sodium ascorbate (mg)	500																500																
Calcium pantothenate (mg)	20																															4	15
Calciferol (i.u.)																																	
Calcium gluconate (mg)																																	200
Zinc sulphate (monohydrate) (mg)								61.8		61.8																	61.8						
[Zn equivalent (mg)]								[22.5]		[22.5]																	[22.5]						
Copper sulphate (mg)																																2.5	
Manganese sulphate (mg)																																2.5	100

P = Prescription only. X = not available on NHS.

GENERAL DIETETIC PRINCIPLES AND PRACTICE

Table 2.77 *contd.*

	Givitol (Galen)	Imferon (Fisons)	Irofol C (Abbott)	Ironorm (Wallace)	Jelcofer (Astra)	Kelferon (MCP)	Kelloate (MCP)	Meterer (Sinclair)	Meterfolic (Sinclair)	Niferex (Tillots)	Niferex tablets (Tillots)	Niferex-150 (Tillots)	Plesmet (Napp)	Pregaday (Duncan Flockhart)	Pregnavite Forte F (Bencard)	Sidros (Arun)	Slow-Fe (Ciba)	Slow-Fe Folic (Ciba)	Sytron (Parke-Davis)
	per capsule	per ml (2, 5 and 20 ml ampoules)	per tablet	per ml (2 ml ampoule)	per ml (1 ml ampoule)	per tablet	per tablet	per tablet	per tablet	per 5 ml	per tablet	per capsule	per 10 ml	per tablet	per tablet	per tablet	per tablet	per tablet	
	PX	P	PX	P	P		P		P					P	PX	X	P	P	
Ferrous sulphate (mg)	305		325														160	160	
Ferrous fumarate (mg)														✓	84				
Ferrous gluconate (mg)																300			
Ferrous succinate (mg)						225	225												
Ferrous glycine sulphate (mg)													✓						
Iron dextran complex		✓		✓															
Iron sorbitol/citric acid complex					✓														
Polysaccharide iron complex										✓	✓	✓							
Sodium iron edetate								✓	✓										✓
[Fe equivalent (mg)]	[100]	[50]	[105]	[50]	[50]	[40]	[40]	[100]	[100]	[100]	[50]	[150]	[50]	[100]	[25.2]	[36]	[50]	[50]	[55]
Thiamin mononitrate (mg)	2																		
Thiamin hydrochloride (mg)															0.5				
Riboflavin (mg)	2														0.5				
Nicotinamide (mg)	10														5				
Folic acid (µg)	500		350				150		350					350	120			400	
Pyridoxine hydrochloride (mg)	4														0.33				
Ascorbic acid (mg)			500												13.3	30			
Sodium ascorbate (mg)	56																		
Calcium pantothenate (mg)																			
Vitamin A (i.u.)															1333				
Calciferol (i.u.)															133				
Calcium gluconate (mg)																			
Calcium phosphate (mg)															160				
Zinc sulphate monohydrate (mg) [Zn equivalent (mg)]																			
Copper sulphate (mg)																			
Manganese sulphate (mg)																			

P = Prescription only; X = not available on NHS.

Table 2.78 Potassium, sodium calcium phosphorus and zinc supplements. Compiled from MIMS, February 1986

	Dioralyte (Armour) per sachet	Kay-Cee-L (Geistlich) per ml	K-Contin (Napp) per tablet	Kloref (Cox) per tablet	Leo-K (Leo) per tablet	Micro-K (Merck) per capsule	Nu-K (Consolidated) per capsule	Rehidrat (Searle) per sachet	Sando-K (Sandoz) per tablet	Slow-K (Ciba) per tablet	Slow sodium (Ciba) per tablet	Calcimax (Wallace) per 5 ml	Chocovite (Medo) per tablet	Calcium Sandoz syrup (Sandoz) per 15 ml	Calcium Sandoz ampoules (Sandoz) per 10 ml ampoule P	Ossopan 800 (Labaz) per tablet	Phosphate Sandoz (Sandoz) per tablet	Sandocal (Sandoz) per tablet	Solvazinc (Thames) per tablet	Z-Span Spansules (Smith, Klein and French) per capsule
Sodium chloride (mg)	200							440			600									
Sodium bicarbonate (mg)	300							420									350 137 mg Na			
Sodium saccharin (mg)									22.5											
Docusate sodium (mg)									1											
Potassium chloride (mg)	300	75	600	140	600	600	600	380	600	600										
Potassium bicarbonate (mg)				455					400								315 176 mg K			
Glucose (g)	8.0							4.09												
Sucrose (g)								8.07												
Laevulose (mg)								70												
Citric acid (mg)								440												
Betaine hydrochloride (mg)				740																
Calcium glycine hydrochloride (mg)												76 mg Ca								
Calcium gluconate (mg)													500							
Calcium lactate gluconate (mg)																		400 mg Ca		
Calcium glubionate (g)														3.27	1.375					
Calcium galactogluconate (g)														2.17						
Hydroxyapatite compound (mg)																830				
Sodium acid phosphate (mg)																	1936			
Zinc sulphate (mg)																				61.8
Zinc sulphate monohydrate (mg)																			200	
Calciferol (i.u.)												400	15 µg							
Thiamin (mg)												0.5								
Riboflavin (mg)												0.125								
Pyridoxine (mg)												0.125								
Cyanocobalamin (µg)												0.125								
Ascorbic acid (mg)												5								
Nicotinamide (mg)												2								
Calcium pantothenate (mg)												0.125								

P = prescription only

Table 2.79 Vitamins with minerals for general use (excluding those designed for parenteral nutrition). (X = not available on NHS)

Gevral capsules (Lederle) per capsule	X	Forceval (Unigrig; Vestric) per capsule	X	Octovit (Smith, Klein & French) per tablet	X	Minamino compound (Consolidated Chemicals) per 100 ml syrup	X
Vit A acetate	5000 i.u.	Retinol	5000 i.u.	Vitamin A	2500 i.u.	Liver extract	70 g
Vitamin D	500 i.u.	Cholecalciferol	600 i.u.	Cholecalciferol	100 i.u.	Fresh spleen	15 g
Tocopheryl acetate	10 i.u.	Tocopheryl acetate	10 mg	Tocopheryl acetate	10 mg	Fresh gastrie mucosa	7 g
Cyanocobalamin	1 µg	Cyanocobalamin	2 µg	Cyanocobalamin	2 µg	Cyanocobalamin	100 µg
Nicotinamide	15 mg	Nicotinamide	20 mg	Nicotinamide	20 mg	Nicotinamide	400 mg
Pyridoxine HCl	0.5 mg	Pyridoxine HCl	0.5 mg	Pyridoxine	2 mg	Pyridoxine HCl	35 mg
Riboflavin	5 mg	Riboflavin	5 mg	Riboflavin	1.5 mg	Riboflavin	40 mg
Thiamin mononitrate	5 mg	Thiamin mononitrate	10 mg	Thiamin	1 mg	Thiamin HCl	300 mg
Ascorbic acid	50 mg	Ascorbic acid	50 mg	Ascorbic acid	30 mg		
Ca pantothenate	5 mg	Ca pantothenate	2 mg				
Inositol	50 mg	Inositol	60 mg				
Choline bitartrate	50 mg	Choline bitartrate	40 mg				
Ca [as Ca hyd. phos.]	145 mg	Ca	70 mg	Ca [as Ca. hyd. phos.]	100 mg		
Fe [as fumarate]	10 mg	Fe	10 mg	Fe [as sulphate]	10 mg	Ferric. am. citrate	410 mg
Cu [as oxide]	1 mg	Cu	0.5 mg			Cu sulphate	2.8 mg
P [as Ca hyd. phos.]	110 mg	P	55 mg				
Mg [as oxide]	1 mg	Mg	2 mg	Mg [as hydroxide]	10 mg		
K [as sulphate]	5 mg	K	3 mg				
Zn [as oxide]	0.5 mg	Zn	0.5 mg	Zn [as sulph. monols.]	5 mg		
I [as KI]	100 µg	I	100 µg				
Mn [as dioxide]	1 mg	Mn	0.5 mg			Mn sulphate	1.7 mg
L-lysine HCl	25 mg	L-lysine HCl	60 mg				

Metatone (Warren Lambert)
Tonivitan A (Medo)
Tonivitan B (Medo)
Verdiviton (Squibb)

Preparations of vitamins with glycerophosphates. The latter are alleged to have "tonic" effects but there is little evidence to support this claim.

Table 2.80 Over-the-counter vitamin and mineral preparations. Compiled from Martindale. The Extra Pharmacopoeia. 28th edn. The Pharmaceutical Press (1982)

Preparation	Dosage unit	Vitamin A (i.u./mg)	Vitamin B1 (mg)	Vitamin B2 (mg)	Vitamin B6 (mg)	Vitamin B12 (µg)	Nicotinamide (mg)	Pantothenate (mg)	Biotin (µg)	Folic acid (µg)	Vitamin C (mg)	Vitamin D (i.u./µg)	Vitamin E (i.u./mg)	Other ingredients
Alcovite (Booker Health)	Tablet		20		5						500			Cysteine 10 mg; Zn 2 mg (as amino acid chelate)
Aluzyme (Phillips Yeast)	Tablet		0.16	0.21			2.5			14				Plus other vitamins natural to brewer's yeast.
Aryton's IVY Tablets (Aryton, Saunders)	Tablet		0.17							4				Ferrous gluconate 98 mg; dried yeast 195 mg
Bemax (Beecham Foods)	Ounce		0.4	0.16	0.27		1.5						6.3 mg	Mn 3.6 mg; Fe 1.9 mg; Cu 0.18 mg; carbohydrate 10.1 g; protein 7.2 g
Biovital Liquid (Radiol)	20 ml		0.6	2.6	1.0	2	10.0				20			Fe 12 mg as sodium ferric citrate; Mn 60 µg as manganese citrate; alcohol 2.341 g.
Biovital Tablets (Radiol)	Tablet		0.6	0.6	1.0	2	10.0				20			Fe 32.5 mg; Mn 0.15 mg.
Boots Children's Vitamin Syrup (Boots)	5 ml	2500 i.u.	0.5	0.6			5				15	250 i.u.		
Boots Effervescent Vitamin C (Boots)	Tablet										1000			
Boots Iron Tonic Tablets (Boots)	Tablet		3											Ferrous fumarate 25 mg; dried yeast 300 mg.
Boots Vitamin and Iron Tonic (Boots)	Tablet		0.7	0.4			6							Ferrous gluconate 225 mg; calcium gluconate 200 mg manganese glycerophosphate 6 mg; caffeine 32 mg
Boots Vitamin Yeast Tablets (Boots)	Tablet		0.19	0.22			2.1							Yeast 300 mg
Boots Vitamin E Tablets (Boots)	Tablet												100 mg	
Box's Multivitamin Capsules	Capsule	5.5 mg	3.13	2.75	0.55	1.25	22	8.75		550	50	0.63 µg	2.2 mg	
Celaton CH3 Plus (Celaton)	Tablet	2 mg	0.6	0.6	0.7	1.0	6	2.5	1.0		25	5 µg	1.4 mg	Rutin 1 mg; methionine 1 mg; procaine hydrochloride 15 mg; ginseng powder 2 mg.
Celaton CH3 Strong and Calm Tablets (Celaton)	Tablet	0.5 mg	0.6	0.6	0.7	0.1	6	2.5	1.0		25	2.5 µg	10.5 mg	p-amino benzoic acid 7.5 mg; sucrose 141 mg; acacia 3 mg; methyl p-hydroxy benzoate 0.22 mg; Na propyl p-hydroxy benzoate 0.11 mg; povidone 6.25 mg
Celaton CH3 Tri-plus Tablets (Celaton)	Tablet	0.5 mg	0.6	0.6	0.7	2.5	6	2.5	1.0		25	2.5 µg	10.5 mg	p-amino benzoic acid 7.5 mg; ginseng 2 mg; heart powder 30 mg; brain powder 30 mg; intrinsic factor 20 mg
Citramins (Minnesota UK)	Tablet	750 µg									25	5 µg		
Crookes Multivitamins (Crookes Products, UK)	Tablet	5000 i.u.	2	2	1	2	20				50	400 i.u.		Fe 15 mg; Cu 0.75 mg
Delrosa syrups	Fluid ounce										110			Sucrose-free

Table 2.80 *contd.*

	Dosage unit	Vitamin A (i.u./mg)	Vitamin B1 (mg)	Vitamin B2 (mg)	Vitamin B6 (mg)	Vitamin B12 (µg)	Nicotinamide (mg)	Pantothenate (mg)	Biotin (µg)	Folic acid (µg)	Vitamin C (mg)	Vitamin D (i.u./µg)	Vitamin E (i.u./mg)	
Efavite (Britannia Health)	Tablet				25		7.5				125			Zn sulphate 25 mg
Effer-C (Cox)	Tablet										1000			(Effervescent)
Emlab Brewer's Yeast Tables (Minnesota)	Tablet													Dried yeast 300 mg
Emlab Iron and Brewer's Yeast Tablets (Minnesota)	Tablet													Ferrous fumarate 15 mg; dried yeast 300 mg
Gamma Formula (Booker Health)	Capsule													Evening primrose oil
GEB6 (Booker Health)					50								400 i.u.	Ginseng root 400 mg
H3 Plus (Eucomark)	Capsule	2850 i.u.	5	5	0.5	0.5	12	3	0.5	25	40	250 i.u.	10 i.u.	Choline dihydrogen citrate 42 mg; inositol 30 mg; *p*-amino benzoic acid 25 mg; lysine 24 mg; Fe 10 mg; I 150 µg; Ca 46.5 mg; P 37 mg; Cu 1 mg; Mn 1 mg; K 5 mg; Zn 0.5 mg; Mg 1 mg
Haliborange Tablets (Farley)	Tablet	2500 i.u.									25	200 i.u.		
Hip-C (Paines and Byrne)	1 ml										3			Rose-hip syrup
Iron Jelloids (Beecham Proprietaries)	Tablet		0.17	0.29			1.67				4.17			Ferrous sulphate 65 mg; Cu carbonate 170 µg; dried yeast 138 mg
Ironplan (Menley and James)	Tablet		3											Ferrous sulphate 150 mg (sustained release)
Ladybird (Booker Health)	Capsule			5	20	5				25	200			Zn 4 mg (as amino acid chelate)
Maw's Orange Halibut Tablets (Ashe)	Tablet	2500 i.u.									25	250 i.u.		
Multone Iron Vitamin Tonic (Cupal)	Tablet		0.5	0.3			3				5			Ferrous gluconate 150 mg
Neovita Capsules (Savoy Laboratories)	Capsule	2400 i.u.	2.5	2.5	1	4.9	20	10		40		240 i.u.	2 mg	Ginseng 100 mg; lecithin 9.5 mg; Ca phosphate 100 mg; Mg oxide 10 mg; Cu sulphate 2 mg; Zn oxide 5 mg; Mn sulphate 2 mg; ferrous sulphate 33 mg
Omega-H3 (Vitabiotics)	Capsule	2000 i.u.	15	3	1	20	15	3	3	500	60	200 i.u.	25 mg	Choline 100 mg; inositol 100 mg; *p*-amino benzoic acid 50 mg; wheat germ oil 100 mg; lecithin 20 mg; rutin 10 mg; Fe sulphate 13.25 mg; Fe fumarate 32 mg; Ca hydrogen phosphate 180 mg; Mg sulphate 3.32 mg; Zn oxide 1.26 mg; Cu sulphate 2.84 mg; Mn sulphate 3.32 mg

Table 2.80 *contd.*

	Dosage unit	Vitamin A (i.u./mg)	Vitamin B1 (mg)	Vitamin B2 (mg)	Vitamin B6 (mg)	Vitamin B12 (μg)	Nicotinamide (mg)	Pantothenate (mg)	Biotin (mg)	Folic acid (μg)	Vitamin C (mg)	Vitamin D (i.u./mg)	Vitamin E (i.u./mg)	Other ingredients
One-a-day Tablets (Crookes Laboratories)	Tablet	5000 i.u.	2	2	1	2	20				50	400 i.u.		Fe carbonate 15 mg; Cu carbonate 0.75 μg
Orange and Halibut Vitamins (Kirby-Warrick)	Tablet	2500 i.u.									25	200 i.u.		
Pharmaton (Pharmagen)	Tablet	4000 i.u.	2	2	1	1	15	10			60	400 i.u.	10 mg	Choline ?; inositol ?; ginseng 200 mg; rutin 20 mg; Fe 10 mg; Ca 90.3 mg; P 70 mg; Fl 200 μg; Cu 1 mg; K 8 mg; Mn 1 mg; Mg 10 mg; Zn 1 mg linolenic acid; linoleic acid; di-methylamino ethanol bitartrate 26 mg
Phillips Iron Tonic (Phillips Yeast)	Tablet		0.16	0.3			2				10			Fe 20 mg as saccharated ferrous carbonate; dried yeast 170 mg
Phillips Tonic Yeast (Phillips Yeast)	Tablet		0.11	0.20	0.009		1.4	0.012						Plus other vitamins natural to brewer's yeast
Phyllosan (Beecham Proprietaries)	Tablet		0.166	0.333			8.5				5			Fe fumarate 35 mg
Plurivite M Tablets (Boots)	Tablet	5000 i.u.	2	2	1	2	20				50	400 i.u.		Fe 15 mg as ferrous carbonate; Cu 0.75 mg as copper carbonate
Plurivite Tablets (Boots)	Tablet	4000 i.u.	2	2	1	2	20	5			50	400 i.u.	5 mg	
Redelan Effervescent Tablets (Roche)	Tablet	5500 i.u.	1.2	1.8	1.6	1.4	15	13			75	400 i.u.	10 mg	
Redoxon (Roche)	Tablet										√			25, 50, 200, 500 or 1000 mg
Sanatogen High-C (Fisons)	Tablet			0.3							1020			Tartaric acid; adipic acid
Sanatogen Junior vitamins (Fisons)	Tablet	2500 i.u.									50	200 i.u.		
Sanatogen Multivitamins (Fisons)	Tablet	4000 i.u.	1.2	1.8			12				30	400 i.u.	2 mg	KI 130 μg
Sanatogen Multivitamins plus iron (Fisons)	Tablet	4000 i.u.	1.2	1.8			12				30	400 i.u.	0.5 mg	KI 130 μg; Fe fumarate 45.6 mg
Sanatogen Vitamin C tablets (Fisons)	Tablet										75			
Sanatogen Vitamin E tablets (Fisons)	Tablet												100 mg	
Scotts Cod liver oil capsules (Beecham Proprietaries)	Capsule	625 i.u.										62.5 i.u.		In 315 mg cod liver oil

Table **2.80** *contd.*

	Dosage unit	Vitamin A (i.u./mg)	Vitamin B1 (mg)	Vitamin B2 (mg)	Vitamin B6 (mg)	Vitamin B12 (µg)	Nicotinamide (mg)	Pantothenate (mg)	Biotin (µg)	Folic acid (µg)	Vitamin C (mg)	Vitamin D (i.u./mg)	Vitamin E (i.u./mg)	Other ingredients
Selenium-ACE (Christy)	Tablet	500 i.u.									100		50 i.u.	Selenium yeast 50 mg (Se 50 µg)
Seven Seas Capsules (British Cod Liver Oils)	Capsule	600 i.u.										60 i.u.	0.3 i.u.	
Seven Seas Orange Syrup (British Cod Liver Oils)	10 ml	4000 i.u.			0.7						35	400 i.u.	3 mg	Cod liver oil with concentrated orange juice and polyunsaturates
Smokers Supplement (Booker Health)	Tablet		20		5						500			Cysteine 10 mg
Super Plenamins (Minnesota)	Tablet	5000 i.u.	2.25	2.25	0.1	2	20				40	300 i.u.	2 mg	Ferrous sulphate 51 mg; Ca 75 mg; P 58 mg; Mg 10 mg; I 150 µg; Cu 750 µg; Mn 1.25 mg; K 3 mg; Zn 1 mg; vitamin B3 500 µg
Totavit Capsules (Cupal)	Capsule	5000 i.u.	1.5	1.2	0.5		10				30	400 i.u.	1 i.u.	Cu 0.1 mg (as copper sulphate); Fe 15 mg (as ferrous sulphate); Ca 24 mg; P 18.5 mg; DL-methionine 30 mg
Vitaplus Multivitamins (Farley)	Tablet	2500 i.u.	1.1	1.5	1.0	4	17			25	30	100 i.u.	5 mg	
Vitaplus Multivitamins with iron (Farley)	Tablet	2500 i.u.	1.1	1.5	1.0	4	17			25	30	100 i.u.	5 mg	Fe 15 mg (as ferrous fumarate)
Vitocee Tablets (Boots)	Tablet	750 µg									25	5 µg		
Vitrite Multivitamin Syrup (British Cod Liver Oils)	5 ml	2000 i.u.	0.7	0.85	0.35		9				17.5	200 i.u.	1.5 mg	
Vykmin E (Beecham Proprietaries)	Tablet	2000 i.u.	1.2	1.8	0.1	1.0	12	1.0			40	200 i.u.	100 mg	Mn 500 µg; K 3 mg; Zn 1 mg; I 150 µg; Mb 100 µg; Fe 15 mg; Ca phosphate 92.34 mg
Vykmin Fortified (Beecham Proprietaries)	Tablet	5000 i.u.	1.2	1.8	0.1	1.0	12	1.0			40	350 i.u.	2 mg	Fe sulphate 51 mg; K molybdate 340 µg; Mn sulphate 2.2 mg; K sulphate 6.68 mg; K iodide 200 µg; Zn sulphate 4.4 mg; Ca phosphate 92.34 mg
Wigglesworth Rapid Energy Release Tablets (Wigglesworth)	Tablet		1	1			5							Caffeine 50 mg
Wigglesworth Vitamin Tablets (Wigglesworth)	Tablet	4000 i.u.									25	550 i.u.		
Yeast-Vite (Beecham Proprietaries)	Tablet		0.167	0.167			1.5							Salicylamide 162 mg; caffeine 50 mg

Table 2.81 Substances used in vitamin preparations

Vitamin	Names	Formula	Molecular weight	Notes
Vitamin A	Vitamin A; retinol	$C_{20}H_{30}O$	286.5	Generally used in the form of esters
	Vitamin A acetate; retinyl acetate	$C_{22}H_{32}O_2$	328.5	1.15 g $\simeq$ 1 g retinol
	Vitamin A palmitate; retinyl palmitate	$C_{36}H_{60}O_2$	524.9	1.83 g $\simeq$ 1 g retinol
Vitamin B1	Thiamin hydrochloride	$C_{12}H_{17}ClN_4OS$ HCl	337.3	
	Thiamin mononitrate	$C_{12}H_{17}N_5O_4S$	327.4	
Vitamin B2	Riboflavin	$C_{17}H_{20}N_4O_6$	376.4	
	Riboflavin sodium phosphate	$C_{17}H_{20}N_4NaO_9P$ $2H_2O$	514.4	1.37 g $\simeq$ 1 g riboflavin
Vitamin B6	Pyridoxine hydrochloride	$C_8H_{11}NO_3$ HCl	205.6	
Vitamin B12	Cyanocobalamin	$C_{63}H_{88}CoN_{14}O_{14}P$	1355.4	
	Hydroxocobalamin	$C_{62}H_{89}CoN_{13}O_{15}P$	1346.4	
	Liver extracts			No longer recommended for routine treatment
Other vitamins of the B group	Biotin	$C_{10}H_{16}N_2O_3S$	244.3	
	Folic acid; folacin; pteroylglutamic acid	$C_{19}H_{19}N_7O_6$	441.4	
	Calcium folinate	$C_{20}H_{21}CaN_7O_7$ $5H_2O$	601.6	
	Nicotinic acid; niacin	$C_6H_5NO_2$	123.1	
	Nicotinamide; vitamin PP	$C_6H_6N_2O$	122.1	
	Pantothenic acid	$C_9H_{17}NO_5$	219.2	Usually used as the calcium salt
	Calcium pantothenate	$(C_9H_{16}NO_5)_2Ca$	476.5	
	Dexpanthenol; pantothenol; pantothenyl alcohol	$C_9H_{19}NO_4$	205.3	
	Aminobenzoic acid; p-amino benzoic acid (PABA)	$C_7H_7NO_2$	137.1	
	Choline	$C_5H_{15}NO_2$	121.2	Used as acid tartrate, acid citrate or chloride
	Choline bitartrate; choline acid tartrate	$C_9H_{19}NO_7$	253.3	
	Choline chloride	$C_5H_{14}ClNO$	139.6	
	Choline dihydrogen citrate; choline acid citrate	$C_{11}H_{21}NO_8$	295.3	
	Inositol	$C_6H_{12}O_6$	180.2	
	Dried yeast (Contains >0.1 mg thiamin hydrochloride, >0.3 mg nicotinic acid; >0.04 mg riboflavin, also pyridoxine, pantothenic acid, biotin, folic acid, vitamin B12, aminobenzoic acid and inositol per 1 g)			
Vitamin C	Ascorbic acid	$C_6H_8O_6$	176.1	
	Sodium ascorbate	$C_6H_7NaO_6$	198.1	
Vitamin D	Alfacalcidol; $1\alpha OHD_3$; 1α hydroxy cholecalciferol	$C_{27}H_{44}O_2$	400.6	
	Calcifediol; $25(OH)D_3$; 25 hydroxy cholecalciferol	$C_{27}H_{44}O_2$ H_2O	418.7	
	Calcitriol; $1\alpha,25(OH)_2D_3$; 1,25 dihydroxy cholecalciferol	$C_{27}H_{44}O_3$	416.6	
	Cholecalciferol; vitamin D_3	$C_{27}H_{44}O$	384.6	
	Dihydrotachysterol	$C_{28}H_{46}O$	398.7	
	Ergocalciferol; calciferol; vitamin D_2	$C_{28}H_{44}O$	396.7	
Vitamin E	d-alpha tocopherol	$C_{29}H_{50}O_2$	430.7	1 mg = 1.49 units
	dl-alpha tocopherol	$C_{29}H_{50}O_2$	430.7	1 mg = 1.1 unit
	d-alpha-tocopheryl acetate	$C_{31}H_{52}O_3$	472.8	1 mg = 1.36 units
	dl-alpha tocopheryl acetate	$C_{31}H_{52}O_3$	472.8	1 mg = 1 unit
	d-alpha tocopheryl acid succinate	$C_{33}H_{54}O_5$	530.8	
Vitamin K	Phytomenadione; vitamin K_1	$C_{13}H_{46}O_2$	450.7	Natural vitamin K
	Acetomenaphthone	$C_{15}H_{14}O_4$	258.3	
Vitamin P	The name given to a substance claimed to increase the resistance of the capillaries and reduce their permeability to red blood cells. All substances claimed to have vitamin P acitivity are flavone derivatives. They include hesperidin, rutin and troxerutin.			

Table 2.82 Some mineral salts used in pharmaceutical preparations

Salt	Formula	Molecular weight	Notes
Calcium glubionate	$(C_{12}H_{21}O_{12}, C_6H_{11}O_7)Ca\ H_2O$	610.5	
Calcium gluconate	$C_{12}H_{22}CaO_{14}\ H_2O$	448.4	1 g $\simeq$ 2.2 mmol (4.5 mEq) Ca
Calcium hydrogen phosphate	$CaHPO_4\ 2H_2O$	172.1	Ca 23%, P 18%
Copper sulphate	$CuSO_4, 5H_2O$	249.7	
Ferric ammonium citrate	Complex		About 21.5% Fe
Ferrous fumarate	$C_4H_2FeO_4$	169.9	About 32.5% Fe
Ferrous gluconate	$C_{12}H_{22}FeO_{14}\ 2H_2O$	482.2	About 70 mg Fe in 600 mg dihydrate
Ferrous glycine sulphate	Chelate		About 40 mg Fe in 225 mg
Ferrous succinate	$C_4H_4FeO_4$	171.9	34−36% Fe
Ferrous sulphate	$FeSO_4\ 7H_2O$	278.0	About 60 mg Fe in 300 mg
Ferrous sulphate, dried	80−90% $FeSO_4$		About 60 mg Fe in 200 mg
Iodide, potassium	KI	166.0	1 g = 6 mmol (6 mEq) I
Iron dextran injection			About 50 mg Fe per ml
Iron sorbitol citric acid	Complex		About 50 mg Fe per ml
Sodium ironedetate	$C_{10}H_{12}FeN_2NaO_8\ 2H_2O$	385.1	
Hydroxyapatite	$3Ca_3(PO_4)_2, Ca(OH)_2$	1004.6	Used in a proteinaceous base, 1 g = 176 mg Ca and 82 mg P
Glycerophosphates	of Ca, Mn, K and Na		Have been widely used as 'tonic' but there is little evidence to support this.
Manganese sulphate	$MnSO_4\ 4H_2O$	223.1	Use for their supposed effect in increasing the haematinic effect of iron in microcytic anaemia
Magnesium sulphate	$MgSO_4\ 7H_2O$	246.5	1 g $\simeq$ 4.1 mmol (8.1 mEq) Mg
Magnesium sulphate dried	62−70% $MgSO_4$		
Potassium bicarbonate	$KHCO_3$	100.1	1 g $\simeq$ 10 mmol (10 mEq) K
Potassium chloride	KCl	74.55	1 g $\simeq$ 13.4 mmol (13.4 mEq) K
Potassium citrate	$C_6H_5K_3O_7\ H_2O$	324.4	1 g $\simeq$ 9.25 mmol (9.25 mEq) K
Potassium sulphate	K_2SO_r	174.3	1 g $\simeq$ 11.5 mmol (11.5 mEq) K
Sodium bicarbonate	$NaHCO_3$	84.01	1 g = 11.9 mmol (11.9 mEq) Na
Sodium chloride	NaCl	58.44	1 g = 17.1 mmol (17.1 mEq) Na
Sodium acid phosphate	$NaH_2PO_4\ 2H_2O$	156.0	1 g = 6.4 mmol (6.4 mEq) Na; 6.4 mmol (6.4 mEq) PO_4; 198.5 mg P
Zinc sulphate	$ZnSO_4\ 7H_2O$	287.5	1 g = 3.5 mmol (7 mEq) Zn; about 50 mg Zn in 220 mg
Zinc sulphate monohydrate	$ZnSO_4\ H_2O$		

Atomic weights: Ca = 40.08; Cl = 35.45; Cu = 63.55; Fe = 55.85; I = 126.9; P = 30.97; Mn = 54.94; Mg = 24.30; K = 39.10; Na = 23.0; Zn = 65.38.

2.13 Diabetic Foods

2.13.1 History of usage

Foods made specially for people with diabetes have been available in the UK since the early 1950s. The use of such foods by diabetics has always been a source of concern to the majority of dietitians and medical advisors, but undoubtedly for many diabetics and their families their availability was perceived as helpful. Many parents of diabetic children who found it difficult to limit their child's intake of ordinary confectionery were delighted to find diabetic products available and made use of them. However, over the year the nutritional composition of these specialist products, and the groups purchasing and using them, became increasingly out of step with the dietary guidelines being given to diabetics. As a result, most dietetic departments were forced to urge the diabetic to avoid all diabetic products (with the exception of non-nutritive sweeteners and low calorie drinks). Despite these warnings, extensive use was still being made of 'diabetic' biscuits, cakes, boiled sweets and chocolate confectionery, as indicated by a study of 700 diabetics (Metcalfe 1981). This showed that over 80% of the sample who were regularly purchasing these products were meant to be on reduced energy diets as the main treatment of their diabetic condition. The majority of products they were selecting, while offering a saving in sugar and total carbohydrate content, were actually providing more energy and fat than the sucrose-containing product they were designed to replace. Furthermore, the majority of these patients did not have precise carbohydrate or energy allowances to follow and were taking these products in *addition* to the foods that they were eating as part of their main diet.

Careful comparison of all the products available in 1982–3 showed that over 70%, while offering savings in sugar and total carbohydrate content, had equal or greater energy densities than the products they were designed to replace. Therefore the use of such products could only be substantiated for lean diabetics on carbohydrate-restricted diets.

Increasingly, dietitians and physicians were recognizing that total energy intake could have a major influence on diabetic control and that carbohydrate restriction should be replaced by carbohydrate regulation, with an emphasis on fibre-rich diets. This further emphasized the unsuitability of the majority of 'diabetic' foods.

2.13.2 Recent changes in legislation governing the composition of diabetic foods

With the publication of the new Dietary Recommendations for the Diabetic (British Diabetic Association 1982), the time to challenge diabetic products was right. The British Diabetic Association first notified companies of a new and stricter code of advertising, which virtually eliminated half the products entitled to appear in their journal 'Balance'. This had a considerable impact on total sales, since many outlets would not consider stocking products which were not approved for advertising by the British Diabetic Association. While this measure was reasonably successful, a number of the larger companies refused to consider changing their products and, instead, moved their marketing strategies directly to the consumer

Table 2.83 Summary of legislation relating to diabetic claims. (Applies to products claiming suitability for diabetics.)

Nutritional criteria	Products must not contain more energy or fat than comparable non-diabetic products.
	Products must offer at least a 50% reduction in rapidly absorbable carbohydrate. [For the purposes of legislation, all sugar alcohols and fructose are defined as carbohydrates *but not* rapidly absorbable.)
	Products must not contain unnecessary amounts of mono or disaccharides (including fructose).
Labelling	A full nutritional statement must be given e.g. protein, fat, total available carbohydrate, the proportion of bulk sugar substitute and the remaining carbohydrate. This information must be given per 100 g of product and, where practicable, per item. There is no statutory requirement for fibre content to be included on the label but the British Diabetic Association encourages manufacturers to do this voluntarily.
	Products *not* offering a 50% saving in total energy must carry a clear warning 'Not suitable for the overweight diabetic'.
	Products containing a bulk sugar substitute must include a warning statement 'Best eat less than 25 g (name of substitute) a day'. Products containing a combination of sugar substitutes must say 'Best eat less than 25 g of a combination of (names of substitutes)'.

Table 2.84 Products making diabetic claims

Type of product	Nutrition composition	Suitable for the overweight?	Other claims	Comments
Beverages Cordials for dilution, soft drinks.	Virtually free of rapidly absorbable carbohydrate (CHO) and very low in energy	Yes	Slimming claim. Low energy claim, i.e. less than 40 kcal/100 ml	Ideal for the whole family. Sweetener usually saccharin and/or aspartame. Increasing trend towards reduced content of artificial colourings/flavourings
Alcoholic drinks e.g. Beer, lager, wine.	Low in rapidly absorbable CHO. No reduction in energy. May be higher in alcoholic strength than equivalent products*	Not usually and only as part of energy allowance	None	*Usually, the CHO content is reduced by conversion of residual glucose to alcohol. The alcoholic strength is therefore increased. Some 'lite' beers, etc. have slightly less carbohydrate, energy and alcohol
Dessert mixes	Low in sugar but still using simple starches (relatively rapidly absorbed) with bulking agents. Some are reduced in energy content but many contain similar amounts of energy to non-diabetic dessert mixes	Varies — only some are suitable	Reduced energy claim in some instances, e.g. 25% less energy. Very few contain 50% less energy	Need to be used with care. Products using fructose or sorbitol to replace starch should be avoided. Products reduced in sugar with sweetness provided by an intense sweetener may be suitable
Jellies	Some exclude all sugars and use an intense sweetener for sweetness. Many use sorbitol or fructose	Yes, if not using sorbitol or fructose	Slimming, low energy claim made when no sorbitol or fructose has been used	Ideal for the whole family if sugar and all bulk sweeteners are absent
Preserves	Available as specific diabetic formulations where energy savings range from 5%—50% with virtually no added sugar Alternatively, diabetics can use a reduced sugar formulation where a 50% or more saving in energy is made by use of a high fruit content. The remaining CHO is simple sugar from the fruit juice or added sugars	Varies — best to recommend reduced sugar formulations	Some make reduced energy claim	Best to advise the use of reduced sugar products for the whole family
Sauces, salad creams, etc.	Very few available now. Previous formulation replaced sugar with sorbitol or used fruit juice	Not usually	None	Better to use ordinary ones in small quantities. If overweight, products making a reduced energy claim should be selected (or better still, not used at all)
Biscuits	All have reduced sugar content, but some use bulk sweeteners and fat to replace the sugar. Not all are high in fibre. None contains over a 50% saving in energy	No — unless taken as part of daily energy allowance	None	Newer formulations use more high fibre ingredients and less fat, but older established products only offer less total CHO and are not recommended
Cakes	All have reduced sugar content but some use bulk sweeteners and fat to replace the sugar. Not all high in fibre. None over 50% energy saving	No — unless taken as part of daily energy allowance	None	Newer formulations use more high fibre ingredients and less fat. Older established products only offer less total CHO and are not recommended
Confectionery a) Pastilles	All have reduced sugar content. Most offer an energy saving, though not usually 50%	Yes, in moderation	None	Useful for occasional use. If taken with care unlikely to add significant energy to usual diet
b) Boiled sweets/mints	Low in sugar but use bulk sweeteners, therefore no energy saving	No	None	Not useful for the majority of patients. Risk of being used in excess, particularly by older patients
c) Chocolates/ chocolate assortments	Reduced sugar content but use sorbitol/ fructose, so virtually no energy saving. Previously manufactured products higher in fat and energy	No	None	Products offer a 50% saving in rapidly absorbed CHO so they are beneficial for occasional use. Risk of being used in excess. Warn patients against eating the whole product as this will easily exceed the 25 g/day limit of bulk sugar substitutes

through the national press and women's magazines, etc. As a result the British Diabetic Association brought pressure to bear at a legislative level and was successful in achieving much stricter legislation covering both nutritional content and labelling. The legislation (Statutory Instruments 1984, No 1305) came into force in September 1984.

The legislation is summarized in Table 2.83. Companies had until 1st July 1986 to comply with the legislation; after this date, all products which are on sale must conform.

2.13.3 Products currently available

Clearly, products now making diabetic claims will be offering compositional benefits when compared with ordinary sucrose-sweetened products. However, it is vital that both consumers and professionals recognize that, while there are benefits of a reduction in rapidly absorbable carbohydrate, the overall composition of 'diabetic' foods may not be markedly lower in carbohydrate or energy than their equivalent products and must therefore be used with care and as part of the diet. Patients must be made aware that even products not requiring the warning statement 'Not suitable for the overweight diabetic' may still provide significant amounts of carbohydrate and total energy.

Table 2.84 shows the type of products available and indicates their nutritional advantages, and any precautions which must be taken.

2.13.4 Likely future developments

There is growing recognition that the nutritional needs of diabetics are very similar to those of the general population, i.e. the dual goals of less fat and sugar and more fibre. This will mean that products adapted along these lines and intended for the general public may also be suitable for diabetic use but not necessarily labelled as diabetic products. This trend is to be encouraged. Careful liaison with manufacturers will lead to the availability of a wider range of products with the added benefits of fewer preservatives and colourings, exclusive use of polyunsaturated vegetable fats, more use of fibre-rich ingredients and fewer total simple sugars.

References

British Diabetic Association (1982) Dietary recommendations for diabetics for the 1980s. *Hum Nutr: Appl Nutr* **36A**, 378–94.
Metcalfe J (1981) Do you use diabetic foods? *Balance* (British Diabetic Association) October issue.

2.14 Artificial and Substitute Sweeteners

Alternative sweeteners, to be used either within the home or within industry to replace sugar, are of two types, namely
1 Intense non-nutritive sweeteners.
2 Bulk nutritive sweeteners.

Under legislation passed in 1983, a range of sweeteners in each category were confirmed to be permissible for use by the consumer and industry as a partial or total replacement for sugar in the diet.

2.14.1 Intense non-nutritive sweeteners

Under existing legislation in the UK there are four intense non-nutritive sweeteners permitted for use. They are
1 Saccharin
2 Aspartame
3 Acesulfame Potassium (Acesulfame K)
4 Thaumatin.

There are a number of new intense sweeteners currently undergoing extensive testing and it is likely that before 1990 at least one new product will receive a safety clearance.

Throughout Europe, legislation regarding sweeteners involves clearance for use in one or more of the following three categories
1 As a simple table top sweetener.
2 As a sweetening agent in beverages.
3 As a sweetening agent in any food, with the exception of baby foods.

In Britain, all four intense sweeteners have been permitted for all three categories.

The term 'intense non-nutritive sweetener' clearly indicates that the products themselves have a very pronounced sweetness, usually hundreds of times sweeter than sugar (sucrose). Hence the amounts used at any one time are very small, so they will not add appreciable amounts of carbohydrate, protein or total energy to the daily intake.

Saccharin

Saccharin is approximately 300 times sweeter than sucrose. It has been in use in the UK since the 1900s.

Concern regarding its safety arose in the 1970s, but pressure, both from consumers and manufacturers, led to its continued availability. Recently this decision has been validated, since a number of major long term studies have failed to identify any significant toxicological problems. As a result, saccharin is now once again securely established as a widely available, inexpensive, non-nutritive replacement for sugar, suitable for use in a range of applications. Its most notable use is as a table top sweetener and a sweetener in beverages, although a number of food items, particularly those created for the dietetic or diabetic market, do incorporate small quantities.

The current maximum Acceptable Daily Intake (ADI) is 2.5 mg/kg body weight.

Availability

Saccharin is widely available in tablet or liquid formulations (see Table 2.85) and in this form it provides very intense sweetness.

It can also be mixed with sugar, lactose or maltodextrin in which case some consideration must be made to the nutritional contribution of the mixer substance.

Advantages

1 Widely tested.
2 Inexpensive. Widescale production and use within industry has kept costs low. Saccharin, when used to establish the same level of sweetness as sucrose, costs aproximately a quarter of the price of table top sugar.
3 Soluble and stable in a wide range of applications. It can be used with success in beverages and chilled foods.

Disadvantages

1 Noticeable 'back-taste'.
2 Does not tolerate a high temperature. Exposure to heat will result in a pronounced bitter, metallic aftertaste. This limits its application in industry and within the home. It is usually necessary to add saccharin at the end of any cooking or baking process.

Aspartame

Aspartame was discovered in 1965 and it consists of two amino acids L-phenylalanine and L-aspartic acid which when combined together produce a substance of intense sweetness (approximately 200 times sweeter than sucrose).

Aspartame was first approved for use in the UK in 1983. Since its introduction, both consumers and industry have adopted it enthusiastically. It is available as a table top sweetener (currently under the name of Canderel) with formulations including tablets, sachets and more recently a volumetric sprinkle form where the aspartame has been combined with maltodextrin. Despite some technical limitations, aspartame is being used increasingly in the manufacturing industry as a sweetener, particularly in beverages (currently under the brand name 'NutraSweet').

Because of the presence of phenylalanine, this product is not suitable for those on low or controlled phenylalanine diets. Therefore all products which incorporate aspartame should have a warning to this effect on the packaging (however, this is not a statutory requirement).

Concern has been expressed regarding the safety of aspartame. However, repeated re-evaluation of the product by Safety Committees in both the USA and UK have not identified any proven side effects. Industry and the consumer continue to use the product in increasing amounts.

The current ADI maximum is 40 mg/kg body weight (EEC Scientific Committee on Foods 1985).

Availability

Currently available in tablet or powder formulations for use in the home and in a powder formulation for industry.

Advantages

1 A clean, sweet taste.
2 It can be used alone or, most effectively, in combination with one or more of the other approved intense sweeteners, when a synergistic effect occurs.

Disadvantages

1 Expensive, due to small volume production and limited use, but with growing utilization by industry costs may fall.
2 Limited solubility leads to potential problems with long term shelf life when used in beverages.

3 Labile to heat, particularly in solution, which further restricts its use in the manufacturing industries.

Acesulfame K

Acesulfame K is the potassium salt of 6-methyl-1,2,3, oxathiazine-4 (3H)-one-2,2 dioxide. It was discovered in 1967 and passed for use in the UK in 1983. It is approximately 200 times as sweet as sucrose. It has potential widespread use within the home and in manufacturing processes where its property of maintaining its sweet taste in both solution and dry state has much to commend it.

The current ADI maximum is 9 mg/kg body weight (WHO/FAO 1983; EEC.SCF 1985).

Availability

For use in the home it is mostly available in tablet form, but it can be obtained in a powder form in combination with either maltodextrin or cellulose. It is provided for industry as a powder.

Advantages

1 Tolerates heat and cold equally well, hence it has potential widespread applications in both the baking and freezing industries. Its use in biscuits, ice creams, and ice desserts is likely.
2 Has a clean, sweet taste.
3 Can be used alone or in conjunction with other non-nutritive or bulk sweeteners.

Disadvantages

1 Expensive.
2 In limited supply at the present time.

Thaumatin

This is extracted from a West African fruit and has very intense sweetness (2000 times as sweet as sucrose). Its application is therefore primarily in food industry as a flavour enhancer or in combination with other less sweet intense sweeteners.

There is no established ADI as yet.

Availability

Only to food or medicine manufacturing industries as a powder (mixed with maltodextrin, mannitol or gum arabic) or a liquid (dissolved in propylene glycol or glycerol).

Advantages/disadvantages

Only used in very limited application at present, mostly in conjuction with other sweeteners. Found in yoghurts, cold beverages and one proprietary sweetener.

Brand names and composition of the intense, non-nutritive sweeteners currently available in the UK are listed in Table 2.85.

Table 2.85 Intense non-nutritive sweeteners currently available in the UK

Brand name	Manufacturer	Sweetener used
Canderel Powder	Searle	Aspartame
Canderel Sachets		Aspartame
Canderel tablets		Aspartame
Hermesetas (liquid)	Hermes Sweeteners	Saccharin
Hermesetas (tablets)		Saccharin
Hermesetas Gold (tablets)		Acesulfame K
Natrena (liquid)	Bayer UK Ltd	Saccharin
Natrena (tablets)		Saccharin
Saxin (tablets)	Ash Consumer Products	Saccharin
Shapers (tablets)	Boots	Saccharin
		Aspartame
Sweet 'n' Low (tablets) (1)	Dietary Foods	Saccharin
(2)		Acesulfame K
Sweetex (liquid)	Crookes Products	Saccharin
Sweetex (tablets)		Saccharin
Sweetex Plus (tablets)		Acesulfame K

2.14.2 Nutritive sweeteners

The term 'nutritive sweetener' refers to sugar substitutes which make some contribution to individual energy, protein and/or carbohydrate intakes. Currently nutritive sweeteners fall into two categories

1 Compound mixtures of an intense non-nutritive sweeteners and either a sugar e.g. sucrose, lactose, or a bulk sugar substitute such as sorbitol, or an inert starch such as maltodextrin.
2 A pure bulk sugar substitute.

Compound mixtures

Products in this category need to be used with care since their nutritional contribution varies. The nutritional analysis per 100 g and the likely quantities of the product to be used by the consumer must both be considered.

Availability

The two most common formulations are
1 Intense sweetener + a sugar (sucrose or lactose).
2 Intense sweetener + bulk sugar substitute.

The most widely available combination of intense sweetener + a sugar is saccharin and sucrose, resulting in a product which is about four times as sweet as sucrose alone. Thus one teaspoon of this mixture replaces four teaspoons of sucrose, resulting in a 75% saving in energy intake.

Currently the most widely available combination of an intense sweetener with a bulk sugar substitute is a mixture of saccharin and sorbitol. However, in the near future, saccharin with fructose, acesulfame potassium with fructose, or aspartame and fructose are all likely to become commercially available. Care must be taken in selecting the products used since equivalent sweetness (which affects quantities and thus nutritional intake) varies considerably (see Table 2.86).

Advantages

1 Some may help reduce total energy intake.

Table 2.86 Compound nutritive sweeteners (mixtures of intense sweeteners and bulking agents) currently available in the UK

Brand name	Sweetener formulation	Suitability for use in baking	Sweetening power compared with sucrose	Energy saving
Boots Sweetener (Powder)	Sorbitol and saccharin	Limited	4 times as sweet	Yes
Canderel Spoonful	Maltodextrin and aspartame	Limited	10 times as sweet	Yes
Diamin Powder	Acesulfame K and cellulose	Limited	11 times as sweet	Yes
Hermesetas Sprinkle Sweet	Maltodextrin, saccharin and thaumatin	No	10 times as sweet	Yes
Sionon	Sorbitol and saccharin	Yes	Equal	No
Sweet 'n' Low (1)	Saccharin and lactose	No	10 times as sweet	Yes
Sweet 'n' Low (2)	Acesulfame K and lactose	No	10 times as sweet	Yes
Sweetex Granulated	Maltodextrin and saccharin	Limited	10 times as sweet	Yes
Sweetex Powder	Sorbitol and saccharin	Yes	4 times as sweet	Yes

2 They can be useful to reduce consumption of simple sugars (e.g. to help prevent dental caries).

Disadvantages

1 Products which contain sucrose must be used with care by some individuals, e.g. diabetics.
2 Not all products are suitable for use in cooking. They cannot be used to replace sugar in recipes where bulk or the reaction of sugar with fat and flour is important in the final product, i.e. in sponge cakes and some biscuits.

Bulk sugar substitutes

Availability

The following are all approved for use in the UK as sugar substitutes
1 Sorbitol
2 Mannitol
3 Xylitol
4 Hydrogenated glucose syrup e.g. Malbit, Lycasin.
5 Maltitol
6 Isomalt.

Fructose (a natural sugar) is widely used to replace sucrose and glucose but is not required to feature in the permitted list of sugar substitutes.

Sorbitol is a sugar alcohol of which at least 90% is metabolized after conversion to fructose. Sorbitol and fructose are widely available, used in the preparation of 'diabetic products' and can be purchased in powder form for use within the home.

Xylitol and mannitol, which are sugar alcohols, are used in limited amounts, where their particular properties of mild sweetness and mouth cooling are required, e.g. chewing gum, toothpaste, pastilles and mints.

Maltitol and isomalt, although approved, are not yet in full scale manufacture and their applications in commercial, manufacturing processes have yet to be firmly established.

Hydrogenated glucose syrups are available in a range of formulations and have a potential use in the production of sucrose-free products, where the main pur-pose of replacing the sucrose is dental protection. Hydrogenated glucose syrups and the sugar alcohols have all been shown to be markedly less cariogenic than sucrose.

Diabetic and slimming use

Diabetics as a group are the most avid users of sorbitol and fructose. However, while single test meals and some mixed meal studies indicate that these substances are less glycaemic than sucrose or glucose, the extent to which they offer benefits on a day to day basis, particularly since the introduction of the higher fibre diet now advocated for the treatment of diabetes, is currently under review. Until new and better controlled studies are available, dietitians are advised to permit patients to use these sweeteners if they want to, but only in limited quantities (<25 g/day) and preferably in a high fibre context. The insulin independent pathway is limited and intakes exceeding 25 g/day of either fructose or sorbitol, or a combination of the two, are likely to lead to a deterioration in glycaemic control. To further reduce this risk, diabetics should be educated not to use sorbitol or fructose for simple sweetening purposes but instead to use one of the intense non-nutritive sweeteners. Sorbitol and fructose should only be used where bulk and/or a degree of preservation is required, e.g. for cake or jam making. In this way it is believed that the effects exerted by the accompanying ingredients or foods (ideally high in fibre) will help to reduce the rate at which these sweeteners are absorbed and metabolized.

Provided the 25 g level is not exceeded, the carbohydrate contribution from sorbitol and fructose can be ignored but the energy contribution must always be considered.

No convincing evidence exists for the use of any of the bulk sugar substitutes for those patients who require reduced energy intakes. All the bulk sweeteners provide approximately 3.75–4 kcal/g, i.e. the same as mono- and disaccharides. All except fructose (which is 1.3–2 times as sweet as sucrose, depending on the application) are *less* sweet than sucrose, so in fact will provide more energy than sucrose if used to provide the same degree of sweetness.

Isomalt and certain formulations of hydrogenated glucose syrup have been claimed to have reduced energy availability, but these claims have yet to be substantiated and are not accepted by the legislative authorities in the UK or industry at present. Nevertheless, these products are, under current legislation, permitted for use in diabetic or dietetic foods despite probably not being suitable for these purposes. Fortunately, the paucity of medical data in support of this usage has restricted the marketing of these sweeteners. Until controlled long term studies are available, dietitians should not regard products containing these sweeteners as offering any advantage over sucrose-sweetened products for diabetics or patients requiring reduced energy intakes.

Advantages of bulk sugar substitutes

Dental caries. With the exception of fructose (for which only weak data exists) all the other bulk substitutes have been shown to be less cariogenic than sucrose. Indeed there is some indication that xylitol and Lycasin may actually be protective against the cariogenic action of other accompanying foods.

Food processing. The poly alcohols and hydrogenated glucose syrups do not crystallize at high temperatures so they can be used very succesfully to replace sucrose in confectionery such as boiled sweets. Fructose tends to be hydroscopic so it helps in baking processes where staleing or drying can be a problem.

Disadvantages of bulk sugar substitutes

Cost. All are substantially more expensive than sucrose or glucose. This limits their use in industry and in the home. For example, fructose costs approximately 55 p for 250 g compared with the current supermarket cost of sucrose which is approximately 45 p for 1000 g.

Low relative sweetness. With the exception of fructose, all are less sweet than sugar, so, unless they are combined with intense sweeteners, greater quantities will be needed to obtain equivalent sweetness.

Gastrointestinal side effects. All the poly alcohols, hydrogenated glucose syrups, maltitol and isomalt have pronounced affects on the gastrointestinal tract. Individual tolerance varies and to a certain extent depends on dosage and previous exposure, but diarrhoea, flatulence and unpleasant stomach cramps can all be experienced on relatively low intakes of less than 25–50 g/day. Some individuals, particularly children, may exhibit pronounced symptoms following the ingestion of very small quantities and this must be borne in mind.

Browning effect. Fructose-sweetened products tend to brown more quickly, so care must be taken in any baking processes if fructose has been used.

Summary

Although many bulk sugar substitutes are currently available, their use at present is limited. At the moment their most effective and proven role appears to be as a substitute for sugar as part of the campaign to prevent dental caries. Even so, until they can be successfully combined with an intense sweetener their applications will be limited by both their cost and gastrointestinal effects.

References

EEC Scientific Committee for Food (1985) Reports (16th Series) Ref EUR 10210EN. Directorate Senesal — Internal market and Industrial Affairs.

WHO/FAO (1983) Report of the Joint Expert Committee on Food Additives (JECFA).

2.15 Food Additives

2.15.1 The E number system for food additives

The E numbers code a list of permitted food additives, generally regarded as safe, for use within the European Economic Community. From January 1 1986, all food labels have to give the E numbers or the actual name of the additives in the ingredients list.

It is important to note that flavourings are exempt from this ruling and have no E number. All that is required by law is that 'flavouring' is included in the ingredient list on the food label. This means that many chemicals of potential interest (such as salicylates or caffeine) which are used in a wide range of foods (e.g. sweets, ice cream, soft drinks, cake and dessert mixes) cannot be identified.

Many food additives are natural in origin, but many of the synthetic additives are being viewed with care, especially in the area of symptoms which may be provoked by sensitivity to a food additive.

The E number classification is summarized in Table 2.87.

2.15.2 Food additives and their uses

Permitted colours

Food is coloured
1   To restore losses occurring during processing and storage.
2   To reinforce colour to meet consumer expectations.
3   To give colour to otherwise colourless foods.
4   To ensure similar products look the same.

Table 2.87 Summary of E numbers

E number	Type of additive	Example
E100−180	Permitted colours	E102 Tartrazine
E200−290	Preservatives	E210 Benzoic acid
E300−321	Permitted antioxidants	E320 BHA
E322−495	Emulsifiers/stabilizers	E322 Lecithin
E420−421	Sweeteners	
E422	Solvents	
E905−907	Mineral hydrocarbons	
E170−927	Miscellaneous additives	E170 Calcium carbonate

Some additives are under consideration by the EEC and have a number but no E prefix, e.g. 621 Monosodium glutamate.

98% of all food colour is caramel (E150) (Denner 1984).

Natural colours

These are not as concentrated or as stable as the artificial colours, but are used in specific foods. Some examples of natural colours are given in Table 2.88.

Artificial colours

These are all derived from coal tar and are commonly known as azo dyes although not all of them have an azo group in their chemical structure (see Table 2.89). Artificial colours have been implicated in food-sensitive urticaria and hyperactivity in children. The most frequently used colour is tartrazine (E102).

Foods commonly containing one or more azo dyes include
1   Sweets and ice lollies.
2   Cakes and biscuits.
3   Packet jelly mixes and trifles.
4   Soups and sauces.
5   Tinned fruits and fruit pie fillings.
Permitted artificial colours are listed in Table 2.89.

Preservatives

The current methods of food production mean that it is not possible to produce safe food without the addition of preservatives. They are added to increase the shelf life of a product and its life on opening, and act

Table 2.88 Examples of natural permitted colours

Name	E number	Typical food uses
Caramel (brown)	E150	Brown bread, cakes, biscuits, soups, gravy mixes, sauces, shandy and soft drinks
Riboflavin (yellow)	E101	Processed cheese
Chlorophyll (green)	E140	Fats, oils, canned and dried vegetables
Carbon (black)	E153	Jams and jellies
Alpha carotene (yellow/orange)	E160(a)	Margarine and cakes

Table 2.89 Artificial permitted colours

Name	E number	Specific food use
Tartrazine (yellow)*	E102	Smoked fish
Quinoline Yellow	E104	Scotch eggs and smoked fish
Yellow 2G*	107[a]	
Sunset Yellow*	E110	Orange squash
Carmoisine (red)*	E122	Swiss roll
Amaranth (red)*	E123	Blackcurrant products
Ponceau 4R (red)*	E124	Tinned red fruits
Erythrosine (red)	E127	Glace cherries
Red 2G*	128[a]	Sausages and cooked meats
Patent Blue V	131[a]	Tinned vegetables
Indigo Carmine (blue)	E132	Savoury food mixes
Brilliant Blue	133[a]	
Green S	E142	Tinned peas, mint jelly and sauce
Black PN*	E151	Brown sauce and blackcurrant products
Brown FK*	154[a]	Kippers and smoked fish
Brown HT*	155[a]	Chocolate flavoured products

[a]Waiting consideration for E prefix by EEC.
*Contain azo group in their chemical structure

Tables 2.90 a, b Commonly used permitted preservatives

a)

Name	E number	Specific food use
Sorbic acid and its derivatives	E200–E203	Cheese, yoghurt and soft drinks
Acetic acid	E260	Pickles and sauces
Lactic acid	E270	Margarine, confectionery and sauces
Propionic acid and its derivatives	E280–E283	Bread, cakes and flour confectionery
Carbon dioxide	E290	Fizzy drinks

b) Permitted preservatives with additional nutritional interest

Name	E number	Specific food use
Benzoic acid and its derivatives	E210–E219	Soft drinks, pickles, sauces, fruit products and jams
Sulphur dioxide	E220	Widely used in soft drinks, fruit products, beer, cider and wine
Nitrites	E249, E250	Cured meats, cooked meats and meat products
Nitrates	E251, E252	Bacon, ham and cheese (not Cheddar or Cheshire)

by preventing the growth of moulds, bacteria and yeasts.

The Preservatives in Food Regulations 1979 (amended 1980 and 1982) (MAFF) give detailed information on the use of preservatives including

1 The current permitted preservatives.
2 The foods in which a preservative may be used.
3 The maximum permitted level of preservative in parts per million (ppm).

Some commonly used preservatives are given in Tables 2.90 a and b. Those of particular interest to nutritionists include:

Benzoic acid

This has been implicated in asthma and chronic urticaria. It occurs naturally in peas, bananas and berry fruit (see Table 2.58), but is widely used as a synthetic food preservative. The latter can be eliminated from the diet by avoiding foods with E210–E219 on the food label, looking especially at soft drinks, fruit products, jams, pickles and sauces.

Sulphur dioxide

This chemical is known to destroy thiamin. It is not permitted in any food which is considered to be a significant source of this vitamin.

Nitrates and nitrites

These preservatives act against the potentially lethal bacterium *Clostridium botulinum*. They also preserve the red colour of meats by reacting with myoglobin. They are used in a whole range of meat products and in some cheeses (not Cheddar, Cheshire or soft cheese).

Food is not the only source of nitrates and nitrites. These chemicals are used in fertilizers and the consequent leaching from the soil into the water supply has increased the levels available to the body.

There is considerable research into their alleged role as carcinogens. Nitrites may react with secondary amines in the gastrointestinal tract to produce nitrosamines which have been shown to be carcinogenic in experimental animals. There is no evidence, as yet, in man to substantiate the role of these preservatives in the causation of cancer.

Permitted antioxidants

As with preservatives, our current methods of food production would not produce goods with satisfactory

Table 2.91 Permitted antioxidants

Name	E number	Specific food use
Ascorbic acid and its derivatives	E300−E305	Beer, soft drinks, powdered milks, fruit products, (e.g. jams) and meat products (e.g. sausages)
Tocopherols (vitamin E and its derivatives)	E306−E309	Vegetable oils
Gallates	E310−E312	Vegetable oils and fat, margarine
Butylated hydroxyanisole (BHA)	E320	Margarine, fat in baked products, e.g. pies, sweets and convenience foods
Butylated hydroxytoluene (BHT)	E321	Crisps, margarine, vegetable oils and fats and convenience foods

Tables 2.92 Examples of emulsifiers and stabilizers

Name	E number	Specific food use
Lecithins*	E322	Chocolate and chocolate products, powdered milk, margarine and potato snacks
Citric acid and its derivatives	E330−E333	Pickles, bottled sauces, dairy and baked products
Tartaric acid and its derivatives	E334−E336	Baking powder
Alginic acid and its derivatives	E400−E401	Ice cream, instant desserts and puddings
Agar	E406	Tinned ham (jelly), meat glazes and ice cream
Carrageenan	E407	Ice cream
Gums		
locust bean gum	E410	
guar gum	E412	
tragacanth	E413	Ice cream, soups, bottled sauces and confectionery
gum arabic	E414	
xanthan gum	E415	
Pectin	E440	Preserves, jellies and mint jelly
Sodium and potassium phosphate salts (polyphosphates)	E450	Frozen poultry and meat products, e.g. sausages

*Also used as an antioxidant.

shelf life without the use of antioxidants. The most important use of antioxidants is to prevent the unpleasant taste and smell which occur if fats or oils go rancid. Table 2.91 lists permitted antioxidants.

BHA and BHT (butylated hydroxyanisole and butylated hydroxytoluene)

These antioxidants have been linked to urticaria and behavioural problems (hyperactivity) in children and are two of the many food additives avoided in the dietary treatment of these conditions. They are both widely used in manufactured foods.

Emulsifiers and stabilizers

These additives are used to affect the texture and consistency of food. They are often needed because of the long shelf life of some manufactured foods, e.g. anticaking agents added to ensure that powders, such as salt, flow freely. They constitute the largest group of additives and many are natural substances. The most controversial additives in this group are the polyphosphates, whose use as a meat tenderizer also enables water to be retained, so increasing product weight, e.g. frozen poultry, cured meats.

Some examples of emulsifiers and stabilizers are given in Table 2.92.

Sweeteners (see Section 2.14)

The UK regulations allow the use of four artificial sweeteners — acesulfame potassium, aspartame, saccharin and thaumatin. In addition, sorbitol (E420) and mannitol (E421) are permitted.

Sucrose, glucose, fructose and lactose are all classified as foods rather than as sweeteners.

Solvents

Alcohol is the most common solvent use to enable the incorporation of a substance into a food product.

Mineral hydrocarbons

These are used as glazing agents, e.g. confectionery.

Miscellaneous additives

These include
1 Anti-foaming agents, to prevent frothing during processing.
2 Propellant gases, e.g. in aerosol cream.
3 Flavour modifiers, e.g. monosodium glutamate.

Many of these additives have a number but no E prefix as they are under consideration by the EEC.

Further reading

Amos HE and Drake JJP (1965) Problems posed by food additives. *J Hum Nutr* **30**, (3), 165−78.
British Dietetic Association manufactured foods lists (but see p 615):
1 *Additive free*. Excludes all E numbers and all foods with added vitamins but does not exclude natural sources of salicylates and benzoates.

2 *Added preservative free.* Excludes E200–299 inclusive but does not exclude natural sources of salicylates and benzoates or preservatives carried over into a product in one of the ingredients.

3 *Colour free.* Excludes E100–199 inclusive, but riboflavin and carotene are included.

4 *Colour and preservative free.* A combination of 2 and 3.

Food and Agriculture Committee (1972) *Interim report on the review of preservatives in food regulations*. HMSO, London.

Food and Agriculture Committee (1979) *Interim report on the review of colouring matter in food regulations*. HMSO, London.

Hanssen M (1984) *E for additives — the complete E number guide.* Thorsons, Wellingborough.

Joint Report of the Royal College of Physicians and the British Nutrition Foundation (1984) Food intolerance and food aversion. Reprinted from the *J Roy Coll Phys* **18**, (2), 3–41.

Ministry of Agriculture, Fisheries and Food (1973) *Colouring matter in food regulations*. HMSO, London.

Ministry of Agriculture, Fisheries and Food (1979) *Preservatives in food regulations*. HMSO, London.

Ministry of Agriculture, Fisheries and Food (1983) *Look at the label*. HMSO, London.

Reference

Dinner WHB (1984) Colourings and preservatives in foods. *Hum Nutr: Appl Nutr* **38A**, (6), 435–50.

2.16 Health Foods and Fad Diets

2.16.1 Health foods

A fundamental problem with health foods is their name. The term 'health food' implies something which is necessary for, or improves, health. A more realistic view is the one offered by Bender (1985), that there is no such thing as a health food, only a health food industry.

While dietitians are fully aware of this fact, it is important to recognize that large numbers of the general public are not. Everyone wants to feel fit and healthy and the idea that this can be achieved quickly and easily via pills and potions has considerable appeal. People want health foods to work and are ready to believe the apparently scientific claims made for them. They are also perhaps impressed by the price; if something costs that much, it *must* be beneficial.

Not all products sold in health food shops are undesirable. 'Wholefoods' such as brown rice, dried fruit, wholewheat pastas and muesli can certainly form part of a healthy diet (but can also be obtained, probably at less cost, from supermarkets).

The availability of *organically grown* produce also has its supporters on the alleged grounds of safety, higher nutrient content and taste. If people are convinced that these supposed benefits justify the economic cost of using them then they are perfectly entitled to do so. But people should not be coerced into thinking they are necessary. Despite having been looked for, there is no satisfactory evidence to support any of these claims (Jukes 1974; White 1974; Bender 1979; Williams 1985). People's fears are easily aroused by the thought of 'chemicals' in their food, not realizing that some of the 'chemicals' naturally present in food (e.g. solanine, haemagglutinins, oxalic acid and cyanide) present a far greater health hazard than traces of agricultural residues many of which are in any case removed by washing or peeling. There is certainly no justification for using organically grown produce on the grounds of better nutritional content; even if true (and there is little evidence that it is) the additional nutrients would probably be insignificant in terms of total dietary intake. Any superiority noted in taste (rarely supported by double blind tasting trials) is perhaps more likely to be due to their relative freshness (due to their small-scale production and local marketing) rather than to the fact that they are 'organically' grown.

It is the use of *dietary aids and supplements* from health food shops which is the area of greatest concern. A vast array of substances are available for a variety of different purposes (Table 2.93). Some of them may even appear to work owing to the power of the placebo effect; if you expect product *x* will make you feel better, then it probably will. But these supplements must not be dismissed as placebos in the sense of being inert pieces of chalk. These substances are what they say they are, and many of them have powerful pharmacological effects (though not necessarily those claimed for them). The dangers of hypervitaminosis is an obvious example (see Section 2.6 Vitamins). The effects of excess quantities of isolated amino acid supplements, minerals such as selenium and substances such as ginseng have never been fully explored and may be no less hazardous.

Even if consumed at a level which is not harmful, their use is still undesirable. In most instances they are unnecessary; either providing nutrients which are surplus to requirements or supposed nutrients which are probably not needed at all. Their use as remedies for various ailments may have little scientific justification and may lead to a delay in seeking, or even abandonment of, proper medical attention.

Of fundamental concern is the fact that their use depends on dietary ignorance and tends to reinforce such ignorance. This tends to hamper efforts to explain the genuine tissues of healthy eating. Furthermore, those who are most susceptible to health food claims are perhaps those who can least afford to be, and the money spent on these products could be better directed elsewhere.

2.16.2 Fad diets

From time to time, a new fad diet which is supposed to improve health, aid slimming or cure illness receives publicity via books, magazines or the broadcasting media. As with health foods, the use of these products largely depends on people's hopes, fears and ignorance.

Table 2.93 Health food supplements and remedies

Reasons for use	Products used	Comments
To correct dietary deficiencies	Vitamins ⎫ Minerals ⎬ in isolated form or in combination Amino acids ⎭ Kelp (a source of minerals) Spirulina (vitamins and minerals) Aloe vera (sugars, vitamins and minerals)	Probably surplus to requirements in most cases. Considerable dangers from over-use
To supply 'nutrients' deficient in a normal diet	Vitamins B13, B15 and B17 Flavanoids Inositol Selenium Lecithin	No evidence that supplements of these are necessary. 'B17' (laetrile) has now been banned from sale
To restore vigour/induce feelings of well-being	Ginseng Honey Kelp Pollen Bee's royal jelly Spirulina	Ginseng has certain pharmacological effects although these are variable and unpredictable, perhaps because Ginseng itself is of variable composition. Extremely expensive. Problems with over-use have been reported (Dukes 1978; Palmer *et al* 1978; Bender 1985). The remaining substances may provide traces of vitamins and/or minerals (at a price) but little in the way of magic
Rejuvenation/to retard ageing	DNA and RNA	The body makes all the DNA and RNA it needs. Dietary excess can cause hyperuricaemia
To 'cleanse' the body of toxins	Cider vinegar Garlic	In the absence of severe liver or renal disease, the body is quite capable of doing this for itself
To aid digestion or metabolism	Enzymes	Cannot possibly act in this way. Are denatured on reaching the stomach and then treated as any other protein
As a slimming aid	Spirulina Cider vinegar Honey Lecithin	Claims that substances can burn up fat or stimulate metabolism are nonsense; if true, obesity would be a thing of the past. Honey and lecithin are significant sources of calories
As a cure	Aloe vera (arthritis) Green lipped mussel (rheumatism) Kelp (healing) Herbal remedies	It should be borne in mind that chronic disorders such as arthritis and rheumatism tend to have periods of partial remission in any case. A skilled herbalist may well be able to relieve minor ailments via the pharmacological effects of some plants. But these effects can be powerful, and sometime toxic (e.g. hemlock, strychnine) and indiscriminate use of these remedies by the uninformed can be dangerous
Because they are 'natural'	'Natural' as distinct from 'synthetic' vitamins Sea salt	By definition, a synthetic vitamin must be identical to a natural one or it wouldn't be a vitamin. Sea salt is, in effect, dirty salt. People often assume that anything 'natural' is automatically superior to anything manufactured. They should be reminded that some of the most toxic substances known to man (e.g. certain plant alkaloids or botulinus toxin) are 'natural'

Some fad diets quickly fade into obscurity, others persist for longer; most are useless.

Some of the fad diets which may be encountered by dietitians among their patients are summarized below.

Elimination and cleansing diets

Elimination diets carried out under qualified medical and dietetic supervision have a proper place in the diagnosis and management of food intolerance (Section 5.9). But alongside this has grown the belief among the general public that 'elimination' or 'cleansing' diets can remove 'toxins' from the modern day diet and can relieve ailments such as catarrh or arthritis. In some instances, genuine food intolerance may indeed be responsible for some of these symptoms, but this possibility should be explored with qualified dietetic help and not on a do-it-yourself basis. The latter course of action may well

1 Be expensive.
2 Be ineffective.
3 Result in nutritional deficiencies as a result of prolonged dietary imbalance.
4 Offer false hope.

In recent years a cleansing diet purportedly of help to cancer sufferers (the Bristol diet) has received considerable publicity. While there is no scientific evidence to support the benefit of this diet, dietitians who encounter patients following this regimen should be careful not to destroy any hopes of its effectiveness which may have been built up, whether or not these are justified. However, by means of tactful enquiry and suggestions, dietitians should at least try to ensure that the diet consumed by the patient is nutritionally adequate (see Section 5.1.4).

Food combining diets

It has been claimed that some modern degenerative diseases are the result of eating the wrong combination of foods, e.g. carbohydrate- and protein-containing foods at the same meal. Followers of food combining regimens observe various rules governing the types of foods which may be eaten at any one time. The system has no scientific support.

Raw food diets

These regimens are based mainly on items such as uncooked fruits, vegetables, sprouted beans and seeds and fruit and vegetable juices. Consequent nutritional deficiencies are highly likely.

Macrobiotic diets

This is an extreme form of vegetarianism which has profound nutritional and even fatal consequences (see Section 3.9).

Fad reducing diets

There is a multiplicity of diets which are claimed to be of benefit in achieving weight reduction. Most fall into two categories

Distorted nutrient composition

Diets such as the 'Mayo Clinic' diet, the 'Chicago' diet or 'Beverley Hills' diet are based on a severe distortion in the nutrient composition of the diet, e.g. a severe carbohydrate restriction sometimes in association with a high protein intake. Many of these diets claim to have discovered the secret of 'speeding up metabolism' or 'burning up fat' more effectively than any other type of diet. In reality, whether they achieve weight loss will depend solely on whether an individual's energy intake is less than his requirement. Their effectiveness depends on the length of time the diet can be tolerated (which is not usually very long).

Restricted food group diets

Women's magazines are particularly fond of recommending diets based on a few foods, e.g. the 'grapefruit' diet. While these diets may achieve short term weight loss (much of which is due to the loss of body water), they are obviously nutritionally unsound and of no value whatsoever in the long term treatment of obesity.

Further reading

Bender AE (1985) *Health or hoax*. Elvendon Press, Reading.

References

Bender AE (1979) Health foods *Proc Nutr Soc* **38**, 163--1.
Bender AE (1985) In *Health or hoax*. Elvendon Press, Reading
Dukes MN (1978) Ginseng and mastalgia. (Letter) *Br Med J* **1**, 1621.
Jukes TH (1974) The organic food myth. *J Am Med Assoc* **230**, 276–7.
Palmer BV, Montgomery ACV and Monteiro JCMP (1978) Ginseng and mastalgia (Letter) *Br Med J* **1**, 1284.
White PL (1974) Organically grown foods. *Nutr Rev* [Suppl] **32**, 1–73.
Williams CA (1985) Health foods. *Midwife, Health Visitor and Community Nurse* **21**, 328–32.

2.17 Food Legislation

2.17.1 Background and current regulations

The earliest record of food legislation in this country was an Act passed in 1266 which protected the purchaser against sale of unsound meat and short weight in bread. Whilst apparently far sighted, the enforcement of the Act left a lot to be desired and was largely ineffective. However, Guilds, which played a very important role at that time, helped to ensure that the commodities were as pure as possible. This meant checking the pepper to ensure there was no added gravel, leaves or twigs, checking the coffee to ensure there was no added grass, acorns or lard and checking bread to ensure that no mashed potato, sand or ashes had been added.

As the population grew, the industrial revolution caused a massive shift from country to town; more people needed to be fed and a larger proportion of them were no longer able to grow their own food and became dependent on others for its supply.

By the middle of the 19th century the abuses were appalling. Increased publicity was now being given to the problem of food adulteration in both the scientific journals and popular press of the day and as a result public pressures led to the establishment of a Select Committee on Food Adulteration. After much dissatisfaction concerning its effectiveness, another Committee was set up, the result of which was the 1875 Sale of Food and Drugs Act. This Act is the basis of present UK law and includes the statement fundamental to current practice

> 'No person shall sell to the prejudice of the purchaser any article of food or any food thing which is not of the nature, substance or quality demanded by such purchasers.'

By the turn of the century, significant improvements had been made to the purity of basic commodities — bread, flour and coffee were no longer adulterated. The 1875 Act remained in force until 1928 when it was replaced by the consolidated Food and Drugs (Adulteration) Act. It was at this time that regulations pertaining to composition and labelling were first introduced.

In 1943 the Food and Drugs Act combined *all* legislation concerning the retailing of foodstuffs. This Act was the basis of Government control during the war years.

In 1955 the Food and Drug Act came into being and was to remain the basis of food legislation until general legislation covering the composition, labelling, hygiene and safety of food in the UK was introduced in 1984 by the Food Act. (The 'drug' aspect was superseded by the Medicines Act in 1968 and from 1974 has no longer been included in this schedule).

At present, there are three separate food Acts: in England and Wales the Food Act 1984, in Scotland the Food and Drugs (Scotland) Act 1956 and in Northern Ireland the Food and Drugs Act (Northern Ireland) 1958.

In view of the considerable changes which have occurred in both food production and eating habits in the past 40 years, current legislation is being increasingly criticized for being out of date and in need of amendment. As a result the Government has proposed a number of major amendments which are the subject of wide consideration among interested parties. It is anticipated that these changes would be welcomed by both the consumer and the food industry and the remainder of this section is written on the understanding that the amendments proposed will be agreed and ratified in the near future.

Table 2.94 details the current regulations for food standards, additives and contaminants. Regulations for Scotland and Northern Ireland may be administratively different.

Whilst the Food Acts provide the basic legislation, the making of new regulations is divided between the Ministry of Agriculture Fisheries and Food in matters dealing with composition and labelling and the Secretary of State for Social Services in matters relating to hygiene. Figure 2.8 shows how a substance, e.g. a food additive, is dealt with by MAFF when referred for approval.

2.17.2 Enforcement

Within the UK

Responsibility for food law enforcement is allocated

Table 2.94 Current regulations for food standards, additives and contaminants

Subject	England and Wales		Scotland		Northern Ireland	
	Regulations	Amendments	Regulations	Amendments	Rules	Amendments
Baking powder	1944/46	1946/157	1944/46		1960/160[1]	
Mustard	1944/275	1948/1073	1944/275	1948/1073	1960/160[1]	
Self-raising flour	1946/157		1946/157		1960/160[1]	
Curry powder	1949/1816	1979/1254	1949/1816	1979/1641	1960/160[1]	
Tomato ketchup	1949/1817	1956/1167	1949/1817	1956/1353	1960/160[1]	
Infestation of food	1950/416					
Fish cakes	1950/589		1950/589		1960/160[1]	
Suet	1952/2203		1952/2203		1960/160[1]	
Offals in meat products	1953/246		1953/246		1960/165	
Milk (Channel Islands, etc.)	1956/919					
Milk and dairies (general)	1959/277	1973/1064				
		1977/171				
		1979/1567				
		1982/1703				
Ice cream (heat treatment)	1959/734	1963/1083				
Arsenic	1959/831	1960/2261	1959/928	1960/2344	1961/98	1964/72
		1963/1435		1963/1461		1972/275
		1972/1391		1972/1489		1973/197
		1973/1052		1973/1039		1973/466
		1973/1340		1973/1310		
Fluorine	1959/2106	1975/1484	1959/2182	1975/1594	1961/110	1975/276
Skimmed milk (with added fat)	1960/2331	1976/103	1960/2437	1976/294	1961/190	1976/70
	1981/1174	1980/1849	1981/137		1981/305	1981/305
		1981/1174		1981/1319		1982/43
Meat inspection	1963/1229	1966/915	1961/243	1963/1231		
		1976/882		1966/967		
		1981/454		1976/874		
		1983/174		1979/1563		
				1981/996		
				1981/1034		
				1983/702		
Bread and Flour	1984/1304					
Liquid egg (pasteurization)	1963/1503		1963/1591		1963/244	
Meat (treatment)	1964/19		1964/44		1964/6	
Soft drinks	1964/60	1969/1818	1964/767	1969/1847	1976/357[2]	1977/182
		1972/1510		1972/1790		1980/28
		1976/295		1976/442		1981/194
		1977/927		1977/1026		1981/305
		1980/1849		1981/137		1983/265
		1983/1211		1983/1497		
Hygiene (markets, etc.)	1966/791	1966/1487				
Salad cream	1966/1051	1966/1206	1968/1206	1968/263	1966/192	1967/282
Butter	1966/1074	1973/1340	1966/1252	1973/1310	1966/205	1973/466
		1980/1849		1981/137		1981/305
Irradiation	1967/385	1972/205	1972/388	1972/307	1967/51	1972/68
Meat pies, sausage rolls	1967/860	1970/400	1967/1077	1970/1127	1967/155	
Canned meat	1967/861	1968/2046	1967/1079	1969/326	1967/157	1968/282
		1970/400		1970/1127		1981/305
		1980/1849		1981/137		
Sausages and other meat products	1967/862	1968/2047	1967/1078	1968/139	1967/156	1968/281
		1970/400		1969/1327		1981/305
		1980/1849		1970/1127		
				1981/137		
Solvents	1967/1582	1967/1939	1968/263	1980/1887	1967/282	1981/192
		1980/1832		1983/1497		1983/265
		1983/1211				
Ice cream	1967/1866	1980/1849	1970/1285	1981/137	1967/13[3]	1981/305
		1983/1211		1983/1497		1983/265
Margarine	1967/1867	1980/1849	1970/1286	1981/137	1967/3	1981/305
Imported food	1967/97	1973/1351	1968/1181	1973/1471	1968/98[4]	1973/1350[4]
		1979/1426		1979/1537		1979/1427[4]
		1981/1085		1981/1035		1981/1084[4]

Table 2.94 *contd.*

Subject	England and Wales		Scotland		Northern Ireland	
	Regulations	Amendments	Regulations	Amendments	Rules	Amendments
Fish and meat spreads	1968/430	1970/400 1980/1849	1970/1065	1970/1127 1981/137	1967/103	1981/305
Cheese	1970/94	1974/1122 1976/2086 1980/1849 1982/1729 1984/649	1970/108	1974/1337 1976/2232 1981/137	1970/14	1974/177 1976/382 1981/305
Food labelling (claims, etc.)	1984/1305	1975/1485 1980/1849 1982/1700	1984/1305	1975/1596 1981/137 1982/1779	1984/1305	1972/318 1981/305 1982/398
Cream	1970/752	1975/1486 1980/1849	1970/1191	1975/1597 1981/137	1970/194	1976/15 1981/305
Milk (skimmed, heat treatment)	1973/1064	1982/1358 1982/1702 1983/1511 1983/1563				
Colours	1973/1340	1974/1119 1975/1488 1976/2086 1978/1787 1979/1254	1973/1310	1974/1340 1975/1595 1979/107 1979/1641	1973/466	1975/283 1976/328 1979/49
Specified sugar products	1976/509	1980/834 1980/1849 1982/255	1976/946	1980/1889 1981/137 1982/410	1976/165	1980/28 1981/193 1981/305 1982/311
Cocoa and chocolate	1976/541	1980/1833 1980/1834 1980/1849 1982/17	1976/914	1980/1888 1980/1889 1981/137 1982/108	1976/183	1981/193 1981/194 1981/305 1982/349
Poultry meat (hygiene)	1976/1209	1979/693 1981/1168	1976/1221	1979/768 1981/1169		
Honey	1976/1832	1980/1849	1976/1818	1981/137	1976/387	1981/305
Milk (drinking)	1976/1883				1977/8	
Milk (bottle caps)	1976/2186					
Erucic acid	1977/691	1982/264 1980/1849 1982/1311	1977/1028	1982/18 1981/137 1982/1619	1977/135	1982/184 1981/305 1983/48
Fruit juices and nectars						
Condensed and dried milk	1977/928	1980/1849 1982/1066	1977/1027	1981/137 1982/1209	1977/196	1981/305 1981/26
Milk (special designation)	1977/1033	1980/1863 1982/1359 1982/1702 1983/1510		1982/1209		
Antioxidants	1978/105	1980/1831 1983/1211	1978/492	1980/1886 1983/1497	1978/112	1981/191 1983/265
Coffee and coffee products	1978/1420	1980/1849 1982/254	1979/383	1979/137 1982/409	1979/51	1980/28 1981/305 1982/298
Materials for food contact	1978/1927	1980/1838 1982/1701	1978/1927	1980/1838 1982/1701	1982/285	1982/144 1983/28
Preservatives	1979/752	1980/931 1981/1063 1982/15 1982/1311 1983/1211	1979/1073	1980/1232 1981/1320 1982/516 1982/1619 1983/1497	1980/28	1980/380 1982/105 1982/297 1983/48 1983/265
Lead	1979/1254		1979/1641		1979/407	1981/194
Chloroform	1980/36		1980/289		1980/75	
Emulsifiers and stabilizers	1980/1833	1982/16 1983/1211 1983/1810	1982/1888	1982/514 1983/1497 1983/1815	1981/194	1982/257 1983/265
Miscellaneous additives	1980/1834	1980/1849 1982/14 1983/1211	1980/1889	1980/137 1982/515 1983/1497	1981/193	1981/305 1982/258 1983/165

Table 2.94 *contd.*

Subject	England and Wales		Scotland		Northern Ireland	
	Regulations	Amendments	Regulations	Amendments	Rules	Amendments
Food labelling	1980/1849	1982/1311	1981/137	1982/1619	1981/305	1982/398
		1982/1700		1982/1779		1983/48
		1983/1211		1983/1497		1983/265
Jam and similar products	1981/1063	1982/1700	1981/1320	1982/1779	1982/105	1982/398
		1983/1211		1983/1497		1983/265
Poultry meat (water content)	1982/1602		1983/1372		1982/386	
Sweeteners	1983/1211		1983/1497		1983/265	
Milk Based (hygiene and heat treatment)	1983/1508					
Cream (heat treatment)	1983/1509					
Imported milk	1983/1563		1983/1545		1983/338	

[1] Several amendments have been made removing other products but not affecting the products listed.
[2] Revoked 1964 rules (as amended).
[3] Includes heat treatment.
[4] Statutory instrument (EEC regulation).

Section II: Regulations specific to Scotland

	Regulations	Amendments
Milk (sale of)	1914/175	
Milk and dairies	1934/675	1956/2110
Ice cream	1948/960	1948/2271
Food hygiene	1959/413	1959/1153
		1961/622
		1966/967
		1978/173
Meat (preparation and distribution)	1963/2001	1967/1507
Milk (skimmed, heat treatment)	1974/1356	1983/940
		1983/1526
Milk (labelling)	1983/938	
Milk-based drinks (hygiene, heat treatment)	1983/1514	
Cream (heat treatment)	1983/1515	

Section III: Rules and regulations specific to Northern Ireland

	Rules	Amendments
Food hygiene	1964/129	
Marketing of milk products	1966/204	1983/336
Shellfish (public health)	1973/453	
Milk	1981/234	1983/337

between the two tiers of local Government as follows

1 'Food and Drug Authorities', i.e. London boroughs and non-metropolitan *county* councils have responsibility for all areas relating to food composition and labelling*.

2 'Local Authorities', i.e. metropolitan and non-metropolitan *district* councils have responsibility for all matters relating to food hygiene and unfit food.

There is only one enforcement tier in Scotland and Northern Ireland.

*Abolition of the GLC and the six metropolitan county councils has resulted in their food and drug function devolving to the district councils. In London there is be no change as the boroughs are already the food and drug authorities.

Internationally

Food is both imported into and exported from the UK, so legislation on standards of composition and on labelling should attempt to comply with international standards.

Codex

The Codex Alimentarius Commission is the main international food standards organisation. It is the front body of the two United Nation bodies — the Food and Agriculture Organisation (FAO) and the World Health Organisation (WHO). Codex sets out to es-

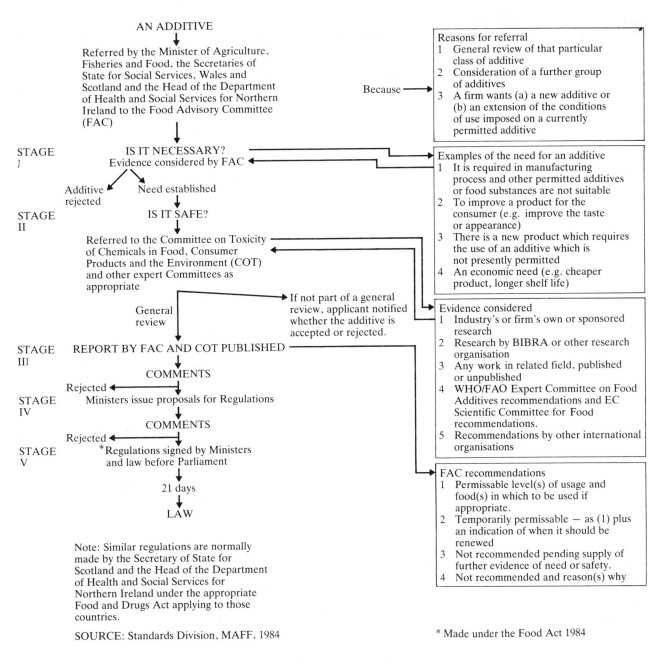

AN ADDITIVE

Referred by the Minister of Agriculture,
Fisheries and Food, the Secretaries of
State for Social Services, Wales and
Scotland and the Head of the Department
of Health and Social Services for Northern
Ireland to the Food Advisory Committee
(FAC)

Because

Reasons for referral
1 General review of that particular
class of additive
2 Consideration of a further group
of additives
3 A firm wants (a) a new additive or
(b) an extension of the conditions
of use imposed on a currently
permitted additive

STAGE I
IS IT NECESSARY?
Evidence considered by FAC

Additive rejected   Need established

Examples of the need for an additive
1 It is required in manufacturing
process and other permitted additives
or food substances are not suitable
2 To improve a product for the
consumer (e.g. improve the taste
or appearance)
3 There is a new product which requires
the use of an additive which is
not presently permitted
4 An economic need (e.g. cheaper
product, longer shelf life)

STAGE II
IS IT SAFE?

Referred to the Committee on Toxicity
of Chemicals in Food, Consumer
Products and the Environment (COT)
and other expert Committees as
appropriate

General review

If not part of a general
review, applicant notified
whether the additive is
accepted or rejected.

Evidence considered
1 Industry's or firm's own or sponsored
research
2 Research by BIBRA or other research
organisation
3 Any work in related field, published
or unpublished
4 WHO/FAO Expert Committee on Food
Additives recommendations and EC
Scientific Committee for Food
recommendations.
5 Recommendations by other international
organisations

STAGE III
REPORT BY FAC AND COT PUBLISHED

COMMENTS

Rejected   Ministers issue proposals for Regulations

STAGE IV

COMMENTS

Rejected   *Regulations signed by Ministers
and law before Parliament

STAGE V

21 days

LAW

FAC recommendations
1 Permissable level(s) of usage and
food(s) in which to be used if
appropriate.
2 Temporarily permissable — as (1) plus
an indication of when it should be
renewed
3 Not recommended pending supply of
further evidence of need or safety.
4 Not recommended and reason(s) why

Note: Similar regulations are normally
made by the Secretary of State for
Scotland and the Head of the Department
of Health and Social Services for
Northern Ireland under the appropriate
Food and Drugs Act applying to those
countries.

SOURCE: Standards Division, MAFF, 1984

* Made under the Food Act 1984

Fig. 2.8 The process of evaluating food additives.

tablish procedures and principles which are acceptable to member countries in relation to meeting agreed standards for food in international trade and to help lower trade barriers.

European Economic Community

Membership of the EEC requires the Government to take into account regularities and directives of the EEC. Two major objectives underlie the legislation in member countries

1 To protect the health of the consumer.

2 The prevention of fraud.

Harmonization of legislation is therefore essential if goods such as foodstuffs are to be able to move as freely as if in a simple market. The original aim of the EEC therefore was to introduce common standards for those products currently controlled by food regulations.

Harmonization can be achieved by either Regulations or Directives.

Regulations. These are applicable directly to all market

Table 2.95 EEC directives relating to foodstuffs in the UK

Subject	Directive number	Amendments		UK implementation (SI number)
Colours				
General	1962/2645	65/469	67/653	1973/1340, 1980/1834
		68/419	70/358	(as amended)
		76/399	78/144	
		81/20*		
Analysis	81/712*			
Preservatives				
General	64/54	65/569	66/722	1980/1834, 1979/752
		67/427	68/420	(as amended)
		70/359	71/160	
		72/2	72/444	
		74/62	74/394	
		76/462	76/629	
		78/145	79/40*	
		81/214*	83/585*	
			83/636*	
			84/86*	
Fresh meat (health)				
Inspection, etc.	64/433	66/601	69/349	1970/1172, 1963/1229
		75/379	81/476	(as amended), 1981/454
Diseases, etc.	72/461	75/379	77/98	(as amended)
		80/213	80/1099	
		81/476	82/893	
Antioxidants				
General	70/357	74/412	78/143	1978/105, 1980/1834,
		81/962		1980/1833 (as amended)
Poultry meat (health)	71/118	74/387	75/379	1976/1209 (as amended)
		75/431	80/216	
		81/476	81/578	
		82/532		
Cocoa and chocolate	73/241	74/411	74/644	1976/541 (as amended)
		75/155	76/628	
		78/609	78/842	
		80/608		
Sugars				
General	73/437			1976/509
Purity criteria	79/796			1982/255
Emulsifiers, stabilizers, thickeners and gelling agents				
General	74/329	78/612	80/597	1980/1833 (as amended)
Honey	74/409			1976/1832
Volumes of pre-packaged liquids	75/106	78/891	79/1005	1979/1613
Fruit juices	75/726	79/168	81/168	1877/927 (as amended)
Dehydrated preserved milk				
General	761/118	78/630(1)	83/635*	1977/928
Analysis	79/1067*			
Weights of pre-packaged products	76/211	78/891		1979/1613
Erucic acid in oils and fats				
General	76/621			1977/691
Analysis	80/891			1982/264
Materials and Articles for food contact	76/893	80/1276		1978/1927 (as amended)
Food for special nutritional uses	77/94			
Meat products (health)				
General	77/99	80/214	81/476	
Expections	83/201			
Coffee and chicory extracts				
General	77/436			1978/1420
Analysis	79/1066			1982/254
Vinyl chloride monomer in food contact materials				
General	78/142	80/590	80/766	1980/1838
Analysis	81/432			1982/1701

Table 2.95 *contd.*

Subject	Directive number	Amendments	UK implementation (SI number)
Labelling, presentation and advertising	79/112		1980/1849 (as amended)
Jams, Jellies Marmalades and chestnut purees	79/693		1981/1063
Prescribed weights	80/232		1981/1780, 1981/1781, 1981/1782
Mineral waters	80/777*		Proposal under discussion
Migration of constituents of plastic materials	82/711*		
Caseins and caseinates	83/417*		
Ingredients' labelling (temporary list)	83/463*		Proposal under discussion

*Directive yet to be implemented.

countries and whilst they may need additional measures to help in enforcement, no national enactment is required. To date regulations exist only for milk and milk products (Reg no 1411/81) and for water content of frozen poultry (Reg nos 2967/76 and 2985/80).

Directives. This is the more usual method used for harmonization of food laws. The directive, once adopted by the EEC Council of Ministers, lays down the ultimate objective for a particular food law, but leaves each member country free to decide how it will be implemented. Table 2.95 details the directives relating to harmonization of laws for foodstuffs in the UK.

Useful addresses

EEC Commission (London Office), EEC Commission, 8 Storey's Gate, London SW1P 3AT.

Enforcement

1 Trading standards — Local Authorities Co-ordinating Body on Trading Standards (LACOTS), PO Box 6, Fell Road, Croydon CR9 1LG.
2 Weights and measures — National Metrological Co-ordination Unit (NMCU), PO Box 6, Fell Road, Croydon CR9 1LG.

(LACOTS and NMCU were established after the 1979 Trading Standards Act.)

Her Majesty's Stationery Office

Copies of the legislation may be obtained from
1 By post — HMSO, PO Box 569, London SE1 9NH.
2 By personal visit — HMSO, 49 High Holborn, London WC1V 6HB.
3 Through local branches of HMSO or through booksellers. HMSO Enquiries: 01-211-5656.

Government departments

Food standards (England and Wales)

Ministry of Agriculture, Fisheries and Food, (Standards Division), Horseferry Road, London SW1P 2AE.

Milk (England and Wales)

Ministry of Agriculture, Fisheries and Food, (Milk and Milk Products Division), 10 Whitehall Place (East block), London SW1A 2HH.

Food standards (Scotland)

Scottish Home and Health Department, St Andrew's House, Edinburgh EH1 3DE.

Milk, imported meat, etc. (Scotland)

Department of Agriculture and Fisheries for Scotland, Chesser House, 500 Gorgie Road, Edinburgh EH11 3AW.

Food and milk (Northern Ireland)

Department of Health and Social Services (Medicines and Food Control Branch), Annexe A, Dundonald House, Upper Newtonards Road, Belfast BT4 3SF.

Trade descriptions (HK)

Department of Trade, (Consumer Affairs Division), Millbank Tower, Millbank, London SW1P 4QU.

Hygiene (England and Wales)

Contact local authority or
Department of Health and Social Security, (Health Services Division), Alexander Fleming House, Elephant and Castle, London SE1 6BY.

Imported Food (England and Wales)

Ministry of Agriculture, Fisheries and Food, (Meat Hygiene Division), Tolworth Tower, Surbiton, Surrey KT6 7DX.

Weights and Measures (UK)

Department of Trade, (Consumer Affairs Division), 26 Chapter Street, London SW1 4NS.

2.18 Food Labelling

The Food Act 1984 (and the regulations made under it) is the main legislation governing the labelling of food in the UK.

The most important *regulation* is The Food Labelling Regulations 1984 which became fully operative in September of that year. In addition, there are regulations which are specific to certain foods, for example, the Meat Regulations which came into force in July 1986. Two Weights and Measures Acts and the Trade Descriptions Act also have an impact on what information is given on a food label.

Because the UK is a member of the EEC, Community Regulations and Directives have to be adopted. EEC Regulations are effective in all member states as soon as they are adopted by the EEC Council. Directives, on the other hand, do not become effective until they are written into a country's legislation.

2.18.1 The Food Labelling Regulations

Almost all food sold to the 'ultimate consumer' or to a catering establishment has to comply with these regulations. Exemptions include certain sugar products, cocoa and chocolate products, honey, condensed and dried milk and cheese. These, and some other foods, have their own special regulations.

Almost all the foods covered by The Food Labelling Regulations must be marked with the following information

1 The name of the food.
2 A list of ingredients.
3 An indication of minimum durability.
4 Any special storage conditions or conditions of use.
5 The name and address of the manufacturer or packer or seller.
6 The place of origin (if omitting this information would mislead the purchaser).
8 Instructions for use (if omitting them would make it difficult to use the product properly).

Ingredients

Nearly all foods which come within the scope of the Food Labelling Regulations must carry a list of ingredients. The few exceptions include fresh fruits and vegetables which are not cut in pieces, carbonated water to which nothing except carbon dioxide has been added, vinegar to which nothing has been added, most cheeses, butters and fermented milks, flavourings, alcoholic drinks with an alcohol content of less than 1.2% by volume and foods which consist of a single ingredient.

When ingredients are listed they must appear in descending order of weight. With the exception of added water, the weight of each ingredient is the amount used during preparation of the food. Water is now generally considered as an ingredient (in the same way as flour, sugar or beef are) but its position in the ingredients list depends on the amount in the final product. Water need not be declared if it is used solely to reconstitute a dried or concentrated ingredient, nor if it is part of a medium not normally consumed, such as the brine in canned vegetables. Water need not be listed if it is 5% or less of the finished product. There are specific EEC regulations governing water in frozen poultry.

If a compound ingredient is used, such as pasta in lasagne, the ingredients may be listed in one of two ways. Either all the consituents of the pasta, meat sauce and cheese sauce are given in one list or the compound ingredient may appear in the appropriate position followed by a list of its ingredients. Thus, in lasagne the ingredients panel may be: water, beef, tomato, semolina, skimmed milk powder, cheese, pork, etc. *or* pasta (semolina, water, egg white), skimmed milk, beef, tomato, vegetable stock, etc.

Additives

All categories of additives must be listed in the ingredients. In every case except flavours the additive must be described by its generic name, for example, acidity regulator and either the specific name, e.g. 'sodium citrate', or the EEC code number or other serial number, e.g. 'E331'. All flavours are covered by the single word 'flavouring(s)'.

Although the current Food Labelling Regulations require more information on the food label than any of the preceding labelling regulations, there may still be ingredients in foods which do not appear on the label.

If an additive is present in an ingredient rather than being added as such to the food it may not need to be listed. For example, sulphite is often added to fruit to preserve it, and if the fruit is made into jam some sulphite may remain in the finished product. If, however, the amount carried over is too small to have any preservative effect on the jam, it need not be declared. Additives used solely as processing aids, for example, tin-greasing agents, do not have to be listed, neither do solvents or carriers of flavours.

If a compound ingredient constitutes less than 25% of the finished product, only its additives, not the main ingredients, need be listed. The other exemption which may be important to dietitians is bread and bread flour. Flour is considered as a single ingredient food and, provided only the additives stipulated in the Bread and Flour Regulations (1984a) are used, they need not appear on the label.

Special emphasis

If one ingredient in a product is given special emphasis, for example, 'with extra fresh cream', the minimum amount of that ingredient (as a percentage of the total product weight) must appear close to the name or in the list of ingredients. Just using the word 'cream' in the name of the food does not constitute special emphasis. Similarly, if particular attention is drawn to the *small* amount of an ingredient, the maximum amount of that ingredient which could be present must be stated.

Minimum durability

Nearly all foods have to be marked with a date up to and including that which the food can reasonably be expected to 'retain its specific properties' if properly stored. The time that any food will keep in good condition depends very much on the storage temperature. This is especially true of frozen and chilled/fresh foods. If a manufacturer is not too sure about the temperatures his food will encounter during distribution and retail display he is going to be very cautious about the 'life' he claims for the food. So, the vast majority of foods are likely to be perfectly edible after the date marked on the packet.

Foods which are exempt from date marking include: foods which are not pre-packed, foods with a shelf life of more than 18 months, eggs, very long life foods such as vinegar and sugar, cheese intended to ripen after it is packed, most alcoholic drinks, fresh fruit and

vegetables which are not peeled or cut, frozen foods and ice cream which carry star marking, flour confectionery and bread intended to be eaten within 24 hours.

The date which appears on the packet depends on the expected 'life' of the food. If it is less than six weeks the label must show either 'sell by' followed by a day and month and an indication of the time the food may be stored in the home *or* 'best before' followed by a day and month.

Foods with an expected life of six weeks to three months must show 'best before' followed by a day and month. Those with a life of three months to 18 months must state either 'best before' followed by a day, month and year *or* 'best before end' followed by a month and year. Foods with an expected shelf life of more than 18 months do not *have* to carry any date but they *may* show a 'best before' or 'best before end' date. In all cases, if any special storage conditions such as refrigeration are necessary, these must be shown close to the date.

Weight

Nearly all packaged foods have to show the net weight in g, the volume in ml or some other approved measure. The imperial measure may also be given. Where a weight is given, it must be the average contents of packs provided that no pack has an unreasonable deficiency. 'Unreasonable deficiency' is defined and the tolerances allowed are so tight that far more than half the packs have to contain more than the declared weight if the regulations are to be met. So the move from declaration of minimum weight to average weight which might appear to be against the consumer's interest has not had any detrimental effect.

Claims

The Food Labelling Regulations make provision for certain claims on labels and elsewhere. They do not state precisely what constitutes a claim, but many enforcement authorities regard any statement as a claim and, therefore, subject to the provisions of the regulations. But the regulations do say that a statement of the energy content of a food is not a claim.

A special schedule in the regulations specifies the criteria which must be met if certain words or descriptions are to be used. Of special interest to dietitians are the criteria for use of the words 'dietary' and 'dietetic'. They may be applied to food which

'has been specially made for a class of person whose

digestive process or metabolism is disturbed or who, by reason of their special physiological condition, obtain special benefit from a controlled consumption of certain substances'.

Also, the food has to be

'suitable for fulfilling the particular nutritional requirements of the class of person'.

A food may be described as 'starch reduced' if less than 50% of the dry food is anhydrous carbohydrate and the starch content is substantially less than that of the same weight of similar food to which the description is *not* applied.

A drink may be described as 'tonic wine' only if the words 'the name tonic wine does not imply health-giving or medicinal properties' appear close by.

Diabetic claims

Diabetic claims may be made only if a number of conditions are met (see Section 2.13). Among them are that the food must not normally be higher in fat or energy than a similar food not carrying a diabetic claim, and it must not contain more mono or disaccharide (other than fructose) than is necessary.

A diabetic food must state that it is not suitable for overweight diabetics unless the energy value is 50% or less than that of an equivalent food for which no diabetic claim is made.

If a diabetic food contains fructose, sorbitol, mannitol, xylitol, isomalt or hydrogenated glucose syrup, the label must make the recommendation that a total of no more than 25 g of these substances should be eaten daily. It must also show the amounts of these carbohydrates, total carbohydrate content and 'other' carbohydrates present.

Slimming claims

Slimming claims may be made only if the food is 'capable of contributing to weight loss'. The claim must be accompanied by the words 'Can help slimming or weight control only as part of a calorie (or joule or energy) controlled diet'.

If a food is claimed to be reduced energy it must have an energy value of no more than 75% that of the same weight of an equivalent food which does not carry a reduced energy claim.

To qualify for a *low* energy claim a food must contain no more than 167 kJ (40 kcal)/100 g or 100 ml and the energy value of a normal portion must be no more than 167 kJ (40 kcal).

Nutrition labelling

The current Food Labelling Regulations make provision for food producers to give some nutrition information. But the whole subject of nutrition labelling is in a state of flux following the publication of the COMA report on Diet and Cardiovascular Disease in 1984. It seems likely that new legislation will be passed to supplement the 1984 Food Labelling Regulations.

The 1984 these regulations do not in any way seek to prevent food producers giving nutrition information on labels which is intended 'exclusively for persons qualified in dentistry, medicine, nutrition, dietetics or pharmacy'. In contrast, the information which COMA recommended should be on packs would be for consumers to use to help them select a nutritionally better diet.

Under current regulations, if a nutrition claim is made it must be accompanied by a statement of the energy (kJ and kcal), fat, protein and carbohydrate value of the food as sold and expressed per 100 g or 100 ml of food. Additional information for a quantified portion may also be given.

The 1984 Regulations also stipulate conditions which must be met if a protein, vitamin or mineral claim is made and if a food is claimed to be high in energy or polyunsaturated fats or low in cholesterol.

The regulations forbid claims that a food has tonic properties or that an artificial baby food is superior to breast milk from a healthy mother.

Fat labelling

The draft proposals for fat labelling, based on the 1984 COMA Report on Diet and Cardiovascular Disease, will make it compulsory for most foods to show the total fat in g/100 g or 100 ml and the amount of saturated fatty acids in g/100 g or 100 ml of food as sold. Whether trans fatty acids will have to be included in the saturated fat figure is being debated. The only foods which would be exempt from the need to declare fat content, it is proposed, would be those with less than 0.5% fat, fresh fruits and vegetables, herbs, spices, seasonings, milk in bottles and bread, flour and cereals as defined in the Bread and Flour Regulations 1984(a). Food for immediate consumption would also be exempt.

Although data would have to relate to food as sold, manufacturers would probably have the option of giving information about cooked food provided the cooking method was stipulated on packs.

Much remains to be resolved about the details, but it is to be hoped that legislators do not lose sight of the objective, namely, to help ordinary, non-expert people choose and eat food which is lower in fat.

Full nutrition labelling

At the same time as the draft Fat labelling Regulations were published, guidelines for fuller nutrition information were issued by the Ministry of Agriculture, Fisheries and Food. It is not intended that these should be mandatory but it is recommended that, if manufacturers do give fuller information, they should follow the proposed format. This, it is hoped, will enable shoppers to compare products and reduce the confusion which might result if many different formats were used.

Views about how much information should be given on labels vary. Some authorities believe that, unless people have the complete nutrition picture, including vitamins and minerals, they will be misled. Others believe that such a large amount of information is both unnecessary and confusing and will detract from the main issues which, they argue, are to prevent or correct obesity and reduce total and saturated fat intake.

After much debate and some consumer research, draft guidelines suggest formats for three levels of nutrition information beyond the basic fat labelling which will be mandatory.

1 At the first level it is suggested that manufacturers could declare fat and saturated fat, protein, carbohydrate and energy.

2 At the second level they could declare fat and saturated fat, protein, carbohydrate and sugar, energy and sodium. Dietary fibre may also be stated if the manufacturer wishes. He may also declare any or all of the following — monounsaturates, polyunsaturates and starch.

3 The third level would allow specified vitamins and minerals to be added to the nutrients stipulated in the second level.

As well as giving information in numerical form and figures relating to food as sold, it is suggested that some pictorial device could be included as an optional extra. The one proposed is based on a bar chart and shows only fat, protein and carbohydrate content. Manufacturers will probably be free to give nutrition information about cooked or ready-to-eat products as well as food as sold if they wish to do so.

Undoubtedly, legislation affecting nutrition labelling and claims will change far more in the late 1980s and the remaining years of the 20 the century than it did in the preceding decades. What these changes will be is speculation, but it seems very likely that the draft proposals for Fat Content of Food (Labelling) Regulations published in 1986 will be adopted.

Further reading

Committee on Medical Aspects of Food Policy (1984) *Diet and Cardiovascular Disease*. HMSO, London.
The Food Labelling Regulations (1984) SI 1305. HMSO, London.
Weights and Measures Acts (1985; 1985(a)). HMSO, London.
The Food Act (1984). HMSO, London.

Section 3 **Nutritional Needs of Population Sub-groups**

3.1 Pregnancy

3.1.1 Preconceptional and periconceptional nutrition

Preconceptional nutrition in men

The preconceptional effect of diet in men is a poorly researched area. Most studies relating to this subject have been carried out in animals and the relevance of this to humans is unclear. It is however known that gross dietary inadequacies or excesses in men can affect either the likelihood of and/or the outcome of conception. For example, undernutrition delays puberty and in adults reduces sex drive and performance, while both undernutrition and gross obesity alter sex hormone production (Calloway 1983). Zinc deficiency can reduce sperm numbers while iodine deficiency lessens libido and androsterone production (Calloway 1983). Cadmium, boron, titanium and excess molybdenum can all injure the gonads (Calloway 1983), and postnatal mental development can be adversely affected by preconceptual exposure to lead which produces abnormal sperm while still permitting conception (Bryce-Smith 1985). Alcohol increases zinc loss and may interfere with vitamin A metabolism (Calloway 1983).

The effects of lesser degrees of dietary imbalance are unknown. The most prudent preconceptional nutritional advice for men at the present time would therefore appear to be to consume an adequate and varied diet, to correct grossly abnormal body weight and to moderate alcohol intake. Any such changes should probably be made at least 2−3 months before the intended time of conception.

Preconceptional and periconceptional nutrition in women

Nutrition and fertility

In female adolescents undernutrition delays the onset of menstruation and interferes with ovulation and the maturation required for best reproductive outcome (Wishik 1977). Amenorrhoea and infertility is a well recognized complication of the excessive weight loss induced by anorexia nervosa. Milder degrees of weight loss in women following slimming regimens can also cause amenorrhoea (Fries 1974). As the Body Mass Index (BMI) falls, the risk of infertility increases, as do other forms of reproductive failure, until at an index of 18 only 10% of women are still fertile. Maximum fertility appears to occur with a BMI at the higher end of the normal range. However, even at this level, infertility can still occur if other dietary inadequacies exist, e.g. pyridoxine induced amenorrhoea (Wynn and Wynn 1981). Underweight women should be encouraged to gain weight prior to conception with the emphasis placed on dietary quality.

Nutrition and early foetal development

The foetus is most susceptible to nutritional imbalance during the first trimester of pregnancy since this is the time of most rapid cell differentation and establishment of embryonic systems and organs (Basu 1981). The time of greatest nutritional vulnerability is possibly before a woman even suspects she is pregnant, and certainly before the first antenatal appointment. Dietary advice should therefore be targeted preconceptionally so that the appropriate nutritional safeguards have been adopted by the time pregnancy occurs.

Much remains to be learnt about the intricacies of nutrition and early foetal development. However, several areas can be highlighted as being of particular relevance

Undernutrition. During the Dutch 'hunger winter' of October 1944−May 1945 there was significantly increased perinatal mortality and low birth weight (LBW) among babies born in the latter half of the period, but even greater perinatal mortality and LBW among babies *conceived* in the latter half of this period (Wynn and Wynn 1981). There were also significantly increased rates of infertility and malformations, the latter persisting among babies conceived in the four months immediately after the end of the food shortage. During this period women who were infertile, and thus protected from pregnancy in adverse circumstances, gradually regained their fertility. This transition period between infertility and fertility (called the penumbra) appears to be associated with a high rate of malformations.

Although overt food shortage is rare in the UK, its consequences are seen in the sufferer from anorexia nervosa. Pregnancy is of course unlikely to occur during the anorexic state itself, but fertility will return during the recovery phase and pregnancy at this time is perhaps inadvisable.

Mild undernutrition, however, is relatively common. Poor eating habits may be due to factors such as ignorance or low income. However, 'slimming' is perhaps the greatest hazard. Large numbers of women spend periods of time following 'diets' of dubious nutritional quality. Additionally, overweight women trying to start a family are often encouraged to lose weight because of the increased risks of late pregnancy complications and perinatal mortality in overweight mothers (Naeye 1979; Edwards et al 1979). It is preferable for weight to be reduced well in advance of conception in order to lessen the likelihood of nutritional inadequacy. If this is not practicable, then efforts should be made to ensure that the diet is adequate in terms of quality for at least 3–4 months prior to the intended time of conception.

Vitamins. An adequate intake of folate may be important in preventing neural tube defects (NTD) in a minority of women. Periconceptional supplements of folic acid, either alone or in conjunction with other vitamins, given to mothers who have previously given birth to a child with NTD appears to reduce the risk of having another NTD birth (Smithells et al 1980, 1981a, 1981b; Holmes-Siedle et al 1982; Laurence et al 1981). Since mothers already delivered of a child with NTD may in some way differ from the rest of the population, it is not yet clear whether such measures would produce similar benefits in the general population. Since the lower socioeconomic groups have both poorer diets and the highest incidence of NTD (Bennett 1982; Doyle et al 1982), it would seem advisable to target preconceptional dietary advice at these groups, emphasizing foods which are good sources of vitamins, especially folic acid. If an improved diet is to be effective it must be altered at least 28 days before conception, since depleted folate stores have to be restored before any significant rise in serum folate can occur (Smithells 1983).

Oral contraception. It has been suggested that the prolonged use of oral contraceptives may be associated with altered plasma levels of trace elements, vitamins and proteins, in particular zinc, folate and B6 (Prasad et al 1977). Couples should be advised that for three or four months before trying to conceive they should use an alternative contraceptive method (not the coil since small amounts of copper from them may prevent embryogenesis) to allow regulation of the woman's body. If glucose tolerance has been impaired since beginning oral contraception, improvement may result from vitamin B6 supplements of 2–3 times the recommended daily intake (Belsey 1977).

Alcohol. Excessive drinking in early pregnancy can cause the foetal alcohol syndrome, characterized by mental and physical retardation. Whether more moderate levels of alcohol intake are harmful at this stage is unknown. However, alcohol is known to affect the absorption, metabolism and excretion of a number of nutrients, particularly zinc, magnesium, copper and iron (Mendelson 1984) and it could therefore compromise trace element status at a vital stage.

To err on the safe side, pre and periconceptional advice should probably recommend alcohol exclusion. However, once pregnancy is established, the occasional 'drink' is unlikely to cause harm (see next section).

The nutritional aspects of preconceptional counselling for women are summarized in Table 3.1.

Table 3.1 Nutritional aspects of preconceptional counselling for women

1	Make dietary changes at least 3–4 months before attempting conception.
2	Achieve acceptable body weight for height.
3	Eat a diet with adequate energy.
4	Eat a varied diet to ensure intake of all nutrients.
5	Restrict, or preferably exclude, alcohol.
6	Seek advice from a doctor before taking any dietary supplements.

3.1.2 Nutritional considerations during the second and third trimesters of pregnancy

Nutritional requirements

During the second and third trimesters of pregnancy, rapid growth of the foetus inevitably imposes increased nutritional demands on the mother. However, the extent to which these increased needs must be met by dietary adjustment is less clear. Although RDAs can be calculated which take the nutritional cost of pregnancy into account, these figures cannot be applied indiscriminately to all pregnant women for two reasons

1 RDAs are set at a level which should prevent nutritional deficiencies in the vast majority of the population (see Section 1.3). The *actual* requirement of many individuals will be considerably less than the RDA.

2 As a physiological response to pregnancy, there is considerable adaptation to the increased nutritional needs. The absorption of many nutrients is increased and their excretion decreased, and metabolism is generally more efficient. In general, RDAs do not take these factors into account and thus may be unnecessarily high.

Nevertheless, there will be some pregnant women in whom the nutritional needs will not be met. The dietitian's role is to identify those who are nutritionally at risk and to recommend appropriate dietary measures.

The most important aspects to consider are

Energy

Hytten (1980) calculates the total energy cost of pregnancy to be about 84,000 kcal. This is the energy cost of the extra protein and fat in maternal tissues and in the product of conception, plus the extra energy cost of maintaining the maternal tissues and the foetus. The daily extra energy requirement is calculated to be about 100 kcal in the first quarter of pregnancy and 300–400 kcal in the remaining three quarters.

However, there are energy savings in terms of physical and metabolic activity. 'The pregnant woman...is relatively listless, spends more time at rest and performs tasks with more economy of effort...there is a general relaxation of voluntary muscle, and a reduction in free thyroid hormone...(which) possibly allows all maternal tissues to metabolize at a slightly reduced tempo' (Hytten 1980). Evidence to support this latter hypothesis has come from recent studies in the Gambia, where Lawrence et al (1984) have shown the actual cumulative cost of resting metabolism to be considerably below the theoretical cost calculated by Hytten. In women eating the normal Gambian diet the cumulative cost was only 1000 kcal; in women receiving food supplements it was 13,000 kcal, whereas Hytten calculated a need for 36,000 kcal.

Earlier dietary surveys suggested that pregnant women might eat about 200 kcal/day more than non-pregnant women. On this basis the RDA for pregnancy has been set at an extra 250 kcal/day (DHSS 1979) with the assumption that the remainder of the energy costs would be covered by reductions in activity. More recent dietary surveys, summarized by Black et al (1986) suggest that pregnant women may not increase their intake even by this much.

In practical terms, the best guide to individual energy requirements during pregnancy is the rate of weight gain (see p 250). If this remains within desirable limits, there is no need to adjust the energy intake. Instead, attention should be focused on the nutrient density of the diet to ensure sufficiency of all other nutrients.

Protein

The protein requirements specific to pregnancy are estimated at 900 g in total, or 5 g/day during the last two trimesters (Hytten and Leitch 1971). The majority of UK diets provide more than enough protein. However, it is possible for protein intakes to fall below the estimated minimum requirement of 44 g in those women habitually taking low energy diets which have low nutrient density. For example, a diet of 1500 kcal containing 10% protein energy, contains only 37.5 g protein. Individuals in 'at risk' groups (see p 250) may need special guidance.

Minerals and trace elements

Iron. Typical iron losses incurred as a result of pregnancy comprise

Iron transferred to the foetus	300 mg
Placenta and cord iron	50 mg
Postpartum blood loss	200 mg
Total	550 mg

Offset against this is the saving of 200 mg due to the absence of menstruation, making a net iron cost to the body of 350 mg. This represents a theoretical extra requirement over the non-pregnant state of 1.8 mg iron/day during the second and third trimesters.

In addition to this, the body requires approximately 500 mg iron for the expansion in red cell mass which occurs after 12 weeks. Normally this is met from internal reserves and creates no extra requirement. However, if iron stores are depleted at the start of pregnancy then, theoretically, an additional 2.6 mg/day will be required from dietary sources throughout the last two trimesters.

While these estimates of additional daily needs are convenient, they are not totally realistic. They assume that the requirement for iron remains constant throughout the last two trimesters whereas, in fact, proportionally less is needed at 12 weeks and correspondingly more as term approaches.

Nevertheless, provided that habitual iron intake is adequate, it seems likely that the extra requirement to cover iron *losses* can be met through physiological adaptation and without the need for a dietary increase. Iron absorption not only increases during pregnancy, but increases progressively as pregnancy advances, therefore meeting the rising demand (Bowering et al 1979). Furthermore, a greater percentage increase in absorption will occur in anaemic than in non-anaemic women. Apte and Iyenger (1970) showed that iron absorption rose from 7.4% at the 16th week of pregnancy to 25.7% in the third trimester; in those who were anaemic, iron absorption rose to 37.9%. Even a lower than average dietary iron intake is not necessarily an indication for supplementation since this too will tend to be offset by an increased absorption (Bowering et al 1979).

However, in women who start pregnancy without adequate iron stores, the situation may be rather different. Low reserves in conjunction with a low iron intake will inevitably result in iron deficiency. It is this group of women who require dietary intervention and, probably, iron supplementation. The problem is that this sub-group is not easy to identify. Some indication of iron stores can be derived from the serum ferritin level but this is rarely carried out as a routine measure. Conversely, regular measurements are usually made of the blood haemoglobin level, although this is not a sensitive reflector of iron status. A fall in haemoglobin during pregnancy does not necessarily indicate iron insufficiency; more usually it is simply a dilution effect caused by the expansion in plasma volume. On the other hand, if iron deficiency is present, few clinicians would wish to wait until frank anaemia (a low haemoglobin coupled with reduced red cell size) appears before instituting corrective therapy. It is for this reason that routine iron supplementation to all pregnant women is so common even though for the majority it is unnecessary.

However, some antenatal clinics do now adopt a more discriminatory approach to iron supplementation. Iron supplements are not always well tolerated and significant numbers of women suffer from nausea, diarrhoea or constipation (Bennett 1982; Lind 1983). There is also some evidence to suggest that unnecessary supplementation may do more harm than good; Lind (1983) showed that iron supplements resulted in an increased mean cell volume (MCV) compared with that in unsupplemented pregnant women. This increased red cell size may be highly undesirable since it could affect blood flow in small capillaries and impair oxygen and/or nutrient supply to the placenta. It has also been suggested that the level of iron supplement commonly used may adversely affect maternal zinc status (Solomons and Jacob 1981; Hambidge et al 1983).

Ideally, rather than routine supplementation, iron insufficiency should be diagnosed and corrected preconceptionally or at an early stage of pregnancy before physiological changes make the usual laboratory indices difficult to interpret.

If women are not seen until pregnancy is more advanced, efforts should be made to identify those who appear to have a habitually low iron intake. If subsequent screening then reveals either a haemoglobin of 10.0 g/dl in association with a MCV of 82 fl or less, or a progressive fall in MCV, dietary intervention or supplementation is indicated.

In women who have neither evidence of nor a history of anaemia, the advice to include some meat in the diet every day is probably sufficient (haem iron from animal sources is better absorbed than inorganic iron from vegetable sources). In those who are vegetarian, care should be taken to ensure that the diet is high in vitamin C (which improves the absorption of inorganic iron) and that phytate intake from cereals which impairs absorption is not excessive.

Calcium. The metabolism of calcium in pregnancy has been summarized by Reeve (1980). A baby at birth contains 25–30 g calcium, most of which is laid down in the last ten weeks of pregnancy. The requirement specific to pregnancy is for approximately 260 mg (6.5 mmol)/day at this time.

However, absorption from the diet increases early in pregnancy and is doubled by 24 weeks (Heaney and Skillman 1971). Thus, in the presence of adequate supplies of vitamin D, the increased requirement is almost certainly met by increased absorption. Although the RDA for pregnancy is set at 1.2 g (30 mmol), there is no evidence to suggest that the UK intakes of 0.8–1.0 g (20–25 mmol) are inadequate.

There is also evidence that even in populations with habitual intakes as low as 400 mg/day (10 mmol), increased absorption can compensate for the increased requirements of pregnancy (Shenolikar 1970; Walker et al 1972).

Calcium absorption is lower in the presence of high fibre intakes, therefore it would be wise, in view of widespread advice to increase fibre intakes, to ensure that pregnant mothers have an intake of at least 800 mg/day.

Special attention should be given to Asian mothers who may have a low vitamin D status and consume diets low in calcium and high in fibre. The addition of any one of the following to the usual diet will provide approximately an additional 300 mg calcium

1 Half a pint of milk.
2 One small piece (30–40 g) cheddar cheese.
3 One small carton yoghurt.
4 Two teaspoons dried milk powder (mixed to a thick cream and added to soups, mashed potato or porridge *or* added dry when baking).

5 One 50 g scone.

6 One 90 g serving of sardines or similar fish with soft bones.

7 One 90 g serving of custard or other milk pudding or dessert.

Zinc. Zinc is of current interest because levels of both plasma and white cell zinc (the latter indicative of zinc stores) fall during pregnancy and many women appear to consume less than the amounts thought to be required. In addition, some of the dietary measures adopted by pregnant women (in particular increased intakes of iron and cereal fibre) may impair zinc absorption. It has been suggested recently that zinc status may be significantly lower in mothers delivered of small-for-dates babies (Truswell 1985).

The significance of these observations, and whether dietary intervention is necessary, remains to be evaluated by further research. But it is possible that dietary zinc may become an issue of some importance in the future.

Dietary sources of zinc are discussed in Section 2.8

Vitamins

Although routine multivitamin supplementation is common, it is probably unnecessary other than in those in high risk groups (see below) or where there is evidence of dietary inadequacy. Most pregnant women can meet their vitamin needs by consuming a diet of adequate quality. Vitamins which may be particularly important in pregnancy are

Folate. The requirement for folate is increased during pregnancy (Chanarin *et al* 1968) and, if looked for, evidence of megaloblastic changes can be found in substantial numbers of women in late pregnancy (Truswell 1985). However, the actual requirement is a matter of some debate and the DHSS has recently withdrawn folate from its table of RDAs owing to insubstantial data (DHSS 1985).

Pregnant women should be encouraged to include good sources of folate in their diet (e.g. yeast extracts, liver and green leafy vegetables). In some women folate supplements may be necessary.

Vitamin D. Vitamin D is important in order to sustain the heightened calcium absorption and utilization which occurs in pregnancy. Normally, the body's requirement for vitamin D is supplied through exposure to sunlight, but whether the increased needs during pregnancy can be met via this route is unclear. In France (where food

is not supplemented with vitamin D) vitamin D deficiency is common in mothers and neonates especially during winter and spring in areas where sunlight is scarce (Salle 1982). Brooke (1983) showed that vitamin D supplemented Asian women gained more weight than unsupplemented controls, and had fewer small-for-dates infants.

For most women, diets which regularly contain vitamin D-enriched margarines or butter, full fat milk or cheese, fatty fish and eggs are probably adequate in vitamin D. All pregnant women should be encouraged to get out of doors as much as possible. Supplements may be necessary for at risk individuals, especially Asian women, and should be accompanied by clear written instructions in the appropriate language to avoid any possibility of vitamin D overdose.

Vitamin C. There is little evidence to suggest that vitamin C intakes below the RDA for pregnant women present any hazard, and the RDA is probably rather high. Nevertheless, because vitamin C adequacy can so easily, and safely, be achieved by the inclusion of a glass of fruit juice each day, this is usually recommended to mothers. If this is disliked as being 'too acid' it may be more acceptable if mixed with soda water or lemonade. For those who dislike citrus fruit in any form, a vitamin C-fortified drink such as blackcurrant cordial or rose-hip syrup are possible alternatives. Particular attention should be paid to the vitamin C intake of women who continue to smoke during pregnancy.

Alcohol

Although alcohol avoidance may be a wise precaution in the early stages of pregnancy (see Section 3.1.1), whether this needs to continue throughout pregnancy is debatable. While it has been suggested that the regular consumption of 1−2 drinks a day may increase mid-term abortion rates (Harlap and Shiono 1980) other studies have shown no significant difference in pregnancy outcome between those with light and heavy prepregnancy drinking habits (Wright *et al* 1983). In the light of present evidence it seems appropriate to caution women against regular or heavy drinking during pregnancy but total abstinence appears unnecessary.

Dietary guidelines for pregnant women not in at risk groups are summarized in Table 3.2. However, these are only guidelines and will vary according to individual energy needs, food preferences and socioeconomic circumstances.

Table 3.2 Dietary guidance for the last 2 trimesters of pregnancy. The diet of pregnant women *without* special nutritional needs will probably be adequate if it includes the following foods on a daily basis

---

1 serving of meat* (preferably red).
1 serving of fish or cheese or eggs or pulses.
2 servings of bread, breakfast cereals, pasta or rice (preferably wholemeal or wholegrain varieties).
1 serving of potatoes.
2 servings of other vegetables (including a green leafy vegetable).
1 glass fruit juice (or 2 portions of fruit, one of them citrus).
1 pint of milk (or its calcium equivalent in yoghurt, cheese or scones).
Some butter or vitamin D-fortified margarine or low fat spread.

---

*Vegetarians need special dietary guidance (see Section 3.8)

Non-nutritional factors

Environmental toxins

It has been found that the higher the placental cadmium and/or lead levels, the lower the foetal birth weight and head circumference (Bryce-Smith 1985). Placental tissue lead levels have also been correlated with malformations, stillbirth and neonatal death (Bryce-Smith 1985).

Smoking

Smoking causes premature ageing of the placenta, leading to damaged blood vessels which increase the risk of stillbirth due to placental haemorrhage and prematurity. Smokers may have an elevated serum copper level which increases the need for vitamin C and can antagonize zinc absorption. Smoking also results in the production of cyanide which requires vitamin B12 for its metabolism; smokers therefore tend to have low serum B12 levels. If these increased requirements, caused by smoking, are not met, foetal development may be impaired.

Factors implicated in a poor outcome to pregnancy

Parents who fall into one or more of the following categories should be monitored closely and the foetus considered at risk. Dietary counselling is particularly important for the following groups:

1 Adolescent mothers. If pregnancy follows soon after menarche, those with a late menarche are likely to be more developed and therefore less at risk than those with an early menarche (Beal 1981). Thomas (1984) recommends a pregnancy weight gain of around 14 kg for the normal weight teenager.

2 Women more than 20% above or 10% below ideal body weight (Pitkin 1981).

3 Immigrant women who may be consuming an inadequate diet in this country.

4 Vegans or vegetarians who follow an inadequate diet.

5 Women with bizarre eating habits such as those suffering with bulimia nervosa.

6 Families with a limited food budget or food management problems.

7 Women with closely spaced pregnancies.

8 Parents with pre-existing medical complications, such as diabetes mellitus or gastrointestinal disease.

9 Women with a poor obstetric history including low birth weight babies (less than 2500 g), spontaneous abortion, prolonged labour, and abruptio placenta.

10 Exposure of either parent to high levels of cadmium or lead via water supplies, food, occupation or place of residence (Stephens 1981).

11 Parents with alcohol or drug problems.

12 Parents who smoke or are constantly exposed to cigarette smoke (Grant 1981).

Weight gain during pregnancy

Desirable weight gain during pregnancy

Naeye (1979) has shown that the lowest incidence of foetal and neonatal death is associated with a weight gain of

1 9 kg (for those who commence pregnancy at 80−120% of ideal weight).

2 7.5 kg (for those who are overweight at the start of pregnancy).

3 13.5 kg (for those who are underweight at the start of pregnancy).

For all three groups, perinatal mortality rates increased with gains less or more than these values.

However, assessing 'desirable' weight gain during pregnancy is complicated by the fact that it is difficult to distinguish between weight gain caused by fat deposition and weight gain due to fluid retention. Hytten and Leitch (1971) found that overweight women tended to gain more water and less fat than thin women, while Campbell (1983) found that primigravidae who restricted their food intake gained less weight than those who ate to appetite. However, the difference was mainly due to reduced fluid retention in the restricted group. Young teenage mothers may have high weight gains but these have been attributed to increased fluid volume and fluid retention rather than additions to body mass (Garn *et al* 1984).

Excessive weight gain

In obese pregnant women, limitation of weight gain has been and still is practiced in order to reduce high blood pressure, pre-eclampsia and gestational diabetes, to prevent the birth of large babies, to ease delivery and to prevent long term obesity. However, the benefits of limiting weight gain are questionable and it may have adverse effects. In some studies dietary restriction has failure to lower blood pressure or reduce pre-eclampsia, but it has reduced birth weight Campbell and MacGillivray 1975; Campbell 1983). Although it has been suggested that this is unimportant as the baby is merely deprived of optional fat reserves (Hytten 1983), any fall in birth weight is undesirable since neonatal mortality rates increase at birth weights less than 3400 g (van den Berg 1981). In addition, Campbell (1983) found that gestation was longer in a diet-restricted group of women, i.e. 32% delivered later than 40 weeks compared with 15% of controls.

Inadequate weight gain

Poor weight gain may be a result of prolonged nausea and vomiting. Some women cope with nausea by eating small starchy meals and as long as they eat frequently, weight gain should be maintained.

Many women may fear what they consider excessive weight gain and thus follow a self-imposed energy restricted diet. They should be encouraged towards accepting a realistic weight gain and advised that weight loss after birth is aided by breast feeding.

If the diet is suspected of being low in energy it should be checked for all nutrients and if necessary suggestions made for improving the quality, if not quantity, of food consumed.

If financial problems are a cause of the poor intake, some suggestions for eating well on a low income may be helpful (see Section 3.7). The social worker may also be able to offer advice regarding social security benefits.

3.1.3 Nutrition-related problems in pregnancy

Nausea and vomiting

Estimates of the incidence of nausea and vomiting in pregnancy vary between 50−86% (Taggart 1961; Soules *et al* 1980; Bennett 1982; Pickard 1982; Doyle *et al* 1982). Psychological factors, hormonal or endocrine changes, vitamin deficiencies and altered carbohydrate metabolism have all been proposed as explanations for the condition but it is still poorly understood.

The symptoms may start before the first missed period or sometimes not until well into pregnancy. They are most common around the 6−9th week and usually worst around the 9th−10th weeks, subsiding generally around the 12−16th week, but occasionally lasting throughout pregnancy. Either weight gain or weight loss may occur during this period.

Nausea can be either slight or extreme. It often becomes worse when the stomach is empty and is usually relieved by eating. This relief may be temporary or last for several hours. It may be triggered by long journeys or some smells such as food, perfume or cigarette smoke. Hunger may occur at the same time as nausea and can be relieved if the mother can eat a meal without having to prepare it herself. Appetite is often increased but may be decreased. Some women may experience retching first thing in the morning and before meals.

Morning sickness is a common problem. Some women feel that they need to vomit to cure the associated nausea and then feel better for the rest of the day. Morning sickness can be minimized by keeping the bedroom well ventilated and free of smoke. A bedtime snack and a dry biscuit or toast 10−15 minutes before getting up, followed by a light breakfast soon after rising, can help. Vomiting may also occur both during and after meals and when travelling.

Nausea and vomiting may be aggravated by iron supplements or other tablets. Other symptoms occurring in conjunction with nausea and vomiting can include unquenchable thirst, a metallic taste and excessive salivation.

All of these symptoms may be partially relieved by plenty of rest, fresh air and avoidance of long journeys, but nutritional advice is also important. Carbohydrate foods, particularly if taken in snack form and at frequent (e.g. two hourly) intervals, provide the most relief although the reason for this is not clear. Some suitable snacks are listed in Table 3.3. The mother should be reassured that snacks can be as nourishing as conventional meals and encouraged to feel she is still eating 'properly.' Some women worry that frequent

Table 3.3 Snacks which may help alleviate nausea and vomiting during pregnancy

Toast and jam (no butter).
Sandwiches (low fat filling).
Plain biscuits and cheese spread.
Breakfast cereals with low fat milk.
Milk puddings with low fat milk.
Soup and crackers.
Cold instant puddings, yoghurt (low fat varieties).
Jacket potatoes with a low fat filling (e.g. cottage cheese or baked beans).
Hot or cold low fat milky drinks.
Lean cold meat or poultry with a potato or roll.
Fruit salad and cottage cheese.

carbohydrate snacks will cause excessive weight gain. They should be reassured that whatever minimizes their symptoms is best for them and that they will probably return to their normal eating pattern within 14–15 weeks of pregnancy (Pickard, personal communication).

If long journeys are unavoidable, the mother may take fruit, sandwiches, biscuits or boiled sweets with her and use them to help ward off nausea.

Hyperemesis gravidarum

Hyperemesis gravidarum is the condition of excessive or uncontrollable vomiting during pregnancy. The aetiology is unknown but it may occur in about 0.2% of all pregnancies (Pickard, personal communication). Early intervention is important and should follow an approach similar to the management of nausea and vomiting but with additional use of low osmolality fluids such as Hycal.

Pickard (personal communications) reported that mothers found the only way to prevent hospitalization was to force themselves to eat and, more importantly, to drink to try to prevent dehydration. If the vomiting is severe enough to cause dehydration, electrolyte imbalance, urinary ketones of 4+, and a total body weight loss of more than 5% of prepregnancy weight, then hospitalization is essential.

Once hospitalized, initial attention must focus on intravenous rehydration, correction of electrolyte imbalance and energy provision. Vitamins, minerals and trace elements should also be supplied as these may be severely depleted. As soon as is practical, a diet history should be taken with particular reference to foods and flavours tolerated or disliked and any special nutritional problems experienced by the mother in the past. Small frequent feeds of clear fluids should be introduced initially and continued for at least 24 hours. Once these are well tolerated, small quantities of liquid energy, or preferably complete food, supplements should be taken at frequent intervals. As tolerance improves the amounts can be increased gradually until intake approaches the mother's daily requirement. She can then be given three small meals a day. Small supplemental drinks should still be given between meals but phased out gradually as the meals increase in size. The mother's body weight, electrolytes, urinary ketones, fluid balance and food consumption should be monitored throughout and she should be discharged once she is tolerating her oral regimens and progressively gaining weight. She should be instructed to have at least three meals a day at home. There should be frequent follow-up with immediate readmission and initiation of supplementary feeds if there is any decrease in weight.

Taste alterations and pica

Estimates of altered taste preferences vary from 45% in Japan to 65% in Scotland and 85% in the USA (Taggart 1961; Sugiura et al 1983; Schwab and Axelson 1984) and many women find their experience differs considerably between pregnancies. Preferences for fruit, salad vegetables, starchy foods and strong tasting foods are frequently reported, and increased milk consumption is not uncommon even among those who disliked it before pregnancy. Aversions to fried or fatty food, alcohol and smoking are the most common, to hot meat dishes and coffee fairly frequent and to tea less frequent. Tea and coffee may be reported to have an odd taste. Other foods and drinks may be the subject of either cravings or aversions, e.g. cheese, eggs, ice cream or confectionery.

Brewin (1980) has found similar appetite changes in men and women with tumours. In both situations there is a rapid return to normal taste perception with delivery of the baby or removal of the tumour.

Pica refers to the habit, often obsessional, of consuming substances not usually classified as food, e.g. clay, coal or chalk. It is most commonly reported in children and pregnant women.

The true incidence of pica during pregnancy is unclear as women are naturally reluctant to admit to eating items such as coal, disinfectant, soap, toothpaste, spent matchheads and laundry starch (Hytten and Leitch 1971). Schwab and Axelson (1984) reported an incidence of 7% and Taggart (1961) only 1%. It appears that the incidence has diminished in recent years, although the reason for this is unknown.

Heartburn

Gastro-oesophageal reflux can start as early as the third month but is generally worse in the third trimester and occurs in 30–50% of women (Taggart 1961; Seymour and Chadwick 1979). Davison et al (1970) found that women with heartburn had slower gastric emptying times than those without.

Small, frequent meals or snacks are usually tolerated better than infrequent large ones. Milk and yoghurt help relieve the symptoms in some people but antacids tend to be widely used. Spicy and fatty foods, fizzy drinks, citrus fruit and fruit juices and bananas may exacerbate the problem.

Constipation

During pregnancy the gastrointestinal tract shows a general reduction in motility, and transit times are prolonged (Hytten 1983). If constipation is a problem while the mother is on iron supplements, the doctor should be asked to consider reducing or stopping them if frank iron deficiency anaemia is not present. In other respects, management of constipation requires the usual high fluid/high fibre regimen suitably modified if the mother is nauseated.

Pre-eclampsia

The cause of pre-eclampsia (pregnancy induced hypertension) is unknown. Excessive weight gain, general undernutrition and inadequate intakes of specific nutrients such as protein, vitamin B6, folic acid, calcium, magnesium and essential fatty acids have all been suggested as causative factors but there is no conclusive evidence implicating any of them (Horrobin 1981).

In the past, restricting weight gain or reducing sodium intake have both been used as treatment, but again there is no evidence that either reduces the development or progress of the condition (Campbell and MacGillivray 1975; Hurley 1980). Indeed, energy restriction may exacerbate the situation by further reducing cardiac output (Rosso 1983) which is already decreased in pre-eclampsia (Llewellyn-Jones 1982). Reduced cardiac output may reduce uterine blood flow and so compromise foetal development.

Though pre-eclampsia is more common among obese pregnant women, it is possible that the incidence of mild pre-eclampsia among them has been overestimated since its diagnosis is largely dependent on blood pressure measurements. Normotensive obese subjects are often misclassified as hypertensive owing to the use of a standard adult blood pressure cuff rather than a large cuff which gives more accurate results in those with a large arm circumference (Maxwell et al 1982). The presence of oedema in face or hands does not necessarily indicate pre-eclampsia (Naeye 1979).

Although diet does not seem to have a role in the treatment of pre-eclampsia, the best method of prevention is probably weight reduction for obese women *well in advance* of conception.

Third degree perianal tear

During the delivery of the baby the mother's vagina may be torn and if the tear extends as far as the anal sphincter or occasionally even the rectum then this is called a 'third degree tear'.

Dietary management of this condition has been conflicting and no comparative trials of alternative management methods appear to have been carried out. In the past, a low residue diet has been used in conjunction with an olive oil enema around the 5–6th day after delivery to avoid 'straining' which could re-open the wound (Donald 1971). Myles (1975) recommends a high fibre diet with Milpar from the second day onwards. However, Milpar contains liquid paraffin and Donald (1971) recommends that this should be avoided as it can seep through any available crevices in the surgical repair, thus encouraging non-union. A normal diet together with Fybogel, a bulking agent, taken with meals or 10 ml Dorbanex (a laxative) given at 10 pm for three days have proved to be satisfactory regimens.

Urinary tract infection

The glycosuria which often accompanies pregnancy predisposes to urinary tract infection in some women. A high fluid intake is recommended for all pregnant women to discourage urinary stasis (Donald 1971).

Gestational diabetes and pregnancy in diabetics

See Section 4.4.6.

Support Organisations

A large stamped addressed envelope should accompany all requests for information.

1 Foresight (The Association for the Promotion of Preconceptual Care) The Old Vicarage, Church Lane, Witley, Godalming. Surrey GU8 5PN.
   Booklets include *Environmental factors and foetal health — the case for preconceptual care* and *Guidelines for future parents* and other information.
2 National Childbirth Trust, 9 Queensborough Terrace, Bayswater, London W2 3TB.
   General information about pregnancy, breast feeding and local groups.
3 Maternity Alliance, 59–61 Camden High Street, London NW1 7JL. Regular bulletin and leaflets.
4 The Alfawap Trust Fund Ltd, 4 Woodchurch Road, London NW6.
   Leaflets and information on the effects of alcohol preconceptually and during pregnancy.
5 Foundation for Education and Research in Childbearing 27 Walpole Street, London SW3.
   Publications by Wynn M and Wynn A
   a) *Nutrition counselling in the prevention of low birth weight*: some conclusions on antenatal care following a visit to Canada, 1975.
   b) *Prevention of handicap of perinatal origin*: an introduction to French policy and legislation, 1976.

c) *The Prevention of preterm birth and an introduction to some European developments aimed at the prevention of handicap, 1977.*

Useful leaflets

Babies and benefits. DHSS FB8
Pregnant at work. 8350573-3/81, HMSO, London.
**Be fit and healthy before you start a baby*
**Nausea and vomiting in early pregnancy*
**Price list on application with SAE to Dr BM Pickard, Department of Animal Physiology and Nutrition, The University, Leeds, LS2 9JT.
Good foods for mothers-to-be. Dietetic Dept, Brighton Health Authority, Royal Sussex County Hospital, Eastern Road, Brighton, BN2 5BE.
Planning to have a baby? and *Genetic counselling*
Greater Glasgow Health Board, 13 Woodside Place Glasgow G3 7QW.
Planning a family? Produced by the Dietetic Departments of Glamorgan and Gwent available from Health Education Unit, St David's Hospital.
A guide for the pregnant woman and *A guide for the nursing mother and her baby* by the National Dairy Council, John Princes Street, London W1M 0AP.
Keeping well with Diabetes — pregnancy. Novo Laboratories Ltd, Ringway House, Bell Road, Daneshill East, Basingstoke, Hampshire, RG24 0QN.

Further reading

Aebi H and Whitehead R (1980) *Maternal nutrition during pregnancy and lactation.* Published for Nestle Foundation by Hans Huber, Berne.
Bennett CA (1982) *Health awareness and practices among pregnant women in Glasgow.* Department of Child Health and Obstetrics, University of Glasgow, Oakfield Avenue, Glasgow.
Bryce-Smith D and Dickerson JWT (1981) Environmental influences on pre- and post-natal development — special issue. *Int J Environ Stud* **17**, 1–98.
Campbell DM and Gillmer MDG (Eds) (1983) *Nutrition in pregnancy.* Proceedings of the Tenth Study Group of the Royal College of Obstetricians and Gynaecologists, September 1982. Royal College of Obstetricians and Gynaecologists, London.
Committee on Nutrition of the Mother and Pre-school Child (1978) *Laboratory indices of nutritional status in pregnancy.* National Academy of Sciences, Washington DC.
Dobbing J (Ed) (1981) *Maternal nutrition in pregnancy — eating for two?.* Academic Press, London.
Hurley LS (1980) *Developmental nutrition.* Prentice Hall, London.
Moghissi KS and Evans TN (Eds) (1977) *Nutritional impacts on women: throughout life with emphasis on reproduction.* Harper and Row, London.
Pickard B (1984) *Eating well for a healthy pregnancy.* Sheldon Press, London.
Worthington-Roberts BS, Vermeersch J and Rodwell-Williams S (1981) *Nutrition in pregnancy and lactation* 2e. CV Mosby Co, London.
Wynn M and Wynn A (1979) *The prevention of handicap and the health of women.* Routledge and Kegan Paul, London.
Workshop on Nutrition of the Child: Maternal nutritional status and foetal outcome. Proceedings of conference sponsored by US Dept of Agriculture and the National Institute of Child Health and Human Development, October 1979, Houston Texas. *Am J Clin Nutr* **34**, 651–817.

References

Apte SV and Iyenger L (1970) Absorption of dietary iron in pregnancy. *Am J Clin Nutr* **23**, 73–7.
Basu TK (1981) The significance of vitamins in pre-natal life. *Int J Environ Stud* **17**, 31–5.
Beal VA (1981) Assessment of nutritional status — 11. *Am J Clin Nutr* **34**, 691–6.
Belsay MA (1977) Hormonal contraception and nutrition. In *Nutritional impacts on women.* Moghissi KS and Evans TN. (Eds) Harper and Row, London.
Bennett CA (1982) *Health awareness and practices among pregnant women in Glasgow.* Department of Child Health and Obstetrics, University of Glasgow.
Black AE, Wiles SJ and Paul AA (1986) The nutrient intakes of pregnant and lactating mothers of good socioeconomic status in Cambridge, UK: some implications for recommended daily allowances of minor nutrients. *Br J Nutr* In press
Bowering J, Sanchez AM and Irwin MI (1979) A conspectus of research on iron requirements of man. *J Nutr* **106**, 985–1074.
Brewin TB (1980) Can a tumour cause the same appetite perversion or taste change as a pregnancy? *Lancet* **ii**, 907–8.
Brooke OG (1983) Vitamin D supplementation and pregnancy outcome. In *Nutrition in pregnancy* Campbell DM and Giller MDG (Eds). pp 167–170. Royal College of Obstetricians and Gynaecologists, London.
Bryce-Smith D (1985) Elemental nutrients and anti-nutrients in pre-natal development. To be published.
Calloway DH (1983) Nutrition and reproductive function of men. *Nutr Abst Rev* **53**, (5), 361–77.
Campbell DM and MacGillivray I (1975) The effect of a low calorie diet or a thiazide diuretic on the incidence of pre-eclampsia and birth weight. *Br J Obstet Gynaecol* **82**, 572–7.
Campbell DM (1983) Dietary restriction in obesity and its effect on neonatal outcome. In *Nutrition in pregnancy* Campbell DM and Gillmer MDG (Eds) pp 243–50. Royal College of Obstetricians and Gynaecologists, London.
Chanarin I, Rothman D, Ward A and Perry J (1968) Folate status and requirement in pregnancy. *Br Med J* **2**, 390–4.
Davison JS, Davison MC and Hay DM (1970) Gastric emptying time in late pregnancy and labour. *J Obstet Gynaecol Brit Commonw* **77**, 37.
DHSS (1979) *Recommended daily amounts of food energy and nutrients for groups of people in the United Kingdom.* Report on Health and Social Subjects No 15. HMSO, London.
DHSS (1985) *Recommended daily amounts of food energy and nutrients for groups of people in the United Kingdom.* Report on Health and Social Subjects No 15, third impression. HMSO, London.
Donald I (1971) *Practical obstetric problems* 5e. Lloyd-Luke Medical Books, London.
Doyle W, Crawford MA, Laurance BM and Drury P (1982) Dietary survey during pregnancy in a low socioeconomic group. *Hum Nutr: Appl Nutr* **36A**, 95–106.
Edwards LE, Alton IR, Barrada MI and Hakanson EY (1979) Pregnancy in the underweight woman. *Am J Obstet Gynaecol* **135**, 297.
Fries H (1974) Secondary amenorrhoea, self-induced weight reduction and anorexia nervosa. *Acta Psychiatr Scand* [Suppl] **248**, 1–70.

Garn SM, Lavelle N, Pesick SD and Ridella SA (1984) Are pregnant teenagers still in rapid growth? *Am J Dis Childh* **138**, 32−4.

Grant ECG (1981) The harmful effects of common social habits, especially smoking and using oral contraceptive steroids, on pregnancy. *Int J Environ Stud* **17**, 57−66.

Hambidge KM, Krebs NF, Jacobs MA, Favier A, Guyette L and Ilke DN (1983) Zinc nutritional status during pregnancy: a longitudinal study. *Am J Clin Nutr* **37**, 429−42.

Harlap S and Shiono PH (1980) Alcohol, smoking and incidence of spontaneous abortions in the first trimester of pregnancy. *Lancet* **ii**, 173−6.

Heaney RP and Skillman TG (1971) Calcium metabolism in normal human pregnancy. *J Clin Endocrinol Metab* **33**, 661−70.

Holmes-Siedle M, Lindenbaum RH, Galliard A and Bobrow M (1982) Vitamin supplementation and neural tube defects. *Lancet* **i**, 276.

Horrobin DF (1981) Nutrition and pregnancy toxaemia (pre-eclampsia). In *The Kamen plan for total nutrition during pregnancy*. Kamen B and Kamen S (Eds) pp 186−7. Appleton Century Crofts, New York.

Hurley LS (1980) *Developmental nutrition*. Prentice Hall, London.

Hytten FE (1980) Nutrition. In *Clinical physiology with obstetrics* Hytten FE and Chamberlain G (Eds). Blackwell Scientific Publications, Oxford.

Hytten FE (1983) Nutritional physiology during pregnancy. In *Nutrition in pregnancy*. Campbell DM and Gillmer MDG (Eds) pp 1−8. Royal College of Obstetricians and Gynaecologists, London.

Hytten HE and Leitch I (1971) *The physiology of human pregnancy* 2e. Blackwell Scientific Publications, Oxford.

Laurence KM, James N, Miller MH, Tennant GB and Campbell (1981) Double-blind randomized controlled trial of folate treatment before conception to prevent recurrence of neural tube defects. *Br Med J* **282**, 1509−11.

Lawrence M, Lawrence F, Lamb WH and Whitehead RG (1984) Maintenance energy cost of pregnancy in rural Gambian women and influence of dietary status. *Lancet* **ii**, 363−5.

Lind T (1983) Iron supplementation during pregnancy. In *Nutrition in pregnancy*. Campbell DM and Gillmer DG (Eds) pp 181−91. Royal College of Obstetricians and Gynaecologists, London.

Llewellyn-Jones D (1982) *Fundamentals of obstetrics and gynaecology*, Vol 1, 3e. Faber and Faber, London.

Maxwell MH, Waks AV, Schroth PL, Karam M and Domfield LP (1982) Error in blood pressure measurement due to incorrect cuff size in obese patients. *Lancet* **ii**, 33−5.

Mendelson RA (1984) Foetal alcohol syndrome: a possible role for nutrition. In *Proceedings of the 9th International Congress of Dietetics*, Toronto.

Myles MF (1975) *Textbook for midwives* 8e. Churchill Livingstone, London.

Naeye RL (1979) Weight gain and the outcome of pregnancy. *Am J Obstet Gynaecol* **135**, 3−9.

Pickard B (1982) Vitamin B6 during pregnancy — a review. *Nutr Health* **1**, 78−84.

Pitkin RM (1981) Assessment of nutritional status of mother, foetus and newborn. *Am J Clin Nutr* **34**, 658−68.

Prasad AS, Moghissi KS, Lei KY, Oberleas D and Stryker JL (1977) Effect of oral contraceptives on micronutrients and changes in trace elements due to pregnancy. In *Nutritional impacts on women*. Moghissi ILS and Evans TN (Eds) pp 160−88. Harper and Row, London.

Reeve J (1980) Calcium metabolism. In *Clinical physiology in obstetrics*. Hytten FE and Chamberlain G (Eds) pp 257−269.

Blackwell Scientific Publications, Oxford.

Rosso P (1983) Nutrition and maternal−foetal exchange. *Am J Clin Nutr* **34**, 744−55.

Salle BL, David L, Glorieux FH, Delvin E, Senterre J and Renaud H (1982) Early oral administration of vitamin D and its metabolites in premature neonates. Effect on mineral homeostasis. *Paediatr Res* **16**, 75−8.

Schwab EB and Axelson ML (1984) Dietary changes of pregnant women: compulsions and modifications. *Ecol Food Nutr* **14**, 143−53.

Seymour CA and Chadwick VS (1979) Liver and gastrointestinal function in pregnancy. *Postgrad Med J* **55**, 343−52.

Shenolikar IS (1970) Absorption of dietary calcium in pregnancy. *Am J Clin Nutr* **23**, 63−7.

Smithells RW (1983) Diet and congenital malformation. In *Nutrition in pregnancy*. Campbell DM and Gillmer MDG (Eds). The Royal College of Obstetricians and Gynaecologists, London.

Smithells RW, Sheppard S, Schorah LJ, Seller MJ, Nevin NC, Harris R, Read AP and Fielding DW (1980) Possible prevention of neural tube defects by periconceptual vitamin supplementation. *Lancet* **ii**, 339−40.

Smithells RW, Sheppard S, Schorah LJ, Seller MJ, Nevin NC, Harris R, Read AP and Fielding DW (1981a). Apparent prevention of neural tube defects by periconceptual vitamin supplementation. *Arch Dis Childh* **56**, 911−8.

Smithells RW, Sheppard S, Schorah LJ, Seller MJ, Nevin NL, Harris R, Read AD, Fielding DW and Walker S (1981b) Vitamin supplementation and neural tube defects. *Lancet* **ii**, 1425.

Solomons NW and Jacob RA (1981) Studies on the bioavailability of zinc in humans: effects of haem and non-haem iron on the absorption of zinc. *Am J Clin Nutr* **34**, 475−82.

Soules MR, Hughes LL, Garcia JA, Livengood LH, Prystowsky MR and Alexander LE (1980) Nausea and vomiting of pregnancy: role of human chorionic gonadotrophin and 17-hydroxy-progesterone. *Obstet Gynaecol* **55**, 696−705.

Stephens R (1981) Human exposure to lead from motor vehicle emissions. *Int J Environ Stud* **17**, 7−12.

Sugiura K, Tanuma J, Inomata Y, Nakajima Y, Hatakeyama M, Higuchi K, Matsuda M, Okuba T et al (1983) Study on dietary habits of pre-natal class attendants at health centres of Yokohama City. *Jap J Nutr* **44**, 111−20.

Taggart N (1961) Food habits in pregnancy. *Proc Nutr Soc* **20**, 35.

Thomas MR (1984) Nutritional recommendations for pregnant and lactating teens. In *Proceedings of the 9th International Congress of Dietetics*, Toronto.

Truswell AS (1985) Nutrition for pregnancy. *Br Med J* **291**, 263−6.

Van den Berg BJ (1981) Maternal variables affecting foetal growth. *Am J Clin Nutr* **34**, 722−6.

Walker ARP, Richardson B and Walker F (1972) The influences of numerous pregnancies and lactations on bone dimensions in South African Bantu and Caucasian mothers. *Clin Sci* **42**, 189−96.

Wishik SM (1977) The implications of undernutrition during pubescence and adolescence on fertility. In *Nutritional impacts on women throughout life with emphasis on reproduction* Moghissi RS and Evans TN (Eds) pp 23−9. Harper and Row, London.

Wright JT, Toplis PJ and Barrison IG (1983) Alcohol and coffee consumption during pregnancy. In *Nutrition in pregnancy* Campbell DM and Gillmer MDG (Eds) pp 195−205. Royal College of Obstetricians and Gynaecologists, London.

Wynn M and Wynn A (1981) *The prevention of handicap of early pregnancy origin*. Foundation for Education and Research in Childbearing, London.

3.2 Infants

In this country, mothers can exercise considerable choice over how to feed their infants. However, many are ill informed about the implications and practicalities of the feeding method chosen. Prenatal information is therefore important.

The following section provides some facts about infant feeding, which may be helpful to dietitians when asked to advise parents or health professionals.

3.2.1 Breast feeding

To some mothers, breast feeding is a natural progression of pregnancy, but others find the idea repulsive. The mother who breast feeds is likely to need practical and emotional support from her family, the midwife and health visitor. Experienced friends, local mother-child support groups and National Childbirth Trust breast feeding counsellors can also be invaluable.

Advantages and disadvantages of breast feeding

Advantages

1 Breast milk provides complete nutrition, when feeding is successfully established. Additional vitamins may be necessary after one month (DHSS 1980a).
2 Breast milk provides protection against infection, both bacterial and viral. Human milk contains macrophages (which produce lysozymes and lactoferrin), lymphocytes (which secrete interferon and secretory immunoglobulin A), bifidus factor (which inhibits growth of *Lactobacillis bifidus*) and antibodies (Downham *et al* 1976; Ogra and Ogra 1978; Adinolfi and Glynn 1979; Pittard 1979; and Yap *et al* 1979; Brock 1980).
3 Breast milk has a lower allergenicity than other milks. The breast fed infant is thus less exposed to potential allergens at a time when they may be most likely to provoke a reaction. However, some allergens can be secreted in breast milk and sensitization in fully breast fed infants has been reported (Chandra 1979; Kjellman and Johansson 1979; Warner 1980 and DHSS 1980s).
4 There is no risk of solute overload. Unlike powdered milks, breast milk cannot be reconstituted incorrectly.

5 Breast milk is immediately available. No kitchen preparation is required.
6 It helps emotional bonding. Bonding between mother and baby is important for the normal emotional and physical development of the child (Klaus and Kennell 1976). Suckling ensures frequent contact between the mother and infant.
7 It has maternal benefits. It assists uterine involution, it utilizes surplus body fat deposited in pregnancy, aiding a return to previous body weight and it has a limited contraceptive effect (Although this effect of breast feeding should not be relied upon as a method of contraception, the reduction in fertility may be advantageous in developing countries.)
8 It is relatively economical. Breast feeding is cheaper than bottle feedings, even when the 'hidden' cost of the additional nutritional needs of the lactating mother are taken into account.

Disadvantages

1 It makes demands on the mother's time. The mother has to be available day and night to feed the baby, especially in the early weeks while breast feeding is being established.
2 There can be problems in establishing and maintaining the milk supply. Physical discomfort, in the early days, from engorged breasts, sore, blistered or cracked nipples, or uterine involution contractions (in second and subsequent pregnancies) may discourage some mothers. Mastitis and breast abscesses may necessitate a temporary or permanent cessation of breast feeding.
3 The mother cannot see the volume of milk taken. Many mothers need continual reassurance that their milk supply is adequate and are unhappy that they cannot see how much the baby obtains. They need to be taught that the infant itself provides the best guide; a baby who is contented and is gaining weight is adequately fed.
4 The milk supply may be inadequate. Poor weight gain and an unsettled baby may be due to an inadequate supply of breast milk. Milk supply can be increased (see p 261), but instead, supplementary bottle feeding

is often advised and once this is started, breast feeding is frequently abandoned altogether.

5 There may be a reaction to the mother's diet. Bouts of gastrointestinal pain may occur in the infant as a consequence of foods eaten by the mother. Foods commonly implicated in this way include onions, green vegetables, milk and dairy products and alcohol. The offending item(s) can usually be identified fairly readily and then avoided while breast feeding continues.

6 It can be embarrassing in the presence of other people. Some mothers are embarrassed to breast feed even within the home, particularly those in lower socio-economic groups (Martin and Monk 1982). Many women find that the attitude of other people to breast feeding in public, coupled with the frequent lack of facilities to feed in private, make prolonged excursions outside the home very difficult.

7 It can create jealousy. Husbands, relatives and siblings may, in different ways, resent the exclusive role of the mother in breast feeding. These problems can be overcome by involving everyone in all other aspects of caring for the infant.

8 It may be incompatible with the mother's return to work. Owing to the lack of suitable child-care facilities in most places of work, returning to work shortly after giving birth makes continuing with full breast feeding almost impossible. However, partial breast feeding (e.g. in the mornings and evenings) can usually be continued and should be encouraged.

Contraindications to breast feeding

1 Serious chronic maternal illness which necessitates drug therapy. Many drugs are passed into the breast milk which may have adverse effects on the baby. These effects have been reviewed by Wilson et al (1980) and White and White (1980). Maternal diabetes mellitus should not preclude lactation.

2 Severe physical problems. These can occur in either the baby (e.g. cleft lip or palate) or the mother (e.g. inverted nipples).

3 Low birth weight. Breast milk may not be suitable for low birth weight infants. (See Section 5.4)

4 The baby is to be adopted. Breast feeding is discouraged on psychological grounds.

5 Illness in the baby. Breast-feeding may not be possible for the infant with acute illness requiring nasogastric feeding (it may be possible to use expressed breast milk as the feeding regimen if the illness is of short duration) or chronic illness necessitating milk exclusion, e.g galactosaemia or lactose intolerance.

Breast feeding may be possible in certain inborn metabolic errors of metabolism (e.g. phenylketonuria) provided that certain precautions are observed (see Section 4.7).

Maternal nutritional needs for lactation

The amounts of food energy and nutrients required for lactation have been summarized by the DHSS (1979). However, as with all RDAs, these figures are designed to cover the needs of all lactating women and the in-built safety factor inevitably means that they will be too high for some individuals.

For most lactating women, increased quantities of a normal and varied diet, based on 'healthy eating' principles, will provide adequate nutrition. In addition, the body will, to some extent, signal its requirements via the sensations of hunger and thirst which are often particularly intense during the lactating period. Mothers should be encouraged to respond to these signals and increase their food or liquid consumption without pangs of guilt.

Energy

The energy cost of milk production is considerable (Thomson et al 1970). The RDA is for 400–600 kcal above the pre-pregnant intakes (DHSS 1979; NRC 1980; FAO/WHO/UNU 1985) and dietary studies among well nourished UK women have shown an intake of 500 kcal above a pre-lactation intake (Black et al 1986).

However, the lactation process appears to be remarkably efficient even in the face of low energy intakes. The milk output by Gambian mothers with an energy intake of 1500–1800 kcal/day is very similar to that of Cambridge mothers with an energy intake of 2330 kcal/day (Whitehead et al 1980). Giving the Gambian mothers a dietary supplement of 1000 kcal daily, thus bringing their intake to the Cambridge level, had no effect on the amount of milk taken by their babies (Prentice et al 1983). The results of these and other studies have been comprehensively reviewed by Prentice et al (1986). The most important factor correlating with the amount of milk taken by a Cambridge baby was the baby's current weight; birth weight, social class, and maternal energy intake were the next most important factors, in that order. It seems probable therefore that a large baby takes more milk and that this drives an increase in maternal appetite rather than the other way round.

The mother's appetite is thus the best guide to energy requirements. Deliberately attempting to limit food intake in order to lose weight is inadvisable; this will only exacerbate any feelings of stress or tiredness being experienced by the mother and, if severe enough, these factors may in turn lead to a decrease in milk production.

Protein

Although lactation will result in an increased requirement for protein, in most cases this will be met easily by a diet which provides 10% of protein energy. However, if the total energy requirement appears to be significantly lower than the RDA, efforts should be made to ensure that sufficient protein-containing foods are included in the diet.

Carbohydrate and fat

There are no specific recommendations concerning these nutrients but, in practice, many lactating women will need to consume more of them in order to met their energy needs.

Dietary fibre

Fibre intake should be relatively high, especially if constipation has been a problem in pregnancy or remains so post partum.

Fluid

An adequate fluid intake is essential to establish and maintain lactation. It will also help prevent constipation. Excessive quantities of strong coffee, tea or alcohol should, however, be avoided.

Vitamins

The requirements for thiamin, riboflavin and nicotinic acid are increased in proportion to the increased energy intake. The requirements for vitamin D and ascorbic acid are similar to those in the third trimester of pregnancy (10 µg/day and 60 mg/day respectively). An increase in vitamin A to 1200 µg/day is recommended. Provided that the additional energy needs are met by means of a varied and balanced diet, vitamin supplementation is probably unnecessary in most individuals. However, many women are advised to take these as a precautionary measure.

Minerals

Calcium intake should be similar to that taken in the third trimester of pregnancy (1200 mg/day). The recommended intake of iron is even higher (15 mg/day) than that for pregnancy (13 mg/day), though some would argue that both these figures are unrealistic and unphysiological.

Possible dietary exclusions

The maternal diet influences the composition of breast milk (Craig-Schmidt et al 1984), and breast milk may contain a number of non-nutritive substances (DHSS 1980a). Alcohol is excreted in breast milk, (Binkiewicz et al 1978), and is ideally avoided, or at least restricted, during breast feeding. Other items which can pass into breast milk include caffeine, nicotine, senna and other amines and alkaloids. Consumption of coffee and other caffeine containing beverages should be watched. Foods which contain alkaloids, e.g. green potatoes, should be avoided. Drugs, including oral contraceptives, should only be taken on medical advice.

It has been suggested that the consumption of dairy products, in particular milk, yoghurt and cheese, may be linked with infantile 'three month' colic in breast fed babies. While this remains to be scientifically proven, many mothers discover from personal experience that reduction or avoidance of these foods result in a dramatic improvement in their babies. If these foods are excluded from the diet, care must be

Table 3.4 General dietary guidelines for lactation

Food

1 Eat regularly
2 Let your appetite dictate how much you eat. If you are hungry, eat more.
3 Do not attempt to slim
4 Eat a variety of foods. Try to include the following in your diet every day
    milk, cheese or yoghurt
    meat, fish or eggs
    yellow or green leafy vegetables
    fruit or fruit juice
    wholemeal bread, or high fibre breakfast cereals
    potatoes
5 If you think some foods in your diet are upsetting your baby, avoid them for a few days and see if it helps. If it does, ask your health visitor for advice as you may need to eat more of other foods to compensate
6 Only take vitamin supplements on medical advice

Fluids

1 Drink plenty of fluids
2 If you are thirsty, drink more
3 *Do not* drink much alcohol, strong coffee or strong tea

taken to obtain adequate calcium from other sources such as pulses, fish and cereals.

General dietary guidelines for lactating mothers are summarized in Table 3.4.

Establishing and monitoring breast feeding

Antenatal advice

The provision of advice about the pros and cons of breast feeding will help the mother decide how she wants to feed her baby. Those who choose to breast feed generally do so on the grounds of convenience and being 'best for the baby' (Martin and Monk 1982). Breast feeding is most common amongst mothers

1 With first babies.
2 Educated beyond the age of 18 years.
3 In higher social classes.
4 Aged 25 years or more.
5 Residing in England and Wales.

Practical advice on care of breasts is usually given by the midwife during antenatal visits.

Initiation of lactation

Studies show that putting baby to the breast immediately after delivery assists in developing the suckling reflex which is particularly strong for a short while after delivery.

The supply of breast milk is determined largely by demand and is stimulated by frequent (rather than prolonged) suckling. Therefore feeding 2–3 hourly for a few minutes at each breast will help the milk supply to become established by the third or fourth day post-partum. Complementary feeds are *not* necessary at this stage and will hinder the establishment of breast feeding. The changes in the composition of breast milk in the early post partum period are summarized in Table 3.5.

Table 3.5 Changes in breast milk

Day	Milk	Description
1–3	Colostrum	Thick, yellowy milk, high in protein, antibodies and some vitamins and minerals
3–7+	Transitional	Thinner, white appearance. Composition approaching mature milk
7–10+	Mature	More watery appearance, almost blue in colour as the feed begins and becoming white by the end of a feed as the fat content increases

It takes 3–6 weeks for lactation to become fully established; it is during this period that frequent feeding round the clock (every 3–4 hours) is most valuable. One lactation is well established, feeds can be spaced further apart without diminishing the milk supply.

If the baby is unable to suckle at birth, the mother can use an electric pump to simulate suckling and the baby can be fed expressed breast milk until normal breast feeding can commence.

Milk supply can be reduced by tiredness and tension, so practical and emotional support is very important at this time. Establishing lactation is more difficult to achieve with some babies than others. Some infants seem to fight at the breast or may be irritable and scream or cry. This is often a result of the very rapid initial flow of milk which overwhelms and frustrates the baby. Expressing a little milk before the feed often resolves the problem.

Mothers should be made aware that crying in their infant does not always signal a demand for food. It may also be because the baby is uncomfortable, over-tired, thirsty or just bored or lonely.

Maintaining lactation

Support for the lactating mother from family, friends, midwife, health visitor, National Childbirth trust local group, etc. is important if breast feeding is to continue. Martin and Monk (1982) found one-third of mothers in their study stopped breast feeding within six weeks. The most common reason given was 'insufficient milk'. Few had been offered or received any guidances as to whether this really was the case.

The breast feeding mother needs to feed on demand, day and night and may find herself feeding every 3–4 hours for several weeks. Practical help in the house and with other children will help the mother get as much rest as possible. The importance of eating properly cannot be over-emphasized. Regular meals or snacks will keep up energy levels during this busy and demanding period.

Once the milk supply is established, the mother may get a break from her responsibilities by expressing breast milk for someone else to feed to the baby in a bottle. Not all babies co-operate with this occasional bottle feed.

Some mothers complement breast feeds with a suitable milk formula from a bottle. This may be done for reasons of

1 Convenience (e.g. a return to work).

2 Acute illness in the mother.

3 Inadequate breast milk supply.

If done for the latter reason, care must be taken to ensure that the natural milk supply cannot be increased (see below). Once some bottle feeding is instituted, the mother's own milk supply will diminish further and a return to complete breast feeding is almost impossible. Assuming the mother wants to persevere with breast feeding, complementary feeding should be introduced only when other efforts to improve the milk yield have failed.

If complementary feeds are used, the bottle feed should be given *after* the breast feed.

Additional nutritional requirements of the infant

Vitamins. Provided that the maternal diet is adequate, breast milk will meet the vitamin needs of the baby. In practice, the following vitamin supplements are usually given

1 Vitamin K (1 mg) given by intramuscular injection at delivery to prevent haemolytic disease of the newborn.

2 DHSS children's vitamin drops (five drops daily) are often recommended for breast fed infants over the age of one month and continued until the age of two or preferably five years of age. Five drops provide 200 μg vitamin A, 20 mg vitamin C and 7 μg vitamin D.

Vitamin supplements are more important when the child is being weaned. Mothers must be warned not to give more than the recommended dose.

Minerals. Provided that the maternal diet is adequate, breast milk will meet the mineral requirements of the baby. However, in order to offer protection to the developing teeth, a daily intake of 0.25 mg fluoride is recommended by the British Dental Association for infants and young children. This amount cannot be obtained from breast or infant milk formulae. However, the level of fluoride in water supplies varies greatly and local levels, together with the infant's water consumption, must be taken into account when deciding whether or not to use fluoride supplements (Dowell and Joyston Bechal 1981). As a general guide, fluoride drops providing 0.25 mg fluoride daily should be given if the water supply contains less than 0.3 ppm fluoride. If the fluoride content of the water supply is between 0.3–0.7 ppm, no additional supplement should be given until 2 years of age. After this age, only half the recommended daily supplement should be given (see p 384; Section 4.8)

Fluid. Additional fluid is not usually necessary for breast fed infants (DHSS 1980a). However, in hot weather, or even over-heated houses, thirst may occur in some babies and should be remedied with cool boiled water from a sterilized bottle or feeding beaker.

Monitoring the progress of a breast fed baby

Most breast fed babies gain weight and thrive. Weight loss during the first few days postpartum should not exceed 10% of birth weight. This loss of weight usually ceases by days 4–7 and birth weight has been regained by 7–10 days. Over the first three months, weight gain averages approximately 200 g per week, then 150 g per week for the 3–6 month period. A normal, full term neonate doubles its birth weight by about five months and trebles it by the end of the first year of life. A meaningful assessment of a baby's growth can only really be made by the regular use of percentile growth charts (see p 43).

If the infant's progress is in doubt, the adequacy of breast feeding can be established by

1 General observation of the mother, including factors such as contentment, undue tiredness or breast discomfort.

2 General observation of the baby, including general health, sleeping, waking and crying patterns, bladder and bowel habits.

3 Recording feeding pattern, i.e. the times and duration of feeds (although duration of feed is not a good indication of quantity taken).

4 Recording the baby's weight gain in relation to length.

5 Test weighing the infant (recording weight before and after several feeds). This will provide an indication of the volume of feed being taken. However by itself, this is not a particularly meaningful figure and since obtaining it tends to be rather traumatic for the mother, the anxiety provoked may even reduce the milk supply and give a false picture.

Failure to thrive at the breast

Poor weight gain and growth and an unsettled baby are clear indications of an inadequate milk intake. However, there are a number of possible reasons for this and the factors responsible — in either the mother and/or the child — must be identified before they can be remedied. They may include

1 In the mother, inadequate milk production due to
  a) Illness.
  b) Tension (Can cause failure of the 'let down' reflex which brings in the hind milk).

Table 3.6 Composition of highly modified infant milk formulae suitable for full term, newborn babies (all values are expressed per 100 ml prepared feed)

Nutrient	DHSS guidelines[1]	Mature breast milk (range)[1,2]	Mature cows' milk (mean)[3]	Cow and Gate Premium	SMA Gold Cap (Wyeth)	Aptamil (Milupa)	Osterfeed (Farleys)
Energy (kJ)	270 −315	270 −315	264	275	275	281	284
(kcal)	65 − 75	65 − 75	63	66	65	67	68
Protein	1.2 − 2.0	1.2 − 1.4	3.2	1.5	1.5	1.5	1.45
casein (g)	As for }	0.5§	2.6	0.6	0.6	0.6	0.58
whey (g)	human milk }	0.8§	0.6	0.9	0.9	0.9	0.87
Fat (g)	2.3 − 5.0	3.7 − 4.8	3.7	3.6	3.6	3.6	3.82
Carbohydrate (g)	4.8 − 10.0	7.1 − 7.8	4.6	7.3	7.2	7.2	6.96
Calcium (mg)	30 −120	32 − 36	117	54	44.5	59	35
Phosphorus (mg)	15 − 60	14 − 15	93	27	33	35	29
Ca:P ratio	1.2:1−2.2:1	2.3:1§	1.3:1	2:1	1.3:1	1.6:1	1.2:1
Sodium (mg)	15 − 35	11 − 20	49	18	15	18	19
Potassium (mg)	50 −100	57 − 62	146	65	56	85	57
Chloride (mg)	40 − 80	35 − 55	93	40	40	38	45
Magnesium (mg)	2.8 − 12	2.6 − 3.0	12	5	5.3	6	5.2
Iron (µg)	70 −700	62 − 93	49	500	670	700	650
Zinc (µg)	200 −600*	260 −330	341	400	500	400	350
Iodine (µg)	ns	2 −12	26†	7	7	4	4.5
Manganese (µg)	ns	0.7 − 1.5	na	7	16	4.2	3.4
Copper (µg)	10 − 60*	37 − 43	20	40	50	46	43
A Retinol equivalents (µg)	40 −150	40 − 76	38	80	79	69	100
D3 Cholecalciferol (µg)	0.7 − 1.3	na	0.03	1.1	1.05	1.0	1.0
E dl-α Tocopherol (mg)	0.3 −ns	0.29− 0.39	97	1.1	0.95	0.7	0.48
K1 Phytomenadione (µg)	1.5 −ns	ns	na	5	5.8	4.0	2.7
B1 Thiamin (µg)	13 −ns	13 − 21	40	40	80	40	42
B2 Riboflavin (µg)	30 −ns	31	185	100	110	50	55
B6 Pyridoxine (µg)	5 −ns	5.1 − 7.2	39	40	51	30	35
B12 Cyanocobalamin (µg)	0.01−ns	0.01	0.02	0.2	0.11	0.15	0.14
Nicotinic acid (µg)	230 −ns	210 −270	840	400	1000	400	690
Pantothenic acid (µg)	200 −ns	200 −330	340	300	210	400	230
Biotin (µg)	0.5 −ns	0.52− 1.13	2.0	1.5	1.5	1.1	1.0
Folic acid (µg)	3 −ns	3.1 − 6.2	4.9	10	5.3	10	3.4
C Ascorbic acid (mg)	3 −ns	3.1 − 4.5	1.5	8	5.8	6	6.9
Choline (mg)	ns	na	na	7	4.75	na	na
Renal solute load (mosmol/l)		78§	224.6	96	92.1	101	93

[1]DHSS 1980b; [2]DHSS 1977; [3]Paul and Southgate 1978.

ns = Not specified.
na = Not available.
*Tentative guideline.
§Average figure.
†Content varies with the diet of the cow.

c) Fatigue.
d) Lack of confidence.

2 In the baby, inadequate milk intake due to
a) Not being fed frequently enough. Some babies need to be fed more often than others. In addition, some babies will require more feeds on some days than others, especially during growth spurts. Rigid feeding schedules should therefore be discouraged and the baby allowed to feed as often as appears to be necessary.
b) Suckling difficulties from temporary nasal obstruction caused by infection, poor suckling position causing the breast to block the baby's nose, breast engorgement making feeding difficult or inverted nipples.
c) Sleepiness or apparent disinterest.

Correcting inadequate milk intake. Most of the above problems can be overcome with help and advice from midwives, health visitors and counsellors from breast feeding support groups.

Improving the maternal milk supply. The cardinal rules for improving the maternal milk supply are
1 Increase the frequency of breast feeding.

Table 3.7 Composition of modified infant milk formulae (all values are expressed per 100 ml prepared feed)

Nutrient	DHSS guidelines[1]	Mature breast milk (range)[1,2]	Mature cows' milk (mean)[3]	Cow and Gate Plus	SMA White Cap (Wyeth)	Milumil (Milupa)	Ostermilk Complete (Farleys)	Ostermilk Two (Farleys)
Energy (kJ)	270 −315	270 −315	264	275	275	298	273	260
(kcal)	65 − 75	65 − 75	63	66	65	69	65	62
Protein	1.2 − 2.0	1.2 − 1.4	3.2	1.9	1.5	1.9	1.7	1.8
casein (g)	As for	0.5§	2.6	1.5	1.23	1.52	1.31	1.39
whey (g)	human milk	0.8§	0.6	0.4	0.27	0.38	0.39	0.41
Fat (g)	2.3 − 5.0	3.7 − 4.8	3.7	3.4	3.6	3.1	2.6	2.4
Carbohydrate (g)	4.8 − 10.0	7.1 − 7.8	4.6	7.3	7.2	8.4	8.6	8.3
Calcium (mg)	30 −120	32 − 36	117	85	56	71	61	65
Phosphorus (mg)	15 − 60	14 − 15	93	55	44.5	55	49	53
Ca:P ratio	1.2:1−2.2:1	2.3:1§	1.3:1	1.5:1	1.3:1	1.3:1	1.3:1	1.2:1
Sodium (mg)	15 − 35	11 − 20	49	25	20	24	31	31
Potassium (mg)	50 −100	57 − 62	146	100	74	85	70	79
Chloride (mg)	40 − 80	35 − 55	93	60	47	44	56	58
Magnesium (mg)	2.8 − 12	2.6 − 3.0	12	7	4.1	6	6	6.4
Iron (µg)	70 −700	62 − 93	49	500	670	400	650	650
Zinc (µg)	200 −600*	260 −330	341	400	500	400	330	310
Iodine (µg)	ns	2 −12	26†	7	3.4	2.1	10	11
Manganese (µg)	ns	0.7 − 1.5	na	7	16	13	3.3	3.1
Copper (µg)	10 − 60*	37 − 43	20	40	50	27	39	38
A Retinol equivalents (µg)	40 −150	40 − 76	38	80	79	65	97	95
D3 Cholecalciferol (µg)	0.7 − 1.3	na	0.03	1.1	1.05	1.0	1.0	1.0
E dl-α Tocopherol (mg)	0.3 −ns	0.29− 0.39	97	1.1	0.95	0.8	0.46	0.45
K1 Phytomenadione (µg)	1.5 −ns	ns	na	5	5.8	4.0	2.6	1.5
B1 Thiamin (µg)	13 −ns	13 − 21	40	40	80	32	39	38
B2 Riboflavin (µg)	30 −ns	31	185	100	110	49	53	51
B6 Pyridoxine (µg)	5 −ns	5.1 − 7.2	39	40	51	42	33	32
B12 Cyanocobalamin (µg)	0.01−ns	0.01	0.02	0.2	0.11	0.21	0.13	0.13
Nicotinic acid (µg)	230 −ns	210 −270	840	400	1000	240	650	640
Pantothenic acid (µg)	200 −ns	220 −330	340	300	210	240	220	220
Biotin (µg)	0.5 −ns	0.52− 1.13	2.0	1.5	1.5	1.1	0.97	0.95
Folic acid (µg)	3 −ns	3.1 − 6.2	4.9	10	5.3	5	3.2	3.1
C Ascorbic acid (mg)	3 −ns	3.1 − 4.5	1.5	8	5.8	7.5	6.4	6.2
Choline (mg)	ns	na	na	7	4.75	na	na	na
Renal solute load (mosmol/l)		78§	224.6	130	100.8	121	115	122

[1]DHSS 1980b; [2]DHSS 1977; [3]Paul and Southgate 1978. ns = Not specified. na = Not available.
*Tentative guideline.
§Average figure.
†Content varies with the diet of the cow.

2 Encourage the mother to relax, both physically and mentally.

3 Ensure the maternal diet is adequate, especially in respect of fluid and energy content.

Common problems in breast fed infants

'Wind'

'Wind', i.e. air taken in with the feed, may make the baby miserable and uncomfortable. If so, the surplus air will be expelled if the baby is moved to a vertical position and the back gently rubbed. However, most babies will either burp when they need to, or not at all. If the baby is not bothered by any residual air in his stomach then neither should his mother be, and prolonged 'winding' will be just an unnecessary ritual.

'Winding' a baby does not appear to have any influence on colic ('three month colic') which is unrelated to air intake. This is discussed further on p 265.

'Posseting' or vomiting

Many babies regurgitate small amounts of milk at the end of a feed. This is of no consequence. However, repeated vomiting both after and between feeds must e reported immediately to a doctor or health visitor.

Table 3.8 Sources of macronutrients in infant milk formulae compared with breast milk

Product	Protein (casein: whey)	Fat	Carbohydrate
Breast milk	(40:60)	Related to maternal diet	Lactose (100%)
Cow and Gate Premium	Skimmed milk + modified whey* (40:60)	Vegetable oils + milk fat	Lactose (100%)
SMA Gold Cap (Wyeth)	Skimmed milk + modified whey* (40:60)	Vegetable oils + beef fat	Lactose (100%)
Aptamil (Milupa)	Skimmed milk + modified whey* (40:60)	Vegetable oils + milk fat	Lactose (100%)
Osterfeed (Farley)	Milk + modified whey (39:61)	Vegetable oils + milk fat	Lactose (100%)
Cow and Gate Plus	Milk + skimmed milk (80:20)	Vegetable oils + milk fat	Lactose (100%)
SMA White Cap (Wyeth)	Milk + skimmed milk (82:18)	Vegetable oils + beef fat	Lactose (100%)
Milumil (Milupa)	Milk + skimmed milk (80:20)	Vegetable oils + milk fat	71% lactose 16% maltodextrin 13% amylose
Ostermilk Complete (Farley)	Milk + skimmed milk (77:23)	Vegetable oils + milk fat	33% lactose (approx) 67% maltodextrin (approx)
Ostermilk two (Farley)	Milk + skimmed milk (77:23)	Vegetable oils + milk fat	66% lactose (approx) 34% maltodextrin (approx)

*Modified whey = demineralized.

Irregular bowel habits

The stools will normally be bright yellow and loose or soft. A breast fed baby may pass several stools on one day and then several days may elapse before another one. Even after 4–5 days without a bowel movement, the breast fed baby is not constipated if the stool, when passed, is soft.

3.2.2 Bottle feeding

Infant milk formulae are manufactured from cows' milk or soya beans. Despite continuing advances in technology, such formulae cannot wholly mimic the composition of human breast milk. However, today's formulae are much better than those produced 10–15 years ago. The DHSS (1980b) have produced comprehensive guidelines on the nutritional composition of

Table 3.9 Other infant formulae available

Product	Protein	Fat	Carbohydrate
Progress (Wyeth)[1]	Whole milk plus demineralized whey	Vegetable oils	77.5% lactose 22.5% maltodextrin
Special formula HN25 (Milupa)[2]	Caseinate skimmed milk (lactose reduced)	Vegetable oils	24.1% starch 10.6% maltodextrin 9.4% glucose 8.6% sucrose 7.4% fructose 5.8% galactose 0.6% lactose
Wysoy (Wyeth)[3]	Soya protein isolate + L-methionine	Vegetable oils Beef fat	Sucrose Corn syrup solids
Formula S (Cow and Gate)[4]	Soya protein isolate + L-methionine	Vegetable oils	Glucose syrup

[1]For babies over 6 months.
[2]For short term replacement in recovery phase of acute diarrhoea, i.e. low lactose formula.
[3]Available 'over the counter'; used in cases of cows' milk allergy.
[4]As 3. Also suitable for vegetarians, vegans and certain ethnic groups.

Table 3.10 Advantages and disadvantages of bottle feeding

Advantages
1 Creates no additional nutritional requirements in the mother
2 No problems in establishing the milk supply
3 The volume of milk given is visible
4 Feeding in public is acceptable
5 Less jealousy may be incurred because other members of the family can feed the baby
6 Creates no problems for the working mother
7 Provided the correct amount is given, it will be nutritionally adequate

Disadvantages
1 Formulae are not identical to human breast milk
2 Confers no protection against infection
3 Subjects the infant to potential allergens*
4 Requires careful preparation and storage
5 Mother-baby emotional bond is not always strengthened
6 No maternal benefits relating to uterine involution, utilization of body fat or contraceptive effect
7 More expensive than breast feeding

*Savilanti (1981) suggests that 1–2% of children become allergic to cows' milk. Soya milk formulae can be used instead but many infants who are allergic to cows' milk will also be allergic to soya-based products (see sections 5.9; 2.11)

artificial infant feeding formulae, based on the composition of pooled samples of mature human milk. There are many different products available, each with a slightly different composition (Tables 3.6–3.9). Infants of low birth weight will require a milk formula specially adapted for their requirements (see Section 5.4). The feeding of infants with chronic illness (e.g. galactosaemia or phenylketonuria) is discussed in Section 4.7.

Table 3.11 Typical feeding guide for the bottle fed infant

Weight of baby		Age	Number of feeds per 24 hours	Level scoops per feed	Quantity of water per feed	
(kg)	(lb)				(fl oz)	(ml)
3.5	7¾	Up to 2 weeks	6–7	3	3	85
4.0	8¾	2–8 weeks	6	4	4	115
4.5	10	2 months	5	5	5	140
5.4	12	3 months	5	6	6	170
6.5	14	4 months	5	7	7	200
7.2	16	5 months	4–5	7	7	200
8.0	18	6 months +	4	8	8	225

Preparation of infant milk formulae

Instructions are given on the tins and boxes in words and pictures, and emphasise the need for care and skill. Errors in reconstitution, making the feed either too dilute or too concentrated, are a cause for concern. Contributory factors may be ignorance, illiteracy, financial or social problems. These factors may also affect the standard of hygiene in feed preparation and storage. Demonstrations of good practices can be given in parentcraft classes, during hospital postnatal care and by midwives and health visitors.

Many of the advantages of bottle feeding tend to be the disadvantages of breast feeding and vice versa (see Section 3.2.1). They are summarized in Table 3.10.

Establishing and monitoring bottle feeding

Many maternity units use 'ready-to-feed' infant milk formulae. Some offer a choice of product. Mothers often try several different milks on their own initiative or after professional advice. A limited range of infant milk formulae will be available at baby clinics. There is a token system for free milk for those on a low income.

Few babies seem to refuse the feed from a bottle. Occasionally a baby will show frustration by crying, refusing the teat or feeding reluctantly and this is usually due to an inappropriate flow rate of milk from the bottle. This can be altered by varying the number and size of holes in the teat. A teat which resembles the human nipple in size and shape may be more successful than the traditional bottle teat. Some teats have an automatic vacuum release which ensures a continuous flow of milk from the bottle.

The correct feeding technique is also important. The bottle should always be angled so that the teat is full of milk thus minimizing the amount of air consumed.

The tins and boxes of infant milk formulae have

feeding guides suggesting the size and number of feeds to be given. These guides are based on average nutritional requirements and are summarized in Table 3.11. However, as with breast feeding, in practice mothers are being advised to feed 'on demand' rather than adhering to a rigid timetable.

Additional nutritional requirements of the infant

Vitamins and minerals. All the infant milk formulae are supplemented with vitamins and minerals during production to meet DHSS guidelines (DHSS 1980b). With the exception of fluoride (see p 270), additional supplements are therefore not required.

Fluid requirements. An average fluid intake in early infancy is 150 ml/kg/day. Actual needs vary depending on fluid losses. Many professional advisors recommend offering cooled, boiled water after or between feeds to safeguard against dehydration. If the baby is healthy, it does not matter if this extra fluid is refused. However, it is important to give additional fluid to a baby with a temperature, diarrhoea or vomiting in order to replace the fluid losses.

Monitoring progress of a bottle fed infant

Monitoring the progress of the baby in general terms has been discussed on p 260. The most important factors to consider in the bottle fed infant are the growth rate (weight gain in relation to length) and the contentment of the child.

Because the volume of feed consumed is known, it is easier to assess the nutrient intake of the bottle fed than the breast fed infant. However, this assumes that the feed is being made up correctly, and this factor must be borne in mind when either an inadequate or excessive weight gain is being investigated.

Inadequate weight gain. This may be due to
1 Feeds being either too few or too small.
2 Feed being over-diluted.
3 Undercurrent illness.
4 Intolerance to a component of the feed (usually evidenced by gastrointestinal symptoms).

Excessive weight gain. This may be due to
1 Feeds being either too frequent or too large.
2 Feeds being over-concentrated.
3 Rusk or cereal being added to the bottle. Although this practice, once common, is now discouraged by health professionals it still occurs, mainly because it is often recommended by well-meaning grandmothers

(particularly as a way of getting the child to sleep through the night).

4 Encouraging the baby to empty the bottle at every feed instead of letting him stop when he appears to have had enough.

Problems associated with bottle feeding

Wind, posseting and vomiting

Bottle fed babies tend to take in more air with their feed than breast fed infants and are therefore more likely to suffer discomfort. For the same reason, regurgitation during or after a feed is also more common. Both can be minimized by allowing the baby to rest from feeding at intervals in a vertical position so that the surplus air can escape. Reducing the flow rate of the milk may also help.

If a considerable proportion of the feed is being persistently regurgitated, medical advice should be sought. A thickening agent to add to the feed (e.g. Carobel or Nestagel) can be prescribed.

Colic

Colic, often termed 'three month colic' is not the same as wind. It also occurs in breast-fed infants (see p 262). It is a distressing condition (for the mother as well as the child) characterized by bouts of severe abdominal pain with accompanying crying or screaming which the mother is powerless to either prevent or treat. It usually starts within three or four weeks of birth and ceases at around the age of three months. The attacks frequently start at the same time of day, often in the early evening. The causes of the condition are unknown. Future research may reveal whether dietary factors (colic often disappears in breast fed infants when their mothers avoid dairy produce) or physiological factors (such as unequal gut pressures occurring in an immature gastrointestinal tract) can explain its onset. Anti-spasmodic drugs can help in some cases but for most parents it is simply an unpleasant phase which has to be endured.

Stool appearance

Artificial feeding results in stools which are often greenish in colour and these are not always easily distinguished from the green stools seen when a gut infection is present. Loose stools or diarrhoea may be normal for a particular baby but can also be indicative of intolerance to a feed component. The sudden appearance of loose stools suggests the presence of infection.

Constipation

This is more likely to occur in bottle than breast fed infants and may reflect an inadequate fluid intake. Bottle fed infants should be offered cooled boiled water at intervals, particularly in hot weather.

Incorrect reconstitution of the milk formula

Over-concentrated feeds can be prepared either by tight packing of powder in the measuring scoop or by deliberately adding more powder or less water than recommended. This will clearly exacerbate the risk of obesity and in addition may lead to the life-threatening problems of hyperosmolar dehydration and hypernatraemia (see below).

Hyperosmolar dehydration and hypernatraemia

The immature kidneys of the young infant can only produce a maximum osmolarity of 700 mmol/l. A high solute load may therefore result in hyperosmolar dehydration and hypernatraemia. Fortunately these conditions are much more rare than they used to be owing to modifications in infant milk formulae. However, they can still arise from a combination of factors such as over-concentrated feeds, high extra-renal fluid losses (e.g. due to diarrhoea or excessive sweating), a reduced renal output and no additional fluid.

Hypocalcaemia and hyperphosphataemia

As with the above, modern milk formulae are less likely to cause these problems. The ratio of calcium: phosphorus in breast milk is 2.3:1 and this is now copied in the artificial formulae. Hypocalcaemia/ hyperphosphataemia can still be a problem in low birth weight infants.

Intolerances

Cows' milk protein (see Sections 2.11 and 5.9).
Disaccharide intolerance (see Section 2.4).
Inborn errors of metabolism (see Section 4.7).

3.2.3 Weaning

Weaning is 'the process which begins when breast or bottle milk starts to be replaced by a mixed diet'

(DHSS 1980a). Weaning is a gradual process taking six months or more, during which time the baby becomes accustomed to food, initially sieved, in addition to milk and the baby changes from sucking from either breast or bottle to swallowing liquids from a feeder beaker and, eventually, an ordinary cup. Infants need to be weaned because

1 Nutritional requirements cannot be met by milk alone. Infants' stores of, for example, iron are depleted by about six months of age and milk is not a good source. In addition, the volume of milk required to meet energy needs becomes too great for an infant's capacity. Although many of the alternative foods offered initially are no more energy-dense than milk, their consumption will lead to a more solid, more energy-dense diet.

2 Feeding behaviour progresses from sucking to swallowing, chewing and biting once teeth are present. As the baby develops it is keen to experience new things, including new foods, tastes and textures. The maturing digestive tract (for example, the increase in amylase at 3−4 months) also enables the infant to tolerate a wider range of foods.

Starting weaning

When to start weaning

The current view (DHSS 1980a) is for a flexible approach to the age of weaning but that it should start somewhere between the ages of 3−8 months. Considerable individual variation must be recognized (Whitehead *et al* 1981). If the baby still seems hungry after a good milk feed this is an indication to introduce solids. The age at which mothers choose to start weaning is affected by

1 Social factors
  a) Social class differences in the age of weaning.
  b) Bottle fed infants tend to be weaned earlier than breast fed infants.
  c) Influence of family and peers.
2 Medical factors
  a) Professional advice.
  b) Growth rate considerations.
  c) Medical conditions.
3 Cultural factors
  a) Delayed weaning in some cultures.
  b) Availability of suitable weaning foods.
  c) Different methods of weaning.

How to start weaning

1 Decide which foods are to be offered (see below)

and have them in readiness.
2 Obtain the equipment needed
  a) Protective clothing for both mother and baby. Weaning is a messy process.
  b) Plastic spoon.
  c) Plastic dish. Initially the top of a feeding bottle or small plastic container will be large enough.
  d) Liquidizer, blender or sieve if fresh foods are to be prepared.
3 Choose a quiet time of day to start weaning when the baby is not tired and other members of the family are not demanding meals.
4 Offer the weaning food either after or during a milk feed so that the baby is not frustrated by hunger.
5 Stay relaxed and be patient. It can take time — days or weeks — for the baby to accept food from a spoon.

Suitable early weaning foods

Factors to be considered include

Nutrient content. This is relatively unimportant at this stage because of the small quantity of food involved. But since the ultimate aim of weaning is to ensure a healthy, balanced diet, the child should be introduced to a wide range of nutritious foods. However, new foods should be introduced one at a time to make it easier to identify any reaction to them.

Flavour. Bland foods with a mild or neutral flavour are preferred to strongly flavoured or spiced foods. No salt or sugar should be added during food preparation, or be added to manufactured baby foods. The food is designed to suit a baby's palate, not an adult's.

Consistency. A thin smooth consistency is necessary initially so that the baby can use the sucking reflex to take food from the spoon. At about the age of 4−6 months, the baby develops a swallowing ability, transferring food from the spoon to the back of the mouth, and can progress to food in the form of a thicker lump-free paste.

Manufactured 'first stage' weaning foods are either ready made or can be reconstituted to a smooth texture. Home-made weaning foods require liquidizing or sieving to achieve a suitable texture and consistency.

Preparation. Dried manufactured weaning foods are particularly useful in the early stages as very small quantities can be made up. Manufactured baby foods in tins and jars are also useful but once opened must be consumed within 24 hours and there may be some wastage initially.

Home-made baby food can be prepared and frozen, initially in ice cube trays and later in small pots, e.g. empty yoghurt cartons. A large freezer is not necessary; the small freezer compartment in a fridge is adequate for storing several days meals.

Expressed breast milk or infant milk formulae should be used to prepare foods where milk is needed.

Allergenicity. The DHSS recommend that children with a strong family history of allergy should avoid potential food allergens until beyond six months of age (DHSS 1980a). Food to be avoided are cows' milk, eggs and some fruits (especially those producing pips). In addition, all infants should avoid gluten-containing foods for the first six months of life.

Suitable early weaning foods are listed in Table 3.12.

Progression of weaning

The main steps in the progression of an infant's diet from milk to family meals are outlined in Table 3.13. However, the timescale over which they are achieved will vary considerably.

Table 3.12 Suitable early weaning foods

Food	Comments
Cooked rice cereal	Because of the small quantities required at this stage, it is usually easier to use a manufactured dried baby rice cereal
Dried manufactured baby foods	Very convenient in the early stages. Use 'Stage 1' varieties (i.e. those which reconstitute to a smooth texture). Introduce the savoury flavours before the sweeter ones. Ensure the product chosen is gluten-free
'Ready-made' manufactured baby foods	Available in cans or jars. Jars are more convenient as a can opener is not required and are particularly useful if the baby has to be fed away from home. Stage 1 or 'strained' gluten-free varieties should be used
Cooked pureed vegetables	No salt should be added or used in cooking. Carrots, potatoes, swede or peas are often well accepted
Pureed fruit	Cooked without sugar or canned in fruit juice e.g. apples, pears, apricots
Additional fluids	Cooled boiled water is sufficient

Table 3.13 Progression of weaning

Approximate age* of infant	Timescale* from starting weaning	Stage of feeding
4 months	Weeks 1 and 2	One teaspoon of different single foods of a thin, smooth consistency at one meal
	Weeks 3 and 4	1–2 teaspoons at two meals, increase consistency to a smooth paste.
5 months	1 month	Gradual increase in quantity and variety of foods offered. Maintain milk intake (breast or bottle). Additional fluid from bottle or feeder cup
6–8 months	2–4 months	Food at three meals, gradually changed to minced/mashed consistency. Suitable finger foods offered. Number and quantity of milk feeds may be reduced. Additional fluid from feeder cup
8–10 months	4–6 months	Diversification of minced/mashed foods at family meal times Milk minimum 1 pint daily Additional fluid from feeder cup Baby uses hands to feed self
1 year	6–8 months	Chopped family meals Milk 1 pint daily (or suitable alternatives) Feeder cup for fluids Learning to feed self with a spoon

*This will vary according to the age at which weaning starts and the rate at which it progresses.

Suitable foods for later stages of weaning

The same considerations of nutritional content, flavour and allergenicity apply as in the early stages. However, at about the age of six months the baby will welcome food of a more interesting texture. A mincer or baby Mouli is a useful piece of equipment. Vegetables may be mashed instead of pureed, and meats can be minced instead of liquidized. Flaked bone-free fish and scrambled egg can also be introduced. By the age of one year, the child will be able to chew chopped foods.

As soon as the child can sit up unsupported, he should be fed in a high chair and given a spoon so he can gradually learn to feed himself. A feeding bowl with a suction base helps to limit the amount of food deposited on the floor. Some finger foods can also be introduced.

Suitable foods at this stage are listed in Table 3.14.

Table 3.14 Suitable weaning foods for later stages of weaning

Food	Comments
Finger foods	Because of the risk of choking, these foods should be given under close supervision. Initially finger foods should be those which soften easily in the mouth.
Cereals	Breakfast cereals without added sugar, including wheat based cereals, e.g. porridge, Weetabix, baby mixed cereals. Cereals to make milk puddings or custard, e.g. rice, cornflour, custard powder, sago. Pasta, e.g. spaghetti, lasagne.
Meats, poultry, offal	Cooked without spices, salt or additional fat and minced.
Fish	Grilled, steamed or baked white fish, carefully checked for bones and then flaked. Later, canned fish such as sardines or tuna can be used.
Eggs	Egg yolk — soft or hard boiled from 6 months of age. Egg white — from about 9 months of age e.g. as scrambled egg or as part of other dishes.
Milk	If required as a drink, an infant milk formula should be used as an alternative to breast milk in infants under the age of 1 year. Cows' milk may be used in cooked dishes (e.g. milk puddings or custard).
Yoghurt	Preferably use low sugar varieties.
Cheese	Cottage cheese or grated mild cheese.
Vegetables	All except those with a stringy texture (e.g. celery) or which are spicy (e.g. chillis or peppers).
Fruits	All should be grated or chopped (with skins) until whole pieces of fruit can be eaten.
Nuts	Babies must *never* be given whole nuts but nut spreads and paste can be useful, especially for vegetarians.
Fluid	Diluted natural fruit juice and baby fruit juices add variety of flavours. Water is always a good source of fluid.

General considerations

Assessing whether a child is getting sufficient to eat and drink

Although a satisfactory growth rate is the most obvious sign of an adequate diet, the baby's general contentment, sleeping pattern and bowel habits are also valuable indicators. Some mothers worry over the apparently minute quantities of food eaten by their child. They should be discouraged from trying to force the child to eat more and be reassured that a healthy baby will not go hungry.

Additional vitamins and minerals

Additional vitamins may be needed at the weaning stage when nutritional requirements are likely to be increasing faster than the rate of dietary supply. The DHSS recommends the use of children's vitamin drops for all children between the ages of one month and two years (and preferably until the age of five) (DHSS 1980a). However, since many manufactured baby foods are already fortified with vitamins (and some minerals) the need for vitamin drops should be assessed individually by a health care professional.

Children living in areas with a low water fluoride content should be given fluoride supplements (see p 270).

Salt and fluid intake

Once the baby is a few months old, the kidneys are able to excrete excess sodium more readily. However, to ensure that too great a liking for salty food in later life does not develop, highly salted food should still be avoided.

As solids replace milk, it is important to offer adequate fluid to the baby so that its thirst may be satisfied. Serious imbalances may occur as a result of

1 Excessive sweating due to hot weather or a fever.
2 Gastroenteritis.
3 Vomiting and/or diarrhoea.

Home made versus manufactured baby foods

Mothers often ask whether they should use home made or manufactured baby foods. Either type is adequate; it is simply a matter of personal preference. Some mothers like to prepare all their infant's food and have the satisfaction of knowing exactly what their baby is eating. Others find it frustrating to take time and trouble preparing a suitable puree only for it to be rejected after one spoonful. In theory, home made baby foods are more economical than manufactured ones although this is not always the case in practice if they have to be prepared separately from the family meals (e.g. to avoid the use of salt or sugar thus incurring extra fuel costs) or if the baby then dislikes what has been produced. In the early stages, many mothers opt for the convenience of dried manufactured foods which can be made up in minute quantities and gradually introduce suitably modified items from the family meals when these are available. Ready made baby foods (especially those in jars) are also a useful adjunct to the diet, particularly when travelling or eating away from home.

Balance between sweet and savoury foods

All babies have a natural tendency to prefer sweet food. They have taste buds which make them respond positively to sweetness and this is probably connected with the fact that breast milk is a relatively sweet product. This preference for sweetness gradually declines with maturity as other taste sensations develop.

Because eating habits developed during weaning form the basis of life-long eating habits, it is important that there is a balance between sweet and savoury foods in the diet. The liking for sweet food by children should be recognized but not over-indulged. Where possible, sweetness should come from items such as fruit or fruit juice and added sugar kept to a minimum.

Age at which bottled cows' milk can be introduced

The DHSS has recommended the use of infant milk formulae rather than cows' milk until the age of one year (DHSS 1980b). However, while it is reasonable to use infant formulae for drinking purposes, avoiding cows' milk completely makes transition to the family meals very difficult. Provided that cows' milk is boiled to help its denaturation, there seems no reason why it should not be given to infants over the age of 6 months in the form of milk puddings, custards or similar dishes. Many commercial baby foods contain cows' milk.

Ideally, any cows' milk used should be pasteurized or UHT. Because of the risk of microbiological contamination, unpasteurized milk is best avoided but if used, it MUST be boiled.

Problems associated with weaning

Risk of choking

It is essential that a baby is never left alone while feeding. Care with the size of lumps in meals and the type of finger food offered will reduce the risk. Initially, finger foods should be those which soften easily in the mouth, e.g. rusk, bread or banana; harder foods such as apple or carrot should only be given when the child has learnt to chew well.

Rejection of solids

It takes time for a baby to become accustomed to feeding from a spoon and to each new taste. There will inevitably be some rejections, but provided that weaning coincides with the baby's development, solids will be taken. Late weaning, e.g. after nine months, may present more problems. Babies with mental or physical handicaps or emotionally deprived children with developmental problems may also be more difficult to wean. Force feeding, hurrying or anxiety in the mother transmitted to the baby can also lead to refusal of solids. Illness may cause a baby to regress to the previous stage of weaning foods but this will soon correct itself.

Faddy children

It is important for parents to recognize that babies, as well as adults, have genuine likes and dislikes which will affect acceptance or rejection of food. Furthermore, babies have variable appetites and should not be labelled as 'faddy' too readily. However, if a child persistently rejects all but a very limited range of foods, advice should be sought to prevent nutritional inadequacies.

The older child can use food rejection as a way of establishing independence and getting attention. This is less likely to become a problem if, at the outset of weaning, the parent learns to become detached from any food refusals and

1 Does not try to force-feed any food.
2 Tries a rejected food again a few days later.
3 Offers a rejected food prepared in a different way.
4 Replaces a disliked food with another food of similar nutritional value.
5 Does not over-indulge a preference for sweet foods.

Poor weaning practices

These may arise if developmental problems are not acknowledged. More common causes include ignorance, child neglect, economic and social problems.

Some ethic groups tend to delay weaning, and allow the child to remain almost exclusively on cows' milk until 2–3 years of age. This problem requires tactful handling.

Over-zealous application of NACNE recommendation to infants (especially high fibre diets) can cause a number of nutritional problems, particularly too low an energy intake and impairment of trace element status (Francis 1986).

Self-diagnosis of food allergy and the use of goats' milk or plant-based milks, and over-restriction of foods offered at weaning can also result in nutritional inadequacies.

Restrictive diets followed for religious, social or cultural reasons

Vegetarian and vegan diets are discussed in Section

3.19. Some ethnic groups, e.g. Asians may also offer restrictive diets at weaning (see Section 3.2.3).

Failure to thrive

The points noted above can, if left, result in the baby failing to thrive. Medical attention is essential to eliminate a functional cause, e.g. coeliac disease or cystic fibrosis (see Sections 4.11 and 4.12).

Constipation and diarrhoea

Constipation can occur if the fluid or fibre intake is inadequate. Some babies are more prone to constipation than others. Encouraging the intake of fruit and vegetables will assist bowel action and higher fibre cereals (e.g. Weetabix and wholemeal rusks) can be introduced at about the age of eight months.

Diarrhoea can be due to
1 Infection.
2 Reaction at teething.
3 Excessive fibre intake.
4 Food intolerance.
Prolonged diarrhoea should receive medical advice.

Dental caries

Dental hygiene should begin as soon as the first tooth appears, using a suitable soft toothbrush and a mild fluoride-containing baby toothpaste.

Dental caries is influenced more by the *frequency* of sugar consumption rather than the total amount of sugar consumed. All sources of sucrose should be minimized, but the frequent use of sugar-rich drinks or dummies filled with syrupy liquids must be strongly discouraged.

No fluoride supplements should be given to children under the age of two years if the fluoride content of the local water is above 0.3 ppm. If the water fluoride content is below 0.3 ppm, a daily supplement of 0.25 mg fluoride can be given from the age of two weeks (Editorial 1981). The role of fluoride in the prevention of dental caries is discussed in Section 4.8.1.

Obesity (see Section 4.1)

Infants are at greater risk of becoming obese if
1 One or both parents is obese.
2 Weaning is started early, before the age of three months.
3 They have certain mental or physical disabilities.
If both the weight and length of babies are regularly

recorded, height-weight percentile charts will show any deviations from desirable weight gain.

Strict reducing diets must never be imposed at this age and instead the aim should be to let the baby 'grow into' its weight. General measures such as minimizing the use of added sugar and sweet drinks, increasing the content of fruit and vegetables in the diet and reducing milk intake once weaning is established are usually sufficient to achieve this.

Food allergy and intolerance (see Section 5.9)

Eczema (see Section 4.30)

Rickets (see Section 4.26 and DHSS (1980c))

Predisposing factors include
1 Inadequate vitamin D intake.
2 Insufficient exposure to sunlight.
3 Delayed weaning or prolonged use of doorstep milk with few weaning foods.
4 Vegetarianism or a high fibre/phytate intake.
5 Poor maternal diet during pregnancy.
Rickets is still most commonly found among infants of Asian parents.

Inconsistent advice from professionals, the mass media, baby food manufacturers and lay groups

The new mother is usually bombarded with advice, some of which may be contradictory. Further confusion may arise with the healthy eating guidelines recommended in the NACNE (1983) and COMA (1984) reports and, for example, mothers may give their children skimmed milk in the belief that its low fat content is beneficial.

The implementation of a local food policy which endeavours to introduce some degree of uniformity to the advice given by health professionals within a particular area may help to reduce these problems. It is also important that the dietitian is a prominent member of the health care team which looks after mothers with young babies, not only to give advice directly to mothers if needed, but also to advise the advisers.

Support organisations

National Childbirth Trust, 9 Queensborough Terrace, London N2 3TB. Tel: 01-221-3833

La Leche League (Great Britain), PO Box BM 3424, London WC1V 6XV. Tel: 01-404-5011

National Association for Maternal and Child Welfare (NAMCW), 1 South Audley Street, London   W1Y 6JS.

Health Education Authority, 78 New Oxford Street, London WC1A 1AH.

(Leaflets include *Breast and bottle feeding* and *Weaning*)

Further reading

Francis DEM (1986) *Nutrition for children*. Blackwell Scientific Publications, Oxford.

Goldfard J and Tibbetts E (1980) *Breast feeding handbook*. A practical reference for physicians, nurses and other health professionals. Enslow Publishers, Hillside, New Jersey. (Distributed in the UK by Johy Libbey and Co).

Gunther M (1973) *Infant feeding*. Penguin, London.

Poskitt EME (1983) Infant feeding: a review. *Hum Nutr: Appl Nutr* **37A**, 271–86.

Stanway P and Stanway A (1978) *Breast is best*. Pan Books, London.

Wood CBS and Walker-Smith JA (1981) *MacKeith's infant feeding and feeding difficulties* 6e. Churchill Livingstone, Edinburgh.

References

Adinolfi M and Glynn A (1979) The interaction of antibacterial factors in breast milk. *Devel Med Child Neurol* **21**, 808–10.

Binkiewicz A, Robinson MJ and Senior B (1978) Pseudo-Cushing syndrome caused by alcohol in breast milk. *J Paediatr* **93**, 965–7.

Black AE, Wiles SJ and Paul AA (1986) The nutrient intakes of pregnant and lactating mothers of good socioeconomic status in Cambridge, UK: some implications for recommended daily allowances of minor nutrients. *Br J Nutr* **56**, 59–72.

Brock JH (1980) Lactoferrin in human milk: its role in iron absorption and protection against enteric infection in the newborn infant. *Arch Dis Childh* **55**, 417–22.

Chandra RK (1979) Prospective studies of the effect of breast feeding on the incidence of infection and allergy. *Acta Paediatr Scand* **68**, 691–4.

Committee on Medical Aspects of Food Policy (1984) *Diet and cardiovascular disease*. Report on Health and Social Subjects No 28. HMSO, London.

Craig-Schmidt M, Weete JD, Fairdoth SA, Wickwire MA and Livant EJ (1984) The effect of hydrogenated fat in the diet of nursing mothers on lipid composition and prostaglandin content of human milk. *Am J Clin Nutr* **39**, 778–86.

DHSS (1979) *Daily amounts of food energy and nutrients for groups of people in the United Kingdom*. Report on Health and Social Subjects No 15. HMSO, London.

DHSS (1980a) *Present day practice in infant feeding*. Report on Health and Social Subjects No 20. HMSO, London. (Reprinted with minor revisions 1983).

DHSS (1980b) *Artificial feeds for the young infant*. Report on Health and Social Subjects No 18. HMSO, London.

DHSS (1980c) *Rickets and osteomalacia*. Report on Health and Social Subjects No 19. HMSO, London.

Dowell TB and Joyston-Bechal S (1981) Fluoride supplements, age related doses. *Br Dental J* **150**, 273–5.

Downham MAPS, Scott R and Sims DG (1976) Does breast feeding protect against respiratory syncytial virus? *Br Med J* **2**, 274–6.

Editorial (1981) Dental caries and fluoride *Lancet* **i**, 1351.

FAO, WHO/UNU (1985) Energy and protein requirements. Report of a joint FAO/WHO/UNU expert consultation. *World Health Organisation Technical Report Series* **724**. WHO, Geneva.

Franus D (1986) *Diets for Sick Children*. Blackwell Scientific Publications, Oxford.

Kjellman NIM and Johansson SGO (1979) Soya versus cows' milk in infants with a biparental history of atopic disease: development of atopic disease and immunoglobulins from birth to 4 years of age. *Clin Allergy* **9**, 347–58.

Klaus MH and Kennell JH (1976) *Maternal infant bonding*. The CV Mosby Co, St Louis.

Martin J and Monk J (1982) *Infant Feeding 1980*. Office of Population Censuses and Surveys, St Catherine's House, 10 Kingsway, London WC2 6JP.

National Research Council (1980) *Recommended dietary allowances*. Ninth revised edition. National Academy of Sciences, Washington DC.

National Advisory Committee on Nutrition Education (1983) *Proposals for nutritional guidelines for health education in Britain*. Health Education Council, London.

Ogra SS and Ogra PL (1978) Immunological aspects of human colostrum and milk. *J Paediatr* **92**, 550–5.

Pittard WB (1979) Breast milk immunology. *Am J Dis Childh* **133**, 83–7.

Prentice AM, Paul AA, Prentice A, Black AE, Cole TJ and Whitehead RG (1986). Cross-cultural differences in lactational performance. In *Human Lactation 2: Maternal and environmental factors*. Proceedings of an international workshop held at Oaxaca, Mexico 1986. Plenum Publishing Corporation, New York.

Prentice AM, Roberts SB, Prentice A, Paul AA, Watkinson M, Watkinson AA and Whitehead RG (1983) Dietary supplementation of lactating Gambian women. 1. Effect on breast milk volume and quantity. *Hum Nutr: Clin Nutr* **37C**, 53–64.

Savilanti (1981) Cows' milk allergy. *Allergy* **26**, 73–88.

Thomson AM, Hytten FE and Billewicz WZ (1970) The energy cost of human lactation. *Br J Nutr* **24**, 565–72.

Warner JO (1980) Food allergy in fully breast fed infants. *Clin Allergy* **10**, 133–6.

White CJ and White MK (1980) Breast feeding and drugs in human milk. *Vet Human Toxicol* **22** [Suppl 1], 1–43.

Whitehead RG, Paul AA and Cole TJ (1981) A critical analysis of measured food energy intakes during infancy and early childhood in comparison with current international recommendations. *J Hum Nutr* **35**, 339–48.

Whitehead RG, Paul AA and Rowland MGM (1980) Lactation in Cambridge and The Gambia. *Br Med Bull* **37**, 77–82.

Wilson JT, Brown RD, Cherek DR, Dailey JW, Hilman B, Jobe PC, Manno BR, Manno JE, Redetz HM and Stewart JJ (1980) Drug excretion in human breast milk. *Clin Pharmokinetics* **5**, 1–66.

Yap PL, Pryde A, Latham PJ and McLelland DB (1979) Serum IgA in the neonate. Concentration and effect of breast feeding. *Acta Paediatr Scand* **68**, 695–700.

3.3 The Pre-school Child

3.3.1 Food and eating in the pre-school child

The pre-school child is a changing individual. The developments which take place between one and five years of age are numerous and directly or indirectly affect eating habits.

The pre-school child is almost totally dependent on others for its food. The parents, and other carers, should be aware that their own eating habits, likes and dislikes, will be the ones that the child imitates and acquires.

Food and eating are wonderful sources of learning for children, e.g. via cooking, shopping and eating out. Food can also be a source of frustration and a cause of arguments between parents and child, e.g. regarding sweets or 'eating up the greens'.

The most useful advice concerning food which can be offered to a parent of a small child is never to let eating problems become 'an issue'. In an attempt to produce a well-behaved, non-fussy child, meal times can very easily turn into a battle ground. It is also easy for parents to fall into the trap of using food (especially sweets) as a means of punishment or reward. Arguments over food are always counter-productive and ultimately are fights which the parent cannot win — a stubborn toddler cannot be *forced* to eat something if he is determined not to. Instead meal times should be governed by calm common sense. Children should be offered a variety of food which they can enjoy and cope with according to their level of development (Table 3.15). Food not eaten should be removed without comment and the impulse to fill the child up with biscuits or sweets strongly resisted.

However, it is also important to consider food from the child's point of view. Small children are not designed to eat large quantities of food at infrequent intervals. The typical adult eating pattern of 2 or 3 substantial meals a day with nothing between is not necessarily appropriate for a toddler and, not surprisingly, may lead to hunger, bad temper and belligerent demands for biscuits, crisps and sweets. Offering the child smaller meals (or nutritious snacks such as a sandwich or a crispbread with cheese) at more frequent intervals may help avert this problem and also improve the overall nutritional intake.

Furthermore, while food faddism as such should not be indulged, it should be recognized that children, like adults, may have genuine likes and dislikes, 'off days' and the occasional desire to eat for comfort. Adults readily alter their food intake in response to these feelings so it is not unreasonable that children should, on occasions, be able to do the same.

Other factors also affect a child's eating pattern. Minor illnesses are common in this age group and can markedly reduce appetite. Major illness such as diabetes or renal disease can also arise and if a therapeutic diet is needed, this will add considerably to the stress experienced by both the child and his family.

Phases of eating patterns are common in the pre-school years. These may have an obvious cause such as illness or stress arising from the parents' marriage break-up or the arrival of a sibling, but more usually they simply reflect the child's developing independence and the need to assert his or her own individuality. These phases may take the form of

1 Eating very little of anything.
2 Eating well from a very narrow range of foods.
3 Eating a bizarre combination (to an adult's taste) of foods (e.g. baked beans and cornflakes).
4 Sudden likes or dislikes.
5 Demanding a particular pattern of eating for security.

Parents often worry a great deal about their child's

Table 3.15 Practicalities of eating for the pre-school child

Age	Seating	Feeding	Utensils	Behaviour
1 year	High chair	Learning to feed self	Fingers, teaspoon. Dishes with sides. Feeder beaker	Messy
2 years	At the table (sitting on a raised seat or cushion if necessary)	Feeds self with help in cutting up foods, etc.	Spoon, small fork, fingers. Dishes with sides. Cup	Some accidents
3 years	At the table	Feeds self	Spoon, small fork, learning to use knife. Plates. Cup	Generally tidy
4–5 years	At the table	Feeds self	Child-size cutlery. Plates. Cup	Competent eaters

apparently meagre or strange diet but most can be reassured that these problems are common, that they won't last very long (although it may *seem* like a long time) and that no lasting harm will result. If the child appears to be fit and active then there is little to worry about. Furthermore, a relaxed attitude on the part of the parent will help the problem resolve itself more quickly.

3.3.2 Healthy eating and the pre-school child

Current guidelines on healthy eating (as given in the COMA (1984) or NACNE (1983) reports) are not intended to be applied to this age group. This is not to say that healthy eating habits cannot be started. The pre-school child's food intake in later years will be greatly influenced by what he or she is offered, and sees other people eating, in the early years. It is therefore the *family* eating habits which are important and should be modified if inappropriate.

Fats

Eating less fat poses no nutritional problems for the adult but, in the small child, such a measure can result in a diet of insufficient energy content. This is because the carbohydrate foods needed to replace the energy from fat are more bulky and a young child may not be able to cope with this volume, especially if the carbohydrate is high in fibre. Moderate reduction in fat, especially saturated fat, can be achieved, while still allowing some high fat (preferably polyunsaturated) foods. Visible meat fat should be discarded and lean meat, poultry and fish offered in preference to fatty cuts of meat. Butter, hard margarines and lard should be replaced by polyunsaturated fats and oils.

The most contentious area is milk, which is usually a major contributor to dietary fat intake. The COMA report (1984) recommends that families opting for skimmed or semi-skimmed milk should 'continue to provide whole cows' milk for children below the age of five'. This is because whole milk usually makes a significant contribution to a child, energy intake. However, many nutritionists feel that the type of milk which a child drinks will not affect nutritional status provided that the child has a good appetite and eats a varied diet. The decision on the type of milk is best left to the family and the health professionals advising them, and based upon the eating habits, growth pattern and health of the child.

Fibre

Healthy eating advice encourages more dietary fibre in the form of whole-grain cereals, bread, fruit and vegetables. This bulky food can result in the child being full before sufficient energy and nutrients have been consumed. Encouraging the consumption of these foods as between-meal snacks rather than with main meals may be a more satisfactory alternative.

There are no recommendations for the amount of fibre which is appropriate for small children. It is perhaps best judged by the quality of the stools. If hard and small, the dietary fibre could usefully be increased. If soft but formed, the diet is correct. Young children must *not* be given unprocessed bran which may cause intestinal blockage.

Sugar

There are no nutritional problems in minimizing the sugar in the diet of this age group.

Salt

Adding salt to the diet of babies is discouraged because of the risk of kidney damage. The pre-school child should therefore already be accustomed to the taste of a relatively low salt diet and, as far as possible, this should be maintained by using very little salt in cooking and not adding salt to food at the table. Unfortunately, many of the popular savoury snacks such as crisps have a high salt content but salt-free forms are becoming available and should be used in preference.

3.3.3 Nutritional problems in the pre-school child

Undernutrition

The growth of the pre-school child is often very uneven and characterized by static periods interspersed with sudden increases in height and weight. Assessment of a child's growth, by means of height and weight percentile charts, should therefore be made over a period of time. An experienced health visitor or a dietitian can then assess whether there is a problem and, if necessary, recommend an appropriate solution.

An inadequate total diet may be due to

1 an inadequate diet being offered to the child, owing to nutritional ignorance, low income (see Section 3.7) or other social problems.

2 an inadequate diet being eaten by the child, due to food refusal or food dislikes, or because the diet is too

high in fibre and low in fat and consequently insufficiently energy-dense.

Specific nutritional inadequacies are often the result of specific food dislikes. For example, refusal to eat fruit or vegetables can lead to an inadequate fibre intake and problems such as constipation and soiling.

Obesity

Because the pre-school child is totally dependent on other people for his food, obesity in this age group is entirely the fault of the parents (or carers) rather than the child. It is easy for high energy foods such as sweets, biscuits, crisps to figure to excess in the diet of a fussy eater, but it is the parents who have allowed this situation to develop. Treatment of childhood obesity is discussed in Section 4.1.4.

Food faddism

The pre-school child will have genuine food likes and dislikes, but these may be difficult to distinguish from food faddism. The latter is characterized generally by a sudden refusal to eat food which was previously considered to be acceptable.

The child may become more faddy before and after an illness or during a traumatic period such as the birth of sibling, moving house or the death of a relative or a pet.

It is important not to force the child to eat, and also not to offer alternatives or give into demands for biscuits or desired treats before the next meal. Once the child realizes that attention and favours will not be gained by these strategies, the faddism will gradually disappear.

Some pre-school children become sensitive to the use of animals for their food and refuse all meats. Sympathetic parents will offer alternative sources of protein and no problem will arise.

A number of tactics such as eating out at a friend's home can be employed to help the fussy child (see p 277).

Hyperkinesis (see Sections 5.9 and 2.15)

Sources of help include child welfare clinics, health visitors and mother and toddler groups.

Further reading

Elliot R (1982) *Vegetarian baby book*. The Vegetarian Society Altrincham.
Lewis C (1984) *Growing up with good food*. Unwin, London.
The Open University (1977) *The pre-school child*. Open University Press, Milton Keynes.
Richardson R (1981) *Cooking for kids*. Jill Norman Ltd, London.

References

DHSS (1984) Committee on Medical Aspects of Food Policy *Diet and cardiovascular disease*. Report on Health and Social subjects No 28 HMSO, London.
National Advisory Committee on Nutrition Education (1983) *Proposals for nutritional guidelines for health education in Britain*. Health Education Authority, London.

3.4 The School-age Child

3.4.1 Healthy eating and the school-age child

The general principles of a healthy diet (see Section 1.1) apply to healthy school-age children. However, the child's eating patterns and taste preferences will have been established by the family eating habits in the pre-school years. Any poor eating patterns acquired during these years will only be changed with difficulty. The child likes familiar foods and concepts of long term health carry no weight at all.

Because of the child's ability to forage for himself, the possible freedom to choose food at school solely according to his own preferences and, in some households where both parents work, the necessity of getting his own food after school, some children may end up with particularly poor eating habits.

At school, education in healthy eating will be standard in home enconomics classes and it is built in to the new GCSE examination syllabus. However, the child may not see this education as relevant to himself if home eating patterns are very different and if school meals run counter to the teaching. Programmes to improve the diet of school children need to be directed at the school meals and tuck shop provision, and to the parent (perhaps through parent teacher associations) as well as to the child. Messages will be reinforced if nutrition topics can also be included in the general curriculum, e.g. study of food plants in biology, trade in food in geography or economics.

The Inner London Education Authority (1985) produced, in collaboration with members of the British Dietetic Association, nutritional guidelines with sound nutrition information, a framework for a balanced diet which suits the eating patterns of all ethnic groups, background information on eating patterns and a teaching plan which can operate at different levels of age, ability or knowledge.

3.4.2 School meals

The 1980 Education Act which became law in April 1980 made major changes in the laws governing the provision of school meals. It removed the statutory obligations of local education authorities to provide meals of a certain nutritional standard at a fixed price in maintained schools. Prior to 1980, a school meal was expected to provide one-third of the child's daily requirement of protein, energy and some vitamins and minerals. The 1980 Act simply requires local education authorities to provide a meal for children in receipt of free school meals and to provide a place for children to eat sandwiches brought to school. Local education authorities therefore do not have to provide meals at all (except for free school meal recipients) and can charge whatever price they feel appropriate.

These changes were introduced by the government in an attempt to curtail the growth in public expenditure. This was to be achieved by a reduction in the working hours of the catering staff; hours are worked out on the basis of the number of meals to be provided and divided between cooks and kitchen assistants. This in turn led to the need to make savings in preparation and cooking time which resulted in more convenience foods being used. It was also believed that by offering foods popular with children, a good cash-return could be guaranteed. The rules governing the provision of free school meals were also altered so that local education authorities need only provide free meals to children from families in receipt of family income supplement and supplementary benefit — it has been suggested that this has resulted in up to 30% of children losing their entitlement. Changes in the system of benefits due to be made in April 1988 will result in some children's entitlement to free school meals being replaced by direct cash payments to the family (which may or may not be spent on food).

There are several nutritional consequences of these changes

1 There is potential for a greater variety of foods to be offered thereby increasing the acceptability of school meals. However it is important that

    a)   A wide choice of food is offered.

    b)   'Healthy' alternatives are included.

    c)   Children are guided in their choice of food.

2 Now that local education authorities are released from their statutory duties to provide a meal of a certain nutritional standard there is no guarantee that children will receive an adequate meal.

3 School meals were always seen in the past as being

good tools for nutrition education; in many cases they are now in direct conflict with current nutritional recommendations.

4 The new menus can result in high intakes of fat and sugar and low intakes of fibre and vitamins.

5 Children may choose to spend dinner money on items other than food.

6 A number of children may now be nutritionally at risk, in particular

a) Those who used to receive free school meals but no longer do so.

b) Those who receive free school meals and who make inappropriate choices.

c) Those whose parents rely on shcool meals to provide the main meal of the day.

d) Those who spend dinner money out of school on sweets or other items.

e) Those who opt to take a packed lunch of an inappropriate content.

It must be remembered that school meals only provide five out of 21 meals per week in term time — parents are responsible for the rest. The midday meal is not just a stop-gap between breakfast and the evening meal. For many children lunch is their first meal of the day as breakfast is often omitted. It is therefore vital that the midday meal is nutritionally adequate and if it is not, this factor must be considered when other meals are being planned.

Types of school meals

These vary according to the type of school and the local education authority (Table 3.16). Prices also vary depending on the system and the local education authority.

Table 3.16 School meal services in common use

Primary schools cafeteria service	No choice or sometimes a choice from two items. Price fixed for meal; there is an upper limit of what the child can spend. Choice may be guided by a 'unit choice' system which gives a limited amount of guidance.
Middle schools cash-cafeteria system	A wider choice of foods is available. Items are individually priced. There may be some guidance in choice.
Secondary schools cash-cafeteria system	Many foods are available. The variety in nutritional terms depends on the caterer. Items are individually priced. Children may spend as much as they wish. Choice generally not guided.

Guidance with food choice

'Unit choice' system

This is designed to help children choose a balanced meal and is often used in primary schools. Pupils are allowed to choose a maximum of five units for each meal in the following way: protein part of meal = 0 units and *must* be included, other items of the meal carry either 1 or 2 units depending on the nutritional desirability of the food, e.g.

Chips	2 units
Jacket potato	1 unit
Steamed jam pudding	2 units
Fresh fruit	1 unit

By allotting the least units to the most healthy foods, children are, in theory, tempted to choose these items because they can have more of them. The system does not guarantee a healthy choice but it does at least encourage healthy eating.

Colour-coded menus

This is another system with can guide food choice. It is based on one of two ideas

1 Food groups. Each of the four basic food groups (milk, meat, fruit and bread) is assigned a colour and items on the menu are colour-coded according to which group they belong to. Pupils are encouraged to choose at least three different colours. An example of this system is shown in Table 3.17

Table 3.17 Example of a colour-coded menu system to guide food choice

Food groups used	Dairy = Blue Meat/fish/pulses = Red Fruit/vegetables = Green Cereal/potato = Orange
Food choice	Pupils are encouraged to choose a meal comprised of at least three different colours.
Menu available	Soup and roll = Orange Beefburger = Red Fish finger = Red Peas = Green/red Salad = Green Jacket potato = Orange Bread roll = Orange Fresh fruit = Green Apple pie = Orange/green Yoghurt = Blue Fruit juice = Green Milk = Blue
Possible meal chosen	Beefburger = Red Jacket potato = Orange Salad = Green Yoghurt = Blue

2 Traffic light system. The NACNE recommendations can be reflected by a system using traffic light colours or similar symbols. No food is labelled as 'bad', instead
a) Foods high in fat, sugar and salt are coded as RED 'stop and think' foods, i.e. items in the diet which should be reduced.
b) Foods high in fibre are coded GREEN 'go' foods, i.e. foods which should be encouraged and which should be eaten to replace foods for the red group.
c) All other foods are coded AMBER 'go carefully' foods, i.e. items which should be eaten in moderation.

Pupils are encouraged to choose their lunch mainly from the green and amber groups, and to limit the number of items chosen from the red group. On the menu board and/or the service counter, foods are coded with red, amber or green labels to help pupils select their lunch wisely.

Milk

Whole milk and whole milk yoghurts are available to schools at a reduced price as a result of EEC subsidies. Milk can also be purchased in $\frac{1}{3}$ pint bottles and many schools offer this for sale at break-time. Milk is available free to 'deprived children' who are identified by the medical authorities and is also free for pupils in special schools. Milk and biscuits are often served by schools as an alternative to dessert.

Problems remaining with the school meals service

Lack of suitable foods. The composition of a protein dish may result in the child selecting a nutritionally inadequate meal.

Lack of guidance in food choice. More help needs to be given to pupils to help them identify the content of a meal. School meals supervisors need to be better informed on nutritional matters so that they can also offer guidance on food choice.

Lack of parental awareness. Parents should know
1 The types of food offered to their children.
2 Which nutrients are lacking in the school meals.
3 Which foods should be included at home.
4 Which foods to provide for packed lunches.

Inadequate time and choice available for lunch. This is a particular problem for young children especially those who are slow eaters. Also, if a child has to queue for a long time to obtain his meal, there may be little time left in which to eat it. The choice may also be limited for the children who are last in the queue.

Lack of suitable meals for minority groups. Minority groups, such as Asian children, may not be well catered for. Many authorities are, however, reviewing their policies in order to provide more suitable foods for these groups. More liaison is also required with the Asian community to remove suspicion of the meals.

3.4.3 Nutritional problems in the school-age child

Undernutrition

This is generally characterized by poor growth rates which can be demonstrated by plotting a child's height and weight on percentile charts (see Section 1.8). However it should not be assumed that maximal growth rates can be equated with optimal nutritional status; other factors besides nutritional intake (e.g. genetics) affect weight.

In order to obtain an adequate nutritional intake, children need to consume a wide variety of foods. This is not always easy to achieve in practice since children are naturally conservative. However, they are also imitators and will tend to adopt the family's eating patterns and likes or dislikes. It is therefore important that the whole family has sensible eating habits; for example, one cannot expect children to eat breakfast if their parents do not.

Various tactics can be employed to encourage the poor eater
1 Anticipating trouble before a meal is served: new or unfamiliar foods should be produced without comment.
2 Serving food in different and novel ways may help a child to eat and enjoy otherwise unpopular food for example
    a) Vegetables can be served raw and attractively arranged rather than always cooked, e.g. a cartwheel presentation of raw sticks carrot, celery, cucumber, with nuts, fruit and raisins.
    b) Meat can be minced and formed into sausage or beefburgers.
    c) Liver can be made into liver paté or sausage.
3 Allowing children to serve themselves often encourages them to try different foods.
4 Not allowing children in a 'bad mood' to get the better of a parent — an untouched plate should simply be removed and no other food (especially not biscuits or sweets) offered until the next meal time.

5 Unfamiliar foods which are rejected when first offered can be left for a few weeks and then offered again, maybe in a different form, but without comment.
6 Eating out or with friends at home often helps a fussy child to eat better.

Obesity

The prevalence of obesity in childhood is hard to assess but is somewhere between 5–15%. Obesity in children is usually obvious but can be confirmed by measurement of skinfold thickness and by plotting height and weight on percentile charts.

Overweight children, in contrast to overweight adults, tend to be taller than average due to advanced bone ages and this reflects their generally increased growth rates, both upwards and outwards. The aetiology and treatment of obesity in children is discussed in Section 4.1.4; p 344.

Rickets

Nowadays, rickets tend to be found mainly in Asian families, but can also occur following growth spurts in borderline vitamin D deficient white British children (see Section 4.26).

Anaemia (see Section 4.18.1)

This may be a problem amongst children from low income families or where a poor diet is eaten. Furthermore, iron-rich foods (e.g. liver and red meats) are not always popular with children, and some children eat few green vegetables or fresh fruit, resulting in low vitamin C intakes and poor iron absorption.

Anaemia may also be due to low folic acid intakes as a result of low intakes of liver, fruit, vegetables or wholegrain cereals.

With a little ingenuity, alternative ways of providing these nutrients can usually be found. Unpopular foods can sometimes be disguised or presented in a way which is more acceptable, e.g. liver turned into a paté or red meat transformed into a hamburger.

Poor meal habits

Omission of meals, notably breakfast, is likely to result in reduced nutrient intakes.

Lunch among many school children may be inadequate due to poor choice of foods or a lack of guidance and supervision. Sometimes, money for school lunches is spent on non-food items. Packed lunches may be inadequate in nutritional composition. These problems are compounded if parents are unaware that the child's lunch is inadequate and that a nutritionally adequate meal is required later at home.

Frequent consumption of snacks may also result in a reduced appetite at meal times with a consequent poor nutrient intake.

Dental disease

Causation, treatment and prevention of dental disease are discussed in Section 4.8.1.

Diet-linked behavioural problems

Hyperkinesis (see also Section 5.9, p 578)

Many different terms are used in the literature for this condition. Hyperkinesis or 'the hyperactive child syndrome' has also been referred to as hypersensitivity, overactivity, hyperactive change syndrome, attention deficit disorder, minimal brain damage, minimal brain dysfunction and learning disorders.

The symptoms as described in the British Medical Journal (1975) are

'a chronic sustained level of motor activity relative to the age of the child, occurring mainly in boys between one and 16 years, but characteristically around six years, accompanied by short attention span, impulsive behaviour or explosive outbursts and causing substantial complaints at home or in school.'

Other symptoms include social, learning and behavioural problems, thirst, anxiety, aggression, poor eating and sleeping habits and temper tantrums. Some hyperactive children may suffer from headaches, catarrh, asthma and hayfever. A few have low IQ, but this is not a general feature. The causes of hyperactivity are unknown but several factors are suggested to have an influence, e.g. food allergies, parental attitudes, smoking in pregnancy and genetic factors.

The incidence of hyperactivity has recently been suggested to be in the region of 0.99% in the UK and 1.9–5% in the USA. However, the reported incidence does vary widely due to different diagnostic criteria and a joint UK/USA study has been set up to try to establish the most suitable criteria for the diagnosis of this condition (MacGibbon 1983). However, irrespective of its true characteristics, 'hyperactivity' is, unfortunately, an increasingly popular 'diagnosis' among the lay-public. Often the problem is simply one of difficult family relationships which express themselves in the child's antisocial behaviour. The problem can also be exacerbated by parental worry over dietary habits or by the child himself who exploits the situation to his advantage.

Treatment of the condition where a true diagnosis is made is by drugs, diet or behaviour therapy and very often a combination of all three.

The use of the Feingold (1975) diet has been extensively encouraged by many lay organisations. The basis of his dietary modification is the avoidance of naturally occurring salicylates and the avoidance of food and drink containing additives and colouring. Scientists and nutritionists have remained equivocal about the benefits of this diet as it has little hard evidence to support it. However, a number of studies are emerging which lend support to the theory that some children are sensitive to some food additives, and in these cases removal of the offending substances can produce dramatic improvements in behaviour and other symptoms, particularly asthma and severe headaches (Freedman 1977; Weiss et al 1980; Egger et al 1985). (See also Section 5.9.)

In many cases of hyperactivity it may be beneficial to give the child a diet free from food additives and colourings for one month to see whether any improvement occurs. If it does, further tests can then be carried out to identify the additive components responsible. However, it should not be forgotten that the extra attention given to the child as a result of the effort involved in providing an additive-free diet may in itself cause an improvement in behaviour. If no improvement occurs, the parents can then be assured that the problem is not a dietary one and thereby one element of worry is removed. This may help to improve relations with the child leading to a general improvement.

In addition to the possible effects of food additives, other causative theories put forward in recent years include a link with essential fatty acid metabolism, abnormality of carbohydrate metabolism and effects of other food allergies. However, as with any behavioural disorder where the benefits of treatment can only be evaluated subjectively, and therefore carry an inherent risk of bias, proof is difficult to obtain.

The idea of Feingold-type dietary treatment is frequently advocated in the media but is generally not recommended by the medical profession. Many families may therefore be trying out dietary treatment on a purely anecdotal and trial-and-error basis. As the diet is very restricted there is a very real danger of nutritional inadequacy in growing children, particularly among children from families who use large amounts of processed and packaged foods or if the dietary measures are imposed for a long period of time. Advice from a qualified dietitian is really needed by anyone who wishes to place their child on a diet of this type. Unfortunately, dietitians are not allowed, at present, to give advice of this nature unless it is accompanied by a medical referral and this may well not be forthcoming. Liaison with the family's health visitor can sometimes resolve this very difficult problem. If parents are determined to embark on dietary experimentation in their children without medical approval, then perhaps they can at least be persuaded to keep it of short duration so that no nutritional damage is done.

Sources of help and support organisations

1 Local dental officers, school nurses, health visitors.
2 The Hyperactive Children's Support Group, Sally Bunday (Secretary), 59 Meadowside, Angmering, West Sussex.

Further reading

British Dietetic Association Community Nutrition Group, Information sheets. No 1 *Changes in school meals — for better or worse?* No 2 *Rickets and osteomalacia — what are we doing?* No 5 *Dental health* and No 11 *Hyperactivity*.

References

Editorial (1975) Hyperactivity in children. *Br Med J* **4**, 123−4.
Education Act (1980) *Section 22 School Meals: England and Wales.*
Education Act (1980) *Section 23 School Meals: Scotland.*
Egger J, Carter CM, Graham PJ, Gumley D and Soothill JF (1985) Controlled trial of oligoantigenic treatment in the hyperkinetic syndrome. *Lancet* **i**, 540−5.
Feingold B (1975) *Why your child is hyperactive.* Random House Publishing,
Freedman BJ (1977) Asthma induced by sulphur dioxide, benzoate and tartrazine contained in orange drinks. *Clin Allergy* **7**, 407−15.
Inner London Education Authority (1985) *Nutritional guidelines.* Published for the ILEA Learning Resources Branch by Heinemann Educational Books, London.
Inner London Education Authority (1985) *ILEA Nutrition guidelines teaching matrices.* Available from Inner London Education Authority Learning Resources Branch, Television and Publishing Centre, Thackeray Road, London SW8 3TB.
MacGibbon B (1983) Adverse reactions to food additives. *Proc Nutr Soc* **42**, 233−40.
Weiss B, Williams JH, Margen S, Abrams B, Caan B, Citron LJ, Cox C, McKibben J, Ogar D and Shultz S (1980) Behavioural response to artificial food colours. *Science* **207**, 1487−9.

3.5 The Adolescent

Adolescence is a time of change to adult behaviour. The eating habits of childhood gradually change into those typical of an adult. Adolescence is therefore an important time for health and nutrition education. However, as part of this process of change, some or even all of such advice is likely to be ignored, at least on a temporary basis, and experimentation with new foods, new tastes and new eating patterns generally will be the norm.

Eating habits may be erratic; large quantities may be eaten one day and very little the next. Teenagers also have a profound wish to exert their independence and make their own decisions and food choice is likely to be one of the first targets. There is also a need to conform within the peer group.

Tact, patience and understanding are required in large measures by both parents and professional advisers so that the adolescent is gently steered towards a pattern of sensible healthy eating and away from extreme diets with potentially harmful consequences.

3.5.1 Nutritional considerations in the adolescent

Energy

Because adolescence is a time of rapid growth, the requirement for energy is relatively high, especially in adolescent boys who may be consuming 3000–4000 kcal/day and are often described by mothers as having 'hollow legs'. The frequent consumption of snack foods, in addition to substantial meals, is not necessarily of nutritional concern; for some, it is the only way to obtain sufficient energy. For the same reason, strict adherence to low fat, high fibre foods may lead to a diet which is unacceptably bulky.

Iron

Iron requirements are increased in girls with the onset of menstruation. Iron deficiency anaemia is not uncommon in this age group and is quite likely in teenagers who become pregnant.

Calcium

Calcium requirements are increased during growth spurts although this is offset by adjustments in calcium absorption. Overt calcium deficiency is rare.

Dietary advice

Dietary advice to the adolescent should follow the principles of a healthy diet as outlined in Section 1.1 as far as foods are concerned. However, the advice must take into account the individual's life style and peer pressures. Advice may well be best given in terms of fast foods, snacks, takeaways and burger bars rather than 'proper' meals. There is nothing inherently wrong with an unconventional meal pattern, if the overall balance of foods chosen is satisfactory.

3.5.2 Nutritional problems in the adolescent

Food faddism

The desire to experiment and express novel views may lead to bizarre eating practices or the adoption of cult diets. Factors such as suspicion, fear, morality, religious beliefs or just misconceptions about food may lead to inappropriate food choice. Sometimes large amounts of money are spent on products from health food shops. Food fads are usually short term crazes but in some cases may become permanent ways of eating.

Food fads which may lead to serious problems include:

Vegetarianism (see also Section 3.9)

This is not in itself a problem and can be a healthy way of eating, but its adoption by teenagers frequently causes problems. Many try to follow vegetarian practices without any guidance and, while they are usually successful at omitting animal products, teenagers are usually not very adept at replacing them with appropriate vegetable ones. Deficiencies of iron, vitamin B12 and protein often result.

An additional problem is that parents may view their child's vegetarianism as an indication of juvenile delinquency or a desire to 'drop out'. They therefore exert parental pressure which inevitably causes friction and may lead to even more restrictive eating. If instead, parents offer the child support and help them obtain reliable information, the problem — if it is a problem — usually just fades away.

Wholefood diets (see also Section 3.9)

As with vegetarian eating, there need be nothing wrong with this way of eating. However, it is essential that a wide variety of foods is consumed if an adequate nutrient intake is to be obtained. A limited choice of foods nearly always leads to nutritional deficiencies.

Macrobiotic diets (see Section 3.9)

Food cults (see also Section 2.16)

Sometimes, particular foods (as distinct from diets) have certain properties attributed to them. They may therefore be either included in large quantities or avoided. Such foods likely to be
1   Honey and raw sugar. These are often believed to be healthier than sugar. Such claims are unsubstantiated.
2   Grapefruit. This is erroneously believed by many to 'burn up fat'.
3   Organically grown products. These are believed to be superior in terms of taste, nutrient content and freedom from pesticide residues compared with traditionally grown products. Usually the main difference is in the price.
4   Vitamin and mineral supplements. Many people spend a lot of money on these products in the belief that their health will be improved whereas they are usually unnecessary and some, if consumed to excess, will be harmful.

Slimming regimens

About half of the adolescent girls in Western society attempt at some time to lose weight. Some of the slimming methods adopted are very restrictive. The diet may be comprised of only two or three items, e.g. fruit and black coffee which will obviously lead to nutrient deficiencies. Sometimes inappropriate foods are eaten in large quantities due to mistaken beliefs about their food value; cheese is a common example. Teenagers are also tempted to buy various slimming aids and gimmicks. Apart from being very expensive,

many of these are undesirable in nutritional terms and are of no help in achieving long term weight loss.

Sound advice on appropriate slimming methods is essential together with encouragement to take adequate exercise. When teenagers leave school, their activity level frequently decreases dramatically and consequently their weight may increase. Dietary advice must be practical to fit in with normal adolescent lifestyle otherwise it is only counterproductive. Guidance is more appropriate than rigid rules.

In this age group there is a particular risk that attempts to slim will lead to anorexia nervosa (see Section 4.24.4). If the slimming appears to be becoming an obsession and weight is falling rapidly, professional help should be sought quickly.

Athletic training (see also Section 3.8)

Many teenagers involved in extensive training schedules adopt bizarre eating patterns. Some consume high protein diets in a mistaken belief that this is essential for stamina. Others take high doses of vitamin and mineral supplements, a practice which should be strongly discouraged. Eating times are often limited due to training schedules and there is a temptation to use products such as complete-liquid diets; however these are expensive and inappropriate. Alternatively, quick snacks may replace proper meals and provide inadequate nutrition.

Advice needs to be given about healthy eating for these circumstances — large quantities of protein are not necessary and adequate minerals and vitamins can be obtained from dietary sources. A relatively high level of carbohydrate is essential to boost muscle glycogen stores, particularly before endurance tests. Adequate fluid intake is very important, both prior to and during sporting events. Rest days should be part of a training schedule in order to allow time to eat and replenish body stores.

Skin disorders in adolescents

Acne vulgaris is common in teenagers and is often attributed to eating excess sweets, chocolates and fried foods but there is no evidence to support the view that dietary factors are responsible. However, since it is of general health benefit to consume less fat and sugar and more fibre-rich foods and fluid, it is still valuable to encourage teenagers to modify their diet along these lines.

Further reading

General

Winick M (1982) *Adolescent nutrition*. John Wiley, Bristol.

Dietary studies

Bull NL (1985) Dietary habits of 15–25 year olds. *Hum Nutr: Appl Nutr* **39A**, [Suppl 1] 1–68.

Cresswell J, Busby A, Young H and Inglis V (1983) Dietary patterns of third-year secondary schoolgirls in Glasgow. *Hum Nutr: Appl Nutr* **37A**, 301–6.

Durnin JVGA (1984) Energy balance in childhood and adolescence. *Proc Nutr Soc* **43**, 271–9.

Durnin JVGA, Lonergan ME, Good J and Ewan A (1974) A cross-sectional nutritional and anthropometric study, with an interval of seven years, on 611 young adolescent schoolchildren. *Br J Nutr* **32**, 169–79.

Hackett AF, Rugg-Gunn AJ, Appleton DR, Eastre JE and Jenkins GN (1984) A two-year longitudinal nutritional survey of 405 Northumberland children initially aged 11.5 years. *Br J Nutr* **51**, 67–75.

Hackett AF, Rugg-Gunn AJ, Appleton DR, Allinson DI and Eastoe JE (1984) Sugars — eating habits of 405 11–14 year old English children. *Br J Nutr* **57**, 347–56.

Woodward DR (1985) What sort of teenager has high intakes of energy and nutrients? *Br J Nutr* **54**, 325–33.

Woodward DR (1985) What sort of teenager has low intakes of energy and nutrients? *Br J Nutr* **53**, 241–9.

Sociological studies

Curry KR (1984) Cultural aspects of food habits: teenager awareness in New Zealand, England and the United States. *J NZ Dietet Assoc* **38**, 38–50.

McGuffin SJ (1983) Food fashions. *Nutr Food Sci* **81**, 6–7.

Special considerations

Heald FP and Jacobsen MS (1980) Nutritional needs of the pregnant adolescent. *Paediatr Ann* **9**, 95–9.

O'Hare AE, Uttley WS, Belton NR, Westwood A, Levin SD and Anderson F (1984) Persisting vitamin D deficiency in the Asian adolescent. *Arch Dis Childh* **59**, 766–70.

3.6 The Elderly

In the UK the term 'elderly' generally refers to persons of pensionable age, i.e. men 65 years and over, women 60 years and over. All will be keen to maintain their health and independence for as long as possible. Many newly retired will be facing some 30+ years ahead. One of the cornerstones for their future health will be the attention which is paid to diet.

There are 9.5 million elderly in the UK and, in 1985, they accounted for nearly 17% of the total population, and numbers are increasing. The greatest increase in the future is likely to be in the over-80s age group. At the age of 80 years the present ratio of women:men is 2:1, at the age of 85 years, the ratio is nearly 3:1. These 'elderly elderly' are among those most in need of nutritional or social support. Thus nutritional problems relating to the elderly will be of increasing importance.

It is a myth that the majority of old folk are in residential or institutional care; most of them live in 'other households'. Numbers in institutional care equal approximately 2.6% in hospitals and less than 3% in other establishments such as residential homes. Therefore, by far the majority will need community support and practical suggestions if they are to retain their independence.

3.6.1 Principles of healthy eating for the elderly

Sound nutritional principles apply to all age groups but an over zealous attempt to apply present healthy eating guidelines to the elderly can result in a backlash of other problems — increased anxiety among elderly people over issues concerning diet, disinterest in food and inappropriate dietary restrictions.

Therefore, before expounding on the virtues of dietary change for older individuals several important points should be considered

1 Dietary change is often equated to dietary restriction. For the elderly one of the greatest risks to health is to lose interest in food — neglect your diet: neglect your health. Imposing unrealistic rules or grading foods as 'good', 'bad' or 'forbidden' is counter-productive and not based on sound scientific principles. For the older person 'a little of what you fancy' really is beneficial if it stimulates an interest and pleasure in eating.

2 Some individuals may have seemingly small or poor intakes yet often there is adaptation to this level of nutrient intake. If such people are managing adequately, maintaining weight, retaining independence and unwilling to change, why should they? A 94 year old who enjoys a sugary cup of tea is, after all, 94.

3 Some changes may inadvertently be for the worst. For example, encouraging a reduction in total fat consumption unless carefully explained, may result in the omission of valuable foods from the diet such as cheese or fatty fish. The former decision could affect total calcium intake, the latter omitting an excellent dietary source of vitamin D. Furthermore, trying to retard the development of atherosclerosis in the over-80s by reducing fat intake is inappropriate as any arterial damage will have already been done.

Care should therefore be taken not to discourage foods unless there is a special reason. Wherever possible, the *positive* aspects of nutrition should be stressed. It has been demonstrated that the elderly are not necessarily set in their ways (Bilderbeck *et al* 1981) and will try new foods. Dietary changes, when they occur, are often motivated by taste preference, ease of preparation or for purported 'health' reasons. It is this latter factor which can make elderly people vulnerable to cranky health messages and can tempt them to turn to expensive 'wonder' foods or supplements.

The overall message should be to keep up an interest in and enjoyment of food and be aware that nourishing foods are of prime importance to health. This can be a strong motivating force to encourage the preparation and cooking of simple, tasty, nutritious meals and snacks. A monotonous menu or a dependence on dried instant foods of the 'just-add-boiling-water' type should be discouraged. Pureed or liquid meals are a textural travesty to the palate and should be used only for short-term exceptional circumstances. Such regimens can lead rapidly to disinterest in food and the slippery slope to malnutrition.

Appropriate nutrition guidelines for the elderly are urgently needed. Some of the suggestions made in the COMA Report (1984) and NACNE discussion document are too restricting. These guidelines concentrate mainly on the excesses in the diet, whereas most of the problems confronting a dietitian dealing with the elderly will be related to loss of appetite. Deficiency states are more common than 'excess states' among the elderly.

3.6.2 General nutritional considerations

Nutrient intakes and Recommended Dietary Allowances (RDAs)

There is a need for RDAs which are more appropriate for the elderly. Nevertheless, nutritional studies on different groups of elderly people in the UK have revealed that intakes of vitamin C, folate, riboflavin and other water soluble vitamins, vitamin D, iron, potassium and other trace elements and fibre are almost certainly lower than is desirable (DHSS 1972, 1979; Exton-Smith *et al* 1972, 1978; Vir and Love 1979; Davies 1981).

The elderly, as a group, can therefore be considered to be especially at risk from deficiencies of these nutrients. However, caution must be exercised when comparing the intake of an individual to a recommended standard such as the RDA. A low intake will not always be a deficient one owing to variations in individual requirements or adaptation. Conversely, some nutrient intakes may seem adequate when compared with RDAs, but may in fact be inadequate for those individuals with extra requirements due to short term trauma (e.g. burns or after surgery) or due to long term changes (e.g. bone loss).

Individual intakes must therefore be considered in conjunction with other factors such as the general eating habits, health and activity of the person concerned.

Energy

The consumption of sufficient energy to maintain satisfactory body weight is important. It has been suggested that low weight may be a biological marker for persons more likely to end up in institutions (Morgan and Hullin 1982). A diet low in energy is also more likely to be deficient in other nutrients.

Vitamin D

Where sunlight exposure is poor, for example in the housebound or institutionalized, vitamin D status is also likely to be poor (Corless *et al* 1979; Sheltawy *et al* 1984; Dattani *et al* 1984). Elderly people should be encouraged to venture out of doors even if only to make use of a balcony. In the UK, the best time of day for sunlight exposure is between 11 am–4 pm during the months May–September. Those at retirement age have been found to have an excellent mean vitamin D status (Holdsworth *et al* 1984) and this needs to be maintained following retirement by encouraging sunlight exposure.

Dietary sources of vitamin D are often those which the elderly find difficult to eat; fatty fish, for example, is often ignored because of the bones. More suitable alternatives such as fish patés or softer canned fatty fish should therefore be suggested.

Minerals

Potassium. As most foods contain moderate amounts of potassium there should be no shortage of this essential mineral. However, diets based on highly refined foods, with an excess of sugar, may be potassium deficient. Depletion of potassium has been associated with depression, muscle weakness and mental confusion (Judge and Cowan 1971; Dall and Gardiner 1971). Conversely, depression may cause some individuals to lose their appetite and to turn to a convenient but high sugar diet (Davies 1981).

Sodium. In order to avoid the risk of sodium depletion, salt restrictions recommended for the general population are inappropriate for most elderly persons, especially those over 85 years of age (Brown *et al* 1984).

Calcium. Milk is an important source of calcium for the elderly and if nutritional supplementation is to be given, milk-based food has been demonstrated to improve nutritional status (Katakity *et al* 1983).

Zinc. Some features of old age such as delayed wound healing, decreased taste acuity and anorexia are also findings associated with zinc deficiency (Hsu 1979). However, healthy elderly subjects have been shown to be in zinc balance despite an apparent low dietary intake (Bunker *et al* 1982), suggesting that there is at least some degree of adaptation.

Fibre

Constipation is a common complaint in the elderly. There is great enthusiasm to encourage the consumption of fibre-containing foods but any increase should be gradual otherwise bowel discomfort, distention and flatulence will result. An excess of fibre may compromise the absorption of iron and certain trace elements. Adequate fluid intake should be encouraged simultaneously.

Fluid

Some elderly individuals may have a fading sense of thirst and may go for long periods without fluid. Others avoid liquid for fear of incontinence or to prevent urgency when away from home.

Dehydration can result in mental confusion, headaches and irritability. If a normally alert elderly person complains of phases of confusion, the fluid intake should be checked. Extra fluids can be taken earlier in the day and bedtime drinks can be avoided by those concerned about nocturnal incontinence. Elderly persons should be advised to consume some fluid at regular intervals even if they are not thirsty.

Physical activity

It has been suggested that, for the elderly, maintenance of physical activity should be the principal objective of nutrition education (NACNE 1983). Where there is reduced physical activity this may be a key factor leading to muscular atrophy. Physical activity and the prevention of immobilization are also important in the prevention of osteoporosis.

Deterioration in physiological function

Changes in physiological function with age must not be ignored. Deterioration in renal function may have profound implications for drug therapy (see p 286). Changes in digestive function may have several nutritional consequences, including malabsorption. The subject of digestive function and ageing has been comprehensively reviewed by Bowman and Rosenberg (1983). However, these authors (Rosenberg and Bowman 1984) also state that 'although changes in swallowing, gastric secretion, fat digestion or calcium absorption may have a significant influence on the nutritional status of certain elderly people, the impact of these functional alterations is modest relating to the far more pervasive influence of social and economic factors on food intake and dietary habits in the elderly population'.

Illness

Illness, which is generally more common among the elderly than the young, may affect both nutritional intake (via effects on appetite and access to food), nutritional requirement and nutrient absorption. Protein turnover has been shown to be significantly increased in ill geriatric patients as a response to tissue trauma, inflammation or sepsis and further infuenced by factors such as nutrition or physical activity (Phillips 1983).

Adapting therapeutic diets for the elderly

Where therapeutic diets are essential for the older person, they can tax the skills of even the most experienced dietitian. As well as knowledge of the appropriate therapies for different disease states, there are invariably other conditions which need to be considered. There may be evidence of multiple diseases, including stroke, Parkinson's disease, arthritis and the physical disabilities which may accompany ageing, e.g. hearing defects, poor sight or poor dentition. Mental states need to be considered; there may be confusion, depression, loneliness, apathy, a recent bereavement or recent loss of will to live. Social factors such as isolation or poverty also need to be recognized.

Drug-nutrient interaction and the elderly

Special attention needs to be paid to drug-nutrient interaction (Section 5.10). Many elderly individuals, whether institutionalized or not, are on drugs — either prescribed or as self-medication. Multiple medication and over-medication is not uncommon.

Specific considerations

When dealing with the elderly, dietitians need be aware that poor nutritional status can impair drug metabolism, and drug treatment can have a detrimental effect on nutritional status. This subject has been reviewed by Roe (1976), Dickerson (1978) and Hyams (1981).

Drug-nutrient interaction is disscussed in more detail in Section 5.10 but drugs which may be of particular relevance to the nutritional status of the elderly are those which

1 Impair absorption, e.g. cytotoxic drugs and antibiotics. Other drugs which can cause malabsorption in geriatric patients include alcohol, cathartics, cholestyramine, clofibrate, certain diuretics, liquid paraffin, mannitol, para-amino salicylic acid, anticoagulants such as phenindione and certain antimetabolites.

2 Affect mineral and vitamin metabolism, e.g.

 a) Anticonvulsants (affect vitamin D metabolism and folate abosorption).

 b) Biguanides (reduce B12 and folate status).

c) Tetracycline (depresses leucocyte levels of ascorbic acid and increases urinary excretion of ascorbic acid).

d) Prolonged aspirin treatment (produces tissue depletion of ascobic acid and can also induce chronic bleeding in the gastrointestinal tract, resulting in iron deficiency anaemia).

e) Thiazide diuretics (can result in potassium depletion and magnesium and zinc deficiency).

f) Anti-cancer drugs (can affect thiamin status).

Other drug categories affecting mineral and vitamin metabolism include anti-arthritics, anticoagulants, cerebrovascular preparations, hypotensives, drugs for the treatment of diabetes, hormones, steroids and barbiturates.

3 Decrease appetite, e.g. anti-cancer drugs such as cyclophosphamide; non-steroid anti-inflammatory drugs such as indomethacin; biguanides, glucagon; morphine and the digitalis group.

4 Increase appetite, e.g. alcohol, insulin, thyroid hormone, steroids, some antihistamines, sulphonylureas, psychotropic drugs.

General considerations

Other important points relating to drugs and the elderly are

1 The lower total body water content in the elderly increases the likelihood of dehydration and necessitates adjustment of the water soluble drug dosage to a smaller volume per unit weight.

2 With ageing, there is a diminished ability to metabolize and to excrete drugs, thus some physicians give paediatric doses. Renal function in particular may be impaired. The glomerular filtration rate and tubular function have been shown to be reduced by 30% in the majority of otherwise healthy people over the age of 65 years when compared with normal young adults, and at 90 years the functional capacity of the 'normal' kidney may be only half what it was at 30 years of age (Agate 1970). This means that less of a drug can be excreted via the kidney and hence a greater risk of toxicity. In addition, kidney function may be further impaired by disease states.

3 Lower percentage of body water results in greater alcohol effects per unit of body weight.

4 When energy and protein intakes are low, there is often a reduced capacity to metabolize drugs.

5 The timing of drug taking and food consumption is important. Some drugs are more rapidly absorbed in the fasting state (e.g. ethanol, aspirin, barbiturates, penicillin and tetracycline) and should be taken on an empty stomach either to attain an effective concentration in the blood (e.g. some antibiotics) or to avoid drug-food interactions (tetracycline should not be taken simultaneously with milk, or with antacids or mineral supplements containing salts of calcium, magnesium or iron, because of the formation of non-absorbed complexes.) Other drugs should be taken *with* food in order to increase bioavailability or to minimize side effects.

6 The longer the period a drug is administered, the greater will be the effect on nutritional status and a poor nutrient status will alter drug requirements.

7 Drugs can cause confusion states due to side effects, thus patients can forget whether they have recently eaten or been without food. They may also forget whether they have taken medication or even exchange drugs with other people.

3.6.3 Malnutrition in the elderly

Although it may be relatively easy to diagnose overt malnutrition, the identification of marginal or subclinical malnutrition is beset with difficulties. The condition can be disguised by disease states, biochemical results can be influenced by factors other than nutritional status (such as dehydration), or there may be low stores but no clinical indication of disturbed form or function until the full manifestation of nutritional crisis occurs.

The prime objective of nutrition policies and practices concerning the elderly should be directed towards the *prevention* of malnutrition. This calls for a wider definition to our concept of malnutrition so that risk factors can be identified in order that appropriate policies, both for groups and for individuals, can be established and appropriate action taken.

Recognizing different types of malnutrition in the elderly

Davies (in press) has defined four main types of malnutrition which are distinct, yet which may be interrelated

Type 1 — 'long-standing'. For some people there can be a long latent period between nutritional deficiency and its clinical appearance. For these people there needs to be recognition of warning signs so that early preventive action can be taken.

Type 2 — 'sudden'. For some elderly men or women a medical or social stress (e.g. a bereavement) can tip marginal, or even perfectly adequate, nutrition swiftly over into poor nutrition. For these people prompt action needs to be taken at that critical stage.

Type 3 — 'specific'. This is defined as the occurrence of a deficiency disease, such as scurvy, or nutrition-related diseases such as diabetes, arthritis, osteoporosis and atherosclerosis. These call for diagnosis, followed by treatment which may include medication and/or dietary manipulation.

Type 4 — 'recurrent'. In some cases there is a repeated return of malnutrition accompanied by a weakening resistance to disease. For these people, monitoring and support must follow the previous episode of acute malnutrition.

Risk factors to identify those at risk of malnutrition

Exton-Smith (1971) recognized primary and secondary causes of malnutrition in the elderly (see Table 3.18) which call for improved social and public health measures or appropriate medical/dietetic treatment.

Table 3.18 Causes of malnutrition in the elderly

Primary causes	Secondary causes
Ignorance	Impaired appetite
Social isolation	Masticatory inefficiency
Physical disability	Malabsorption
Mental disturbance	Alcoholism
Iatrogenic disorder	Drugs
Poverty	Increased requirements

The DHSS Report (1979) associated the incidence of undernutrition with the following social and medical 'at risk' factors

Living alone	Chronic bronchitis
Housebound	Emphysema
No regular cooked meals	Gastrectomy
Supplementary benefit (i.e. poverty bracket)	Poor dentition
Social classes IV and V	Difficulty in swallowing
Low mental test score	Smoking
Depression	Alcoholism

Active measures for those at risk

The elderly living in the community

By far the majority of our elderly UK population is community based (over 94%) but many are in need of nutritional support in order to prevent Type 1 (long-standing) or Type 2 (sudden) malnutrition and unnecessary institutionalization. To identify those in need of nutritional support, such as meals-on-wheels or other services, ten main risk factors have been highlighted (Davies 1981)

1 Fewer than eight main meals, hot or cold, eaten in a week.
2 Very little milk consumed.
3 Virtual abstention from fruits and vegetables.
4 Wastage of food — even that supplied hot and ready to eat.
5 Long periods in the day without food or beverages.
6 Depression or loneliness.
7 Unexpected weight change, either a significant gain or loss (this is a more valuable index of risk than either obesity or underweight).
8 Shopping difficulties.
9 Poverty.
10 Indication in medical record of disabilities, including alcoholism.

Elderly individuals vary widely in their ability to cope with difficulties; a risk factor in isolation does not therefore necessarily indicate the need for intervention. Each risk is only a potential danger sign and must be considered in relation to the others. Thus depression or loneliness in themselves may not affect nutrition, but when found in combination with wastage of food and weight loss, the danger is apparent. Almost without exception it was found in the DHSS survey that when *four or more* risk factors were evident, an individual was likely to be malnourished (DHSS 1979).

Those delegated to take action need to be provided with a simple technique. An assessment kit, making use of risk factors and suggesting appropriate local services has been devised by the Gerontology Nutrition Unit (GNU 1981) for use by dietitians and meals-on-wheels organisers (see Sources of help, p 290). Much of the action to be taken is simple and basic such as help with shopping, good neighbour services, help with food preparation (especially for those who are housebound or handicapped). Even non-nutritional intervention such as the provision of a walking frame can encourage mobility and independence.

The elderly living in residential homes

Research on nutrition and catering in old people's homes has led to the identification of 26 risk factors, any of which may affect nutritional intake. Many of these are social factors known to influence food intake

Table 3.19 An A–Z check list of potential risk factors in residential homes

A   Weekly cyclic menu *or* monotony of menu.
B   Difficulties with tea/supper meal menus. (This highlights lack of experience in menu planning and recipe ideas, and may affect costing).
C   Tea/supper meal at or before 5 pm. (This frequently occurs in the UK, mainly because of staffing difficulties. Biscuits often have to be supplied later in the evening because some residents become hungry before bedtime).
D   Lack of rapport between head of home and cook, or the cook resists and resents suggestions.
E   Residents' suggestions (e.g. for recipes) unheeded. Residents' needs for special diets ignored. Inadequate contact between the residents and the home's decision-making committee or board.
F   Residents not allowed choice of portion size *or* poor portion control *or* no second helpings available.
G   No heed taken of food wastage.
H   Very little home-style cooking. (Residents frequently express a desire for familiar foods they have been used to eating, rather than institutional type catering).
I   No special provision for food treats from the local community or from the home, apart from Christmas dinner.
J   For active residents: poor or no facilities for independence in providing food and drink (e.g. tea making).
K   Hot foods served lukewarm or poorly flavoured.
L   Poor presentation of food, including table setting and appearance of the dining room.
M   Unfriendly or undignified waitress service. Meal too rushed.
N   No observation of weight changes of the residents. (Significant changes in weight can be used as an early diagnostic tool for illness, depression or other conditions which can affect nutritional status).
O   No help in feeding very frail residents. No measures taken to protect other residents from offensive eating habits.
P   Head of home and cook lacking basic nutritional or catering knowledge. Isolation from possible help.
Q   Lengthy period between preparation, cooking and serving. Time lag between staff meals and resident meals.
R   Lack of vitamin C-containing foods or risk of destruction of vitamin C due to poor cooking procedures.
S   Few vitamin D-containing foods used, combined with lack of exposure of residents to sunlight.
T   Low fibre diet and complaints of constipation.
U   Possible low intake of other nutrients, e.g. iron, folate and vitamin B12.
V   Preponderance of convenience foods of poor nutritional content.
W   Disproportionate expenditure between animal protein/fruit and vegetables/high energy foods may lead to a nutritionally imbalanced menu.
X   Obvious food perks to staff to detriment of residents' meals. High proportion of food served to others.
Y   Conditions conducive to food poisoning. Lack of cleanliness.
Z   Recommendations may not be implemented.

(Davies and Holdsworth 1979) and are listed in Table 3.19.

A 'homes' assessment kit (GNU 1982) is available for use by dietitians. It contains three interview questionnaires for the officer in charge, cook/chef and residents, plus an observations questionnaire. (See p 290.)

The answers to those questions indicate whether there is a high, moderate or low risk for each factor. By surveying the homes in a particular area using this technique, the ideas on the solutions to problems in one home can be exchanged with other homes where problems still exist.

The elderly in hospital

It is pitiful to see an elderly, ill, frail patient struggling to reach a tray of food placed insensitively out of reach. Such events should not occur. In busy wards, however, unless there is close supervision, problems like this do arise. Constant attention must therefore be paid to meal service. It is especially in geriatric wards that Type 3 (specific) and Type 4 (recurrent) malnutrition may be evident.

Evaluating the meal service and identifying the problems. A dietitian confronting the problems in a geriatric ward firstly needs to know what happens at meal times. This may necessitate several visits to each ward before action is taken and the ward sister should be consulted beforehand. The following points should be observed

1   At meal times, are the patients in bed, in chairs by their beds, or communally dining at small tables?
2   Are patients sitting in positions where they can eat comfortably?
3   Who serves the meals?
4   Who delivers the food and beverages to the patients?
5   What do the meals look like?
6   Is the food appetising?
7   Are portion sizes appropriate for individual appetites?
8   Are needs for special diets met and are the appropriate diets being given to the right people?
9   What is the reaction of the patients to the food?
10   Can patients handle crockery and cutlery?
11   Is there help with feeding when necessary? If so, how is this done?
12   Is there much food wastage? If so, which food or dish is it?
13   Are meal times rushed or is there adequate time to eat?
14   Is the food kept appetising if the patient is interrupted by a visit?
15   Are dentures available — or are they hidden away in a drawer?
16   Are sufficient staff around at meal times to cope with the patients' extra needs?
17   Is there an over-emphasis on pureed foods?
18   How would you react to being served this food on a long term basis?
19   Other general comments or complaints.

Diplomatic enquiries should be made regarding
1   Whether the patients have any suggestions concerning the food.
2   What the staff on the ward think of the food.

3 Whether weight checks are made at least monthly and what action is taken if there is a loss or gain of 2 kg or more.

4 Whether staff are getting patients into the sunlight in summer.

Taking action. An important use of a dietitian's time is to educate those already involved in food preparation and service

1 Arrange meetings for nursing, ancillary and catering staff to discuss the service of beverages and food and to inspire enthusiasm regarding the importance of their work. Remind them that patients need to be able to help themselves; if patients are unable to reach the meals the frustration may lead to anorexia or depression. Suggest ways of motivating those disinterested in food or who have lost the will to live — perhaps a change in menu is required, some home-style cooking or even a series of small treats. Where appetites are small, a large meal can be off-putting. Watch out for monotony of the menu and inflexibility of meal size due to standardized servings. Discuss the observations made over the previous weeks and discuss ways to correct poor practices.

Discuss what the staff would most like to eat or drink if they were destined to be a patient in a long stay ward. Try some practical exercises: get a staff member to volunteer to be a patient, then immobilize in a chair and feed an unidentified puree at a brisk pace. Try getting them to drink out of a feeding beaker. Note the reaction.

2 Keep up good liaison with the catering manager and make sure that he accompanies you to the wards from time to time and discusses any problems with you and the nursing staff. Do likewise with a member of the diet kitchen staff, keeping these visits short but informative.

3 With the catering manager, arrange refresher courses in dietetic practices for chefs and cooks. These need be for only an hour each week for, say, a six week period. Subjects could include theoretical topics and practical sessions related to the elderly.

4 Medical staff also need up-dating in dietetic practice. This is often best conducted informally in quieter moments on the ward.

5 Contribute as part of the team in ward rounds and in case conferences where appropriate.

6 Work closely with the physiotherapist or occupational therapist on any nutritional problems which they are involved in treating.

7 Where special diets are required for the elderly, much the same principles apply as for pathological conditions at younger ages, but see p 285.

8 Set up a 'patients' food group' in long stay wards. This allows patients to contribute ideas to the menu and encourages valuable comments on the total meal service.

New admissions undernourished through self-neglect. When an elderly man or woman is admitted to hospital with undernourishment through self-neglect, the stay in hospital should be used to teach the patient the importance of diet. Discuss with the doctor whether the patient's condition is caused primarily through self-neglect or a disease state. If the former, encourage the patient to regard *food*, not just vitamin or mineral supplements, as the main treatment. Monitor the diet carefully checking that extra food supplements including fresh fruit juices are provided when necessary.

In order to prevent recurrence of the malnutrition, the cause of the pre-existing condition, i.e. a poor diet, must also be tackled. When alcohol has tended to replace meals, emphasizing the importance of food in relation to health is of particular importance.

The anorexic patient will need encouragement to eat especially if loss of appetite is due to drug administration. The patient's food preferences should be considered and meals should be small, dainty and served frequently. Such individual care can motivate the patient to eat. Lowered intakes are not inevitable with ageing (Davies 1984).

Rehabilitation. The main aim in rehabilitation is to enable the individual to retain sufficient independence to prevent constant readmissions to hospital. Where there is risk of Type 4 (recurrent) malnutrition, special support outside the hospital environment will need to be arranged.

Support services. The social worker will be able to suggest local support services which may assist the patient. These may include

Meals-on-wheels	Community centres
Home helps	Social clubs
Luncheon clubs	Cookery classes
Visits to a day hospital	Local church facilities
Day visits to a residential home	Street wardens
Day centres	Good neighbour schemes
	Shops with delivery services

Most elderly people living at home will not be totally dependent on these services for their meals. Most will still need to cook a few times a week and to prepare breakfasts. They may therefore need advice on meal planning and preparation, together will recipe suggestions which are easy to prepare, economical, tasty and nourishing. Ideally suitable are two paperback books by Louise Davies: *Easy cooking for one or two* (1972) and *More easy cooking for one or two* (1979). These books contain chapters on 'Nutrition on your own', 'Recipes for non-cooks', 'Store-cupboard cookery' and 'Cooking for companionship'. The print is large and clear for fading eyesight and the recipes are tested and approved by the elderly themselves.

If recommending other books, consider the size of the print. If designing leaflets, make sure the print is large and clear (see Section 3.12, p 320, concerning the visually handicapped).

Nutrition education

With the changing nutrition scene there is an increased need for updating other health professionals regarding the nutritional needs of elderly people. These professionals include doctors, medical students, nurses, occupational therapists and other hospital staff, especially ancillary staff who can influence a patient's food intake. Those outside the hospital setting, e.g home helps, health visitors, officers in charge of old people's homes, meals-on-wheels organisers and wardens of 'sheltered housing' will also benefit from nutrition education.

Teaching sessions should be conducted informally in small groups or on a one to one basis. Alternatively, they can be in the form of one day seminars where 20–30 people with a common interest (e.g. officers in charge or cooks/chefs of old people's homes, cooks in luncheon clubs or hospital based staff) can gather to hear a series of short talks on relevant topics, followed by a discussion or questions and answers session. Topics could include menu planning, how to improve the diet, getting the elderly out of doors, fibre in the diet, costing and budgeting, nutritional risk factors in residential homes, use of freezers, prevention of food poisoning, or special diets (where relevant). Such seminars can also involve discussion groups, demonstrations (especially on cookery techniques and recipes for supper ideas), recipe exchanges or slide or film sessions.

For the elderly themselves, ideal venues for teaching 'eating for health and pleasure' are luncheon clubs, day hospitals, Darby and Joan clubs and cookery classes for the over 60s.

For those approaching retirement, talks and demonstrations can be given to groups within pre-retirement courses. Here the overall message should be 'keep interested in food and if you can't be bothered to cook at any time, turn to the nourishing easy-to-prepare foods rather than neglecting your diet'. Appropriate topics have been reported elsewhere (Davies *et al* 1985). A nutrition survey on a pre-retirement sample has indicated the need for nutrition education at this age (Holdsworth and Davies 1984).

Teaching aids and assessment kits

Leaflets

An updated list of leaflets is available for dietitians from the British Dietetic Association's Nutrition Advisory Group for the Elderly (NAGE)

Booklets

National Dairy Council in conjunction with the Gerontology Nutrition Unit (1985) *Take something simple.* pp 23. Free from the National Dairy Council, John Princes Street, London W1M 0AP.

Potato Marketing Board in conjunction with the Gerontology Nutrition Unit *Catering for the elderly.* Available from the PMB, 50 Hans Crescent, London SW1X 0NB.

Homes Advice Guide Card No 6 *Catering and nutrition.* A card giving the A–Z at risk factors in residential homes.

Homes Advice Guide Card No 11 *Suggestions for supper variety when menu-making in residential homes.*
Both free from the Centre for Policy on Ageing, Nuffield Lodge, Regent's Park, London NW1 4RS.

Slide lecture kits

The Gerontology Nutrition Unit produces four slide lecture kits
1 Set A *An emergency food store for the elderly.* Comprises 12 colour cartoon slides, full lecture notes and 30 leaflets for the audience.
2 Set B *Keeping foods fresh without a refrigerator.* Comprises 21 black and white cartoon slides, full lecture notes, 30 leaflets on keeping foods fresh, and 30 leaflets on how to store left-overs.
3 Set C *What is a balanced diet?* Comprises 15 colour cartoon slides, full lecture notes and 30 reminder leaflets for the audience. This set has been revised recently to take account of recent nutritional research and NACNE guidelines.
4 Set D *Vitamin D and Calcium.* Comprises 21 colour cartoon slides, full lecture notes and 30 leaflets.
The money raised by the sale of these kits helps to fund nutrition research. Price on application (please send SAE) to Gerontology Nutrition Unit, Royal Free Hospital School of Medicine, 21 Pond Street, London NW3 2PN.

Assessment kits

1 *Meals-on-wheels assessment kit.* Price £20.00. Contents

a) Who needs Meals-on-wheels? (background research paper).

b) Four pages for index card, with details for first and subsequent assessments.

c) The sample four-sided index card — to show the recommended reduction in size.

d) Instructions for Meals-on-wheels organiser
   a) Preliminary fact finding.
   b) The individual cards.
   c) Your instructions to the interviewer.

e) Information for Meals-on-wheels organisers to assess 'at risk' factors.

f) Sample check-list — local services available.

g) 'Three score years...and then? by Louise Davies.

2 *Nutrition and catering in old people's homes assessment kit.* Price £15.00. The kit comprises

a) Questionnaire for officer in charge/matron.

b) Questionnaire for cooks/chefs.

c) General observations.

d) Short questionnaire for residents.

e) List of A−Z 'at risk' factors.

f) Instructions: how to interpret your findings.

Further reading

Albanese AA (1980) Nutrition for the elderly. In *Current topics in nutrition and disease* Vol 3. AR Liss Inc, New York.

Andrews J and von Hahn HP (Eds) (1981) *Geriatrics for everyday practice.* S Karger, London.

Davies L (1981) *Three score years...and then?* A study of the nutrition and well-being of elderly people at home. Heinemann Medical Books, London.

Department of Health and Social Security (1972) *A nutrition survey of the elderly.* Report on Health and Social Subjects No 3. HMSO. London.

Department of Health and Social Security (1979) *Nutrition and health in old age.* Report on Health and Social Subjects No 16. HMSO, London.

Exton-Smith AN and Caird FI (Eds) (1980) *Metabolic and nutritional disorders in the elderly.* John Wright and Sons, Bristol.

Isaacs B (1985) *Understanding stroke illness.* A Chest, Heart and Stroke Association Publication, Tavistock House North, London WC1H 9JE.

Rosenberg IH and Bowman BB (1984) Gastrointestinal function and ageing. In *The role of the gastrointestinal tract in nutrient delivery.* Bristol-Myers Nutrition Symposia Vol 3 Green M, Greene HL (Eds). Academic Press, London.

Sheltawy M, Newton H, Hay A, Morgan DB and Hullin RP (1984) The contribution of dietary vitamin D and sunlight to the plasma 25-hydroxyvitamin D in the elderly. *Hum Nutr: Clin Nutr* **38C**, 191−4.

Vir SC and Live AHG (1979) Nutritional status of institutionalized aged in Belfast, Northern Ireland. *Am J Clin Nutr* **32**, 193−207.

References

Agate J (1970) *The practice of geriatrics* 2e. Heinemann, London.

Bilderbeck N, Holdsworth MD, Purves R and Davies L (1981) Changing food habits among 100 elderly men and women in the UK. *J Hum Nutr* **35**, 448−55.

Bowman BB and Rosenberg IH (1983) Digestive function and ageing. *Hum Nutr: Clin Nutr* **37C**, 75−89.

Brown JJ, Lever AF, Robertson JIS, Semple PF, Bing RF, Heagerty AM, Swales JD, Thurston H, Ledingham JGG, Laragh JH,

Hansson L, Nicholls MG and Espiner EA (1984) Salt and hypertension. *Lancet* **ii**, 1333−4.

Bunker VW, Lawson MS, Delves HT and Clayton BE (1982) Metabolic balance studies for zinc and nitrogen in healthy elderly subjects. *Hum Nutr: Clin Nutr* **36C**, 213−21.

Committee on Medical Aspects of Food Policy (1984) *Diet and cardiovascular disease.* Report on Health and Social Subjects No 28. HMSO, London.

Corless D, Gupta SP, Salter DA, Switala S and Boucher BJ (1979) Vitamin D status of residents of an old people's home and long stay patients. *Gerontology* **25**, 350−5.

Dall JLC and Gardiner HS (1971) Dietary intake of potassium by geriatric patients. *Geront Clin* **13**, 119−24.

Dattani J, Exton-Smith AN and Stephen JML (1984) Vitamin D status of the elderly in relation to age and exposure to sunlight. *Hum Nutr: Clin Nutr* **38C**, 131−7.

Davies L (1972) *Easy cooking for one or two.* Penguin Handbooks, London.

Davies L (1979) *More easy cooking for one or two.* Penguin Handbooks, London.

Davies L (1981) *Three score years...and then?* Heinemann Medical Books Ltd, London.

Davies L (1984) Nutrition and the elderly: identifying those at risk. *Proc Nutr Soc* **43**, 295−302.

Davies L (in press) Nutritional risk factors for disease in the elderly. In *Malnutrition in the Elderly.* WHO Publication, USA.

Davies L, Anderson JP and Holdsworth MD (1985) Nutrition education at the age of retirement from work. *Health Education* **44**, (4), 187−92.

Davies L and Holdsworth MD (1979) A technique for assessing nutritional 'at risk' factors in residential homes for the elderly. *J Hum Nutr* **33**, 165−9.

Department of Health and Social Security (1972) *A nutrition survey of the elderly.* Report on Health and Social Subjects No 3. HMSO, London.

Department of Health and Social Security (1979) *Nutrition and health in old age.* Report on Health and Social Subjects No 16. HMSO, London.

Dickerson JWT (1978) The interrelationships of nutrition and drugs. In *Nutrition in the clinical management of disease.* Dickerson JWT and Lee HA (Eds) pp 308−31. Edward Arnold Ltd, London.

Exton-Smith AN (1971) Nutrition of the elderly. *Br J Hosp Med* **5**, 639−45.

Exton-Smith AN (1978) Nutrition in the elderly. In *Nutrition in the clinical management of disease* Dickerson JWT and Lee HA (Eds) pp 72−104. Edward Arnold Ltd, London.

Exton-Smith AN, Stanton BR and Windsor ACM (1972) *Nutrition of housebound old people.* King Edward's Hospital Fund for London, London.

Gerontology Nutrition Unit (GNU) (1981) *Meals-on-wheels* assessment kit.

Gerontology Nutrition Unit (GNU) (1982) *Catering and nutrition in residential homes* Assessment Kit.

Holdsworth MD, Dattani J, Davies L and Macfarlane D (1984) Factors contributing to vitamin D status near retirement age. *Hum Nutr: Clin Nutr* **38C**, 139−49.

Holdsworth MD and Davies L (1984) Nutrition at retirement age. *Proc Nutr Soc* **43**, 303−13.

Hsu JM (1979) Current knowledge on zinc, copper and chromium in ageing. *World Rev Nutr Diet* **33**, 42.

Hyams DE (1981) Drugs in the elderly. In *Geriatrics for everyday practice* von Hahn and Andrews (Eds). Karger, Basel.

Judge TG and Cowan NR (1971) Dietary potassium intake and grip strength in older people. *Gerontol Clin* **13**, 221−6.

Katakity M, Webb JF and Dickerson JWT (1983) Some effects of a food supplement in elderly hospital patients: a longitudinal study. *Hum Nutr: Appl Nutr* **37A**, 85−93.

Morgan DB and Hullin RP (1982) The body composition of the chronic mentally ill. *Hum Nutr: Clin Nutr* **36C**, 439–48.

National Advisory Committee on Nutrition Education (1983) *Proposals for nutritional guidelines for health education in Britain.* Health Education Council, London.

Phillips P (1983) Protein turnover in the elderly: a comparison between ill patients and normal controls. *Hum Nutr: Clin Nutr* **37C**, 339–44.

Roe DA (1976) *Drug-induced nutritional deficiencies* pp 272. The AVI Publishing Company Inc Westport, Connecticut.

3.7 Low Income Groups

3.7.1 The size and nature of the problem

Is there a problem?

'Homeless in diet alert' — 'malnutrition is being found again among London children, for the first time in probably 50 years, claims a GP' (Evening Standard, 20th May 1985). The nutritional status of the poor in the UK has improved little in the last ten years and for many has probably declined. 'It is not uncommon for a social worker to visit homes where the refrigerator is empty and turned off, or the cupboards are bare' (Stiles and Cameron 1974). These alarming statements could just be the tip of the iceberg. A recent survey in the north of England (Lang *et al* 1984) has highlighted the problems facing people on low incomes. The survey of 1,000 people on low incomes (two-thirds of whom were living on less than £50 a week), shows that a third of the participants were eating inadequate diets. Counting a 'meal' as anything eaten for breakfast, midday or in the evening, nearly two people out of every five did not have something to eat at all three meal times. A quarter said they did not have what they considered to be a 'main meal' every day, of whom one third said they couldn't afford to — that is 10% of the sample. 37% of the unemployed participants in the survey had gone without food at some time in the last year because they could not afford it and 10% of all the people interviewed (25% of those unemployed) said that they usually did not have enough money for food all week. Food was one of the first items they cut back on when short of cash, despite the fact the main budget priorities for most people were housing, fuel and foods. Alcohol, cigarettes, going out and clothes for oneself were the least important. Lang *et al* (1984) confirm that in the ten years since two community health workers in Inner London (Stiles and Cameron 1974) interviewed 35 families in north Lambeth, the situation for people on low incomes has not improved. What *has* changed is the number of people who have low incomes (the unemployed and those receiving low wages) and this state of affairs is unlikely to improve significantly in the immediate future.

What is the problem?

The unemployed and those on low incomes suffer significantly more ill health and early death than the better-off (Townsend 1982). Many of the health problems experienced can be partially attributed to diet. The problems are particularly acute for the unemployed (Lang *et al* 1984). It is now well established that low birth weight, perinatal mortality and morbidity rates and birth abnormalities are relatively high amongst the disadvantaged groups of people in the population (Brotherston 1979; Goel 1979; Townsend 1982; Cole 1983; Doyle *et al* 1983). Also, dental health has been shown to be poorest (French *et al* 1984), children are generally shorter (Brotherston 1979) and obesity most common (Garman *et al* 1982; Royal College of Physicians 1983) in these groups. A similar trend is shown in diseases of the circulatory system, including coronary heart disease, hypertension and stroke, particularly amongst women (Townsend 1982).

An analysis of National Food Survey Data from 1982 (MAFF 1984) shows that food intake is closely related to both income level and the number of children in the household. Households on low incomes eat considerably less cheese, carcass meat, meat in total, butter, cooking oils, fresh and frozen vegetables, fresh fruit and wholemeal bread. This effect is sometimes compounded by the presence of children. For example, households with three or more children in the lowest income group eat less than one-quarter the amount of fruit of similar households in the highest income group. In households with adults only, the low income groups still eat significantly less fruit but the difference is not as great. In the larger low income households, intake per person per week is as little as 6 oz — equivalent to one large orange. In wealthier households with adults only it is 31 oz — five times as much.

Low income households also eat significantly more of relatively cheap foods which tend to be energy dense and relatively high in fat and sugar (Table 3.20). This suggests that the diets of people with low incomes are likely to be lower in dietary fibre, vitamin C, β-carotene, folic acid, vitamin E and possibly zinc, and higher in sugar than the diets of people from higher

Table 3.20 Relative amounts of different foods eaten by low income households compared with high income households in 1982 (MAFF 1984)

	Relative consumption	
More	Less	No consistent difference*
Meat products	Cheese	
Margarine	Carcass meat	Milk
Lard	Total meat	Poultry
Sugar	Butter	Fish
Jam	Cooking oils	Total fat
Potatoes	Fresh and frozen vegetables	Cakes and biscuits
Canned vegetables (including baked beans)	Fresh fruit	
White bread	Wholemeal	
Total bread	bread	

*Although there were differences, in some sized households they were higher, and in others lower.

income groups. Some of these and other concerns have been highlighted by recent research. Hackett et al (1984) showed that children from social classes IV and V (partly skilled and unskilled workers — the lowest income groups), would have a daily intake of calcium below the RDA if bread was not fortified. French et al (1984) showed that children from these social classes had the poorest dental health and Poh Tan et al (1984) showed that folic acid content of household diets was related both to social class and the number of children in the household. Lang et al (1984) also found that there were differences in the consumption of different foods depending on whether the people were unemployed, employed or living on a pension. On the whole the diets of employed people were better than the unemployed and pensioners. For example, 15% of the unemployed and pensioners 'never or hardly ever' ate fresh fruit and vegetables whereas only 5% of those employed claimed the same.

Changes in buying patterns with changes in income have also been reported by the Market Research Bureau, Mintel. In 1981/2 the consumption of sausages by households on low incomes rose by 4% whereas for well-off households it dropped by 9% (Mintel 1983). Sausages are, of course, relatively cheap, but also relatively high in saturated fats.

The problems of availability and price

The potential problems of poor nutrition amongst people from disadvantaged households are likely to be primarily connected with the relative price and availability of healthy food; people can only eat the food available in accessible shops and at a price they can afford (see Section 1.14.2). These problems will be compounded by other needs and priorities as well as lack of access to relevant useful information. On average the highest income groups recorded in the National Food Survey 1982 (MAFF 1984) spent $1\frac{1}{2}$ times as much on food as the low income households.

In some large cities there is rapid expansion by major retailing chains of 'Superstores' (London Food Commission 1985). These are increasingly situated away from local shopping centres and in areas of relative affluence. At the same time smaller supermarkets owned by these retailing chains are being run down. The result is that in deprived inner city areas the main food shops are the smaller, relatively expensive supermarkets and grocer's shops. Some of the retailing chains actually have pricing policies which result in prices for some products being higher in small, local shops than in large superstores (London Food Commission 1985).

At the same time the type of foods currently encouraged for a healthy diet are often relatively expensive. For example wholemeal bread can be 25% more expensive than white; reduced fat cheese, wholewheat pasta, brown rice, fresh fruit and many fresh vegetables are all comparatively expensive. Table 3.19 has shown that these are the types of food lacking in the diets of people on low incomes. The availability of these foods in many small shops is also often limited.

Cheaper foods are not necessarily better value for money. For example, cheap cuts of meat tend to be fattier than more expensive cuts and use more fuel in cooking. Similarly, even though many beans and pulses are considerably cheaper than meat, and have the added advantages of being low in fat and high in fibre, the fuel costs involved in cooking them must be taken into consideration. Chips cook more quickly than boiled potatoes and take considerably less fuel than jacket potatoes, while crisps present no fuel costs at all.

A study which examined individual diet histories from people on low incomes in the North of England, revealed diets which could well lead to nutritional problems (Lang 1984). Blaxter and Paterson (1982) when discussing their work into social class, poverty and nutrition concluded:

'Thus cultural, commercial and practical pressures dictated dietary habits.... This study suggested that poverty can be defined in terms of constraints upon choice, and powerlessness over the environment. In the circumstances of deprived lives, certain behaviours — from early childbearing to patterns of eating —

are inevitable. The 'culture of poverty' is a concept now largely discredited, if it implies simply persisting subcultural beliefs and behaviours. However, the very practical constraints of poverty remain.'

3.7.2 Practical advice from dietitians

Often the main items of expenditure in the household food budget of low income groups are processed foods such as meat pies, fish fingers, sausages, bacon, breakfast cereals, biscuits, cakes and other convenience and canned foods. The price of foods such as these varies widely, but the cheaper ones are usually high in fat, sugar or salt and low in dietary fibre.

With very careful shopping and the use of relatively cheap foods such as dried pulses and larger amounts of potatoes instead of bought pies, etc. it is possible for a healthy diet to cost no more, and sometimes less than an unhealthy one (Leverkus et al 1985). But this may not be the case if food expenditure is already low, however carefully menus are planned or budgeted. A NACNE diet costed by the London Food Commission cost 50% more than the average diet consumed by households with low incomes (Cole-Hamilton and Lang 1986). If people are asking for this type of advice then it should, of course, be given. For some people, however, these concepts are totally inappropriate and of little interest. Like many people, they do not want to spend time shopping round, preparing cheap foods which take longer to cook, and eating the sort of diet which has long been associated with poverty. There is no justifiable reason why poverty should force a person to eat differently from anyone else.

Social Security benefits

The most important thing a dietitian can do to help people on low incomes is to help them find out if they are receiving all the welfare benefits to which they are entitled. Millions of pounds in benefits go unclaimed every year. Dietitians cannot be expected to investigate in detail whether every individual is receiving their full entitlement of benefits, but should have some knowledge of available benefits and be able to tell people where they can get more help.

Currently, benefits are available as 'one-off' payments for such things as furniture, bedding, baby wear, clothing (if the need arises as a result of sudden weight change) and footwear. There can also be weekly payments for laundry, heating, special diets and people suffering from bedwetting and incontinence. It is not always easy to get these benefits and they have to be asked for specifically. Nevertheless, they can make a difference to a household with a low income. It may also be possible for pregnant women to receive extra payments of 'whole cost' diet additions and they should be encouraged to try (Cohen 1985).

The current system of benefits is extremely complicated and people can receive detailed advice at Citizen's Advice Bureaux and local Law Centres where they exist. Two useful books are produced annually by the Child Poverty Action Group (CPAG) (CPAG 1985a, 1985b) These books are available through bookshops or direct from the CPAG, are inexpensive and give detailed accounts of all benefits available, eligibility and how to apply for them. The Department of Health and Social Security also produces a leaflet (DHSS 1984); they also have individual leaflets detailing each type of benefit. More detailed information is given in *The law relating to supplementary benefits and family income supplement* (HMSO) which is kept by most reference libraries and is up-dated regularly.

The social security and welfare benefits system is currently under review. Dietitians should be aware of changes in the system, and their implications, and look for ways of helping households with low incomes to ensure they receive their maximum entitlement.

Dietary advice

The type of dietary advice given to individuals and groups will depend very much on their own needs and interests.

Dietitians must be aware of what foods are available in the local shops and their relative prices. They must also assess the individuals cooking skills and interest in food preparation.

Ideally, *everyone* should be able to afford healthy, convenience foods. This unfortunately is not the case at present and until it is dietary advice has to be realistic and sensitive. As stated previously fuel costs are an important consideration and both the gas and electricity board provide leaflets and information about economizing on fuel during cooking. Supplies of these leaflets could be held in dietetic departments. Some foods being recommended may be unfamiliar and involve new cooking practices. Demonstrations and tasting sessions are useful if the facilities exist.

Lang et al (1984) showed that parents, newspapers and magazines were important for the role they played in teaching people 'how to manage' and 'what was good for them'. Dietitians should use these media when possible. Interesting, quick, easy, cheap recipes and meals in a regular column in a local free newspaper could reach thousands of people. Lang *et al* (1984) also found that when people were really short of money they tended to eat, firstly, sandwiches, toast or bread (white bread); then eggs; then beans and chips. Dietitians could provide information about inexpensive sandwich fillings and spreads.

Lean meat is considerably more expensive than fatty meat and in the past dietitians have often advised that cheap meat is 'just as good for you' as expensive meat. This advice should now be turned on its head and people advised that a small amount of lean meat is 'much better for you', and more economical to cook, than a larger amount of fatty meat costing the same.

Ways of increasing the nutritional quality of the diet, which may save money as well, include

1 Using less meat and more vegetables in stews and casseroles.

2 Using as little fat or oil in cooking as possible.

3 Using natural yogurt instead of cream.

4 Using skimmed or semi-skimmed milk instead of whole milk.

5 Using lentils, peas and dried beans to replace some of the meat in mince dishes.

6 Having larger portions of potatoes, rice or starchy vegetables with smaller portions of meat or meat products.

7 Spreading butter or margarine thinly on thick slices of bread (rather than the other way round).

8 Making stale bread into breadcrumbs which can be used for meat loaves, rissoles and stuffings.

9 Grating cheese for salads and sandwiches. Grated cheese goes much further than sliced.

10 Using a small amount of a very strong cheese in a cheese sauce rather than a larger amount of a mild cheese.

11 Buying fruit and vegetables in small quantities to avoid storing them.

12 Being careful not to buy too many sweets, cakes and biscuits.

13 Avoiding convenience foods with little nutritional value such as instant meals in pots, sweet dessert mixes and sweet drinks.

These need to be offset against increased costs such as wholegrain products, reduced fat cheeses, extra fresh fruit and more vegetables.

Shopping advice

When giving advice about shopping it is important to remember that people with low incomes not only have a limited amount to spend on food each week, but also that this problem is compounded by the fact that small quantities are often relatively more expensive, local shops are usually dearer than superstores, transport facilities are often poor in deprived areas and there is insufficient money to buy in the quantities needed to justify a trip to a big, cheaper shop. These problems are not easily resolved but a few tips which may be useful are

1 Make a list of all the most important items and buy those first.

2 Try to think ahead to avoid wastage and to make sure there is no need to go to more expensive shops outside normal opening times.

3 Share shopping trips with friends and neighbours to make better use of transport.

4 If it is cheaper to buy in larger quantities, share products with friends and neighbours and split the costs between you. Setting up small buying co-operatives can be a useful form of social contact as well as making food cheaper.

5 Be careful not to buy bruised or damaged fruit or vegetables as, although these may be cheaper, they deteriorate more quickly and the vitamin content is lower.

6 Shopping last thing in the afternoon (especially on a Saturday) often means the price of perishable goods is reduced.

Food preparation

Time and fuel costs are as important to most people as maintaining the nutritional quality of the food. Cost can be kept down by

1 Eating more raw fruit and vegetables.

2 Cooking vegetables very rapidly in a small amount of water.

3 Stir frying vegetables in a small amount of oil.

4 Grilling tender lean meat rather than stewing tough fatty meats.

5 Sharing meals with friends and neighbours. This cuts costs and increases social contact.

Therapeutic diets

Advising people with low incomes with special dietary requirements is not an easy task. However, some people on special diets are entitled to extra social security allowances. At the time of writing (1986) these are patients with: diabetes, peptic ulcers (including stomach and duodenal), ulcerative colitis, tuberculosis, serious difficulty in swallowing, or an illness requiring a

NUTRITIONAL NEEDS OF POPULATION SUB-GROUPS

similar diet to one of these, and patients requiring dialysis. Furthermore, convalescence after a serious illness or operation or any *illness which requires a special diet* (e.g. high protein or low fat) may also qualify for extra benefit. Theoretically, therefore, anyone in receipt of supplementary benefit or housing benefit supplement who has been referred to a dietitian by a doctor and is, by definition, in need of a 'special diet' is entitled to extra payments. With the introduction of the new social security changes (1986) special dietary additions and therapeutic diets are to be covered by flat rate 'premiums'. The application of these is not clear at present.

Dietitians should make it their responsibility to make sure the patient is aware of these facts and to provide the appropriate back-up as required. Payments will differ depending on the type of diet required (Cohen 1985).

Summary

Dietitians cannot alleviate poverty directly but they can, by means of sensitive and appropriate advice, help to minimize some of its likely nutritional consequences. In addition, dietitians have a general responsibility to highlight the nutritional problems which can result from a low income to the policy makers and planners.

Further reading

Child Poverty Action Group (1985) Poverty and food in *Poverty*. Newsletter No 60.

The London Food Commission (1986) *Low income and Food*. A report by the London Food Commission. PO Box 291, London N5 1DU.

References

Blaxter M and Paterson E (1982) Social class, poverty and nutrition. In *Food and people*. Turner M (Ed). John Libbey, London.

Brotherston J (1979) Inequality, is it inevitable? In *Equalities and inequalities in health*. Carter CO and Peel J (Eds). Academic Press, London.

Cohen (1985) What is so special about a healthy diet? In *Poverty*: Child Poverty Action Group No 60. pp 31–4.

Cole (1983) Unemployment, birth weight and growth in the first year. *Arch Dis Childh* 58, (9), 717–21.

Cole-Hamilton IM and Lang TML (1986) *Low Income and food*. A report by the London Food Commission. PO Box 291, London N5 1DU.

Child Poverty Action Group (1985a) *National welfare benefits handbook* 7e. Unwins

Child Poverty Action Group (1985b) *Rights guide to non means-tested benefits* 14e. Unwins

Department of Health and Social Security (1984) *Which Benefit?* Leaflet FB2.

Doyle W *et al* (1983) Maternal nutrition in pregnancy: the special role of dietary fats and socioeconomic interactions. *Nutrition and Health* 1, (3/4), 209–12.

French AD, Carmichael CL, Furness JA and Rugg-Gunn AJ (1984) The relationship between social class and dental health in 5 year old children in the north and south of England. *Br Dent J* 156, (3), 83–6.

Garman AR, Chinn S and Rona RJ (1982) Comparative growth of primary school children from one and two parent families. *Arch Dis Childh* 57, (6), 453–8.

Goel KM (1979) *Nutrition survey of immigrant children in Glasgow*. Scottish Health Service Studies No 40. Scottish Home and Health Department, Edinburgh.

Hackett AF, Rugg-Gunn AJ, Allinson M, Robinson CJ, Appleton DR and Eastoe JE (1984) The importance of fortification of flour with calcium and the sources of calcium in the diets of 375 English adolescents. *Br J Nutr* 51, (2), 193–7.

Lang *et al* (1984) *Jam tomorrow*. Food Policy Unit, Hollings Faculty, Manchester Polytechnic, Manchester 14.

Leverkus C, Cole-Hamilton I, Gunner K, Starr J and Stanway A (1985) *The Great British diet*. The British Dietetic Association. Century Publishing, London.

London Food Commission (1985) *Access to food stores in London: a pilot study of three large retailers*. A report commissioned from CES Ltd. The London Food Commission PO Box 291 London N5 1DU.

Ministry of Agriculture, Fisheries and Food (1984) *Household food consumption and expenditure 1982*. HMSO, London.

Market Intelligence Reports (1983) Special report — British Market Research Bureau September 1983. Mintel.

Poh Tan S, Wenlock RW and Buss DH (1984) Folic acid content of the diet in various British households. *Hum Nutr: Appl Nutr* 38A, (1), 17–22.

Royal College of Physicians (1983) Obesity. *J Roy Coll Physicians Lond* 17, (1), 3–58.

Stiles J and Cameron D (1974) Food budgeting and the economic crises. *Nutrition* 25, (1), 22–4.

Townsend (1982) *Inequalities in health — The Black Report*. Townsend P and Davidson S (Eds). Penguin, London.

3.8   Nutrition and the Athlete

Whenever the potential role of nutrition in improving athletic performance is considered, the majority of sportsmen and women immediately think of vitamin supplementation and a vast array of other pills, powders and potions. However, the primary dietary consideration must undoubtedly be the maintenance of substrate supply in order to ensure that the high rates of energy utilization associated with exercise can be maintained. Yet very few athletes or coaches are aware of the way in which personal beliefs, likes and dislikes result in eating habits which can seriously influence performance (Wootton 1986).

Owing to the wide diversity of different sporting activities and the vastly differing demands placed upon the individual by their particular sport of their own level of performance and commitment, it is clearly beyond the scope of this chapter to provide detailed guidelines for every sport. However, there are two specific nutritional themes which are applicable to most sports, irrespective of the standard of the participant

1   The intake of sufficient dietary carbohydrate to maintain muscle energy reserves during training and competition.

2   The intake of fluids during exercise to maintain normal thermoregulatory function.

3.8.1   Carbohydrate and exercise

In order to appreciate the relationship between nutrition and performance, it is helpful to summarize the effects of exercise on energy metabolism.

Energy metabolism during exercise

Whenever muscular work is performed, the energy needs of the muscle are covered by accelerating the rate of adenosine triphosphate (ATP) resynthesis to match the rate at which ATP is being utilized. The greater the intensity of exercise, the greater the rates of both ATP utilization and resynthesis. Fatigue can be considered simply as a mismatch of the rates of ATP utilization and resynthesis in the working muscle, either through the reduced availability of substrate for ATP resynthesis or the accumulation of end product (for review see Williams 1985).

The resynthesis of ATP can be derived from either the simultaneous oxidation of glycogen, glucose and free fatty acids when the rate of energy demand can be met primarily from aerobic metabolism, or from the conversion of glycogen to lactate (anaerobic metabolism) when the rates of energy demand are very high. The resynthesis of ATP from deaminated amino acids or from other sources (e.g. ketones) is considerably less, yet becomes increasingly important when low-intensity exercise is maintained for prolonged periods. The relative utilization of the various substrates as fuels depends upon the intensity and duration of exercise, the type of exercise (either continuous or intermittent) as well as the training status and preceding diet of the individual (Williams 1985).

The effective culmination of the many metabolic adaptations to training serves to reduce the dependency on these limited glycogen reserves by a greater fractional utilization of alternative substrates (particularly free fatty acids) or a relatively greater oxidative glycogenolysis (less anaerobic utilization of glycogen). Both adaptations could be thought of as glycogen-sparing (Williams 1985).

What is important to appreciate is that whatever exercise is performed, some carbohydrate will always be used — the longer or harder the exercise, the greater the demands placed upon the carbohydrate stores of the body. One of the primary limitations to maintaining high rates of energy expenditure is the availability of glycogen to maintain the desired rate of ATP resynthesis. Without the contribution made by glycogen utilization, the rate at which ATP can be resynthesised is markedly reduced. The only way in which the imbalance in the rates of demand and supply can be redressed is by decreasing the demand for ATP (e.g. by slowing down the rate at which work is performed). Consequently, without adequate muscle glycogen reserves, the ability to perform high levels of work is markedly impaired.

The role of carbohydrates in training

Whilst the significance of this observation will be readily appreciated during competition, the necessity of maintaining glycogen reserves during training is probably less clear. Every time an individual trains, the amount of glycogen within the working muscle will fall.

Unfortunately, as these stores are limited, they must be repleted adequately prior to the next training session, or it will be started with lower than normal glycogen reserves. If the reserves are lower than normal, the point at which glycogen could become limiting may be attained more rapidly, impairing both the quality and quantity of training which can be accomplished within a training session.

If the process of incomplete refuelling is repeated over successive days of training, a progressive depletion of glycogen stores within the working muscles will result and even the lightest exercise will become extremely difficult to complete (Costill and Miller 1980). The feeling of continual lethargy and heavy tired muscles or incomplete recovery between training sessions and the over-training phenomena may all be related to trying to train with insufficient repletion of muscle glycogen.

Factors influencing the rate of glycogen repletion

The principle factor limiting the rate at which glycogen is repleted within skeletal muscle is time. Complete repletion of muscle glycogen reserves following prolonged exercise which totally depletes muscle glycogen may take 48 hours — irrespective of the intake of carbohydrate over that period (Piehl 1974). Moreover, it appears that the trauma associated with hard heavy sessions (such as speedwork, gymnasium/weights work and hill running) or competition will result in even longer delays in restoring normal muscle glycogen stores. The cellular damage inflicted upon the muscle appears to impair the process of glycogen resynthesis and it may take seven days or more to fully refuel after the rigours of a marathon, irrespective of carbohydrate intake (Sherman et al 1983).

However, other studies have shown that consumption of a diet high in carbohydrate will increase the rate of refuelling following exercise-induced glycogen depletion (Costill et al 1981). Moreover, consumption of a high carbohydrate diet has been shown to reduce the progressive depletion of muscle glycogen normally associated with repeated training sessions (Costill and Miller 1980). A diet high in carbohydrate could therefore be beneficial to the athlete by supporting intensive and consistent training. Without adequate energy reserves, the degree of stimulus afforded by each training session would be reduced as would the ensuing adaptation. Without the adaptation, the improvements in performance will be minimal.

Dietary recommendations for training

Whilst the exact relationship between the amount, type and frequency of carbohydrate consumption and glycogen repletion has yet to be established (Costill et al 1981), it is generally agreed that the diet should be high in carbohydrates (approximately 50–60% of the total energy intake or greater than 500 g for adult male athletes with a high energy expenditure) with a corresponding reduction in total fat and protein intake. As this is essentially the same advice as would be given to all members of the population, there is no conflict between eating for performance or health. Moreover, an interest in sport may present the opportunity to introduce healthy eating to an otherwise non-compliant population, particularly, the young adolescent.

However, from the evidence available it would appear that the majority of athletes consume the same sort of diet as non-athletes and fail to consume a diet rich in carbohydrate (Brotherhood 1984). One possible explanation for this observation is the relative degree of nutritional naivety amongst athletes and coaches in the UK (Wootton 1986). Another factor contributing to the low carbohydrate intake may be that the practical constraints placed upon the individual by their lifestyle make it extremely difficult for the athlete to achieve a balanced, healthy diet high in carbohydrates. These are specific to each individual athlete and should be taken into consideration when advising an athlete — a single standardized set of dietary guidelines will result in poor compliance!

For example, one of the greatest difficulties facing the athlete is simply fitting in the purchase, preparation and consumption of relatively large amounts of food with training, travel, competition and employment/education. Many athletes rely heavily on the use of confectionery and convenience foods to satisfy their appetite. If athletes remove such foods from their usual diet in order to improve the overall quality of the diet, alternative sources of carbohydrate of comparable density must be included (e.g. muesli bars for confectionery, pizza for beefburger, etc.) or total carbohydrate intake will fall considerably. Ease and speed of preparation of meals are important considerations.

General recommendations during preparation for competition

The most important nutritional consideration is ensuring that the athlete starts the competition fully recovered from training with at least normal muscle glycogen stores. Training will result in substantially lowered glycogen stores — thus, the first consideration is to taper the training load over the week preceding competition to allow repletion. Consumption of a normal diet (350–450 g carbohydrate per day) combined with rest should result in normal muscle glycogen stores within 3–4 days; whilst consumption of a high carbohydrate diet will result in significantly greater than normal increases in muscle glycogen (Sherman 1983). Such increases are comparable to those increases in glycogen achieved using the traditional 'carbohydrate-loading' or 'bleed-out' regimen of prolonged exhaustive exercise and three days carbohydrate-restriction followed by three days of a high carbohydrate diet. The latter technique can result in inadequate glycogen repletion through poor dietary management (Wootton et al 1981). Therefore, the best approach would be for the athlete to consume a high carbohydrate diet at all times and then simply taper their training in preparation for competition.

Whilst the endurance capacity of an individual appears to be related to the size of the initial glycogen stores (for review see Wootton et al 1981), there is little evidence to suggest that greatly elevated stores of glycogen will improve performance in every sport. However, in tournament situations where competition is over several days, starting the competition with high glycogen stores may help offset the progressive depletion of muscle glycogen stores with each bout of competition. One possible disadvantage of increasing glycogen stores is the commensurate increase in body weight through the associated storage of water with glycogen — this may be an important consideration where weight classes are in operation.

The pre-competition meal should be carbohydrate-based and readily digested. The ideal timing of the meal will vary greatly between individuals and should be determined on the basis of experience; a meal taken 2–3 hours beforehand is usually appropriate. Anxiety greatly reduces gastric emptying and in extreme cases where the situation may arise several times a week over long periods, a commercial liquid meal (e.g. Build-up or Ensure) may be useful. Fluid intake over the preceding days before competition must be encouraged in order to ensure complete rehydration.

The ingestion of carbohydrate solutions either before or during exercise can supplement the limited glycogen reserves and enhance performance — but can also be detrimental if used incorrectly (for review see Costill and Miller 1980). The presence of a hyperosmolar solution in the stomach can retard fluid absorption and

carbohydrate solutions can cause hyperglycaemia followed by rebound hypoglycaemia and also hyper-insulinaemia which will inhibit fat mobilization (thereby increasing glycogen utilization) — all these will impair performance. Thus the use of glucose tablets and confectionery immediately prior to or during exercise should be discouraged.

However, very weak glucose and electrolyte solutions (less than 2–5% w/w) such as diluted Maxijul, XLI, Mineral Plus 6 may actively promote hydration and supply exogenous carbohydrate during exercise. The electrolytes are not present to replace those lost in sweating, but to help promote fluid absorption. Similarly, glucose polymers (e.g. maltodextrins) which allow greater concentrations (up to 10% w/w) of carbohydrate to be delivered whilst maintaining low osmolality can also be useful, particularly during prolonged low-intensity activities or between bouts of competition in tournaments. However, care must be taken to ensure that fluid absorption is never compromised.

3.8.2 Fluid balance

Thermoregulation during exercise

Man is very inefficient when it comes to converting the energy stored in food into mechanical work. Only about 20–25% of the available energy stored in carbohydrate or fat is actually converted into a form which the muscles can actually use to contract and generate force. The remaining 70–80% is lost as heat. During exercise, when the rate of energy utilization increases, the rate of heat production will also increase. In order to prevent an excessive rise in body temperature (hyperthermia) the body must lose this additional heat. It can do this by several mechanisms, the most important of which is through the evaporation of sweat on the surface of the skin.

Although sweating is a very effective way of losing heat, care must be taken to ensure that this process is not impaired through dehydration. Sweat is simply a dilute version of blood. Thus when sweating is prolonged or pronounced, the body loses both water and electrolytes. The loss of electrolytes is much less than the loss of water and does not represent an immediate problem. It does not appear to be necessary to replace these electrolytes during exercise — if anything the concentration of the major electrolytes in plasma tend to increase during exercise. However, the water loss will cause serious problems if no attempts are made to replace the lost fluid. Losses of fluid corresponding to as little as 2% of body weight can result in pronounced impairment of the capacity to perform muscular work (see Costill and Miller 1980).

The body needs to balance the losses and intake of fluids in order to maintain the capacity to regulate body temperature. In man where sweat losses greatly exceed replacement, the circulatory system is unable to cope and skin blood flow falls. With this comes a reduction in sweating and a reduction in the ability to lose heat — thus, body temperature will rise with potentially fatal consequences.

Therefore, considerable care should be taken to ensure adequate hydration before, during and after exercise so as to avoid thermal distress. These principles apply equally to both training and competition as progressive depletion of the body water can occur over several days of insufficient fluid intake in the same way as the progressive depletion of glycogen. It should also be remembered that these points apply equally to all sportsmen and women — not just marathon runners — and especially to those exercising indoors.

Dietetic advice concerning fluid balance

Before exercise

The athlete should be fully hydrated prior to taking any exercise; sporting activities should never be started in a dehydrated condition. Large amounts of alcohol the night before should be avoided. Some fluid (e.g. 400–600 ml water) should be taken about 30 minutes before the activity commences.

During exercise

Small amounts of fluid should be taken little and often. Drinking should be encouraged at an early stage and *before* thirst has developed; in some sports, a cyclist's water bottle may be a useful piece of equipment. Where possible, regular water breaks should be planned and the athlete should be encouraged to drink even if not thirsty.

Since cold fluids leave the stomach faster than warm or hot ones, drinks should ideally be between 8–13°C. Larger volumes of fluid also empty from the stomach more quickly than smaller volumes; however, too much fluid in the stomach can have unfortunate consequences!

Salt tablets are unnecessary (an ordinary diet contains more than sufficient salt for any athlete) and

should be avoided at all costs since they will exacerbate dehydration.

Heat build-up can be minimized by splashing water on the skin during exercise which will cause heat loss via evaporation. Sporting activities in warm climates require careful preparation and sufficient time for acclimatization before competition.

Following exercise

The rehydration process should start immediately, and not some hours after the event. Athletes should always carry their own supply of fluid in their kit bag; the coach or organiser of the event cannot be relied on to have fluids available.

Athletes must condition their bodies to ingesting fluids during exercise and thus must drink during training as well as in competition.

3.8.3 Other considerations

Protein

Endurance exercise results in a protein catabolic state characterized by decreased protein synthesis, increased amino acid oxidation and increased conversion of amino acids to glucose. Conversely, the adaptive response to strength exercise results in an anabolic state in hypertrophying muscles, and the accretion of protein is the result of an increased protein synthesis. Because of changes in protein metabolism there is an increased dietary requirement for protein in both endurance and strength exercise. However, the normal dietary intake of protein is adequate for athletes as long as the energy intake is sufficient to maintain body weight. There is little scientific evidence that consumption of large protein supplements will have any beneficial effect on muscle hypertrophy, muscular strength or physical performance (for review see Dohm 1984). The consumption of large amounts of protein-rich foods may also establish abnormal eating habits which will serve to limit the intake of carbohydrate-rich foods thereby limiting glycogen repletion and the extent of adaptation.

Weight control

The aim of all reducing diets is to reduce the body's fat store. However, most traditional weight reduction regimens in sport exert a more profound influence on the carbohydrate and water stores of the body. Chronic weight reduction by exclusion of carbohydrate-rich foods from the diet (e.g. 'starchy and sugary' foods) would limit the repletion of muscle glycogen, thereby making it difficult to train and lose weight simultaneously. Acute reductions in body weight by fasting, diuretics and exercise in plastic body suits commonly used to 'make the weight' will simply result in dehydration and glycogen depletion — both of which have been shown to severely impair performance (for review see Smith 1984).

Vitamins and minerals

Whilst there is little evidence that vitamin or mineral supplementation enhances athletic performance when added to the diet of an athlete who is well nourished, there may be certain instances where specific attempts to increase intakes through alterations in diet or supplementation may be warranted (Williams 1984; Bruce *et al* 1985). For example, the poor eating habits of some athletes may give rise to limited intakes and sub-optimal stores of certain nutrients in the same way as in many other young people (Brotherhood 1984). More specifically those participating in combat sports, lightweight rowers and jockeys competing at specific weights as well as young female endurance runners, gymnasts and ballet dancers may all be continually restricting their food intake in order to maintain low body weights. In these circumstances the consequences of hyponutrition limiting nutrient intakes (particularly iron) over prolonged periods require intervention.

Sources of help

1 Dr SA Wootton, Department of Nutrition, Southampton University, Southampton, Hants SO9 3TU. Tel: (0703) 559122 ext 4315.
2 Prof C Williams and Ms Moya Walker SRD, Dept of Physical Education and Sports Science, Loughborough University, Loughborough, Leics LE11 3TU. Tel: (0509) 263161 ext 664.

3 National Coaching Foundation Information Service, National Coaching Foundation, 4 College Close, Beckett Park, Leeds LS6 3QH. Tel: (0532) 744802.

References

Brotherhood JR (1984) Nutrition and sports performance. *Sports Med* **1**, 350−89.

Bruce A, Edblom B and Nilsson I (1985) The effect of vitamin and mineral supplements and health foods on physical endurance and performance. *Proc Nutr Soc* **44**, 283−95.

Costill DL and Miller JM (1980) Carbohydrate and fluid balance. *Int J Sports Med* **1**, 2−9.

Costill DL, Sherman WM, Fink WJ, Maresh C, Witten M and Miller JM (1981) The role of dietary carbohydrates in muscle glycogen resynthesis after strenuous running. *Am J Clin Nutr* **34**, 1831−6.

Dohm GL (1984) Protein nutrition for the athlete. In *Nutritional aspects of exercise. Clinics in sports medicine* Hecker AL (Ed). pp 595−604. WB Saunders Co, Philadelphia.

Piehl K (1974) Time course for refilling of gycogen stores in human muscle fibres following exercise-induced glycogen depletion. *Acta Phys Scand* **90**, 297−302.

Sherman WM (1983) Carbohydrate metabolism. In *Ergogenic aids in sport*. Williams MH (Ed). pp 3−26. Human Kinetics Publishers, Champaign.

Sherman WM, Costill DL, Fink WJ, Armstrong LE, Hagerman FC and Murray TM (1983) The marathon: recovery from acute biochemical alterations. In *Biochemistry of exercise* Int Series on Sports Sciences vol 13. pp 312−7. Knuttgen HG, Vogel JA and Poortmans JR (Eds). Human Kinetic Publishers, Champaign.

Smith NA (1984) Weight control in the athlete. In *Nutritional aspects of exercise. Clinics in sports medicine* Hecker AL (Ed). pp 693−704. WB Saunders Co. Philadelphia.

Williams C (1985) Nutritional aspects of exercise-induced fatigue. *Proc Nutr Soc* **44**, 245−56.

Williams MH (1984) Vitamin and mineral supplements to athletes: do they help? In *Nutritional aspects of exercise. Clinics in sports medicine* Hecker AL (Ed). pp 623−38. WB Saunders Co, Philadelphia.

Wootton SA, Shorten MR and Williams C (1981) Nutritional manipulation of metabolism for the purpose of sport. In *Applied Nutrition I* Bateman EC (Ed). pp 60−4. John Libbey, London.

Wootton SA (1986) Eating habits and nutritional beliefs of British athletes and coaches. In *Proceedings of National Symposium on Nutrition in Sport* D Shrimpton (Ed). In press.

3.9 Vegetarianism and Veganism

3.9.1 Definitions

A *vegetarian* is 'one who lives wholly or partially on vegetable foods, a person who on principle, abstains from any form of animal food or at least such as is obtained by the destruction of life' (Oxford English Dictionary). *Lactovegetarians* include milk and milk products in their diets. Meat, poultry, fish and eggs are excluded. *Lacto-ovovegetarians* eat milk, dairy products and eggs but no flesh foods. *Vegans* are those who consume no animal products at all; their diets are comprised totally of vegetables, vegetable oils and cereals.

Partial vegetarians exclude some groups of animal foods but not others. For example, people who consume no red meat but do eat fish and/or chicken. This sort of diet is often adopted for 'health' rather than 'moral' reasons.

Zen macrobiotic diets. This is a Japanese way of eating based on the 'Yin Yang' theory. It aims to keep the balance between Yin and Yang (positive and negative) aspects of life for optimal spiritual, mental and physical welfare. Foods are divided into Yin and Yang, and a spiritual goal is aimed for by working through ten levels of diet. These gradually eliminate all animal produce, fruit and vegetables towards the final goal which is only cereal (brown rice). Fluids are also severely restricted. Many nutritional deficiencies may develop and death can result. Infants and children subjected to these restrictions are particularly at risk.

Not all 'macrobiotic' diets however are taken to extremes. Some are equivalent to balanced vegan diets.

3.9.2 Guidelines for formulating nutritionally balanced vegetarian and vegan diets

A wide variety of foods should be chosen from the following groups
1 *Milk* 1 pint (children) or $\frac{1}{2}$ pint (adults) of milk or a milk substitute (e.g. soya milk, yoghurt). Milk products such as cheese and/or yoghurt if eaten daily can also be a substitute for milk.

Milk or milk products should be consumed *in addition to* 2–3 portions of protein listed below.
2 *Proteins.* 2–3 portions daily of any of the following: pulses and beans — in casseroles, rissoles and soups; nuts — in salads, rissoles and roasts; cheese and eggs; soya products, e.g. textured vegetable protein in casseroles and Tofu in stir fry, flans and dips.
3 *Cereals.* 3–5 portions daily of any of the following: bread, breakfast cereals, rice, pasta, flour, crackers (ideally wholegrain) or other cereals such as millet, bulghar wheat, wheat grain and buckwheat.
4 *Fruit.* 2–3 portions daily of: fruits (fresh, dried or juice). This should include 1 citrus fruit or glass of citrus fruit juice daily.
5 *Vegetables.* At least 2 portions daily, lightly cooked or raw, of a variety of vegetables which includes both dark green and root vegetables.
6 *Fats.* Butter (if permitted), margarines and oils should be consumed as required.

In contrast to most of the population, the diets of vegetarians and vegans are naturally low in fat. It is therefore unnecessary to restrict the amounts of fats and oils used in cooking or to recommend the use of low fat spreads. Furthermore, some vegetarians may need to be advised to *increase* their consumption of fats and oils in order to meet their energy requirements.

3.9.3 Possible nutritional problems and remedies

Nutritional deficiencies can occur, particularly when an individual decides to become vegetarian and simply stops eating meat or animals products, without considering what can be eaten instead. It is particularly important to check the vegetarian diet of people who are nutritionally at risk, e.g. pregnant women, infants and children, teenagers and the elderly. Particular features to look for are summarized in Table 3.21.

3.9.4 Vegetarian or vegan infants and children

Weaning

Breast milk or modified baby milk should provide sufficient nutrients for the baby until the age of 4–6

Table 3.21. Checklist to assess the nutritional adequacy of a vegetarian or vegan diet

Nutrient	Comments
Protein	In order to obtain an adequate mixture of amino acids (and consequently protein of high biological value) it is essential that there is a mixture of vegetable protein foods at each meal, i.e. 1 Beans, pulses or nuts *and* cereal (e.g. bean stew with rice or nuts and breadcrumbs made into a nut roast). 2 Cheese or egg *and* cereal (e.g. egg on toast). 3 Seeds *and* cereal (e.g. chickpeas and sesame seed spread (tahini) which makes a dish called Hummus).
Energy	For those with small appetites and for children there must be an adequate intake of concentrated energy sources such as nuts, nut butters, margarine, oil, milk or milk substitute, yoghurt, cheese or sunflower seeds.
Vitamins B group	Wholegrain cereals, bread and green vegetables should be consumed daily. The intake of B group vitamins can be increased by the addition of yeast extract to soup and stews and wheatgerm to cereals and flour.
B12	This is only found in animal foods, so vegan diets in particular *must* contain vitamin B12 fortified foods (e.g. Barmene or Tastex (yeast extracts), Plamil, Protoveg or Grapenuts). Vitamin B12 supplements are needed if these foods are not eaten.
D	Exposure to sunlight is important. Margarine and fortified soya milk (e.g. Plamil), fortified breakfast cereals (e.g. Kellogg's cereals) are the best sources of dietary vitamin). Eggs (if acceptable) can also boost vitamin D intake.
Minerals	Pregnant and lactating women and vegans are particularly at risk of deficiencies.
Iron	To ensure an adequate iron intake, the following should be consumed: Pulse vegetables (at least daily). Egg (if eaten) 5–7 times weekly. Wholegrain bread and cereals at least twice daily. Wheatgerm, nuts, dried fruit, green vegetables, cocoa, molasses and curry powder also contain iron. A vitamin C-containing food or drink should ideally be consumed at each meal to aid absorption of non-haem iron. Iron supplements are likely to be required during pregnancy.
Calcium	Extra sources are required during pregnancy and lactation and can be obtained from 1 Fortified soya milks, e.g. Plamil and Granolac. 2 Sesame seeds — sprinkled on soups, cereals, stews and desserts, or added to pastry or biscuit mixes or made into a spread (tahini). 3 Nuts, particularly almonds. 4 Hardwater. 5 Cereals, particularly millet (which can be eaten instead of rice or in the form of rissoles). If the dietary intake is inadequate, calcium supplements are needed.

months. Solid food should then be introduced gradually. Vitamin drops should be given from the age of one month to two years and preferably until five years of age.

If no foods of animal origin are to be eaten, either vitamin B12 supplement or a food fortified with vitamin B12 (such as soya milk) should be given. Tastex and Barmene are too high in salt for an infant but are suitable for children over the age of two years.

Starting weaning at 4–6 months

Foods should be introduced one at a time, and the quantities gradually increased. Suitable first foods include

1 Baby rice and water (or baby milk).
2 Smooth puree of vegetables, e.g. carrot.
3 Smooth puree of fruit, e.g. apple, pear or apricot.

If the baby is thirsty it can be given boiled cooled water or very dilute unsweetened fruit juice. No sugar or salt should be added to food.

Continuing weaning at 5–7 months

New foods may be introduced one at a time. Suitable foods include

1 Well cooked pureed pulses, e.g. lentils and split peas.
2 Pureed root vegetables.
3 Pureed brown rice, brown rice flour and water or baby rice.
4 Mixtures of pulses, vegetables and/or rice puree.
5 Pureed stewed fruit or well mashed banana.

No sugar or salt should be added to food and salt-free stock (e.g. Vecon) should be used in cooking.

At about six months the baby can be given, under *close* supervision, wedges of apple, sticks of carrot or baked wholemeal bread to encourage chewing.

Some commercial baby foods, e.g. baby rice and vegetables main courses are suitable for vegetarian and vegan babies. These will be fortified with some vitamins and minerals.

7–9 months

The baby should still be having 1 pint of milk or equivalent each day. If cows' milk is not taken, boiled goats' milk or a soya milk substitute (e.g. Plamil or Granogen) may be used, but NOT UNTIL the baby is eating a variety of other foods and not without first consulting a doctor or health visitor. Formula S is a suitable soya milk for infants. Foods can now be minced or finely chopped and new foods can be introduced. Suitable foods include

1 Wholegrain breakfast cereals, e.g. Weetabix, porridge.
2 Cheese (grated or finely chopped, cottage or curd cheese).
3 Eggs (if eaten).
4 Yoghurts.
5 Wholemeal bread.
6 Brown rice.
7 Well-cooked pasta.

8 A variety of vegetables.
9 Fruit (grated, chopped or stewed including cooked dried fruit).
10 Soya bean curd (Tofu).
11 Pulses and beans — well cooked and mashed or pureed, given with cereal food such as rice, rice flour or bread.
Suitable dishes to try include:

Savoury dishes. Pureed bean and vegetable stew with rice; lentil rissole mashed with a little stock: finely ground nuts or nut butters; pureed nut roast or cutlets; savoury egg custard and cheese sauce with vegetables.

Desserts. Rice pudding made with brown rice flour; wholemeal semolina and custard or egg custard.

9–12 months

At this stage most babies will be eating three meals a day.

Most of the family's foods will be suitable and a wide variety of foods, flavours and textures should be encouraged. However, spicy, fatty foods and whole nuts should avoided. At least 1 pint of milk or milk substitutes should be consumed daily.

In order to get the best nutritional value from foods, it is essential that a mixture of foods is eaten at each meal. For example

Breakfast. Wholegrain breakfast cereal
and milk or milk substitute
and wholemeal bread or toast and margarine
and egg (if eaten).

Lunch. Mashed bean stew and rice
or cauliflower cheese and pasta
or mashed potato with cheese and egg
or lentil and vegetable soup and bread
or mashed nut roast
and vegetables, cooked or raw
and fruit, yoghurt or milk pudding.

Tea. Wholemeal bread and margarine
and cheese or egg or lentil paté or peanut butter
and vegetable or bean soup (if desired)
and salad, vegetables
and fruit, yoghurt or milk pudding.

Feeding vegetarian and vegan children

The guidelines for formulating vegetarian diets for children are the same as those for adults (see p 303). However, the following factors should also be considered
1 A wide variety of foods must be given in order to meet nutritional requirements.
2 One pint of milk or its equivalent in yoghurt or rennet-free cheese, or a soya milk, should be given daily.
3 Some vegetable margarine (approximately $\frac{1}{2}$–1 oz daily) should be included.
4 If no animal foods are eaten, vitamin B12-fortified soya milk, Tastex or Barmene should be used.
5 Sugar and sugary foods should be kept to a minimum. Dried fruit, molasses and black treacle will help to sweeten foods and provide extra iron.
6 Because the diet is bulky, some children will find it difficult to consume sufficient energy. An adequate supply of energy-dense foods such as margarine, cheese or milk should be included.

Support organisations

Literature, including menu ideas, recipe sheets and books are available from
1 The Vegetarian Society, Parkdale, Denham Road, Altrincham, Cheshire.
2 The Vegan Society, 47 Highlands Road, Leatherhead, Surrey.
3 Friends of the Earth, 377 City Road, London BC1U 1NA.
Locally, literature can also be obtained from wholefood and vegetarian shops and restaurants. The Vegetarian Society and some education authorities may also run vegetarian cookery classes.

Further reading

American Academy of Pediatrics: Committee on Nutrition (1977) Nutritional aspects of vegetarianism, health foods and fad food diets. *Paediatrics* **59**, (3), 460–4.
Bull NL and Barber SA (1984) Food and nutrient intakes of vegetarians in Britain. *Hum Nutr: Appl Nutr* **38A**, 288–93.
Community Nutrition Group of British Dietetic Association. Information sheet No 3 *Vegetarian and vegan diets*. Information Sheet No 8 *Wholefoods*.
Ellis FR (1967) The nutritional status of vegans and vegetarians. *Proc Nutr Soc* **26**, 205–12.
Gear JS, Mann JI, Thorogood M, Carter R and Jelfs R (1980) Biochemical and haematological variables in vegetarians. *Brit Med J* **1**, 1415.
Roshanai F and Sanders TAB (1984) Assessment of fatty acid intakes in vegans and omnivores. *Hum Nutr: Appl Nutr* **38A**, 345–54.
Sanders TAB (1978) Vegan diet — a remedy for diseases of affluence? *Getting the most out of food* **13**, 15–51. Van den Berghs and Jurgens Ltd, Burgess Hill, W. Sussex.
Sanders TAB (1979) Vegetarian diets. *British Nutrition Foundation Bulletin* **27**, 137–144. British Nutrition Foundation, London.
Tripp JH, Francis DEM, Knight JA and Harries JT (1979) Infant feeding practices; a cause for concern. *Br Med J* **2**, 707–9.

General books

Elliot R (1982) *The vegetarian baby book*. Fontana, London.
Moore Lappe F (1978) *Diet for a small planet*. Ballantine Books, New York.

Recipe books

Brown S (1984)·*Vegetarian kitchen*. BBC Publications, London.

Duff G *Vegetarian cookery*. Pan Books, London.
Elliot R *Not just a load of old lentils*. Fontana, London.
Elliot R *The bean book*. Fontana, London.
Liddell C *The wholefood cookbook*. Coronet, London.
The Sainsbury's wholefood cookbook. Available from Sainsbury's supermarkets.

3.10 Cultural Minorities

3.10.1 General considerations

Many factors affect what we eat. People arriving in a country and to a culture to which they are not accustomed, will, for some time, wish to follow their normal eating pattern which will have been influenced by

1 Religious beliefs or other strongly held principles.
2 Cultural background and customs in their country of origin.
3 Foods available in their country of origin and with which they are familiar.

Whilst it is possible to give general information on the food habits of different groups it is important to be aware of individual variations. It is equally important to respect the wishes of those (normally older people) who adhere to their known way of life, including dietary constraints. Change should not be imposed or suggested for the sake of conformity: although foods eaten or the meal pattern may be unfamiliar in Britain, most of the diets are nutritionally adequate provided that sufficient of the food is eaten. Where change is nutritionally desirable, any alterations should fit in with the tenets on which the customary diet is based.

The influence of the society in which we live on our eating habits is considerable. Amongst cultural minorities in Britain, school children, young adults who are out at work, and indeed all but those leading a sheltered life within their homes begin to include local dishes in their diet. The degree and speed of change varies and it is this which makes it essential to consider each person individually. The difficulties of adapting to life in a new community should not be increased by pressure to change to local feeding patterns, especially when the individual is ill at home or in hospital.

Health workers can contribute much to their patients welfare by acquiring a real understanding of the culture and religion which govern their lives and tailoring the treatment to fit.

3.10.2 Asian diets

General features

Restrictions on what may be eaten due to religious beliefs are part of the Asian way of life. The three main religions are Hinduism, Islam (the religion of Muslims) and Sikhism. Each has its specific restrictions but there are some points in common.

'Hot' and 'cold' foods

This is nothing to do with the temperature or spiciness of the food; rather it is the concept that certain foods will either cool or heat the body. Generally, 'hot' foods are avoided in pregnancy and fever and 'cold' foods when breast feeding or when suffering from a cold or cough.

Foods usually considered 'hot' are brown sugar, chilli, carrots, dates, eggs, egg plant, fish, ginger, honey, lentils, meat, onions and tea.

Foods usually considered 'cold' are cereals, chick peas, most fruits, green and red grain, milk and dairy products, nuts, potatoes, most vegetables and white sugar.

Food preparation

1 Vegetables are cooked in fat or water.
2 Spices are used individually or in specific combinations. Curry powder, as used in Britain, is not comparable.
3 Homemade pickles and chutneys often accompany main course dishes.
4 Yoghurt is used in cooking and to serve with other food.
5 Homemade curd cheese is quite unlike the cheese used in Britain. The nearest equivalent is cottage cheese.
6 Eggs are usually eaten hard boiled or fried.
7 Considerable use is made of pulses, seeds and nuts.
8 Side salads, especially of raw onion and tomato, are frequently eaten at main meals.
9 Even where the diet permits their use, meat, chicken and fish are eaten in relatively small quantities.

Customs associated with meals

1 Hands are always washed before and after meals.
2 Many people like to rinse their mouths with water after a meal.

3 It is customary in Asia to use the right hand for picking up food at table.

4 Strict vegetarians will not wish to use china or utensils which may have been in contact with meat or fish.

Many Asian cookery books give useful information on the food habits and customs of the country concerned.

The meal pattern

Breakfast: yoghurt with rice or chapattis *or* egg with bread *or* cereal with milk. Tea with hot milk and sugar.

Main Meals: rice or chapattis; meat or fish dish if acceptable; several vegetable or pulse dishes; pickles and side salad.

Variations occur within this pattern but in general the variety of dishes used is less than in a typical British menu cycle.

Hindus

Hinduism is founded on reverence for life, non-violence and a belief in reincarnation. Because they will not kill, most Hindus are strict vegetarians.

Most Hindus in Britain have come from Gujerat on the north-west coast of India; some come from the Indian Punjab and East Africa. Their first language is likely to be Gujerati, but those from East Africa may speak and understand some English.

Naming system

The Hindu naming system consists of: *first name*, used by family and friends; *complementary name*, used only with the first name, never on its own, and *subcaste name* which is used like a British surname.

It is the subcaste name which indicates the religion. The most frequently used Hindu subcaste name in Britain is Patel.

Food restrictions

1 Most Hindus will not eat meat or fish of any kind. Less strict Hindus may eat lamb, chicken or white fish. It is most unusual for a Hindu to eat beef or pork.
2 Very strict Hindus may not eat eggs since they are potentially a source of life.
3 Fats such as dripping, margarine or lard are not acceptable. Ghee and vegetable oil are used in cooking.

4 Strict Hindus will be unwilling to eat food unless they are certain that the utensils used in preparation and service have not been in contact with meat or fish.

Festivals and fasting

Three festivals in the Hindu calendar are observed as fast days
1 Mahashivrati — the birthday of Lord Shiva (March).
2 Ram Naumi — the birthday of Lord Rama (April).
3 Jan Mash Tami — the birthday of Lord Krishna (late August).

Additionally, some devout Hindus will fast on one or two days a week. The fast is observed from dawn to sunset. During this time some Hindus will eat foods considered to be pure, such as yoghurt and fruit, whilst others forego all food but may take fluids. It is a matter for individual decision.

Muslims

The religion of Muslims is Islam. There are five main principles, known as the pillars of Islam, one of which is to fast during the month of Ramadan. The Muslim community in Britain come mainly from Pakistan, Bangladesh and East Africa, with smaller numbers from the Middle East, Malaysia and Indonesia. Many of Indian origin will speak Punjabi or Bengali, but some speak Urdu or Gujerati.

Naming system

This is complex and needs detailed study for a full understanding.* The personal name, which has its origin in religion, is not usually the first name listed. Each person also has a Muslim title which is never a personal name. The principle Muslim titles are Abdul, Allah, Mohammed, Shah, Syed and Ullah (spellings may vary). Khan and Chaudry are frequently used titles amongst Muslims from Pakistan. It is quite usual to use the title followed by the personal name when addressing someone. Bibi, Begum and Khatoon occur in some female names and signify the sex of the bearer. Members of the same family may not share a common family name, nor does a woman always take her husband's name on marriage.

Food restrictions

In the Islamic tradition all wholesome things may be

*See Asian names and records training pack.

used for food and the general rule is that every food is lawful (Halal) unless it is declared unlawful (Haram).

Unlawful foods are
1 Foods from the pig or any carnivorous animal.
2 All meat which has not been ritually slaughtered (Kosher meat is acceptable).
3 Alcohol, including that used in cooking.

It should be noted that a Muslim may refuse a food if he cannot be sure that it does not contain an unlawful ingredient. Similarly, a devout Muslim will be concerned that the dishes used for cooking have not been in contact with unlawful foods.

Festivals and fasting

There are two major festivals in the Muslim calendar
1 Id-al Fitr marks the end of the month of Ramadan, and celebrations in the community and at home last for two days.
2 Id-al Adha commemorates the pilgrimage to Mecca and is celebrated, by those who can afford it, by the sacrifice of a lamb and sharing the meat amongst family, friends and the poor.

Muslims are required to fast from dawn to sunset during the month of *Ramadan*, which is the ninth month of the Muslim calendar. The date varies slightly each year. Fasting involves abstinence from all food and all drink. Feelings of weakness and lethargy often occur as a result of this abstinence and, to help overcome this, most Muslims rise early and eat a good meal before dawn. another meal is taken after sunset. Old people and children under 12 are exempt from fasting. Women who are pregnant, breast feeding or menstruating and people who are ill or travelling during Ramadan are exempt from fasting then, but are expected to compensate by fasting at some other time. Special exemption can be granted for chronically ill people for whom fasting would be physically harmful.

Sikhs

Sikhism began as an offshoot of Hinduism and Islam and has developed into a religion in its own right. Sikhs believe in one personal God, with whom each Sikh must make his own relationship and through that lead a virtuous, useful life in the community. Most Sikhs in Britain come from the Punjab, but some come from East Africa. Their first language is Punjabi but many speak English.

Naming system

All Sikh men have a first or personal name plus Singh.

All Sikh women have a first or personal name plus Kaur. Additionally a Sikh family may adopt a hereditary family name.

Food restrictions

For Sikhs this is a matter for each individual's conscience. As a group they are less strict than Hindus and Muslims, but for each Sikh their own self-imposed restrictions are binding. Some Sikhs, especially women, are vegetarian, but many eat chicken, lamb and fish. They are unlikely to eat beef and even less likely to eat pork. Alcohol is forbidden, but some less devout Sikh men do drink some alcohol.

Festivals and fasting

There are three main festivals in the Sikh calendar
1 Baisakhi — the Sikh New Year's Day (April).
2 Diwali — the festival of Light — (October/November).
3 Birth of Guru Nanak — the founder of Sikhism (November).

Additionally, some devout Sikhs fast once or twice a week.

3.10.3 **Jewish diets**

Judaism is an ancient religion. Many people of the Jewish faith have been born in Britain in families which have been here for several generations; some have come from Europe and some from the Middle East. For many, English is their native language.

Naming system

This is the same as that used in Britain.

Food restrictions

Jews observe the Laws of Kashrut or the Jewish food laws. These laws are imposed as an act of discipline and contribute towards the Jewish way of life. Maintenance of health and food hygiene underlie the laws, especially in hot countries. The laws are
1 Pork and all products of the pig are forbidden.
2 Meat of animals with a cloven hoof and which chew the cud is allowed, e.g. deer, goat, ox, sheep.
3 Permitted birds are chicken, duck, goose, partridge, pheasant, pigeon and turkey. Birds of prey, which are more prone to disease than herbivorous birds, are forbidden.

4 Fish with scales and fins are allowed. Shellfish are not allowed as they are considered to be a source of disease.

5 Meat and milk must not be served at the same meal or cooked together.

6 Animals and birds must be slaughtered by the Jewish method; this procedure, which must be carried out by a trained and authorized person, entails a rapid cut with a sharp knife to sever the jugular vein and carotid artery. The meat is then salted and soaked in water to remove the blood and render it Kosher (permitted).

Festivals and fasting

1 The Jewish Sabbath is celebrated on Saturday each week with ceremonies and rituals both in Synagogues and Jewish homes.

2 Passover, which commemorates the Exodus of Jews from Egypt, is celebrated over eight days in April. Unleavened bread (Matsos) and cakes and biscuits made from Matso-meal are eaten in place of leavened bread.

3 The Jewish New Year (Rosh Hashanah) is celebrated in September.

4 The Day of Atonement (Yom Kippur) is a fast day in September or October.

3.10.4 Vietnamese diets

Three doctrines of Chinese tradition are practised in Vietnam; these are Buddhism, Confucianism and Taoism, each of which influence the conduct of daily life.

Many of the Vietnamese community in Britain are ethnic Chinese and speak Cantonese. Some also speak Vietnamese or French; many now speak English.

Naming system

In Vietnam the family or surname is the first name listed, and is followed by one or more personal names. Amongst these personal names, many men include Van and many women have Thi. The last personal name is usually the one used by family and friends. Women do not take their husband's family name on marriage.

Food habits

1 No specific foods are forbidden in Vietnamese culture, but some foods which are unfamiliar are un-

likely to be acceptable. These include lamb, ox liver, tinned or cooked fruit and some root vegetables.

2 Fresh milk is not available in Vietnam, but some use is made of evaporated and sweetened condensed milk. Lactase deficiency is fairly common amongst the Vietnamese, and may account for the limited use of milk and milk products in the traditional diet.

3 Rice is the main staple and is served either boiled or fried at main meals. Rice grown in Vietnam is a useful source of iron and calcium.

4 Meat and fish are used in small quantities, augmented with pulses, nuts and seeds. A combination of vegetable dishes with rice and soup may constitute a nutritionally adequate meal, as the traditional mix of pulse, rice and nut dishes makes good use of limited resources.

5 Vegetables are usually stir-fried or steamed and only lightly cooked. The average British boiled vegetable is not comparable.

6 Raw fruit is used in great variety.

7 Spices and seasoning are widely used; monosodium glutamate, soy sauce, fish sauce, chilli sauce and vinegar are popular flavourings.

8 Vegetable oil or lard are used in stir-fry cooking. Butter and margarine are expensive and used sparingly and cheese, which is only eaten in small amounts, is processed. Hence the Vietnamese diet is fairly low in fat.

9 Roasted nuts, sweet potato, rice or noodle soup, rice with shreds of meat, spring rolls and fresh fruit are popular snacks between meals eaten by the more affluent.

10 Tea, coffee and fruit juice are the usual drinks, with alcohol kept for special celebrations.

Possible dietary problems

A lack of calcium

Calcium may be low in the diet of Vietnamese people in Britain because

1 Rice grown in Vietnam contributes much more calcium than is available from the rice imported into Britain.

2 Fruit and vegetables in this country contain less calcium than some tropical varieties.

3 Milk and cheese are taken in small amounts, if at all.

An inadequate intake of vitamin D

Low vitamin D intake has been identified in some Vietnamese children; in Vietnam their principle source of this nutrient is sunlight and oral supplements may be necessary for those in Britain.

Yin and Yang

This is the Chinese version of the concept of 'hot' and 'cold' foods. A balance between the two is considered necessary for good health. Yin equates to cool, female energy, and yang to hot, male energy. If the body is hot and fevered, an increase in yin will help to cool it; in cold conditions an increase of yang is required.

The specific foods which come into each category will vary but Table 3.22 is a guide.

Table 3.22 Yin and Yang foods

'Hot' or Yang	'Cold' or Yin
Red meat, duck, goose	Chicken
Oily fish	Green vegetables
Spices	Fruit
Coffee	Vegetable soup
Nuts	Barley water
Potatoes	Boiled or steamed food
Fried foods	

Rice and bread are considered neutral foods. The concept of yin and yang is particularly relevant in illness and pregnancy.

Diet in pregnancy

This is thought of as a 'hot' condition and a pregnant woman may cut down on red meat and fish. A traditional stew, Keung Chow, made from pigs' trotters, boiled eggs soaked in vinegar and ginger is given to a woman after childbirth to help recovery, and in celebration of the birth of a child. For several weeks after childbirth a woman is encouraged to eat 'hot' foods to regain her strength.

Festivals and fasting

Fasting in the terms of abstinence from food and drink is not practised amongst the Vietnamese, but the calendar includes a number of festivals with associated traditional foods and meals. The main festival of New Year, early in February, is celebrated over seven days. Rice cakes, soyabean soup, fruit and seeds are enjoyed, and the end of the celebrations is marked with a special feast.

Within the family, special ritual meals are associated with births, weddings, anniversaries and funerals.

3.10.5 Chinese diets

The Chinese community in Britain is well established; Chinese food is popular with many of the indigenous population although the majority confine their sampling to a few better known 'westernized' dishes.

Food habits

Rice is the staple in much of China and is eaten at all meals. It is served boiled or steamed except at breakfast, when Congee or soft rice (a form of thin porridge) is eaten with salted eggs, fried salt fish or Chinese cheese. Fried rice is regarded as a snack and not normally eaten by Chinese as part of a meal.

In Northern China wheat, maize and corn are used more than rice. They are made into Chinese bread, which is steamed and white and formed into small buns which are used in place of rice with other dishes at main meals.

Noodles are another important staple; fried noodles or Chow Mein are popular and may be served with other ingredients such as chicken. Soup and noodles can be a substantial meal as the 'soup' contains pieces of meat, fish, egg and vegetables.

Communal dining is usual and a Chinese main meal consists of rice or Chinese bread plus several dishes cooked by different methods and using different ingredients to produce a variety of textures and flavours. These dishes are served simultaneously, each diner taking a serving of rice and adding a small amount of each of the other dishes one at a time. Thin soup will often accompany the meal as a drink. A sweet course is unusual.

Vegetables are an important part of the meal and are often quick-fried and served with a sweet and sour or soy sauce. Braised vegetables are popular, and a mixture of vegetables cooked in different ways may be served. Vegetables are always lightly cooked.

Chinese food is not highly spiced, but salt is used in abundance. Garlic, fresh ginger and soy sauce are used as flavourings. Food may be marinated in wine before cooking.

Cooking methods

1 Quick stir-frying of food which has been diced or shredded is common, and a small amount of sauce may be added.
2 White braising is cooking in chicken stock.
3 Red braising is done in soy sauce.
4 Steaming in a closed pan is used for whole birds or larger pieces of meat.

5 Roasting may be done on a barbecue.

6 Salting, smoking and drying are used as methods of food preparation.

Possible dietary problems

The high salt content of their diet may give cause for concern.

3.10.6 Rastafarian diets

As part of their religious beliefs, Rastafarians follow a diet known as I-tal. This is fundamentally vegetarian but details and the degree of strictness vary amongst the community. Young, male Rastafarians tend to be very strict.

In some cases meat, fish, eggs, canned foods, processed foods and salt are excluded. In Jamaica, fish forms an important part of the diet but the types of fish available in Britain are not usually acceptable.

Possible dietary problems

Little is known of the effect of this diet but rickets has been identified in some children of black Rastafarians in Britain. Difficulties may arise during weaning, in the pre-school child and during pregnancy.

Sources of help

1 Local community leaders may help with information, translation and establishing contacts with individuals or groups.

2 Dietetic departments in districts with specific cultural groups locally develop diet sheets and nutrition education material for their use. Many are willing to have their material used in other districts. Details cannot be given as publications change, but an approach to dietitians in relevant districts is worthwhile.

3 The Commonwealth Institute in Kensington High Street, London has an excellent reference library and many publications on Commonwealth countries.

4 Individual embassies will often be helpful in sup-plying information on their own national diet, and some offer translation facilities.

Food tables

Immigrant Foods. Second Supplement to *McCance and Widdowson's The composition of foods*. HMSO, London.

Training packs

Henley A and Taylor C *Asian names and records.*
Henley A *Asian foods and diets.*
  Both these training packs are available from the National Extension College, 1 Brooklands Avenue, Cambridge CB2 2HN.

Further reading

Brissenden R *South-east Asian food*. Penguin, London.
Henley A *Asian patients in hospital and at home*. King Edwards Hospital Fund for London, London.
Lazarus HM *The ways of her household*. Jewish Memorial Council.
Lo K *The Chinese cookbook*. Penguin, London.
McDermott MY *The Muslim guide*. The Islamic Foundation, Leicester.
Mares P *The Vietnamese in Britain*. National Extension College, Cambridge.
Ortis E *Carribean cookery*. Penguin, London.
Singh D *Indian cookery*, Penguin, London.

3.11 The Mentally Handicapped

3.11.1 Background information

Incidence

Three in a 1000 of the population are severely mentally handicapped (i.e. have an IQ less than 50) (DHSS 1971). In 1984, it was estimated that, in England, there were 38,600 mentally handicapped persons resident in hospitals and 102,300 at home. If this distribution is applied throughout the British Isles, the total number of mentally handicapped persons in the UK in 1984 was probably in the region of 170,000.

Location

Long stay hospitals

These are large institutions often situated in countryside remote from towns, villages and communities and normally surrounded by many acres of land. Residents are usually housed in lodges rather than wards which are divided into living, dining and sleeping areas. Most residents leave the lodge during the day for work or some kind of activity. Each lodge has a fairly static population and could be the individual's home for 30−40 years.

Some degree of menu choice has recently been introduced by some Health Authorities but menus may still be limited and food selection made by ward staff rather than by the residents. Timing of meals is sometimes inappropriate; the evening meal is usually served very early as a result of the shift hours of the catering, portering and nursing staff. Sometimes meal helpers are employed just to help out at meal times.

Hostels

These are medium-sized homes with an institutionalized style of living and are either the responsibility of the Health Service or Social Services. They are usually situated in communities so have better access to shops, libraries and transport. Sometimes they are used as a stepping stone to more independent living.

Smaller hostels found in the public or private sector are often converted houses, accommodating small groups of mentally handicapped individuals. These are also occasionally used as a stepping stone but are more often a permanent home run by appropriately qualified people.

Group homes and sheltered housing

These are houses in the community owned by local authority (council houses) with the rent often paid by the Health Authority. Small family-sized groups of individuals live together as a unit, probably supported by social workers and other agencies working in the community. There may be a resident Community Service Volunteer on a temporary basis.

At home

Nowadays most younger mentally handicapped people remain with the family unit supported by agencies from community services.

Adult Training Centres/Social Education Centres/ Sheltered Workshops

These are run by Social Services with the trainees recruited from hospitals/hostels or directly from the community. They learn life-skills and are trained in various activities. The trainees are anxious to work, as other people, and not merely to be kept occupied.

These centres are not controlled by any legislation so each one differs and is autonomous.

Adult Further Education Centres

These run a variety of courses some of which are appropriate for the mentally handicapped.

Staff who care for the mentally handicapped

Medical

General Practitioners are responsible for the day to day medical care of residents and often hold surgeries on a regular basis.

Psychiatrists will probably be the best contact for dietitians wishing to learn about medical/psychiatric conditions and treatment. Most psychiatric units organise multidisciplinary study days, lectures and seminars.

Nursing

Averaged throughout the country, the percentage of qualified to unqualified staff working in this field is about 30:70; this is lower than that nationally recommended.

Nurses are trained either as Registered Nurse Mental Handicap (RNMH) or Enrolled Nurse Mental Handicap (ENMH). With the help of regular study days, nursing auxiliaries can also play an important role teaching patients the basic skills relating to food.

Other paramedical personnel

Psychologists are involved in behaviour modification and are instrumental in deciding which residents are placed or housed where. The advice of psychologists can be enlisted to help suggest rewards and treats other than food and they can also help to enforce this throughout the system.

Speech and occupational therapists have an established place in the health care team and need to be involved to ensure 'healthy nutrition'. The speech therapist will be helpful with feeding problems.

Dentists and dental hygienists visit the institutions regularly and are interested in preventing dental decay as well as ensuring well-fitting and suitable dentures.

Social workers provide support, assistance and information about entitled benefits and budgeting, etc. They also bridge the gap between the health service and the community.

The pharmacist can provide valuable information about which drugs are commonly used in treatment and whether they have any effect on the gastrointestinal tract or if there is an interaction with any nutrient (see section 5.10).

Mentally handicapped patients and the staff looking after them are still a very close knit population though this is gradually changing as integration into the community becomes a priority. This is illustrated by patients being rehoused in hostels or family houses and by the development of support services such as

1 Advocacy alliance. This is a developing network to recruit lay people to act as a resident's representative so that the legal and other rights of those who are mentally handicapped can be assured. In the long term it is hoped that the individual will be able to manage by himself.
2 Respite Care/Help the family/Family support schemes. These are organised locally to give support and relief to the family of the handicapped member living at home. The family is usually paired with another and help is given on a 'baby sitting' type of arrangement for a weekend 'off'.
3 Multidisciplinary Community Mental Handicap Teams. A core member/key worker is assigned to each individual to co-ordinate any necessary resources or services to ensure prevention of illness and maintenance of health. The dietitian could be the key worker if nutrition was the major problem and the psychologist, speech or occupational therapist, etc. would be involved as required.

3.11.2 The role of the dietitian in the care of the mentally handicapped

In 1975 when district-based dietetic departments were first established, there were few dietitians who had any responsibility to provide a service for the mentally handicapped. At the present time it is still probably the cinderella of the dietetic service as our expertise is unknown to most members of health and social service personnel working in this field. This is illustrated by Kekstadt and Primrose (1983) whose book includes the statement 'the diet is ordered by the physician and prepared in the kitchen by a dietitian who will supply the ward with the meal the patient requires'!

Nutrition education

Many of those caring for the mentally handicapped will have had little, if any, nutritional training. They may be unaware of the nutritional needs of their residents or the dietetic services which are available or can be realistically provided. Requests for obsolete therapeutic regimens such as gastric diets are not uncommon. Educating the *carers* is therefore a vital part of a dietitians's work in the field of mental handicap. Some of the ways this can be achieved include
1 Nurse education. Since the new syllabus for nurse training was introduced in September 1985, it is easier for dietitians to participate in the educational programme as it includes four direct references to nutrition.

2 In-service training. This is becoming more regular and broader in content and information related to nutrition and diet can frequently be included in seminars or study days. Since a higher proportion of the staff are unqualified when compared with District General Hospitals, teaching methods should take this into account; workshops or informal discussion groups may be more appropriate than formal lectures.

3 Educating social services personnel. Social services responsible for adult training centres and other day care facilities also have staff who require training and support to ensure that the approach to dealing with nutritional problems, and the information given, is consistent.

Improving the quality of the diet

The ultimate objective of the dietitian's work is to ensure that each individual's nutritional needs are met in a way which is compatible with healthy eating guidelines. The quality and adequacy of the food provided in residential institutions will need to be assessed and practical ways to improve it may need to be suggested (see pp 3, 287, 327).

There will be therapeutic referrals but these will be a minimum rather than a maximum commitment. The therapeutic problems will be similar to those found in the rest of the population but regimens may need to be modified. Opportunities abound for improving the nutrition of these individuals so that a healthy diet is assured.

Specific measures which may help to improve the quality of the diet offered to mentally handicapped patients include

1 Creating a District Food Policy. This will help to provide a healthier diet which will in turn help to educate those eventually rehabilitated into the community. Hopefully it will also lessen the regular use of enemas and laxatives.

2 Improving the type of consumable items available for purchase. Many hospitals have their own shop run by the WRVS or other volunteer service which probably sells food and beverages. This may provide a good opportunity to introduce a change in the variety and type of products available.

3 Advising schools for children with moderate or severe learning difficulties. Many of these children have special dietetic needs (see below). The home economics teacher can be enlisted ot help and informal 'round the table' discussions with health, education and school catering service personnel can be very beneficial.

3.11.3 Possible nutritional problems of the mentally handicapped

Mental handicap does not in itself pose nutritional problems in the majority of residents. Most are physically normal and likely to suffer the same ailments as non-handicapped people, e.g. diabetes or hypertension. When mental handicap is coupled with institutional life, physical handicap, behaviour disturbances, some syndromes or certain medication, problems can arise. These may include

1 Undernutrition. This may result from bizarre eating habits or a poor feeding ability. Investigation of vitamin status may be a useful way of providing evidence of undernutrition.

2 Obesity. This is a widespread problem and not aided by the use of sweets/chocolates as rewards, or sugar being added to drinks as a routine. It is often difficult to motivate the resident to lose weight. Help can be sought from psychologists who may be able to introduce behaviour modification programmes.

3 Feeding and swallowing problems. These can present nutritional hazards and liaison with a speech therapist may be helpful.

4 Down's syndrome. Parents of children with Down's syndrome need advice as early as possible so that sensible eating patterns are developed from the beginning. There have been many studies investigating the vitamin requirements of these children (Harrell *et al* 1981) but the findings have not been consistent (Smith *et al* 1984). Current research may resolve the situation. The leaflet *'Healthy eating for your child'* produced by the Down's Children Association in conjunction with the Paediatric Group of the British Dietetic Association gives very useful advice. Local branches of the Down's Children Association can often assist in disseminating information to their members.

5 Hyperactivity. The possible involvement of diet in this syndrome is a topical subject. Dietetic advice may be requested but should only be given when baseline studies of behaviour have been made so that the effect of any dietary modifications can be evaluated. Dietitians should ensure that patients receive adequate nutrition throughout any dietary exclusion trial (see also Section 5.9).

A high energy intake is sometimes prescribed for the hyperactive or behaviourally disturbed. Supplements, extra snacks or larger portions may need to be programmed into what is sometimes a rather rigid catering system. There are occasional problems with induced vomiting, rumination and regurgitation; these need to be treated on an individual basis.

3.11.4 Communicating with the mentally handicapped

The art of communication is the main skill needed with the mentally handicapped. Motivation and enthusiasm are also required, together with the ability to work with and through colleagues of several disciplines.

It would be wrong to assume that the mentally handicapped have the same concepts as ourselves. They may not necessarily understand a picture and are often unable to conceive the idea of size or weight. They do not necessarily read from left to right or from top to bottom. Some may not be able to read at all and others have little or no speech.

As far as food is concerned, obvious links between food items may not be at all obvious to those with a mental handicap. Chips and mashed potatoes, for example, may be regarded as totally unconnected items because they may never have seen the original potato as purchased and watched its alteration by different methods of cooking. Similarly, an omelette may not be connected with a poached egg; some residents will not have seen an egg broken out of its shell.

In order to convey concepts and ideas about food, *non-verbal communication* may be appropriate. Several systems have been evolved over the years. 80% of schools for learning difficulties in Britain use the British Sign Language and the majority use it in conjunction with the *Makaton vocabulary* which uses signs to teach words. This vocabulary is used in the mental handicap unit of many Health Authorities and can be used alone or in conjunction with speech, depending on the individual needs. It has been useful in some situations for dietitians to learn this means of communication. *Bliss symbols* use nine shapes to form the basis of all symbols, so combinations can be built into a complete language. *Makaton symbols* have been introduced recently. There are many other means of communication — suitable programmes are being developed for use on a computer, and videos are used extensively. (Further information is available in the British Dietetic Association's Mental Health Group information Booklet No 1).

3.11.5 Developments in the care of the mentally handicapped

Child assessment units

In most Health Authorities these units are being set up for children with a handicap (mental or physical) to ensure that all facilities and agencies are made available for the individual.

Hopefully, paediatric dietitians will make regular visits to these units and, provided that good liaison with the staff is achieved, many potential problems can be prevented if identified early.

The National Development Team for mentally handicapped people

This team responds to invitations to visit individual units and is responsible directly to the Secretary of State for Health. It is independent of the DHSS but the latter provides support and resources. The team has two main functions
1 To advise individual health and social services authorities and voluntary bodies on the development and operation of their mental handicap services within the overall resources available to them.
2 To inform the DHSS about the provision of mental handicap services within the Health and Personal Social Services. As from 1985, the team's reports have been published and are a valuable source of information.

The British Dietetic Association's Mental Health Group (MHG)

As a response to the inadequacies of current training for dietitians in this field, the First Post-Registration Course in Mental Health was held in February 1986.

The MHG has also produced an information booklet on working with the mentally handicapped. This includes sections on the mental handicap unit, training, practical information, organisation, non-verbal communication methods, menus, dietary treatment and commonly used drugs.

Health Education Projects

These are being developed for mentally handicapped children and adults in the hospitals and the community (e.g. the Forth Valley Health Board project). The Open University is also preparing a short course on mental handicap in collaboration with The Royal Society for Mentally Handicapped Children and Adults (MENCAP). (Course P555 Mental Handicap: Pattern for Living, November 1986.) The Spastics Society runs courses at Castle Priory College for adults with profound handicaps.

Improved care of the mentally handicapped including, where possible, their integration into the community, is a current priority of the Health Service. As a result, there are many new opportunities for implementing dietetic skills and for making a real impact on nutritional health of mentally handicapped people via research, therapeutic dietetics, ensuring adequate nutrition, communication, and the provision of visual aids. It is thus a particularly stimulating and challenging time for a dietitian to become involved in this field. It is also very satisfying to help individuals cope with the transition from institutional life to living in the community.

Patient support organisations

1 The Royal Society for Mentally Handicapped Children and Adults (MENCAP), 123 Golden Lane, London EC1Y ORT.
2 Down's Syndrome Association, 12/13 Clapham Common Southside, London SW4 7AA.
3 The Hyperactive Children's Support Group (HACSG). S Bunday, 59 Meadowside, Angmering, Littlehampton, West Sussex BN16 4BW.
4 The National Autistic Society (NAS), 276 Willesden Lane, London NW2 5RB.
5 The Spastics Society, 12 Park Crescent, London W1N 4EQ.
6 Association for Spina Bifida and Hydrocephalus, Tavistock House North, Tavistock Square, London WC1H 9HJ.

Other useful addresses

1 British Dietetic Association — Mental Health Group, Daimler House, Paradise Circus, Queensway, Birmingham B1 2BJ.
2 British Institute of Mental Handicap (BIMH) Current Awareness Services, Wolverhampton Road, Kidderminster, Worcs DY10 3PP.
3 Castle Priory College, Thames Street, Wallingford, Oxfordshire OX10 0HE. (Courses run by The Spastics Society)

4 The Open University, PO Box 188, Milton Keynes MK7 6DH.
   Visual Aids *You see you can cook* — first edition from: Seargeant Brothers Ltd, Unit 9, Pontyfelin Road Industrial Estate, New Inn, Pontypool, Gwent, NP4 0DQ. Second edition available from: Martin Robinson, Assistant Administrator, Brentry Hospital, Charlton Lane, Brentry, Bristol.

Further reading

Anderson CA *A guide to assessment and intervention with handicapped children.* Jordonhill College of Education.
British Dietetic Association *Working with the mentally handicapped.* BDA Mental Health Group Information Booklet No 1. Available from the secretary of the Mental Health Group, c/o BDA.
Clarke D *Mentally handicapped people: living and learning.* Balliere Tindall, Eastbourne.
Craft M, Bicknell J and Holling S *A multidisciplinary approach — mental handicap.* Balliere Tindall, Eastbourne.
Nurse Training Syllabus — Registered Nurse Mental Handicap.
Simon GB (Ed) *The community team, the community unit and the role and function of the community nurse, social worker and some other members of the community health team.*
The Down's Children's Association *Healthy eating for your child.*
Warren J *Helping the handicapped child with early feeding.* Winslow Press,

References

DHSS (1971) *Better services for the mentally handicapped* (Reprinted 1979). HMSO, London.
Harrell RF, Capp RH, Davis DR, Peerless J and Ravitz LR (1981) Can nutritional supplements help mentally retarded children? An explanatory study. *Proc Nat Acad Sci* **78**, 574–8.
Smith GF, Spiker D et al (1984) Use of megadoses of vitamins with minerals in Down's Syndrome. *J Pediatr* **105**, 228.

3.12 The Physically Disabled

The United Nations (1975) has defined 'disabled person' to mean any person unable to ensure by himself or herself, wholly or partly, the necessities of a normal individual and/or social life, as a result of a deficiency, either congenital or not, in his or her physical or mental capabilities. This section considers the physically disabled.

3.12.1 General considerations

The physically disabled can have many feeding difficulties. They may exhaust themselves from the effort of feeding, or even be unable to get food into the mouth. The limitations of income, shopping, mobility or motivation may militate against the preparation of a varied and interesting diet. Depression and/or the above problems can cause lack of appetite. There may be difficulties in masticating or swallowing. Badly positioned for eating, the disabled person can suffer discomfort from distension.

In institutions food may be given which is unattractive in appearance, cold or of unsuitable consistency. There may be a lack of feeding helpers, or helpers can be too fast or too slow, or the disabled person may not be given adequate time to complete a meal.

Feeding abilities can often be improved by attention to the above problems. Depression can be treated. Helpers can have a positive and realistic attitude. Small, frequent meals may be better for some with small capacity or distorted bodies. A conventional appetite stimulant such as a glass of sherry before a meal can also help. Attention to a good position for eating is important. Support for arms can be given by arms on chairs or by pillows. The right shape of chair for the patient is also important and for some, such as spastics, individually designed chairs may be necessary. Modified cutlery, non-slip cups and plates, and flexi-straws can all play their part. The use of a bain-marie plate can be useful for slow eaters to keep the food hot.

For the disabled at home, budgetary advice and help with obtaining benefits should be given. If necessary, patients can be referred to social workers or they, or their relatives, encouraged to seek advice from them or relevant voluntary organisations. Home helps or volunteers can assist with shopping and food preparation, or use can be made of luncheon clubs, day centres and meals-on-wheels. Kitchens and kitchen equipment can be adapted.

Within institutions, training of all staff and helpers, skilled and unskilled, regarding feeding and nutrition and the matters listed above is important. Attention should be paid to the quality of food and its presentation. The company, physical surroundings and atmosphere at meal times should be considered and improved if necessary. There should be sufficient helpers at meal times.

3.12.2 Possible nutritional problems of the physically handicapped

1 Undernutrition. The degree of undernutrition can be assessed by observation, talking with the patient and by blood chemistry. High energy supplements may be required. Patients may be undernourished when there are not enough feeding helpers (Bergstrom and Lundberg 1969; Comerford 1978).
2 Dehydration. This is often caused by a reluctance to drink, particularly if bladder problems are present, for example in cases of multiple sclerosis (MS).
3 Constipation. This can be caused by immobility, lack of fibre and/or fluids or changes in gut mobility with spinal injury and conditions such as MS.
4 Anorexia. This can result from depression, uninteresting food, boredom, bedsores or the inability to take exercise. Anorexia may also be secondary to constipation.
5 Over dependence on laxatives, which can result in nutrient deficiency.
6 Excess weight, which may result from compensatory over-eating and from badly balanced diets.
7 Vitamin C deficiency is a high risk due to the use of soft, processed foods and the avoidance of fresh fruit.

3.12.3 Problems and treatment of specific physical disabilities

Rheumatoid arthritis

Rheumatoid arthritis is the most common type of inflammatory arthritis. The role of diet in its treatment is discussed in Section 4.28.1.

Osteo-arthritis

Osteo-arthritis is a disease in which erosion of the joint cartilage is accompanied by the production of new bone, and is a major cause of disability in the elderly (see Section 4.28.2).

Ankylosing spondylitis

This is a rheumatic disease affecting the spine and sacroiliac joints. In severe cases the spine becomes completely rigid, through fusion of its joints, and the back becomes hunched.

Spinal injuries

These are caused by injuries to the spinal column or by disease which damages the spinal cord. There may be *paraplegia*, no feeling or movement of the legs or *tetraplegia* (quadriplegia), no feeling or movement below the neck or limited sensory and motor functions of arms and hands but none in the legs. Patients are initially treated by immobilization, being nursed flat, sometimes under traction until vertebrae and ligaments have healed. There is passive (and, if possible, active) physiotherapy of limbs. This is followed by an intensive programme of rehabilitation including bladder and bowel training for control, prevention of pressure sores and mobilization.

Dietary problems

These are likely to arise as a result of a number of factors.

The metabolic response to trauma. As with other types of accidental trauma, there will be a metabolic response to the injury (see Section 5.1). This is likely to result in rapid and significant weight loss (Kleinman 1953; Daignault-Gelinas and Roy 1984; Kaufman *et al* 1985) and compounded by emotional factors affecting appetite. Paralytic ileus may occur for about a week after the injury and normal bowel function may be lost permanently. Stress ulcers may also develop following the injury.

Physical difficulties in eating. Eating and drinking whilst lying flat and under traction is awkward. The consistency of the food must be such that it is easy for the staff to administer; very sloppy food tends to get spilt on the patient.

Paralysis of the intercostal muscles increases the dependence on the diaphragm for breathing. Abdominal distension from large meals, constipation or flatulence can cause respiratory distress and should be avoided.

Emotional problems. Patients need to mourn the loss of use of limbs (Lambert 1985) and sometimes the death of relatives or others in the same accident. They need to adjust to a new lifestyle and often a change of role within the family. This can have a profound effect on the attitude to food, often contributing to significant weight loss.

Pressure sores. Spinal injury patients are particularly susceptible to pressure sores. These are caused by the loss of sensation of pressure and concomitant ischaemia of the skin; patients' inability to change position; changes in the flow of blood to the skin caused by the spinal injury; and impaired nervous control of the bladder, leading to urinary incontinence. Obesity may also aggravate these problems (Pierce and Nickel 1977). Pressure sores may need prolonged expensive hospitalization to heal and are a serious threat to life. Treatment includes a high energy, high protein diet. If bedsores are present, obesity should not be treated until they are well healed.

Renal and bladder stones. Spinal injury patients are particularly susceptible to renal and bladder stones (see Section 4.17). The chief factor causing their formation is the rise in urinary pH caused by infection (Smith *et al* 1969). Impaired nervous control of the bladder leads to incomplete emptying, and the risk of infection. The use of catheters also encourages infection.

Immobilization also tends to cause resorptive hypercalciuria as does the catabolic response to trauma (Kleinman 1953). The relationship between the calcium intake, in particular milk intake, of spinal patients and stone formation needs clarification. Patients with resorptive hypercalciuria have a raised 24-hour urine calcium *at all intakes of dietary calcium* (Howard *et al* 1945; Peacock and Roberston 1979). However, there seems to be no published work relating specifically to spinal injury patients, investigating the relationship between calcium intake and stone formation. It is possible that the very high calcium intakes achieved when spinal injury patients are given milk-based high protein, high energy supplements may be significant when the combination of infection and resorptive hypercalciuria is present.

Renal failure. This can occur secondary to stones and/or recurrent urinary tract infections (see Section 4.16).

Nutritional assessment of spinal injury patients

Ideal weight. Normal ideal body weight tables are not applicable to spinal patients because of the disuse and consequent atrophy of muscles. Recommended weight guidelines have been established for spinal patients (Peiffer *et al* 1981). These are
1 For paraplegia 4.5–6.5 kg below normal ideal weight.
2 For quadriplegia 6.5–9.0 kg below normal ideal weight.

Energy requirements. These can be calculated using the modified Harrison-Benedict Equation (Lagger 1983). (see Section 1.11.)

Serum albumin. Spinal patients have a high elimination rate of serum albumin (Ring *et al* 1974). It therefore seems reasonable to expect healthy spinal patients to have a slightly lower serum albumin concentration than the general population (Peiffer *et al* 1981).

Stroke

See Section 4.22.

Spastics — cerebral palsy

This is a developmental abnormality of the brain resulting in weakness and inco-ordination of movement affecting posture, head control and use of limbs, tongue and lips.

Correct feeding techniques must be taught and encouraged from an early age. Different techniques and flavours should be continually introduced. Improvement in the use of the tongue, lips and teeth can be made by exercises, e.g. licking a lollipop, blowing bubbles or sucking through a polythene straw.

Multiple sclerosis

See Section 4.25. Food preparation and shopping present particular problems because of the nature of the disabilities caused by multiple sclerosis.

Epilepsy

See Section 4.23. Some anti-epileptic drugs may cause nausea and consequent loss of appetite.

The visually handicapped

In the UK the common causes of visual handicap are cataracts, glaucoma, trauma and diabetic retinopathy. Diabetic retinopathy is the commonest cause of blindness in people of working age (Sorsby 1972). A survey (Cullinan 1977) suggests that, in the UK, 2 people per 1000 are registered as blind and a further 1 per 1000 is registered as partially sighted. A further 3 per 1000 have difficulty reading. Seventy five percent of the visually handicapped are over retirement age.

The particular problems of dietary significance for the visually handicapped are the preparation of food and their inability to use normal educational material about diet and nutrition. Obviously their needs must be met by material produced specifically for them.

Preparation of food

Details of special equipment available can be obtained from occupational therapists or technical officers for the blind employed by local social services departments or voluntary organisations.

Communication

Talking to a blind person
1 Before you start, gain the blind person's attention by using his/her name and by touching the person on the shoulder. Say who you are.
2 Before you leave, make sure the blind person knows you are going.
3 Do not shout.

Reference material for the blind

Cookery books. On cassette
1 Davies L (1972) *Easy cooking for one or two.* Ada Reading Services, Salisbury. Also in Magna Large Print Books, Skipton.
   In braille
1 Sainsbury's Food Guides No 1 *Food for One,* and No 8 *Cooking made easy for disabled people.* Available from the RN1B.
2 Elliot R (1976) *Not just a load of old lentils.* Available from the RNIB.

3 HM Prison — Wakefield *Whole meals in minutes* and *High fibre diet sheets — 100 quick and easy recipes.*

The RNIB list '*A feeling for food: cookery books for visually handicapped people*' gives details of books in Braille, in Moon, on tape and in large print (details from the RNIB Customer Liaison Officer).

Diet and nutrition information

On cassette

1 Matthews W and Wells D (1982) *A second book of nutrition* 4e.

2 Ministry of Agriculture, Fisheries and Food (1976) *Manual of nutrition* 8e. HMSO, London.

In Braille

1 British Heart Foundation (1976) *Cooking for your heart's content.* Dyson K (Ed)

2 Flora Project for Heart Disease Prevention *Eating for a Healthy Heart*

3 Matthews W and Wells D (1967) *A first book of nutrition* 3e.

The Students Tape Library, Students Braille Library and the National Library for the Blind have a good selection of both cookery and diet and nutrition information.

Weight reduction

In Braille

1 Sandwell Area Health Authority *weight reducing diet — 1000 calories: hints on cutting down calories.* Available from the RNIB.

2 Slimming Magazine (1983) *The flexible 1000 calorie diet.* (from Slimming Magazine).

3 Which? Magazine *Which? way to slim.* Available from the RNIB.

Diabetes

Food values list for diabetics and Balance magazine are both available on cassette from the British Diabetic Association. The following BDA leaflets available in Braille:

Diet and Health (1983) DH210, *Diet during illness* (1983) DH217, *Food values — list for diabetics* (1983) DH223 and *Hypoglycaemia and diet* (1983) DH211.

These leaflets can be obtained from the RNIB. A Braille pamphlet *Living with diabetes — a guide for insulin dependent diabetics* is also available.

Other sources of information

Student Tape Library

1 British Diabetic Association, *Simple diabetic cookery.*

2 Metcalfe J (1983) *Cooking the new diabetic way.*

Hypoguard produce *Understanding diabetes* — an hour long cassette with Dr Arnold Bloom and Helen Desmond SRD.

Eastbourne Health Authority produce *Sugar-free diet for mild diabetics* (large print).

Various other aids, such as pre-set syringes, are available. Diabetic consultants and specialist diabetic nurses will have information.

Transcribing your own material for the visually handicapped

Relative merits of Braille, Moon and tapes. Only some of the visually handicapped learn Braille. People who lose their sight in later years find it particularly hard to learn. Many elderly learn 'Moon' which consists of simplified Roman letters.

Tapes are easy to carry and store and can also be understood by sighted helpers. They tend to be used mainly by the young because some of the elderly are discouraged by the technicalities of using them. Tapes can distract others whereas Moon and Braille can be read silently.

Organisations which will transcribe material. Transcription services are offered by the RNIB, HM Prison Wakefield and The Braille Unit, Aylesbury Youth Custody Centre.

Producing your own large print material. The size of the print is not the only criterion on which the readability depends (Gardiner 1979). Other criteria include

1 Contrast. Black on a white background with high density print is best. Photocopied material is often hard to read.

2 Spacing. Letters should be spaced so that the area between them is similar; the width of an 'o' should be left between words; and at least half the height of a letter should be left between lines (Russell 1984).

3 Case. Words produced in lower case can be recognized by their shape more readily than those in upper case.

4 Style of print. There needs to be sufficient contrasting background within the letters.

An enlargement service in offered by the Partially Sighted Society who, for a small charge will enlarge material (subject to copyright).

Communicating with those who are deaf or hard of hearing

Listening through a hearing aid is rather like listening over a very bad telephone line. Sounds are distorted and there may be a lot of background noise. People with a hearing aid often lip-read as well. This requires a great deal of concentration.

When interviewing someone who is deaf or hard of hearing use the following techniques to help the person understand you

1 Speak clearly and slowly and raise your voice slightly. Never shout. Do not over-exaggerate lip movements.
2 Try to ensure privacy and absence of distracting voices and sounds.
3 Face the deaf person directly. Make sure your face is well lit.
4 Do not hide your mouth with your hand or anything else.
5 Use gestures to make your meaning clear.
6 Do not expect a deaf person to listen to you and look at a diet sheet or other paper at the same time.

Sources of help and support organisations

1 Speech and occupational therapists.
2 Appropriate societies for specific problems, e.g. The Chest, Heart and Stroke Association for stroke patients and Action for Research with Multiple Sclerosis for multiple sclerosis patients. *With a little help* by Phillipa Harpin lists appropriate societies for the handicapped as well as the addresses of manufacturers of various aids (and is available from the Muscular Dystrophy Society, Natrass House, 35 Macauley Road, London SW4 0QP). Details about the societies should also be held in the reference section of Public Libraries.
3 Disabled Living Foundation, 380–384 Harrow Road, London W9.
4 *Disability rights handbook* from 25 Mortimer Street, London W1N 8AB.
5 Boots the Chemists have a large selection of eating and cooking aids for the disabled. They produce a catalogue giving full details and cost of the items.
6 Some branches of the Red Cross and St John's Ambulance Brigade have eating and cooking aids available for hire.

Useful addresses

1 Royal National Institute for the Blind (RNIB), (Also Student Braille and Student Tape Libraries), 338 Gowell Road, London EC1V 7JE. Tel: 01 834 9921. (RNIB main headquarters are at 224 Great Portland Street, London W1N 6AA, Tel: 01 388 1266)
2 Magna Large Print Books, Magna House, Long Preston, nr Skipton, N Yorks BD23 4ND. Tel: 072 94 225.
3 Ada Reading Services, Mrs Artus, 6 Daleword Rise, Laverstock, Salisbury, Wiltshire SP1 1SF. Tel: 0722 26987.
4 HM Prison Wakefield (Braille Unit), 5 Live Lane, Wakefield WF2 9AG. Tel: 0924 378282.
5 Hypoguard Ltd, Dock Lane, Melton, Woodbridge, Suffolk IP12 1PE.

6 Department of Nutrition and Dietetics, Eastbourne Health Authority, Avenue House, Eastbourne, East Sussex BN21 3XY.
7 The Braille Unit, Aylesbury Youth Custody Centre, HM Prison, Brerton Road, Aylesbury, Bucks.
8 The Partially Sighted Society, 40 Wordsworth Street, Hove, Sussex BN3 5BH.

Further reading

General

Blackley Last J and Miller G *Feeding techniques with cerebral palsy children*
Devlin R (1985) *Coping in the kitchen. Nursing Times* (Community). March issue.
Home management 5e. Equipment for the Disabled. Nuffield Orthopaedic Centre, Headington, Oxford OX3 7LD.
Ryan M *Feeding can be fun.* Spastics Society

Arthritis

Community Nutrition Group of the British Dietetic Association (1986) *Diet and arthritis*. CNG Nutrition Group Information. Sheet
Swinson DR and Swinburn WR (1980) *Rheumatology.* Unibooks,

Spinal injuries

Burke DC and Murray DD *Handbook of spinal cord medicine.* Macmillan Press, London.

The visually handicapped

Ford Mand Hesher T *In touch — aids and services for blind and partially sighted people* 3e. BBC Publications, London.
Hocken S *Emma and I.* Sphere Books Ltd, London.

References

Bergstrom S and Lundberg A (1969) Dietary intake in physically disabled students. *Nutritio et Dieta* (Basel) **11**, 173–83.
Comerford P (1978) Dietary intake and nutritional problems of the disabled — Unpublished.
Cullinan T (1977) *Health Services Research Unit Report* No 28 University of Kent, Canterbury.
Daignault-Gelinas M and Roy H (1984) Nutritional assessment in spinal cord injury patients. In *Abstracts, Dietetics in the global village.* IX International Congress of Dietetics. Toronto, Canada.
Gardiner PA (1979) *ABC of Ophthalmology.* BMA Publications, London.
Howard JE, Parson W and Bigham RS (1945) Studies on patients convalescent from fracture, III: The urinary excretion of calcium and phosphorus. *Bull Johns Hopkins Hosp* **77**, 291.
Kaufman HH, Rowlands BJ, Stein DK, Kopaniky DR and Gildenberg PL (1985) General metabolism in patients with acute paraplegia and quadriplegia. *Neurosurgery* **16**, 309–13.
Kleinman AM (1953) Problem of nutrition. In *Injuries of the spinal cord* Prather and Mayfield (Eds) Chapter IV. Blackwell Scientific Publications, Oxford.
Lagger L (1983) Spinal cord injury: Nutritional management. *J Neurosurg Nurs* **15**, 310–2.

Lambert J (1985) Adjusting to tetraplegia. *Nursing Times* **81**, 32−3.

Peacock M and Robertson WG (1979) The biochemical aetiology of renal lithiasis. In *Urinary calculous disease* Wickham JEA (Ed) pp 69−95. Churchill Livingstone, Edinburgh.

Peiffer SC, Blust P and Leyson JFJ (1981) Nutritional assessment of the spinal cord injured patient. *J Am Diet Assoc* **78**, 501−5.

Pierce DS and Nickel VH (1977) *The total care of spinal cord injuries*. Little Brown and Company, Boston.

Ring J, Seifert J, Lob G, Stephan W, Probst J and Brendel W (1974) Elimination rate of human serum albumin in paraplegic patients. *Paraplegia* **12**, 139.

Russell GJ (1984) *Teaching in further education*

Smith PH, Cook JB and Robertson WG (1969) Stone formation in paraplegia. *Paraplegia* **7**, 77.

Sorsby A (1972) The incidence and causes of blindness in England and Wales 1963−1968. *HMSO Reports of Public Health Medical Subjects* No 28 pp 33−51. HMSO, London.

United Nations (1975) Declaration of the rights of disabled persons. Annex IV. *General Assembly Resolution* 3447 (XXX)

3.13   Institutional Feeding

The first two sections in this chapter generally apply to the hospital environment as this is the familiar situation for most dietitians. However, many of the points are also relevant to other institutions. School meals are specifically discussed in Section 3.4.2.

3.13.1   Meeting the nutritional needs of mixed groups

Role of the caterer

The caterer should

1   Ensure that there is an adequate choice on the menu to cover the majority of people. A common core of familiar foods should form the basis of menu planning. Regional dishes can be included.

2   Be aware of the nutritional requirements of the group being catered for (see Recommended Daily Allowances, section 1.2). He should be able to distinguish, for example, between the requirements of those in the maternity unit, the long stay geriatric ward and the children's ward. In particular, portion control at kitchen or serving level should be appropriate for that particular group.

3   Be aware of current nutritional views regarding healthy eating and apply those appropriately to the groups being catered for. For example, at present this might include implementing NACNE recommendations or fulfilling a role within a district food policy.

4   Consider if special provisions are necessary for particular groups. For example

a)   Some patients may require food outside normal meal times (e.g. new admissions or those who have missed meals due to investigations).

b)   The children's ward will often eat at different times and have a different menu to the rest of the hospital.

c)   The pregnant woman in hospital may need a snack available other than at set mealtimes.

d)   Ethnic groups may form part of the local population and will need to be considered when menus are planned.

e)   If no choice of vegetarian dish is possible on the basic menu, there should be the facility to provide a vegetarian dish on request.

5   Revise menus regularly. This is particularly important in long stay hospitals to avoid menu fatigue.

Popularity of dishes may be assessed by uptake over a period of time. The caterer should look for feedback by making ward visits to hear patients' views, and attending unit meetings with nursing staff. A questionnaire to a sample of patients may answer any specific issues.

Role of the dietitian

The dietitian
1   Should liaise with the caterer in menu planning.
2   Can help the caterer to be aware of the nutritional requirements of specific groups. The dietitian can also provide information and assist in staff training.
3   Can assess if the menu is varied enough to fulfil the requirements of the majority of patients.
4   Should be responsive to the needs of particular wards and inform the catering department of any further requirements. For example, extra milk may be required for wards (such as geriatric or ear, nose and throat (ENT)) making their own milky supplements, or extra fibre in the form of bran may be needed on geriatric or maternity wards.
5   Should ensure that basic therapeutic diets can be supplied from the main hospital menu wherever possible.

Role of the nursing staff

The nursing staff should
1   Help the patient make a suitable choice of foods from the dishes available, either by filling in a menu card with them or choosing the appropriate foods.
2   Be aware of the appetite of their patients and select the appropriate meal portions. This can be done either by selecting an appropriate portion size on a menu card or by serving the appropriate amount of food to the patient.
3   Monitor the patient's food intake, so that any individual difficulties with food are spotted and any necessary supplements to, or modifications of, the diet can be made.
4   Inform the kitchen of any requirements not covered by the normal menu, e.g. kosher or milk-free diets, so that a suitable diet can be provided.

3.13.2 Achieving the balance between nutritional desirability and food preferences

1 There should be adequate choice or variety on the menu. In order to be acceptable to the majority of people, this may mean providing foods other than those considered nutritionally desirable.

2 The patient should be given information on how to choose a healthy diet. This can be incorporated into the hospital admissions booklet, or be available on the ward as a separate leaflet. Printed menus can either be coded to indicate food suitability or advice can be printed on the back of the menu.

3 A healthier diet can be provided by ingredient manipulation of popular dishes. For example

a) The use of skimmed or semi-skimmed milk in sauces and puddings.

b) The use of a proportion of wholemeal flour in baking.

c) Reducing the amount of sugar in cakes and puddings or, if appropriate, using an artificial sweetener.

d) Adding less salt to recipes which already contain stock cubes and convenience mixes.

e) Replacing part of the meat in a recipe with pulse vegetables.

f) Where possible, using wholegrain rice and pasta in place of the refined equivalents.

4 It is possible to manipulate food choice to some extent by the positioning of foods on the menu — there is a tendency to favour the first item in a selection. Thus, selection of wholemeal bread can be increased by putting it before white bread on the menu.

5 Artificial sweeteners, low calorie drinks and low fat milks may be provided on the wards as an alternative to sugar, sugar-containing drinks and full fat milks.

6 The patient's opinion of the menu choice (and the food provided) should be sought, particularly where menus are being modified in line with current nutritional guidelines.

7 The caterer and the dietitian should co-operate in selecting nutritious and acceptable convenience foods. For example

a) Fish canned in brine, not oil.

b) Fruit tinned in fruit juice or water, not syrup.

c) Sausages with a lower fat content.

In the future, caterers may ask manufacturers to fulfil nutritional specifications before tendering their products for contract.

8 It should be recognized that diet is also part of the medical treatment. Some patients may need a high fat and sugar intake to achieve the required energy intake.

9 Regional preferences should be taken into account.

Some may be healthy options, e.g. tripe, porridge, oatcakes; others, such as adding salt to porridge, may not.

10 Hospital shops, trolleys and vending machines should be encouraged to offer more nutritionally desirable items, e.g. sugar-free drinks, low fat milk for drinks and low salt soups.

3.13.3 Particular problems of catering in hospitals

Administration and catering problems

Budget limits

The catering manager must always work within his budget. In menu planning, he has to compromise between cost, nutritional value and popularity. He may also have to consider special diets when planning the main menu, particularly light and soft diets. The average stay in a District General Hospital is ten days but patients may stay much longer, or permanently, in other hospitals.

Solution — the catering manager can offset a more expensive popular dish at one meal against a cheaper popular dish at another. Alternatively, a cheap popular dish may be offered against a more expensive, but less popular item. Putting cheap unpopular dishes on the menu achieves nothing!

Unsuitable kitchens

Kitchens may be out of date or have outgrown the purpose for which they were originally designed. Equipment may be inadequate or no longer appropriate.

Solution — is there any money available for new development? If not, could the kitchens be rearranged and existing equipment re-sited to give a better working arrangement? Menu planning should allow for these problems.

Inappropriate catering-sized packs

Certain products may not be available in the appropriate size. For example, a low calorie spread may not be available on the menu where an individual tray system operates. On the other hand, fruits tinned in natural juices are not usually available in anything larger than an A4 tin which is unsuitable for bulk use.

Solution — if there were sufficient interest among catering managers, and a big enough market, manufacturers might be willing to produce the product in the appropriate size.

Nutritional problems

Undesirable cooking practices

Cooking practices may reduce the nutritional quality of the food. Food may be prepared too far in advance with resultant nutrient losses. For example, vegetables may be cooked and then kept warm for some hours before being served, or cauliflower for a cauliflower cheese may be prepared 24 hours in advance; these practices will result in loss of vitamin C. Meats may be roasted and sliced in advance and then reheated in gravy, causing loss of B vitamins. In addition to the loss in nutritional value, overcooking and/or reheating food tends to make it flavourless and less appetising.

There may also be conflict between established catering practices and good nutrition as illustrated by the use of large quantities of butter on cooked vegetables, on 'grilled' fish and in jacket potatoes; the decorative use of cream on desserts; traditional methods of making sauces or the preliminary preparation of meats and vegetables by frying.

Solution — kitchen staff should be encouraged to observe good cooking practices by in-service training where necessary, and discussion at unit meetings. Preparation ahead of time may be cut down by co-operation between the manager and kitchen staff over menu and work planning. The use of steamers for batch cooking can help to reduce overcooking and ensure that vegetables are not kept warm for long periods of time. Staff and managers could look at ways of amending catering practices to arrive at a more nutritionally sound product without reducing its acceptability. Some changes in practice may lead to financial savings.

Over-use of convenience foods

The use of more convenience foods to reduce labour costs may not always be nutritionally desirable as it may include the use of packet soups and stock powders with a high sodium content or the use of dessert mixes with a high sugar and fat content. A possible solution to this problem is illustrated in Fig. 3.1.

Remember that the Health Service has spending power and in the future may make nutritional specifications with which a manufacturer must comply before tendering for contract.

Nutritional needs of particular groups of patients not being met

Certain groups of patients may have particular nutritional problems of which the catering manager must

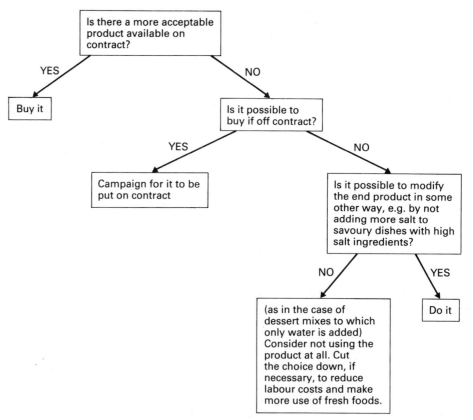

Fig. 3.1 A possible solution to the over-use of convenience foods in hospital catering

NUTRITIONAL NEEDS OF POPULATION SUB-GROUPS

be aware. Post-operative, and other groups of patients, may have high energy and nutrient requirements. Geriatric patients may not choose sufficient vitamin C-containing foods. Other patients may be constipated due to lack of fibre in the diet. Long stay patients lacking exposure to sunlight may not receive adequate vitamin D.

Solution — the catering manager should have good communication with the nursing staff, dietitians and patients so that he is aware himself, or through his staff, of the needs of particular groups of patients. Inadequate vitamin C intake could be compensated for by providing natural or vitamin C-enriched fruit juices and cordials. Extra fibre from wholemeal flour, bread and cereals could help to relieve constipation and save money on laxatives. Long stay patients should be encouraged to take vitamin D-enriched foods such as cornflakes, evaporated milk or Ovaltine.

No dietitian within the hospital

The catering manager, in the absence of a dietitian, may have to be aware of the specific nutritional requirements of some patients. He may be required to supply a special diet, differing from the standard menu, and also supply special dietetic foods.

Solution — ask for dietetic advice. This should be available within the district. Ask for basic up-to-date information on common therapeutic diets as a source of reference.

Environmental problems

Meals not able to be chosen in advance

Ideally a patient should be able to choose one meal in advance, e.g. at breakfast time, he chooses his lunch. However, this is not always the case. Meals not chosen in advance may also pose problems for special diets where the work sheets need to be drawn up in advance for the cook. In some hospitals or wards the staff or relatives may be making menu choices for the patient for reasons of speed and convenience rather than because the patient is incapable of doing so.

Solution — look at the present system. Could it be improved by alterations of work practices? Take the opportunity in lecturing and in-service training to stress the importance of the patient making his own choice.

Lack of choice in portion size

Although in theory, there may be a choice of portion size, this may not operate in practice. With a bulk trolley system, the nurse in charge will be able to exercise portion control at ward level. However, with a plated system, portion control may depend on the speed of service. Staff may be unable to distinguish between the smaller portions required for a female geriatric ward and the large portions required for young male orthopaedic patients.

Solution — ideally staff should be instructed on standard sizes available (e.g. small/standard, or small/medium/large, etc.) and the speed of service should be such that they can recognize the appropriate choice and respond accordingly. Ward staff should be encouraged not only to help the patient choose the appropriate food, but also to select the appropriate quantity.

Poor presentation of food

Presentation and delivery of food may not be ideal. Presentation of food is particularly important when the patient is anorexic. If food is not at the correct temperature, e.g. lukewarm soup, cold chips or melted ice cream, it will certainly not be enjoyed and probably not eaten.

Solution — the use of appropriate garnishes, good portion control and attractive arrangement of food on the plate all help to improve presentation and should be emphasised during in-service training. If trolleys and equipment are at the correct temperature, the portering service is delivering the food quickly and the nursing staff or ward orderlies are serving the meal promptly there should be no problem. It requires co-operation and co-ordination between the links in the chain.

3.13.4 Problems of catering in institutionalized homes (see also Section 3.6, p 287).

Administration and catering

Budget limits

The manager may be working to a limited budget with insufficient catering and nutritional knowledge to cope with the problems that arise.

Solution — provide training for the manager to acquire the necessary basic skills. Where appropriate, he should be aware of, and be able to call on, help either within the organisation or from the community dietitian, district catering adviser or other relevant bodies.

Purchasing difficulties

Private organisations may buy where they can find the best deal but government institutions may be restricted to buying from contract holders. Storage facilities may be insufficient to take advantage of discount on bulk orders. Convenience foods may not be available in a suitable pack size. There may be excessive use of convenience foods in an effort to reduce labour costs, although these products may not always be acceptable either nutritionally or to the consumer.

Solution — shop around for the best deal either with a wholesaler or retailer. Don't be afraid to go elsewhere for better quality or price. It may be convenient to buy locally and build up a relationship with your supplier but reassess the position regularly. Those having to buy on contract should ensure that food meets contract specifications or be prepared to send it back. Look at the feasibility of creating extra storage space or buying extra freezer capacity. In the private sector, it may be possible for a group of homes to work together as a co-operative and buy in bulk. Consider whether convenience foods are labour saving, or whether better work schedules and menu planning would be more effective. If possible, don't just buy a brand name, but look at the range of a particular convenience food available. Ask for tasting samples (perhaps involving the residents), compare the nutritional quality (or take advice on this) and consider the best value for money.

The 'system'

Kitchens may be outdated, badly planned with inadequate equipment. The staff may be poorly trained and resistant to change.

Solution — is it possible to plan the kitchen better by rearrangement of moveable equipment? Is there any money available to buy new equipment? If so, what are the priorities? What are the particular problems and restrictions of the existing equipment? Could these be taken into account or overcome when planning menus and work schedules? Involve the cooks in these discussions. Organise a basic programme of in-service training. Arrange for short talks by outside speakers, e.g. environmental health officers, dietitians or caterers. Encourage staff to communicate. Compile a standard procedure book including recipes, relevant information on kitchen practice, equipment, hygiene and safety.

'Menu fatigue'

Lack of variety on the menu and no change of menu will inevitably result in complaints from the residents.

Solution — Take time to plan a menu cycle. Fill in first the midday meal, then supper and breakfast and choose suitable puddings and vegetables last. Try to vary the menus with the seasons to take advantage of gluts of cheap fruit and vegetables. Incorporate local dishes, e.g. tripe and onions, into the menu and ask residents for suggestions or favourite recipes. Remember that for some people in long stay institutions, the home is the only source of food. A resident representative could be appointed to forward suggestions and grievances regarding catering. In some homes it may be possible to offer a choice and others may have another choice available for definite dislikes. Remember high days and holidays and treat them as special occasions.

Nutritional problems

Lack of awareness of the specific nutritional problems of the group being catered for

For example, insufficient or excess energy, lack of vitamin C, lack of vitamin D for the elderly, constipation and special diets.

Solution — observe the portion sizes served — does this vary with residents' requirements? Keep a regular check on residents' weight. Monitor the uptake and wastage of food. Pure fruit juice, vitamin-enriched squashes and freshly prepared raw vegetables and fruit salads should be available. Fresh fruit may need to be pre-peeled or chopped for handicapped residents. Elderly residents should be encouraged to sit or walk outside in reasonable weather to boost their vitamin D status. Vitamin D-rich foods, e.g. margarine, oily fish, malted milks and dried milks should be incorporated into the menu. High fibre foods (e.g. appropriate breakfast cereals, wholemeal bread) should be available.

Poor cooking practices

Solution — see p 326.

Unbalanced menus

Menus may not be in line with recent nutritional guidelines.

Solution — rectify over-reliance on fried foods and pastry or sweet foods. Use methods of cooking other than frying. Consider providing only cereals, bread and toast at breakfast time, so that eggs, bacon, sausages and mushrooms may be used in more supper dishes. Increase the fibre content of the diet by providing high fibre cereals, wholemeal bread and using wholemeal flour in bread and baked products. Pulses can be used to thicken soups and stews. Residents may respond to some simple nutrition education.

Unsatisfactory evening meals

These are often high in fat and sugar; in some homes, only cold food may be available due to staffing rotas.

Solution — it may be possible to employ staff for a short period in the evenings at residential homes, or to rearrange rotas so that more help is available for evening meals.

More imaginative menu choices may also help alleviate the problem. Nourishing soup, thickened with pulses, can be made and reheated to serve with sandwiches; cheese may be used in sauces, flans and pasta dishes. Jacket potatoes with a variety of fillings can be a tasty snack meal.

Environmental problems

The surroundings are not conducive to enjoying food

Solution — is the dining area clean? Is the service suitable for the type of resident? Is presentation attractive, including crockery and cutlery?

The dining area should have a cheery atmosphere — new curtains and table cloths can transform a room. 'Family service' (i.e. residents served at the table in groups of 4–6) may be most suitable for the very young and the elderly. Those with feeding difficulties, which may upset other residents, may benefit from sitting together. The same applies with slow eaters. Special feeding aids should be provided where ap-

propriate. Young adults may prefer a cafeteria-type system.

No facilities for self-catering

Some residents may miss the facility of being able to cook or make a cup of tea.

Solution — investigate the feasibility of having tea and coffee making facilities and the possibility of residents doing some of their own cooking/baking for therapy or interest.

Sources of help

1   Catering and Dietetic Branch, Department of Health and Social Security, Hannibal House, Elephant and Castle, London SE1.
2   Hospital Caterers Association, 43 Royston Road, Penge, London SE20 7QW.
3   The Gerontology Nutrition Unit, Royal Free Hospital School of Medicine, 21 Pond Street, London NW3 2PN.
4   Health Education Authority, 78 New Oxford Street, London WCA 1AH.
5   Centre for Policy on Ageing, Nuffield Lodge, Regent's Park, London NW1 4RS.
6   The local college/polytechnic may have a catering/institutional management department.

Further reading

Department of Health and Social Security guides: *Catering in community homes*, *Catering for patients in long stay hospitals*, *Nutrition and modified diets* and *Nutrition and modified diets* (teaching pack).
All available from Catering and Dietetic Branch at the above address.
DHSS (1979) *Recommended daily amounts of food energy and nutrients for groups of people in the United Kingdom.* Report on Health and Social Subjects No 15. HMSO, London.
Catering for a healthy diet. Conference Report 1985. The Coronary Prevention Group, 60 Great Ormond Street, London WC1N 3HR.

Section 4 **Therapeutic Dietetics for Disease States**
A: Metabolic and Endocrine Disorders

4.1 Obesity

4.1.1 Energy intake and expenditure

Obesity results from an excess of energy intake over expenditure. However, this simple statement, although correct, does not begin to reveal the complex nature of this condition, the many factors which contribute to its causation and the notorious difficulty in treating it successfully.

The requirement for energy varies enormously. Two people, similar in terms of age, sex and level of physical activity, can have widely different energy requirements, i.e. can maintain their body weight on very different energy intakes. Conversely, differences in energy requirement mean that, on the same energy intake, one person can become obese while another can remain lean. Thus, obese people do not necessarily eat more than those who are lean, but all obese people have at some time consumed more energy than their individual requirement.

Energy requirements

Measuring energy expenditure as a means of assessing the energy requirements of obese people is more reliable than assessing energy intake but less accessible to the dietitian. It involves measurements generally only utilized in specialist units such as direct calorimetry, which is the measurement of heat production using a whole body calorimeter, or indirect calorimetry which is the measurement of oxygen uptake and carbon dioxide production by means of a ventilated hood system.

The components of energy expenditure are

1 Basal metabolic rate (BMR) or resting metabolic rate (RMR).

.2 Energy expended above the resting metabolism due to physical activity, i.e. sitting, standing, walking, running, etc.

3 Energy expended above the resting metabolism due to heat production (thermogenesis), i.e. as a response to food intake, cold, drugs and psychological influences.

Figure 4.1 shows the contribution made by these three components to the 24-hour energy expenditure of normal weight subjects and the factors which affect them (Jéquier 1984).

Resting metabolic rate (RMR)

There has been extensive research into the metabolic causes of obesity. As the RMR contributes the greatest percentage to total energy expenditure, many workers have tried to establish whether there is a lower RMR in obese people. There is certainly a wide variation between individuals of average body weight. Absolute values of RMR have been found to be higher in the obese (James et al 1978; Halliday et al 1979; Ravussin et al 1982; Prentice et al 1986) and this is related to the increase in lean body mass (muscle mass) which accounts for some of the acquired weight gain. Garrow et al (1978) showed that under strictly controlled metabolic conditions there were large variations of weight loss between obese individuals on the same energy intake (1.6–9.8 kg lost on an 800 kcal/day (3.4 MJ) diet over a three week period). These differences could not be explained by 'cheating' on the diet. This study showed the best single predictor of weight loss to be the RMR of the individual. This lends some credibility to those patients who claim that friends or relatives are losing more weight than they are on the same reducing diet. There is a very wide individual variation in energy requirements.

Resting metabolic rate falls during periods of weight loss. This is due, in part, to the metabolic adaptation of the tissues to reduced energy intake as well as a decrease in lean body mass (Keys et al 1950). This fall in RMR obviously poses enormous problems to the obese patient whose weight loss will inevitably decrease with time on the same energy intake. With any degree of weight loss there needs to be a permanent reduction in energy intake to maintain the body weight at a lower level. This is the reason why most people find it so difficult and are unable to maintain weight loss in the long term.

Physical activity

This is not, as often supposed, just the 'sporting' type activities (which in fact only contribute a small percentage to total energy expenditure) but, instead, the everyday activities such as sitting, standing, talking, walking, i.e. any activity which involves the body

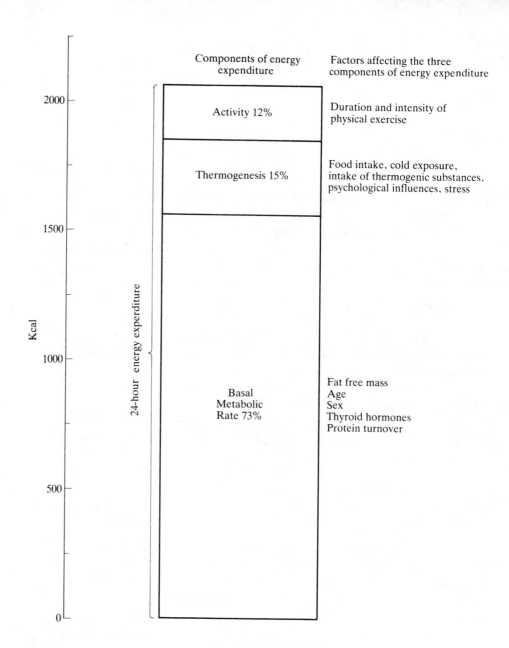

Fig. 4.1 Factors affecting the three components of energy expenditure.

moving from its resting position. The energy cost of performing these simple activities varies enormously between individuals. Warwick *et al* (1978) showed in subjects matched for age, weight, surface area and level of physical activity, who differed greatly in energy intake and expenditure, that the differences between them mainly lay in the different energy costs of performing the same tasks.

Thermogenesis

Thermogenesis is defined as the energy expenditure above RMR due to the effects of food intake, drugs, cold and psychological influences. The contribution of an impaired thermogenesis to the development of obesity remains controversial and further research is needed in man.

4.1.2 Obesity in adults

Identifying the problems

Classification of obesity

The Quetelet index or body mass index (BMI) is a useful way of classifying obesity

$$BMI = \frac{weight\ (kg)}{height^2\ (m)}$$

(measured in indoor clothing and without shoes).

Garrow (1981) proposes that grades of obesity be defined as follows

		BMI
1	Grade O	20–24.9
2	Grade I	25–29.9
3	Grade II	30–39.9
4	Grade III	>40

Grade O indicates a 'desirable' weight range and Grade III indicates severe obesity.

The equivalent of the 1983 Metropolitan Height and Weight tables in terms of BMI over the range from the minimum for 'small frame' to the maximum for 'large frame' is 21.0–26.0 for men and 19.7–26.0 for women.

The aim of any treatment regimen is initial weight loss and future weight maintenance. Active treatment should be geared towards those people in obesity Grades II and III as they are likely to have the most serious medical and psychological problems. It is recommended that Grade I obesity be treated if any of the following factors are present

1 Adult below 50 years of age.
2 Hypertension.
3 Hyperlipidaemia.
4 Diabetes.
5 Distribution of fat is central.

When calculating an obese patient's 'target weight', although Grade O represents 'desirable' or 'acceptable healthy' weight, it is worth considering the age of onset of obesity. Those patients whose obesity stems from childhood may have grown through the 'desirable' weight range during late childhood and early adolescence and only ever been at an obese weight since that time. Attempts at dieting may have resulted in weight loss only to have been followed by rapid weight gain. This presents a problem in that these patients have no concept of themselves at normal body weight and therefore have unrealistic expectations of such. Patients who becomes obese in adult years and have maintained a normal weight previously do, at least, have a mental picture of themselves and therefore more realistic expectations. Frequently these patients will carry photographs of themselves at their own 'target' weight. So, by taking a weight history, a realistic 'target' weight (or weight range) can be established which, although perhaps not in Grade O, can be seen to be achievable by the patient.

However, the BMI only indicates the degree of severity of the obesity, it does not reveal what the underlying problems are. There are many reasons why energy intake may have exceeded requirement (poor eating habits, behavioural and psychiatric problems, low energy requirements) and disentangling the relevant factors in each individual case are fundamental for ultimate success in achieving and maintaining weight reduction.

Obtaining background information

It is useful to try to include some of the following questions at the first appointment

1 Why does the patient want to lose weight? Is it for him/herself or because of pressure from other family members? Are there health reasons?
2 What is the patient's own target weight? Has it ever been achieved? Is the presenting weight the highest weight the patient has been? Is there a weight which the patient has maintained for any period of time?
3 What are the previous attempts at dieting? Why have previous diets failed? What is the maximum length or time the patient has been 'on a diet'? What is the maximum weight loss which has been achieved? Has any weight loss ever been maintained?
4 What rate of weight loss is the patient expecting or hoping for?
5 What are the patient's expectations of the anticipated weight loss?
6 Is the patient working? Is it full time/part time/shift work? Does the job involve travelling/living away from home?
7 What is the family structure? Are other members of the family overweight? Do the family eat regular meals together or is there a casual attitude towards food or meal times creating a more erratic pattern? Who does the shopping/cooking? Are the other family members interested in the patient losing weight?

Obtaining dietary information

Careful investigation into a person's usual eating habits will provide many valuable clues to the cause of the energy imbalance and hence give indications of how this may best be tackled. It is thus well worth the investment in time.

Methods of obtaining dietary information, and the problems associated with them, have been discussed in detail in Section 1.4. Points which are particularly relevant to the assessment of the intake of obese people are summarized below.

Dietary history/24-hour recall. Though a dietary history cannot be totally relied upon, careful and skilful questioning can provide a reasonable estimate of energy intake and a picture of eating habits in obese patients.

The simplest method of finding out what people have been eating is to ask them what food and beverages they have consumed over the past 24-hours. This relies upon the facts that

1 People will remember what they have eaten.
2 A 24-hour period is representative of their general energy intake.
3 They are willing to disclose what they eat.

It is the latter point which must, in particular, be watched when assessing the intake of obese people; most of them will be very sensitive about the amount and type of food they eat (even if there is no reason to feel guilt). In order to help distinguish between a genuinely low intake and a fabricated one, the 24-hour recall must be substantiated with information which acts as a cross-check (e.g. weekly food shopping, family meal patterns and meals eaten away from home). Questions relating to eating habits must be phrased in an open rather than a suggestive manner, for example 'Do you eat breakfast?' rather than 'what do you eat for breakfast?'.

Assessment of portion size must also be done with care. Some obese people may have a different concept of an 'average' portion compared with non-obese people. Food models are useful as they present the patient with a visual picture.

The dietitian must also enquire whether the patient's weight is static or changing (either decreasing or increasing) at the time of the interview since this is obviously relevant to the assessment of energy requirement.

Food diary. This involves patients in recording their own food and beverage consumption for a number of days. It has the advantage of not being dependent on memory and covering a longer time span than the 24-hour recall, but carries the risk of a reduced or unrepresentative food intake as a result of having to record everything consumed (Black *et al* 1985; Prentice *et al* 1986).

Obese patients should be given (rather than supplying their own) record sheets, ideally divided into columns for recording the quantity and type of item consumed since this gives a clearer idea of the sort of information required. Additional guidelines on how to measure food intake (by means of scales, household measures, packet or can size) should also be given. It must be emphasized that the record should be made *at the time* of consumption and not at the end of the day (or even several days!). At the end of the recording period, the patient's weight should be checked; sudden weight loss is strongly suggestive of dietary alteration.

It must be remembered that neither the dietary recall nor the food diary will provide a totally accurate measure of dietary intake. Both methods are subject to distortion and atypicality and probably underestimate 'true' intake (Acheson *et al* 1980), especially in obese people. Nevertheless, providing that the limitations are borne in mind, they are useful indicators of energy intake (and in fact the *only* readily available indicators of energy requirement). Whichever method is used it is essential that obese patients are urged to give as accurate a picture as possible of their usual food intake — however 'bad' they might think this is — since it is only by being truthful that the dietitian will be able to help them.

Behavioural aspects of food intake

Most people do not eat to satisfy hunger, but in response to other feelings. This may be particularly so in people who are overweight. A group of twenty women at a slimming club (BMI 26−34) were asked why they ate and gave the following reasons: hunger, boredom, comfort, stress, tiredness, habit, availability, anger and to be sociable. On further discussion the majority of them decided that hunger came at the bottom of the list (Bowyer, personal communication).

Food diaries can be used to explore why and where people eat as well as what they are eating. A record sheet suitable for recording this information is shown in Table 4.1. Patients can be asked to describe how they feel before and after eating and with accurately kept records patients can begin to learn about their own eating behaviour. The dietitian must take time to discuss with the patient methods of dealing with some of the reasons given, e.g. boredom, socializing or habit.

Table 4.1 Suggested format for recording eating patterns

Day Date Time	Where	Who with	Food and drink consumed	Comments and feelings e.g. hunger, anxiety, enjoyment, anger.

Any change of behaviour of this type could help towards long term weight maintenance.

This type of record keeping may or may not identify the patient who is 'bingeing', i.e. consuming large quantities of food at one time, generally secretly, in response to emotional feelings and problems. Obesity caused by psychiatric disturbance of this type should be differentiated from other forms of obesity. If necessary, dietitians should feel able to refer the patient back to the consultant or General Practitioner (GP) with the recommendation for psychological or psychiatric assessment. Problems of this type may require psychological counselling before the obesity itself can be tackled; the dietitian can become involved in the treatment at a later and more appropriate time.

Tackling the problem

A standardized diet sheet handed out to all obese patients irrespective of their problems is of no therapeutic value whatsoever. Instead, the dietitian must work from a basic dietary outline and employ different strategies in order to create an individualized treatment programme tailored to the needs of the patient. Dietitians must also be prepared to educate their obese patients, not only in nutrition, but in relevant basic physiology, i.e. how their bodies work. Some patients have strong preconceived ideas about their obesity and may believe that no diet will work for them because their body 'defies the laws of physics' or 'has a slow metabolism' or because of their 'glands'. These are beliefs patients carry with them as they are referred from professional to professional and create a barrier to effective action by them.

The basis on which any obesity treatment should be planned is one of change; the concept of being 'on a diet' should be discouraged as it is the time of being 'off the diet' which causes the damage. The long term goal is to change habits, attitudes and behaviour by encouraging the patient to maintain the short term goals which have been achieved.

Responsibility

So often a patient's 'weight problem' is presented in such a way as if it is the responsibility of the professional and not the patient to solve the problem. In part, this is due to the manner in which obesity is managed and patients wanting someone else to cure it. Typically, a patient goes to the GP who provides a low energy diet sheet and on a return visit, if the patient has lost no weight, the GP refers the patient to a dietitian on the patient's insistence that the diet didn't work. If the dietitian's advice 'doesn't work' then the patient goes back to the GP for the next referral on to an obesity clinic and so the situation continues. The end result of these referrals is reaffirmation for the patient that his/her 'weight problem' cannot be solved by any dietary intervention given by any professional. Many chronic dieters have a long list of diets they have tried which 'didn't work'. However, in many of these patients, little attempt will have been made to help them discover the fundamental reasons for their weight problem.

The emphasis with any obesity treatment programme should be on permanent change — change of eating habits, attitudes, behaviour and perhaps even lifestyle — if patients are to have any chance of losing weight effectively and then maintaining the weight achieved. Health professionals should take time and effort to uncover the real nature of the problem and advise on how this can be remedied; the responsibility for acting on this advice then lies with the patient alone.

The reducing or low energy diet

There is an extensive amount of literature continually trying to provide the avid obese reader with the 'reducing diet that works' published as books (many reaching the best seller list), in women's magazines and in national newspapers. Many rely on gimmicks, and most food constituents in the nation's diet have been the focus of restraint at some time. However, ultimately the only reducing diet which works is one which achieves a sustained reduction in energy intake and such a reducing diet will only be beneficial if it provides a balanced nutrient intake.

General considerations. When prescribing a reducing diet, the following factors must be borne in mind

1 The diet must provide the body with all the essential nutrients, vitamins and minerals necessary to maintain health, without meeting the patient's total energy requirements.

2 The diet must be sufficiently flexible to take into account a patient's taste, financial status and religious restrictions and must be adapted to their lifestyle.

3 The diet must be acceptable to the patient, but the patient must also understand that if the present energy intake is maintaining the obesity there must be substantial change initially, in order to lose weight, and permanently to maintain a lower weight.

4 The diet must be presented to the patient as a basis for long term change of eating habits and *not* a short term crash diet.

5 An energy deficit of 1000 kcal (4.2 MJ)/day below requirement will achieve an approximate weight loss of 1 kg/week. For many patients this will be the maximum, practical deficit achievable and for most it will be less than this.

6 The physiological responses of the body to weight loss such as sensitivity to cold and increased tiredness are frequently reported by patients and they need to be reassured that this will resolve.

Energy content and dietary composition

1 Many obese patients claim to be unable to lose weight on a daily intake of either 1000 kcal (4.2 MJ) or 800 kcal (3.4 MJ). James (1983) reports not to have yet found a single value for total energy expenditure over 24 hours below 1200 kcal (5 MJ) using whole body calorimetric studies on adults whether of normal weight, obese or underweight. The lowest oxygen uptake recorded by Pilkington (personal communication) is 161 ml/min which equates to an RMR of approximately 1100 kcal (4.7 MJ)/24 hours. The usual energy intake of each individual will provide the best guide to what the energy content of the weight reducing diet should be.

2 Protein content must be adequate to meet daily requirements. Although weight loss may be faster if protein intake is restricted, this will be achieved at the expense of loss of lean body mass, rather than adipose tissue (Garrow *et al* 1981). All energy restricted diets should contain approximately 15% of energy in the form of protein. Guidelines are needed for recommended portion sizes of the protein-rich foods, e.g. meat, fish, cheese, eggs, milk, yoghurt and pulses to be included in the low energy diet.

3 With an energy value of 9 kcal (38 KJ)/g, fat is a very concentrated source of energy in any person's diet. Reduction in fat intake is vital if a significant energy saving is to be made. The percentage of energy from fat in a reducing diet should be as low as is achievable for palatability. All fat-rich foods should be avoided. Low fat spread can be used instead of butter or margarine and should be included in a measured quantity. Patients often find it more useful to know what quantity of fat will last a period of time, e.g. 1 week, rather than a daily amount. Adding fat to food (e.g. butter on vegetables), cooking in fat (e.g. frying or roasting) or consuming fat-containing sauces, gravies or batter should be avoided. However, ideas for alternative foods or cooking methods should also be given.

4 The importance of a regular meal pattern should be emphasized and most people should consume a minimum of three meals per day. This is partly because the metabolic rate is increased after each eating episode (thermogenic effect of food) but also because an unstructured meal pattern lends itself to erratic eating and the likelihood of consuming excess food. Many obese patients feel they are doing themselves good by missing a meal whereas in practice the energy saving is usually more than compensated for by nibbling throughout the day. Many patients accommodate between-meal snacks by cutting down at their next meal which in turn does not satisfy them sufficiently leading to further between-meal eating. At the onset of treatment the meal pattern, as well as the content of the meals themselves, should be arranged to suit the patient's lifestyle and once agreed should not be altered.

5 Bread, cereals and potatoes are still thought to be 'fattening' by many people and this misconception must be clarified. Fibre-rich sources of carbohydrate such as wholemeal bread, cereals and potatoes have a low energy density, are inexpensive, easily available, good sources of protein, vitamins and minerals and help provide satiety. They should be included with every meal. The use of carbohydrate exchange lists is sometimes useful — not so much for the purpose of restricting intake but to ensure that adequate amounts of these foods are consumed.

6 Fruit and vegetables should be included daily as they are valuable sources of fibre, vitamins and minerals.

7 Although energy-rich foods such as sweets, chocolates, cakes, etc. cannot be recommended for inclusion on a low energy diet, the use of the words 'fattening' 'bad' or 'forbidden' as a means of describing them should be avoided. Obese patients frequently regard these foods in this way and the guilt feelings produced by one lapse in this direction can lead patients to assume that they have 'failed' and that their dietary efforts have been in vain.

It should be stressed to patients that, for example, one bar of chocolate or one cake will not cause uncontrollable weight gain; it will only add the equivalent energy intake to that day's total intake. Weeks or even months of effort must not be abandoned simply because of lapses on one day. Dietary restrictions of any kind create craving for those foods 'not allowed'. Only the most superhuman will be able to resist totally the constant temptations.

8 It should be impressed clearly upon patients that short term (daily) fluctuations in weight are due to changes in *water* balance and that the changes in fat weight are small and slow. They should not therefore allow a sudden increase in weight after a dietary indiscretion to discourage them from continuing with the attempt to lose *fat*.

9 Lists of both 'foods which can be eaten freely' and 'foods to avoid' based on low and high energy dense foods respectively are helpful to patients. However, these lists should be practical and reasonably balanced in length; a long list of pleasant-tasting 'foods to avoid' accompanied by an 'unrestricted' list comprised only of items such as salt, pepper, mustard and low-calorie squash will not help the patient's morale.

Motivation

Adequate motivation is a vital component of a successful weight loss programme. The reasons people give for wishing to lose weight are numerous and range from purely aesthetic reasons to very defined medical reasons. The associated complications and risks of obesity include diabetes mellitus, coronary heart disease, hypertension and premature death. Conditions exacerbated by obesity include osteoarthritis and respiratory disease. All of these complications can be improved by weight loss (Royal College of Physicians 1983).

Motivation may initially be very high, but within a very short period of time the resolve fades because these ultimate goals concerning health or appearance seem to be so far into the future and so out of reach. It becomes difficult to balance the long term benefits with the immediate satisfaction of eating.

Support from a partner, spouse or other family members can increase motivation substantially. Re-educating the eating habits of the whole family often secures a better chance of change rather than focusing solely on the individual who is 'on a diet'. Dietitians should involve other family members more often as ideas about supportive behaviour vary enormously. Many obese female patients feel their husbands/partners continually 'nag' them about their weight and about any food eaten which is considered 'fattening'. This can drive them to begin eating secretly. Hence a further problem arises of the husband/partner only then seeing the patient eat correctly and frugally yet losing no weight! So, the patient should be encouraged to define what behaviour from other family members will be supportive to the patient's own motivation, e.g. compliments, non-food treats, change of family eating behaviour. Every overweight patient must want to lose weight for him/herself and this must be the prime motivation. The situation where a patient claims to be losing weight for the dietitian should be avoided. Time and effort should be put into helping obese patients to find and secure their own motivational goals.

Rate of weight loss

Excess energy is stored in the body predominantly as adipose tissue. Any weight losing programme should result in the utilization of these adipose tissue stores with minimum loss of other important body tissue such as the lean body mass.

Many obese patients who seek treatment view a successful outcome as one which produces the 'greatest weight loss in the shortest period of time'. The following facts provide evidence as to why this may be impossible or undesirable

1 Adipose tissue has an energy value of approximately 7000 kcal (29 MJ)/kg therefore a deficit of 1000 kcal (4.2 MJ)/day below requirement will achieve a weight loss of approximately 1 kg per week.

2 Garrow (1980) has shown that a more rapid weight loss than this, for example, over 3 kg/week, is effected by increased loss of lean body mass.

3 The RMR, (which contributes the greatest percentage to total energy expenditure) falls during weight loss as an adaptive response to a reduced energy intake. Therefore the rate of weight loss decreases with time for the same reduction in energy intake.

4 The initial rapid weight loss which patients experience when first reducing their energy intake, particularly from restricting carbohydrate, is due to the utilization of the body's glycogen stores and consequent loss of water. This can create motivation and resolve at the beginning of a reducing diet, but as the body begins to utilize its adipose tissue stores a decrease in the rate of weight loss is inevitable. Patients can become disillusioned very easily by this and the expected pattern of weight loss, and if possible the reason for it, should be clearly explained by the dietitian at the onset of dietary treatment.

Exercise

It is generally acknowledged that some exercise is beneficial to general health and well-being and people are being encouraged to include regular exercise in their lives. To many obese people 'exercise' means either stripping down to a minimum of clothing in a gymnasium or swimming pool or jogging around the park and, not surprisingly, most are unwilling to contemplate any of these. However, most are unaware that significant amounts of 'exercise' can be performed by means of ordinary daily tasks, e.g. walking up the stairs rather than using a lift; walking to the shops instead of taking the bus or car and finding some household task to do instead of watching television.

The severely obese have particular problems because they have difficulty with breathing, joints and balance. Increasing the level of activity should be taken slowly and the type of activity geared to each patient's capabilities. Once the patient starts to lose weight and adapts to the level of activity, the amount and degree of difficulty of the tasks performed can be increased, e.g. walking briskly, walking further and using the stairs more.

Although exercise will not in itself contribute a great deal to weight loss directly, it undoubtedly increases a sense of well-being and helps divert attention from food and hence is a valuable part of any weight reducing regimen. Some patients enjoy, as well as benefit from, a formalized exercise programme and this can be planned with the help and advice of a physiotherapist.

Realistic goals and expectations of treatment

Successful weight loss often brings its own problems. Far too often obese patients view every difficulty in their lives as a consequence of their obesity which will disappear completely with weight loss. They may have an unrealistic view of normal weight people leading problem-free lives and are dismayed to discover that this is not the case. Furthermore, many obese patients fail to realize that achieving their target weight does not mean the end of their dietary efforts. Although most are confident that they will never regain weight, in practice this is not easy, as follow-up studies show. The difficulties arise as a result of lowered energy requirements and the psychological readjustment to a new body shape. A new eating pattern needs to be learned to match the lowered energy requirements and patients must also learn that life difficulties are still there and have to be faced.

Apart from unrealistic expectations of what target weight will mean, most obese patients feel that only when this ultimate goal is reached will they be able to obtain any real benefit from their efforts. Unfortunately, there are more people who falter along the way than reach this goal and although the achievement may have brought benefits, these are blocked out because the target weight is not reached. Patients may give up totally, rapidly regaining the lost weight and frequently even more. As well as long term goals, patient's should be encouraged to set themselves short term achievable goals as they progress.

The benefits in daily living can often be the motivating force. For the patients with severe obesity it may be the desire to pass through ticket barriers at underground stations, sit in cinema or theatre seats, walk one flight of stairs without becoming breathless or to buy 'off the peg' clothes, which have most effect. Patients can be asked to list their desired goals for defined weight bands (e.g. 6 kg or 1 stone) as part of the monitoring process (see Table 4.2). Copies of the goals should be kept by both patient and dietitian and the patient should use them constantly as a reminder of progress being made.

Regular follow-up visits should be incorporated into a weight reducing programme where the patient's overall progress can be monitored in addition to their weight loss. Some people can gain motivation and support from a slimming club (see p 345).

Table 4.2 Example of the goals and aims of a 19 year old female. Initial weight 111 kg (BMI = 40). Personal target weight 64 kg (BMI = 23).

Weight		Goals and aims
102 kg	(16 st)	Treat body with more respect. Wake up earlier Walk faster and more often. Start light exercise.
95.5kg	(15 st)	Start keep fit class. Buy new clothes.
89 kg	(14 st)	Swimming.
83 kg	(13 st)	Buy first ever pair of jeans. Have a ride on everything at a Fun Fair.
76 kg	(12 st)	Try for promotional course at place of work. Ride a bicycle without feeling self-conscious. Wear shorts.
70 kg	(11 st)	Run for bus. Buy size 12–14 clothes.
64 kg	(10 st)	*Main goal* 'my coming out'. Plan a holiday to show real me.

4.1.3 Radical treatment approaches to obesity

Several radical approaches have been used in the treatment of severe obesity. All present problems to the medical and surgical teams involved and require skilled dietetic help.

Jejuno-ileal bypass

This long established surgical procedure involves the anastamosis of a short length of the proximal jejunum to a short length of the terminal ileum, hence bypassing a large segment of the small intestine. The most recent operations include a cholecystjejunostomy, in which the end of the excluded segment is anastomosed to the gall bladder. It has been found that the length of small intestine remaining in continuity and therefore available for the digestion and absorption of food should be less than 50 cm.

The operation carries many medical and surgical complications which include 'bypass enteritis', electrolyte disturbances, renal stones, liver damage, inflammatory skin and joint disease and mineral and vitamin deficiencies (e.g. iron, folic acid, vitamin B12 and vitamin D). Many of the complications are severe enough to warrant reversal of the operation and are not always confined to the early post-operative period. There is a mortality rate of 3–4% (Bray et al 1977; McFarland et al 1985).

The weight loss after bypass approximates 35% of pre-operative weight, the majority of which occurs during the first year (Pilkington 1980). After this time body weight is maintained but there may be some weight regained. It is frequently assumed this weight loss occurs due to severe malabsorption and many obese patients request the operation thinking they can eat as much as they like and still lose weight. However, it has been shown that the weight loss is due largely to a self-imposed reduction in food intake in order to avoid the unpleasant side effect of diarrhoea which tends to occur after an over-liberal fat and fluid intake (Pilkington et al 1976; Bray et al 1976). Patients who are unable to alter their food intake may have such severe complications that reversal becomes essential in order to prevent death.

The procedure also carries a risk of renal stone formation arising from the increased formation of calcium soaps with unabsorbed fatty acids in the gastrointestinal tract. The consequent reduction in intraluminal calcium ions results in less oxalate being bound and passive oxalate absorption being increased, particularly in the colon (Stauffer 1977). A high calcium, low oxalate, low fat (<40 g/day) intake can prevent excessive oxalate excretion via the kidneys.

Jejuno-ileal bypass is now virtually obsolete as a method of treating severe obesity due to the serious side effects and consequent life-long follow-up.

Gastric surgery

Because of the side effects associated with the jejuno-ileal bypass, surgeons have searched for another operation to offer to the severely obese. Mason introduced the gastric bypass in America in 1966 which was based on the Billroth II gastrectomy. Modifications of this bypass have been performed over the years and recent techniques in gastroplasty (leaving a passage along the greater or lesser curvature of the stomach without bypassing it) now involve stapling the stomach to create a very small upper pouch with a reinforced stoma through the staple line. Foods and fluids then pass from the upper pouch through to the remainder of the stomach. As there is no interruption of the gastrointestinal tract food is digested in the normal way. The aim of the procedure is to limit the quantity of food and fluids taken at any one time by producing early satiety. The size of the upper pouch is important if maximum weight loss is to be achieved and Mason (1980) suggested 50 ml as the optimum capacity. Complications associated with large upper pouches include vomiting, stomal ulcer and inadequate weight loss. The other criterion for successful outcome of gastric bypass and gastroplasty is a reinforced small stoma to prevent its dilatation. Mason (1980) reported an average weight loss of 30% of initial weight if the specifications of upper pouch size and reinforced stoma are met.

To allow the staple line to heal and prevent its disruption, all patients need to follow a strict regimen of small volumes of fluids for at least eight weeks post-operatively, progressing slowly to solids via stages of carefully liquidized foods, again in very small quantities. This strict regimen demands highly motivated patients. American workers teach pre- and post-operatively both the patient and the family using multidisciplinary teams which include dietitians.

However, the end result of this operation is not without problems. A 'normal' eating pattern with regular meals is difficult to achieve. Instead patients have to eat small, frequent snacks throughout the day to meet all their nutritional requirements except for energy. Some foods cause problems such as a feeling of the food being stuck, nausea or discomfort and the items causing these often seem to be those with a valuable nutrient content such as meat, fruit and vegetables. Conversely, the foods which are often best tolerated are items such as chocolate, biscuits and cakes.

To ensure an adequate nutritional intake and the adoption of new eating habits, the involvement of a dietitian during the period of weight loss and subsequent weight maintenance is essential. Patients should be advised to consume 3–5 small meals per day, avoiding high fibre, high fat and spicy foods. Patients also need to be educated to eat slowly, chew food thoroughly and learn to acknowledge feelings of fullness, at which time they should stop eating. If too much food and/or fluid is taken too quickly the patient experiences severe pain which may result in vomiting with subsequent disruption of the staple line.

Gastric surgery does not seem to result in the severe metabolic side effects seen after jejuno-ileal bypass. However, the long term effectiveness of this method of treating severe obesity has yet to be evaluated.

Jaw wiring

Jaw wiring is a simple and effective procedure aimed at limiting the dietary intake in severely obese patients. Methods used are modifications of those used by oral surgeons for fractured jaws. Provided that patients attend for regular dental check-ups and maintain a good standard of personal oral hygiene there are few dental problems and complications.

The first two to three days after jaw wiring are the most difficult — patients feel very uncomfortable and anxious and speech may be impaired. However, after this time patients are able to speak quite normally and all fluids are drunk successfully by sucking them through the teeth. Patients awaiting jaw-wiring benefit enormously from talking to a patient who has already been wired as worries about the practical difficulties can be discussed in advance. All jaw-wired patients must be given the instruction that in the event of vomiting, they must lean over a bowl and allow the vomit to escape from the mouth and nose. Also that they must carry wire cutters (in the form of toe nail clippers) with them at all times in case the wires need to be cut in an emergency.

Dietary management

Patients should be prescribed a low energy fluid diet. This could for example be achieved by

    1200 ml full cream milk
    300 ml fruit juice
    1 teaspoon Marmite/Bovril
    Unlimited low calorie fluids

This would provide approximately 900 kcal (3.8 MJ).

The total daily fluid intake should be in the region of 1800–2400 ml (3–4 pints). Liquid multivitamin supplements and iron should also be given. The diet will then be nutritionally adequate in all but energy and fibre. Recipes for low energy soups may be helpful to patients.

The fluid diet should be used as a meal replacement with the majority of it being drunk as three 'meals'. This is to establish a meal pattern throughout the jaw wiring period and to encourage patients to continue sitting with their partners and/or families at mealtimes.

Most patients report having a small bowel movement every other day without discomfort. If constipation becomes a problem, ensure that the daily fluid intake is adequate (1800–2400 ml; 3–4 pints) and, if necessary, a bulking agent such as Cologel (liquid methycellulose) can be prescribed.

Regular follow-up visits should be made to both the oral surgeon and dental hygienist. The maximum length of time any patient is wired is 12 months.

Effectiveness

Weight loss following jaw wiring has been shown to be comparable to that of both jejuno-ileal bypass and gastric bypass (Rodgers *et al* 1979; Garrow and Gardiner 1981), yet it is still not a widely used procedure in the treatment of obesity. This may be due to its one drawback which is failure to maintain the weight loss after the wires are removed. Kark (1980) found that 13 of 14 patients not only failed to maintain their initial weight loss over a two year follow-up period, but also regained most of the weight lost. Fordyce *et al* (1979) reported that patients showed better maintenance of their weight loss if the period of jaw wiring was followed by a gastric bypass and suggested that this operation should be recommended to patients who regain more than 5 kg in the first three months after jaw wires were removed. Garrow and Gardiner (1981) found that the simpler measure of fastening a nylon cord around the waist of patients when their jaw wires were removed was also effective in limiting weight gain.

Patients' expectation of jaw wiring is a rapid rate of weight loss enabling them to reach their personal target weights which they will then maintain without difficulty. The latter part of this statement does not appear to be borne out in practice. Jaw wiring must not be seen as a simple procedure to be offered to the severely obese patient without taking this problem of weight maintenance into account. The Adelaide Obesity Group feel that the key to successful management of jaw wiring is a multidisciplinary team approach, utilizing the skills of physicians, dietitians, social workers and nurses in consultation with oral surgeons and psychiatrists (Goss 1979).

Very low calorie formula diets

The very low calorie diet (VLCD) is a method of weight reduction in which conventional meals are replaced with a formula diet which is nutritionally complete but low in energy (usually providing less than 500 kcal/day). The VLCD is designed to produce rapid loss of body fat but without the loss of lean body tissues or the harmful metabolic consequences of fasting *per se*.

In recent years, the VLCD has become an increasingly popular slimming method among the general public in the UK and other countries. The reaction of the medical and dietetic professions has been more cautious, and at times hostile, but many health professionals now believe the VLCD has a place in the treatment of some cases of obesity, in particular the chronically failed dieter who lacks the resolve to achieve weight loss by traditional dietary means.

Safety and contraindications

Initially, concern was expressed over the safety of the VLCD largely as a result of the unhappy experiences with some of the early formula diets pioneered in the USA, some of which produced severe electrolyte disturbances and some fatalities (Isner *et al* 1979). However, experimental studies and controlled clinical trials on the modern version of the VLCD (Contaldo *et al* 1981; Howard 1981; Wadden *et al* 1983) have shown that it is safe provided that it is used with medical approval and in accordance with the manufacturer's instructions. The VLCD is not suitable for children, adolescents or those who are pregnant and must not be used by persons with any of the following conditions
1 Cardiovascular disease or cardiac arrhythmius.
2 Cerebrovascular disease.
3 Renal disease.
4 Hepatic disease.
5 Hyperuricaemia.
6 Overt psychosis (or treatment involving lithium therapy).

Effectiveness

In the short term, the VLCD is undoubtedly very successful in producing weight loss. Side effects such as headaches, nausea, dizziness, halitosis and postural hypotension can occur, but are usually of short duration and can be alleviated by an increase in fluid intake.

The long term success of the VLCD is less well-established. It can be argued that, unlike conventional weight reducing diets, the VLCD makes no contribution to the re-education of the eating habits which caused the obesity in the first place. On the other hand, the VLCD has enabled some obese patients to achieve a body weight which seemed unattainable by other dietary means, and the consequent morale boost can generate a strong resolve to eat sensibly in order not to revert to a former size and shape.

Risk of misuse

Perhaps the main concern about the VLCD remaining among doctors and dietitians is not so much the concept of the VLCD itself but more the fear that it may be misused. VLCDs are not controlled by medical prescription and are sold directly to the general public either by pharmacies or by agents (often termed advisors or counsellors) of the manufacturers. While the literature which accompanies these products states quite clearly that intending users of them should obtain medical approval beforehand, there is no guarantee that everyone will do this. It is also conceivable that a person who has already spent a considerable sum of money in purchasing the product may be tempted to use it anyway, even if subsequently advised not to do so.

There is also a risk that the VLCD may be followed for an inappropriately long period of time. Again, reputable manufacturers give clear guidelines regarding the maximum period of time (usually 3–4 weeks) for which the VLCD should be the sole source of nutrition. Although VLCDs have been used under supervision for longer periods of time without apparent ill-effect, the possible dangers from people doing so on their own initiative and without any monitoring checks being carried out are obvious — especially if they shouldn't be using the product in the first place.

No matter what steps the manufacturers of VLCDs take to point out the safeguards and contraindications in the use of their products, there is, at present, no way of ensuring that the users will be equally responsible in observing them. Since it seems likely that the VLCD is likely to remain, and probably become an increasingly popular option in the treatment of obesity, the medical and dietetic professions should perhaps be taking steps to ensure that VLCDs are used correctly rather than, as happens in some instances, to ignore their existence.

4.1.4 Obesity in children

Aetiology

As with adults, there are many factors contributing to obesity in children

1   Hormonal causes. These are rare.

2   Hereditary tendency. Obesity tends to run in families, possibly due to lifestyle and eating habits, but also as a consequence of genetic factors. Eating habits should be watched closely in these families so that any potential problem can be diagnosed and corrected at an early stage.

3   Feeding habits in infancy. Breast fed babies are thought to be less likely to become overweight children than those who are bottle fed (although with the introduction of more modified feeding formulae in recent years, this difference may be less likely to occur). However, the incorrect use of artificial formulae, early weaning and inappropriate weaning foods may contribute to the development of obesity.

4   Emotional factors. Food for many children is a source of comfort; unhappy children may therefore eat more than happier children. Food is often used as a bribe or reward or as a replacement for love and attention and the least nutritious foods are usually chosen. Grandparents and separated parents tend to use sweets or chocolates to gain a child's confidence, favour and love.

5   The general lifestyle. This may exacerbate a tendency to acquire excess weight, e.g. lack of exercise resulting from travelling everywhere by car, watching television for prolonged periods and not participating in any active leisure pursuits. Children who are already obese often try to avoid games and sports at school because they are embarrassed by their physique.

Treatment

This will only be successful if the child wants to lose weight. Co-operation of the parents and other close family members is essential to ensure success.

Explaining *why* a child should achieve a more normal weight is important, i.e. the health risks attached, attitude of peers.

Dramatic weight loss is not desirable for children and, in general, it is better if a child 'holds' or 'grows into' his weight. This must also be carefully explained to the parents and child who can otherwise become very discouraged by the absence of any weight loss and apparent lack of progress.

Children still require a healthy varied diet whilst reducing weight. A high fibre diet may help achieve

satiety in addition to its other benefits. During growth spurts, and with the onset of menstruation in girls, adequate intakes of calcium, protein and iron are essential. Very low energy diets are not suitable for any child.

It is very important that overweight children are not made to feel any more different than is necessary either at home or at school.

At home

Children and parents should be encouraged to look at the family lifestyle and eating habits generally and make modifications for the whole family. As well as benefiting the family's health, such measures may also help prevent other members of the family becoming overweight. All members of the family should be encouraged to

1   Not add sugar to drinks and cereals.

2   Use a low calorie sweetener if necessary.

3   Choose a high fibre breakfast cereal and avoid sugar-coated varieties.

4   Choose wholemeal bread.

5   Eat more fruit and vegetables.

6   Only eat chips once a week at most — jacket potatoes with or without fillings are often just as popular with children.

7   Only eat crisps once or twice a week at most and to try the wholewheat varieties.

8   Eat fewer cakes, biscuits, puddings and sweets.

9   Choose low calorie squash and soft drinks.

10   Choose tinned fruits in natural juice and natural fruit juices instead of sweetened varieties.

At school

Snacks taken to school ideally should be fruit, but this is not always popular or practical; the occasional bag of wholewheat crisps or a muesli-type bar may be more acceptable to a child and are preferable to chocolate or sweets.

School meals present problems as many items are fried, but discussion with school cook or head teacher may result in a better choice of foods being offered generally; the health visitor or community dietitian may be able to exert some influence if the school is unresponsive to a request from the parents. Packed meals brought from home may be a better alternative in some cases.

Tuckshops in school could be encouraged to offer healthier alternatives for children to purchase, e.g.

fresh fruit, muesli bars, plain biscuits and low calorie drinks.

Overweight children are often reluctant to participate in sports due to teasing, but should be encouraged to take some form of regular exercise. This can be in the form of walking, cycling or swimming as well as the traditional sporting activities.

Guidance on spending pocket money may be necessary and children should be advised not to spend it on sweets or crisps but to save it up to buy a book, toy or game instead. Relatives and friends should be encouraged to give gifts other than sweets.

Birthday parties

Parties can be regarded as a permissible treat but it is still possible to include plenty of suitable foods, for example

1   Wholemeal bread used in the sandwiches.
2   Low calorie squash or soft drinks.
3   Natural fruit juice.
4   Various interesting salads using fruit, nuts, raw vegetables, pulses, brown rice and pasta in attractive presentations.
5   Dried fruit, nuts and raisins.
6   Fresh fruit salad.
7   Yoghurt-based desserts.
8   Birthday cake — this could contain a fruit filling or be a fruit flan or fruit cake.
9   Savoury flans with wholewheat pastry.
10 Filled jacket potatoes.

Group therapy

This may be helpful with some children but this option is not available in every locality. Topics for discussion can include all aspects of healthy living and eating and not just slimming, i.e. exercise, dental health, hygiene and general healthy eating habits. They should also provide plenty of activities which involve the child and hold his interest, e.g. food diaries, scrap books, paintings and posters, practical cookery, games or quizzes.

Overweight children are often fussy eaters who require a great deal of encouragement. Attractive presentation of food and the choice of a wide variety of foods are essential. It is important for the child to realize that healthy eating is interesting and enjoyable.

4.1.5   Setting up a slimming club

The following information is directed towards setting up a slimming club within the structure of the National Health Service. The guidelines could also be adapted to apply to a private or commercial slimming club.

Advantages and disadvantages of slimming clubs

Advantages

They are an efficient use of dietitians' time because more patients are advised more regularly. This is especially true if the club is run by a non-dietitian with occasional input from the dietitian. Another advantage is that members of the group gain more support from sharing a common aim.

Disadvantages

The patient has less individual dietetic attention. There is a risk that some members will attend for solely social reasons rather than in a serious attempt to slim.

Aims and target group

It is important to be clear about the aims of the club. As well as the general aims of weight loss and improved health, there may be others, such as off-loading out-patient commitments or all GP referrals. Any planning will also depend on the target group. It may be all those with a weight problem or a more specific group, e.g. children or men. These points should be clarified so that they can be referred to while planning and used for evaluation later.

Type of club

Most commercial slimming clubs operate an open club; this runs indefinitely and members can join at any time. It has the advantage that a constant supply of new members will replace defaulters. Closed courses are more suitable for a structured educational programme (Seddon et al 1981), possibly including behavioural modification techniques (Long et al 1983). These have a set number of sessions (usually between ten and sixteen) and every member joins at the same time. This helps bond the group together and enables the leader to have a specific short term commitment. The disadvantages of set courses is that some members may default, decreasing the size of the group, and some may wish to rejoin every subsequent course preventing the input of new applicants. The answer may be to provide another course which follows on with less frequent, shorter sessions. As there is usually a higher drop-out rate, a central club taking members from several courses is one way of keeping numbers fairly steady.

Management backing

Consultation at an early stage with the District Management Team, Board, or equivalent, is essential to discuss finance, personnel, premises, publicity and policy decisions. Further meetings will be needed to approve more definite plans.

Finance

For a club run as part of the NHS dietetic service, financial allocations must be approved and monitored by the District Management Team or equivalent. Charging a fee may be necessary either to cover sundry expenses such as refreshments, leaflets and film hire, or for substantial funding of the project including hire of premises, payment of leader, speakers' fees and possibly insurance. If the club is aimed at health education, it is usually permissable to charge even if it is held on health service premises. A self-financing, but non-profit-making club can still charge considerably less than commercial organisations. Paying a fee in advance will also encourage attendance.

Club membership

A club membership of approximately 20 is a manageable size, but allows for some defaulting. The method of publicizing to potential members will depend on the target group. Some clubs only enrol members with a medical referral. It would not be regarded as a breach of professional conduct for a State Registered Dietitian to give general nutritional and dietetic advice to a group without individual referral (CPSM Dietitians Board Statement, item 2). In the event of a dietitian actually being the club leader, it would obviously be their professional responsibility to ensure that individual patients' GP's are aware of their membership of the slimming club (Bond 1983). The GP could be notified by a standard letter asking if there is any medical contraindication to their patient's enrolment or any health details affecting diet (e.g. diabetes), suggesting that if no reply is received within ten days then it will be assumed that there is no objection.

The club can be publicized by notifying relevant personnel, and by notices in GP surgeries, health clinics, out-patient departments and non-NHS premises such as libraries. The local newspaper might also mention it in a slimming feature.

Club leaders

Dietitians from the local dietetic department may be interested in being club leaders. The advantage of the closed course system is that there can be more than one leader, each running a different course. Some health visitors or clinic nurses welcome the opportunity to run a club but may benefit from an instruction course beforehand. Alternatively, the leadership could be shared, with a dietitian only taking certain sessions. Another possibility is to charge a fee and use it to pay dietitians who are looking for part time or evening work. Long *et al* (1983) also describe a group led by a dietitian/clinical psychologist team.

Organisation

The organisation of a slimming club can be time-consuming. Telephone enquiries, enrolling members, publicity, planning programmes, booking films and speakers, ordering leaflets can add to the load of a busy dietetic department. It may be worthwhile to pay an organiser to do this (e.g. one of the leaders), possibly using a home telephone as a base for enquiries.

It may also be helpful to form a small planning group including dietetic, medical, nursing, health education and administrative input. Once the club is established this group can be convened periodically to review progress and report to the District Management Team.

Premises and timing

Most people prefer an evening club due to work and family commitments, though some mothers and senior citizens may favour the daytime.

Evening clubs need well-lit premises with adequate public transport. Health centres, clinics, the hospital or rented halls may be suitable.

It is essential to have accurate scales, preferably the bar type, which are serviced regularly. Health clinics are usually equipped with these and may have other useful equipment such as audio visual aid facilities and floor exercise mats.

It is usually best to plan weekly sessions of around $1\frac{1}{2}$–2 hours duration on a convenient day, allowing six to eight weeks before the commencement date for publicity, enrolment and programme planning.

Programme planning

Whether a structured course or an open club is decided upon, planning the sessions is important to ensure variety and a balance of topics.

The first half of the session should concentrate on recording member's weights and discussing their problems. It should be remembered that weighing a group of people takes time, 20 people take at least half an hour and much longer on the first session when height is measured and the target weight is determined as well. The second half of the session should be devoted to a different topic each week — films, quizzes and talks including some by outside speakers such as a doctor, physiotherapist, psychologist or beautician. As well as visual aids such as films, videos, posters and slides, use real food where possible, e.g. a demonstration of the pros and cons of various slimming products borrowed from a local chemist or a tasting session of favourite low calorie recipes.

Giving members their own copy of the programme will encourage attendance. In addition to the diet sheet and a weight record card, the teaching should be endorsed with leaflets on recipes, exercise, calorie counting, a week's menu and helpful hints. Home made handouts are improved by using a cartoon picture or logogram on coloured paper; alternatively, there is a choice of printed material available (refer to BDA list of leaflets and posters). Instead of a comprehensive diet sheet at the first session, step-by-step advice cards can be given out for the first few weeks. Although financial limitations will influence the use of visual aids and leaflets, their cost per head is usually relatively small compared to other expenses.

Some useful suggestions for improving the programme content may come from members, especially if a questionnaire is circulated.

Evaluation

It is important to evaluate whether the original aim is being achieved and to review weight loss and attendance rates. It can be useful to refer to published studies of slimming clubs in the UK showing average weight loss — 9.7 kg in 25.7 weeks (Ashwell and Garrow 1975), 4.4 kg in 10 weeks (Seddon et al 1981), 4.6 kg in 16 weeks and 6.9 kg in 16 weeks with behavioural modification (Long et al 1983). The leaders should keep clear records of weight and height (in metric units), age and possibly occupation for evaluation or for use in research studies.

References

Acheson KJ, Campbell IT, Edholm OG, Miller DS and Stock MJ (1980) The measurement of food and energy intake in man — an evaluation of some techniques. *Am J Clin Nutr* **33**, 1147–54.

Ashwell M and Garrow JS (1975) A survey of three slimming and weight control organisations in the UK. *Nutrition (London)* **29**, 347–56.

Black AE, Prentice AM and Coward WA (1985) Validation of the 7-day weighed diet record by comparison against total energy expenditure. In *Proceedings of the British Dietetic Association Study Conference*, Keele University, April 1985, p 25.

Bond S (1983) *The professional approach*. British Dietetic Association.

Bray GA, Barry RE, Benfield JR, Castelnuovo–Tedesco P and Rodin J (1976) Intestinal bypass surgery for obesity decreases food intake and taste preferences. *Am J Clin Nutr* **29**, 779–83.

Bray GA, Greenway FL, Barry RE, Benfield JR, Fiser RL, Dahms WT, Atkinson RL and Schwartz AA (1977) Surgical treatment of obesity. A review of our experience and an analysis of published reports. *Int J Obesity* **1**, 331–67.

Contaldo F, Dibiase G, Fischetti A and Mancini M (1981) Evaluation of the safety of the very low calorie diets in the treatment of severely obese patients in a metabolic ward. *Int J Obesity* **5**, 221–6.

Council for Professions Supplementary to Medicine, Dietitians Board Statement of Conduct (1987)

Fordyce GL, Garrow JS, Kark AE and Stalley SF (1979) Jaw wiring and gastric bypass in the treatment of severe obesity. *Obesity/ Bariatric Medicine* **8**, (1), 14–7.

Garrow JS, Durrant ML, Mann S, Stalley SF and Warwick PM (1978) Factors determining weight loss in obese patients in a metabolic ward. *Int J Obesity* **2**, 441–7.

Garrow JS (1980) Combined medical-surgical approaches to the treatment of obesity. *Am J Clin Nutr* **33**, 425–30.

Garrow JS (1981) *Treat obesity seriously* Churchill Livingstone, London.

Garrow JS and Gardiner GT (1981) Maintenance of weight loss in obese patients after jaw wiring. *Br Med J* **282**, 858–60.

Garrow JS, Durrant ML, Blaza S, Wilkins D, Royston P and Sunkin S (1981) The effect of meal frequency and protein concentration on the composition of the weight lost by obese subjects. *Br J Nutr* **45**, 5–15.

Goss AN (1979) Management of patients with jaws wired for obesity. *Br Dental J* **146**, (11), 339–42.

Halliday D, Hesp R, Stalley SF, Warwick P, Altman DG and Garrow JS (1979) Resting metabolic rate, weight, surface area and body composition in obese women. *Int J Obesity* **1**, 1–6.

Howard AN (1981) The historical development, efficacy and safety of very low calorie diets. *Int J Obesity* **5**, 195–208.

Isner JM, Sours HE, Paris AL, Ferrans VJ and Roberts WC (1979) Sudden, unexpected death in avid dieters using the liquid protein modified fast diet. Observations in 17 patients and the role of the prolonged QT interval. *Circulation* **60**, 1401–12.

James WPT, Davies HL, Bailes J and Dauncey MJ (1978) Elevated metabolic rates in obesity. *Lancet* **i**, 1122–5.

James WPT (1983) Energy requirements and obesity *Lancet* **2**, 386–9.

Jequier E (1984) Energy expenditure in obesity. *Clinics in endocrinology and metabolism* **13**, (3), 563–77.

Kark AE (1980) Jaw wiring. *Am J Clin Nutr* **33**, 420–4.

Keys A, Brozek J, Henscher A, Mickelson O and Taylor HL (1950) *The biology of human starvation*. University of Minnesota Press, Minneapolis.

Long CG, Simpson CM and Allot EA (1983) Psychological and dietetic counselling combined in the treatment of obesity: a comparative study in a hospital out-patient clinic. *Hum Nutr: Appl Nutr* **37A**, 94–102.

Mason EE (1980) *Surgical management of obesity* pp 29–39. Academic Press, London.

McFarland RJ, Gazet JC and Pilkington TRE (1985) A 13 year review of jejuno-ileal bypass. *Br J Surg* **72**, 81–7.

Pilkington TRE, Gazet JC, Ang L, Kalucy RS, Crisp AH and Day S (1976) Explanations for weight loss after jejuno-ileal bypass in gross obesity. *Br Med J* **1**, 1504–5.

Pilkington TRE (1980) *Surgical management of obesity* pp 171–8. Academic Press, London.

Prentice AM, Black AE, Coward WA, Davies HL, Goldberg GR, Murgatroyd PR, Ashford J, Sawyer M and Whitehead RG

(1986) High levels of energy expenditure in obese women. *Br Med J* **292**, 983–7.

Ravussin E, Burnand B, Schutz Y and Jéquier E (1982) Twenty-four hour energy expenditure and resting metabolic rate in obese, moderately obese and control subjects. *Am J Clin Nutr* **35**, 566–73.

Rodgers S, Burnet R, Goss A, Phillips P, Goldney R, Kimber C, Thomas D, Harding P and Wise P (1977) Jaw wiring in the treatment of obesity. *Lancet* **i**, 1221–2.

Royal College of Physicians of London (1983) Obesity. *J R Coll Physicians Lond* **17**, (1), 3–58.

Seddon R, Penfound J and Garrow JS (1981) The Harrow Slimming Club: analysis of results obtained in 249 members of a self-financing, non-profit making group. *J Hum Nutr* **35**, 128–33.

Stauffer JQ (1977) Hyperoxaluria and calcium oxalate nephrolithiasis after jejuno-ileal bypass. *Am J Clin Nutr* **30**, 64–71.

Wadden TA, Stunkard AJ and Brownell KD (1983) Very low calorie diets: their efficacy, safety and future. *Ann Intern Med* **99**, 675–84.

Warwick PM, Toft R and Garrow JS (1978) Individual differences in energy expenditure. *Int J Obesity* **2**, 396.

4.2 Prader Willi Syndrome

Definition

The Prader Willi Syndrome (PWS) was first described thirty years ago in Switzerland (Prader *et al* 1956) and in England five years later (Laurance 1961). It is characterized by severe congenital hypotonia, poor weight gain and feeding difficulties prior to the age of two years, followed by mild mental retardation, short stature, hypogonadism, a voracious appetite and the rapid development of obesity. Other synonyms such as 'H2O' syndrome (indicating hypotonia, hypomentia and obesity) (Engel and Hogenhuis 1965) and 'HHHO' — adding hypogonadism (Zellweger and Schneider 1968) are now not normally used.

Prevalence

Estimates of the prevalence differ. Holm (1981) suggested an incidence of 1 in 5,000–10,000, an increase on an earlier figure of 1 in 170,000 (Spencer 1968); Laurance (1985) suggests 1 in 40,000 of the population is affected, but also surmises that greater awareness of the syndrome may result in a higher incidence of diagnosis.

The only data available in the UK is membership of the PWS Association (UK) which currently is under 200 and clearly an underestimate.

Clinical features

Some patients display all of the described features, others fewer, but all are severely hypotonic at birth. If the mother has had a previous normal pregnancy she may possibly recognize that foetal movements are less with the PWS pregnancy. The floppiness affects sucking to such an extent that nasogastric feeding is essential. Nevertheless, artificial ventilation is never required and the absence of this feature helps to differentiate PWS from other causes of neonatal hypotonia, e.g. Werdnig Hoffman's disease. Although the PWS infant is grossly hypotonic there is potentially good underlying muscle power and they may be able to lift a limb against gravity, either in response to stimulation or spontaneously.

During the first six to twelve months, PWS babies are often unresponsive to either their own needs or to their environment and may not cry when hungry or when disturbed by a loud noise, painful stimuli or frightening experience. The placid infant usually progresses to a naively charming child who occasionally has temper tantrums. (These may, rarely, become worse when adult.) In addition, during the first 2–3 years of life, the infants fail to thrive. After the age of 3–4 years or sometimes earlier, there is a bizarre change in appetite (probably as a result of disorder in the appetite centre in the hypothalamus) so that the child becomes apparently insatiable. As a consequence, weight increases and obesity eventually becomes the major problem.

Other features include small hands and feet, short stature (usually below the third centile), distinctive facial appearance (high forehead, almond shaped eyes, prominent nasal bridge and slightly open mouth), hypogonadism, scoliosis and strabismus and mild mental retardation. Occasionally there are dental deformities.

A PWS child is rarely able to continue at a normal school after the age of about 7 years and then special schooling (ESN) is usually more appropriate; subsequently most patients continue at training centres.

Aetiology

Usually only one member of the family is affected, but affected identical twins are known (Gellatly, personal communication). Several sources have reported either translocation or deletion of chromosome 15 but only in approximately half the cases. The aetiology of the remainder is unknown.

Dietary management

The dietitian's involvement in the treatment of PWS ranges from advice for the two extremes of the appetite problem of the syndrome: failure to thrive in infancy and hyperphagia gross obesity in later years. The important problems of the physically and mentally handicapped have also to be considered and all these aspects are discussed in general terms elsewhere (see Sections 3.2, 3.11, 3.12 and 4.1.)

In infancy, once tube feeding is no longer required,

it is important that energy intake should not be increased beyond recommended daily requirements. By avoiding an increased food intake at this stage, there is less risk that the child will become accustomed to a higher one — undesirable when he enters the gross appetite/obesity phase.

In addition, there is evidence to suggest that PWS children require a lower energy intake than the normal child; most of them gain appropriate weight on an intake of 10–11 kcal/cm height (Pipes and Holm 1973), and some can maintain their weight on energy levels far below the recommended daily intake (Holm and Pipes 1976; Coplin et al 1976). Energy requirements during exercise are reported to be similar to the non-PWS obese subject for the same level of work (Nelson et al 1973).

There is no evidence that extra energy supplements stimulate the release of growth hormone; such erroneous advice, which has been given in the past, is distressing to parents, many of whom understandably later lose confidence in their advisers.

When the hyperphagic phase commences, early diagnosis and intervention is essential. The literature on PWS generally describes grossly obese, retarded patients with early death from obesity-related diseases. If obesity can be controlled this need not be the case. Crnic et al (1980) reported that early and comprehensive management can not only control obesity but also improve intellectual performance.

Because of the hyperphagia, adherence to a strict dietary regimen is difficult, but if taught early enough, is not impossible. Dietitians should be aware of lack of understanding of this difficulty by doctors, parents or indeed the patients themselves when old enough to have insight into their own problems. Ensuring awareness of this by all concerned avoids misunderstandings and is well worth the dietitian's time.

Many dietary regimens have been tried; strict energy control, an exchange system similar to that used in the treatment of diabetics, ketogenic diets or very low calorie diets. Some parents have attempted to use elimination type diets (dietary-linked behavioural problems have been reported in the USA), but if followed or attempted, energy restriction is also necessary, thus making the diet extremely difficult.

The regimen of choice is that which suits the individual and which provides essential nutrients; the PWS patient has to follow a diet for life so the nearer it is to normal the better.

Parents and patients must accept that diet control is vital; rules must be made and kept. Parents should be advised to weigh all food initially and not rely on guess-work when learning about the diet. Meals should be prepared so that they appear larger than they are (e.g. by using small plates, cutting meat very thinly, or spreading the food out rather than piling it up).

Variety within the diet is essential as are occasional treats — perhaps as a reward or at Christmas or on a birthday. The subject of treats needs to be discussed with the parents — for example, should siblings have them only when the PWS child is not present or will low calorie treats be acceptable to the PWS child as a substitute? Indeed many aspects of food provision for siblings must be discussed with parents. As with any diet, the PWS diet must fit in with family meals and the dietary needs of the non-PWS members of the family should not be overlooked.

Food stealing is a major problem. In one study (Page et al 1983) a behavioural approach reduced it successfully but only when the child was in a controlled setting. Any food left unguarded, including items normally accepted as unappetizing (e.g. food waste in dustbins, pet food, plants, berries, frozen products, packets of butter and margarine and plate waste), may be devoured. For successful management, families have to realize that they must resort to extensive measures which upset their usual routine and normal social behaviour. Food cupboards, freezers and refrigerators must be locked or made inaccessible. It may be easier to keep the kitchen locked which, although inconvenient, can soon become routine; the key should be hidden carefully. Other entries to the food storage areas or kitchens such as back doors, hatches and open windows must also be guarded. Siblings and other members of the family must not keep food in their rooms. Food should only be eaten at meal times so that no crisps, sweets, fruit, etc. are left lying around. A meal being prepared in the kitchen should not be left unattended nor the table set with food unsupervised; it should be cleared and dishes washed immediately. Clearly PWS individuals should not be left unsupervised at meal times. These problems are far less when dietary control has been taught early in life.

Friends, neighbours, relations, school teachers and day centre staff need to have the condition explained so that they co-operate with the diet. As the child grows so do the problems — pocket money, collecting shopping, or attending youth groups and clubs where there is a 'tuck-shop'. Parents of ordinary children often find it a wise measure to let their children have only a limited amount of spending money; PWS parents need even greater wisdom. Unfortunately there have been instances of shoplifting, money stealing or eating large meals in restaurants and cafes without the money to pay for them. It is important for others such as the police, local shopkeepers or assistants to understand and for all to remember how stressful these situations can be for both the individual and family.

Hospital admissions can cause trauma and distress for all concerned, particularly if admission is to a busy medical ward. Other patients, nurses, domestics and porters must be made aware of the management problems. Unfortunately it is common for needs other than that for which the patient is admitted, to be overlooked.

It is imperative that medical advisers, including therapists and dietitians, as well as those caring for the patient (either parents or social service agencies), appreciate the necessity for dietary intervention, while at the same time recognizing the children's mental and physical handicaps and behavioural disturbances. Unfortunately, many parents lose heart because their children are discharged from follow-up by the doctor or dietitian because there is little or no weight loss. This is especially so with the older child; doctors and others may lose patience with the child and their parents for the apparent lack of effort.

The reasons for failing to lose weight are manifold — lack of compliance with a weight reducing regimen, too high an energy intake in the basic diet, or, especially in the older child, the sheer physical impossibility of not eating because the appetite control centre has failed. Laurance (1985) suggests the child really can be kept to a reasonable weight without cruelty, but he also considers the battle is lost if one waits until later in life — say 10—12 years — before embarking on dietary intervention. Dietitians should not be pessimistic; cases have been reported where the teenagers or older patients in a controlled environment (e.g. village or hostel for the mentally handicapped, or one-person flatlet with food sources strictly controlled) have achieved weight loss with an accompanying improvement in morale and the quality of life, but these cases are rare.

A sympathetic and supportive role is essential. With the PWS patient obesity is only part of the problem, it is easy to overlook the slow development of the child. Dietitians need to co-ordinate their work, not only with the parents but with all others caring for the child, e.g. physiotherapists, speech therapists, social workers, medical and nursing staff.

Surgical treatment

Intestinal bypass operations have been tried, both jejuno-ileal and gastric, but such procedures are not always acceptable to parents and are by no means always successful. However, in one reported case, a bypass operation not only produced a loss of 55 kg which aided mobility, but resulted in improvement in mental outlook. This allowed the individual to become more socially acceptable and to develop typing skills not previously thought possible (Gellatly, personal communication).

Support organisation

Prader Willi Syndrome Association (UK), 30 Follett Drive, Abbot's Langley, Herts WD5 0LP.

This is a voluntary parents group which was established in 1980. The subscription (in 1985) is £5.00 per Prader Willi family. Interested professionals can become associate members for the same subscription. The Association publishes a newsletter regularly, arrranges local meetings and an annual meeting, usually in the Autumn. There are close links with the American counterpart (Prader Willi Syndrome Association) which was established in 1975.

The handbook for parents produced by the American organisation has been reprinted by the UK group and is currently available at £1.00. The Association has charitable status. Profits from fund-raising are directed towards research and to the provision of suitable homes for Prader Willi adults.

Further reading

Holm, Sulzbacher and Pipes (1981), *Prader Willi Syndrome*. University Park Press, Baltimore.
Bray GA, Dahms WT, Swerdloff, Fisher RH, Atkinson RL and Carrell RE (1983) The Prader Willi Syndrome: A study of 40 patients and a review of the literature. *Medicine* **62**, (2), 59—79.

References

Coplin SS, Hine JH and Gornican A (1976) Out-patient dietary management in the Prader Willi Syndrome. *J Am Diet Assoc* **68**, 330—4.
Crnic KA, Sulzbacher S, Snow J and Holm VA (1980) Preventing mental retardation associated with gross obesity in the Prader Willi Syndrome. *Paediatrics* **66**, 787—9.
Engel WK and Hogenhuis LAH (1965) Genetically determined myopathies: conditions difficult to classify: H2O syndrome. *Clinical Orthop* **39**, 34—62.
Holm VA (1981) The diagnosis of Prader Willi Syndrome. In *Prader Willi Syndrome*. Holm VA, Sulzbacher S and Pipes PL (Eds). University Park Press, Baltimore.
Holm VA and Pipes PL (1976) Food and children with Prader Willi Syndrome. *Am J Dis Childh* **130**, 1063—7.
Laurance BM (1961) Hypotonia, obesity, hypogonadism and mental retardation in children. *Arch Dis Childh* **36**, 690.
Laurance BM (1985) The Prader Willi Syndrome. *Maternal and Child Health* **10**, 106—9.
Nelson RA, Anderson LF, Gastineau CF, Hayles AB and Stamnes CL (1973) Physiology and natural history of obesity. *J Am Med Assoc* **223**, (6), 627—30.
Page TJ, Finney JW, Parrish JM and Iwata BA (1983) Assessment and reduction of food stealing in Prader Willi Children. *Applied Research in Mental Retardation*. **4**, 219—28.

Pipes PL, and Holm VA (1973) Weight control of children with Prader Willi Syndrome. *J Am Diet Assoc* **62**, 520–4.

Prader A, Labhart A and Willi H (1956) Ein syndrom von adipositas, kleinwuchs, kryptorchismus, und oligophrenie nach myatonieartigem zustand im neugeborenenalter. *Schweiz Med Wschr* **86**, 1260–1.

Spencer DA (1968) Prader Willi Syndrome. *Lancet* **ii**, 571.

Zellweger H and Schneider HJ (1968) Syndrome of hypotonia–hypomentia–hypogonadism–obesity (HHHO) or Prader Willi Syndrome. *Am J Dis Childh* **115**, 558–98.

4.3 Hyperlipidaemias and Hyperlipoproteinaemias

The involvement of the dietitian in the treatment of patients with hyperlipidaemias will differ depending on local practices. This can vary from working as part of a team running a specialized lipid clinic to responding to requests from general practitioners requiring cholesterol-lowering diets for some of their patients. For this reason, it is important to establish a local policy for the treatment of patients with raised blood lipid levels. In either case it is essential that the dietitian receives adequate information on the blood lipid levels of the patient so that the appropriate diet can be tailored to suit the individual.

4.3.1 Terminology

Lipids such as cholesterol and triglyceride are insoluble in water and therefore need to be transported in plasma bound to specific proteins called apolipoproteins (apoproteins). The resulting complexes have the solubility characteristics of proteins and are called lipoproteins. Lipoproteins are classified according to their density

1 Chylomicrons which carry dietary triglyceride from the intestine to peripheral tissues.
2 Very low density lipoproteins (VLDL) which are synthesized by the liver and carry excess triglyceride produced by the liver to other tissues.
3 Intermediate density lipoproteins (IDL) which are short-lived intermediates derived from partial degradation of VLDL.
4 Low density lipoproteins (LDL) which are formed from VLDL and transport cholesterol from the liver to the peripheral tissues.
5 High density lipoproteins (HDL) which transport excess cholesterol from cells to the liver for excretion in the bile.

Each of these lipoprotein fractions contains a different amount of cholesterol and triglyceride (together with smaller amounts of protein and phospholipids) (Table 4.3). Because the lipoprotein component itself is technically very difficult to measure, one of its other components (usually either the cholesterol or the triglyceride) is measured in order to determine the concentration of a particular lipoprotein class. More recently

Table 4.3 Percentage composition of serum lipoproteins

Lipoprotein	Cholesterol (%)	Triglycerides (%)	Protein (%)	Phospholipids (%)
Chylomicrons	5	90	2	3
VLDL	10	60	10	20
IDL	30	40	10	20
LDL	50	10	25	15
HDL	20	5	50	25

it has become possible to measure the apoprotein content of some lipoproteins.

4.3.2 Hyperlipidaemia and hyperlipoproteinaemia

Hyperlipidaemia means a higher than average amount of lipid in the blood. It can be defined as a serum cholesterol and/or triglyceride level which is above the 95th percentile of the level found in a comparable healthy population. *Hyperlipoproteinaemia* is a more precise term which means higher than normal amounts of one or more of the lipoproteins which transport lipid.

Although discussed separately below, hyperlipidaemias and hyperlipoproteinaemias are not different disorders, just different ways of looking at the same disorder. Most hyperlipidaemias (e.g. a raised total cholesterol or triglyceride level) are accompanied by an elevation in one or more lipoprotein fractions and are, in reality, hyperlipoproteinaemias.

There are however, exceptions. A hyperlipidaemia may result from two or three lipoproteins being at the upper end of the normal range. Conversely, a normal total lipid level may disguise an elevated LDL level and an abnormally low HDL.

It is therefore important to remember that measurements of *total* serum cholesterol or triglyceride (i.e. the lipid content of all the lipoprotein fractions) is of only limited value in diagnosing a lipid disorder. While total lipid levels may indicate that some lipid abnormality exists, they are an insensitive way of revealing the type of disorder. The nature of the abnormality, and its dietary and other implications, can only be determined by finding out which lipoprotein fractions are responsible for the raised total lipid level.

Hyperlipidaemias

Hypercholesterolaemia

The normal level of total cholesterol in serum is in the region of 3.8–6.7 mmol/l. This varies according to age and, to a lesser degree, sex. Thus what may be a 'normal' cholesterol level for one person may not be for another.

The total cholesterol level is directly related to the development of coronary heart disease; the incidence of this disease is reduced in populations with a mean total cholesterol level below 5.5 mmol/l. Within a population, the relationship between total cholesterol and arterial disease is less clear, partly because genetic susceptibility to heart disease varies between individuals but also because cholesterol bound in the different lipoprotein fractions has different effects. Approximately 60% of total cholesterol is found in the LDL fraction and it is LDL cholesterol which is most closely associated with heart disease. Most of the remaining cholesterol is found in the HDL fraction en route to the liver for excretion. A *high* level of HDL cholesterol is therefore likely to be beneficial and a negative (or protective) risk factor for heart disease.

However, HDL cholesterol is fairly resistant to dietary manipulation, though it may be affected beneficially by other factors such as regular exercise, cessation of smoking and reducing weight. In contrast, LDL cholesterol (and hence also total cholesterol) can be reduced by dietary measures, in particular a reduction in total (especially saturated), fat intake and to a lesser extent by an increase in polyunsaturated fat intake (i.e. an increase in the dietary P/S ratio).

The majority of patients presenting with a high total cholesterol level will have elevated LDL levels (Type IIA or IIB hyperlipoproteinaemia) and will require dietary treatment. However, in cases where the total cholesterol level is raised only mildly, it should be borne in mind that this may be due to a beneficially high *HDL* cholesterol level, in which case *no* dietary treatment will be needed. In these instances it is very important that an HDL cholesterol measurement is obtained and ideally all estimates of total serum cholesterol should be accompanied by an HDL assessment.

Hypertriglyceridaemia

Total serum triglyceride is composed mainly of VLDL triglyceride and, in the fasting state is usually less than 2.0 mmol/l. It varies with both age and sex.

The relationship between total (and VLDL) triglyceride and the development of coronary heart disease is controversial. Although the triglyceride level is associated with coronary heart disease incidence, it is now generally believed that serum triglyceride is not an *independent* risk factor. The serum triglyceride level is inversely related to the HDL cholesterol level (i.e. if triglyceride is high, then HDL cholesterol will be low) and it is probably the low HDL cholesterol level which enhances the atherosclerotic process and is the real risk factor.

However, high triglyceride levels are still of concern since they may cause acute pancreatitis. Ideally, all patients who present with acute abdominal pain where the cause is not clear should have their triglyceride level measured.

The triglyceride level is most strongly affected by energy restriction and weight loss. Carbohydrate restriction also has a marked effect. Fat restriction has much less effect on triglycerides caused by raised VLDL levels unless the P/S ratio is increased markedly. However, raised triglycerides resulting from chylomicronaemia is directly caused by fat consumption and hence does respond to fat restriction.

Measurement of serum lipids

Measurements of triglyceride must always be made on samples obtained after a 12–14-hour (usually overnight) fast. Chylomicrons can remain in the blood for *at least* eight hours after a fatty meal and, if still present, will severely distort triglyceride measurements.

Chylomicrons have less effect on total cholesterol estimation (chylomicrons contain only small amounts of cholesterol in their structure) so cholesterol can be measured non-fasting. However, alcohol should not be consumed the night before any lipid measurement because of its acute hypertriglyceridaemic effect and hence the risk of it causing misdiagnosis.

Probably the best simple way of examining patients for hyperlipidaemia is by measuring fasting total serum triglyceride and cholesterol and measuring HDL-cholesterol (after chemical precipitation). This strategy identifies patients with a mildly raised total cholesterol level which is in fact due to a high (and beneficial) HDL cholesterol.

Gross hypertriglyceridaemia can be identified without the need for chemical analysis. VLDL and chylomicrons are sufficiently large particles to scatter light and the presence of either or both of them in serum will be visible as turbidity. If a turbid serum sample is stored overnight in a refrigerator, any chylomicrons present will rise to the surface and form a skin. This will indicate either a hyperlipoproteinaemia characterized by the presence of chylomicrons (i.e. Type I or V) *or* that the subject was not in a fasted state!

Before committing a person to dietary (and/or) drug therapy at least two fasting lipid screens should be performed since there is considerable day to day variation in individual lipid levels.

Hyperlipoproteinaemias

Most patients with hyperlipidaemia can be assigned to a specific hyperlipoproteinaemia, if the appropriate measurements (i.e. total cholesterol, triglycerides, HDL cholesterol and chylomicrons) are made.

Hyperlipoproteinaemias are classified in six types (the Fredrickson classification; Beaumont *et al* 1970) depending on which lipoproteins are elevated (Table 4.4). Each hyperlipoproteinaemia is not a single disease but a group of disorders characterized by the same lipoprotein abnormality/ies.

Hyperlipoproteinaemia may be primary (genetically transmitted) or secondary to some other disease (e.g. diabetes, kidney disease and hypothyroidism). It is therefore important to establish the cause of the lipid disorder because, if secondary, treatment of the underlying disease state may fully resolve the lipaemia. Dietary treatment should not be commenced until the

cause is established and, even during treatment, further evidence of the primary cause may emerge and, possibly, necessitate a change of treatment.

Dietary treatment of hyperlipoproteinaemias

The dietary treatment of each type of hyperlipoproteinaemia is outlined below. However, these should not be interpreted as strict rules but as guidelines to be considered in conjunction with the relevant factors (e.g. lipid abnormalities, body weight and any associated disease state) in each case. In practice, different types of hyperlipoproteinaemia (especially IIB, III, IV and V) will require similar dietary measures.

Type I

The aim of treatment is to reduce chylomicron formation. Dietary treatment is as follows
1   Severely restrict fat intake, usually to about 25–35 g/day. As a consequence of the severe fat restriction, the following dietary aspects must also be considered
a)   Energy. The reduction in fat intake inevitably results in a diet low in energy. If the patient is overweight (*not* usually a feature if the disorder is familial)

Table 4.4 Classification and features of hyperlipoproteinaemias

Type	Lipoprotein(s) elevated	Serum cholesterol	Serum triglyceride	Primary (genetic) causes	Secondary causes	Notes
I	Chylomicrons	Normal or slightly raised	Very high	1 Lipoprotein lipase deficiency. 2 Apoprotein C II deficiency.	Alcoholism	Rare
IIA	LDL	Raised	Normal	Familial hypercholesterolaemia 1 Homozygous form is severe. 2 Heterozygous form mild to moderately severe.	1 Hypothyroidism 2 Nephrotic syndrome	1 Heterozygous form relatively common. 2 Enhanced risk of CHD in both types but especially in homozygous form which has a poor prognosis.
IIB	LDL and VLDL	Raised	Raised	Familial combined hyperlipoproteinaemia	1 Hypothyroidism 2 Nephrotic syndrome 3 Affluent living	1 Most common form of hyperlipoproteinaemia. 2 Carries enhanced risk of CHD.
III	IDL ('broad beta')	Raised	Raised	Familial dysbetalipoproteinaemia (Accumulation of partially degraded VLDL)		Uncommon
IV	VLDL	Normal or slightly raised	Raised	1 Mild familial hypertriglyceridaemia 2 Tangier disease	1 Diabetes or glucose intolerance. 2 Obesity 3 Excessive alcohol 4 Renal failure 5 Advanced liver disease.	1 Common 2 May predispose to atherosclerosis.
V	Chylomicrons and VLDL	Moderately raised	Very high	Severe familial hypertriglyceridaemia	1 Diabetes (poorly controlled). 2 Uraemia	Rare

then this does not matter. But in children and normal-weight adults, the energy deficiency may need to be rectified with medium-chain triglycerides (MCT); these do not form chylomicrons.

b) Essential fatty acids (efa). The daily fat allowance should include sufficient quantities of a polyunsaturated fat or oil to prevent efa deficiency.

c) Fat soluble vitamins. Supplementation may be necessary in order to prevent deficiencies.

d) Palatability/acceptability. These are particular problems with a diet of such low fat content. The use of MCT supplements may be helpful.

Type IIa

The aim of treatment is to reduce LDL and total serum cholesterol. Dietary treatment is as follows

1 Reduce total fat intake and in particular the consumption of saturated fat. This measure has the most impact on LDL and total cholesterol levels.

2 Increase the P/S ratio. This measure will help to lower the serum cholesterol but is far less important than total fat restriction. Its main value is that it can help dietary acceptability, in particular by the use of polyunsaturated spreading fats and cooking oils as a substitute for their more saturated equivalents (see Section 2.3).

3 Reduce dietary cholesterol in some cases. Cholesterol is synthesized endogenously hence the influence of dietary cholesterol on serum cholesterol is relatively small. The dietary cholesterol level must be reduced to below 300 mg/day to have any significant effect and this is almost impossible to achieve with other than a vegetarian diet. Restriction of dietary cholesterol is therefore not important in patients with mild or moderate Type IIA hyperlipoproteinaemia. However unusually high intakes of dietary cholesterol (e.g. if large numbers of eggs are eaten per week) should be corrected. In patients with severe homozygous Type IIA, characterized by grossly elevated serum cholesterol levels, complete avoidance of cholesterol-rich foods (see Section 2.3) may be necessary.

Other dietary factors to be considered

1 Energy. In children and normal-weight adults, care should be taken to ensure that the diet contains sufficient energy.

2 Fibre. Some types of fibre may have a mildly hypolipaemic effect and an adequate fibre intake should be encouraged.

Type IIB

The aims of treatment are to reduce LDL and total serum cholesterol and to reduce VLDL and total serum triglycerides. Dietary treatment is as follows

1 The attainment/maintenance of normal weight. If overweight, attainment of normal weight is the first priority. Dietary measures 2 and 3 below will automatically produce a diet of reduced energy content.

2 Reduce fat intake. For those of normal weight, some polyunsaturated fats and oils can be substituted for saturated fats.

3 Modify carbohydrate intake. Refined carbohydrates (e.g. sugar-rich items) should be restricted and, depending on the level of dietary energy required, should be replaced by fibre-rich sources of carbohydrate such as bread, cereals, potatoes and pasta.

4 Reduce alcohol intake if this is excessive.

Type III

The aims of treatment are to reduce total serum cholesterol and total serum triglycerides. Dietary treatment is the same as for Type IIB.

Type IV

The aim of treatment is to reduce the production of endogenous triglycerides. Dietary treatment is as follows

1 Achieve/maintain normal body weight. The majority of these patients are overweight and require energy restriction. This should be achieved primarily by measures 2 and 3 below.

2 Carbohydrate restriction, particularly of refined carbohydrates. A maximum of 45% of dietary energy should be comprised of carbohydrate, principally from fibre-rich sources.

3 Alcohol should be restricted.

Type V

The aims of treatment are to reduce serum chylomicron and VLDL triglyceride. Dietary treatment is as follows

1 Achieve/maintain normal body weight.

2 Restrict fat intake to a maximum of 30% of dietary energy. Where appropriate the energy deficit should be rectified with unrefined carbohydrate.

3 Alcohol should be excluded.

General dietary considerations

Follow up appointments for anyone on a lipid lowering diet are essential. The diets may be complicated and it is important to review the·patient soon after the initial interview to answer questions and give supporting information. An initial individually constructed diet sheet is necessary, and it is sensible to see whoever cooks the family meals to advise on meal suggestions, recipe adaptation, changing cooking methods and eating out.

Support is also available from family self help groups, such as the Familial Hypercholesterolaemia Association, who produce a newsletter and provide recipe ideas. Some very useful literature is also available from commercial companies (e.g. Bristol-Myers and Flora).

In order to monitor and evaluate the success of the diet, it is important that the dietitian has access to regular blood results so that the diet can be adapted accordingly. The regularity of these should be agreed locally, but may be three monthly or six monthly.

Drug therapy may be considered if dietary advice alone is unsuccessful, but diet remains the major approach and continues when drug therapy is introduced.

Support organisation

Familial Hypercholesterolaemia Association, PO Box 133, High Wycome, Bucks HP13 6LF.

Further reading

Lewis B (1976) *The hyperlipidaemias. Clinical and laboratory practice*. Blackwell Scientific Publications, Oxford.

Reference

Beaumont JL, Carlson LA, Copper GR, Feifar Z, Fredrickson DS and Strasser T (1970) Classification of hyperlipidaemias and hyperlipoproteinaemias. *Bull World Health* **43**, 891.

4.4 Diabetes Mellitus

4.4.1 Aims of dietary treatment

The main aims of dietary therapy in the treatment of diabetes are

1 To maintain blood glucose and lipids at as near normal levels as possible while maintaining optimal nutrition.

2 To minimize the risk of hypoglycaemia in diabetics treated with insulin and certain oral hypoglycaemic agents.

3 To achieve weight loss in the overweight diabetic.

The belief that diabetic control can only be achieved by means of carbohydrate restriction is no longer held. It is the energy content of the diet, rather than the amount of carbohydrate *per se*, which has the most influence on long term diabetic control. The traditional diabetic diet, based on severe carbohydrate restriction while all other foods were 'allowed freely', was relatively high in fat and may have increased the risk of cardiovascular disease, a complication to which diabetics are particularly susceptible. As a result of epidemiological evidence and the findings of clinical trials, many countries including Britain, the USA, Canada, Finland, Norway and Australia have recently revised their dietary recommendations for diabetics, now placing more emphasis on the need for control of total energy intake, reduction in fat consumption and a more liberal intake of unrefined carbohydrate.

The dietary recommendations of the British Diabetic Association (1982) are summarized in Table 4.5.

4.4.2 General dietary considerations

The sequence of diet therapy which should be followed is summarized in Fig. 4.2.

Energy

Effective long term diabetic control depends on the energy intake not exceeding (and, in the case of the overweight, being less than) energy requirement. Since

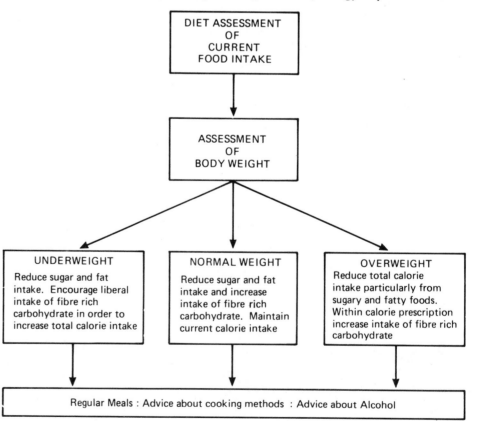

Fig. 4.2 The sequence of dietary therapy in diabetes mellitus.

Table 4.5 Dietary recommendations for diabetics (British Diabetic Association 1982)

Dietary recommendation	Notes
Controlled energy intake	Energy intake must be based on the *individual* need, with suitable adjustment for the overweight.
Increased intake of fibre-rich (slowly absorbed) carbohydrate	Half or more of the energy content of the diet should be obtained from slowly absorbed, fibre-rich carbohydrate foods (e.g. wholemeal bread, wholegrain cereals, pulses and potatoes). Rapidly absorbed carbohydrate (e.g. sugar, sweets, sweetened drinks and fibre-free starches) should only be taken in small quantities as part of a fibre-rich meal, or in cases of illness or a hypoglycaemic emergency or in conjunction with strenuous exercise.
Decreased fat intake	Ideally, fat intake should be reduced to about 35% of the total energy intake. This should be achieved primarily by a reduction in the saturated fat content of the diet, e.g. by limiting the intake of fat-rich meat and dairy products. Partial substitution of the usual fat intake with polyunsaturated fat may be necessary for dietary palatability and practicality.
Balance between carbohydrate intake and medication	In diabetics treated with insulin or certain oral hypoglycaemic agents, the timing of meals is important in order to prevent hypoglycaemia. The carbohydrate exchange/portion system remains a simple method of distributing the daily carbohydrate intake. For diabetics not requiring hypoglycaemic medication, the timing of carbohydrate consumption is not so critical, but regularly spaced meals should still be encouraged.
Weight reduction	Achieving effective weight loss is the most important dietary goal for the overweight non-insulin dependent diabetic. The low fat, high fibre-rich carbohydrate diet is recommended for this as for any other type of diabetic patient, but any dietary strategy, provided that it is nutritionally sound, is acceptable if it produces weight loss.
Salt	Diabetics should not be prescribed a diet which contains more sodium than that consumed by the non-diabetic.
Alcohol	Unless medically contraindicated, diabetics may consume alcohol as long as its energy contribution to the diet is noted.
Sorbitol, fructose and diabetic speciality foods containing them.	These foods should be regarded with caution. In the past, some of these products have been of questionable health benefit in terms of energy and carbohydrate intake and many have been used by diabetics for an unsuitable purpose (e.g. as a slimming aid). However, new legislation governing the composition and labelling of such speciality foods is likely to improve their quality and value (see Section 2.13).
Diet prescription	A diabetic diet will only be effective if it is based on *individual* nutrient needs and eating habits; standardized preprinted diet sheets are of little value. Furthermore, insulin regimens should, where possible, be chosen to fit in with a patient's existing eating habits rather than attempting to adjust the diet to a fixed insulin prescription. Professional dietetic assistance is vital and should be available at a level sufficient to provide individual assessment, counselling, education and follow-up.

individual energy requirements can differ widely from the 'average', energy requirement cannot be determined from tables quoting average energy needs. Instead, the patient's prescribed energy intake should be based on the usual energy intake, as determined by dietary enquiry.

The dietary data so obtained (e.g. regarding meal patterns and general eating habits) should also be used to form the basis of subsequent dietary modification. Obtaining good background dietary information about the patient is thus a pre-requisite for giving appropriate dietary advice.

Carbohydrate

It remains important that the diabetic avoids carbohydrate which is absorbed rapidly and produces undesirable blood glucose peaks. Traditionally, simple sugars (e.g. sucrose or glucose) have been eliminated from the diabetic diet on the grounds that they are absorbed more rapidly. However, this is now known to be incorrect and that, in an isolated form, starch and glucose have an identical rate of absorption and glycaemic effect, while sucrose has *less* effect on blood glucose levels than either of them, owing to the fructose component of the sucrose molecule (Wahlquist *et al* 1978; Bantle *et al* 1983).

This confusion arose because of the effects of dietary fibre. A mixture of carbohydrate and fibre generates a smaller rise in glycaemia than the same type and amount of carbohydrate consumed alone. Thus an apple has less effect on blood glucose than apple juice (i.e. fibre-free apple) (Haber *et al* 1977); a high-fibre cereal such as All-bran has a lesser glycaemic effect than cornflakes, despite containing four times the quantity of sugars (Jenkins *et al* 1983). Such studies, and in particular the work of Jenkins and colleagues have led to the concept of the 'glycaemic index' i.e. the glycaemic response to individual foods in relation to that of glucose. These studies have revealed that, as well as the amount of fibre, the *type* of fibre in a food is important. Different fibres have different effects; foods containing gel-forming fibres, e.g. legumes, have a much lower (i.e. better) glycaemic index than those containing cereal fibre (Jenkins *et al* 1981, 1983; Mann 1984).

The effects of foods in combination is also relevant to glycaemia. Sugar-containing marmalade by itself is a rapidly absorbed carbohydrate but has a negligible effect if consumed on a slice of wholemeal bread (Lean *et al* 1985). The protein and fat content of a meal may further influence the glycaemic effect of its carbohydrate constituents; protein stimulates insulin secretion, while fat can delay gastric emptying. Food form i.e. whether food is intact or disrupted (e.g. whole or pureed vegetables) or raw or cooked may also be relevant.

Much remains to be learnt of this complex subject. Meanwhile, dietitians should encourage their diabetic patients to choose carbohydrate foods predominantly of an unrefined, slowly absorbed type. Complete

Table 4.6 Suitability of carbohydrate for the diabetic (These are only approximate groupings; the glycaemic effect of a carbohydrate food is influenced by many factors including other foods consumed at the same time.)

Food group	Most suitable (slowly absorbed)	Intermediate	Least suitable (rapidly absorbed)
Bread	Wholemeal bread	Brown and white bread	
Flour and baked products	Wholemeal flour Wholewheat pastry High-fibre biscuits, e.g. digestive, oatcakes, crispbread.	White flour White flour pastry Plain biscuits High fibre sugar-containing cakes.	Cornflour Sweet, filled or coated biscuits Low fibre sugar-containing cakes.
Breakfast cereals	High fibre, e.g. All-bran, Weetabix, Shredded Wheat, Bran Flakes, Muesli and Porridge.	Low fibre, e.g. Cornflakes, Rice Krispies and Special K.	Sugar coated, e.g. Sugar Ricicles, Honey Smacks and Sugar Puffs.
Pasta	Wholegrain (brown) pasta	White pasta	
Rice and pudding cereals	Brown rice	White rice	Sago, semolina and tapioca
Vegetables	All, but especially pulses		
Fruit		Fresh, cooked, dried fruit. Fruit canned in natural juice. Fruit juice	Fruit canned in syrup
Beverages		Milk	Sugar-rich drinks e.g. squash and lemonade. Evaporated and Condensed milk.
Miscellaneous		Thickened soups Pizzas (white flour)	Syrup, sweets/chocolates, sugar*, honey*, jam, marmalade* jelly and ice cream.

*If consumed in isolation without a source of fibre.

avoidance of sugar is unnecessary but it should only be used in conjunction with a fibre-containing food or meal; isolated sources of sugars (e.g. a sugar-rich drink) should continue to be avoided (other than in special circumstances such as illness or hypoglycaemia).

Table 4.6 groups some carbohydrate foods according to their suitability for diabetics (i.e. their presumed glycaemic effect). Dietitians should be aware that some patients will be unfamiliar with some of the recommended foods (e.g. pulses or pasta) and may need advice regarding cooking methods and suitable recipes. The energy content of some foods made with 'good' sources of carbohydrate, e.g. wholewheat pizza or wholewheat pastry will usually be unsuitable for those who are overweight.

Fat

The diabetic has an increased risk of arterial disease and so a reduction in dietary fat, particularly from animal sources, is strongly advised. Ways of achieving this can include

1 Replacing full cream milk with skimmed or semi-skimmed milk.
2 Using a low fat spread instead of butter or margarine. If this is unacceptable to the patient, the quantity of full fat spreads used should be markedly reduced and preferably be confined to those of a poly-unsaturated nature.
3 Avoiding obvious meat fat by trimming and skimming stews, casseroles, etc.
4 Eating less lamb, pork and beef and more chicken, turkey, fish, shellfish or offal.
5 Avoiding particularly fatty foods, esepcially meat products such as sausages, paté, salami or meat pies.
6 Replacing full fat or cream cheese with reduced fat hard cheese or, better still, cottage or curd cheese.
7 Limiting cream and oil-based dressings such as mayonnaise, salad cream or french dressing. Yoghurt-based dressings or reduced fat salad cream can be useful alternatives.
8 Avoiding fried foods as much as possible; grilling, baking, boiling or braising are preferable cooking methods. Any fat which is used in cooking should be used sparingly and be of a polyunsaturated nature (e.g. sunflower, safflower or corn oil).

Protein

The diabetic's requirement for protein is no different to that of the non-diabetic. However, diabetics should be made aware that animal protein foods such as meat and cheese contain appreciable quantities of fat and energy and can upset the balance of a diabetic diet if consumed in excess. Patients should be encouraged to include sources of vegetable protein such as beans and lentils in their diet.

Alcohol

The position of alcohol in the diabetic diet has been reviewed recently by the British Diabetic Association (Connor and Marks 1985). Their conclusions can be summarized as follows

1 Unless medically contraindicated, there is no reason why diabetics should not include some alcohol in their diet, up to maximum of three 'drinks' daily (one 'drink' being half a pint of beer, a single measure of spirits or one small glass of sherry or wine). Sweet sherries, wines or liqueurs are best avoided and mixer-drinks (e.g. tonic water) should be sugar-free. 'Low carbo-hydrate' beers, lagers or ciders offer no advantage and are not recommended because of their higher than average alcohol and energy content.
2 Alcohol potentiates the action of insulin and in-hibits hepatic gluconeogenesis and hence there is always a risk, especially in the insulin treated diabetic, of hypoglycaemia and this can be severe or even fatal. For this reason, diabetics should not reduce their food intake by counting the carbohydrate content of alcoholic drinks into their diet. Furthermore, alcohol must never be consumed on an empty stomach but always with or after meals; nor should it be consumed with rapidly absorbed carbohydrate which may trigger reactive hypoglycaemia. Alcohol should not be consumed before driving or operating dangerous machinery; the risk of hypoglycaemia persists for at least four hours after the consumption of alcohol. Patients should also be warned that hypoglycaemia can mimic drunkenness; if the breath smells of alcohol, this may confuse the diagnosis.
3 All alcoholic drinks provide appreciable amounts of energy and, if consumed on a regular basis, their contribution to the total energy intake should be taken into account. Patients on weight reducing diets should ideally avoid alcohol completely; if medical or dietetic advice permits some alcohol, its energy content must be included as part of the diet and, in any event, should not exceed 10% of the total energy intake, i.e. one drink daily.
4 Treatment with oral hypoglycaemic agents is not in itself a contraindication to the use of alcohol provided the recommended maximum limits are observed. Patients should be warned of the possibility of facial flushing when taking chlorpropamide or other first generation sulphonylureas.

4.4.3 Special considerations for insulin dependent diabetics

The diet should be formulated in accordance with the general guidelines outlined in the previous section, i.e. the energy requirement should be determined by dietary enquiry and the appropriate dietary content of carbohydrate and fat can then be calculated from this figure. Fat intake should be reduced to as near to 35% of the total energy as the patient will accept; carbohydrate should comprise half or more of the total energy intake and should be mainly of a fibre-rich type. Some useful daily allowances appropriate for various levels of energy intake are summarized in Table 4.7. However, it should be borne in mind that these are targets to aim for and should not be applied too rigidly. If the dietary history reveals an eating pattern which will make attaining these levels difficult, more realistic targets should be set initially.

Table 4.7 Energy and carbohydrate content of the diet. Fat (and, if necessary, protein) allowances should be individually determined

Daily energy intake (kcal)	Recommended carbohydrate intake (g)	Number of carbohydrate exchanges
1,000 (4,200 kJ)	120	12
1,200 (5,040 kJ)	150	15
1,500 (6,300 kJ)	180	18
1,700 (7,140 kJ)	210	21
2,000 (8,400 kJ)	250	25
2,200 (9,240 kJ)	270	27
2,500 (10,500 kJ)	310	31
2,700 (11,340 kJ)	330	33
3,000 (12,600 kJ)	370	37

In addition, the following factors must also be considered in the insulin dependent patient.

Balance against insulin action

Hypoglycaemic reactions will occur if food is not eaten to cover the times of peak insulin activity, and the blood glucose level will become unacceptably high if food is taken at times when insufficient insulin is available. A regular meal pattern is therefore essential. Usually, food intake is divided into three meals and a bedtime snack with a provision for a mid-morning and mid-afternoon snack if this is necessary. A single daily insulin injection is normally given 30–40 min before breakfast. Twice daily injections are usually given half an hour before breakfast and the evening meal.

Such patterns of meals and insulin injections are convenient but not the only way of achieving good balance. Ideally, the patient's existing meal pattern should be taken into account *before* the insulin regimen is prescribed. If, for example, a light meal is usually eaten at midday and a larger meal in the evening, the type and amount of insulin given should reflect this so that there is minimal disruption to the diet. However, patients whose food intake is variable and sporadic will have to accept that a more regular eating pattern is essential.

Insulins

Figure 4.3 summarizes the activity of the main types of insulin currently available. Figure 4.4 shows a 24-hour regimen of short acting (soluble) and long acting (ultralente) insulins and the dietary pattern which complements these insulins. Figure 4.5 shows the dietary pattern which is more suitable for a combination of short and intermediate acting insulins. If a short acting insulin is given before a meal, the patient often needs a snack of 10–20 g or more of carbohydrate 2–4 hours later to prevent hypoglycaemia. It therefore follows that a mid-afternoon snack is unnecessary for a diabetic taking short acting insulin at breakfast and the evening meal only.

Diabetics who are controlled on long acting insulin alone may, or may not, require snacks between meals;

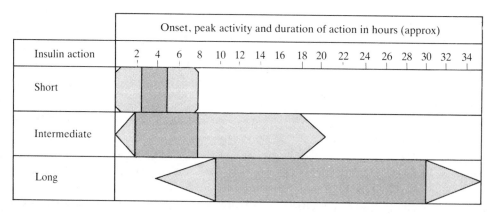

Fig. 4.3 Activity of the main types of insulin.

THERAPEUTIC DIETETICS FOR DISEASE STATES

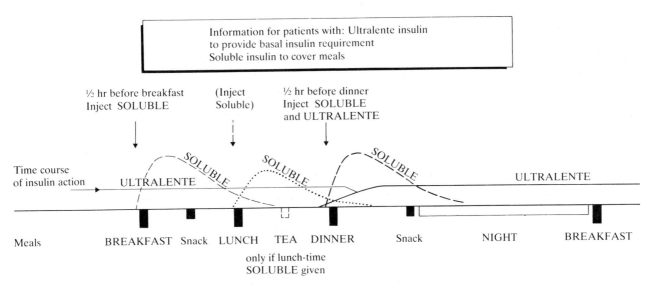

Information for patients with: Ultralente insulin
to provide basal insulin requirement
Soluble insulin to cover meals

½ hr before breakfast
Inject SOLUBLE

(Inject
Soluble)

½ hr before dinner
Inject SOLUBLE
and ULTRALENTE

Time course
of insulin action

ULTRALENTE   SOLUBLE   SOLUBLE   SOLUBLE   ULTRALENTE

Meals

BREAKFAST   Snack   LUNCH   TEA   DINNER   Snack   NIGHT   BREAKFAST

only if lunch-time
SOLUBLE given

Fig. 4.4 Dietary pattern suitable for a combination of short acting (soluble) and long acting (ultralente).

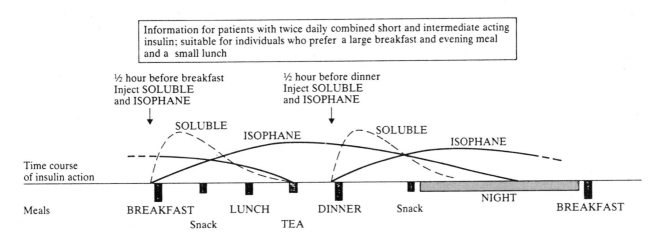

Information for patients with twice daily combined short and intermediate acting
insulin; suitable for individuals who prefer a large breakfast and evening meal
and a small lunch

½ hour before breakfast
Inject SOLUBLE
and ISOPHANE

½ hour before dinner
Inject SOLUBLE
and ISOPHANE

SOLUBLE   ISOPHANE   SOLUBLE   ISOPHANE

Time course
of insulin action

Meals

BREAKFAST   LUNCH   DINNER   Snack   NIGHT   BREAKFAST

Snack   TEA

Fig. 4.5 Dietary pattern suitable for a combination of short and intermediate insulins.

this should be assessed by monitoring the blood glucose level at these times.

An alternative method of giving insulin is via an insulin pump. This continuously injects a basal insulin supply and a bolus of insulin with meals. Such pumps are not yet in general use but have helped the blood glucose control in specific groups, e.g. pregnant diabetics, patients with peripheral neuropathy and brittle diabetics. Although dietary restrictions can be slightly less rigid, the pump does not permit total dietary freedom; avoidance of rapidly absorbed carbohydrate and a high fibre intake remain important.

Insulin can also be given by a system of multiple insulin injections which, like the pump, allows more flexibility in the timing of meals and the quantities of food consumed. Nevertheless, the composition of the diet (i.e. its fat and rapidly absorbed carbohydrate

content) should still be watched and undesirable weight gain (which will increase insulin resistance) avoided. Introduction of the pen injector, which simplifies insulin administration considerably, will make the multiple insulin regimen more acceptable and popular.

Carbohydrate exchange system

The 10 g carbohydrate exchange/portion system (see p 131) remains a useful way of distributing and regulating the daily carbohydrate intake.

Patients should be encouraged to choose carbohydrate foods of a fibre-rich type and those who are overweight should be advised which foods are the least energy-dense.

Many insulin treated diabetics find that slavish attention to the carbohydrate allowance is unnecessary;

with time and experience they become familiar with the amounts and types of food which are suitable for a particular meal.

For others, use of the full exchange system is inappropriate or too complex. With the more liberal recommendations regarding carbohydrate intake, a diet plan can be taught successfully without the exchange system, but simple quantities of staple sources of carbohydrate such as bread, cereals, potatoes and fruit and alternatives must be given. Assignment of a target *total* (or maximum) daily carbohydrate or energy allowance can be useful.

Exercise

Diabetics, like non-diabetics, should be encouraged to take physical exercise and there is no sport which is barred to the diabetic simply on the grounds of diabetes (though some potentially hazardous activities, such as hang-gliding or deep-sea diving, should have medical approval). However, in the insulin dependent patient, the effects of any overt physical activity must be considered. Exercise increases the uptake of glucose by exercising muscles and thus acts, in effect, as an extra dose of insulin. An increase in carbohydrate is therefore needed to counterbalance this effect. The amount of extra carbohydrate needed for a given activity will vary widely between individuals and most patients will learn by experience what is appropriate for them. In the past, diabetics have often been advised to take this additional carbohydrate in the form of sugar-rich drinks or confectionery. However, studies on glucose utilization during exercise have shown that this is rarely necessary or desirable. Particularly strenuous or prolonged forms of exercise may need supplements of rapidly absorbed carbohydrate, but in general an extra 20 g of mixed carbohydrate (e.g. more bread, potatoes or a larger dessert) at the meal beforehand will be

Table 4.8 Carbohydrate for exercise. (Carbohydrate requirements for exercise may vary widely between individual diabetics.)

	Carbohydrate sources
For exercise taken shortly after a meal	20 g carbohydrate additions to a main meal could comprise Extra potato, e.g. 1 medium (100 g) + 100 ml fruit juice. *or* 1 small potato (50 g) + 1 small carton of 'diet' fruit or natural yoghurt. Extra bread e.g. 1 large thick slice or 1 small roll, preferably wholemeal. 1 small carton fruit yoghurt. 2 wholemeal bran biscuits. 1 oat cookie + ⅓ pint milk *or* 100 ml fruit juice. 1 small wholemeal spiced fruit bun.
For exercise taken 2–3 hours after a meal (and before the next meal/snack)	10 g carbohydrate snacks 1 digestive, muesli or bran biscuit. 1 small packet reduced fat crisps. 100 ml fruit juice *or* 1 portion fresh fruit. 1 small carton 'diet' fruit yoghurt. 20 g carbohydrate snacks 1 'no added sugar' fruit bar. 1 oat and nut bar + 100 ml fruit juice. 1 small 'crunch' bar + ⅓ pint milk. 1 small slice fruit malt loaf.
Carbohydrate 'top-ups' to be taken during strenuous or prolonged exercise or when strenuous exercise has ceased	10 g carbohydrate 'top-ups' 100 ml fruit juice. 50 ml Lucozade. 3 Dextrosol *or* 2 boiled sweets *or* 3 small mints. 1 mini-Marathon. 1 cream biscuit. 1 small chocolate wafer, e.g. Bandit. 20 g carbohydrate 'top-ups' 1 *mini* Mars/Picnic/Bounty bar. 100 ml fruit juice + 1 wholemeal biscuit. 1 Penguin bar *or* Wagon Wheel 1 small slice sponge cake. 200 ml chocolate milk drink. 1 fruit yoghurt. 1 mini Swiss roll. 30 g carbohydrate 'top-ups' 1 small scone (preferably wholemeal). 1 fruit bun or muffin.

sufficient. If exercise is taken more than 2—3 hours after a meal, approximately 20 g of carbohydrate in the form of biscuits or a snack bar will be needed. Further top-ups may be needed during the course of the activity, depending on its nature and duration. Some suggested forms of carbohydrate for exercise are summarized in Table 4.8.

Diabetics are often not warned that they may be more at risk from hypoglycaemia *after* the exercise period than during it. This is because, even when the exercise has ceased, the body continues to use glucose at an elevated rate to replete muscle glycogen stores. If a meal is not due immediately, a carbohydrate snack may therefore be needed at this time.

Diabetics should also be warned not to make excessive reductions in their insulin dose as a means of minimizing the risk of hypoglycaemia during exercise. The enhanced glucose utilization of exercise can only occur in the presence of insulin; the combination of exercise and insufficient insulin will lead to rapid deterioration in control. For the same reason, diabetics who are in a state of poor control should temporarily avoid strenuous exercise as this will only exacerbate the problem.

Diabetics who take insulin should be reminded that additional physical activity which is not deliberately intended to be a form of 'exercise' or 'sport', e.g. vigorous housework, shopping or running to catch a bus, will nevertheless have the same effects and can sometimes result in hypoglycaemia. Patients must therefore *always* carry a source of rapidly absorbed carbohydrate (e.g. glucose tablets) with them, wherever they go, in case of emergency.

Illness

During times of illness there is an increased risk of ketoacidosis and extra care must be taken to balance insulin and carbohydrate. Even if the patient cannot, or does not feel like, eating 'normal' food, it is imperative that the usual amount of insulin is taken, and often more insulin than usual will be needed. The effects of the insulin must still be 'covered' by carbohydrate in some form, if necessary in a liquid or semi-solid form. It is not, however, necessary to force feed the prescribed amount of carbohydrate at specific times of day. The total carbohydrate intake can usually be reduced safely by up to one-quarter provided that the remaining carbohydrate is spaced out evenly throughout the day, e.g. via hourly snacks of 10—20 g carbohydrate instead of the customary pattern. If medicines are required, sweetened versions can be used to help meet carbohydrate needs. For a patient who is very nauseated, a few mouthfuls of sweetened fluid every 20—30 min should maintain a satisfactory blood glucose level. Some suitable carbohydrate at times of illness are given in Table 4.9.

Table 4.9 Suitable carbohydrate at times of illness (Some of these forms of carbohydrate are very concentrated and should be measured carefully.)

Food	Portion providing 10 g carbohydrate
Liquids	
Lucozade	50 ml (2 fl.oz)
Grape juice (unsweetened)	50 ml (2 fl.oz)
Fruit juice (unsweetened)	100 ml (4 fl.oz)
Cola	100 ml (4 fl.oz)
Lemonade	150 ml (5 fl.oz)
Milk	200 ml (7 fl.oz)
Soup (thickened, creamed)	200 ml (7 fl.oz)
Soup (tomato, canned)	100 ml (4 fl.oz)
Solids	
Ice-cream	50 g (2 oz)
Natural yoghurt	150 g (5 oz)
Sweetened fruit yoghurt	50 g (2 fl.oz)
Drinking chocolate, Ovaltine or Horlicks	2 heaped teaspoons
Sugar or glucose	2 level teaspoons
Honey, jam or syrup	2 level teaspoons
Glucose tablets	3 tablets
Build-Up (Carnation)	½ sachet

4.4.4 Special dietary considerations for non-insulin dependent diabetics

Body weight

Most non-insulin dependent diabetics are overweight. For these patients, the most important dietary objective is to achieve and maintain a desirable weight; this will reduce hyperglycaemia, hyperlipidaemia and hypertension.

Weight loss can only be accomplished by a reduction of total energy intake below the level of individual energy expenditure; the distribution of the diet is less important than for that of the insulin requiring diabetic. Although any diet which achieves weight loss will be beneficial, a diet with a reduced fat and high carbohydrate content is preferable in terms of blood glucose control, satiety and re-education of eating habits. Standardized printed weight reducing diet sheets are of little value; time and effort is needed to find a suitable slimming strategy for each person.

Oral hypoglycaemic drugs

The distribution and timing of carbohydrate intake depends upon whether oral hypoglycaemic drugs form part of the treatment. These drugs either stimulate the production of insulin or make the body more sensitive to its action. They can cause hypoglycaemic reactions, although these are relatively rare.

In order to prevent hypoglycaemic reactions and maintain good blood glucose control, the carbohydrate intake of patients given hypoglycaemic drugs should be divided fairly evenly between three meals a day (with some of it being consumed as between-meal snacks if necessary). The use of a precise carbohydrate exchange system is usually unnecessary, but some guide to the total carbohydrate for the day, and how this can be obtained, is helpful. In those who are overweight, the emphasis should be on a diet of appropriate energy content together with meal plan advice to ensure a suitable carbohydrate distribution.

Patients treated by diet alone can be more flexible regarding the timing of carbohydrate intake, but the importance of regular meals comprised of the right types of foods (and, if overweight, limited in energy content) should still be stressed.

4.4.5 Dietary management of children with diabetes

Children with diabetes have the same nutritional requirements as non-diabetic children. Dietary advice should aim to encourage good eating habits for the whole family rather than isolating the diabetic child with a separate eating pattern.

Energy intake

Assessment of the child's *usual* energy intake and body weight prior to diagnosis is the best basis for energy prescription because it allows for variation in individual needs. The energy content of the diet must be reviewed regularly (at least annually) as energy needs rise with growth and activity. Undesirably rapid weight gain should be kept in check by dietary regulation, often in conjunction with a change in insulin prescription.

Nutrient composition

A mixed and varied diet should provide all the essential nutrients for a child's growth and development. The British Diabetic Association's dietary recommendations should be the goal to work towards in the dietary therapy of children as well as adults. Since such a diet is also a healthy one for non-diabetics, the dietary guidelines and instruction on cooking methods should be recommended for the whole family. Care should be

taken to ensure that fat regulation in young children does not result in an inadequate intake of either energy or fat soluble vitamins.

Timing and distribution of meals

Minimizing the risk of hypoglycaemia by regulating the timing and distribution of meals is as important in diabetic children as it is in all insulin dependent adults. However, it is much more difficult to achieve this in practice because of a child's variable energy demands. Getting the balance right is largely a process of trial and error. However, in the early stages following diagnosis, the family will require some guidelines about amounts of food to match various activities, e.g. an extra 20 g of carbohydrate before swimming or a sport involving running. With experience and a growing knowledge of food values and insulin action, families become more confident about changing the meal or snack size or altering the insulin dose to suit the circumstances.

Education

If possible, the family with a newly diagnosed diabetic child should be introduced to the dietary aims gradually. During the initial hospital admission or out-patient visit, a dietitian should see the family and child together and give simple advice about avoiding concentrated sources of rapidly absorbed carbohydrates (e.g. sugar-containing drinks) and the need for regular meals and snacks but keeping the child's eating pattern as unchanged as possible. Following this, a further session, preferably within a week, should cover facts about basic nutrition, explanation of the balance between food intake and insulin, and how the diet can be varied using carbohydrate exchanges. Initial weighing of food may be essential until the family are accustomed to portion sizes but handy measures are recommended for routine use. Families and children are more receptive in their own environment and so a home visit by the dietitian is invaluable; this also enables the dietitian to assess the families' understanding of the diet and to see how they have adjusted.

Education must be continued and reinforced in out-patient sessions. It is important to assess the actual *food* intake and not just to enquire how much carbohydrate is being consumed. As children approach adolescence they should be encouraged to take full responsibility for their diet so that when the time comes to leave home they have a full understanding of their diet and can cope with all situations. Diabetic children can benefit greatly by spending time in the company of other diabetics at children's education weekends or summer camps. Dietitians too can learn a lot about childhood diabetes by helping out at one of these camps.

4.4.6 Dietary management of diabetics in pregnancy

The dietary requirements of the pregnant diabetic are no different from those of the non-diabetic (see Section 3.1). The clinical problem of diabetes and pregnancy can be classified into two groups

1 Those who develop diabetes during pregnancy but previously had normal carbohydrate tolerance, i.e. gestational onset diabetes.
2 Those who have diabetes and become pregnant, i.e. pre-gestational diabetes.

In either group, maintaining as near-normal blood glucose levels as possible is essential to ensure normal growth and development of the foetus.

Gestational onset diabetes

Although patients may not have insulin prescribed initially, many are likely to have insulin prescribed in the last trimester of pregnancy. Sulphonylureas and other oral hypoglycaemic drugs are not usually used. Insulin therapy is often prescribed for a patient with a fasting plasma glucose above 5 mmol/l; however, some centres would choose a higher threshold before adding insulin to diet therapy.

The same sequence of dietary therapy should be followed as that of an insulin treated diabetic. Initially, an assessment must be made of the individual's current energy intake and body weight. Strict weight reduction in pregnancy should be avoided, but moderate energy restriction will help normalize the blood glucose levels of those who are overweight. Within the framework of an individual energy prescription, advice about food choice and quantities and timing of meals should be given. Because of the likelihood of insulin therapy in gestational onset diabetes and the strict blood glucose control required, it is essential to teach each patient about the carbohydrate exchange system at an early stage so that the patient is familiar with careful portioning of food at meal and snack times. The diet must be sound in terms of all nutrients, minerals, vitamins and trace elements, and alcohol should be avoided.

Pregestational diabetes

The incidence of major congenital abnormalities is about four times greater in infants of diabetic mothers than in the general population. There is increasing evidence that women who give birth to infants with congenital malformations are drawn mainly from those who have had poor control of their diabetes between the time of conception and about eight weeks of gestation. There is a growing consensus that good diabetic control during this period is necessary to prevent foetal abnormalities. Since pregnancy is rarely confirmed before about six weeks, it follows that an effort to attain good diabetic control should begin *before* conception. This has led to the organisation of pre-pregnancy clinics in some centres, a relatively new idea which will no doubt be taken up by others if resources are available. The main aims of these clinics are to assess the patients' fitness for pregnancy, identify and treat infertility as early as possible and to obtain maximum co-operation from patients and their partners in order to achieve optimum diabetic control before conception and throughout pregnancy. This requires careful tailoring of diet, insulin and physical activity with the help of home blood glucose monitoring. Patients who are not already on a twice daily regimen of short plus an intermediate or long acting insulin will be changed to this type of prescription or sometimes even more frequent injections. The diet should be reviewed, and possibly changed, and patients encouraged to follow it closely, taking care with the energy and carbohydrate content of each meal and snack. Patients are taught to carry out blood glucose monitoring several times daily and to adjust their own insulin dosage to obtain pre-prandial glucose concentrations of approximately 4 mmol/l. The patients are seen regularly by both the doctor and the dietitian. Weight gain should be monitored closely, and attention should also be paid to overall nutrient intake especially calcium, iron, vitamins and trace elements. Ideally, all alcohol should be avoided.

Morning sickness, heartburn and constipation are all problems of pregnancy which require extra dietetic skill if they are to be overcome without upsetting the balance of blood glucose control. Successful management of morning sickness may require an alteration in the size and timing of meals accompanied by a change in insulin prescription.

The use of pure, multiple-dose insulin regimens and a rigid approach to diet, self-monitored and modified by frequent checks on the pre-prandial blood glucose levels, can produce virtual euglycaemia but requires considerable effort by the patient who must be highly motivated. For most, the prospect of a healthy child at the end of the pregnancy is sufficient to achieve this. The attainment of near-normal glycaemic control has resulted in decreased perinatal morbidity and mortality, with more home care and less hospitalization.

4.4.7 Effective diabetic dietary education

Individual needs

Dietary compliance among diabetics has, in the past, often been poor and in part this has been due to the unrealistic and over-restrictive dietary advice which has often been given. All people are highly resistant to dietary change. It is therefore of fundamental importance that dietary advice is tailored to individual needs. Ideally, the patient should see the same dietitian at each consultation so that a rapport from an initial interview can be built upon. Following a diet history, the dietitian must adapt the patient's diet, but only to a degree which is acceptable to the patient, taking into account psychological, physical and socio-economic factors. The dietitian must be approachable, flexible, understanding and advise in a non-judgmental manner. Close liaison with the physicians and other health care professionals is essential.

Where possible, the insulin regimen should be prescribed to fit in with a patient's existing eating pattern and for this reason a preliminary consultation with the dietitian prior to seeing the physician is valuable. Patients should understand the reasons for their diet therapy and, in order to achieve their dietary goals, should be taught about basic nutrition, food selection and preparation, daily food plans and the nutrient content of foods. Education to this degree cannot be achieved in a single consultation; adequate follow-up is essential to reinforce teaching, answer queries and expand awareness.

Diet Sheets

The use of standardized pre-printed diet sheets is strongly discouraged. A variety of printed advice leaflets covering the spectrum of diet therapy should be at the disposal of the dietitian with space for individual diet therapy to be documented.

Printed advice should be given about cooking methods, along with some basic recipes. There are several diabetic cookery books on the market which may be recommended if appropriate. Comprehensive information on manufactured, convenience and takeaway foods is also available.

Teaching aids

Assessing food intake and giving advice about portion sizes and types of food can be made easier and much more interesting with the aid of photographs, food models and examples of food packaging. Some centres have initiated education programmes for diabetics in which a teaching room is allocated for group learning and demonstrations. The facilities and teaching aids offered include blackboards, video equipment and food preparation and demonstration equipment in an effort to create a suitable environment for effective learning.

Many patients can get valuable support and advice by joining the local branch of the British Diabetic Association.

Support organisation

The British Diabetic Association, 10 Queen Anne Street, London W1M 0BD. Tel: 01-323-1531.

Useful books for patients

Longstaff R and Mann J (1984) *The diabetics' cookbook*. Martin Dunitz Ltd, London.
Mann J and the Oxford Dietetic Group (1982) *The diabetics' diet book*. Martin Dunitz Ltd, London.
Metcalfe J (1985) *Cooking for diabetics*. Thorsons, Wellingborough.
Thomas B (1985) *Diet and diabetes*. Churchill Livingstone, Edinburgh.

Video for Asian diabetics

So you have diabetes. How to eat for health
An integrated education programme for Asian diabetics and their families. A 12 min video with dialogue in Hindi but accompanying users notes available in English/Gujerati; English/Urdu; English/Punjabi. Produced by Brent Nutrition and Research Group in association with Brent Health Education Team.

Publications and products available from the British Diabetic Association
(1987 prices are given as a guideline to cost)

Leaflets

1 *Food values list for diabetics* DH223, price 20 p
2 *Diet and diabetes* DH210, price 5 p
3 *Diet during illness* DH217, price 5 p
4 *The diabetic at school* DH127, price 10 p
5 *Exercise and sport* DH133, price 10 p
6 *Hypoglycaemia and diet* DH211, price 10 p
7 *Home preserving* DH220, price 30 p
A wide range of similarly priced leaflets on other aspects of diabetes is also available.

Books

1 *Insulin-dependent diabetes handbook*. Published in conjunction with Thorsons. Wellingborough. Price £7.50.
2 *Non-insulin dependent diabetes handbook* Published in conjunction with Thorsons, Wellingborough. Price £4.50.
3 *Better cookery for diabetics*. Low fat high fibre recipes. Price £2.95.
4 *Cooking the new diabetic way* — the high fibre, calorie conscious cookbook. Price £3.95.

5 *Vegetarian on a diet*. Price £4.30.
6 *The diabetic's microwave cookbook*. Price £1.75.
7 *Packed lunches and snacks*. Price £1.75.
8 *Simple diabetic cookery*. Price 50 p.
9 *Simple home baking*. Price 50 p.
10 *Christmas cookery*. Price 50 p.
11 *Countdown*. A guide to the carbohydrate and calorie content of manufactured foods and drinks. Price £3.95.

Teaching aids

1 *British Diabetic Association diet teaching set* — comprised of 36 pictures which depict a series of foods. Available as slides or photographs and in ethnic or English versions. Price £20 per set with teaching notes.
2 *Countdown* board game. Price £5.75.

Dietary aids

1 Beaker. Made of plastic for measuring exact amounts of fluid and wholefood carbohydrate sources. Price 40 p.
2 Measuring spoons. Set of four plastic spoons for accurate measurement of carbohydrate portions. Price £1.45.
3 BDA food and diabetes pad. Basic dietary advice for GPs to give newly diagnosed diabetics before they have a hospital consultation. These pads are available only to dietitians (for distribution to GPs), and not directly available to doctors.

Further reading

Dietary recommendations for diabetics for the 1980s. A policy statement by the British Diabetic Association (1982) *Hum Nutr: Appl Nutr* **36A**, 378–94.

Nutrition Sub-committee of the Medical Advisory Committee of the British Diabetic Association (1982) The role of the dietitian in the management of the diabetic. *Hum Nutr: Appl Nutr* **36A**, 395–400.

American Diabetes Association (1984) Policy Statement: glycaemic effects of carbohydrates. *Diab Care* **7**, 607–8.

American Diabetes Association (1979) Special report: principles of nutrition and dietary recommendation for individuals with diabetes mellitus. *Diabetes* **28**, 1027–30.

Canadian Diabetes Association Special Report Committee (1981) 1980 guidelines for the nutritional management of diabetes mellitus. *J Canad Diab Assoc* **42**, 110–8.

References

Bantle JP, Laine DC, Castle GW, William Thomas J, Hoogwerf BJ and Goetz FC (1983) Post-prandial glucose and insulin responses to meals containing different carbohydrates in normal and diabetic subjects. *N Engl J Med* **309**, 7–12.

British Diabetic Association (1982) Dietary recommendations for diabetics for the 1980s. *Hum Nutr: Appl Nutr* **36A**, 378–94.

Connor H and Marks V (1985) Alcohol and diabetes. A position paper prepared by the Nutrition Sub-committee of the British Diabetic Association. *Hum Nutr: Appl Nutr* **39A**, 393–9.

Haber GB, Heaton KW, Murphy D and Burroughs LF (1977) Depletion and disruption of dietary fibre. *Lancet* **ii**, 679–82.

Jenkins DJA, Wolever TMS, Taylor RH, Barker H, Fielden H, Baldwin JM, Bowling AC, Newman HC, Jenkins AL and Goff DV (1981) Glycaemic index of foods: a physiological basis for carbohydrate exchange. *Am J Clin Nutr* **34**, 362–6.

Jenkins DJA, Wolever TMS, Jenkins AL, Thorne MJ, Lee R, Kalmusky J, Reichert R and Wong GS (1983) The glycaemic index of foods tested in diabetic patients: a new basis for carbohydrate exchange favouring the use of legumes. *Diabetologia* **24**, 257–64.

Lean MEJ, Tennison BR and Williams DRR (1985) Glycaemic effect of bread and marmalade in insulin dependent diabetes. *Diabetic Med* **2**, 117–20.

Mann JI (1984) What carbohydrate foods should diabetics eat? *Br Med J* **288**, 1025–6.

Wahlquist ML, Wilmshurst EG, Murton CR and Richardson EN (1978) The effect of chain length on glucose absorption and the related metabolic response. *Am J Clin Nutr* **31**, 1998–2001.

4.5   Disorders of the Thyroid Gland

The thyroid gland secretes two hormones — thyroxine (T4) and triiodothyronine (T3). The output of these hormones is regulated by the pituitary by means of thyroid stimulating hormone (TSH).

T3 and T4 have profound effects on the rate of many metabolic activities. Disturbances in thyroid function can therefore affect growth, BMR, energy balance and heat production.

4.5.1   Hyperthyroidism (thyrotoxicosis)

Excessive production of thyroid hormone (usually as a result of Graves disease or an adenoma) results in

1   An increased metabolic rate, tissue catabolism and weight loss.
2   Vasodilation and sweating due to excessive heat production.
3   Muscular atrophy and weakness due to the accelerated protein metabolism.
4   Accelerated absorption of carbohydrate from the gastrointestinal tract resulting in a rapid post-prandial rise in the blood glucose level. However, carbohydrate utilization is also increased.
5   Decreased lipid levels, in particular serum cholesterol, as a result of the enhanced conversion of cholesterol to bile acids.
6   Decalcification of bone owing to an increased rate of bone resorption, sometimes producing hypercalcaemia and hypercalciuria.

Treatment

Treatment may be
1   Surgical. Thyroidectomy may be performed (usually with prior treatment with anti-thyroid drugs or beta-blockers to make the patient euthyroid).
2   Medical. Treatment may be anti-thyroid drugs (e.g. propylthiouracil or carbimazole) or by administration of iodine (which reduces thyroid hormone release).

Dietary implications

Although the treatment for hyperthyroidism is non-dietary, it does have dietary implications

1   Prior to surgery, an attempt should be made to improve the nutritional status of those who have suffered severe weight loss. As well as being high in energy the diet should contain adequate protein and vitamins (especially of the B group).
2   After successful treatment, the patient's appetite may increase but the energy requirement will be lower than during the state of thyrotoxicosis. There is thus a risk of obesity. Weight gain should be monitored so that excessive weight gain can be corrected at an early stage.

4.5.2   Hypothyroidism

Causation

Hypothyroidism may be
1   Idiopathic (cretinism in infants or myxodoema in adults).
2   Iatrogenic (e.g. a consequence of thyroidectomy or chronic consumption of iodine-containing medicines).
3   Dietary (due to iodine deficiency or excessive consumption of goitrogens which impair production of thyroxine).

Dietary causes of hypothyroidism are extremely rare in developed countries.

Features

Features of hypothyroidism may include
1   Reduced BMR.
2   Lowered heat production and consequent intolerance to cold.
3   Obesity. However, in the early stages, anorexia may offset the reduced energy requirements and weight *loss* may be a feature.
4   Mental retardation (in untreated infants) and reduced mental acuity in adults.
5   Reduced protein metabolism leading to retarded growth in children.
6   Delayed gastric emptying and decreased intestinal mobility (leading to nausea, vomiting, abdominal distension and constipation).
7   Mild anaemia due to hypoplasia of bone marrow.

Treatment

Replacement therapy with thyroid hormones reverses all the metabolic abnormalities. No special dietary measures are required other than for the correction of obesity if this persists after treatment.

4.5.3 Goitre

Goitre is the term used to describe an enlargement of the thyroid gland. Endemic goitre is still common in underdeveloped areas of the world and is the result of either a dietary insufficiency of iodine or excessive consumption of goitrogens which interfere with the uptake and utilization of iodide by the thyroid gland. (Iodine is an essential constituent of thyroid hormones T3 and T4.)

In the UK goitre is most likely to be a consequence of thyroiditis, anti-immune disease or a side effect of treatment with certain drugs, possibly in conjunction with a low iodine intake.

Goitre can be symptomless or it can be accompanied by either hypothyroidism or hyperthyroidism. Iodine supplementation can prevent endemic goitre but is not usually an effective way of treating it once established. Treatment usually requires the administration of thyroxine (which reduces the pituitary output of TSH and hence the size of the thyroid gland).

4.6 Disorders of the Parathyroid Glands

Parathormone (PTH), the hormone produced by the parathyroid glands, has a vital role in calcium and phosphorus metabolism. Some of the effects of PTH occur as a result of its influence on vitamin D metabolism.

PTH secretion is regulated primarily by the concentration of ionized calcium in the blood; a fall in the calcium level stimulates PTH release. This results in the following effects which restore the calcium level to normal

1 In the kidney. Tubular reabsorption of calcium is increased and that of phosphate decreased. PTH also stimulates the hydroxylation of 25-hydroxyvitamin D (25-OHD) to the active metabolite, 1,25 dihydroxy-vitamin D (1,25(OH)$_2$D). This in turn promotes calcium absorption and mobilization.

2 In bone. PTH stimulates osteocytes to resorb calcium which can then be released into the circulation.

4.6.1 Hyperparathyroidism

There are two categories

1 Primary hyperparathyroidism. This is a result of parathyroid adenoma, carcinoma or hyperplasia.

2 Secondary hyperparathyroidism. This can be a feature of vitamin D deficiency, states where vitamin D metabolism is altered (e.g. prolonged anticonvulsant therapy or renal or liver disease) or hypocalcaemia.

Symptoms

The main features of hyperparathyroidism are hypercalcaemia and hypophosphataemia. Often the condition is symptomless and discovered by chance, but it may be accompanied by fatigue, weakness, anorexia and weight loss. Hypercalciuria may result in polyuria. Occasionally, severe bone demineralization may lead to bone disease (e.g. osteitis fibrosa cystica).

Treatment

Usually this is by surgical parathyroidectomy. Following surgery, patients with bone disease may require large supplements of calcium (intravenously or orally) in order to meet the high demand for calcium by remineralizing bone. Occasionally, hypocalcaemia may be a post-operative complication and this may require the dietetic measures described for hypoparathyroidism.

4.6.2 Hypoparathyroidism

Idiopathic hypoparathyroidism is rare; it is usually a consequence (sometimes inadvertent) of thyroid or parathyroid surgery.

Symptoms

Hypocalcaemia and hyperphosphataemia may be accompanied by tetany, cataracts and alterations in hair and skin texture.

Treatment

1 As a first step, hyperphosphataemia should be reduced by temporary imposition of a low phosphate diet (see Section 2.7.2).

2 When the serum phosphate level is near normal, vitamin D can then be given. Supraphysiological amounts of vitamin D (e.g. up to 5 mg (200,000 units) per day) will be required, but the precise dose needed will vary according to the patient's age, calcium intake and the degree of severity of the condition. 1.25 mg (50,000 units) per day is often a useful starting dose. Vitamin D preparations such as dihydrotachysterol, alfacalcidol or calcitriol, which act more rapidly than vitamin D, may be useful but they are much more expensive.

3 Calcium supplementation of around 1000−3000 mg/day may be necessary.

THERAPEUTIC DIETETICS FOR DISEASE STATES

4.7 Inborn Errors of Metabolism

4.7.1 Phenylketonuria (PKU)

This is an inherited disorder in which there is a deficiency of the enzymes necessary for the breakdown of the amino acid phenylalanine to tyrosine. This results in a rise in the plasma levels of phenylalanine and a fall in the level of tyrosine. The urine contains abnormal metabolites of phenylalanine. If the condition is not detected and treated in early infancy the majority of affected individuals will become severely mentally retarded. However, because of neonatal screening, early detection and treatment is now general and normal development is usual.

Treatment consists of controlling the phenylalanine levels in the blood by dietary modification. The amount of phenylalanine in the blood must be neither high enough to cause damage nor so low that normal growth and development is prevented. The desirable level is approximately three times the upper limit of normal in infancy but can be rather higher in older children (Table 4.10).

Table 4.10 Acceptable phenylalanine blood levels in children of different ages with phenylketonuria

Age range (years)	Phenylalanine (mmol/l)
0−2	0.2−0.4
2−4	Up to 0.5
4−8	Up to 0.6
8−10	Up to 1.0
Over 10	Up to 1.2

Principles of dietary management

1 Reduce the dietary phenylalanine intake to that amount which maintains the desired level in the blood, remembering that levels should not be allowed to fall below 0.2 mmol/l for prolonged periods.

The amount of phenylalanine tolerated varies greatly from patient to patient. Some children will tolerate only 200 mg, and a few only 150 mg, daily, while others can be well controlled on 500 mg. The amount tolerated daily at six weeks of age will not alter much as the child grows. There may be a slight decrease at around six months when the rate of growth slows down and there may be an increased requirement at periods of rapid growth later in childhood.

2 Supply sufficient protein for normal growth and development. Phenylalanine is present in all proteins and the amount tolerated by the phenylketonuric child will be supplied by a little as 3−10 g protein daily. This amount of protein is clearly not adequate and therefore a phenylalanine-free protein substitute must be given. There are a number of preparations available (Table 4.11).

Table 4.11 Protein substitutes used in the treatment of phenylketonuria

Product	Manufacturer	Vitamin supplements required?	Mineral supplements required?
Minafen	Cow and Gate	Yes	No
Lofenalac	Mead Johnson	No	No
Albumaid XP	SHS	Yes	No
Aminogran food supplement	Allen and Hanbury	Yes	Yes
PKaid I	SHS	Yes	Yes
Maxamaid XP	SHS	No	No

3 The diet must at all times supply all the vitamins, minerals and trace elements necessary. Except for Lofenalac and Maxamaid XP, all the protein substitutes need supplementing with vitamins and, in some cases, minerals. Care must be taken to ensure that the appropriate supplements for the particular protein substitute are consumed (Table 4.11).

4 The diet must provide enough energy for normal growth and activity. Low protein bread, biscuits and pasta as well as fats, sugars and starches are important sources of energy.

The nutritional adequacy of any diet is most easily assessed by monitoring the rate of growth in length and weight. As well as regular blood tests for phenylalanine levels, it is important that PKU children are weighed and measured and the results recorded on centile charts so that any decline in the rate of growth can be spotted and the diet adjusted.

Introduction of the diet in infancy

Before commencing a low phenylalanine diet, a quantitative estimation of plasma phenylalanine must be made in order to confirm the diagnosis and indicate the number of days needed on a diet completely free from phenylalanine. In centres specializing in the treatment of phenylketonuria these results should be available within hours of the blood sample being taken so that if any feed is needed, the baby may continue with either breast or bottle as before. If days elapse before the information is available, the baby should continue to be breast fed or, if bottle fed, be given a whey-based feed such as SMA Gold Cap, Farley's Osterfeed or Cow and Gate Premium.

Bottle feeding

The protein substitutes most suited to infants are those which when made up in 12.5–15% solutions provide a similar concentration of protein and energy to cows' milk-based baby feeding formulae. Preparations available in Britain are Minafen (Cow and Gate) and Lofenalac (Mead Johnson). When the diet is first started, provided that the plasma phenylalanine levels can be measured several times a week, Minafen or Lofenalac *only* should be given for up to four days depending on the initial phenylalanine level (Table 4.12).

Table 4.12 Length of time required on a phenylalanine-free diet

Initial blood phenylalanine level (mmol/l)	Period required on phenylalanine-free protein substitute (days)
Over 3.0	4
2.4–3.0	3
1.8–2.4	1
1.2–1.8	—

After the appropriate period on a phenylalanine-free diet, phenylalanine must be given. This may be in the form of unboiled pasteurized milk (silver or red cap) or a whey-based proprietary baby milk such as SMA Gold Cap. Baby milks are particularly suitable for premature babies, but great care must be taken to make up the formula accurately. Scoops of powder must be levelled carefully and not over compressed. 50 mg phenylalanine will be provided by 30 ml pasteurized milk or 2 level scoops SMA Gold Cap. Full term normal weight babies should initially be given 200 mg phenylalanine daily (Table 4.13).

If the blood phenylalanine level does not fall steadily to the desired level then a reduction in the phenylalanine intake may be necessary. However, some phenylalanine must always be given and a baby will seldom tolerate less than 150 mg daily. Failure to respond to the diet may indicate that the baby is not consuming enough of

Table 4.13 Formulation of a diet providing approximately 200 mg phenylalanine suitable for a normal weight phenylketonuric infant

Phenylalanine-free protein substitute. (quantity required per day)	Phenylalanine source (quantity required per day)
400–500 ml Minafen (150–200 ml per kg body weight)	120 ml cows' milk *or* 8 scoops of SMA Gold Cap + 240 ml water
400–500 ml Lofenalac (200–250 ml per kg body weight)	90 ml cows' milk *or* 6 scoops of SMA Gold Cap + 180 ml water

the phenylalanine-free preparation (Minafen/Lofenalac) to provide the protein and energy required and this will be demonstrated by little or no increase in weight. Alternatively, there may be an underlying infection keeping the baby in a catabolic state.

Breast feeding and phenylketonuria

When a woman has been successfully breast feeding her baby, the diagnosis of phenylketonuria is made more traumatic if it means she has to stop feeding in this way. A certain amount of breast feeding may be possible. However, if the mother is already relying on complementary feeding or is not particularly enthusiastic about breast feeding, it is probably wise to feed the baby exclusively by bottle right from the start, especially if none of those concerned (dietitian, paediatrician and mother) has much experience in the management of PKU. The mother who already has a PKU child and understands the principles of the diet and is keen to breast feed, or a woman who has successfully breast fed previous children, will be more suitable candidates for breast feeding the PKU infant. It must be made clear that breast feeding must be discontinued if satisfactory control has not been achieved within two or three weeks.

Breast feeding regimen for infants. Initially the procedure is as for the bottle fed baby. After confirmation of the diagnosis, a phenylalanine-free diet should be given for an appropriate period (Table 4.14a) during which time the mother must maintain lactation by expressing her milk. When breast feeding is recommenced, the amount of breast milk and hence phenylalanine that the baby receives is regulated by giving carefully measured feeds of Minafen or Lofenalac five times daily followed by breast feeds on demand. (Table 4.14b) If the serum phenylalanine level falls too low the volume of complementary feed is reduced; if it remains high the amount of Minafen/Lofenalac is increased (Table 4.14c).

Appropriate vitamin and mineral supplements should be given, but water and fruit juices should be discouraged as they will reduce the volume of breast milk taken.

Table 4.14a–c Dietary formulation for the breast fed phenylketonuric infant

a) Stage I: Immediately after confirmation of diagnosis

Initial plasma phenylalanine (mmol/l)	Phenylalanine-free protein substitute (ml × number feeds daily)		Breast feeds
	Minafen	Lofenalac	
Greater than 0.2	150–200 ml on demand	150–200 ml on demand	Nil for 3 days
1.2–2.0	150–200 ml on demand	150–200 ml on demand	Nil for 2 days
0.9–1.5	30 ml × 5	40 ml × 5	After each bottle
Less than 0.9	—	—	On demand

b) Stage II: Reintroduction of breast feeding

Initial plasma phenylalanine (mmol/l)	Phenylalanine-free protein substitute (ml × number feeds daily)		Breast feeds
	Minafen	Lofenalac	
Greater than 0.2	60 ml × 5	80 ml × 5	After each bottle
1.2–2.0	45 ml × 5	60 ml × 5	After each bottle

c) Stage III: Adjustment in the light of subsequent blood tests

Plasma phenylalanine (mmol/l)	Phenylalanine-free protein substitute (ml × number feeds daily)		Breast feeds
	Minafen	Lofenalac	
Over 0.45	Increase by 15 ml × 5	Increase by 20 ml × 5	Baby should take less
Less than 0.2	Decrease by 15 ml × 5	Decrease by 10 ml × 5	Baby should take more

Weaning

Bottle fed infants

At around 12 weeks (or when the baby reaches 5 kg if that is later), low protein foods should be introduced with a spoon after one feed, gradually increasing to after three feeds daily. The first food is usually Cow and Gate Aminex biscuit or Aproten Crispbread, crushed and mixed to a porridge with hot water, followed by a fruit dessert. Once the baby is taking a measurable quantity from the spoon (e.g. half a rusk), phenylalanine-containing solids such as baby cereal may be given as a part of the phenylalanine allowance (Table 4.15) mixed with water and/or a measured portion of cows' milk.

Table 4.15 Portions of foods containing 50 mg phenylalanine. More extensive lists including information on the phenylalanine content of manufactured foods are available to dietitians on application to the National Society for Phenylketonuria and Allied Disorders

Food	Quantity
Milk (plain, pasteurized)	30 ml
Cream	
single	40 ml
double	60 ml
Potatoes	
boiled or mashed	75 g
roasted in oven	40 g
chips	30 g
canned new, drained	100 g
jacket weighed with skin	55 g
Brussel sprouts	50 g
Broccoli	45 g
Banana	one
Cornflakes	15 g
Rice Krispies	15 g
Sugar Puffs/Smacks	15 g
Weetabix/Weetaflakes	10 g
Shredded Wheat/Shreddies	10 g
Oatmeal (raw)	7.5 g
Ready Brek	7.5 g
Farleys Rusk	1 rusk
Baby Rice (raw)	15 g
Baby Rice (boiled)	45 g

Once solids are being taken well, the volume of protein substitute should be reduced and the protein increased by adding an amino acid mixture such as PKaid I or Aminogran food supplement so that by the age of 18 months, the child is having 2 g amino acid mixture/kg body weight daily, divided into three doses, together with a mineral supplement (Table 4.16) The amino acids and mineral supplement should be mixed to a paste with water or fat emulsion and flavoured with undiluted orange cordial or milk shake syrup, or taken as a drink according to what is most acceptable to the child concerned. Ketovite (Paines and Byrne) supplementary vitamin tablets and liquid should be given. It is important to ensure that any reduction in energy due to reduction in the amount of Minafen/Lofenalac taken is compensated for by an increased intake of solid foods or by giving measured amounts of glucose polymer and fat emulsion if poor weight gain indicates that more energy is required.

Table 4.16 Example of changing from Minafen or Lofenalac to amino acid supplement*

Minafen/Lofenalac		Amino acid mixture*		Mineral mixture†	
(g/day)	(product scoops)	(g/day)	(product scoops)	(g/day)	(product scoops)
100	(25)	5	(1)		
75	(19)	10	(2)	2.7	(1)
50	(13)	15	(3)	5.4	(2)
—		25	(5)	8.0	(3)

*Aminogran food supplement (Allen and Hanbury) or PKaid I (SHS)
†Aminogran mineral supplement (Allen and Hanbury) or Metabolic mineral mixture (SHS)

Breast fed infants

From 3–4 months onwards solids may be introduced. Initially, a 50 mg phenylalanine portion of cereal (e.g. one Farley's rusk) is mixed with a little boiled water or expressed breast milk and given *before* the Minafen/Lofenalac, with the breast feeds being given last. Gradually the measured solids are increased and the breast feeds decreased.

From approximately six months of age additional protein will be required and should be given as Aminogran Food Supplement or PKaid I mixed with an Aminogran mineral or metabolic mineral in the proportion of 5 g amino acids and 1.3 g ($\frac{1}{2}$ scoop) minerals. This can be given as a paste flavoured with concentrated fruit juice given off a spoon, at first giving one teaspoon a day before one of the feeds, gradually increasing to 1 teaspoon three times daily. Then the amount of the paste is increased so that the baby eventually receives 3 g amino acids/kg/day and a maximum of 8 g minerals divided into three doses. As the amino acid mixture is taken in progressively larger amounts, the phenylalanine-free protein substitute (Minafen or Lofenalac) and breast feeds should be reduced gradually and finally stopped altogether.

Regulation of control

Once a child is established on a diet the amount of phenylalanine tolerated does not alter greatly but blood levels will fluctuate from time to time.

Reasons for high phenylalanine levels

High phenylalanine levels may result from
1 Infection. This is the most usual reason for a high phenylalanine level in a normally well controlled child. Any infection will cause catabolism and hence a rise the amount of phenylalanine in the blood. As soon as the infection is over, the levels will return to normal. During an illness the diet should not be forced. If the infection is a gastroenteritis, clear fluids for 24 hours (as for any other child) are the correct treatment.
2 Dietary error. After the introduction of solids, careless measurement of phenylalanine exchanges or misunderstanding of the concept of exchanges may explain the high level.
3 Dietary inadequacy. If the child is taking insufficient protein substitute or obtaining insufficient energy from the diet, growth will not occur and the phenylalanine consumed will not be taken up.
4 Dietary cheating. Once the child is mobile and not under constant supervision, stealing high protein foods may be a problem. Parents should be advised to keep food out of reach.
5 Contribution from free foods. In older children the larger portions of 'free' foods such as vegetables which they eat to satisfy their increased appetites may contribute considerable amounts of phenylalanine. If this results in a higher blood phenylalanine level than is desirable, a 25 mg or 50 mg phenylalanine portion should be taken off the daily allowance.

Reasons for low phenylalanine levels

Excessively low phenylalanine levels may result from
1 All allowances not being taken. Sometimes a phenylalanine portion will be refused; this should be replaced with another more acceptable food or by an appropriate volume of milk.
2 A growth spurt. At times of rapid growth the requirement for phenylalanine will be increased.
3 Vomiting. Babies who frequently regurgitate some of their feed may lose some of their milk allowance and it is difficult to judge just how much has been lost. If the blood phenylalanine levels are very low the milk intake should be increased by 15 ml increments until a satisfactory level is achieved. Once the baby is on to solids the posseting will stop and then the phenylalanine intake may need to be reduced again.

Vomiting as a result of an infection will usually be for only a short period and the phenylalanine levels will return to normal as soon as the normal diet is resumed.

Diet and pregnancy

Women with PKU who have high phenylalanine levels at the time of conception have a high risk of bearing children with congenital defects (e.g. a small head and mental retardation).

There is now evidence that if diet is introduced before conception and carried on throughout pregnancy a normal child will be born. Women with PKU must be advised to return to a strict diet before stopping any contraceptive measures and to continue on this diet until they conceive. Once pregnancy has been confirmed the diet should be adjusted to provide for the needs of pregnancy. These include

1 Adequate protein. Protein can be supplied by a protein substitute such as the specially modified form of Maxamaid XP — Maxamum XP available from SHS for use in pregnancy with a tyrosine supplement of 4 g daily, or PKaid with added tyrosine. Using Maxamum XP, vitamin and mineral supplements are not required. With PKaid, metabolic mineral mixture and Ketovite tablets and liquid are needed.

2 Appropriate phenylalanine. Before the woman becomes pregnant and during the first part of the pregnancy, the phenylalanine requirement will be similar to the amount needed in childhood to keep the level in the blood at approximately 0.3 mmol/l (i.e. 300–500 mg daily). From the 20th week of the pregnancy the phenylalanine requirement will rise rapidly as the foetus grows, until the diet contains about three times the initial amount.

3 Adequate energy. When pregnant, the phenylketonuric woman should have an energy intake which is sufficient to permit weight gain at the appropriate rate. If overweight, she should be encouraged to lose the excess *before* starting the pregnancy as it is difficult to keep the blood phenylalanine level down during weight loss.

4.7.2 Atypical phenylketonuria

This is a benign form of hyperphenylalaninaemia which does not usually require much dietary modification. Infants with initial phenylalanine levels of less than 0.9 mmol/l should be given SMA Gold Cap at the rate of 2 g protein per kg (125 ml/kg) plus Minafen or Lofenalac on demand. Breast fed babies should continue to be breast fed; if the phenylalanine levels remain above 0.6 mmol/l a small amount of complementary feed of Minafen or Lofenalac may be necessary to reduce the volume taken from the breast.

4.7.3 Homocystinuria

This inborn error of metabolism is due to lack of the enzyme cystathionase which is required for the breakdown of methionine to cystine. Untreated, there is an accumulation of homocystine in the blood and urine,

and the blood level of cystine is low and that of methionine is raised. There are two forms of the disease

1 Pyridoxine responsive. Giving pyridoxine promotes the production of the necessary enzyme.

2 Non-pyridoxine responsive. If pyridoxine fails to improve the biochemical condition within 7–10 days it may be assumed that the child has homocystinuria which must be treated with a low methionine diet. The principles of management are similar to those for phenylketonuria. Methionine is restricted to the amount tolerated by limiting the quantity of natural protein and the deficit made up with a protein substitute free from methionine and supplemented with cystine, e.g. Albumaid RVHB (SHS).

A diet suitable for an infant with homocystinuria can be constructed as follows

1 Albumaid RVHB — 3 g/kg/day.

2 Metabolic mineral mixture — 1.5 g/kg/day to a maximum of 8 g.

3 Glucose polymer and fat emulsion to make up the energy content to 80 kcal/100 ml feed fed at the rate of 150–250 ml/kg/day.

4 Cows' milk — pasteurized silver or red top starting at 120 ml (120 mg methionine) per day and adjusted in the light of blood tests. The baby is eventually weaned on to 20 mg methionine exchanges or 1 g protein exchanges as for PKU. PKU exchanges may be used but a more generous portion of some legumes can be allowed since these foods have a low methionine content in relation to their protein value, e.g. 20 g baked beans will provide one phenylalanine exchange (50 mg phenylalanine) but 35 g baked beans can be consumed to obtain one methionine exchange (20 mg methionine).

5 Vitamin supplements of Ketovite tablets and liquid are needed and extra pyridoxine (200 mg daily) is also advisable.

Those affected by homocystinuria should remain on their diet indefinitely since as well as mental retardation, the condition affects the connective tissue and can cause skeletal deformities and dislocation of the lenses of the eyes. Homocystinuria also causes increased stickiness of the blood platelets, and thrombosis has been the cause of death in untreated cases.

4.7.4 Maple syrup urine disease (MSUD)

MSUD is an inherited condition involving the metabolism of isoleucine, leucine and valine. Affected infants usually become seriously ill in the first few days of life. After the initial treatment of the acidosis by dialysis or by an infusion of dextrose with subcutaneous insulin infusion, a suitable diet is introduced. A formula similar to that for homocystinuria using MSUDaid (SHS) instead of Albumaid RVHB is appropriate with small amounts of cows' milk to provide some leucine, isoleucine and valine starting with 30 ml and increased according to the results of blood tests. It may be necessary to give supplements of either leucine, isoleucine or valine as it is not possible to alter the intake of one of these amino acids on its own using a natural protein. The required amino acid should be given in doses measured in multiples of 25 mg which are added to the daily MSUDaid formula.

A high energy intake is necessary at all times. During infections the protein should be stopped and high energy fluids such as a 25% glucose polymer solution or Hycal, Fortical or liquid Maxijul should be given.

4.7.5 Organic acidaemias (e.g. methylmalonic and propionic acidaemia)

Some forms of these conditions may respond to large doses of vitamins. For example, methylmalonic acidaemia can be treated with vitamin B12 and propionic acidaemia with biotin. However, if there is no response to these vitamins, a high energy, low protein diet is essential. Infants should be given SMA Gold Cap at a rate which initially provides 0.5 g protein per kg body weight, i.e. 30 ml/kg with fluid and energy requirements made up with water, fat emulsion and glucose polymer to provide a volume of 150–200 ml/kg daily and an energy intake of up to 200 kcal/kg daily. When the intake of SMA Gold Cap is very small, Ketovite tablets and liquid should be given and a mineral supplement such as Aminogran mineral supplement or metabolic mineral mixture in sufficient quantities to provide the recommended intake appropriate to the patient's age.

4.7.6 Hyperammonaemia

The dietary management of this condition is similar to that for organic acidaemias, i.e. it is treated with a high energy, low protein diet.

During infections causing catabolism the protein in the diet should be stopped and high energy fluids given freely as in MSUD. Adequate vitamin and mineral supplements are essential.

4.7.7 Galactosaemia

Galactosaemia due to galactokinase deficiency or the very rare diphosphate-4-epimerase deficiency, is treated with a lactose-free diet. Other possible sources of galactose such as raffinoses and stachyoses in fruits and vegetables are unlikely to affect the control since the human gut does not produce the enzymes necessary for the breakdown of these substances (Clothier and Davidson 1983).

The diet must be completely free from cows' and other mammalian milks, milk products such as cheese, cream, butter and yoghurt and foods which have milk added to improve the flavour and texture such as bread and margarine (see Section 2.11.4).

A lactose-free milk substitute such as Formula S (Cow and Gate), Prosobee (Mead Johnson) or Wysoy (Wyeth) should be given to replace breast milk or milk-based formulae. All these preparations are fully fortified with minerals and vitamins. These milk substitutes can also be used to replace milk in cooking.

Lists of lactose-free manufactured foods should be given to patients with the warning that labels on packets must be checked each time and any food said to contain milk, whey, casein, caseinate or lactose should be avoided. Parents should also be warned that medicines, especially tablets, may contain lactose as an extender and therefore the pharmacist should be asked to check that any medicines prescribed are lactose-free.

Control is assessed by monitoring the level of galactose-1-phosphate in the blood at regular intervals.

Support organisation

The National Society for Phenylketonuria and Allied Disorders (NSPKU), 26 Towngate Grove, Mirfield, West Yorkshire.

Further reading

General

Collins JE and Leonard JV (1985) The dietary management of inborn errors of metabolism. *Hum Nutr: Appl Nutr* **39A**, 255.

Forfar JO and Arneil GC Metabolic disorders. In *Textbook of paediatrics* Vol 2, 3e. Longman, Harlow.

Francis DEM (1986) *Diets for sick children* 4e. Blackwell Scientific Publications, Oxford.

Francis D and Smith I (1982) Amino acid disorders. In *Textbook of paediatric nutrition* 2e Burman D and Holton JB (Eds). Churchill Livingstone, Edinburgh.

Sinclair L (1979) *Metabolic disease in childhood*. Blackwell Scientific Publications, Oxford.

Stanbury JB, Wyngaarden JB, Frederickson DS (1983) *The metabolic basis of inherited disease 5e*. McGraw-Hill, Maidenhead.

Phenylketonuria

Frances DEM and Smith I (1981) Breast feeding regime for the treatment of infants with phenylketonuria. *Applied Nutrition I* Bateman C (Ed). John Libbey, London.

Holton J and Tyfield L (1980) *The child with phenylketonuria* 2e. Society for Phenylketonuria and Allied Disorders, Mirfield.

Komrower GM, Sardharwalla IB, Coutts JMJ and Ingham D (1979) Management of maternal PKU: an emerging clinical problem. *Br Med J* **1**, 1383–7.

Neilson K, Wamberg E and Weber J (1979) Successful outcome of pregnancy in a PKU woman after low phenylalanine diet introduced before conception. *Lancet* **i**, 1245.

Smith I, Clayton B and Wolff OH (1975) New variant of phenylketonuria with progressive neurological illness unresponsive to phenylalanine restriction. *Lancet* **17 May**, 1108.

Smith I, Lobascher ME, Stevenson JE, Wolff OH, Grubel-Kaiser S and Bickel H (1978) Effect of stopping low phenylalanine diet on intellectual progress of children with phenylketonuria. *Br Med J* **2**, 723.

Walker V, Clayton BE, Ersser RS, Francis DEM, Lilly P, Seakins JWT, Smith I and Whiteman PD (1981) Hyperphenylalaninaemia of various types among three quarters of a million neonates tested in a screening programme. *Arch Dis Childh* **56**, 759–64.

Organic acidaemias

Laing SS (1985) The dietary challenge of propionic acidaemia in an Asian girl. *Hum Nutr: Appl Nutr* **39A**, 273.

Galactosaemia

Donnell GN, Koch R, Fishler K, Ng WG (1980) Clinical aspects of galactosaemia. In *Inborn errors of carbohydrate metabolism*. Burman D Hilton JB and Pennock CA (Eds) pp 103–15. MTP Press, Lancaster.

Reference

Clothier CM and Davidson DC (1983) Galactosaemia workshop report. *Hum Nutr: Appl Nutr* **37A**, 483.

B: Disorders of the Mouth and Gastrointestinal Tract

Diseases of the gastrointestinal tract and changes in gut function will inevitably have profound effects on nutritional and metabolic processes. Treatment of gastrointestinal disease by drugs, surgery or radiotherapy can also result in decreased appetite and changes in the normal mechanism for the digestion and absorption of food.

Loss of body weight is often a reflection of gastrointestinal disease and a diet history may reveal obvious nutritional deficiencies associated with the underlying disease, eating problems, psychological problems and surgical conditions.

4.8 Diseases of the Mouth

Healthy teeth and gums are important for good digestion. Dental caries, periodontal disease and poorly fitting dentures are often implicated in malnutrition and indigestion. When giving dietary advice it is important to ensure that the patient can masticate his/her food adequately.

4.8.1 Dental caries

Dental caries results from demineralization of the enamel surface of the tooth by acids produced from dietary sugars by microbial action. Initially mineral disappears from the sub-surface of the tooth and if this process is not checked or reversed, a cavity will develop in which more bacterial growth can occur causing further dissolution of enamel and progression of the lesion into the dentine and towards the pulp. Eventually the tooth may be lost.

Causation

The factors which determine the extent of dental caries are

The bacterial flora of the mouth

Dental caries does not occur in the absence of the appropriate bacteria. *Streptococcus mutans* is probably the most significant organism for initiating lesions. It converts sucrose into glucan, a viscous and sticky polymer which adheres to the surface of the tooth. This enables other acid-forming bacteria such as lactobacilli to colonize the tooth and once the critical pH of 5.5 is reached, the enamel will begin to dissolve.

Substrates for acid production

The presence in the mouth of fermentable sugars, such as sucrose and glucose, is essential for the development of dental caries. Within minutes of their consumption, such sugars cause the pH in dental plaque to fall below the critical pH (5.5) for enamel dissolution. This fall in pH will occur irrespective of the amount of sucrose consumed (or whether it comes from an apple or a bar of chocolate) and the normal oral pH of 7.0 will only be restored about 30 min after the sugar has been finally swallowed. The quantity of sugar eaten is therefore less important than the time taken to consume it and the interval before more is taken. Normal pH will return sooner if an item is consumed quickly rather than sipped or sucked slowly. For example, a sugar-rich drink consumed rapidly will cause less damage than one containing less sugar but sipped over a period of time. A packet of sweets eaten at frequent intervals during the day will result in acid conditions in the mouth for most of that period; if the same sweets are eaten all at once, the normal pH can be restored within half an hour. The type of sugar-containing food eaten is also relevant to caries formation; items which are sticky and can leave residues in the teeth (e.g. toffees, dates or raisins) can also result in cariogenic conditions persisting in the mouth for extended periods of time.

The acidity of foods eaten

Acid foods (such as citrus fruits or juices) inevitably lower the mouth pH and hence produce cariogenic conditions. Cola drinks are particularly acidic and thus even sugar-free cola is still potentially damaging to teeth (but to a lesser extent than the sugar-containing type). Finishing a meal with an alkaline food (such as cheese, milk or peanuts) can help to raise the pH of the mouth.

The resistance of the teeth

There is considerable variability in the resistance of tooth enamel to decay. Those with crowded teeth or poorly developed enamel are most vulnerable. Fluoride can markedly increase enamel resistance since it results in the formation of fluorhydroxyapatite crystals in the tooth matrix which are more resistant to acid erosion than unfluoridated hydroxyapatite. The maximum benefit from fluoride is obtained if it is available during the period of tooth formation, i.e. before the tooth erupts through the gum. Once the tooth has emerged, further protection can be obtained from topical or dietary fluoride.

Oral hygiene

Proper cleansing of the teeth and gums by means of brushing and flossing is essential to remove plaque and accumulation of debris at the base of the teeth which can lead to gum inflammation (gingivitis). Patients undergoing radiotherapy to the head and neck or chemotherapy may be more susceptible to dental caries and good oral hygiene is essential throughout their treatment.

Treatment and prevention of dental caries

Fillings

Fillings do not prevent caries but merely repair the damage caused. Caries can still occur around or alongside fillings if preventative measures are not observed.

Oral hygiene

Correct and regular brushing and flossing of the teeth and gums is essential to help prevent both caries and gum disease.

Diet and fluoride supplementation.

Complete exclusion of fermentable sugars from the diet is neither practical nor desirable since they are present in many nutritious foods (e.g. fruits) as well as in manufactured confectionery. However, children should be discouraged as far as possible from consuming sugar-rich drinks and sweets and ideally these should only be eaten at meal times and the teeth cleaned afterwards. In practice, most children do eat sweets at other times and if this cannot be prevented then they should at least be taught to avoid the sticky or slowly sucked items and that their intake of all sweets should be 'few and far between'.

The availability of adequate fluoride, either systemically or topically, is important. This can be obtained in several ways

Drinking water.
Some parts of the country have a naturally high level of fluoride in the drinking water; other areas add fluoride artificially to the water supply. A water fluoride content of 1.0—1.5 ppm has been shown to reduce significantly the incidence of dental caries.

Fluoride supplements.
These are available in either tablet or liquid form, the latter being especially useful for babies and young children who will benefit most from fluoride supplementation. However, before these supplements are given it is essential to check the local fluoride water content since too high a fluoride intake can cause mottling of the teeth. Local dentists are usually the best people to advise as to whether supplements would be beneficial. If the fluoride content of the local water supply is less than 0.3 ppm, the fluoride supplements given in Table 4.17 should be given.

Table 4.17 Recommended levels of fluoride intake.

Age	Fluoride supplement (mg/day)
2 weeks—2 years	0.25
2 years—4 years	0.5
4 years—6 years	1.0

If the fluoride content of the local water supply is between 0.3—0.7 ppm, no supplements should be given below the age of 2 years. Thereafter, only half of the recommended levels of supplementation described in Table 4.17 should be given.

If the fluoride content of water exceeds 0.7 ppm, additional fluoride supplements are probably unnecessary.

Fluoride toothpastes.
Tooth enamel will accrue fluoride from toothpaste to some extent and thus be strengthened further, but the benefit will be less if fluoride was not already available systemically during the stage of tooth formation.

Topical fluoride.
Fluoride can be 'painted' on to teeth in the form of a varnish or, more commonly, a gel and this can be a useful way of remineralizing enamel in the pre-cavitation stage of decalcification. Routine applications can be beneficial to children, particularly those on long term medication which is syrup-based.

Fluoride mouth rinses.
These also arrest decalcification, encourage remineralization and will increase the benefit from a fluoride toothpaste. Mouth rinses are more suitable for adults than children (who tend to swallow them).

Fissure sealing

In children, the vulnerable biting surfaces of the teeth

can be coated with a thin layer of plastic sealant. This is a very effective way of preventing decay especially on molars where the deep grooves readily accumulate plaque and are not easily accessible to the toothbrush. This procedure can only be carried out by a dentist and should ideally be performed as soon as the crown of each permanent tooth emerges (i.e. around the age of six years). If left later than this, the coating will also seal in any decay process which has already commenced and this may cause more damage than if the tooth is left alone.

4.8.2 Periodontal disease

Healthy gums can withstand hard usage. The massaging effect of chewing unrefined foods helps to keep both the teeth and gums healthy. A soft diet, rich in refined carbohydrate, tends to stick round the teeth and forms an ideal medium for bacterial growth causing the gum margin to become red and inflamed (gingivitis). Histological changes in the gingival crevice can be seen within 2–4 days after stopping normal oral hygiene. It is therefore particularly important that the teeth and gums of those who are acutely ill or unable to care for themselves are cleansed regularly.

Deficiencies of certain vitamins, particularly vitamin C, may produce similar inflammation and the teeth may become loose from the lack of cement which normally holds them to the jaw. However, lack of vitamin C is not usually a common factor in the cause of periodontal disease. The disease is treated by improved oral hygiene and antibiotic therapy if necessary. The amount of refined carbohydrate eaten should be reduced and unrefined carbohydrate increased as the condition of the gums improves.

Periodontal disease and dental caries are frequently seen together, though this is not always the case. Both can be prevented if children are taught how to care for their teeth as part of the foundation of good eating habits. It is most important that dentists, doctors, dietitians, health educators and school teachers work together to provide sound advice in antenatal clinics, children's clinics and schools.

4.8.3 Mouth lesions related to nutritional deficiencies

Deficiencies of practically all the vitamins of the B group have an effect on the soft tissues of the mouth. A sore mouth and pain on eating may lead to anorexia and result in multiple nutritional deficiencies.

Angular stomatitis

Angular stomatitis is an infection of the skin at the corners of the mouth and responds rapidly to large doses of riboflavin and sometimes pyridoxine. It also occurs in iron deficiency anaemia. A common cause of angular stomatitis is ill-fitting dentures! Radiotherapy to the head and neck can also cause angular stomatitis and lesions of the oral mucosa (see Section 5.1.4).

Cheilosis

Cheilosis is a zone of red denuded epithelium at the line of closure of the lips. It is seen in people with pellagra and often associated with angular stomatitis. It is not likely that a lack of one specific vitamin or nutrient is the sole cause and a good mixed diet with multi-vitamin therapy should help to improve the condition.

Scurvy

A lack of vitamin C causes weakening of periodontal fibres and the teeth may become loose and fall out. The gums become tender and bleed easily. Treatment is by vitamin therapy and sources of vitamin C should be included in the diet regularly.

Vitamin A deficiency

Deficiency of vitamin A may cause hypoplasia in the enamel and dentine of the teeth of children.

Vitamin D deficiency

Deficiency of vitamin D causes defective calcification of the dentine of the teeth and may increase susceptibility to dental caries. Eruption of the teeth may be delayed in children with rickets. Vitamin D therapy should be given and good sources of vitamin D taken in the diet, together with exposure to sunlight where possible.

Patients with lesions of the mouth resulting from vitamin deficiencies should find a soft or even liquid diet more acceptable to take. Very hot, cold, salty or spicy foods should be avoided until the lesions have healed (Table 4.18).

Anaemia

Iron deficiency and pernicious anaemia both result in changes in the tongue causing it to become very red, sore and smooth. The deficiencies should be corrected by iron and vitamin B12 as appropriate and a soft diet taken until the condition improves.

4.8.4 Disorders of the salivary glands

Inflammation of the parotid glands due to either the mumps virus or bacterial infection may make chewing and swallowing painful and difficult. A high protein, high energy fluid diet using either commercially available sip feeds, liquidized foods or a combination of both should be given until the inflammation subsides (see Section 1.12.2).

Salivary calculi cause pain and difficulty on eating. A soft or high protein, high energy fluid diet should be consumed (see Section 1.12.2). Removal of the stones is usually by surgical excision and the diet gradually regraded to normal as the mouth heals.

4.8.5 Fractured jaws and oral surgery

Patients with fractured jaws are likely to require wiring of the jaws. Jaw wiring may also be required in some cases of oral surgery. In both cases nutritionally complete commercially available liquid feeds are the most suitable means of providing nutrition (Section 1.12.2). If patients can sip these through a straw and consume adequate fluid, energy and protein, they should be encouraged to do so. In most cases the jaws remain wired for approximately 6–8 weeks. Many patients can be managed successfully at home taking a high protein, high energy fluid diet. Variety is important and a range of savoury and sweet nourishing fluids should be recommended together with liquidized meals if the patient wishes and is able to take them. However if they are unable to suck or unwilling to take adequate amounts, a nasogastric tube may need to be passed to provide nutritional support until oral fluids can be taken (see Section 1.12.3).

As the wires are relaxed and ultimately removed, the diet should be regraded from nourishing fluids to a liquidized, soft or semi-solid diet, with protein and energy supplements if indicated, until a normal diet can be taken.

Careful attention should be given to oral hygiene as protein and energy-containing fluids are an ideal medium for bacterial growth.

Patients whose jaws are wired for the treatment of frank obesity obviously do not require a high energy intake. This use of jaw wiring in obesity is discussed in Section 4.1.3; (p 342).

4.8.6 Cancer of the mouth and pharynx

Cancer of the mouth and pharynx causes difficulties in chewing and swallowing food and many patients experience anorexia and weight loss. These tumours are treated by surgical excision and/or radiotherapy. Chemotherapy may also be used.

Prior to treatment a soft, semi-solid or fluid diet should be given. If the mouth is sore, very hot, cold, salty and spicy foods should be avoided (Table 4.18). Protein and energy supplements may be required to help prevent further weight loss and maintain nutritional status (see p 74). If an inadequate oral diet is consumed, nasogastric feeding may be required (see Section 1.12.3).

Table 4.18 Advice for patients with a sore mouth or throat

1 Meals should be small and frequent.
2 A soft, semi-solid diet or nourishing fluids may be better tolerated than solid foods.
3 Very hot, salty and spicy foods such as pepper, curries or bottled sauces should be avoided.
4 Food should be eaten lukewarm or cold rather than hot.
5 Well chilled foods and drinks may be soothing.
6 Acid fruits and fruit juices (such as orange, grapefruit, lemon or tomato juice) should be avoided as they may sting the mouth and throat.
7 Dry meals should be avoided; plenty of sauce or gravy should be added to meals.
8 Strong alcoholic drinks (such as spirits and sherries) should be avoided.
9 Protein and energy supplements should be used as directed.
10 Ill-fitting dentures should be removed when eating.
11 Care should be taken with oral hygiene; teeth should be brushed with a soft brush and the mouth rinsed with a mouthwash after each meal.
12 Smoking and smoky atmospheres should be avoided.
13 All medications should be taken as directed.

The benefit of pre-operative feeding is debatable and early surgery may be preferred with nutritional support provided post-operatively. Where surgery is required it may necessitate extensive reconstruction of the face and mouth (e.g. Commandos procedure) resulting in severe disfiguration. At the time of surgery a nasogastric tube should be inserted and feeding using a commercially prepared enteral feed commenced post-operatively once gastric emptying is established (see Section 1.12.3). A soft, high protein, high energy light diet should be introduced when oral diet is tolerated and enteral feeding via the nasogastric tube phased out. These patients require regular and practical dietetic advice in order to encourage their interest in, and adequate consumption of, food.

Radiation of the mouth will cause tender, swollen tissues and management should be by either nasogastric feeding or sip feeding using nutritionally complete enteral feeds (Section 1.12.3). There are many side effects and problems associated with radiotherapy (see Section 5.1.4). Radiotherapy to the mouth may damage the taste buds and alter taste sensitivity. It may also result in a dry mouth due to lack of saliva. The resistance of the teeth to dental caries is also reduced and particular attention should be given to oral hygiene and the protection of the teeth. The treatment can also have profound psychological, physiological and nutritional side effects. 'Post-irradiation mouth blindness' (Macarthy Leventhal 1959) may persist for some time after the completion of treatment.

4.8.7 Cancer of the larynx

As well as causing difficulty in speaking and hoarseness of the voice, carcinoma of the larynx may also result in difficulty in eating and swallowing solid foods.

At the time of laryngectomy, a nasogastric tube should be inserted and nutritional support provided using a nutritionally complete enteral feed (see Section 1.12.3). Nasogastric feeding is usually continued for a minimum of ten days. Once healing has taken place a soft, light diet plus protein and energy supplements should be introduced as nasogastric feeding is phased out. Patients requiring radiotherapy may need to continue with this diet, but most should be encouraged to resume a normal diet. Some patients may still experience difficulty in swallowing and require dilatation to improve the situation. A frequent check should be kept on nutritional intake as some patients may exist on a very limited range of soft foods and drinks. Patients in whom the parathyroid gland is also removed will need appropriate calcium and vitamin D therapy.

4.8.8 Oral Crohn's disease

Crohn's disease is primarily an inflammatory disorder of the small bowel, (see p 416) though lesions can occur anywhere along the gastrointestinal tract from the mouth to the anus. Crohn's disease of the

Table 4.19 Dietary management of disorders of the oral cavity

Oral condition	Eating difficulty	Treatment	Dietary management
Dental caries	Pain on eating, loss of teeth	Dental treatment ? Fluoride protection Oral hygiene	Reduction of sugar in diet, especially sugary snacks between meals. General nutrition education
Periodontal disease	Pain on chewing and eating	Oral hygiene ? Antibiotics	Gradual increase in unrefined foods and reduction in soft, sugary foods. General nutrition education
Vitamin deficiencies Associated dental/oral problems.	Sore, painful mouth, poorly developed or loose teeth	Vitamin replacement therapy	Regular intake of vitamins in diet to achieve RDA. Soft, semi-solid diet if mouth is sore
Anaemias — iron — vitamin B12	Red, inflamed tongue, pain on eating	Iron and vitamin B12 therapy	Increase iron and B12 content of the diet to achieve RDA. Pharmaceutical supplements may still be required.
Inflammation of the salivary glands	Pain on eating	Antibiotic therapy if required	Soft, semi-solid or liquidized diet, protein, and energy supplements as indicated
Salivary stones	Pain on eating	Surgical excision	Protein and energy supplements as indicated.
Fractured jaws and oral surgery	Unable to eat	Jaw wiring	High protein, high energy fluids, plus liquidized meals if desired, sipped through a straw. May require nasogastric feeding
Cancer of the mouth, pharynx and larynx	Difficulty and pain on eating. Dysphagia, anorexia	Surgery, radiotherapy and chemotherapy	Pre-treatment — sip feeding or nasogastric feeding. Post-operation — nasogastric feeding and then gradual introduction to soft diet plus protein and energy supplements
Crohn's disease of the mouth	Sore, painful mouth	Steroid therapy	Soft, semi-solid or liquidized diet. Protein and energy supplements as required. Sip feeding or nasogastric feeding if indicated

mouth may result in multiple lesions in the oral mucosa and on the lips either as part of a generalized condition or without other gut involvement (Tyldesley 1979). The mouth is sore, making eating painful and difficult. During an acute attack, a soft or fluid diet should be advised and hot, salty and spicy foods should be avoided (Table 4.18). Nutritional support provided by supplementary sip feeding or nasogastric tube feeding may be needed if the oral diet is inadequate (see Section 1.12).

General dietary advice for patients with oral disorders is summarized in Table 4.19.

Further reading

Davidson S, Passmore R, Brock JF and Truswell AS (1979) *Human nutrition and dietetics* pp 304; 389−96. Churchill Livingstone, Edinburgh.

Dickerson JWT and Lee HA (1978) *Nutrition in the clinical management of disease* pp 161−2. Edward Arnold, London.

Mason DK and Chisholm DM (1975) *Salivary glands in health and disease*. WB Saunders, London.

Levine RS (1985) *The scientific basis of dental health education. A policy document*. Health Education Council, London.

Stones HH (1962) *Oral and dental disease* pp 47−71. E and S Livingstone, Edinburgh.

References

MacCarthy-Leventhal EM (1959) Post-radiation mouth blindness. *Lancet* ii, 1138−9.

Tyldesley WR (1979) Oral Crohn's disease and related conditions. *Br J Oral Surg* 17, 1−9.

4.9   Disorders of the Oesophagus

The oesophagus is a muscular tube about 25 cm in length. The function of the oesophagus is relatively simple, i.e. the transport of food from the mouth to the stomach. The upper oesophageal sphincter lies below the pharynx, and the lower oesophageal sphincter at the gastro-oesophageal junction. Various mechanical factors help to prevent the reflux and regurgitation of food from the stomach (Fig. 4.6) though reflux of acid gastric contents occurs in most people from time to time without causing undue discomfort.

4.9.1   Acid reflux, oesophagitis, heartburn and hiatus hernia

Acid reflux, oesophagitis and heartburn

The refluxed contents of the stomach may contain partly digested foods, acid, pepsin and possibly bile and pancreatic enzymes (Fig. 4.7). It is probably this combination which causes mucosal damage and oesophagitis. Symptoms develop if reflux becomes frequent and the mucosa of the oesophagus becomes sensitive to the acidic reflux.

Symptomatic reflux may occur after operations in the gastro-oesophageal region, e.g. truncal vagotomy and proximal partial gastrectomy. The main symptom of reflux is heartburn which is felt sub-sternally and may be accompanied by regurgitation of acid fluid into the mouth. Heartburn occurs after meals and may be aggravated by bending, lying flat, lifting or straining. A gain in body weight will also aggravate heartburn. Meals which are high in protein increase sphincter pressure and reduce the likelihood of reflux and heartburn. Fatty meals, chocolate, coffee, alcohol, spicy foods and citrus juices lower the sphincter pressure and may induce reflux.

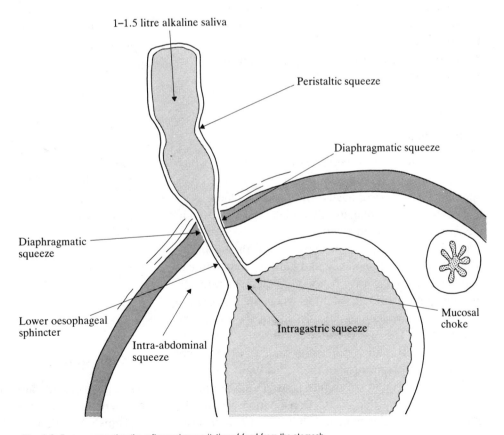

Fig. 4.6 Factors preventing the reflux and regurgitation of food from the stomach.

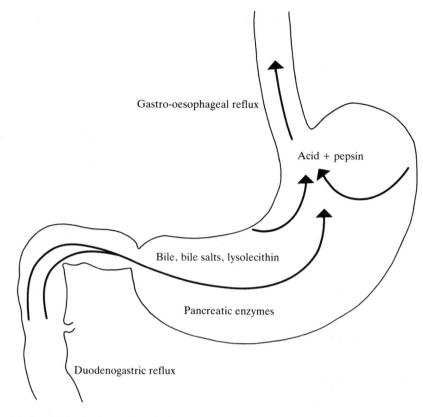

Gastro-oesophageal reflux

Acid + pepsin

Bile, bile salts, lysolecithin

Pancreatic enzymes

Duodenogastric reflux

Fig. 4.7 Constituents of gastro-oesophageal reflux.

The aims of the drug treatment of reflux are as follows

1 To reduce acid by use of antacids.
2 To reduce reflux by increasing sphincter tone.
3 To increase mucosal resistance.

Hiatus hernia

The diaphragm has several openings through which the abdominal viscera can enter the thorax. The opening for the oesophagus, the hiatus, is loosely attached to the oesophagus. In middle age this attachment weakens and in overweight patients additional abdominal weight puts an extra strain on the hiatus which herniates. Pregnancy and chronic coughing can also act in a similar way. A low fibre diet which results in constipation causes straining when the bowels are opened and weakening of the hiatus (Burkitt and James 1973). The major symptoms of hiatus hernia are those of reflux and oesophagitis and patients might complain of the sensation of food 'sticking'.

The management of reflux and hiatus hernia is summarized in Table 4.20. Constipation should be avoided and a high fibre diet advised. Certain foods may cause more discomfort than others and 'stick'. These often include salad items, new bread and rich,

heavy cakes and puddings. If pain and discomfort persists, surgical treatment may be required to correct a hiatus hernia.

Table 4.20 The management of hiatus hernia and acid reflux

Measures which may help	Things to avoid
1 Losing weight, if overweight	1 Smoking
2 Eating small, frequent meals	2 Eating large meals
3 Eating foods which are known to be well tolerated	3 Eating late at night
4 Standing upright and bending correctly	4 Eating very hot, very cold or very spicy foods, fatty foods, chocolate, onions, cucumber
5 Propping up the bed by approximately 4 inches, e.g. a household brick under each leg at the head end	5 Strong coffee and alcohol
	6 Stooping, bending from the waist or lying completely flat
6 Taking all medicines regularly as prescribed by the doctor	7 Tight fitting underwear, skirts or trousers

4.9.2 Dysphagia

Dysphagia is a difficulty or a discomfort in swallowing and may be due to oropharyngeal or oesophageal problems. A number of benign conditions as well as malignant lesions make the swallowing of food difficult or painful.

Benign stricture

Chronic persistent gastro-oesophageal reflux may result in a benign peptic stricture. Strictures may at first be due to muscular spasm following mucosal injury. Intubation with wide bore nasogastric tubes may predispose a patient to benign stricture.

The first symptom is usually difficulty in swallowing solid foods. The foods which usually cause problems include white bread, beef and roast potatoes. Dysphagia with solid foods may soon progress to dysphagia with semi-solids and liquids (Table 4.21). Appetite is usually reduced and severe weight loss may be reported. Sadly, many patients seem to suffer these difficulties for some time before seeking or obtaining help and may be dehydrated and malnourished on presentation. Some patients who are very depleted may need intravenous fluid replacement and nutritional support prior to treatment which is usually by oesophageal dilatation. Following dilatation, swallowing should be improved though most patients still need to choose their foods carefully. Some patients may require repeated dilatations and should be observed closely for possible oesophageal perforation. Younger patients fit for surgery may undergo thoracic surgery to reduce reflux and dilate the stricture.

As with many gastrointestinal disorders, dysphagia is often affected by anxiety. Anxious patients should be helped to relax and encouraged to discuss their problems with the appropriate counsellors.

It is important to treat gastro-oesophageal reflux adequately to prevent recurrence of the stricture.

Table 4.21 The dietary management of dysphagia

Stages of dysphagia	Dietary management
Dysphagia to solids	Small, frequent meals. Soft to semi-solid foods. Day-old wholemeal bread and crispbreads or biscuits may be tolerated. Protein and energy supplements if necessary (see Section 1.12.2)
Dysphagia to semi-solids	Liquidized meals or liquid meal replacement preparations. Protein and energy supplements. If severely depleted or intake nutritionally inadequate, may require fine bore nasogastric tube and enteral nutrition (see Section 1.12.3)
Dysphagia to liquids	May need rehydration with intravenous solutions. Enteral nutrition via a fine bore nasogastric tube if intubation possible. If severely depleted and completely dysphagic, TPN prior to treatment may be needed (see Section 1.13)

Sideropenic dysphagia

(Patterson-Kelly or Plumber-Vinsom Syndrome) Sideropenic dysphagia results from iron deficiency. The condition is relatively rare, occurs more commonly in women and may be associated with hiatus hernia, oesophagitis or partial gastrectomy. Relief is gained by medicinal iron and advice on an iron-rich diet to maintain body iron stores.

Malignant stricture of the oesophagus

Carcinoma of the oesophagus is more common in the elderly and is seen more frequently in men than in women. The lower third of the oesophagus is the most common site and the upper third is the least common site.

Patients may present with loss of body weight, dysphagia and chest pain on eating. The extent of weight loss is related to the degree and duration of the dysphagia.

The diagnosis of cancer of the oesophagus is by barium swallow, endoscopy, biopsy and brush cytology. When patients present with symptoms, the disease is often advanced. Once symptoms have developed deterioration may occur rapidly, changing from dysphagia with solids to dysphagia with liquids. Patients may appear poorly nourished and cachectic. The dietary management of the dysphagia is the same as for benign peptic structure of the oesophagus.

A brief diet history will reveal the recent changes in dysphagia and highlight which particular foods are most difficult for the patient to chew and swallow. There is seldom need for an accurate nutritional analysis of food intake to be calculated. Patients who are severely depleted and dehydrated will need rehydration with intravenous fluids. If a soft diet can be taken, protein and energy supplements should be used (see p 74). If fluids only can be taken, nutritional support should be provided by sip feeding or nasogastric feeding using a fine bore tube (see Section 1.12.3). In patients who are dysphagic to fluids, it may not be possible to pass a fine bore tube and total parenteral nutrition (TPN) may be required to provide pre-operative nutrition (see Section 1.13).

In the majority of patients with cancer of the oesophagus, palliative therapy is all that can be offered. The controversy about the relative value of surgery and radiotherapy continues (Earlam 1980) and treatment is by radiotherapy, chemotherapy, laser therapy, surgery or the insertion of a prosthetic tube (Celestin or Atkinson tube, see Fig. 4.8) through the tumour.

Disagreement also exists about the relative value of pre- and post-operative nutrition. Whilst pre-operative nutrition may reduce the risk of post-operative complications (Moghissi 1977), some surgeons may operate shortly after diagnosis has been confirmed and provide nutritional support either enterally or parenterally in the early post-operative period (Russell 1984). Whichever method of treatment is to be offered to the patient, the dietitian should be available to give advice as early as possible. Contact with the gastric clinic in the hospital allows the dietitian to meet the patient at the time of suspected diagnosis and advise accordingly. Details of the dietary advice given should be clearly stated in the patient's notes and the appropriate diet provided on admission to hospital.

Surgical treatment

Surgical treatment of carcinoma of the oesophagus may be by limited or total oesophagectomy or oesophago-gastrectomy, depending on the site and extent of the lesion. In some cases, a length of colon may be substituted for the excised oesophagus.

Post-operative nutrition is required to promote wound healing and maintain nutritional status. This has been achieved successfully by either jejunostomy feeding or TPN. Assessment of nutritional requirements should be made and most patients will require approximately 2,500 kcal and 12−14 g of nitrogen, together with adequate vitamins, minerals and trace elements (see Section 1.11).

The integrity of the anastamosis should be confirmed before an oral diet is introduced. Oral fluids followed by a light diet should be phased in as enteral nutrition or parenteral nutrition is phased out. Regular dietetic advice and supervision should be offered, both during hospitalization and following discharge.

Post-operative nutritional problems can include
1 Poor appetite.
2 Early satiety.
3 Fear of eating, particularly foods which were difficult to eat pre-operatively.
4 Difficulty in maintaining body weight.
5 Nausea.
6 Reflux.
Dietary treatment of these problems is summarized in Table 4.22.

Table 4.22 Dietary advice for post-oesophagectomy patients

1 Meals should be small and frequent
2 Fluids should be consumed separately from meal times, e.g. 1 hour before or 1 hour after eating
3 Protein intake can be increased with supplements such as Build-up, Complan or Fortimel taken between meals (see also Section 2.12). Skimmed milk can be incorporated into foods such as sauces, milks and custards
4 Energy intake can be increased by supplements of glucose polymers, sugar, Hycal and Fortical
5 Patients should be encouraged to relax before and after eating
6 Food should be chewed well
7 Reflux can be minimized by avoiding eating late in the evening and by sleeping with two to three pillows or with the head of the bed raised on household bricks

As with all carcinomas it is very difficult to regain body weight. Patients should not be expected to achieve their pre-illness weight. The dietary aims should be to prevent further weight loss and maintain the quality of life. A gain in weight should be regarded as a bonus.

Treatment by radiotherapy

Radiation of oesophageal carcinoma may be used as the sole treatment, in combination with chemotherapy or following surgery. During a course of radiotherapy, the tissues will become oedematous, inflamed and swollen, making dysphagia worse and the patient possibly unable to swallow liquids. This stage is usually temporary. but as these patients are already often malnourished and may have lost a lot of body weight it is best to pre-empt the situation. The passing of a fine bore nasogastric tube at the start of treatment when there is sufficient space to do so enables nutritional support to be given if dysphagia worsens and nutritional intake is inadequate. The tube need not be used if the patient can achieve an adequate intake orally.

Reintroduction of a normal diet should be gradual and protein and energy supplements should be used. Most patients continue on a soft diet as they will often still experience some difficulties with swallowing and may be afraid to try foods with which they associate problems.

Insertion of prosthetic tubes

When radical surgery is contraindicated because of metastatic spread or because the patient is elderly and too frail, a palliative procedure should be considered. The establishment of satisfactory swallowing will enable the patient to be managed at home. A prosthetic tube may be inserted at laparotomy or by an endoscopic technique using light sedation. The tubes most commonly used are the Celestin tube or the Atkinson tube (short, medium or long length) (Fig. 4.8).

These tubes provide an opening through the tumour but the diameter of the tubes is relatively small (approximately that of the index finger). The insertion of these tubes carries with it a risk of perforation of the oesophagus and death. If perforation is suspected, introduction of an oral diet should be delayed and TPN may need to be instigated until the site has healed and an oral diet can be introduced. The internal lining of the tubes is specially coated to facilitate the passage of food through them but care should be taken when eating. Dietary guidelines for patients will a prosthetic tube are summarized in Table 4.23.

More and more patients are seeking the help of

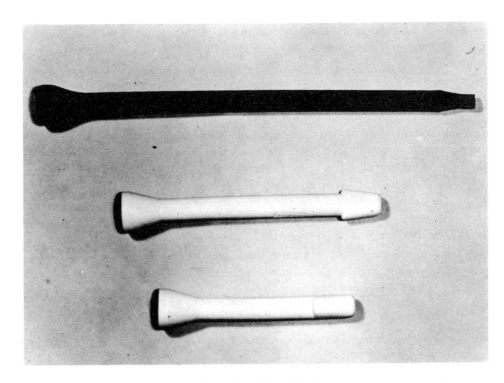

Fig. 4.8 Prosthetic tubes. 1. Celestin tube; 2. Medium length Atkinson tube; 3. Short length Atkinson tube.

alternative methods of treating their cancer. These methods usually involve a vegetarian diet consisting largely of raw fruits, vegetables and cereals. Any patients who have prosthetic tubes inserted must be advised of the hazards of eating such a diet which will undoubtedly block their tube.

Table 4.23 Dietary guidelines for patients with a prosthetic tube

1 Meals should be small and frequent and, if necessary, soft, semi-solid or liquidized
2 Meat should be very tender, minced or liquidized
3 Food should be chewed well. If the patient has dentures, ensure that they fit properly
4 Meals should be accompanied by plenty of sauces, gravy or custard
5 New bread should be avoided. Day-old wholemeal bread and crispbreads crumble more easily and are usually better tolerated
6 Nourishing fluids (such as milk, Horlicks, Ovaltine and Bournvita) should be taken between meals
7 Protein and energy supplements (such as Complan, Fortimel, Build-up, Maxijul, Fortical or Hycal) should be used
8 A good source of vitamin C (such as Ribena) should be included in the diet
9 After eating a meal, a fizzy drink (such as soda water or lemonade) should be consumed to help clear the tube of any food particles
10 Should the tube block, the patient should be advised NOT to panic but to take sips of fizzy drinks, walk around, jump up and down and take more fizzy drinks. If the blockage persists, the hospital gastric clinic or casualty department will be able to clear it. Patients should be reassured that if their tube does block, they will come to no harm

Radiotherapy following the insertion of a prosthetic tube

This combination of treatment is occasionally used. During radiotherapy, dysphagia may recur and a fine bore tube can be passed through the oesophageal prosthetic tube to provide nasogastric feeding throughout the period of treatment, until an oral diet may be resumed.

Occasionally the prosthetic tube may need to be replaced if the tumour has grown and obstructed the entrance or the exit of the tube. This procedure carries a high risk of mortality.

4.9.3 Other disorders of the oesophagus

Perforation and caustic burns

If the oesophagus perforates spontaneously or is perforated as a result of dilatation, intubation or oesophagoscopy, any foods consumed would enter the thoracic cavity which would need to be drained by suction. The perforation may be allowed to heal naturally or may need surgical repair. Patients should be 'nil by mouth' and an alternative means of feeding instituted, e.g. TPN, nasogastric feeding or jejunostomy feeding (see Sections 1.12 and 1.13). If a nasogastric tube is to be used it should be inserted at the time of surgical repair.

Household cleaning agents such as caustic soda or industrial acids or alkalis taken accidentally or deliberately destroy the oesophageal mucosa and may also damage the muscle coats of the oesophagus. The area must be totally rested and intravenous fluids provided. If an oral diet has to be withheld for more than six or seven days, enteral feeding from a site below the level of damage (if necessary via a gastrostomy or jejunostomy) or TPN should be commenced.

Pharyngeal pouch

The mucosa of the pharynx may protrude through the triangular space formed by the cricopharyngeus and the inferior pharyngeal constrictor muscles. A pharyngeal pouch may occur and cause symptoms of dysphagia with regurgitation, particularly of fluids. This may occur some hours after a meal and especially when lying flat which increases the risk of pulmonary aspiration. Surgical correction and post-operative nasogastric feeding is the usual treatment.

Achalasia

Achalasia is characterized by the inability of the lower oesophageal sphincter to relax after a swallow, and weak peristalsis of the oesophagus. It is relatively uncommon. Food collects in the oesophagus, causing discomfort and eventually may pass through the sphincter by the action of gravity and the weight of food consumed. Regurgitation of food is common but lacks the bitter taste of acid or bile which is typical of reflux. Aspiration of food from the oesophagus may lead to pneumonia. As food collects it can irritate the mucosa and cause oesophagitis and pain. Loss of weight is uncommon unless the patient becomes afraid to eat. Relief may be obtained by following a typical gastric regimen (Table 4.25). A semi-fluid diet can also be beneficial and the patient may find that standing up several times during a meal, drinking a glass of water and exhaling hard may help to force food into the stomach. If these measures are ineffective, surgical myotomy or mechanical dilatation may give permanent relief.

Further reading

Atkinson M (1983) The oesophagus. In *Recent advances in gastroenterology* 5 Bouchier IAD (Ed) pp 1–20. Churchill Livingstone, Edinburgh.

Davidson S, Passmore R, Brock JF and Truswell AS (1979) *Human nutrition and dietetics* 7e pp 396–7. Churchill Livingstone, Edinburgh.

Dickerson JWT and Lee HA (1978) *Nutrition in the clinical management of disease* pp 163–6. Edward Arnold, London.

Hunt RH (1981) *Disorders of the oesophagus*. Update Post-Graduate Centre Series. Update Publications, London.

References

Burkitt DP and James PA (1973) Low residue diets and hiatus hernia. *Lancet* **ii**, 128–30.

Earlam R and Lunha-Melo JR (1980a) Oesophageal squamous carcinoma i: A critical review of surgery. *Br J Surg* **67**, 381–90.

Earlam R and Lunha-Melo JR (1980b) Oesophageal squamous carcinoma ii: A critical review of radiotherapy. *Br J Surg* **67**, 457–61.

Moghissi KN, Hornshaw J, Teasdale PK and Dawes EA (1977) Parenteral nutrition in carcinoma of the oesophagus treated by surgery: nitrogen balance and clinical studies. *Br J Surg* **64**, 125–8.

Russell CA (1984) Fine needle catheter jejunostomy in patients with upper gastrointestinal carcinoma. *Appl Nutr* **11**, 1–7.

4.10   Disorders of the Stomach and Duodenum

Diseases of the gastrointestinal tract account for almost one-third of the medical referrals to hospital and disorders of the stomach and duodenum constitute a large proportion of these.

The stomach functions as a reservoir for food received from the oesophagus and plays a role in the digestion and absorption of nutrients. It is sensitive to pain and thermal sensations. Gastric disease, and particularly the surgical treatment of gastric disease, are likely to have considerable effects on gastric function and nutritional intake.

4.10.1   Gastric and duodenal ulcer

It has been common practice to describe gastric and duodenal ulcers as peptic ulcers and include them under this one heading. However, there is much to suggest that they are separate diseases and have a different aetiology.

Gastric ulcers are less common than duodenal ulcers. Normally, there is a balance between factors which attack the gastric mucosa and those which protect it (Table 4.24). Ulcers may be single or multiple, acute or chronic, large or small. They are usually associated with normal or reduced gastric acid and pepsin output. Confirmation of diagnosis is made by upper gastrointestinal endoscopy.

Table 4.24 Factors affecting the gastric mucosa

Destructive factors	Defensive factors
Hydrochloric acid	Epithelial cell barrier
Pepsin	Mucus
Psychogenic factors	Gastric blood flow
Gastric irritants, e.g. alcohol	Cell regeneration
Duodenal and biliary reflux	Regulation of acid secretion
Nicotine and tobacco tars	
Analgesics and anti-inflammatory drugs	

A duodenal ulcer, like a gastric ulcer, is a defect in the mucosa. It may be single or multiple, superficial or deep. The majority of duodenal ulcers occur in the duodenal cap and duodenitis is invariably present. Ulceration may also occur in the pyloric antrum which may, in time, cause pyloric stenosis.

The cause of duodenal ulcers is not fully understood. Hypersecretion of acid, nocturnal acid secretion and the rapid delivery into the duodenum of acid contents which are inadequately buffered by pancreatic secretion of bicarbonate, are all precipitating factors. It has been suggested that certain occupations may predispose to peptic ulcers and factors such as stress, irregular meals, eating quickly and inadequate mastication may contribute to ulcer development.

Treatment of gastric and duodenal ulcers

Relief of symptoms

Many different dietary regimens have been used. In the past, very strict diets consisting of frequent milk drinks interspersed with antacids sometimes resulted in patients becoming severely malnourished. Other patients have spent years on boiled fish and milk with very little benefit. Ingelfinger (1966) recommended a more normal diet to 'let the ulcer patient enjoy his food'. A bland or gastric diet comprised of small, frequent meals interspersed with snacks may relieve the symptoms of dyspepsia (Table 4.25). However, such a regimen may not necessarily accelerate the healing of an ulcer.

Table 4.25 The general principles of a gastric diet

1   Meals should be small, frequent and regular
2   Fried foods should be avoided
3   Strong tea, coffee and alcohol should be avoided
4   Mucosal irritants such as spices, pickles, black pepper, vinegar or mustard should be avoided
5   Any food known to cause dyspepsia should be avoided
6   Very hot or very cold foods should be avoided: air is swallowed which may aggravate dyspepsia
7   Smoking must be stopped
8   Aspirin should not be taken. Paracetamol will provide analgesia without acting as a gastric irritant

Healing of the ulcer and prevention of recurrence

The drug treatment of gastric ulcer and duodenal ulcer may include antacids, anticholinergic drugs or histamine H_2 receptor antagonists (e.g. Cimetidine, Ranitidine). H_2 receptor antagonists have now become the routine treatment for benign gastric and duodenal ulcers. Their widespread use has enabled ulcers to heal whilst allowing patients to eat a more normal diet. However certain guidelines should be followed

1 Regular meals should be eaten, preferably little and often.

2 Strong tea and coffee should be taken in moderation only.

3 Any food known to cause dyspepsia should be avoided.

4 Alcohol and aspirin should be avoided.

5 Smoking must be stopped.

Complications of gastric and duodenal ulcers

The most common complications are

1 Haemorrhage.

2 Perforation.

3 Penetration into adjacent tissues or organs.

4 Obstruction, e.g. pyloric stenosis and gastric outlet obstruction.

These complications will require surgery, either as an emergency or, in some cases, electively. Surgery, for patients who have failed to respond to medical treatment, prevents recurrence in most cases. A number of gastric reconstructions may be undertaken depen-

dent on the site and extent of the ulcer. Partial gastrectomy (Billroth I, Billroth II or Polya operations) (see Fig. 10) may result in two-thirds to three-quarters of the stomach being removed and may have a higher incidence of post-operative mechanical or nutritional problems (see p 398). These operations are however rarely performed nowadays for peptic ulcer. Truncal vagotomy (Fig. 4.9a) may be combined with gastro-enterostomy, gastro-jejunostomy or pyloroplasty. Patients may suffer problems of gastric stasis and delayed stomach emptying, dumping syndrome or diarrhoea. Highly selective vagotomy (HSV) or proximal gastric vagotomy (PGV) is a refinement of selective vagotomy (Fig. 4.9b,c). In this operation the parietal cell mass alone is denervated and the mobility and drainage of the stomach is preserved. There are a number of advantages of this procedure; the stomach itself is not opened or reconstructed and diarrhoea, dumping, nausea and vomiting are relatively rare. The nutritional status of the patient is better and oral intake may be resumed in the early post-operative period.

The different vagotomies

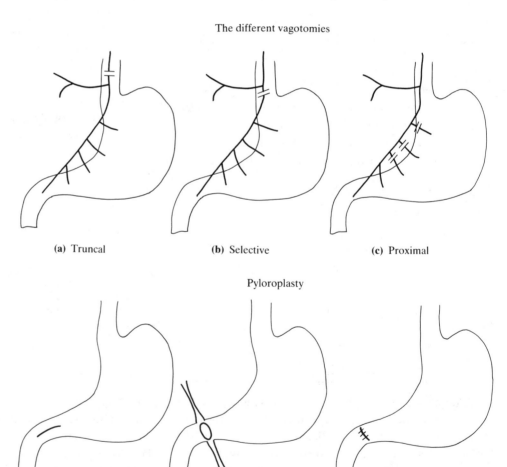

(a) Truncal   (b) Selective   (c) Proximal

Pyloroplasty

(d) Incision   (e) Splitting   (f) Re-Suture

Fig. 4.9 The different vagotomies.

Pyloric stenosis

Pyloric stenosis stems from scar tissue resulting from duodenal ulcers around the pyloric channel. Gastric emptying is delayed and food debris collects in the stomach, obstructing the pylorus. Retained food in the stomach tends to ferment and cause the characteristic bad breath associated with pyloric stenosis.

Patients complain of discomfort, nausea, vomiting and anorexia. Food debris must be removed from the stomach by gastric lavage. Once the stomach has been emptied, a high protein, high energy fluid diet, taken either orally or administered via a nasogastric tube, may be well tolerated prior to surgery. Occasionally, if the stenosis is severe and the patient nutritionally depleted, TPN may be instigated pre-operatively (see Section 1.13).

Post-operatively, gastric retention may still occur for some days. If the introduction of oral fluids and diet has to be withheld for more than about seven days post-operatively, nutritional support should be provided by nasojejunal, jejunostomy or parenteral feeding (see Sections 1.12, 1.13).

4.10.2 Carcinoma of the stomach

Carcinoma of the stomach affects mainly middle-aged or elderly people and is seen more often in men than in women. Unfortunately, most treatments are palliative as a permanent cure can only be achieved by radical surgery before metastasis has occurred. Early diagnosis is difficult and on presentation most patients complain of pain on eating, nausea, vomiting, anorexia and severe weight loss.

If the carcinoma is resectable, a total or partial gastrectomy may be performed (Figs 4.10, 4.11). Lesions in the cardia of the stomach will be treated surgically

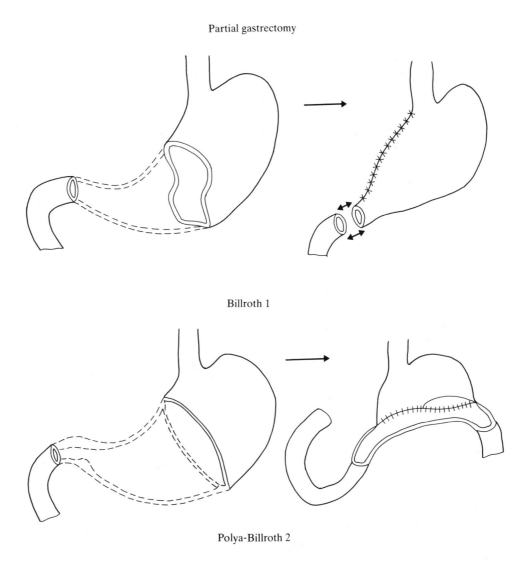

Partial gastrectomy

Billroth 1

Polya-Billroth 2

Fig. 4.10 Partial gastrectomy.

(a) Jejunojejunostomy

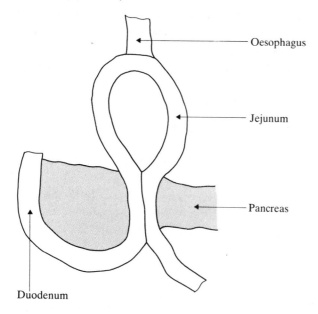

(b) Roux-en Y Jejunojejunostomy

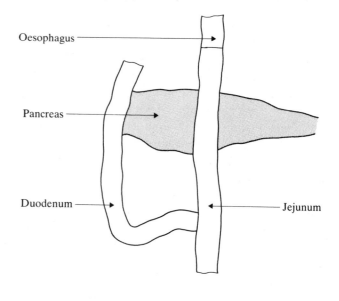

Fig. 4.11 Anatomy after a total gastrectomy.

by an oesophago-gastrectomy. When gastrectomy is contraindicated, a gastroenterostomy may relieve symptoms and allow the patient to be managed at home eating such foods as he can tolerate with the addition of protein and energy supplements.

Pre-operative feeding may be undertaken in severely malnourished patients. Enteral feeding via fine bore nasogastric tube may be tolerated; if not, parenteral nutrition should be considered (see Sections 1.12, 1.13).

4.10.3   Nutritional problems following gastric surgery

Disturbances in gastric function (Table 4.26) often occur following gastric reconstruction and have an effect on nutritional intake and nutritional status. Some of these problems occur soon after eating and may be described as early or post-cibal syndromes; others develop later due to long term effects of disturbed gastric function. These may be described as late symptoms (Table 4.27).

Early symptoms

Small stomach syndrome

The majority of patients experience early satiety and may feel distended and uncomfortable during or after eating. This occurs particularly after total and partial gastrectomy. It may also occur after vagotomy and

Table 4.26 Changes in gastric function following gastric resection and reconstruction (Celestin 1981)

Rapid emptying of the stomach remnant
Rapid secretion of hydrochloric acid and pepsin
Reduced secretion of intrinsic factor
Reduced secretion of pancreatic enzymes
Inadequate mixing of food with enzymes and bile
Reduced absorption of certain food substances, especially protein and fat
Rapid absorption of glucose
Abolition of the normal pH gradient in the alimentary canal
Increased intestinal mobility
Altered bacteriological state of the intestine (occasionally)
Effects related to the creation of the afferent loop

Table 4.27 Post-gastrectomy syndromes

Early symptoms	Late symptoms
Small stomach	Weight loss and malnutrition
'Dumping syndrome'	Calcium malabsorption
Diarrhoea	Anaemia
Bile vomiting	

pyloroplasty. Small, frequent meals should be eaten and fluids should be consumed separately from solid food.

'Dumping syndrome'

Early dumping. This occurs soon after eating and the symptoms include hypotension, tachycardia, diminished pulse volume and giddiness. The cause is thought to be due to the rapid and early delivery of a hyper-osmolar meal into the jejunum. The symptoms usually settle 2–3 months after surgery, but in the meantime may be relieved by avoiding liquids at meal times and taking limited amounts of refined sugars. A glucose polymer is often better tolerated as an energy supplement than sucrose or glucose. Small meals containing protein and fat also help to reduce the incidence of dumping.

Late dumping. Some patients may experience symptoms about two hours after a meal either in addition to early dumping or alone. The symptoms are similar to those of hypoglycaemia, i.e. feeling weak, faint, cold and sweaty and are usually corrected by eating carbohydrate. The cause of late dumping is probably due to an over-production of insulin by the pancreas in response to elevated blood glucose levels following rapid absorption from the upper small intestine. Again, symptoms can be relieved by eating less sugar and refined carbohydrates at meal times and consuming fluids separately from solid foods.

Diarrhoea

Diarrhoea frequently occurs following vagotomy or total gastrectomy. The problem may be allevitated by codeine phosphate or Imodium ® and should disappear 1–2 months after surgery.

Vomiting

Pancreatic and biliary secretions may accumulate in the afferent loop and, after a meal has left the stomach, can enter the gastric remnant causing nausea and vomiting. Treatment is surgical and involves reducing the size of the afferent loop.

Late symptoms

Following gastric reconstruction, long term follow-up of patients is important to identify early signs of nutritional disturbances and to ensure that an adequate diet is being taken.

Weight loss and malnutrition

Weight loss is a well known consequence of gastric surgery and is a result of reduced food intake. Patients are often afraid to increase their food intake and frequently experience early satiety. Such patients should be reassured and encouraged to take small,

frequent meals with protein and energy supplements (see p 74). Malnutrition and malabsorption resulting in steatorrhoea may be due to poor mixing of food with pancreatic enzymes and bile, or possibly pancreatic insufficiency or bacterial overgrowth in the afferent loop. Reduction in dietary fat content may be beneficial.

Calcium malabsorption

Significant malabsorption of calcium occurs after gastrectomy and can cause osteomalacial bone changes (Eddy 1971). Inadequate intake of calcium will aggravate the situation and calcium and vitamin D supplements should be given.

Anaemia

Iron deficiency anaemia occurs in almost half the patients following partial gastrectomy. It may be due to a poor iron intake, inadequate conversion of ferrous iron to ferric iron or the bypassing of the duodenum and upper jejunum in patients with gastroenterostomies.

Megaloblastic anaemia due to vitamin B12 deficiency may occur in partial or total gastrectomy due to reduction or loss of intrinsic factor. This may only be severe in patients who survive five years after total gastrectomy but can be prevented by vitamin B12 therapy.

Impaired absorption of folate occurs in some gastrectomy patients (Elsbourg 1974) though folate deficiency is a much less important cause of anaemia. However, routine folic acid supplements are given occasionally.

General dietary advice following gastric reconstruction is summarized in Table 4.28.

Table 4.28 Dietary advice following gastric reconstruction

1	Small, frequent, regular meals should be eaten
2	Fluids should be taken between meals
3	Excess quantities of sugar, glucose and sweet sugary foods should be avoided
4	Excess fat should be avoided
5	Small amounts of vegetables and fruit should be eaten — these are bulky and may result in early satiety. A vitamin C supplement should be taken
6	Eating late at night should be discouraged
7	Protein and energy supplements should be advised as indicated
8	Good sources of calcium and vitamin D should be advised
9	Iron, folic acid and vitamin B12 supplements should be prescribed as appropriate

4.10.4 Gastritis

Gastritis is an inflammatory lesion of the gastric mucosa and may be an acute, erosive gastritis or a chronic, atrophic gastritis. Alcohol, drugs such as aspirin, other chemical irritants and occasionally foods infected with pathogens may be associated with acute gastritis. Chronic gastritis may follow repeated attacks of acute gastritis and is more common in patients who smoke and drink alcohol heavily.

Iron deficiency anaemia may result from repeated bleeding, and pernicious anaemia may result from reduced production of intrinsic factor and consequent reduced absorption of vitamin B12.

The symptoms of acute gastritis are nausea, pain and vomiting. The treatment should concentrate on resting the stomach, preventing dehydration and restoring electrolyte balance. Water, with or without glucose, or diluted fruit juices may be taken hourly if tolerated. Regeneration of healthy mucosa should occur in 2−5 days.

Chronic gastritis is relieved by resting the inflamed gastric mucosa and removing or correcting the cause of gastritis, such as faulty eating habits, smoking, drinking and drugs. Iron and vitamin B12 deficiencies should be corrected and once symptoms have disappeared, patients may return gradually to a normal diet. They should be urged to correct bad eating habits and to stop smoking and drinking.

Further reading

Davidson S, Passmore R, Brock JF and Truswell AS (1979) *Human nutrition and dietetics* 7e, pp 398−402. Churchill Livingstone, Edinburgh.

Dickerson JWT and Lee HA (1978) *Nutrition in the clinical management of disease* pp 166−170. Edward Arnold, London.

Hunt R (1981) *Disorders of the stomach and duodenum.* Update Post-Graduate Centre Series. Update Publications, London.

References

Celestin LR (1981) Postgastrectomy and postvagotomy problems. In *Basic gastroenterology 3e* Read AE, Harvey RF and Naish JM (Eds), pp 104−14. Wright, Bristol.

Eddy RL (1971) Metabolic bone disease after gastrectomy. *Am J Med* **50**, 442−9.

Elsborg L (1974) Malabsorption of folic acid following partial gastrectomy. *Scand J Gastroenterol* **9**, 271−4.

Ingelfinger FJ (1966) Let the ulcer patient enjoy his food. In *Controversy in internal medicine.* Saunders, Philadelphia.

4.11 Disorders of the Pancreas

Inflammation of the pancreas causes impaired secretion of pancreatic enzymes leading to a failure of digestion and absorption. Weight loss and steatorrhoea are common symptoms and the problem may be further complicated by the onset of diabetes mellitus.

4.11.1 Pancreatitis

Acute pancreatitis

The aetiology of this serious disorder is not clear. It may occur in association with biliary tract disease (such as obstruction of the pancreatic duct by gallstones) or it may be associated with a history of alcoholism.

Autodigestion of the cells and the blood vessels of the pancreas occurs and a serosanguinous exudate passes into the peritoneal cavity causing peritonitis and hydrolysis of the fat in the omentum and mesentery.

The main symptom is severe pain which often follows the consumption of a heavy meal or alcohol. Nausea and vomiting frequently occur. Treatment of acute pancreatitis consists of the relief of pain and the control of shock. The pancreas must be rested and oral nutrition completely withheld. Total parenteral nutrition (TPN) (see Section 1.13) may be commenced to provide nutritional support until the acute inflammation has settled and an oral intake can be resumed. The dietary management should then be the same as for chronic pancreatitis.

Chronic pancreatitis

This may follow repeated attacks of acute pancreatitis or be associated with chronic inflammation of the biliary tract or the penetration of duodenal ulcers into the pancreas. Fibrosis destroys the epithelial cells but the cells of the islets of Langerhans are spared for longer.

Symptoms include recurrent attacks of mid-abdominal and lumbar pain, nausea, vomiting and pyrexia. Steatorrhoea may be present and loss of body weight is often apparent. Glucose tolerance may be abnormal and ultimately the malabsorption syndrome and diabetes mellitus may develop.

Dietary management of chronic pancreatitis

1 Alcohol must be prohibited.
2 Fat must be reduced and a low fat, light diet commenced. Medium chain triglycerides (MCT) may be given.
3 Protein must be adequate. Most protein-containing foods also contain fat and the protein intake may need to be supplemented using preparations such as Maxipro or Casilan (see Section 2.12).
4 Carbohydrates need to be increased to ensure adequate total energy intake. Blood glucose should be monitored closely and controlled accordingly.
5 Vitamins and minerals. Fat soluble vitamins should be regularly administered parenterally and calcium supplements should be given to all patients with long standing steatorrhoea.
6 Pancreatic enzymes (see p 405) should be taken with all foods and the amount taken at each meal adjusted according to the quantity of foods eaten and the fat content of the meal.
7 Elemental diets have been used successfully in the management of patients with chronic pancreatic insufficiency or other pancreatic disease, such as cystic fibrosis, pancreatic abscess or pancreatic fistulae (Russell 1981). Care must be taken that the high carbohydrate content of these preparations does not aggravate existing hyperglycaemia. Elemental diets may also be useful as an intermediary stage in acute pancreatitis between TPN and the introduction of oral diet.

4.11.2 Cancer of the pancreas

Diagnosis is made by ultrasound, endoscopic retrograde cholangiopancreatography (ERCP), fine-needle biopsy and/or cytology. Treatment is usually surgical excision with or without radiotherapy.

Pancreatic surgery

Early surgery for patients with acute pancreatitis is associated with a high rate of mortality (Ransom 1979) but it may be the only hope for patients with acute necrotizing pancreatitis. Surgical resection may result in partial pancreatectomy (e.g. Whipple resection) or a total pancreatectomy with resulting pancreatic enzyme insufficiency and diabetes mellitus.

Post-operative nutrition should be provided initially by TPN or enteral nutrition using an elemental diet (see Sections 1.13, 1.12). A low fat, high carbohydrate diet with pancreatic enzyme replacement and control of blood glucose by hypoglycaemic agents or insulin may then be introduced. The nutritional status of these patients may be improved by the use of an elemental diet as a supplement to their low fat diet.

4.11.3 Cystic fibrosis

Cystic fibrosis (CF) is a generalized hereditary condition in which there is widespread dysfunction of the exocrine glands. It is characterized by chronic pulmonary disease, reduced secretion of water and bicarbonate, pancreatic enzyme deficiency and abnormally high concentration of electrolytes in the sweat. The incidence is approximately 1 in 2000 (Evans et al 1981). It is usually symptomatic in the first year of life and, with modern management, 80% survival up to 20 years can be expected (Phelan et al 1979). Progressive malnutrition and poor growth are common features of CF and they represent a serious problem. A wide range of nutritional deficiencies has been described. The most common include energy malnutrition, vitamins A and E and essential fatty acid deficiency (Dodge 1983).

Dietary problems

Dietary problems are the result of
1 Pancreatic insufficiency.
2 Poor appetite.
3 Increased nutrient requirements due to pulmonary infection.

Pancreatic insufficiency (present in the majority of the patients) can result in severe malabsorption. Even with replacement of the pancreatic enzymes, a high proportion of patients have significant malabsorption of fat, nitrogen and fat soluble vitamins (Forstner et al 1980). The anorexia which so commonly accompanies a chest infection contributes to a low nutrient intake (Shepherd et al 1980) and, in addition, pulmonary infection increases the energy requirement (Hubbard 1980). In practice, loss of weight may be the first sign that the patient's respiratory condition is deteriorating. It has been suggested that the combined effects of the poor appetite and increased nutrient requirements due

to pulmonary infection may be as important a determinant of undernutrition and growth failure as nutritional losses due to malabsorption (Sproul and Huang 1964).

Dietary therapy

It is important to provide the CF patient with the optimum diet for the potential for growth to be fulfilled and resistance to infection maximized. Specific diet therapy should be determined individually, taking into account age, activity, weight, clinical condition, food preferences and tolerances.

Energy

Energy requirements are generally increased due to steatorrhoea and pulmonary infection (MacDonald 1984). As a general guideline, it has been arbitrarily suggested that energy intake be increased at least 50% above the Recommended Daily Amount (RDA) in patients with CF (Hubbard 1980). However, because of the heterogeneity of these patients, it is difficult to give precise recommendations and patients need to be assessed individually. Occasionally, a patient can grow in a normal fashion by consuming no more than the RDA for energy for normal healthy people. On the other hand, patients with advanced pulmonary disease may need as much as twice the normal intake of energy.

In contrast to the usual textbook description of the voracious appetite of CF patients, dietary surveys indicate that the average energy intakes are well below the RDA (Chase et al 1979; Hubbard and Mangnum 1982). There is no correlation between energy intake and severity of malabsorption, i.e. patients with severe steatorrhoea do not necessarily compensate by eating more food (di Sant'Agnese and Hubbard 1984).

In order to achieve an adequate energy intake, effective use should be made of suitable energy supplements (Table 4.29 and see also Tables 1.43 (p 77) and

Table 4.29 Useful energy supplements in the treatment of cystic fibrosis

Product category	Product (manufacturer)
Glucose polymers	Caloreen (Roussel), Maxijul (SHS), Liquid Maxijul (SHS), Polycal (Cow and Gate), Polycose (Abbott)
Glucose drinks	Hycal (Beechams), Fortical (Cow and Gate)
Enteral feeds in the form of supplementary drinks (appropriate enzyme preparations should be taken simultaneously).	Clinifeed (Roussel), Ensure (Abbott), Isocal (Mead Johnson), Fortison (Cow and Gate), Triosorbon (Merck)

2.70 (p 198). Fat intake should, if tolerated, be normal and frequent snacks should be encouraged. Occasionally, it may be necessary to resort to nocturnal nasogastric feeding to achieve the required energy intake.

Protein

Although the exact protein requirements are unclear, it is generally accepted that the protein intake should be increased to compensate for excessive loss of nitrogen in the faeces and to support the accretion of amino acids in growing tissue (Beddoes *et al* 1981). It has been suggested that at least 15–20% of the energy intake should come from protein sources (Farrell and Hubbard 1983). In practice, the protein intakes are usually high and do not need special supplementation.

Fat

Traditionally, fat restriction has been widely advocated for CF in order to reduce steatorrhoea, increase protein absorption and improve the character of the stools. However, there is no objective data supporting this practice and fat restriction reduces the intake of energy and essential fatty acids. There is now evidence that patients who consume normal fat intakes exhibit better growth and that fat malabsorption is not exacerbated by an increased intake (MacDonald *et al* 1984). It is now widely accepted in CF centres that the majority of patients can tolerate normal fat intakes (Walker-Smith *et al* 1983; di Sant'Agnese and Hubbard 1984) and a liberal fat intake should be encouraged. Fat restriction is only indicated if a patient complains of foul smelling stools, flatulence and abdominal pain and if this is not improved either by an increased dose of pancreatic enzymes or by changing the enzyme preparation. The addition of histamine (H2) antagonists such as Cimetidine or Ranitidine which reduce gastric acid secretion and preserve the enzyme activity may be helpful (Chalmers *et al* 1985).

Medium chain triglycerides (MCT)

MCT oil has been used as a supplement in patients with CF because shorter chain fatty acids (less than 12 carbon atoms) can be absorbed in the absence of pancreatic lipase and bile salts (Dodge and Yassa 1980). Although it has been shown to improve the character of the stools, a consistent improvement in weight gain has not been demonstrated (Gracey *et al* 1969). Pancreatic enzymes should be administered concurrently with MCT oil (Durie *et al* 1980). In practice, many patients find the oil is unpalatable and inconvenient to use. If normal fat intakes are tolerated, the use of this supplement is unnecessary.

Elemental and artificial diets

Artificial diets have been tried with variable success (Allen *et al* 1973; Berry *et al* 1975; Yassa *et al* 1978). The diets usually consist of a casein hydrolysate, a glucose polymer, MCT oil, vitamins and minerals and have been used to replace or to supplement normal nutrient intake. It has been claimed that the growth and general health of CF children on such diets improve. However, if the diet is continued for any length of time, patient acceptance of this monotonous and relatively unpalatable mixture is poor. It is doubtful that such regimens will play a significant part in future dietary management.

Fat soluble vitamins

Deficiencies of vitamins A, D, E and K are well documented. Biochemical deficiency is not always accompanied by clinical effects, but it is reasonable to correct it when demonstrated (Dodge and Yassa 1980).

Vitamin A. Daily supplementation of 8000 µg (2400 i.u.) is currently advised (Congdon *et al* 1981). Monitoring of blood levels ensures that adequate supplementation has been prescribed. However, if this is not possible, 8000 µg/day usually restores the plasma levels to normal (MacDonald, unpublished observation).

Vitamin D. Although rickets is rarely seen in CF, subclinical deficiency has been noted (Littlewood *et al* 1980) and a daily supplement of 20 µg (800 i.u.) is advisable for patients with pancreatic insufficiency.

Vitamin E. Plasma levels of vitamin E are generally low, but can be corrected by giving a daily supplement varying from 50 mg for infants to 200 mg for adults.

Vitamin K. Deficiency of this vitamin has been noted in patients with liver disease and in young infants with CF, causing bleeding due to hypoprothrombinaemia (Farrell and Hubbard 1983). A supplement is only necessary if deficiency has been demonstrated.

Water soluble vitamins

Although there is little evidence of water soluble vitamin deficiency (Littlewood *et al* 1980), twice the recommended dose of a multivitamin preparation is usually given.

Minerals

Low plasma iron levels are common but the reason for this is uncertain (di Sant'Agnese and Hubbard 1984). Low plasma zinc levels have also been reported (Dodge 1983). Appropriate supplementation of these minerals should be given when deficiency is demonstrated.

Salt

In patients with CF, it is clear that salt supplements may be required in hot environments when exposure to the sun and/or physical exertion causes increased sweating (di Sant'Agnese and Hubbard 1984). However, the problem of salt loss is only of major concern during heat waves and in hot climates and there is no good rationale for the traditional practice of recommending routine consumption of salty foods and aggressive use of the salt-pot (Farrell and Hubbard 1983).

Feeding infants with CF

Breast feeding has been associated with the develop-ment of hypoproteinaemia, oedema and anaemia in untreated CF infants (di Sant'Agnese and Hubbard 1984). It should be allowed only on the understanding that adequate weight gain must be maintained. In addition, an increased incidence of electrolyte depletion has been recognized in CF babies being fed on breast milk and the normal modified infant formula milks (Laughlin *et al* 1981).

A useful high protein formula feed for CF babies, based on an infant milk, skimmed milk powder and a glucose polymer is summarized in Table 4.30 (Francis 1986). If infants fail to thrive on this preparation, or have other complications, they may benefit from a formula based on hydrolysed casein and MCT oil such as Pregestimil (Mead Johnson). Infants should be given 200 ml/kg body weight of fluid daily.

Although early weaning (at three months) is encouraged, solid foods are introduced into the diet in much the same way as for any other baby.

Pancreatic enzymes

Exogenous pancreatic enzymes are available in powder, tablet or capsule form (see Table 4.31). There is no standard dose of pancreatin. The optimal dose varies for each patient and does not necessarily bear a relationship to the intake of dietary fat. Although faecal fat estimations can help to determine the enzyme dose, in practice it is usually decided by bowel habits and abdominal discomfort. Enzymes should be administered

Table 4.30 Formula and analysis of a special milk for feeding infants with cystic fibrosis

Formula*	Analysis per 100 ml						
	Energy (kcal)	(kJ)	Protein (g)	Fat (g)	CHO (g)	Sodium (mmol)	Potassium (mmol)
Using SMA Gold Cap (Wyeth)							
6.5 g SMA Gold Cap	33	138	0.8	1.8	3.6	0.3	0.7
4.3 g Marvel (Cadbury's)	16	65	1.6	0.1	2.2	1.0	1.8
6.5 g glucose polymer + water to 100 ml	26	104	Nil	Nil	6.5	0.1	Tr
Total	75	307	2.4	1.9	12.3	1.4	2.5
Using Premium (Cow and Gate)							
6.2 g Premium	33	138	0.8	1.8	3.7	0.4	0.9
4.6 g Marvel (Cadbury's)	16.5	69	1.7	0.1	2.4	1.1	1.9
6.5 g glucose polymer + water to 100 ml	26	104	Nil	Nil	6.5	0.1	Tr
Total	75.5	311	2.5	1.9	12.6	1.6	2.8

*Both formulae can be made as follows
  2 level scoops of SMA Gold Cap or premium ⎫
  2 level scoops of glucose polymer   ⎬ Using SMA Gold Cap or Premium scoop
  2 level scoops of Marvel   ⎭
  + 4 oz (120 ml) water.

Table 4.31 Pancreatic enzyme preparations available in the UK

Product (Manufacturer)	Composition (per g of powder/ granules or per capsule/tablet) BP units		
	Lipase	Protease	Amylase
Powder			
Pancrex V (Paines and Byrne)	25,000	1,400	30,000
Capsules			
Cotazym (Organon)	14,000	500	10,000
Pancrex V '340 mg' (Paines and Byrne)	8,000	430	9,000
Pancrex V '125 mg' (Paines and Byrne)	3,300	160	3,300
Tablets			
Enteric-coated tablets			
Nutrizym (Merck)	9,000	400	9,000
Pancrex V (Paines and Byrne)	1,900	110	1,700
Pancrex V Forte (Paines and Byrne)	5,600	330	5,000
Enteric-coated granules			
Pancrease (Johnson and Johnson)	4,000	350	4,000
Creon (Duphar)	8,000	210	9,000

Table 4.32 General guidelines for the use of pancreatic enzyme preparations*

1 Give with every meal; during rather than all before or after
2 Give extra enzymes (e.g. 1—2 capsules or tablets) with fatty or large snacks and milky drinks
3 Do not give enzymes with squash, lemonade, fruit or boiled and jelly sweets
4 Do not add enzymes to raw food which requires cooking (e.g. raw batter mix) or add to very hot food
5 Mix powdered enzyme either with a little soft food or jam or honey. Do not sprinkle over a complete meal
6 The new enteric-coated microsphere, e.g. Pancrease (Johnson and Johnson) and Creon (Duphar) can be swallowed whole. Where swallowing is difficult, they may be opened and the contained microsphere taken with liquids or mixed with jam or honey. They should not be crushed or chewed
7 Increase the enzyme dose (e.g. by 1—2 capsules or tablets) if the stools are loose, fatty or more than twice daily

*The correct dose of pancreatic enzymes is that which controls bowel symptoms and not necessarily the dose recommended by the manufacturers

with all meals and substantial snacks. Guidelines for using pancreatic enzymes are summarized in Table 4.32. The new enzyme preparations, Pancrease (Johnson and Johnson) and Creon (Duphar) which consist of microspheres of pancreatic enzymes with a pH-sensitive coating, have enabled the number of enzyme capsules taken to be reduced. Another advantage is that they can be mixed with food without changing the taste or consistency although the capsules themselves should not be chewed.

Support organisation

The Cystic Fibrosis Research Trust, 5 Blythe Road, Bromley, Kent BR1 3RS.

Further reading

Cushieri A and Wormsley KG (1983) The pancreas. In *Recent advances in gastroenterology* 5, Bouchier IAD (Ed) pp 183—99. Churchill Livingstone, Edinburgh

Davidson S, Passmore R, Brock JF and Truswell AS (1979) *Human nutrition and dietetics* 7e pp 419—21. Churchill Livingstone, Edinburgh.

Dickerson JWT and Lee HA (1978) *Nutrition in the clinical management of disease* pp 185—6. Edward Arnold, London.

Hodson Margaret E, Norman AP, Battern JC (Eds) (1983) *Cystic fibrosis*. Bailliere Tindall, London.

Lloyd-Still, JD (1983) *Textbook of cystic fibrosis*. John Wright and Sons Ltd, Bristol.

Taussig LM (Ed) (1984) *Cystic fibrosis*. Thieme-Stratton, New York. Inc, New York.

Sturgess JM (Ed) (1980) *Perspectives in cystic fibrosis*. Imperial Press Ltd, Mississauga.

References

Allan JD, Mason A and Moss AD (1973) Nutritional supplementation in treatment of cystic fibrosis of the pancreas. *Am J Dis Childh* **126**, 22—6.

Beddoes V, Laing S, Goodchild MC and Dodge JA (1981) Dietary management of cystic fibrosis. *Practitioner* **255**, 557—60.

Berry HK, Kellogg FW, Hunt MM, Ingberg RL, Richler L and Gutjahr C (1975) Dietary supplement and nutrition in children with cystic fibrosis. *Am J Dis Childh* **129**, 165—71.

Chalmers DM, Brown RC, Miller MG, Clarke TNC, Kelleher J, Littlewood JM, Losowsky MS (1985) The influence of long term Cimetidine as an adjunct to pancreatic enzyme therapy in cystic fibrosis. *Acta Paediatr Scand* **74**, 114—7.

Chase HP, Long MA and Lavin MH (1979) Cystic fibrosis and malnutrition. *J Paediatr* **95**, 337—47.

Congdon PJ, Bruce G, Rothburn MM, Clarke PCN, Littlewood JM, Kelleher J and Losowsky MS (1981) Vitamin Status in treated patients with cystic fibrosis. *Arch Dis Childh* **56**, 708—14.

di Sant'Agnese PA and Hubbard VS (1984) The pancreas. In *Cystic fibrosis* Taussig (Ed) pp 230—95. Thieme-Stratton Inc, New York.

Dodge JA (1983) Nutrition. In *cystic fibrosis* Hodson ME, Norman AP and Batten JC (Eds) pp 132—43. Bailliere Tindall, London.

Dodge JA and Yassa JG (1980) Food intake and supplementary feeding programmes. In *Perspectives in cystic fibrosis* Sturgess JM (Ed) pp 125—36. Imperial Press, Mississauga.

Durie PR, Newth CJ, Forstner GG and Gall DG (1980) Malabsorption of medium chain triglycerides in infants with cystic fibrosis: correction with pancreatic enzyme supplements. *J Paediatr* **96**, 862—4.

Evans RT, Little AJ, Steel AE and Littlewood JM (1981) Satisfactory screening for cystic fibrosis with the BM meconium procedure. *J Clin Path* **34**, 911—3.

Farrell PM and Hubbard VS (1983) Nutrition in cystic fibrosis: vitamins, fatty acids and minerals. In *Textbook of cystic fibrosis* Lloyd-Still JD (Ed) pp 263—92. John Wright and Sons Ltd, Bristol.

Francis DEM (1986) *Diets for sick children* 4e. Blackwell Scientific Publications, Oxford.

Forstner G, Gall G, Corey M, Durie P, Hill R and Gaskin K (1980) Digestion and absorption of nutrients in cystic fibrosis. In *Perspectives in cystic fibrosis* Sturgess JM (Ed) pp 137—48. Imperial Press, Mississauga.

Gracey M, Burke V and Anderson CM (1969) Assessment of medium chain triglyceride feeding in infants with cystic fibrosis. *Arch Dis Childh* **44**, 401—3.

Hubbard VS (1980) Nutrient requirements of patients with cystic fibrosis. In *Perspectives in cystic fibrosis* Sturgess JM (Ed) pp 149—59. Imperial Press, Mississauga.

Hubbard VS and Mangnum PJ (1982) Energy intake and nutritional counselling in cystic fibrosis. *J Am Diet Assoc* **80**, 127—31.

Laughlin JJ, Brady MS and Eigen H (1981) Changing feeding trends as a cause of electrolyte depletion in infants with cystic fibrosis. *Pediatrics* **68**, 203—7.

Littlewood JM, Congdon PJ, Bruce G, Kelleher J, Rothburn M, Losowsky MS and Clarke PCN (1980) Vitamin status in treated cystic fibrosis. In *Perspectives in cystic fibrosis* Sturgess JM (Ed) pp 166—71. Imperial Press, Mississauga.

MacDonald A (1984) The adequacy of current nutritional therapy in the treatment of cystic fibrosis. In *Applied nutrition* II Bateman EC (Ed) pp 67—72. John Libbey, London.

MacDonald A, Kelleher J, Miller MG and Littlewood JM (1984) Low, moderate or high fat diets for cystic fibrosis. In *Cystic Fibrosis: Horizons.* Lawson D (Ed) p 395. John Wiley and Sons, Chichester.

Phelan PD, Allan JL, Landau LI and Barnes GL (1979) Improved survival of patients with cystic fibrosis *Med J Aust* **1**, 261—3.

Ransom JHC (1979) The time of biliary surgery in acute pancreatitis. *Ann Surg* **179**, 654—63.

Russell RI (1981) *Elemental diets* pp 152—4. CRC Press, Florida.

Shepherd R, Cooksley WGE and Cook WD (1980) Improved growth and clinical, nutritional and respiratory changes in response to nutritional therapy in cystic fibrosis. *J Paediatr* **97**, 351—7.

Sproul A and Huang N (1964) Growth patterns in children with cystic fibrosis. *J Paediatr* **65**, 664—76.

Walker-Smith JA, Hamilton JR and Walker WA (1983) Disorders of the exocrine pancreas. In *Practical paediatric gastroenterology* pp 316—32. Butterworth, London.

Yassa JG, Prosser R and Dodge JA (1978) Effects of an artificial diet on growth of patients with cystic fibrosis. *Arch Dis Childh* **53**, 777—83.

4.12   Disorders of the Small and Large Intestine

4.12.1   The malabsorption syndrome

There are a number of reasons why a defect in absorption of one or more nutrients may occur and these are summarized in Table 4.33. Although dietary therapy or nutritional supplementation may be indicated it is important that the primary disorder is recognized and treated.

Table 4.33 Causes of malabsorption

Reduced absorptive surface	Intestinal or gastric resection. Villous atrophy, e.g. coeliac disease, tropical sprue. Gastro-colic and jejuno-colic fistulae. Inflammatory bowel disease. Infiltration — amyloid, scleroderma, lymphoma. Protein-energy malnutrition. Vascular insufficiency. Mucosal damage by drugs or irradiation.
Intra-luminal causes	Pancreatic insufficiency — chronic pancreatitis, cystic fibrosis, (a deficiency of pancreatic lipase and pancreatic bicarbonate are implicated). High pH in duodenum — achlorhydria. Low pH in duodenum — Zollinger-Ellison syndrome. Bile salt deficiency — obstructive jaundice.
Infection	Blind loop syndrome — bacterial deconjugation of bile salts resulting in steatorrhoea. There may also be some competition by bacteria in the small intestine for available nutrients. Bacterial growth may also lead to secondary disaccharide and monosaccharide intolerance. Parasitic infestations. Acute enteritis.
Enzyme deficiencies	Disaccharidase deficiency Primary alactasia and primary sucrose-isomaltose deficiency. A permanent lactose or sucrose-free diet is required. Secondary lactase deficiency and occasionally sucrose–isomaltose deficiency. A temporary lactose-free diet is required. The primary disorder must also be treated. Typical causes include gastrointestinal infection, reduced absorptive surface, gastrointestinal tract trauma, protein intolerance and protein-energy malnutrition.

Table 4.33 *contd.*

Enzyme deficiencies (*contd*)	Racial or late-onset lactase deficiency is common in certain ethnic groups, e.g. Africans, American negroes, Indians, Chinese and others. The incidence in UK caucasions is small at around 6%. There is a variable degree of tolerance to lactose and a symptomatic approach to treatment should be taken. Specific deficiency of one or more pancreatic enzymes including isolated lipase deficiency, combined lipase and proteolytic enzyme deficiency and trypsinogen deficiency. Enterokinase deficiency
Impairment of fat transport and clearance	Congenital lymphangectasia, retroperitoneal fibrosis, congestive heart failure, lymphoma. Abetalipoproteinaemia.
Impairment of monosaccharide transport	Primary — a rare congenital malabsorption of monosaccharides has been reported involving a disturbance in the active transport of glucose and galactose. Strict adherence to a diet free of all carbohydrates other than fructose is necessary throughout infancy. Secondary — Malabsorption of all monosaccharides may occur in infants following surgery, protein-energy malnutrition or gastroenteritis.

Diagnostic features

Principal clinical features of the malabsorption syndrome include diarrhoea, abdominal distension, flatulence and nutritional deficiencies, although not all of these need be present. In steatorrhoea the stool is pale, malodorous, greasy and unformed whereas in carbohydrate malabsorption the diarrhoea tends to be watery and frothy due to the presence of fermented sugars. The nutritional features may include those of fluid and electrolyte loss, weight loss and other specific nutritional deficiencies.

In the diagnosis of fat malabsorption, a measured faecal fat greater than 7% of dietary fat intake is indicative of impaired fat absorption (Losowsky *et al*

1974). Unless the steatorrhoea is severe, the loss of faecal fat is of little nutritional importance compared with the concomitant loss of other nutrients, particularly the fat soluble vitamins A, D, E and K as well as calcium and magnesium. Specific nutritional deficiencies may also occur as a result of disease or resection of a specific part of the gastrointestinal tract as will be appreciated from Fig. 4.12 which shows absorption sites.

Dietary treatment

Whatever the cause of malabsorption the principles of dietary therapy remain the same

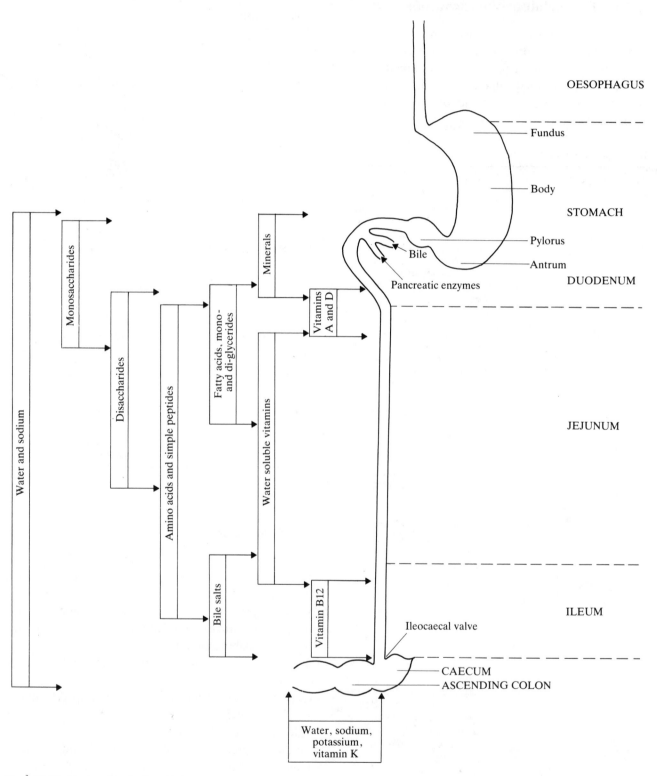

Fig. 4.12 Principle absorption sites for nutrients.

1 Dietary treatment of the primary disorder, e.g. coeliac disease.
2 The daily replacement of large losses of fluid and electrolytes.
3 The restoration of optimal nutritional state, by supplementation if necessary.

Fat malabsorption

Restriction of dietary fat should not be pursued too enthusiastically in patients with steatorrhoea as energy deficiency is a common consequence of severe malabsorptive disorders. Fat restriction is indicated when
1 The patient finds the symptoms socially and personally unacceptable despite optimum drug therapy for steatorrhoea.
2 The steatorrhoea is severe enough to lead to electrolyte disorders or mineral deficiencies.
3 There is a defect in fat transport and clearance from the lymphatic system as in abetalipoproteinaemia, intestinal lymphangectasia, chylouria or chylothorax.

Figure 4.13 shows the major steps involved in fat absorption and metabolism. Where fat restriction is indicated but adequate energy provision is also desirable, medium chain triglycerides (MCT) and glucose polymers may be used (see Section 2.12). Long chain triglycerides (LCT) should continue to provide 10−20% of energy requirements in a form which will ensure an adequate provision of linoleic acid. In the absence of pancreatic lipase and bile salt activity, absorption of MCT is about one-third of normal. A proportion of MCT is able to enter the mucosal cell directly as a triglyceride, where it can be hydrolysed by a mucosal lipolytic system. The medium chain fatty acids then pass into the portal vein.

In some individuals, rapid intraluminal hydrolysis of MCT may result in osmotic diarrhoea; if this is the case then the MCT should be administered at a slower rate. Although as an energy substrate MCT may have some metabolic advantages over LCT there appears to be no clinical advantage to be gained, in terms of absorption, from the use of MCT in the LCT tolerant patient.

When a LCT fat restriction is employed, particularly for the malnourished individual, it must be ensured that the resultant diet is adequate in protein, minerals, vitamins and trace elements. Suitable low fat supplements may be needed.

Carbohydrate malabsorption

Treatment of carbohydrate malabsorption centres on the avoidance of the relevant carbohydrate in the diet, although in the case of a secondary carbohydrate malabsorption, the primary cause must also be recognized and treated, e.g. milk protein intolerance, enteritis, intestinal surgery. The osmotic diarrhoea of untreated carbohydrate malabsorption is dose-related and usually most severe in infants, who will require a milk formula free of the sugar concerned, e.g. lactose or sucrose.

Lactase deficiency is the most common carbohydrate malabsorption state. It is necessary to identify the cause (Table 4.33) to estimate the severity and likely duration of the dietary lactose restriction. For adults with late onset or 'racial' lactase deficiency, dietary restriction may need to be permanent but the restriction should relate to the individual's level of tolerance of lactose. *Sucrose−isomaltase deficiency* may also be primary or secondary in origin and a sucrose-free diet is required. Starch, however, is tolerated.

Congenital malabsorption of monosaccharides is rare. It involves a disturbance in the active transport of the monosaccharides glucose and galactose. The diet must be free of all starch, disaccharides, glucose and galactose. For infants a fructose-based formula such as Galactomin 19 (Cow and Gate) may be used. All oral medicines must be carbohydrate-free. The diet should be nutritionally adequate in all other respects and vitamin and mineral supplementation may be necessary. Strict adherence to the diet is required during infancy though in later years limited quantities of milk and sucrose may be added.

Secondary malabsorption of all monosaccharides may occur in infants following surgery, protein-energy malnutrition or gastroenteritis. An initial period of intravenous fluids is often necessary to correct water and electrolyte imbalances. This will be followed by a carbohydrate-free formula during which there should be careful monitoring for signs of hypoglycaemia. The problem is thought to be one of monosaccharide malabsorption, since disaccharidase activity is normal. The ability to tolerate carbohydrates slowly recovers and a monosaccharide such as glucose or fructose may be added to the diet in increasing increments of 1% of normal carbohydrate intake. These children are often underweight and gravely ill and parenteral nutrition may be life saving if resumption of adequate oral nutrition is delayed. The detailed dietary management of carbohydrate malabsorption in infants and children is discussed by Francis (1974 and 1986).

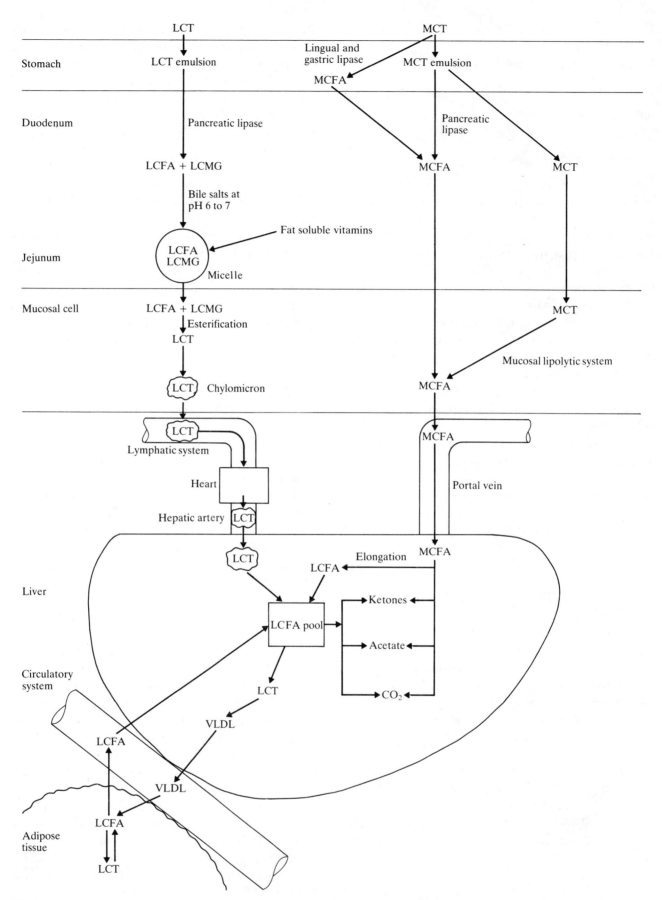

Fig. 4.13 Absorption and metabolism of long chain and medium chain triglycerides. LCT = long chain triglyceride; MCT = medium chain triglyceride, LCFA = long chain fatty acids; LCMG = long chain monoglycerides; VLDL = very low density lipoprotein.

Protein malabsorption

Malabsorption states in which there is a deficiency of enzymes involved in protein digestion, e.g. pancreatic proteolytic enzyme, trypsinogen, or enterokinase deficiency are not indications for the dietary restriction of protein.

4.12.2 Coeliac disease

Coeliac disease is a condition in which the lining of the small intestine is damaged by gluten, a protein found in wheat and rye. Coeliacs are also affected by similar proteins present in barley and possibly oats. The damage which occurs considerably impairs the absorption of nutrients from the small intestine causing wasting and ultimately severe illness resembling malnutrition.

Causation

Despite a great deal of research, exactly why or how gluten harms the intestine is unknown. It is known that the fraction of gluten responsible for the damage is gliadin, but gliadin is itself a mixture of proteins. Work is in progress to identify the toxic elements and it is now known that the alpha, beta, gamma and omega fractions are all harmful to coeliacs.

There are several theories about the pathogenesis of gluten intolerance in coeliac disease. Enzyme deficiency has been suggested in the past but it is now thought that an abnormal immunological response is the most likely cause. A number of studies have shown that in spite of running in families, the disease is not inherited as a dominant characteristic. Although the mode of inheritance is not clear, susceptibility to coeliac disease is thought to have a genetic basis related to the HLA type. Whether a particular individual then develops the condition probably depends on a wide variety of environmental factors, including the actual gluten content of the diet (Swinson and Levi 1980).

It has been estimated (McCrae 1969) that the coeliac condition affects approximately one person in 1,850 in the UK, but it is likely that many cases remain undiagnosed and that the true incidence is higher (Swinson and Levi 1980). There are known variations in the incidence of coeliac disease in different populations. A very high incidence of one in 300 has been reported in the West of Ireland (Mylotte *et al* 1973), whereas the condition is virtually unknown in Negro and Oriental populations.

History of the condition

The word 'coeliac' is derived from the Greek word koiliakos which means 'suffering in the bowels'. The coeliac condition was first described nearly 1,800 years ago in the writings of the Roman physician, Aretaeus of Cappadocia. He mentioned fatty diarrhoea, loss of weight, pallor and food passing undigested through the body. He also said 'that bread is rarely suitable for giving (coeliac children) strength'. It was not until 1888 that Samuel Gee of St Bartholomew's Hospital in London gave the second classic description and a clear clinical account of the condition.

Early this century a few physicians drew attention to the harmful effect or carbohydrate in coeliac disease and the 'banana diet' — a diet low in carbohydrate except for ripe bananas — was recommended. However, no real progress in recognizing and treating the disease was made until after the Second World War. In 1950, Professor Dicke, a Dutch paediatrician, described how coeliac children had benefited dramatically during the war when wheat, rye and oat flours, which were unavailable, were replaced by maize or rice; while at the end of the war, the children relapsed when wheat flour was air-lifted into Holland. This work was confirmed and extended by Professor Charlotte Anderson in Birmingham, who extracted the starch from wheat flour and found that the remaining gluten was the harmful part.

Since the 1950s, therefore, a gluten-free diet has been the treatment for coeliacs. In 1954, Paulley, a physician in Ipswich, described an abnormality of the lining of the small intestine found during an operation on an adult coeliac patient. This abnormality was the existence of an inflammatory condition, resulting in the loss of the villi from the mucosa of the small intestine and hence considerably reducing the surface area available for nutrient absorption. Treatment with a gluten-free diet usually results in the 'flat' lining of the coeliac intestine returning to the normal state as the villi grow again. On the whole, the younger the patient the more dramatic the improvement, provided that the diet is followed rigidly.

The development of biopsy tubes (in particular by Dr Margot Shiner in 1956 and Colonel Crosby, an American army officer, who designed the 'Crosby capsule' (Crosby and Kugler 1957) which removes a small section of intestinal mucosa for microscopic examination of the villi) resulted in jejunal biopsy becoming the standard technique for diagnosis of coeliac disease.

Diagnosis

The coeliac disorder can manifest itself at any age. In children, symptoms usually become apparent between three and five months after eating gluten, although in a few cases this interval may be shorter. After being weaned on to solids containing gluten, a normal baby who has thrived well initially on milk begins to refuse feeds and stops gaining weight. The next stage is actual weight loss and the child gradually becomes irritable, listless and develops a large abdomen or pot-belly. The stools become abnormal and are either large, pale and smell offensive or they may be loose, later developing into diarrhoea. Vomiting may also occur. If this state of affairs continues, the baby will quickly become wasted, especially around the buttocks, and may eventually develop acute diarrhoea and dehydration and become seriously ill.

In a few cases children do not show symptoms until they are older, when they present with a poor appetite and failure to grow. These children are obviously much more difficult to diagnose, as there are many other possible reasons for these symptoms. Various investigations can be undertaken for malabsorption (see p 407), but a definite diagnosis can only be established by an intestinal biopsy. In the hands of experienced operators this is not a traumatic procedure, and can usually be completed within a couple of hours.

Twenty years ago coeliac disease was almost exclusively a paediatric condition. But now it is more prevalent in adults than in children. Figures issued by the Coeliac Society of the UK show that between 1983 and 1985 only 25% of coeliacs joining the Society were children — 75% were newly diagnosed adults. The number of babies affected has decreased considerably, possibly due to the change in infant feeding practices resulting from the recommendation that children under the age of 6 months should not be given gluten-containing foods. The number of adults being diagnosed is continually on the increase as more doctors become aware of the many different ways in which the condition can present itself in later life.

The majority of adult coeliacs consult their doctors not because of gastrointestinal symptoms but because of problems such as breathlessness, fatigue or just because they feel more tired at the end of the day than they used to. The difficulty for the general practitioner is that almost any chronic illness can start in this way. In the case of coeliacs, the fatigue and breathlessness is usually due to the anaemia which results from poor absorption of iron and folic acid. Deficiency of other essential nutrients such as calcium may also occur. The diagnosis is first suspected from the clinical evidence of symptoms or on the results of routine blood tests; it is then confirmed by jejunal biopsy. A smaller proportion of adult coeliacs see their doctors complaining

of symptoms which arise directly from the effects of gluten on the small intestine, such as diarrhoea, abdominal fullness, discomfort, pain or vomiting. The diarrhoea is usually caused by inadequate absorption of dietary fat and the stools are pale, bulky, offensive and may be difficult to flush down the lavatory. It is this last feature which is sometimes more troublesome to patients than the increase in the number of bowel actions.

Treatment

The gluten-free diet always excludes wheat, rye and barley, but the use of oats is controversial. Some coeliacs are undoubtedly intolerant to oats and must avoid them, but others can tolerate them well and suffer neither obvious ill-effects nor microscopic changes on biopsy. Without conclusive evidence as to whether or not oats are harmful, medical opinion is divided but many leading authorities tend to err on the side of caution and exclude oats from the gluten-free diet.

The gluten-free diet must be followed strictly and it is now strongly recommended that it is continued for life. Patients with coeliac disease are at greater risk than the general population for the development of malignant neoplasms, particularly lymphomas (Swinson et al 1983) but no definitive answer can yet be given to the crucial question of whether strict adherence to the gluten-free diet reduces the risk of lymphoma. Nevertheless, it is hoped that by life-long elimination of gluten from the diet, the risk of malignancy may be reduced and chronic nutritional deficiencies, relapse and infertility will be avoided.

Avoidance of gluten

There are two sources of gluten in the diet — the obvious and the less obvious. Firstly, it occurs in foods obviously made from wheat flour such as ordinary bread, cakes, biscuits, pastries and pies (Section 2.11.1). Secondly, it occurs in manufactured or processed foods including a whole range of convenience foods in which wheat flour is used either as an ingredient or as a filler. It is through eating foods in the second category that most dietary indiscretions occur.

To help fill the gap in the diet left by the omission of common gluten-containing foods, excellent gluten-free products are specially manufactured for patients with coeliac disease and dermatitis herpetiformis. Details of these can be found in Section 2.11.1. Many of these products are available to patients on prescription. A current list of prescribable products is given in

Table 2.62 and up-to-date lists can be obtained from the Coeliac Society or found in Monthly Index of Medical Specialities (MIMS) (Borderline Substances Appendix). Coeliac patients are not normally exempt from prescription charges unless they are in the general categories for exemption (such as children, pregnant or lactating mothers or old age pensioners). Since many items are likely to be needed, non-exempt patients may find that a prescription 'season ticket' (prepayment of charges) may be worthwhile. Details of this can be found on form FP95 available from Post Offices.

General dietary considerations

At diagnosis many coeliacs are anaemic and may also exhibit varying degrees of malnutrition. Immediately after treatment has started, there will be a phase of tissue growth and regeneration, and requirements for iron, folic acid and other vitamins will increase. Supplementation will be required and many need to be continued for several months. When full recovery has occurred and the patient is well established on a full and varied gluten-free diet, no further supplementation is usually necessary.

Apart from restriction of gluten the diet must be adequate in all other respects for normal growth and development. In general there need be no restriction of milk or dairy products, eggs, meat, fish, vegetables, fruit, rice or maize (corn).

Role of the dietitian

Following a gluten-free regimen is a life-long measure for the coeliac and it is vital that good dietary foundations are laid at the onset of treatment. Poor teaching or inadequate explanations will leave the patient confused and unable to follow the diet correctly. Months of ill-health can result.

In addition to teaching the essentials of a gluten-free diet to the patient and their family, dietitians are also likely to be asked by patients for further information about coeliac disease or to clarify various points raised during their consultation with the doctor. It is important to reassure the patient or, if it is a child, the parents, that a gluten-free diet will restore normal health.

Patients should be encouraged to adopt a positive attitude to their diet and think about all the foods which they *can* eat instead of dwelling on those which are no longer suitable. Showing patients the 80-page long gluten-free foods list published by the Coeliac Society is a useful way of illustrating this point.

Dietitians should remind their patients to keep up-to-date with information about their diet and in particular to use *only* current gluten-free manufactured food lists since the ingredients of products do change.

It is also important to stress to patients the need for regular follow-up and for them to see a dietitian when they attend an out-patient or coeliac clinic. Patients who have done well initially often become complacent about their diet and do not take so much trouble over it; gradually they become under par, often without realizing it, and an astute dietitian will pick this up.

Complications

Secondary intolerances

In a few isolated cases, secondary disaccharide intolerance may occur and it is necessary to restrict lactose and sucrose as well as gluten (see Section 2.11.1; p 192 and p 134). This is, however, only a temporary condition and usually only affects children who are severely wasted. Special dietetic advice is required and milk substitutes will be required for a period of 2−3 months. In certain areas it has become common place to restrict milk as well as gluten in newly diagnosed coeliac children. There is no scientific support for making this a routine procedure and merely makes the dietary regimen more restrictive and more difficult to follow.

Constipation

Some coeliacs regularly complain to their dietitian that they are constipated and care needs to be taken in assessing whether this is really the case. Many coeliacs do become obsessed with their bowels and may think they are constipated when they are not; others feel that because their diet cannot contain wheat bran, their fibre intake is bound to be lower than it should be.

Fibre intake can be increased by either soya bran or rice bran or by an increase in fruit, vegetable and nut intake, together with the consumption of commercial high fibre gluten-free foods (see Section 2.11.1).

Weight problems

It may seem ironic, when one of the main concerns of the coeliac before diagnosis is weight loss and wasting, that after diagnosis and subsequent treatment, excessive weight gain can become an even greater long term problem. After diagnosis the coeliac usually feels so much better on his gluten-free diet that appetite and interest in food returns. Excessive weight gain is therefore not surprising. A weight reducing diet, in line with an ordinary weight reducing diet, should be advised.

Diabetes mellitus

An increase in the incidence of coeliac disease in diabetics and a more frequent occurrence of diabetes in coeliac patients have been reported (Thain *et al* 1974; Koivisto *et al* 1977). Gluten-free diabetic diets are therefore not uncommon. Gluten-free products have a similar carbohydrate content to ordinary foods and can therefore be substituted easily into a conventional dietary regimen for diabetes.

Special needs of particular groups

The gluten-free diet causes different problems with different age-groups.

Infants

Apart from choosing baby foods which are gluten-free, there is no need for a mother to feed or treat her baby differently from any other baby. Parental attitudes are extremely important, and if the parents accept their child's coeliac condition and gluten-free diet as a way of life, so will the child.

Pre-school children

In this age-group it is generally easier if the whole family eat gluten-free foods; difficulties at meal times are guaranteed if different members of the family have different things on their plate. Other children's parties need not be a problem if the situation is explained to the appropriate mother beforehand and the coeliac child sent to the party with suitable gluten-free food. Food for their own birthday parties should all be gluten-free. Playgroups present few problems since the children are usually only allowed to eat food under supervision so it is not difficult to ensure that the coeliac child is only allowed to eat gluten-free snacks.

Children

Parents should be reassured that they will be able to cope easily with social occasions such as eating out, parties, holidays, school dinners, and all school activities. Invitations to eat at other children's houses should be accepted. The coeliac child, unlike his friends, will soon get used to the idea that he takes his own gluten-free bread, for example, with him, and that this, for him, is a normal procedure. When entertaining at home, gluten-free food can be provided for everyone, which helps the child to feel secure.

A child soon learns to eat only those foods which are familiar which means in effect that they are gluten-free. 'If in doubt, leave it out' should be the child's motto. Occasional dietary accidents and indiscretions may occur (as may also happen with adults!) and cause minor symptoms, but these will usually clear up within a few days. Such episodes can act as a useful warning against further dietary deviations.

Teenagers

During adolescence many children may rebel against their parents and coeliacs are no different; it is important to the coeliac teenager to be one of the crowd and to do the same sort of things as his friends. Many stray off their diet, eating foods such as fish and chips, pies, hamburgers or pizzas. Those who become ill after doing so are usually wary of future indiscretions, but there is a problem with those teenagers who seem to have a high degree of gluten tolerance and can get away with dietary indiscretions without any obvious symptoms, although damage to the intestinal mucosa will still occur (Kumar *et al* 1979). Parents should be advised to keep their wayward children on the straight and narrow as much as possible, but should be warned not to become obsessional about the diet as this is likely to lead to further behaviour problems. Most teenagers have good appetites and may be extremely hungry because of inadequate school lunches; providing extra food from home may help prevent the tendency for their children to fill up with unsuitable foods from nearby shops.

Adults

The motto for adults is to 'be prepared'. They should carry supplies of gluten-free foods in their cars, briefcases and shopping bags.

Some canteens will provide gluten-free meals and most will certainly save or put aside a naturally gluten-free meal for a coeliac *if* they are aware of the person *and* the nature of the diet. In many large companies, food for evening and night shift workers is often left in a cooler to be microwaved by the worker when he takes his meal break. It may be possible for a gluten-free labelled meal to be left for the coeliac; alternatively, the worker concerned may have to provide his own food.

The elderly

Many elderly patients find it difficult to change the eating habits of a lifetime overnight but others do so very successfully, because they find that retirement gives them more time to experiment with cooking.

Some meals-on-wheels services provide gluten-free diets but others do not, patients will need to make enquiries.

General problems which may arise

Eating away from home

Although many coeliacs opt for self-catering holidays, there is no reason why holidays in hotels or guest houses should not be successful if a coeliac is prepared to explain the essence of his diet and to be careful in the choice of his food. The Coeliac Society produces lists of holiday hotels and guest houses in Britain where a gluten-free diet can be guaranteed and also publishes information leaflets for most foreign countries. When away on holiday or just travelling, coeliacs should be encouraged to take supplies of bread, biscuits, wafers or crackers so that they always have gluten-free foods available. Most airlines will supply a gluten-free diet if it is ordered beforehand when the ticket is booked; information about this is also available from the Coeliac Society. Eating in other people's homes can be hazardous and coeliacs should always tell their hosts of their gluten-free diet requirements when the invitation is offered and not when they arrive on the doorstep. Most buffet food is unlikely to be gluten-free and coeliacs should be warned of this and encouraged to eat something beforehand or take food with them; the effects of drinking alcohol on an empty stomach can be disastrous!

Other people's attitudes

One of the greatest problems experienced by coeliacs is the attitude of friends or relatives who cannot, or will not, understand the need for a strict gluten-free diet. Coeliacs should be encouraged to explain their diet simply and briefly to other people. Friends and relatives are often eager to help the patient comply with the diet when the diagnosis is initially made, especially if the person concerned has been obviously ill; problems tend to arise later when a patient becomes fit and well and many relatives then feel that the diet need not be so strictly complied with. Grandparents can often be the most difficult in this respect — 'surely one biscuit won't hurt' said in front of a grandchild, can make life extremely difficult for parents.

Many coeliacs have found that showing the Coeliac Society's video about the condition to their relatives has been helpful.

Ignorance of medical and nursing personnel

Dietitians should explain to coeliacs that, statistically, they are likely to be the only coeliac patient in the care of their GP, and it is therefore a little unfair to expect their doctor to have complete knowledge of all the gluten-free foods or even all those available on prescription. The same argument applies to hospitals and hospital staff (unless the patient attends a children's hospital or one with a coeliac clinic); the nursing and catering staff may only have a very limited knowledge of the condition and its treatment. If a coeliac knows that he has to go into hospital, it is sensible and helpful if he contacts the hospital dietitian and ward sister in advance and then also takes with him into hospital gluten-free bread and biscuits. Coeliacs should be warned that in specialist units such as orthopaedic or obstetric, they may have to fend for themselves and explain the condition and their diet to all personnel, even the doctors.

Minor ailments

Patients should be warned not to blame all their medical problems on their coeliac condition, as coeliacs are not immune to all other disorders. Mothers tend to attribute all incidences of diarrhoea in their coeliac child to dietary indiscretions whereas it is often just a minor tummy upset which is going around.

Pharmaceutical preparations

A few pharmaceutical preparations including some on prescription do contain gluten. This is not a great problem since wheat or wheat flour is rarely used as an excipient by the pharmaceutical industry. A list of pharmaceutical preparations containing gluten is available from the Coeliac Society.

Support organisation

The Coeliac Society

In the UK, the Coeliac Society exists to help those who have coeliac disease or dermatitis herpetiformis. The Society produces a booklet listing brands of gluten-free manufactured foods which is invaluable for all coeliacs. This comprehensive list is published annually and is up-dated every six months via the Society's magazine, and monthly on BBC Ceefax. The Coeliac Society also produces a handbook giving information about the condition and its treatment, recipe books, a magazine *The Crossed Grain*, holiday information, a video about coeliac disease and many other services. There are about 50 local groups of the Coeliac Society The Society's address is: The Coeliac Society, PO Box 220, High Wycombe, Bucks HP11 2HY. Tel: 0494-37278.

4.12.3 Inflammatory bowel disease

Inflammatory Bowel Disease (IBD) is an all-embracing term used for the idiopathic chronic inflammatory disorders of the intestine. It includes conditions such as Crohn's disease, ulcerative colitis, ischaemic colitis and iatrogenic antibiotic-associated colitis. The two more common conditions — Crohn's disease and ulcerative colitis will be discussed in this section. The aetiology of both conditions is unknown and many aspects of their management are controversial. Successful management relies on close co-operation between the physician and surgeon.

Crohn's disease

Crohn's disease is a chronic granulomatous inflammatory condition which can affect any part of the gut from mouth to anus, but which predominantly involves the terminal ileum and the colon. It may occur as single or multiple lesions and involves the whole of the intestinal wall.

Although it may affect any age group, Crohn's disease is most common in young adults — men and women being equally affected. The cause of the disease is still unknown. Epidemiological studies have implicated foods such as cornflakes (James 1977) and an excess of sugar (Thornton *et al* 1979) as possible causative factors. More recently, it has been suggested that Crohn's disease may be due to an intolerance to specific foods (Hunter *et al* 1983) and exclusion diets have been used in the management of the disease.

Symptoms

Depending on the site of involvement, the intestinal inflammation usually produces abdominal pain and diarrhoea. The gut may become narrowed and cause strictures and adhesions resulting in episodes of vomiting and constipation. Bleeding is likely to occur if the disease is present in the colon or rectum. The disease may be complicated by the development of abscesses and fistulae, both internal and external. A small proportion of patients suffer episodes of inflammation affecting the eyes, skin, limb joints or spine. Apthous mouth ulcers may also occur. The disease is characterized by periods of remission and relapse.

The influence of pregnancy

Many women who develop Crohn's disease are young and may wish to have children. Active Crohn's disease may reduce fertility and can cause inflammation and blockage of the Fallopian tubes. The disease can make intercourse painful and therefore reduce the chance of conception. However, the majority of women with Crohn's disease are able to conceive. On the whole, the disease is more likely to improve rather than deteriorate during pregnancy.

Crohn's disease in childhood

Crohn's disease can occur in infancy (Miller and Larsen 1971) but is more likely to occur in childhood between the ages of 12 and 14 years (Hamilton *et al* 1979; Walker Smith 1979). Crohn's disease, like many chronic illnesses, can interfere with a child's normal growth and development. Growth retardation correlates with active disease and growth spurts often occur after effective therapy (Horner *et al* 1977). Nutritional factors also affect growth retardation and acceleration and close attention should be paid to the nutritional requirements of children with Crohn's disease.

Metabolic and nutritional consequences of Crohn's disease

Patients with Crohn's disease are at risk of developing a range of metabolic and nutritional problems. Weight loss and anaemia are frequently observed and the incidence of hypoalbuminaemia, intestinal protein loss and negative nitrogen balance is quite high.

Anaemia may be due to deficiencies of iron, folate or vitamin B12. Sodium and fluid depletion are common in patients with persistant diarrhoea and deficiences of magnesium, zinc, copper and manganese and other trace elements may occur. Following the formation of an ileostomy, the losses of both sodium and potassium can be high, particularly in the early post-operative phase.

Bile salt absorption is often impaired in patients with involvement of the distal ileum and in those patients who have undergone resection of the terminal ileum. This will result in reduced absorption of fat, and fat soluble vitamins, with consequent steatorrhoea.

Considerable losses of fluids and electrolytes can occur in patients with a diseased or absent colon, and an adequate intake should be ensured to avoid dehydration and electrolyte imbalance.

Management of Crohn's disease

Drug therapy may be used in conjunction with, or independently of, nutritional therapy. The drugs most commonly used are sulphasalazine, corticosteroids (e.g. prednisolone) and immunosuppressive drugs (e.g. azothioprine and 6-mercaptopurine [6MP]). Antidiarrhoeal drugs such as codeine phosphate and loperamide may be used to control diarrhoea, but they do not act against the disease itself. It should not be forgotten that the use of some of these drugs may have nutritional consequences, e.g. sulphasalazine impairs folate absorption and utilization and steroids affect protein-energy metabolism (see also Section 5.10).

The aim of the dietary management of Crohn's disease is to meet the nutritional requirements in the face of symptoms which often interfere with dietary adequacy. Whether the nutritional therapy is regarded as a primary or secondary therapy is still debatable. A complete nutritional assessment and estimation of nutritional requirements should be made to establish energy, nitrogen, mineral and vitamin needs and to counteract existing deficiencies. The dietary management will vary depending on the activity of the disease.

Active disease

Methods of nutritional support used in inducing remission of active disease include
1 Total parenteral nutrition.
2 Enteral nutrition using elemental or polymeric diets.
3 Elemental diet followed by the identification of food intolerances.

Total parenteral nutrition (TPN) in conjunction with total bowel rest, has been used in the management of active Crohn's disease (Fischer *et al* 1973; Driscoll and Rosenberg 1978; Dickinson *et al* 1980). Although the technique is of proven value, it is also invasive, expensive and should ideally be supervised by a specialized nutrition team. Peripheral intravenous therapy may maintain fluid and electrolyte balance, but the nutritional requirements of Crohn's disease patients would be difficult to administer via a peripheral line. It may be uncertain whether the clinical improvements and reduction of the activity of the disease are due to improved nutritional state, the removal of some agent from the intestinal environment or simply to bowel rest.

Enteral nutrition has been used both as a complete feed during active disease and as a nutritional supplement for depleted patients during remission. A number of studies have reported encouraging results for the use of elemental diets in achieving remission of active Crohn's disease (Axelsson and Jarnum 1977; Morin *et al* 1982; O'Morain *et al* 1980, 1983, 1984). The elemental diets most commonly used are those containing mainly free amino acids as the nitrogen source (e.g. Vivonex, EO28). The use of feeds containing mainly short chain peptides as the source of nitrogen has not been fully investigated.

Alun Jones and co-workers (1985) compared the use of an elemental diet with TPN as a primary treatment of active Crohn's disease. They reported no significant differences between the two treatment methods.

Elemental diet and the identification of food intolerances. The majority of patients who go into remission following TPN or enteral nutrition are often maintained on steroids and other drugs. They may relapse after a relatively short period of time. Searching for food intolerances which might provoke symptoms has produced excellent results and generated a great deal of interest in the use of exclusion diets in the management of the disease.

Patients with active Crohn's disease are fed artificially using an elemental diet. The diet may be taken either orally or administered via a nasogastric tube. During this period, all medication is tailed off. When patients are symptom-free, foods are reintroduced one by one and the elemental diet is maintained as a supplement until an adequate range of foods can be tolerated. Foods which cause problems are avoided and retested at a later stage. Those foods most frequently found to provoke symptoms include wheat, dairy products, corn, brassicas and citrus fruits (Workman *et al* 1984).

The nutritional management of Crohn's disease during remission. A variety of diets have been tried and tested which might possibly be of long term benefit in Crohn's disease and reduce the incidence of relapse.

Heaton *et al* (1979) studied the effect of a diet high in fibre and low in refined carbohydrates. He found that the patients studied had significantly fewer and shorter admissions to hospital than a group of matched control patients. However, patients known to have intestinal narrowing and strictures should *not* be advised to take a high fibre diet. In Italy Levenstein *et al* (1985) compared a low residue diet with a normal Italian diet and found that the low residue diet offered no advantage.

One cause of nutritional deficiencies in Crohn's disease is the use of over-restrictive diets and care should be taken to ensure that the diets advised are well planned and nutritionally adequate. Supplementary feeding with ready-prepared enteral feeds can significantly increase total energy and nitrogen intake and improve body weight and general well being (Harries *et al* 1983).

Lactose intolerance may occur, particularly if there is involvement of the jejunum, but it is not a common problem. It may be that lactose loads cause problems whereas small quantities of lactose taken quite frequently do not.

Malabsorption of bile salts and vitamin B12 following ileal resection can be controlled by the use of cholestyramine (Questran) and routine vitamin B12 injections.

Patients with Crohn's disease of the small bowel, particularly those who have had bowel resections, may experience fat malabsorption to varying degrees of severity. Increased losses of fat in the stools also result in increased losses of calcium, magnesium and possibly zinc. Benefit may be gained by taking a low fat diet. Care should be taken to ensure that the energy lost by reducing the fat in the diet is replaced by a more readily absorbable source of energy, e.g. carbohydrates and possibly medium chain trglycerides (MCT). Fat soluble vitamins may need to be given.

Ulcerative colitis

Symptoms and prevalence

Ulcerative colitis is a chronic inflammatory disease of the large bowel. Part or all of the mucosa of the bowel becomes diffusely inflamed and ulcerated. The inflammation is haemorrhagic and an excess of mucus (which may contain some pus) is produced. The condition typically manifests itself in acute attacks interposed with periods of remission and freedom from symptoms.

During an acute attack, the patient presents with rectal bleeding and diarrhoea with or without pain. The presence of blood and mucus in the stools, helps to distinguish ulcerative colitis from Crohn's disease in which these features are not usually present (except in Crohn's disease of the colon).

Ulcerative colitis occurs throughout the world but there are enormous variations in its prevalence. It is most common in the USA, Canada, UK, Scandinavia and other North European countries where the occurrence is about 1 in 1,000–1,500. The disease may begin at any age, but most first attacks occur in young adults. It is fairly uncommon in childhood and becomes more frequent at puberty. Throughout the world there is little sex difference, but in England women are more commonly affected than men. The cause of the disease is still unknown.

The onset of symptoms is often more gradual than acute. When an attack is severe the patient may pass up to 20 stools per day. Profuse diarrhoea results in dehydration and loss of electrolytes. Anaemia may develop due to chronic blood loss and patients may complain of malaise, weakness, weight loss, fever and tachycardia.

Complications

These fall into two main groups
1 Local complications — occurring in and around the diseased large bowel.
2 Remote and systemic complications — affecting other organs of the body.

Local complications include
1 Perforation of the colon which requires an emergency colectomy.
2 Toxic megacolon when the colon becomes grossly dilated and may also require emergency surgical treatment.
3 Abscesses and fistulae-in-ano.
4 Cancer of the large bowel.

Remote complications are very diverse and include
1 Angular conjunctivitis in one or both eyes.
2 Ulceration of the mouth.
3 Skin lesions, e.g. erythema nodosum and pyodermia gangrenosum. Skin rashes may also occur in response to drug therapy (sulphasalazine).

Arthritis, ankylosing spondylitis, fatty changes of the liver, sclerosing cholangitis and very occasionally cirrhosis of the liver may also occur.

The influence of pregnancy

Women with ulcerative colitis are usually able to conceive but should not plan to do so if the disease is active. In general, women who conceive when they are symptom-free have fewer problems. Symptoms are most likely to flare-up in the first three months of pregnancy and may also become worse shortly after delivery.

Treatment of ulcerative colitis

The drugs most commonly used are sulphasalazine and corticosteroids. Mild and moderate attacks should be treated promptly by these drugs together with a suitable iron supplement if indicated.

A severe attack will require admission to hospital. Fluid and electrolyte balance must be restored and blood transfusions may be necessary. Nutritional therapy, either TPN or enteral nutrition (if considered appropriate), may be used as an adjunct to the medical treatment. An emergency colectomy may be required. A proctocolectomy with a permanent ileostomy is the standard operation for ulcerative colitis. The entire large bowel is removed which totally eliminates the disease.

Dietary treatment. The main dietary aims in colitis are to ensure that nutrition is adequate and to correct malnutrition, if present. Patients with inflammatory bowel disease are at risk of developing malnutrition due to anorexia, inadequate energy intake, vomiting, diarrhoea, dehydration and pyrexia. In addition, drug therapy may interfere with the absorption of vitamins and minerals.

1 Acute stage. A low residue diet is often advised during mild or moderate attacks of colitis. However, a low residue diet could aggravate problems because of the difficulty in passing hard faeces by those patients with distal colonic or rectal disease. During a more severe attack, enteral feeding using either whole protein feeds or elemental preparations taken either orally or via a nasogastric tube may be prescribed. Whether the therapy is beneficial by allowing bowel rest or simply by providing nutritional support is questionable. If enteral feeding is not tolerated or considered inappropriate (e.g. in severe cases of toxic megacolon) TPN should be prescribed.

2 Lactose intolerance. Anatomical and functional abnormalities of the small intestinal mucosa have been shown in ulcerative colitis (Salen and Truelove 1965) and hypolactasia has occurred during acute attacks of colitis. This usually improves when the patient goes into remission (Cady *et al* 1967). As milk is a good source of protein, minerals and energy, a milk-free diet should only be recommended reluctantly and a suitable milk substitute prescribed (see p 195).

3 Remission. Patients with ulcerative colitis who are symptom-free should be encouraged to eat a normal diet with adequate amounts of protein, energy, vitamins and minerals. A high fibre diet can be prescribed without fear of causing a relapse and may be beneficial in patients with distal colitis who have phases of forming hard stools and may need to strain in order to pass them. Lactose intolerance may only be a problem if a lactose load is taken and most patients can tolerate milk without developing diarrhoea. Patients may have individual food intolerances and may benefit from avoiding certain foods (see Section 2.11). Care should be taken to ensure that such steps do not result in a nutritionally inadequate diet.

4.12.4 Irritable bowel syndrome

Irritable bowel syndrome (IBS) is a very common condition which accounts for 33−70% of gastrointestinal consultations in Britain (Drossman *et al* 1977; Harvey *et al* 1983). It occurs about twice as often in women as in men.

Patients complain of diarrhoea or constipation, or an alternation between the two conditions, and abdominal pain and distention. The condition is usually exacerbated by stress. Patients with IBS have abnormal gut motility which can be demonstrated in the small bowel and oesophagus as well as in the colon. No specific mucosal changes are evident.

Dietary treatment

High fibre diets were advocated for patients with IBS in the late 1970's (Manning *et al* 1977). Patients may find such a diet beneficial and should be advised to consume an adequate quantity of soluble fibre in the form of fruits, vegetables, beans and pulses and wholegrain cereals as well as insoluble fibre (e.g. wheat bran). Patients with diarrhoea may not benefit as much from the diet as those with constipation.

A bulking agent such as methylcellulose or ispaghula may be prescribed (Heaton 1985) and natural laxatives such as lactulose may also be beneficial. Anti-spasmodic drugs can be prescribed to give relief from abdominal pain and distention.

During recent years evidence has emerged which suggests that specific food intolerance may be responsible for some cases of IBS — particularly those with diarrhoea (Cooper *et al* 1980; Lessof *et al* 1980; Alun-Jones *et al* 1982; Hunter *et al* 1985).

Many patients seize upon the idea of 'food allergy' being responsible for their symptoms, a conclusion often greeted with scepticism by their physician. If a food allergy is suspected, it should be investigated under proper medical and dietetic supervision (see Section 5.9) and not on a 'do-it-yourself' basis by the patient at home. The latter course of action is likely to result in an unnecessarily restricted and nutritionally inadequate diet.

4.12.5 Constipation

Constipation is the delayed transit of faeces which results in them becoming hardened and difficult to pass. The consequent straining can precipitate and exacerbate conditions such as haemorrhoids and anal fissure.

In the past, the excessive and inappropriate use of laxatives to regularize bowel function has frequently been counter-productive and has resulted in an atonic, poorly functioning colon. It is now recognized that dietary measures should be the primary form of treatment and laxatives should be used only as an adjunct to dietary therapy where there are complicating factors.

Dietary treatment

Simple constipation can usually be remedied by
1 Increasing the intake of dietary fibre, of both cereal and vegetable origin (see Section 2.5).
2 Increasing fluid intake, both with and between meals.

Dietary fibre acts by absorbing fluid and thus producing a soft bulky stool; it also encourages beneficial bacterial action in the bowel.

Although it is relatively simple to increase the fibre intake of a motivated adult, it can be difficult in those with conservative eating habits, in particular the very young and the very old. Elderly people, especially those with dentures, may reject fibre-rich foods on the grounds that they are too difficult to chew and leave irritating residues in the mouth. Children who live mainly on white bread, tinned spaghetti and refined rice-based breakfast cereals are unlikely to greet the sudden advent of fresh fruit and vegetables, whole meal bread and fibre-rich breakfast cereals with much

enthusiasm. This is one reason why healthy eating habits should be encouraged in children from the time of weaning and, in addition, that the whole family should consume such a diet so that the child sees this as the norm.

In both of these groups, changes should be introduced gradually. If wholemeal bread is disliked, a high-fibre white bread may be more acceptable. Cooked and pureed fruit may be preferred to raw fruit. Vegetables can be 'hidden' in casseroles or pies. Wholemeal flours and cereals can be incorporated into home-baked products.

Bulk-forming preparations and laxatives

Bulk-forming preparations

Patients who cannot, or will not, consume sufficient dietary fibre for adequate bowel function may require an additional bulk-forming preparation. Unprocessed wheat bran, taken either in tablet form or added to foods or liquids, is one of the most effective. Ispaghula, sterculia or methylcellulose are suitable alternatives for those who cannot tolerate bran. However, it is vital that sufficient fluid intake accompanies the use of these bulking agents to avoid the risk of faecal impaction or intestinal obstruction. It is also important to remember that bran impairs the absorption of iron, calcium, zinc and other trace elements and prolonged supplementation should be avoided, especially in children and the elderly.

Laxatives

Faecal softeners (e.g. dioctyl sodium sulphosuccinate) or lubricants (e.g. liquid paraffin) are sometimes useful for the management of haemorrhoids or anal fissure. However, patients should be strongly discouraged from the regular use of liquid paraffin without medical direction as it can cause a number of severe side effects in addition to impairing the absorption of fat soluble vitamins.

Osmotic laxatives, which act by maintaining a volume of fluid in the bowel by osmosis, have occasional medical uses but must never be used on a regular basis. Preparations such as magnesium carbonate, magnesium hydroxide and magnesium sulphate (Epsom salts) all have a very rapid purgative action (the latter within 2–4 hours).

A less drastic and more acceptable laxative effect

can be achieved with lactulose, a disaccharide which is unabsorbed and hence exerts an osmotic effect. Lactulose results in softer, bulkier motions within 1—2 days and is particularly useful for re-establishing bowel habits in constipated children or in patients following treatment for an impacted bowel. Lactulose is also a useful preparation for the elderly when constipation does not respond to fibre supplementation alone owing to deterioration in bowel muscle function. Lactulose should be administered in gradually decreasing doses over a period of a few days, ideally with a concomitant increase in dietary fibre and fluid intake.

Stimulant laxatives (such as senna, fig, castor oil, bis-acodyl or danthron) which act by increasing intestinal motility should not be used routinely, and preferably not at all, without medical direction. Some preparations (e.g. sodium picosulphate) are a useful way of achieving bowel evacuation prior to investigative or surgical procedures (see Section 5.8).

4.12.6 Diverticular disease

Diverticular disease is a common disorder of the large bowel. Early stages of the disease can be identified in 15% of people over the age of 50 years. There is usually a history of constipation which results in increased colonic pressure, straining to pass hard faeces and rupture of the bowel wall to form small pockets — diverticuli. Inflammation and bacterial overgrowth in diverticuli may result in diarrhoea.

Dietary treatment

Patients should benefit from a high fibre diet together with increased fluid intake. The addition of bran or bran products may be particularly beneficial in those patients with constipation.

4.12.7 Colorectal cancer

This common cancer is found predominantly in developed Western nations and has been linked to environmental and dietary factors. There is some inconclusive evidence that diets high in fat or sugar or low in fibre, vitamin A or vitamin C may be causally related to its incidence.

Patients are likely to need surgery, probably resection, and may require a temporary or permanent colostomy.

Dietary treatment

Patients are frequently undernourished and this is of particular concern prior to surgery. Nutritional support, either enterally or parenterally, may be needed. Patients who have a colostomy should be given specific advice (see p 422).

4.12.8 Bowel surgery

Patients who have chronic diseases of the bowel which require surgical intervention are likely to be malnourished and to have higher nutritional requirements than patients admitted for acute or elective surgery.

Intestinal resection

The diseased part of the bowel is removed and the two ends of the unaffected bowel joined. If only a small area is removed, the small intestine will adapt quite quickly and most patients can soon return to eating a normal diet. If extensive resection of the small bowel is required, only a very short length of bowel, 100 cm or less, may be left. The consequent limited absorptive capacity remaining results in the *short bowel syndrome* and this will require dietary intervention until adaptation eventually occurs.

Short bowel syndrome

In the early post-operative phase, such patients will require TPN to provide nutritional support (see Section 1.13). Enteral nutrition should be introduced as early as possible, either as oral or nasogastric feeding using elemental or whole protein enteral feeds (see Section 1.12). During this stage attention should be paid to the fluid and electrolyte requirements of the patients, in particular the sodium content of the feed. Most elemental feeds contain low concentrations of sodium and intestinal absorption of fluid and electrolytes has been shown to improve if at least 70 mmol of sodium/l are administered (Spiller *et al* 1982). Enteral feeding should be gradually replaced by a light, low residue diet. Once oral diet has been introduced, energy and protein intake can be increased by the use of dietary supplements (see Section 2.12). Lactose tolerance may be impaired in the very short bowel syndrome and lactose loads should be avoided.

Malabsorption of fat may aggravate diarrhoea and increase malabsorption of fat soluble vitamins and minerals such as calcium. If a low fat diet is advised, the energy deficit should be corrected by the use of supplementary carbohydrates and possibly MCT (see Section 2.12).

Persistent diarrhoea can result in fluid and electrolyte deficiencies and an adequate intake should be ensured to restore fluid and electrolyte balance. Patients with a permanent ileostomy in whom the absorptive capacity of the colon is bypassed will also have increased requirements for fluid and electrolytes.

Iron, folate supplements and vitamin B12 injections may be required to prevent anaemia, and bile salt malabsorption should be controlled by the use of cholestyramine.

Close dietetic supervision of these patients is important, particularly during the early stages until intestinal adaptation has taken place and the patient is able to take a nutritionally adequate diet.

Colostomy and ileostomy

Following intestinal resection, a colostomy or ileostomy may be performed. The gut is brought out to the surface of the abdomen and a prominent stoma fashioned.

A variety of stoma bags are manufactured and a stoma therapist should be available to advise the best type of appliance for each patient. The bag is fitted over the stoma and the intestinal effluent collected in it and discarded regularly. If the rectum is left *in situ*, a mucus fistula will be formed on the surface of the abdomen to allow drainage.

Dietary treatment. Patients should follow as normal a diet as possible but individuals may find certain foods cause the stool consistency and odour to be unacceptable and these foods should be avoided. Foods which pass through unaltered need not be avoided unless they cause embarrassment to the patient by suddenly filling the bag and causing it to leak. Patients may also prefer to avoid foods which tend to cause flatulence (e.g. onions, lentils, beans and sprouts), but a moderately high fibre intake should be encouraged in order to ensure efficient functioning of the stoma.

Patients with ileostomies may initially lose both electrolytes and fluid and require an increased intake of these for at least 6−8 weeks after which time the ileum appears to adapt and losses decrease. Diarrhoea may exacerbate the electolyte imbalance and extra potassium (via fruit juices) and sodium (via extra salt on food or salty beverages such as soup or Bovril) should be consumed. Alternatively, supplementary electrolytes can be given.

Support organisation

Ileostomy Association of Great Britain and Ireland, Amblehurst House, Chobham, Woking, Surrey GU24 8PZ.

Further reading

Allan RN, Keighly MRB, Alexander-Williams J. and Hawkings C (1983) *Inflammatory bowel disease.* Chrchill Livingstone, Edinburgh.

Alun-Jones V (1985) Irritable bowel syndrome. In *Food and the gut* Hunter JO and Alun-Jones V (Eds). Bailliere Tindall, London.

Bingham S, McNeil NI and Cummings JH (1977) Diet for the ileostomist. *J Hum Nutr* **31**, 367.

Brodribb AOM (1977) Treatment of symptomatic diverticular disease with a high fibre diet. *Lancet* i, 664−6.

Burkitt D (1979) *Don't forget fibre in your diet* (Positive Health Guide). Martin Dunitz, London.

Celestin LR (1974) Ano-rectal disease. In *Basic gastroenterology* Naish JM and Read AEA (Eds). Wright and Sons, Bristol.

Cooper BT (1983) Inflammatory bowel disease. In *Gastrointestinal disease* Roberts CJC (Ed). Springer-Verlang, Berlin.

Davidson S and Passmore R (1986) *Human nutrition and dietetics* Passmore R and Eastwood MA (Eds). Churchill Livingstone, Edinburgh.

Dickerson JWT and Lee HA (1978) Diseases of the alimentary tract. In *Nutrition in the clinical management of disease.* Edward Arnold, London.

Dickerson JWT and Jones MH (1982) Malabsorption. *Nursing* **2**, 113−7.

Francis DEM (1986) *Diets for sick children* 4e. Blackwell Scientific Publications, Oxford.

Gear JSS, Fursdon P, Nolan DJ, Weare A, Mann JI, Brodribb AJM and Vessey MP (1979) Symptomless diverticular disease and intake of dietary fibre. *Lancet* i, 511−4.

Greenberger NJ and Silkman TG (1969) Medium chain triglycerides — physiologic consideration and clinical implications. *N Engl J Med* **280**, 1045−59.

Heaton KW (1983) Dietary fibre in perspective. *Hum Nutr: Appl Nutr* **37C**, 151−70.

Heaton KW (1985) Crohn's disease and ulcerative colitis. In *Dietary fibre, fibre-depleted foods and diseases* pp 205−16. Trowell H, Burkitt D and Heaton K (Eds). Academic Press, London

Heaton KW (1985) Diet and diverticulosis — new leads. *Gut* **26**, In press.

Losowsky MS, Walker BE and Kelleher J (1974) *Malabsorption in clinical practice.* Churchill Livingstone, Edinburgh.

Northfield T, Zentler-Munro P and Fine D (1984) Mechanisms and management of pancreatic steatorrhoea. *Hospital Update* **10**, 489−99.

Rawcliffe P and Rolph R (1985) *The gluten-free diet book.* Martin Dunitz, London.

Truelove SC (1984) *Ulcerative colitis.* Update Publications, London.

Walker-Smith J (1975) *Diseases of the small intestine in childhood* pp 157−84. Pitman Medical Publishing, Tunbridge Wells.

References

Alun-Jones V, McLaughlan PP, Shorthouse M, Wakman E and Hunter JO (1982) Food intolerance: a major factor in the pathogenesis of irritable bowel syndrome. *Lancet* ii, 1115−7.

Alun-Jones V, Dickenson RJ and Hunter JO (1985) Controlled trial of elemental diet and parenteral nutrition in the induction of remission in Crohn's disease. In press.

Axelsson C and Jarnum S (1977) Assessment of the therapeutic value of an elemental diet in chronic inflammatory bowel disease. *Scand J Gastroenterol* **12**, 89−95.

Cady AB, Rhodes J, Littman A and Crane RA (1967) Significance of lactose deficit in ulcerative colitis. *J Lab Clin Med* **70**, 279−86.

Cooper BT, Holmes GKT, Ferguson R, Thompson RA, Alan RN and Cooke WT (1980) Gluten sensitive diarrhoea without evidence of coeliac disease. *Gastroenterology* **79**, 801–6.

Crosby WH and Kugler HW (1957) Intraluminal biopsy of the small intestine; intestinal biopsy capsule. *Am J Dig Dis* **2**, 236–41.

Dicke WK (1950) Coeliackie. MD Thesis, University of Utrecht, The Netherlands.

Dickinson RJ, Ashton MG, Axon AT, Smith RC, Yeung CK and Hill GL (1980) Controlled trial of intravenous hyperalimentation and total bowel rest as an adjunct to the routine therapy of acute colitis. *Gastroenterology* **79**, 1199–204.

Driscoll RH Jr and Rosenberg IH (1978) Total parenteral nutrition in inflammatory bowel disease. *Med Clin North Am* **62**, 185–201.

Drossman DA, Powell DW and Sessides JT (1977) The irritable bowel syndrome. *Gastroenterology* **73**, 811–22.

Fischer JE, Foster JS, Abel RM, Abbot WM and Ryan JA (1973) Hyperalimentation as primary therapy for inflammatory bowel disease. *Am J Surg* **125**, 165–73.

Gee S (1888) On the coeliac affliction. *St Bartholomews Hospital Reports* **24**, 17.

Hamilton JR, Bruce GA, Abdourhaman M and Gall DG (1979) Inflammatory bowel disease in children and adolescents. *Adv Paediatr* **26**, 311–41.

Harries AD, Jones LA, Davis V, Fifield R, Heatly RV, Newcombe RG and Rhodes J (1983) Controlled trial of supplemental oral nutrition in Crohn's disease. *Lancet* **i** 887–90.

Harvey RF, Salih SY and Read AE (1983) Organic and functional disorders in 2000 gastroenterology out-patients. *Lancet* **i**, 632–4.

Heaton KW, Thornton JR and Emmett PM (1979) Tratement of Crohn's disease with an unrefined carbohydrate fibre-rich diet. *Br Med J* **2**, 746–66.

Heaton KW (1985) Role of dietary fibre in irritable bowel syndrome. In *Irritable bowel syndrome* p 203. Grune and Stratton Ltd, New York.

Horner DR, Grand RJ and Colodry AH (1977) Growth, cause and prognosis after surgery for Crohn's disease in children and adolescents. *Paediatrics* **59**, 717–25.

Hunter JO, Alun-Jones V, Freeman AH, Shorthouse M, Workman E and McLaughter P (1983) Food intolerance in gastrointestinal disorders. *Proc 2nd Fisons Food Allergy Workshop*, Harrogate pp 69–72. Medicine Publishing Foundation, Oxford.

Hunter JO, Workman E and Alun-Jones V (1985) Role of diet in the management of irritable bowel syndrome. In *Topics in gastroenterology* Vol 2 Gibson PR and Jewell DP (Eds). Blackwell Scientific Publications, Oxford.

James AH (1977) Breakfast and Crohn's disease. *Br Med J* **1**, 943–5.

Koivisto VA, Kuitunen P, Tiilikainen A and Akerblom HK (1977) HLA antigens in patients with juvenile diabetes mellitus, coeliac disease and both of the diseases. *Diabet Metab* **3**, 49.

Kumar P, O'Donoghue D, Stenson K and Dawson A (1979) Reintroduction of gluten in adults and children with treated coeliac disease. *Gut* **20**, 743.

Lessof MH, Wraight DG, Merrett TG, Merrett J and Buisseret PD (1980) Food allergy and intolerance in 100 patients. *Quart J Med* **195**, 259–71.

Manning AP, Heaton KW, Uglaw P and Harvey RF (1977) Wheat fibre and irritable bowel syndrome: a controlled trial. *Lancet* **ii**, 417–8.

Levenstein S, Prantera C, Luzi C and D-Ubaldi A (1985) Low residue or normal diet in Crohn's disease: a prospective controlled study in Italian patients. *Gut* **26**, 989–93.

McCrae WM (1969) Inheritance of coeliac disease. *J Med Genet* **6**, 129–31.

Morin CL, Railet M, Roy CC, Weber A and Lapointe N (1982) Continuous elemental enteral alimentation in the treatment of children and adolescents with Crohn's disease. *J Parent Nutr* **6**, 194–9.

Mylotte M, Egan-Mitchell B, McCarthy CF and McNicholl B (1973) Incidence of coeliac disease in the west of Ireland. *Br Med J* **1**, 703–5.

O'Morain C, Segal AW and Levi AJ (1980) Elemental diets in the treatment of acute Crohn's disease. *Br Med J* **281**, 1173–5.

O'Morain C, Segal AW, Levi AJ and Valman HB (1983) Elemental diet in acute Crohn's disease. *Arch Dis Childh* **53**, 44–7.

O'Morain C, Segal AW and Levi AJ (1984) Elemental diet as primary therapy of acute Crohn's disease: a controlled trial. *Br Med J* **288**, 1859–62.

Paulley JW (1954) Observations on the aetiology of idiopathic steatorrhoea. *Br Med J* **2**, 1318–21.

Salen SN and Truelove SC (1965) Small intestine and gastric abnormalities in ulcerative colitis. *Br Med J* **1**, 827–31.

Shiner M (1956) Jejunal biopsy tube. *Lancet* **i**, 85.

Spiller RC, Jones BJM and Silk DBA (1982) Influence of sodium content of enteric diets on water absorption from the human jejunum. *JPEN* **6**, 342.

C: Disorders of the Liver and Biliary Tract

4.13 Diseases of the Liver

4.13.1 Acute hepatitis

Hepatitis may be a quite mild, flu-like illness, accompanied by a degree of jaundice or it may be a severe inflammatory disease of the liver causing acute liver failure and coma.

Dietary treatment

This depends on the severity of the condition.

Mild hepatitis

Patients with mild hepatitis should be given a diet which is generally nutritious and high in protein and energy. Jaundice should not be treated by fat restriction as this will lower energy intake and serve no useful purpose. Some patients may be nauseated by very fatty foods, but milk, butter and cheese are usually well tolerated.

Severe hepatitis

If the patient is in a coma, protein must be withdrawn completely and energy requirements met by carbohydrate and fat, initially parenterally, through a peripheral vein. A suitable regimen is shown in Table 4.34. (see also Section 1.13.) In addition to parenteral feeding, a nasogastric feed may be advisable to provide enough energy to prevent tissue breakdown. A suitable formulation is given in Table 4.35 (see also Section 1.12.3). The 'no protein' regimen is usually only required in the very short term as consciousness will return quite rapidly, if death has not intervened. Electroencephalography (EEG) is a useful guide to prognosis and to assess the level of returning consciousness (Kennedy 1973).

As consciousness returns, protein can be added to the diet, either in liquid (Table 4.36) or solid form (see Table 2.5, p 120). Protein should initially be increased in 10 g increments and the patient's tolerance assessed at each stage.

If improvement in liver function is not apparent within approximately three weeks, necrosis may be present and the prognosis is poor.

Table 4.34 Parenteral formula for use in coma due to liver disease

1−2 litres 10% dextrose in 24 hours
Parenterovite I and II
No Intralipid

Blood glucose should be tested hourly

Table 4.35 Minimal protein tube feed for use in liver coma

100 g Maxijul (or other glucose polymer)
200 ml Calogen (or other 50% fat emulsion)
10 ml Crusha milk shake syrup
500 ml sterile water

This formula provides 1300 kcal, 600 ml water and 2 mmol sodium. Vitamins may be added to the feed if required. If a parenteral feed is being given at the same time, complete vitamin cover should be provided with that.

Table 4.36 Low protein liquid feed for use in severe encephalopathy

25 g Maxipro
200 g Maxijul
50 ml Calogen
1 g sodium chloride
500 ml water

This formula provides 1200 kcal, 20 g protein, 22 mmol sodium and 525 ml water.

4.13.2 Chronic active hepatitis

This is an HLA associated disease characterized by exhaustion and fluctuating jaundice. Ascites and bleeding varices are late features of cirrhosis which may result from untreated chronic active hepatitis. Serum transaminase and gammaglobulin concentration are raised. Serum bilirubin is elevated in some, but not all, patients, and any individual may have varying levels in the course of the disease.

Ascites is a common symptom in later stages of this disease. This is due primarily to failure of the liver to synthesise albumin, resulting in a lowered plasma osmotic pressure and portal venous hypertension. More fluid enters the peritoneal cavity than leaves it and ascites develops. Patients with ascites may retain sodium avidly and have low urinary sodium levels. Serum sodium may be below normal, but this does not reflect sodium deficiency; due to the greatly expanded extracellular sodium space, the actual total body stores of sodium are increased.

Treatment of ascites is bed rest, diet, fluid restriction and diuretics. Over vigorous early use of diuretics is contraindicated as this can trigger hepato-renal failure (Sherlock 1981). An initial diuresis may be obtained by confining the patient to bed and giving a low sodium diet. A diet containing no more than 22 mmol (500 mg) sodium is usually effective (see p 151). A fluid restriction is imposed because water excretion is defective. If the ascites is well controlled on this diet plus suitable diuretics, the sodium intake may be increased to 40 mmol sodium (see p 151) when the patient leaves hospital. Cirrhotic patients have been shown to have low levels of serum arachidonic acid, which may lead to reduced prostaglandin production. The resulting impairment of salt and water balance may be a factor in resistant ascites. Sufficient sources of linoleic acid, the metabolic precursor of arachidonic acid, should therefore be provided in the diet (Johnson et al 1985).

Care must be taken to see that other sources of sodium are not added inadvertently. Some drugs may contain sodium and pharmacists should be advised of the need for low sodium versions of certain mixtures. Antacids may be a case in point. It is not unknown for an ascitic patient to be given intravenous sodium by a unit other than that caring for the patient's liver disease. The construction of sodium-restricted regimens is summarized on p 151.

Complications of chronic active hepatitis

Encephalopathy

Encephalopathy may develop as a feature of late stage chronic active hepatitis. Treatment is by lactulose, enemas and restriction of dietary protein to minimize the absorption of protein breakdown products from the gut. Constipation should be avoided, so that the bowel is free from nitrogen-containing materials. The diet should be high in fibre if possible, but for patients on low dietary protein intakes it is difficult to provide enough fibre to affect the encephalopathy. High fibre diets act too slowly to treat the acute condition.

Diabetes

There is an increased incidence of diabetes mellitus in chronic hepatitis, either as a primary condition or secondary to steroid treatment. Dietary treatment of diabetes is here of secondary importance to the liver disease but diabetic ascitic patients may benefit from some dietary control of their diabetes. A low sodium, carbohydrate exchange list is given on p 134.

Other complications of chronic active hepatitis

Coeliac disease (Section 4.12.2) and thyroid dysfunction (Section 4.5) may also occur, as these are also HLA associated conditions.

4.13.3 Alcoholic hepatitis

The clinical signs of alcoholic hepatitis may be a tender liver, jaundice, spider naevi, red palms and bruising. The symptoms include nausea, a raised temperature and general malaise. Patients are not usually encephalopathic and rarely ascitic.

The diet should be high in both protein and energy. The energy intake should be sufficient to replace the energy from alcohol which, hopefully, has been stopped. Additional vitamins, especially a therapeutic multivitamin such as Orovite (Bencard) and thiamine and folic acid, should be given. On admission, the diet may have to be given as a nasogastric feed as nausea may limit oral energy intake (Mezey 1980).

4.13.4 Hepato-renal failure

The prognosis of this condition is poor. Dietary treatment will be symptomatic and depend on the medical treatment. Due to the generally poor results, dialysis has not been considered to be a cost-effective treatment for these patients. Dietary management therefore includes sodium and protein restriction according to the progress of the disease. If dialysis is used, dietary treatment should be guided by blood chemistry. In the future, use of haemofiltration may offer an alternative in specialized centres where intensive nursing can be provided. This technique allows sufficient quantities of fluid, energy and protein to be given to the patient for good nutritional support to be possible during the period of acute illness.

4.13.5 Drug overdosage

Overdosage with paracetamol is a common cause of liver failure, especially in young people (Meredith and Goulding 1980). The patient may appear to recover initially but relapse into coma some days after ingestion of the drug. A 40 g protein diet (see p 120) should be instigated to rest the liver and allow it to metabolize the paracetamol. If a lethal dose has been ingested, protein must be further restricted as the patient becomes more encephalopathic.

4.13.6 Cirrhosis of the liver

Causative factors may include a number of liver toxins

such as drugs, viral toxins, carbon tetrachloride or alcohol but the majority of cases occur as a complication of chronic active hepatitis or alcoholic liver disease.

Clinical signs include vitamin deficiency, encephalopathy, ascites, bleeding and muscle wasting. The biochemical features are a low serum albumin, raised alkaline phosphatase, raised aspartate transaminase (AST) and prolonged prothrombin time.

Dietary treatment

There is no diet which will affect the underlying cause Treatment is to remove the precipitating factor and then treat the symptoms which may include.

Ascites

This will necessitate a low sodium diet, with or without fluid restriction, and the use of diuretics.

Encephalopathy

The intake of dietary protein should be restricted and lactulose given to prevent and treat constipation. Sufficient energy should be given to meet the patient's requirements, but energy from fat and carbohydrate should not be excessive in proportion to protein. Energy from non-protein sources should not exceed 300 kcal/g nitrogen if protein tolerance is only in the range of 10−40 g/day. When protein tolerance is higher, the energy/nitrogen ratio can be decreased to about 200 kcal/g nitrogen. If the patient can tolerate a protein level of 80 g or more, the non-protein energy supply can be further decreased. (A normal diet contains approximately 50 kcal per g nitrogen).

Liver patients with chronic encephalopathy have raised serum levels of the aromatic amino acids (methionine, phenylalanine and tyrosine) and reduced levels of the branched chain amino acids (valine, leucine and isoleucine) (Morgan et al 1978). It has been suggested that better nutritional status and an improved mental state may be achieved in such patients by increasing the intake of branched chain amino acids. Diets with vegetables as the sole protein source have been used for this purpose (Greenberger et al 1977; Shaw et al 1983) but with only limited success, especially in patients in the late stages of liver failure. Such diets are very bulky and it is difficult for very ill patients to eat a sufficient quantity to obtain the desirable amount of protein. A number of commercial supplements with a high concentration of branched chain amino acids

have come on to the market. These should be used with caution as there is limited evidence of their value to the encephalopathic patient, and they could increase the incidence of liver coma (Horst et al 1984).

Oesophageal varices

There is no evidence linking foods which are hard in texture with bleeding. It should be remembered that an episode of bleeding places a protein and sodium load in the gut, which could precipitate encephalopathy or ascites in susceptible patients. It may be necessary to restrict dietary protein, especially if blood transfusions are being given.

4.13.7 Wilson's disease

Wilson's disease is an inherited disorder characterized by failure to handle copper storage, resulting in excessive copper deposition in body tissues. Early and effective treatment should prevent damage to organs. Late diagnosis may result in copper deposition in soft tissues, causing cirrhosis of liver and brain damage. Unfortunately, brain damage may occur before the diagnostic Kayser-Fleischer rings in the periphery of the cornea are apparent. The siblings of any such patients should therefore be screened for the disease by urine copper estimations. Treatment by dietary copper restriction is impractical. Administration of penicillamine, which chelates excessive circulating copper and facilitates its excretion, is much more effective. It should be noted that penicillamine has the side effect of chelating zinc and also alters taste perception which may result in problems of food acceptance. However, zinc supplementation is inadvisable, because penicillamine will preferentially chelate the additional zinc resulting in less copper being removed from the body.

4.13.8 Budd-Chiari syndrome

This arises from obstruction of the hepatic veins and is characterized by hepatomegaly, abdominal pain and ascites. The ascites may be gross and in the chronic condition will require treatment with a low sodium diet and diuretics over a prolonged period. The syndrome is often associated with clotting diseases such as polycythaemia, which may make treatments such as the insertion of a peritoneo-jugular (Leveen) shunt impractical. A low sodium (22 mmol) diet should be advised (see p 151).

Further Reading

Sherlock S (1981) *Diseases of the liver and bilrary system* 6e. Blackwell Scientific Publications, Oxford.

References

Greenberger NJ, Carley J, Schenker S, Battinger I, Stannes C and Bayer P (1977) Effects of vegetable and animal protein diets in chronic hepatic encephalopathy. *Dig Dis Sci* **22**, 845−55.

Horst D, Grace ND, Conn HO, Schiff E, Schenker S, Viteri A, Law D and Atterbury CE (1984) Comparison of dietary protein with an oral, branched chain-enriched amino acid supplement in chronic portal-systemic encephalopathy: a randomized controlled trial. *Hepatology* **4**, (2), 279−87.

Johnson SB, Gordon E, McClain C, Low G and Holman RT (1985) Abnormal polyunsaturated fatty acid patterns of serum lipids in alcoholism and cirrhosis: arachidonic acid deficiency in cirrhosis. *Proc Nat Acad Sci USA* **82**, 1815−8.

Kennedy J (1973) Electroencephalography. *Nutrition* **27**, (5), 325−9.

Meredith TJ and Goulding R (1980) Paracetamol. *Postgrad Med J* **56**, 459−73.

Mezey E (1980) Alcoholic liver disease: roles of alcohol and malnutrition. *Am J Clin Nutr* **33**, 2709−18.

Morgan MY, Milson JP and Sherlock S (1978) Plasma ratio of valine, leucine and isoleucine to phenylalanine and tyrosine in liver disease. *Gut* **19**, 1068−73.

Shaw S, Warner TM and Lieber CS (1983) Comparison of animal and vegetable sources in the dietary management of hepatic encephalopathy. *Am J Clin Nutr* **38**, 59−63.

4.14 Biliary Disease

4.14.1 Cholecystitis and cholestasis

These are usually associated with the presence of stones which block the passage of bile into the duodenum. Treatment may be medical or surgical. If fat is not well tolerated a low fat diet should be advised. Very low fat diets may be contraindicated, as lack of dietary fat may stop the gall bladder contracting vigorously, and encourage the growth of further stones.

4.14.2 Primary biliary cirrhosis

This is a disease of unknown aetiology, arising in the biliary system and causing liver cirrhosis. The condition usually occurs in women between the ages of 40–59 and is characterized by hepatomegaly and skin xanthomas. The biochemical features are raised serum alkaline phosphatase and raised serum bilirubin (stable until the terminal stages).

The symptoms include pruritis which is often insidious in origin but can become a major problem causing great distress to patients. Jaundice may be slight, or absent, at diagnosis, but may increase markedly during the course of the disease. Steatorrhoea, and latterly bone pain, are also persistent problems. Deep jaundice usually indicates a poor prognosis. The terminal stage is indicated by deepening jaundice and disappearance of xanthomas and pruritis.

Dietary treatment

This should be governed by the prevailing symptoms.

Steatorrhoea

If steatorrhoea is troublesome, a low fat diet is advised together with a supplement of medium chain triglycerides (MCT) to keep energy intake up to the daily requirement (see pp 124 and 199). Fat soluble vitamins can be given intramuscularly. Calcium supplements may help to counteract poor calcium absorption (Epstein *et al* 1982).

Malnutrition

Initially patients are usually well nourished, but as the disease progresses the patient may be unable to eat enough to compensate for the impaired absorption. Supplementary drinks made with MCT oil and fruit juice containing glucose polymers (see p 199) should be encouraged between meals.

Pruritis

This can often be controlled by cholestyramine, though this sometimes causes diarrhoea and can be bulky and unpleasant to take. Uncontrolled pruritis is distressing for the patient and can lead to skin breakdown and infection through scratching.

Elevated liver copper levels

The level of copper in the liver may be as high as in Wilson's disease. Use of D-penicillamine helps control liver damage and prolongs survival, but has unpleasant side effects (see Section 4.13.7).

Liver failure

In terminal stages, cirrhosis develops with symptoms of end stage liver disease. These may include ascites, bleeding varices and encephalopathy. Dietary treatment is the same as for chronic active hepatitis (see Section 4.13.2).

4.14.3 Biliary atresia

Biliary atresia is defined as the inability to excrete bile and is associated with malformation of the biliary tree.

The malformation may be congenital, in which case it is usually extrahepatic, but in the majority of cases it results from a progressive obliterative sclerosis of the bile ducts and may be a consequence of rubella, cytomegalovirus or reovirus infection. These lesions usually start intrahepatically but may progress to the extrahepatic ducts. The signs and symptoms include deep jaundice, pruritis, dark urine and pale stools characteristic of lack of bilirubin in the gut. Serum cholesterol is raised and skin xanthomas may be present.

If untreated, either by surgery or transplantation, biliary atresia is always fatal, survival beyond four years of age being exceptional. However, prolonged jaundice-free survival can be achieved if infants are treated with hepatoportoenterostomy before the age of ten weeks (Kamath 1986).

Dietary treatment

A low fat diet should be given to reduce steatorrhoea if present. MCT oil can be added to improve the energy content of diet. Extra calcium in the form of skimmed milk may be an advantage. Special milks with added MCT may be useful, e.g. Portagen (Mead Johnson) or MCT (1) (Cow and Gate). Portagen contains added vitamins and minerals, but fat soluble vitamins should be given intramuscularly since they are not well absorbed. D-penicillamine may be given as a prophylactic measure against organ damage.

Further reading

Sherlock S (1981) *Diseases of the liver and biliary system* 6e. Blackwell Scientific Publications, Oxford.

References

Epstein O, Kato Y, Dick R and Sherlock S (1982) Vitamin D, hydroxyapatite and calcium gluconate in treatment of cortical bone thinning in post-menopausal women with primary biliary cirrhosis. *Am J Clin Nutr* **36**, (3), 426–30.

Kamath KR (1986) *Clin Gastroenterol* **1**, 157–72.

4.15 Liver Transplantation

Patients considered for liver transplantation are either children with congenital defects such as biliary atresia, adults with end stage liver disease who have increasing morbidity and poor prognosis or those with certain types of primary liver tumours. Patients with end stage disease are usually malnourished, and pre-operative nutritional assessment and supplementation is critical (see Sections 1.11 and 1.12). The pre-operative nutritional state is thought to be an indicator of post-operative mortality (Epstein 1985, Personal communication). Weight loss peri-operatively can be up to 20% of body weight and feeding either intravenously or enterally should be commenced as soon as possible after surgery (see Sections 1.12 and 1.13). Often the gut is one of the first organs to recover function after transplant, and it is preferable to feed by this route if possible, as enteral feeding carries less risk of infection.

On recovery, as in all transplant surgery, there is a risk of steroid-induced diabetes developing, due to the necessary large doses of immunosuppressive drugs which must be given.

Further reading

Sherlock S (1981) *Diseases of the liver and biliary system* 6e. Blackwell Scientific Publications, Oxford.

D: Disorders of the Kidney and Urinary Tract

4.16 Renal Disease

The aims of management of the patient with renal failure are to maintain residual renal function, to keep blood chemistry within normal limits and, in the case of children, to promote growth, all with the least possible disruption to family life.

With all patients in renal failure, six aspects of the diet need to be considered

1 Protein
2 Sodium
3 Fluid
4 Potassium
5 Phosphorus
6 Energy

In addition, the carbohydrate intake may need to be adjusted and the diet must be nutritionally adequate in respect of all other minerals and vitamins. In patients with urinary calculi the intake of calcium, oxalate and vitamins C and D must also be considered. It is therefore clear that each patient must be treated individually according to their prevailing nutritional and clinical requirements, and their biochemical and clinical status carefully monitored.

4.16.1 The nephrotic syndrome (NS)

The nephrotic syndrome has four essential features

1 Oedema
2 Proteinuria greater than 5 g/l in adults
3 Hypoalbuminaemia
4 Hypercholesterolaemia and hypertriglyceridaemia. The hypercholesterolaemia is secondary to hypoalbuminaemia (Lewis 1976).

The nephrotic syndrome is not a diagnosis of a particular renal disease and can occur in the following conditions

1 Glomerulonephritis (GN). Patients with GN can present with the nephrotic syndrome, an acute nephritic syndrome (facial swelling, haematuria, hypertension and granular casts in the urine), asymptomatic proteinuria or as acute or chronic renal failure (CRF). Fifty per cent of patients on renal replacement therapy have some form of GN as their underlying aetiology. GN can be subdivided into several different types and since the years of Richard Bright (c.1830) the classification of GN has been the subject of changing concepts. Pathological findings do not always correlate with clinical symptoms (Table 4.37).

Table 4.37 Classification of glomeulonephritis (GN)

Pathological features	Clinical symptoms
Minimal change GN	Most common type of GN in children. Occasionally occurs in adults Selective proteinuria. Good prognosis, rarely progresses to CRF. Usually responds to steroids and/or cyclophosphamide.
Membranous GN	May be associated with malaria, malignancy and drugs such as gold and penicillamine. Often progresses to end stage renal failure (ESRF).
Focal sclerosis	Usually progresses to ESRF
Focal and segmental GN	Occasionally presents as nephrotic syndrome. May progress to ESRF.
Mesangio-capillary GN	Presents as nephrotic syndrome or acute nephritic symptoms
Mesangio-proliferative GN	This may present with a variety of clinical presentations.
Rapidly progressive GN	Rapidly progresses to ESRF. Epithelial crescents in glomeruli seen on biopsy. May be associated following streptococcal infection, polyarteritis nodosa or Wegener's granulomatosis.

2 Renal vein thrombosis. This can be a cause or a complication of the nephrotic syndrome.
3 Systemic lupus erythematosis (SLE). This is a multi-system disease which may present with fever, arthritis, rashes, leucopenia, positive anti-nuclear factor (ANF), positive DNA binding and low complement 3 and complement 4 (C3 and C4). Some patients will develop renal manifestations which usually present initially as the nephrotic syndrome, later progressing to end stage renal failure (ESRF).
4 Amyloidosis. Occasionally patients with amyloidosis will present with the nephrotic syndrome, those who do usually develop ESRF.
5 Congenital nephrotic syndrome. There are several different aetiologies (Barratt 1985).

Clinical presentation of the nephrotic syndrome

The first symptom is usually a rapid increase in body weight (up to 30 kg) due to oedema. In children, facial and abdominal oedema are usual but in adults, leg oedema predominates. White transverse bands develop on the nails if the syndrome becomes chronic.

Patients' urine often froths excessively on micturition owing to the presence of albumin. The proteinuria is caused by an increased permeability of the glomerular basement membrane (GBM) to protein. This may lead to hypoalbuminaemia (the degree of proteinuria and serum albumin levels are only loosely related) and a decreased plasma osmotic pressure causing fluid to be lost from the intravascular spaces thus lowering plasma and blood volumes, cardiac output and blood pressure. This in turn is thought to activate homeostatic responses involving plasma renin and aldosterone which lead to salt and water retention as a secondary response. Many patients with NS do not show the expected drop in plasma volume nor raised plasma aldosterone or renin levels. Dorhout Mees et al. (1984) suggest there may be some other renal abnormality at glomerular level in addition to a protein leak, such as increased reabsorption of sodium and a possible stimulation of renin which is inappropriate for the requirements of the circulation.

Medical treatment of the nephrotic syndrome

One of the main objectives in treating the nephrotic syndrome is to reduce the oedema using diuretics such as frusemide and bumetanide. These can cause potassium to be excreted in large quantities and patients may need potassium supplementation. Spironolactone, a potassium sparing diuretic, can be used but care must be taken to monitor potassium levels. If the oedema is resistant to diuretics, salt-poor albumin is sometimes administered, but this is very expensive. It acts by temporarily increasing plasma osmotic pressure and producing a diuresis. If haemodialysis facilities are available, ultrafiltration may be used to remove fluid. Too rapid fluid removal may induce acute renal failure. If on biopsy there appears to be vascular damage in the glomeruli, the patient may be anticoagulated and given dipyridamole. Patients with minimal change GN invariably respond to steroids. Patients with other forms of GN, depending on biopsy findings, may be given azathioprine, prednisolone, cyclophosphamide and/or plasmapheresis to try to arrest the destructive process.

Dietary treatment of nephrotic syndrome

It has been traditional to put patients with nephrotic syndrome on high protein (> 100 g/day), low sodium ($50-100$ mmol/day) diets. Since patients are often anorexic this diet is very difficult for them to adhere to, especially since the strict sodium restriction limits the choice of protein source.

The rationale behind such diets is based on some patients having urinary losses of up to 20 g protein/day and others having a serum albumin level below 15 g/l. However, little work has been done to prove the effectiveness of these diets and because there is now evidence to suggest that hepatic synthesis of protein may be inhibited by a high protein intake (Lee 1978), many nephrologists no longer prescribe it.

It has been shown that in adult patients with nephrotic syndrome, a diet providing 1 g protein/kg ideal body weight plus 1 g protein for every g of protein lost in the urine combined with 200 kcal (840 kJ)/g of dietary N can achieve nitrogen balance. Some patients maintain nitrogen balance on a lower protein intake (Manos et al 1983).

In GN, even though the initiating process has either remitted spontaneously or been controlled therapeutically, renal failure may still progress. Ad libitum feeding of protein may contribute to the progression of CRF by causing a compensatory hyperfiltration in the less affected glomeruli contributing to further nephron destruction (Brenner et al 1982). In addition, El Nahas (1984) showed that in a group of patients with GN and mean serum creatinine levels of 241 μmol/l (normal range $60-120$ μmol/l), a reduction in protein intake succeeded in reducing the magnitude of proteinuria.

These patients also showed improvement in the slope of reciprocal serum creatinine concentration when plotted against time which has been shown to be a reliable indicator of renal function (Mitch et al 1976). Figure 4.14 illustrates the effect of a low protein diet on the creatinine/time plot of a patient with membranous GN. At the time of starting the diet, the serum albumin was 27 g/l and this rose to 39 g/l after a few weeks on a 40 g protein diet.

The evidence therefore points away from the use of high protein, low sodium diets in the treatment of the nephrotic syndrome in adults except in the case of minimal change GN which rarely progresses to ESRF. The work by Menos et al (1983) shows that energy intake is important in achieving nitrogen balance. Malnourished patients should be encouraged to increase their energy intake. However, in the syndrome of glomerular sclerosis associated with massive obesity, there is evidence to show that weight loss leads to a reduction in proteinuria (Cochran et al 1979). Patients with very large protein losses may benefit from increased protein and energy intakes on a short term

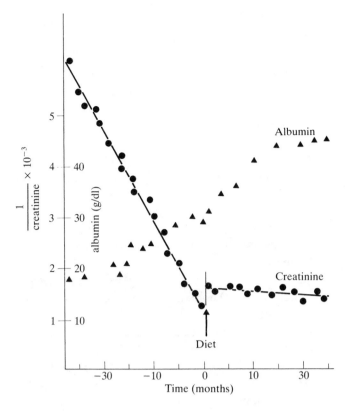

Fig. 4.14 Patient with membranous GN showing 1/serum creatinine and serum albumin versus time. ▲ = serum albumin; ● = serum creatinine (reciprocal).

basis. If oedema remains a problem after treatment with diuretics a 'no added salt' diet (80−100 mmol/day) may be beneficial. (see p 151). In view of the almost universal hyperlipidaemia it is probably wise to reduce animal fat and substitute polyunsaturated fat in the diet.

Until more research is carried out, if renal function tests are normal, 1 g of protein/kg ideal body weight, plus the equivalent to that protein lost in the urine is probably an appropriate intake. The dietary advice must be reconsidered if renal function deteriorates. Most patients with CRF due to glomerulonephritis respond well to a reduction in protein intake, and show a reduced rate of progression of renal failure (Williams *et al* 1985). More research needs to be done on what dietary advice patients with the nephrotic syndrome should receive as many patients achieve serum albumin levels within the normal range without dietary intervention.

4.16.2 Acute renal failure (ARF)

ARF is a syndrome in which the kidneys are unable to excrete the products of metabolism. This leads to a rapid increase in serum urea and creatinine concentrations in patients with previously normal renal func-

tion. Urine output in the majority (98%) of cases drops to less than 400 ml/day and the patient is classed as oliguric. If urine production ceases altogether, the patient is termed anuric. Occasionally patients who present with ARF maintain or even increase urine output (Polyuric ARF). Some patients with ARF may have acute tubular necrosis (ATN). Patients may occasionally be in ARF for as long as six weeks.

Causes of ARF

Many patients will have more than one possible cause
1 Shock, dehydration leading to hypotension, e.g. accidents, surgery or gastrointestinal bleeding.
2 Impaired vascular supply, e.g. renal artery thrombosis or aortic aneurysms.
3 Drugs and poisons, e.g. antibiotics, aminoglycosides, carbon tetrachloride, ethylene glycol, paraquat and paracetamol.
4 Intravascular coagulation, e.g. septicaemia or postpartum ARF.
5 Haemolysis (transfusion reactions or drugs).
6 Myoglobinuria (traumatic and non-traumatic).
7 Intrinsic renal disease.
8 Obstruction, e.g. bilateral renal calculi, bilateral papillary necrosis or malignancy (such as cancer of the cervix or bladder).

Treatment of ARF

This will depend on the facilities available, the aetiology of ARF and the clinical condition of the patient. In the past, the high morbidity and mortality rates were related to infections and inadequate nutrition and negative nitrogen balance often resulted from unnecessarily restricted protein intakes.

IMMEDIATE TREATMENT

1 If the ARF is due to dehydration, rehydration of the patient using intravenous fluids is essential. In dehydration the urinary sodium concentration will be < 20 mmol/l. Patients who, after volume repletion, have a low cardiac output may benefit from a dopamine infusion. If there is no response to all these measures it is likely that ARF has become established.
2 Hyperkalaemia. This is managed initially by administering glucose and insulin intravenously which temporarily pushes potassium back into the cells. Dialysis is needed to remove it. Exchange resins (such as resonium A and calcium resonium) given rectally or orally can reduce further absorption of potassium from

the gastrointestinal tract but act slowly and thus the enteral or parenteral administration of potassium may need to be restricted.

3 Obstruction. This must be relieved by either surgical means or pericutaneous nephrostomies.

Patients with ARF can be divided into three groups in order to assess dialysis requirements and nutritional needs (Lee 1980). Classification of patients with ARF is summarized in Table 4.38.

Table 4.38 Classification of patients with acute renal failure

Group	Daily blood urea rise (mmol/l*)	Protein breakdown (g N/day)
A Normocatabolic (ARF usually due to 'medical' causes)	4–8	10–14
B Moderately raised catabolism ('surgical')	8–12	14–24
C Hypercatabolic (severe multiple trauma/septicaemia)	> 12	> 24

* Gastrointestinal bleeds may make these figures invalid.

a) *Normocatabolic patients (Group A)*

These patients can usually be managed conservatively (i.e. no dialysis).

Dietary considerations

Fluid. Once the fluid balance has been corrected, the daily fluid intake should be 500 ml plus the equivalent of the previous day's urine output and gastrointestinal losses. It is important that patients are weighed daily if possible. Blood pressure and serum electrolytes need to be monitored routinely and adequate nutritional support must be given.

Protein. Patients in this group are non-catabolic so they can be managed on a diet providing 0.6–0.7 g high biological value (HBV) protein/kg ideal body weight (see p 117). This should prevent an excessive rise in the blood urea level. A lower protein intake is not recommended as it will inevitably lead to negative nitrogen balance.

Potassium. The intake should be reduced to 0.6–0.7 mmol/kg ideal body weight unless serum levels are below 4 mmol/l (see p 153).

Sodium. The intake will depend on the patient's state of hydration. If the patient is oedematous, anuric or oliguric, foods with a high sodium content should be avoided as they will make the patient want to drink more. Sodium intake should also be reduced if the patient is hypertensive (see p 151).

Energy. A minimum of 2000 kcal (8400 kJ)/day should be consumed. Glucose polymers either in powder or liquid form or combined with a fat source (e.g. Duocal) will probably be needed to add to beverages and puddings (see Section 2.12). Carbonated glucose drinks (e.g. Lucozade) are also a convenient way of achieving high energy intakes if the fluid allowance permits. Patients should be encouraged to suck boiled sweets or barley sugars. Anorexic patients may require naso-gastric feeding to supplement oral intake.

If serum urea and creatinine levels rise on this therapy, or if the patient becomes fluid overloaded, haemodialysis, continuous haemofiltration or peritoneal dialysis (PD) will be necessary. The latter can be carried out in most hospitals.

Acute peritoneal dialysis

In PD a rigid catheter (as opposed to a soft silastic catheter used for continuous ambulatory PD) is placed in the peritoneal cavity through a stab incision. 1–2 litres of dialysate is then run in and left to dwell for 10–15 min and then drained out. Cycles are carried out continuously over several days. Protein and amino acids are lost during PD to the extent of 25 g protein and 15 g of amino acids per 40 litres dialysis exchange (Lee 1980) and the diet should therefore provide 1 g protein per kg ideal body weight. As potassium is dialysed out continuously, a normal intake can be allowed and it may be necessary to add potassium chloride to the dialysate to prevent excessive losses. The aim should be to keep the serum potassium level within the normal range.

Continuous haemofiltration

Up to 12 litres of ultrafiltrate can be removed daily through a small haemofiltration unit perfused at low blood flow rates. Vascular access is similar to haemodialysis (HD). Care is needed with fluid replacement. It is less efficient than HD in clearing of metabolic toxins (Dodd *et al* 1983).

b) *Mildly or severely hypercatabolic patients (Groups B and C)*

It is very important in these patients that muscle wasting through catabolism and starvation is prevented. A large percentage of patients from Group B and the majority of Group C will have concurrent respiratory failure and require artificial ventilation. Dysfunction of the gastrointestinal tract is common and will determine the initial route of nutrient administration. In addition to these problems, the metabolic consequences of surgery, injuries, sepsis, cardiac dysfunction, pancreatitis or concurrent liver failure may be present. It is therefore not surprising that there is a high mortality rate in these patients. They require dialysis but PD is often difficult or impossible due to abdominal surgery or injuries and it will increase protein/nitrogen losses. These patients therefore require transfer to specialist renal centres.

The first priority is to establish vascular access for administering drugs, replacement fluids and blood, setting up a central venous catheter solely for parenteral nutrition and gaining access for haemodialysis (see p 448) or continuous haemofiltration either by a subclavian catheter, (HD only), catheterization of the femoral vein/artery, or creating an arteriovenous (AV) shunt in the arm or leg. Before any feeding can be contemplated the patient's fluid balance must be corrected.

Group B. Patients who are moderately hypercatabolic will require 9–14 g of nitrogen/day (60–90 g protein). Sodium intake must be tailored for individual patients, but an initial intake of between 25–50 mmol/day is usual. Potassium requirements will also vary, but again an initial intake of 25–50 mmol/day is suitable. A non-nitrogen energy to g nitrogen ratio of 175–200 kcal (730–835 kJ): 1 should be aimed for. Ideally, 2 litres of feeding space is needed but this will depend on the patient's fluid balance status.

Group C. Patients who are severely hypercatabolic will require 14–18 g nitrogen/day. The patient may be losing 40–50 g daily but it is impossible to replace this. The liver is unable to deaminate more than 20 g nitrogen/day (Allison 1984) so this should be the maximum amount given. Potassium and sodium requirements must be calculated on an individual basis. A non-nitrogen energy to g nitrogen ratio of 135–175 kcal (565–730 kJ): 1 should be aimed for. At least 2.5 litres of feeding space is ideally needed.

Patients in Groups A, B and C will need vitamin supplementation (especially B complex, folic acid and vitamin C).

Parenteral feeding (see also Section 1.13)

Nitrogen source. The source of nitrogen should be a crystalline amino acid solution containing a well balanced profile of both essential and non-essential amino acids (Lee 1980). There is little rationale for using essential amino acids alone (Abel 1976). Note must be made of the electrolyte content of the solution used. A wide range of suitable solutions is now available. If fluid space is a problem, using a solution which has 9 or 12 g nitrogen/500 ml may be advantageous.

Energy. This should come from both fat and carbohydrate sources if possible but at least 25% of the energy should be supplied by fat. Blood clearance of Intralipid should be checked. The administration to septic and critically ill patients of glucose in excess of 500–600 g daily causes an increased carbon dioxide production with a consequent rise in respiratory quotient which is a problem for patients on respirators. A maximum of 2000 kcal (8400 kJ) should come from glucose, and insulin administration may be required for its metabolism. Glucose however may have a greater protein sparing effect than fat in patients with burns (Allison 1984). Intralipid may sometimes 'clog' the fibres of hollow fibre dialysers. Few problems have been encountered with flat-plate dialysers.

In renal failure there is an increased risk of lactic acidosis. Energy substrates known to be associated with a risk of inducing lactic acidosis (i.e. fructose, sorbitol, ethanol and xylitol) should therefore be avoided (Woods and Alberti 1972).

Minerals. Most patients will require some supplementation, e.g. Addamel — 1 vial. If the patient is well dialysed, additional phosphate may be needed. Most phosphate supplements have added potassium and therefore close monitoring of serum electrolytes is essential.

Vitamins. If large quantities of glucose are given extra B vitamins will be required. Vitamin B12 should be given on a regular basis.

Other considerations of parenteral regimens (see also Section 1.13)

1 Advantages and disadvantages of '3 litre bags' over bottles. The 'big bag system' allows all the nutrients to be mixed and therefore given at an equal rate as a continual infusion and may reduce the need for insulin. It also provides the electrolytes over a 24-hour period, avoiding sudden fluctuations. If the patient is being dialysed, the amino acids infused will, however, be dialysed out although these losses do not occur with haemofiltration. Problems are rarely associated with giving glucose or Intralipid during dialysis. The electrolyte content of the 'big bag' must be decided in advance whereas a 'bottle system' allows for greater flexibility but also has the disadvantage of not allowing infusion of all the nutrients over 24 hours.

2 Dialysis as a method of feeding. 500 ml of Intralipid can be given slowly into the venous return line over the dialysis period. 500 ml of 9 g/l amino acids solutions can also be given during the last 3 hours of dialysis, ensuring a large percentage retention of the amino acids. Larger quantities or a more rapid infusion will cause nausea, vomiting, flushing and paraesthesia (Lee 1980).

3 Change-over from parenteral to enteral feeding. This should be done gradually. If a patient has had TPN for some time it may take several days before adequate quantities of a full strength feed can be tolerated. Supplemental parenteral feeding should therefore continue over this period and care should be taken to maintain electrolyte balance.

Enteral feeding in renal failure (see also Section 1.12.3)

The composition of the feed will depend on whether and how frequently the patient is receiving dialysis or haemofiltration. Patients being treated conservatively may have a fluid restriction of 1 litre/day and therefore require a concentrated feed. This should be given via a feeding pump over at least 18 hours with the concentration slowly increasing to 2 kcal/ml over several days. Normal strength commercial feeds can be modified by adding a fat emulsion such as Calogen or Prosparol and a glucose polymer. There are amino acid mixtures marketed specifically for patients with renal failure, but these have a high osmotic load even at 1 kcal (4.2 kJ)/ml and it is doubtful whether they have any advantage over conventional feeds (Lee 1980).

As renal function improves dietary restrictions may be lifted and dialysis treatment phased out. Nutritional support is still vital as most patients will have lost muscle mass due to catabolism. Extra sodium, potassium and phosphate will probably be required and an increased fluid intake will also be needed to keep the patient well hydrated. Enteral and parenteral nutritional support can gradually be replaced by oral food. Many patients will not have eaten anything for periods of 4−6 weeks. They should be warned that the taste buds alter during a uraemic state and be given as much choice as possible when selecting their meals.

4.16.3 Chronic renal failure (CRF)

CRF is the irreversible destruction of kidney tissue by disease, eventually resulting in the death of the patient if not treated by dialysis, haemofiltration or transplantation. CRF has a variety of aetiologies, the most common of which are listed in Table 4.39.

Table 4.39 Aetiology of chronic renal failure

Glomerulonephritis (GN) — see Table 4.38 for subdivisions
Pyelonephritis (CPN) (reflux nephropathy)
Polycystic disease of the kidney (PCK)
Hypertension
Diabetic nephropathy
Myeloma
Obstruction (stones, prostatic enlargement)
Analgesic nephropathy
Systemic lupus erthymatosis (SLE)
Unknown aetiology

The treatment of CRF can be divided into several types: conservative management (i.e. prior to needing renal replacement therapy), dialysis, haemofiltration and transplantation. Dietary treatment is discussed in detail in each section but is summarized in Table 4.40.

Conservative management

This is usually a combination of medical and dietary treatment depending on the clinical state of the patient at time of referral and the preferences of the consultant in charge. Policies vary widely. Some patients are referred at a relatively early stage in the course of CRF whilst others may not present until requiring urgent dialysis treatment, either in end stage renal failure or during an 'acute on chronic' episode.

Table 4.40 Dietary management of adults with chronic renal failure

	Protein/day[1]	Sodium/day[2]	Potassium/day[2]	Phosphorus/day[3]	Energy/day[4]	Fluid/day[5]
Conservative management	0.6 g/kg ideal body weight; 70% HBV	Normal unless blood pressure raised or fluid overload then no added salt (NAS) (80–100 mmol). Salt losers require an increased intake.	Unrestricted unless serum level above normal then reduce to 30–40 mmol. Do not encourage excessive intake.	Restricted to < 700 mg (23 mmol)	35 kcal (146 kJ)/kg ideal body weight	Unrestricted unless oedematous or in ESRF and oliguric. Then reduce to 500 ml plus equivalent to previous days urine output (PDUO).
Haemodialysis	1–1.2g/kg ideal body weight	Usually NAS (80–100 mmol)	< 1 mmol/kg ideal body weight	Restricted to < 1000 mg (33 mmol)	35 kcal (146 kJ)/kg ideal body weight. Reduce if obese	500 ml plus equivalent to PDUO
Chronic haemofiltration	1–1.2 g/kg ideal body weight	Usually NAS	< 0.8 mmol/kg ideal body weight	Restricted to < 1000 mg (33 mmol)	35 kcal (146 kJ)/kg ideal body weight	500 ml plus equivalent to PDUO
Continuous ambulatory peritoneal dialysis (CAPD)	1.2–1.5 g/kg ideal body weight	Usually NAS	No restriction unless serum k+ at or above upper limit of normal range. Do not encourage excessive intake.	Restricted to < 1200 mg (40 mmol)	70% absorption of dialysate dextrose therefore reduce to 25 kcal/kg *ideal* body weight. Reduce if obese	700 ml plus equivalent to PDUO
Continuous cyclic peritoneal dialysis (CCPD)	1.2–1.5 g/kg ideal body weight	Usually NAS	Restrict intake on day off CCPD	Restricted to < 1200 mg (40 mmol)	As for CAPD	700 ml plus equivalent to PDUO
Long term intermittent peritoneal dialysis (IPD)	1.2–1.5 g/kg ideal body weight on dialysis	Unrestricted on dialysis unless hypertensive	Normal on dialysis	Restricted on dialysis to < 1200 mg (40 mmol)	As for CAPD on dialysis	Unrestricted on dialysis unless fluid overloaded
	0.7–0.8 g/kg ideal body weight on inter-dialysis days	Usually NAS on inter-dialysis days	40 mmol/day on inter-dialysis days	Restricted on inter-dialysis days to < 600 mg (20 mmol)	35 kcal/kg ideal body weight on inter-dialysis days	500 ml plus equivalent to PDUO on inter-dialysis days

[1]Section 2.2; [2]Section 2.7.1; [3]Section 2.7.2; [4]Section 2.1 and 2.12; [5]Section 2.9.

Aims of conservative management

The aims of conservative management of CRF are
1 To determine the aetiology.
2 To retrieve some or all of the lost renal function by identifying and treating the cause.
a Hypertension. This is both a cause and complication of CRF. The early treatment of it can slow the progression of renal deterioration or lead to an improvement in renal function.
b Treatment of concurrent urinary tract infections (UTI).
c Correction of urinary tract abnormalities: surgery to the ureters may prevent vesicoureteric reflux; lithotomy and prostatectomy will relieve renal obstruction and thus may convert the situation from one of progressive renal destruction to stable renal insufficiency.
d Iatrogenic. The use of certain drugs in renal impairment (such as tetracyclines) may lead to a rapid deterioration in renal function. Some of the loss of renal function may be recoverable.
e Dehydration may lead to a deterioration in renal function which may be reversible.

Monitoring renal function

This can be done in a variety of ways. Creatinine clearance is often measured as there is a good correlation with glomerular filtration rate (GFR). The rate of deterioration in renal function can be calculated by using linear regression analysis of the relationship between time and the reciprocal of serum creatinine concentration (Mitch *et al* 1976). The ingestion of meat causes a slight rise in serum creatinine concentrations (Jacobsen *et al* 1979) but this does not affect the value of long term measurements. Serum urea is not a good marker of renal function. It increases as function worsens but can also be affected by diet, drugs (e.g. steroids and tetracyclines), gastrointestinal bleeds, a catabolic state, blood transfusions and dehydration.

Preventing uraemic bone disease

Hyperphosphataemia has been implicated as a factor causing deterioration in renal function (Maschio 1982) but the main concern is its role in uraemic osteodystrophy. When GFR is less than 15 ml/min (normal adult value is 60–120 ml/min) the calcium and phosphate compensatory mechanisms can no longer maintain normal serum levels. Hyperphosphataemia is usual and can cause mild hypocalcaemia leading to secondary hyperparathyroidism as the body attempts to raise serum calcium by bone resorption. Intestinal calcium absorption may also be reduced due to a failure of the kidney to hydroxylate 25-hydroxy vitamin D3 at the 1 carbon position to produce 1,25 dihydroxy vitamin D3. The latter acts as a hormone on the gut to promote calcium absorption. It is important to correct these abnormalities in calcium metabolism as early as possible in the course of renal failure.

In order to correct hyperphosphataemia, a reduction in phosphorus intake to 600–700 mg (20–23 mmol/day) will be required (see p 156). To some extent this will have automatically occurred due to the reduction in protein intake. The additional use of phosphate binders is usually needed to maintain serum phosphate within the normal range (adults 0.8–1.6 µg/l; girls 7–17 years 0.9–1.7 mmol/l and boys 7–17 years 1.0–1.7 mmol/l (Round 1973). Neonates have higher serum phosphate levels and an excessive phosphate restriction must be avoided. In adults the most effective binder is aluminium hydroxide. There is, however, concern regarding aluminium intoxication especially as binders may have to be taken for many years. The minimum dosage possible should be prescribed and serum aluminium levels monitored. Aluminium hydroxide is available as a gel (Aludrox) (30–50 ml daily), Alucaps (4–16 daily) or aluminium hydroxide tablets (4–16 daily). It is important that the prescribed dosage is divided between meals and snacks and taken just before eating. It acts by combining with dietary phosphate in the gut to form non-absorbable aluminium phosphate. aluminium hydroxide frequently causes constipation. If serum aluminium levels are elevated (> 100 µmol/l) an alternative binder should be used. In children, calcium carbonate is the preferred binder as there have been reports of aluminium bone disease (in adults it has only been noted in dialysis patients). Children on aluminium hydroxide often require an additional calcium supplement, but this is not normally necessary with calcium carbonate (Start et al 1985). In adults, however, the use of calcium carbonate sometimes leads to hypercalcaemia. New alternative phosphate binders are being investigated.

Serum calcium levels should be maintained within the normal range (2.1–2.6 mmol/l in adults). If serum calcium levels are still low after being corrected for albumin level, and in the presence of serum phosphate levels of < 2 mmol/l, vitamin D should be administered.

It should be prescribed in its active form, i.e. 1,25 dihydroxy vitamin D3 (calcitriol) or its analogue one-alpha calcidol and should be introduced gradually (0.25 µg b.d. initially). Serum calcium levels must be monitored as over-dosage leads to hypercalcaemia which can result in a deterioration of renal function and calcification of blood vessels. Calcium supplements may be needed and should be given as calcium carbonate or calcium Sandoz syrup (325 mg calcium/15 ml). These are free from sodium and potassium, unlike many other calcium preparations (Sandocal is high in potassium). Most dietary sources of calcium are also high in phosphate.

Renal bone disease can be monitored by skeletal survey which will reveal signs of uraemic bone disease, e.g. erosions of fingertips, clavicle or Looser's zones. In adults (but not growing children) alkaline phosphatase will rise in active bone disease and fall with successful therapy.

Controlling anaemia

A normal kidney produces erythropoietin which stimulates the bone marrow to produce erythrocytes. With loss of renal parenchyma, insufficient erythropoietin is produced and anaemia develops. The half life of red blood corpuscles is also reduced in uraemia and haemogloblin levels may fall to 5–7 g/100 ml. Asian vegetarian patients may also be vitamin B12 deficient. Red cell folate, serum B12, serum iron and serum ferritin levels should be checked and appropriate supplements given if necessary. Patients are rarely iron deficient.

Correcting acidosis

Acidosis results from the diminished ability of the kidney to excrete the daily quantity of hydrogen ions produced from the metabolism of dietary protein. Protein restriction will obviously help but sodium bicarbonate may be needed if serum bicarbonate levels are very low. Acidosis can sometimes contribute to hyperkalaemia.

Preventing hyperkalaemia

Potassium levels do not normally rise until end stage renal failure when there is often associated oliguria. If hyperkalaemia occurs a check should be made on which drugs are being administered, especially diuretics with added potassium. Blood transfusions may also be a cause. A dietary potassium restriction (see p 153) is necessary if blood levels are above the normal range. Haemolysed blood samples may give falsely elevated results.

Monitoring sodium and water balance

Patients with CRF cannot respond normally to changes in sodium intake. The quantity of sodium excreted each day in CRF is relatively fixed between 60–100 mmol and this amount will continue to be excreted even if dietary sodium is restricted. It is important therefore to prevent negative sodium balance which ultimately leads to dehydration. Some patients are 'salt losers' and require additional sodium which can be given as sodium chloride or sodium bicarbonate. Sodium restriction is necessary only if the patient is oedematous or severely hypertensive.

Most patients with CRF will have nocturia and some polyuria. With the loss of renal parenchyma the remaining nephrons function under a constant osmotic load and the kidney loses its ability to produce concentrated urine. It is important that the patient does not become dehydrated. However, in end stage renal failure the urine volume may drop to less than 1 litre/day and oedema develop. Fluid intake should then be restricted to 500 ml plus the equivalent of the previous day's urine output. Dialysis may soon be required.

Preventing accumulation of nitrogenous compounds

In the 1960s Giovannetti and Maggiore (1964) and Giordano (1963) showed that diets containing 0.24 g protein/kg body weight were successful in diminishing symptoms of uraemia and preventing death by lowering protein metabolism to a minimum. The Italian diets were modified by Berlyne (1966) for use in the UK. These diets were often started in end stage renal failure and many patients went into negative nitrogen balance over a period of time partly due to their inability to take the whole diet and meet the high energy requirements. By the mid 1970s these diets had fallen from favour. An editorial in the *BMJ* (1975) stated that 'the imposition of an unpalatable diet solely in an imperious attempt to improve biochemistry was neither reasonable nor kind'. Thus patients were started on dialysis earlier and dietary management offered only to those not selected. If a protein restriction was given it was rarely less than 40 g protein/day. The aim of the diet was palliative, aimed at the reduction of uraemic symptoms such as nausea, vomiting, pruritis, bone pain, shortness of breath, fatigue, weakness and anorexia. It has been shown recently that low protein diets may slow down the rate of progression of chronic renal failure (Barsoti *et al* 1981; Maschio *et al* 1982; Bennett *et al* 1983b) and such diets are once more in favour although the exact mechanisms responsible for their success are not yet fully established. The underlying aetiology may have an effect but the published data do not agree (El Nahas *et al* 1984; Williams *et al* 1984). The recent studies lend support to Brenner's hypothesis on dietary protein intake and the progressive nature of kidney disease — the hyperfiltration theory (Brenner *et al* 1982).

The initial studies by Barsoti (1981) were carried out using very low nitrogen diets supplemented with amino acids and keto analogues. Work in Sweden (Alvestrand *et al* 1983) has confirmed the beneficial effects of these diets in delaying the progression of renal failure. Recent studies in the UK (Williams *et al* 1984; El Nahas *et al* 1984), Italy (Maschio *et al* 1982) and the Netherlands (Rosman *et al* 1984) have achieved satisfactory results using diets containing 0.5–0.6 g protein/kg body weight. The FAO recommend 0.5 g protein/kg body weight as the minimum protein intake for healthy adults. Kopple and Loburn (1973) showed that patients with CRF maintained on diets containing 0.6 g protein/kg body weight remained in positive nitrogen balance. The latter diets have been shown to be as effective as very low protein diets with keto analogues/amino acid supplements in slowing down the progression of renal dysfunction. There seems little justification for the administration of unpalatable expensive amino acid/keto analogues together with the extra social constraints of a very low protein diet. Long term compliance in patients on 0.6 g protein/kg body weight/day is good (Bennett *et al* 1938b). Figure 4.15 shows the effect of a low protein diet in a typical patient from the study of Williams *et al* (1984). At one time it was customary to allow for urinary protein losses but work by El Nahas *et al* (1984) suggests that this is unnecessary.

Recent research shows that introducing a protein restriction early in the course of the disease may be beneficial (El Nahas *et al* 1984; Rosman *et al* 1984). Patients may, however, respond to diet at any level of renal function (Williams *et al* 1984). It is much easier to establish effective dietary therapy when the patient is not suffering from uraemic symptoms which usually appear when the serum creatinine levels exceed 500–600 µmol/l. Low protein diets should not be used as a substitute for efficient dialysis when it is indicated. Many patients can be maintained successfully on conservative management for periods of up to ten years, but the rate of progression of renal failure depends on individual patients and aetiology.

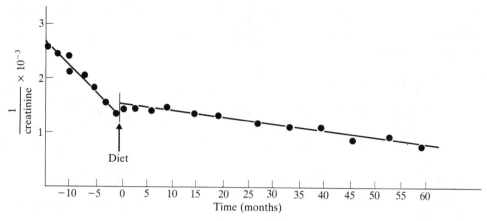

Fig. 4.15 Example of 1/serum creatinine versus time plot in a typical patient (male aged 29) with CRF before and after protein restriction.

Dietary treatment of patients with CRF being managed conservatively

Dietary composition

Protein. At least 70% of the protein should be of high biological value (HBV). Protein should be spaced out evenly over the whole day to allow for better utilization, e.g. one 7 g protein exchange at breakfast (or bedtime), mid-day and evening meal and one 7 g protein exchange for milk. Some milk should be included each day to provide a source of calcium. The remaining protein allowance can be made up from foods providing protein of a lower biological value as given in the protein exchange list (see p 118). Diets should be accurate to within 2 g protein, but should not constantly be over the calculated requirement.

When planning a diet, the milk allowance for drinks can often be tailored to make the diet accurate. The inclusion of nuts/dried beans/chocolate is not normally recommended due to their high potassium and phosphate content. Examples of the calculation of protein exchanges are shown below

1   A 70 kg man
    70 × 0.6 g = 42 g protein/day.

4 × 7 g HBV protein exchanges	= 28 g
6 × 2 g LBV protein exchanges	= 12 g
Fruit and cream	= 2 g
	42 g

2   A 55 kg woman
    55 × 0.6 = 33 g protein/day

3½ × 7 g HBV protein exchanges	= 24.5 g
4 × 2 g LBV protein exchanges	= 8.0 g
Fruit and cream	= 1.5 g
	34 g

Energy. In diets providing 30–45 g protein/day it is unnecessary for most patients to try to consume the very high energy intakes which were essential with the 'Giovannetti' type diets. Positive nitrogen balance can be achieved on 35–40 kcal (146–158 kJ)/kg ideal body weight. Malnourished patients may need initial supplementation and patients with CRF who have undergone surgery or have intercurrent illness may also need to increase their energy intake. Obese patients should be given a diet containing approximately 1500 kcal (6250 kJ)/day. Strict reducing diets will lead to catabolism and a rise in serum urea levels and they should not be used until the patient is on dialysis.

A large percentage of patients with CRF will have hyperlipidaemia and therefore it is probably unwise to encourage an excessive intake of animal fat. Cholesterol intake will automatically be lowered by the protein restriction. Many patients will happily use corn oil for frying and polyunsaturated fat for cooking (White Flora shortens low protein pastry) and most will use a margarine high in polyunsaturated fat instead of butter, but some double cream does help the palatability of the diet. It is wise to leave the final choice to the patient since too many restrictions lead to non-compliance.

Low protein flour is useful for adding variety and energy to the diet. It can be made into extra 'free' bread, biscuits, cakes and crumbles. The choice of low protein biscuits has improved in recent years; the wafer type and low protein crackers being very popular. Low protein pastas are also useful as fillers. Ordinary boiled sweets, barley sugars and glacier mints are good sources of energy. Proprietary low protein products are listed on p 121.

The energy intake can also be increased by making custard, blancmange and 'milk-type' puddings with water and double cream mixed in equal quantities or using coffee creamers such as Coffeemate or Coffee Compliment (1 oz to 10 fl oz water or 25 g to 250 ml water) instead of milk. White sauces can be made in a similar way using cornflour or low protein flour instead of ordinary flour. (Recipes can be found in *Enjoying food on a renal diet* edited by M Vennegoor.)

The use of glucose polymers (see Section 2.12) in either powder or liquid form are only needed in adults if they are acutely ill or underweight.

Sodium. A restriction, if required, should be no added salt (60−100 mmol/day) (see p 151) Patients should be told not to use salt substitutes because of their high potassium content.

Potassium. The change from normokalaemia to hyperkalaemia can be quite sudden and even if a restriction is not needed, excessive intakes should be discouraged since a restriction will probably become necessary at a later date (see p 153) Patients find it difficult to cut down on something they have previously been encouraged to eat in unlimited amounts. Vegetables, as well as containing potassium, also contain appreciable amounts of protein (e.g. cabbage 2 g per 75 g serving) therefore prescribing two normal-sized servings of vegetables and one or two servings of fruit is a sensible guide. If a potassium restriction is necessary because serum levels are raised, fruit and vegetables should be restricted to a maximum of two 4 mmol exchanges of each per day with a restriction on high potassium foods. (See haemodialysis.) This will reduce potassium intake to 35−40 mmol/day.

Phosphorus. The protein restriction will automatically reduce phosphate intake. High phosphorus foods are listed in Table 2.39, p 159 and should only be taken occasionally. Eggs should be limited to one per day.

Fibre. Wholemeal bread is normally encouraged within the protein allowance unless hyperkalaemia is a problem. Bran should be used with caution as the absorption of potassium and phosphorus from it varies between patients. Bran might also affect calcium and iron absorption, the intakes of which are already low. A phytate free 'bran' 'Trifyba' is available which may be useful for constipated renal patients.

Special dietary considerations

Vegetarians. The diet of 'lacto-ovo vegetarians' and 'lactovegetarians' should cause few problems since 70% of protein should be from sources of HBV protein such as eggs, milk and cheese. Phosphate levels should be carefully monitored. Vegans require a more carefully constructed diet to obtain the highest biological value protein possible while keeping phosphate and, if necessary, potassium intakes low. The use of essential amino acids and/or keto analogues may be advantageous.

Asians. The diet should be adapted to use as many of their traditional foods as possible, but unfortunately full analysis of these foods is not always available. Few are vegans so the diet can usually be easily modified. Yoghurt and milk are usually the main protein sources and many will use vegetables other than dhal or beans to make curries if requested. Many eat meat occasionally. The use of gram flour to make poppadums and batters should be discouraged because of its LBV protein and high phosphate and potassium content.

Several problems may arise if a potassium restriction is needed. Asians find it strange to boil vegetables (necessary in order to leech out the potassium) prior to frying with spices. Chilli and ginger, which they commonly use, are high in potassium and Indian sweets often contain condensed milk, a rich source of potassium, protein and phosphate. The use of rice instead of potatoes will reduce potassium intake and should be recommended.

The same problems apply for patients on haemodealysis (see p 448) as for those being managed conservatively.

Dietary compliance

It is important that patients who are advised to follow low protein diets are seen regularly so that changes in biochemistry can be assessed, and any necessary changes in diet (such as potassium intake) made. The importance of adhering to the diet should be reinforced regularly, and patients given help and encouragement to follow what can be a monotonous regimen. They should be given a phone number for contacting the dietitian.

The ratio of serum urea: creatinine is individual for each patient but should fall on commencing a low protein diet and is a useful measure of dietary compliance. An increase in the ratio may indicate poor compliance but can also be due to drug regimens or intercurrent illness. An increase in serum phosphate levels may also indicate non-compliance. Serial 24-hour urine collections for urea estimations may assist in assessing dietary compliance (El Nahas *et al* 1984).

Side effects of diet

1 Protein malnutrition. Serum albumin, protein and transferrin levels should be checked regularly. If any are low or falling, assess whether the patient is consuming an adequate energy intake.

2 Weight loss. Some patients have difficulty in maintaining an adequate energy intake. Without the use of proprietary low protein products it is difficult to increase the energy intake above 1500 kcal (6300 kJ)/day Mid-arm circumference measurements are useful in assessing whether a change in weight is due to fluid or flesh loss or gain (Bennett *et al* 1983a) since patients with CRF can easily become dehydrated or oedematous.

3 Hyperkalaemia. This can result from patients being encouraged to eat large quantities of fruit and vegetables.

4 Dehydration. If a sodium restriction is imposed unnecessarily dehydration can occur.

Further advice can be obtained from the Renal Dialysis Group of the British Dietetic Association.

Management with renal replacement therapy

In the past two decades dialysis facilities have increased allowing most patients with end stage renal failure (ESRF), including the 'over 60s' and diabetics, to be offered treatment. There are various forms of treatment available and, patients can change from one mode of therapy to another as required (Fig. 4.16). Complications on continuous ambulatory peritoneal dialysis (CAPD) may mean temporary or permanent transfer to haemodialysis (HD). Problems of vascular access may lead to transfer from HD to CAPD.

Replacement therapy should start before the patient enters the terminal phase of ESRF (i.e. serum creatinine concentration in the range of 1000 − 1500 μmol/l, depending on the patients size and therefore muscle mass). Children and diabetics normally start replacement therapy at a much lower serum creatinine concentration. The patients clinical condition should be used to determine the exact time.

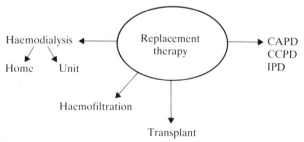

Fig. 4.16 Treatment of end stage renal failure.

Haemodialysis

Over the past 20 years major changes have taken place with the dialysis equipment used. There are now machines with automated proportioning systems for the dialysate, and integral blood and heparin pumps with increased use of microprocessor technology. The non-disposable kiils and coils are now rarely used, being replaced by smaller disposable haemodialysers. The latter are either 'flat-plate' with a multilayer configuration of semi-permeable membranes or 'hollow fibre' — a bundle of cuprophan or cellulose hollow fibre. Both types are available in a range of sizes to suit specific needs, e.g. children or 90 kg men.

The process of haemodialysis requires the transport of bood and dialysate on either side of a semi-permeable membrane. Products of metabolism are removed from the blood by diffusion and fluid by convection through the semi-permeable membrane. If a patient has fluid overload, sequential ultrafiltration may be performed before or after dialysis. An ultrafiltration of plasma is obtained by a pressure gradient across a semi-permeable membrane.

Dialysate contains electrolytes, Na^+, Ca^{2+}, Mg^{2+}, K^+, Cl^-, acetate (or bicarbonate) and dextrose. The concentration of K^+ is lower in dialysate than serum.

Blood access is achieved via an arteriovenous fistula which is normally constructed several weeks before it is needed by joining an artery and vein in the arm, allowing the vein to dilate and thicken. When dialysis is necessary two needles are inserted. One is used to carry the blood from the patient to the dialyser and the other to return blood to the patient. Alternative forms of access are arteriovenous shunts or subclavian catheters; both of which can be used immediately. Subclavian catheters provide temporary access only. Most patients dialyse for 4−6 hours, two or three times per week.

Dietary composition

Patients on regular haemodialysis therapy need to adhere to some dietary and fluid restrictions to prevent the build up of protein metabolites, phosphate, potassium and fluid between each dialysis.

Protein. Most patients are allowed 1−1.2 g protein/kg ideal body weight, of which 70% should be from HBV sources. This will make up for losses of amino acids during dialysis but prevent excessive urea generation between dialysis. Pre-dialysis urea should be < 30 mmol/l.

The diet for a 65 kg man would be made up of 7 × 7 g *or* 8 × 6 g protein exchanges plus 8 − 15 × 2 g protein exchanges. This will provide 65−78 g protein/day. The number of 2 g protein exchanges will depend on the patient's energy needs. The patient's other dietary restrictions (sodium, potassium and phosphorus) will limit the type of HBV protein exchanges taken. No more than two should come from dairy produce. The protein should be spaced out, usually giving one 7 g exchange for milk drinks, one 7 g exchange for breakfast, two 7 g exchanges for a snack meal and three 7 g exchanges for main meals (see p 117)

Phosphorus. The removal of phosphate is less efficient with shorter hours on dialysis. As discussed in conservative treatment, hyperphosphataemia may lead to renal bone disease and soft tissue calcification and therefore phosphate binders are routinely prescribed (see p 444). Aluminium intoxication in dialysis patients was thought to be almost entirely due to the alum added to water supplies but patients dialysed in areas with low aluminium levels in water have also been found to have high serum aluminium levels, indicating absorption from the phosphate binder aluminium hydroxide. Patients should be reminded to take the latter with food for maximum effect and keep to the low dose prescribed. Dietary phosphorus restriction is becoming increasingly important and a list of foods with a high phosphorus content is given on p 159. Serum phosphate should be kept within the normal range 0.8−1.6 mmol/l both pre- and post-dialysis.

Potassium. The risk of hyperkalaemia (serum K > 5.5 mmol/l) is high. This is the most dangerous of all electrolyte disturbances in patients with CRF. Potassium is normally dialysed out efficiently but it does accumulate between each dialysis. Furthermore, the insidious onset of hyperkalaemia without clinical signs is no disincentive to dietary cheating. Hyperkalaemia if untreated will lead to cardiac arrhythmias and cardiac arrest. Patients should be discouraged from eating high potassium foods during dialysis since its shorter duration often means that post-dialysis potassium levels are acceptable, only to rise an hour later when the potassium in the food is fully absorbed.

Potassium intake should be restricted to 1 mmol/kg ideal body weight. This level of intake usually ensures that serum potassium levels remain in the normal range. Patients starting on haemodialysis may still be excreting some potassium in their urine, and should be encouraged to take their full allowance as anorexic patients can become hypokalaemic. Most renal dietitians use an exchange system based on 4 mmol exchanges of fruit and vegetables which allows most of them to be eaten, thus giving the patient variety. It must be remembered that over half the potassium in the diet comes from protein foods. Milk is especially high and contains more potassium per ml than pure orange juice. Section 2.7, p 153 lists high potassium foods which should be restricted and those which can be used on an exchange basis. Foods which are very high are better 'banned' than exchanged (for example, most people cannot restrict themselves to 25 g (1 oz) banana and eat a whole one instead) but each patient must be treated as an individual. The potassium content of vegetables can be reduced by soaking them in cold water for several hours, then boiling in plenty of water and draining them well. Steaming, baking, pressure cooking, frying or microwave cooking do not reduce the potassium content.

It is important that the potassium allowance is spread over the whole day and not eaten all at one meal which could lead to hyperkalaemia despite the patient keeping to the prescribed amount.

Potassium exchange resins, calcium resonin or resonium A are sometimes given on a short term basis.

Sodium. This is normally restricted to control blood pressure which is usually salt and water-related in ESRF, and to prevent undue thirst leading to excessive fluid intake. A few patients, usually those with a maintained urine output may not need a sodium restriction. Most however follow a 'no added salt' diet (80−100 mmol/day). Occasionally patients with severe hypertension require lower intakes than this; these need to be worked out individually. Most patients with severe hypertension are controlled on drugs rather than very low sodium intakes. A list of foods high in sodium which should be avoided is given in Section 2.7, p 151.

Foods with a high sodium and low potassium content are often allowed during dialysis, especially if the patient experiences cramps and hypotension.

Fluid. It is important that the weight gain between dialysis sessions is kept under 2 kg and preferably nearer to 1 kg. In small patients, especially children, it should be kept even lower.

In adults a daily fluid allowance of 500 ml plus the equivalent to the amount of urine passed the previous day will prevent fluid overload. An excessive fluid intake will lead to increased blood pressure, raised jugular venous pressure (JVP), shortness of breath and pulmonary oedema.

Patients should be reminded of hidden sources of fluid in food especially in puddings, gravies and sauces. The patient can be given useful hints to limit fluid intake such as using a smaller cup and rinsing the mouth out without swallowing. During hot weather, pyrexia or diarrhoea and vomiting, an increased fluid allowance will be needed and the patient must be given appropriate advice.

Energy. At one time it was customary to encourage high energy intakes in all renal patients but the majority do not need it and an intake of 35 kcal (146 kJ)/kg ideal body weight is normally adequate. This can come from ordinary bread, biscuits, rice, pasta, potato, sugar and fats. It must be remembered that up to 70% of dialysis patients have lipid abnormalities (Golper 1984) and cardiovascular disease remains a major cause of death in the dialysis population. Patients should therefore be encouraged to use polyunsaturated margarine rather than butter and to use a polyunsaturated oil when cooking. The intake of milk, eggs and cheese should in any case be reduced due to phosphate restriction. The final decision on what type of fat to use is best left to the patient after the facts have been given, since too many restrictions make dietary compliance and eating outside the home very difficult.

Overweight patients should be encouraged to lose flesh weight. Patients who are underweight or acutely ill (for example with appendicitis or septicaemia) may need energy supplements. Glucose polymers and products such as Duocal and Calogen are useful. (For further advice see under Acute Renal Failure, and Section 2.12.) Although a 'free' diet may in theory, encourage an increased nutritional intake in the malnourished, in practice they tend to eat 'forbidden' foods low in energy but high in potassium such as fruit and vegetables. Time spent on individual patient advice is more beneficial than free choice.

Patients with polycystic kidneys may have kidneys weighing up to 5−7 kg and may also be underweight despite apparently being of ideal body weight.

Vitamins and minerals. It is normal practice to supplement patients with water soluble vitamins, i.e. B complex, folic acid and vitamin C. 'Leaching' of vegetables to reduce potassium and small dialysis losses lead to a diet deficient in folic acid and providing only borderline amounts of vitamins B1, B2, B6 and C (Bennett *et al* 1985b). However, large doses of vitamin C should not be given as these may lead to high serum levels of oxalic acid with the possible deposition of calcium oxalate in bones and tissues (Pru *et al* 1985).

Vitamin D if needed should be given in an active form (see conservative management, p 444).

Iron supplements are usually given as ferrous sulphate to make up for blood losses during HD, but patients who have frequent blood transfusions may become iron overloaded (Van de Vyver *et al* 1984). Iron should therefore be prescribed to meet individual patient requirements.

Special dietary considerations

Eating out. Patients on HD should be encouraged to go out for meals as it is extremely important that as normal a life as possible is maintained. Giving advice on how to choose sensibly from a menu is obviously important as they often want to hide the fact that they are on a 'special diet'. Some restaurants and hotels will cater for patients on renal diets and a list is available through the National Federation of Kidney Patients Associations.

Weight fluctuations. Loss or gain of flesh weight and setting of 'dry weight' is often difficult to assess accurately. Serial measurements of mid-arm circumference will reflect changes in flesh weight (Bennett *et al* 1983a). Emphasis should be placed on 'dry weight' if patients have intercurrent illnesses.

Hyperkalaemia. Hyperkalaemia can be a major problem as described previously.

Haemofiltration (HF)

In haemofiltration, blood is pumped from the body in a similar manner to HD but instead of passing through a dialyser with semi-permeable membranes it passes through a haemofiltration column. The ultrafiltration flow is augmented by using high flux membranes, e.g. Polyamide. Metabolic breakdown products are removed by convection. Replacement of water and electrolytes is required to maintain blood volume and composition. There is a large fluid exchange of 20−30 litres. The machine with a microprocessor controls the accurate balancing and monitoring systems which are needed. As haemofilters and replacement fluid are relatively expensive, haemofiltration is often reserved for those patients who do not tolerate haemodialysis, i.e. those with severe hypotension, (HF causes less hypotension than HD) and/or nausea vomiting or muscle cramps. Total peripheral resistance and catecholamine levels are unchanged in HF but decrease in HD. Patients with severe hypertension may also benefit from HF.

Patients are usually on HF 2−3 times per week for approximately 4−5 hours depending on the size of fluid exchange. They require a similar diet to HD patients. Potassium may not be as efficiently lowered during HF so the patient should be advised to restrict dietary intake to 0.8−0.9 mmol/kg body weight/day. Fluid should be restricted to 500 ml plus the equivalent of the previous day's urine output. The eating of forbidden foods should not be encouraged.

A different method of haemofiltration may be used in ARF — continuous haemofiltration (see p 440).

Continuous ambulatory peritoneal dialysis (CAPD)

Since its conception in 1975 by Popovich *et al* (1976) the use of CAPD has grown rapidly as a form of renal replacement therapy. It mimics the normal kidney by providing continuous dialysis with steady state biochemistry. This fact led to patients being allowed an unrestricted diet, fluid overload being prevented by the use of hypertonic (3.86−4.5%) dextrose dialysate. Long term complications of CAPD now include obesity, hypertriglyceridaemia (Oreopolous 1979) and hypoalbuminaemia.

In CAPD a silastic catheter is inserted into the peritoneal cavity. The catheter is attached to a giving set which in turn is connected to a bag of dialysate by means of a spike or luer lock connection. Once the fluid has flowed into the peritoneum, the empty plastic bag and giving set are folded and usually put into a cloth pouch beneath the clothing. Four to six hours later the peritoneum is drained by unfolding the bag and giving set, the fluid is allowed to run out by gravity. Usually four exchanges are carried out each day. Fluid and metabolic toxins are removed by osmosis and diffusion. CAPD is able to remove the toxic breakdown products of metabolism but at a much slower rate than the normal kidney. As the removal is continuous a much more liberal intake of certain foods can be allowed than to patients on HD.

The size of dialysate exchange will vary (1.5−3 litres) depending on the patient's size and biochemistry. Two strengths of dialysate are routinely used, 1.36% and 3.86% dextrose. The more dextrose, the more fluid that can be removed. Seventy per cent of dextrose is absorbed into the blood stream (De Santo *et al* 1979) and uncontrolled use of hypertonic dialysate often leads to unwanted gains in flesh body weight and may lead to accelerated hypertriglyceridaemia because of the carbohydrate absorbed, e.g 2 litres 3.86−4.5% dialysate provides 60 g CHO and 220 kcal (920 kJ) and 2 litres 1.36−1.5% dialysate provides 20 g CHO and 80 kcal (335 kJ). The use of hypertonic dialysate should therefore be controlled (Turgan *et al* 1981).

Dietary composition

Fluid. As it is important to prevent dehydration or fluid overload, weight and blood pressure should be measured daily. Sudden changes in weight reflect changes in fluid balance. Gradual changes in weight may reflect either flesh or fluid gains or losses. The former can be assessed by serial measurements of mid-arm circumference (Bennett *et al* 1983a). Fluid overload is associated with hypertension, oedema, shortness of breath and elevated JVP. If the patient is fluid overloaded it is important that hypertonic dialysate is used to remove the excess fluid. A fluid restriction of 700 ml plus the equivalent to the urine output will usually prevent fluid accumulation. Some patients continue to pass good volumes of urine while others become virtually anuric after 1−2 months on CAPD.

Sodium. Salty foods should be avoided as these create thirst. A more severe sodium restriction may be needed (60−80 mmol) if the patient is hypertensive.

Energy. Many patients lose weight prior to starting dialysis and may need to regain flesh weight initially. However, continued weight gain should be prevented. The oral energy intake should be reduced to 25 kcal (110 kJ)/kg ideal body weight since the patient will absorb approximately 300 kcal (1250 kJ) daily from isotonic dialysate. Reducing the intake of sugar and sugar-containing foods as well as reducing energy intake will also prevent accelerated hypertriglyceridaemia (Bennett *et al* 1981) but overweight patients may need to reduce energy intake further.

Protein. Unfortunately, as well as removing toxic metabolites, CAPD also removes up to 5−12 g protein per day (Rubin *et al* 1981; Blumenkrantz *et al* 1981; Heide *et al* 1983; Sandoz *et al* 1984). Protein losses may double during peritonitis. If these losses are not compensated, hypoalbuminaemia will result. An intake of 1.2−1.5 g/kg ideal body weight should be achieved (Kopple and Blumenkrantz 1983) of which at least 70% should be HBV.

Phosphorus. Uraemic bone disease is a problem in CAPD patients as in other patients undergoing replacement therapy and conservative management for CRF. A dietary phosphorus restriction of < 1200 mg/day (40 mmol) will therefore be needed (Kopple and Blumenkrantz 1983) This necessitates limiting milk to 300 ml/day; eggs to one per day and only occasionally eating hard cheese, offal and shellfish.

Potassium. The risk of hyperkalaemia, although a major problem in HD patients, rarely occurs in patients being treated by CAPD due to continuous dialysis 24 hours a day, seven days per week. Potassium levels should be maintained within the normal range of 3.3–5.5 mmol/l. If levels rise above the upper limit of normal it is wise to cut out high potassium foods (see Section 2.7; p 153) and restrict fruit and vegetable intake.

Vitamins and minerals. The exact requirement for these is unknown in CAPD patients. If the appetite is good, there is probably no need to supplement water soluble B vitamins including folic acid or vitamin C, but anorexic patients should be prescribed them temporarily. Vitamin B12 should be given if serum levels are low as B12 is dialysed out. Vegetarian patients, or those on Cimetidine or Ranitidine, which affect the gastric parietal cells' production of intrinsic factor, are at special risk of B12 deficiency (Bennett *et al* 1985a). If vitamin D is needed to raise serum calcium levels after phosphate levels have been corrected it should be given as 1,25 dihydroxy vitamin D3 or 1-alpha calcidol. Calcium supplementation may be needed in some patients (see p 444). Iron supplementation is probably unnecessary unless the patient has low serum iron and ferritin levels.

Problems of dietary treatment

Vegetarians. Difficulties may be encountered in trying to achieve an adequate protein intake whilst keeping the phosphous intake low. A close check should be kept on serum phosphate levels. Up to two eggs with extra milk, yoghurt and cheese may need to be allowed. Patients who do not eat eggs or cheese should include pulse vegetables daily. These patients will probably need supplementing with proprietary protein products such as Maxisorb or Maxipro HBV. These two products have the advantage of being low in phosphorus. Difficulties will be encountered with vegans, but amino acid supplements such as Dialamine can be useful if

the patient is willing to take them. Serum vitamin B12 levels should be monitored regularly.

Small appetite. Some patients, especially small women, find it difficult to eat normally due to the pressure of 2 litres of dialysate against the stomach. Timing dialysate drainage to coincide with meal times and eating small meals with snacks in between may help.

Constipation. It is important that constipation is prevented as this can lead to poor dialysate drainage. Patients should be encouraged to take wholegrain cereals as part of their diet. 'Trifyba' may be useful for those requiring additional fibre.

Diabetics on CAPD (see also Section 4.16.4). Good control of blood glucose is essential and levels should be maintained between 4–7 mmol/l. Hypertonic dialysate needs to be avoided where possible. Insulin will normally be given by the intraperitoneal route allowing a continuous insulin infusion. The insulin is absorbed directly into the portal circulation. The contribution of dialysis dextrose should be taken into account when planning the diet. Carbohydrate should be evenly distributed throughout the day with snacks being given in between the main meals.

Eating out. Patients on CAPD can go out for a meal and not worry too much what they eat (unless they have difficulty maintaining normal potassium levels). However, it is wise for them to control fluid intake and avoid eating anything in excess. If eating out on a regular basis, dietary guidelines should be followed.

Complications of CAPD and their nutritional implications

Peritonitis. . Peritonitis can cause protein losses to be doubled and lead to anorexia (Heide *et al* 1983), but it is very important that adequate protein intakes are achieved otherwise hypoalbuminaemia will result. The phosphorus restriction may need to be relaxed on a temporary basis to permit the use of fortified milk-based drinks and/or commercial enteral feeds. If sip feeding and oral foods are not tolerated nasogastric feeding or parenteral feeding may be required. High protein enteral feeds should be used (extra energy being provided by dialysate). Hypertonic dialysate may be needed to allow for increased fluid intake. The ultrafiltration capacity of the peritoneum is reduced during peritonitis. Ileus or severe vomiting occasionally occur during peritonitis and parenteral nutrition is then essential. If a peripheral line is used, 1–1.5 litres/day of Vamin 9 glucose (KabiVitrum) can be given, utilizing the glucose supplied via dialysate. Intralipid may be added if an increased energy intake is required. If a central venous line is used, either 1 litre Vamin 14 or Vamin 18 with 500 ml 50% dextrose (and Intralipid if fluid allows) can be administered with electrolytes (70–90 mmol potassium and 50 mmol sodium/day) in most cases. Vitamin supplements will also be needed.

Recurrent peritonitis and/or fungal infections may mean the removal of the catheter and temporary or permanent transfer to haemodialysis with a change in nutritional requirements. Good nutritional support can prevent long term effects of peritonitis (Bennett *et al* 1985a).

Hernias. Hernias are a common complication of CAPD. After the repair of abdominal hernias the CAPD catheter is usually clamped off for 1–2 weeks to allow the surgical incisions to heal. Temporary haemodialysis or conservative management will be given during this time and thus appropriate changes in dietary advice will be needed.

Monitoring patients on CAPD

The following blood parameters should be monitored regularly
1 Urea. If levels are below 10 mmol/l it is likely that the patient is not consuming sufficient protein.
2 Sodium. This should be within the normal range (135–148 mmol/l) and a high level usually indicates dehydration.
3 Potassium. This should be kept within the normal range. Anorexic patients may become hypokalaemic and need supplementation. If levels are high the dietary intake of potassium should be restricted.
4 Phosphate. Levels should be kept between 0.8–1.8 mmol/l. If they are higher the dietary intake should be assessed carefully. If they are low, check that phosphate binders are not being given unnecessarily.
5 Albumin and protein. If either are below the normal range the dietary protein intake should be increased.
6 Transferrin. This is a useful indicator of protein status and responds to improvements or deterioration in nutritional status more quickly than albumin levels as it has a shorter half life.
7 Red cell folate and serum B12. These should be

assessed every few months to check they are within the normal range.

Anthropometric measurements should be carried out on a serial basis. Changes in weight may reflect flesh or fluid fluctuations. The mid-arm circumference is the most accurate marker of flesh weight changes (Bennett *et al* 1983a).

Continuous cyclic peritoneal dialysis (CCPD)

On CCPD a machine cycles 4–8 exchanges of 1.5–2 litres of dialysate overnight, leaving dialysate in the peritoneum (usually 2 litres) during the day. This allows more freedom during the day than CAPD. Often CCPD is only carried out six days a week leaving fluid in the peritoneum for a 36-hour dwell on the seventh day. Care must be taken on the day off to avoid large intakes of potassium and fluid. Patients on CCPD often need more hypertonic dialysate than patients on CAPD to achieve adequate fluid removal. Extra advice may be needed on sodium and fluid intake to keep the use of hypertonic dialysate to a minimum.

Intermittent peritoneal dialysis (IPD)

IPD has become less common since the introduction of CAPD. Patients on IPD are usually dialysed using hourly exchanges for a period of 48–72 hours once a week. A relatively free diet may be allowed during dialysis ensuring that at least 1.2 g protein/kg ideal body weight is consumed to compensate for losses into the dialysate. On non-dialysis days, a diet containing 0.7–0.8 g protein/kg and 0.7 mmol of potassium/kg ideal body weight/day is normally allowed. Fluid will also need to be restricted off dialysis to 500 ml plus the equivalent of the previous day's urine output. Sodium is restricted to avoid thirst and control blood pressure. Phosphorus will also need to be restricted.

Transplantation

Patients look forward to a successful kidney transplant with the relative freedom from dietary and fluid restrictions. Those patients on conventional immunosuppression therapy of prednisolone and azathioprine tend to have increased appetites and may need advice on weight reduction later. Many will also have hyperlipidaemia (usually Type IIb) and remain hypertensive so should be advised to reduce salt intake, increase their fibre intake and eat less fat. Some patients will develop steroid-induced diabetes and require more specific advice.

The use of Cyclosporin A (CyA) as an immunosuppressive

This drug is used either alone or in combination with prednisolone. It is a liquid and is lipid soluble. It should be taken mixed with a small quantity of fluid, e.g. milk with a little drinking chocolate or 'Nesquik' or a fizzy drink such as cola. Some patients on Cyclosporin A have been noted to become hyperkalaemic (Dutton and Adu 1983). It is thought that the hyperkalaemia is due to a combination of hypoaldosteroidism and a tubular defect of potassium and hydrogen ion excretion. A potassium restriction may therefore be needed.

Following transplantation the patient's diet should not be changed until it has been established that the transplanted kidney has good function. This may take several weeks during which time the patient still requires dialysis.

4.16.4 Renal failure and diabetes

About 50% of Type I (insulin dependent) diabetics (IDD) develop renal failure in a mean of 20 years after diagnosis (Friedman 1982). In the USA, aproximately one in four patients starting therapy for end stage renal failure are diabetic (Tai-Ping Shyh *et al* 1985). As techniques of renal dialysis and kidney transplantation improve and become more readily available more diabetic patients in the UK will be treated for end stage renal failure.

Dietary composition

As with all patients in renal failure, six components of the diet need to be considered
1 Protein
2 Sodium
3 Fluid
4 Potassium
5 Energy
6 Phosphate.

In addition, the carbohydrate intake has to be considered and the diet must be nutritionally adequate in respect of all other minerals and vitamins.

Protein

Protein intake in patients with renal failure has been the focus of much discussion (El Nahas *et al* 1984; Rosman *et al* 1984). It would appear that the work of

Brenner *et al* (1982) is being borne out and that renally impaired patients with a reactive renal vascular bed benefit from some degree of protein restriction early on in their treatment. However, the benefit of early protein restriction has yet to be illustrated in diabetic nephropathy since all such patients have some degree of proteinuria and are often cachectic (Comty *et al* 1974). Protein restriction of less than 1 g/kg ideal body weight/day is probably not useful in these patients and early renal replacement therapy is preferable to conservative management involving protein restricted diets. In non-diabetics, dialysis can usually be delayed safely as long as the glomerular filtration rate (GFR) exceeds 5 ml/min but diabetic patients are often severely symptomatic when the GFR falls to 10 ml/min and therapy must be started earlier (Friedman 1982).

Sodium and fluid

Requirements are determined in much the same way as for non-diabetic patients but fluid balance is somewhat more difficult to achieve. The main reason for this is that poor control of blood glucose induces thirst and makes it extremely difficult for patients to comply with their fluid allowance (Comty *et al* 1974; Wauters 1983). Lemon tea, ice cubes and artificial saliva (e.g. Glandosane) can be useful aids for quenching thirst.

Potassium

Requirements for diabetic patients are no different from those of non-diabetics. Diabetics do have a more labile serum potassium than non-diabetics, especially if their glycaemic control is poor. The dangers of hyperkalaemia must be emphasized to the patient and good glycaemic control encouraged.

Energy and carbohydrate

Intake of these must be considered together and must be adequate to prevent malnutrition. Most workers agree that a relatively high carbohydrate intake is to be encouraged, i.e. 150−350 g of carbohydrate/day (Comty *et al* 1974; Wauters 1983). This will need to be covered with an adequate amount of insulin and may necessitate an increase in insulin dosage. Since insulin in an anabolic hormone, an increased insulin requirement is not necessarily a bad thing. An energy intake of 25−35 kcal/kg ideal body weight/day is ideal (Comty *et al* 1974) and should be achieved by increasing carbohydrate rather than fat intake because the incidence of lipid abnormalities in this group of patients is high (Comty *et al* 1974; Chan *et al* 1981; Wauters 1983).

Phosphate

Dietary phosphate considerations are presumed to be the same for the diabetic in renal failure as for the non-diabetic.

Special dietary considerations

There are four main problems which are associated with diabetics in renal failure

1 Gastrointestinal problems
2 Blindness
3 Compliance
4 Complicated dietary regimens.

Gastrointestinal problems

These make feeding particularly difficult, especially during hospital admissions when the patient is likely to be ill or undergoing some investigation which involves periods of starvation. Diabetic neuropathy can affect the gut and leads to an increased incidence of anorexia, nausea, vomiting and constipation (Comty *et al* 1974). If the patient is anorexic, losing weight or has hypoalbuminaemia, the diet should be supplemented with a commercially available liquid feed such as Build-up or nasogastric tube feeding may need to be instituted. These measures often lead to a change in insulin requirements which can be met by more frequent adminstration of short acting insulins or, occasionally, continuous intravenous infusion of insulin. The provision of regular antiemetics such as metoclopramide or prochlorperazine may be useful. A regular prescription rather than a *pro re natum* dose is preferable because these drugs work better as prophylactic measures. When the patient is eating normally, a high fibre diet as recommended for all diabetics (British Diabetic Association 1982) is to be encouraged to help promote better control of diabetes and prevent constipation.

Loss of vision

This is a major handicap and has been linked with the high suicide rate in this group of patients (Shapiro *et al* 1974; Shapiro 1983). It is also a major handicap to patients endeavouring to learn a somewhat complicated diet without the use of a diet sheet. Patients who live alone need their dietary instructions recorded on audio tape so that they can remind themselves of their dietary needs.

Compliance

With a very complicated dietary regimen, compliance is extremely difficult. There is much debate in the literature about whether or not good glycaemic control can prevent or arrest the progress of multi-organ damage, including renal failure. However, until there is evidence to the contrary, normoglycaemia is a reasonable goal to strive for (Friedman 1982; Wauters 1983). Provided that the reasons for dietary adherence are carefully explained, most patients are well motivated and will comply. Some patients find it very difficult to balance the control of diabetes with the control of uraemia, fluid balance and serum potassium and there is no doubt that the renal diabetic diet is one of the most complicated to explain, understand and live with. Patients should be warned that it will take time to understand the dietary modifications and they should be prepared to learn from their mistakes. Patients should not be given too much information too quickly and the initial explanations of the dietary regimen should be limited to that which is necessary to prevent danger to life. In the early stages of following the diet, problems will arise and need to be corrected but most patients eventually find a regimen which suits them medically, nutritionally and socially.

Patients who suffer from both diabetes and renal failure are nutritionally very much at risk and can deteriorate rapidly (Comty *et al* 1974). It is therefore vital that appropriate dietary measures are instituted at an early stage.

4.16.5 Nutritional management of children in end stage renal failure (ESRF)

The aims of management of children with end stage renal failure are to promote growth, to maintain residual renal function and to keep blood chemistry within normal limits with the least possible disruption to family life.

Nutritional consequences of chronic renal failure

Energy

A child's intake of energy, related to body size, is much higher than that of an adult. The increased requirement is determined by the greater proportion of body mass comprised of metabolically active organs including the brain, heart and kidneys. In addition, a child requires not only energy for metabolism but also for growth. It is thought that a child in end stage renal failure requires more than the recommended daily allowance (RDA) of energy, for reasons which are not yet fully understood.

If the diet of infants and children provides sufficient energy it usually provides other nutrients such as protein, electrolytes and minerals, in amounts in excess of requirements, and one of the main functions of the kidney is to excrete these excesses. However, the inability of the diseased kidney to cope with excessive intakes of protein, sodium, potassium and phosphate may exacerbate the metabolic changes found in renal failure. The aim of the dietitian is to provide a diet which supplies the child's energy requirements while minimizing the associated over-provision of other nutrients.

When weaning starts in a baby with ESRF, advice should be given to avoid unmodified cows' milk and products containing it, as these are high in protein, particularly casein which contains sulphur (and is therefore acidogenic), and minerals, especially phosphate. Low protein baby milks which can be used are SMA Gold Cap (Wyeth), Premium (Cow and Gate) and Aptamil (Milupa). Although expressed human milk can be used, it is common for the lactating mother's supply to fail as a consequence of the emotional stress and disruption of life style caused by the diagnosis of ESRF in her baby.

A child's growth velocity is greatest in the first year of life, and this growth rate needs to be sustained by a higher energy intake/kg body weight than at any other stage in life and up to two and a half times that of an adult (Holliday 1972). It is during this period that energy deficiency can have the greatest impact on growth.

The child in ESRF is usually anorexic and difficult to feed. Vomiting is often a major problem. It is important that at least the RDA for energy is consumed so that the child has the optimum chance of growth. A high energy intake will also aid in maintaining other biochemical parameters within normal limits (e.g. blood urea, creatinine and potassium). The use of energy supplements in the form of carbohydrate and fat is invaluable (Table 4.41). Energy supplements (see also Section 2.12) can be used individually or in combination to supplement either an infant milk formula or drinks for the older child. For example, Maxijul or Duocal can be added to a suitable milk such as SMA Gold Cap. Alternatively, for the older child, Hycal may be added to lemonade or frozen into

miniature ice lollies. By means of these supplements, energy intake can be increased to supply up to 150 kcal/kg body weight for patients under one year and 90–120 kcal/kg body weight for those over one year.

Table 4.41 Energy supplements useful for children with end stage renal failure

Energy source	Products (manufacturer)	Description
Carbohydrate alone	Caloreen (Roussel)	A glucose polymer
	Maxijul (SHS)	A glucose polymer
	Polycal (Cow and Gate)	A glucose polymer
	Hycal (Beechams)	A glucose drink
	Maxijul drink (SHS)	A glucose drink
Fats alone	Calogen (SHS)	A 50% fat emulsion
	Liquigen (SHS)	A 50% MCT fat emulsion
	Double cream	
Carbohydrate and fat	Duocal (SHS)	A powder containing 72.7 g carbohydrate and 22.3 g fat (of which 34% MCT and 66% LCT) per 100g.

Full compositional details of these (and other) products in given in Section 2.12 (p 197).

Protein

Protein restriction may or may not be necessary. The advantage of protein restriction is that it may slow the rate of deterioration of renal function (Jones *et al* 1981). The protein intake required will be dependent on age, height and weight and will be determined partly by the blood urea and growth rate. Optimum growth is most likely to occur in children with a blood urea of < 20 mmol/l (120 mg/100 ml). However, a blood urea of up to 30 mmol/l does not necessarily preclude growth. Ideally, the blood urea of an infant newly diagnosed as having ESRF should be lowered to < 20 mmol/l as soon as possible (this can usually be achieved within one week) by reducing the protein intake or increasing the energy intake. As a general rule the energy supplied by protein should not be less than 6% of the total energy intake. If the protein intake falls below this then there is a danger of protein malnutrition. The use of proprietary low protein products (see Section 2.2, p 121) as a means of increasing energy intake is of limited value and the most acceptable diet is one which, as far as possible, incorporates the normal foods preferred by the child.

The use of essential amino acid supplementation or keto analogues (which provide essential amino acids without providing nitrogen) in conjunction with a severe protein restriction is only experimental and has been found to be expensive, difficult in practice and of questionable effectiveness (Jones *et al* 1980; Start and Jones 1983).

A sudden *rise* in blood urea in the absence of a simultaneous increase in creatinine level may be caused by
1 An increased intake of dietary protein.
2 A reduction in energy intake as a result of anorexia and/or decreased patient compliance.
3 The development of a catabolic state due, for example, to infection.

Sodium and potassium

Patients born with obstructive uropathy and/or renal dysplasia often 'leak' sodium and they may require sodium supplementation. This should be given as chloride or bicarbonate or a mixture of the two, according to the need for simultaneous correction of acidosis. The quantity given should be sufficient to achieve a normal blood sodium concentration but avoid fluid overload leading to oedema and hypertension. Patients who are 'salt losers' are often easier to feed because they have a craving for salty foods which can be utilized by the dietitian. In addition they are thirsty and all drinks can be 'laced' with high energy supplements.

Potassium restriction is only necessary when hyperkalaemia is present. This usually only occurs in the late stages of renal failure. A high potassium level (> 5.5 mmol/l) may be caused by either a high potassium intake or an inadequate energy intake. The latter results in a breakdown of body protein for use as an energy source with consequent release of potassium. A low potassium diet or increased energy supplementation may correct a high serum potassium level. If these measures are not effective, then a potassium binder such as resonium in the calcium phase (not resonium A which contains sodium) can be given orally or rectally. However, a persistently high potassium level requiring such measures and accompanied by a high serum creatinine is an indication to start dialysis.

Vitamins and minerals

Vitamin D supplementation is almost always required in end stage renal failure in an active form such as one alpha calcidol or 1,25 dihydroxy vitamin D3. The dose required is usually in the range 10—20 μg/kg body weight/day.

Calcium. Blood levels should be monitored regularly since hypercalcaemia may occur requiring a reduction in the dose of vitamin D.

Other vitamins should be given routinely particularly if the child's diet is restricted either voluntarily, by anorexia, or by prescription. Regular dietary assessment of the child's intake will reveal which vitamins are likely to be deficient.

Pyridoxine and folic acid are required in increased amounts in kidney failure, particularly in patients on dialysis, because of the increased turnover (Kopple 1978) due to loss in the dialysate (Holliday *et al* 1979).

Iron supplementation should only be given when the diet provides less than the recommended daily allowance (RDA). There is a risk of iron overload, particularly if the patient has had blood transfusions, as is common for haemodialysis patients. Thus the patient's iron status should be assessed by periodic measurement of serum ferritin levels and either iron supplements or treatment (desferrioxamine) to remove excess iron given as necessary.

Zinc deficiency frequently causes alterations in taste, exacerbating anorexia. Since zinc deficiency is likely to occur on a very restricted diet, supplementation may be indicated.

Other minerals such as aluminium, fluoride and magnesium are usually present in excess of requirements. Fluoride supplements, although indicated in normal children living in areas where the water fluoride concentration is low, should be avoided in uraemia since its accumulation may contribute to metabolic bone disease. In any case, tooth decay in children in ESRF is rare (Jaffee *et al* 1986). In general tooth decay can best be prevented by topical application of fluoride or by using fluoride-containing toothpaste, but the latter is less desirable as it may be swallowed.

Assessment of the child in renal failure

Anthropometry

Height and weight should be measured monthly and plotted on standard charts for all patients, so that a failure in growth rate and weight gain can be detected at an early stage. In the interests of accuracy it is advisable that measurements should be made by the same person on each occasion using standardized techniques.

Some centres also measure skinfold thickness but this is difficult to interpret, particularly as oedema is likely to be present.

Despite all efforts to ensure an adequate energy intake, the majority of children with long standing renal insufficiency fall below the tenth centile for height and weight. The object of aggressive dietary therapy is to avert, or at least minimize, the reduction in final height consequent to early growth failure. This means that the optimal diet should be established as soon as possible after diagnosis in order to give the child the greatest chance of growth.

Radiological Assessment

The appearance of ossification centres in the small bones of the hand and wrist is a sensitive guide to bone maturation. Bone maturation in children in ESRF is usually retarded.

Clinical evaluation

Close attention should be paid to arterial blood pressure, nutritional status, the presence of oedema and the state of hydration. It must be remembered that the assessment of the child is not confined to these simple clinical measurements. Management is unlikely to succeed unless proper account is taken of the child's family, school and social life. Specific enquiries about the child's activities in these areas are therefore an integral part of the doctor's or therapist's involvement with the child. The participation of a psychologist and a social worker are essential for adequate assessment and treatment of infants and children in ESRF.

Biochemical measurements

Regular monitoring of biochemical parameters is an essential part of management. Blood levels of sodium, potassium, bicarbonate, calcium, phosphorus, alkaline phosphatase, urea, creatinine, cholesterol, triglyceride and proteins (total protein, albumin and transferrin) should be measured regularly. Cholesterol and triglycerides should ideally be fasting measurements, but in the smaller child this is sometimes impossible due to the long distances some of them are required to travel to clinic visits and a 3−4 hour interval since the time of a meal is adequate (Lloyd 1984).

Optimum management of bone mineral metabolism also requires that parathyroid hormone levels be monitored as well as indices of renal phosphate handling, such as estimation of the fractional tubular re-absorption of filtered phosphate (TRP) (Fig. 4.17).

Any abnormalities in any of these parameters can be rectified by dietary manipulation. An up-to-date assessment of the child's dietary intake is required, together with a knowledge of the child's food preferences and an appreciation of what is practicable since it is pointless prescribing a diet which will not be followed.

Dietary assessments

Ideally dietary assessments (recorded by the parents) should be obtained monthly or bi-monthly, for a three

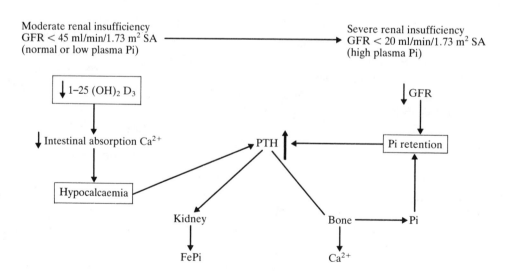

Fig. 4.17 Pathogenesis of secondary hyperparathyroidism. GFR = glomerular filtration rate (normal = 120 ml/min/1.73 m²), 1,25 (OH)₂D₃ = 1.25 dihydroxycholecalciferol; Ca = calcium, PTH = parathyroid hormone; FePi = fractional excretion of inorganic phosphate; Pi = inorganic phosphate. Figure courtesy of SPA Rigden, Consultant Paediatric Nephrologist, Evelina Children's Hospital, Guy's Hospital, London SE1.

day period. Seven day assessments are neither practicable nor accurate. Calculation of nutrient intakes can be most easily made using computerized tables of food analysis. The patient's intake can then be compared with the appropriate RDA together with their biochemistry results and discussed with the dietitian at a clinic visit.

Nutritional management

Pre-dialysis

Each child and family must be treated individually, taking into account the child's age, dietary preferences and the economic and psychological background. The dietitian must be careful not to instil anxiety or guilt in the child or parents when the aims of the feeding regimen are not met; these can only be achieved if realistic goals are set. Sensitivity, tact and the ability to compromise are indispensable to effective dietary and therapeutic counselling. The family should feel that they can communicate freely with all medical staff involved and that they are an important part of the team in the management of their child.

The importance of energy intake in relation to the promotion of growth cannot be over-emphasized. Children in ESRF are often difficult to feed because their appetites are usually poor and they soon learn to manipulate the situation to their own advantage in battles with their parents over feeding. Vomiting is common and some children, particularly older children on dialysis, can make themselves sick at will. Parents should be advised not to worry excessively and encouraged to offer another meal as soon as possible.

If adequate energy intake cannot be achieved orally, or if vomiting persists, nasogastric feeding should be considered. This can be done at home but usually needs to be initiated on the ward. The use of a pump instead of gravity drip feeding will help prevent vomiting or diarrhoea by allowing delivery of the feed at a slow controlled rate.

Nasogastric feeds should usually be based on either a milk formula or a feed low in Na, K, Ca and P (such as Clinifeed 400). Feeds should be individually designed for each child with the aim of correcting any biochemical imbalance and satisfying fluid requirements. For the older child a 'renal feed' may be necessary if the biochemical abnormalities cannot be corrected by ordinary means, if the child's weight is static, or if sufficient energy cannot be consumed. This feed is a variable mixture of protein, fat and carbohydrate similar to a nasogastric feed but palatable and designed to be taken orally and meet the individual child's requirements. An example of a 'renal feed' is given in Table 4.42.

In patients with CRF a low nitrogen, low phosphate diet has been shown to slow the decline in renal function (Walser 1975) and should be considered.

Table 4.42 Example of a 'renal feed' for a child in renal failure

	Protein (g)	Fat (g)	Carbohydrate (g)	Energy (kcal)
1 can Clinifeed 400	15	13.4	55	400
100 g Duocal	—	22.3	70	470
300 ml water	—	—	—	—
	15 g	35.7 g	125 g	870 kcal

Haemodialysis

The same general principles of nutritional therapy for adults on HD apply to the management of children on HD, but there are some specific factors to be considered.

Haemodialysis generally takes place three times a week lasting 3–6 hours. In some units the child is allowed to drink freely and to eat 'forbidden foods' during the first two hours of dialysis. The wisdom of this practice is questionable especially in families already having difficulties with dietary compliance. Regular dietary assessments should also be carried out on this group of patients.

Potassium. Since potassium restriction is usually necessary, potassium levels are measured every other day and potassium intake controlled accordingly.

Fluid. If the patient is anuric or oliguric, fluid restriction is required. The fluid allowed should equal in volume the previous day's urine output plus insensible losses. For the average anuric child the latter is about 400 ml fluid/m²/24 hours. The fluid content of foods and drinks should be discussed with the child who should be taught, as far as possible, the principles underlying their dietary treatment.

Fluid weight gain is often a difficult concept for the patient or parent to understand. Excessive weight gain between dialyses (< 0.5 kg for weekdays or < 0.8 kg for weekends) is caused by excessive fluid intake and should be avoided since fluid overload is a potentially dangerous state. It causes hypertension and may lead to pulmonary oedema, cardiac failure and sudden death. Since the drive to excessive fluid intake is thirst, and the major determinants of thirst are the blood concentrations of sodium and chloride, it follows that the most effective means of reducing fluid intake is dietary salt restriction. It is totally unrealistic to expect a child to refrain from drinking if their plasma is hypertonic.

Protein. This should not be restricted unless there is a persistently high blood urea (> 25–30 mmol/l) and then only if increased energy intake fails to correct the urea concentration.

Peritoneal and continuous ambulatory peritoneal dialysis (PD and CAPD)

The same principles apply as for patients on haemo-dialysis. The child should be weighed when the peritoneal cavity is empty to ensure consistent and accurate readings.

There may be considerable protein and water soluble vitamin losses via the peritoneum which need monitoring and replacing. A check must be kept on the patient's albumin levels as the blood urea level may not accurately indicate total body protein. Depending on their blood biochemistry, children on CAPD may be able to enjoy a more liberal diet and fluid intake than those on haemodialysis but an adequate energy intake must still be ensured. Obesity is not usually seen in the pre-adolescent child on CAPD.

Transplantation

With the recent introduction of the immunosuppressive agent Cyclosporin A and the associated reduction in maintenance steroid dosage, excessive weight gain in the early post-transplant period occurs less frequently and the need for weight reducing diets is therefore less common.

Almost without exception transplanted children will eat a normal diet provided there is good renal function.

Nonetheless obesity is still the major problem in children with well functioning transplants, largely due to the effect of steroids on appetite. An additional factor is that after possibly years of having to be forced to eat when anorexic, the child feels so well that he is actually hungry and wants to eat. It may also be difficult or impossible for parents to execute the necessary about-face from force feeding to food restriction. It is wise to prepare for this situation by discussing it with patient and parents well in advance of transplantation.

Cyclosporin A can be measured in blood and when high levels have been recorded, hyperkalaemia has also been noted. This is usually transient and disappears when correct drug levels are achieved.

Management of children in renal failure poses a challenge to the multi-disciplinary team in which the dietitian plays a vital part. The development of a diet which can enhance the quality of the child's life requires commitment from the dietitian, the parents and the other members of the team. Achieving this aim can be a rewarding task, particularly if it delays the necessity for dialysis and transplantation for as long as possible whilst allowing the child to continue growing and maintaining residual renal function.

Support organisations

1 The British Kidney Patients Association, Bordon, Hants
2 National Federation of Kidney Patients' Association (NFKPA), Chairman Mr B Pearmain, Swan House, The Street, Wickham Skeith, Eye, Suffolk.

Further reading

Cameron S (1981) *Kidney disease 'the facts'*. Oxford Medical Publications, Oxford.
Chantler C (1979) Renal failure in childhood. In *Renal disease* 4e. Black D and Jones NF (Eds). Blackwell Scientific Publications, London.
Fine and Graskin (1984) *End stage renal disease in children*. WB Saunders and Co, Philadelphia.
Gower PE (1893) *Nephrology*. Grant McIntyre Medical and Scientific,
Karran SI and Alberti KGMM (Eds) (1980) *Practical nutrition support*. Pitman Medical, London.
Leading article (1980) Acute renal failure after major surgery. *Br med J* 5, (1), 2–3.
Nursing Times Publication (1982) *Renal nursing*.
Venegoor M (1982) *Enjoying food on a renal diet*. Oxford University Press, Oxford.

References

Abel RM (1976) In *Total parenteral nutrition* Fischer J (Ed) p.143. Little Brown and Co Boston.
Allison SP (1984) Nutritional problems in intensive care. *Hospital Update* Dec, 1001–12.
Alvestrand A, Ahlberg M, Furst P and Bergstrom J (1983) Clinical results of long term treatment with low protein diet and a new amino acid preparation in patients with chronic uraemia. *Clin Neph* 19, (2), 67–73.
Barratt TM (1985) In *Post-graduate nephrology* Marsh F (Ed) pp 467–8. Heinemann Medical Books, London.
Barsoti G, Guiucci A, Ciardella F and Giovannette S (1981) Effects on renal function of a low nitrogen diet supplemented with essential amino acids and ketoanalogues and of haemodialysis and free protein supply in patients with chronic renal failure. *Nephron* 27, 113–7.

Bennett SE, Smith BA, Turgan C, Feehally J and Walls J (1981) Prevention of hypertriglyceridaemia in patients on continuous ambulatory peritoneal dialysis. *Proc Eur Dial Transplant Assoc* **10**, 200–3.

Bennett SE, Russell GI, Williams AJ, Wilson JM, and Walls J (1983a) Accurate assessment of 'dry weight' in haemodialysis and continuous ambulatory peritoneal dialysis patients. *Proc Eur Dial Transplant Assoc* **12**, 137–40.

Bennett SE, Russell GI and Walls J (1983b) Low protein diets in uraemia. *Br Med J* **287**, 1344–5.

Bennett SE, Smith BA, Wilson JM and Walls J (1985a) The effects of peritonitis on the nutritional status of patients on continuous ambulatory peritoneal dialysis. *Proc Eur Dial Transplant Assoc* **13**, 80–84.

Bennett SE, Feehally J and Walls J (1985b) Vitamin and mineral supplementation in chronic haemodialysis patients. *Proc Eur Dial Transplant Assoc* **14**, in press

Berlyne GM, Janabi KM and Shaw AB (1966) Dietary treatment of chronic renal failure. *Proc Roy Soc Med* **665**, 7.

Blumenkrantz MJ, Gahl GM, Kopple JD, Fauder AV, Jones MR, Kessel M and Coburn JW (1981) Protein losses during peritoneal dialysis. *Kidney Int* **19**, 1593–602.

Brenner BM, Meyer TW and Hostetter TH (1982) Dietary protein intake and the progressive nature of kidney disease. *N Engl J Med* **307**, 652–9.

British Diabetic Association (1982) Dietary recommendations for diabetics for the 1980s; a policy statement. *Hum Nutr: Appl Nutr* **36A**, 378–94.

Chan MK, Varghese Z and Moorhead JF (1981) Lipid abnormalities in uraemia, dialysis and transplantation. *Kidney Int* **19**, 625–37.

Cochran ST, Pagani JJ and Barbaric ZL (1979) Nephromegaly in hyperalimentation. *Radiology* **130**, 603–6.

Comty CM et al (1974) Nutritional and metabolic problems in the dialysed patient with diabetes. *Kidney Int* **6**, [Suppl] S51.

DeSanto NG, Copodicass G, Senatore R, Cicchetti T, Cirillo D, Domiano M, Torella R, Giugliano D, Improta L and Giordano C (1979) Glucose utilization from dialysate in patients on continous ambulatory peritoneal dialysis. *Int J Art Organs* **2**, 119–24.

Dodd NJ, O'Donovan RM, Bennett Jones DN, Rylance PB, Bewick M, Parsons V and Weston MJ (1983) Arteriovenous haemofiltration: a recent advance in the management of renal failure. *Br Med J* **287**, 1008–10.

Dorhout Mees EJ, Geers AB and Koomans HA (1984) Blood volume and sodium retention in the nephrotic syndrome. A controversial path of physiological concept. *Nephron* **36**, 201–11.

Dutton J and Adu D (1983) Hyperkalaemia in renal allograft recipients on Cyclosporin A — a dietary problem? *Proc Eur Dial Transplant Assoc.* **12**, 153–5.

Editorial (1975) Low protein diets in chronic renal failure. *Br Med J* **iv**, 486.

El Nahas AM, Masters-Thomas A, Brady SA, Farrington K, Williamson V, Hilson AJW, Varghese Z and Mooorhead J (1984) Selective effect of low protein diets in chronic renal diseases. *Br Med J* **289**, 1337–41.

Friedman EA (1982) Diabetic nephropathy: strategies in prevention and management. *Kidney Int* **21**, 780–91.

Giordano C (1963) Use of exogenous and endogenous urea for protein synthesis in normal and uraemic subjects. *J Lab Clin Med* **62**, 231–40.

Giovannetti S and Maggiore Q (1964) A low nitrogen diet with proteins of high biological value for severe chronic uraemia. *Lancet* **i**, 1000–3.

Golper TA (1984) Therapy for uraemic hyperlipidaemia. *Nephron* **38**, 217–25.

Heide B, Pierratos A, Khanna R, Pettit J, Ogilvie R, Harrison J, McNeil K and Oreopoulos DF (1983) Nutritional status of patients undergoing CAPD. *Peritoneal Dialysis Bulletin* **3.3**, 138–42.

Holliday MA (1972) Calorie deficiency in children with uraemia, effect upon growth. *Paediatrics* **50**, 590.

Holliday MA, McHenry-Richardson K, Portale A (1979) Nutritional management of chronic renal disease. *Med Clin North Am* **63**, 945.

Jacobsen FK, Christensen CK, Mogensen CE, Andreasen F and Heilstov NSC (1979) Pronounced increase in serum creatinine concentration after eating cooked meat. *Br Med J* **1**, 1049–50.

Jaffee I, Roberts G, Chantler C and Carter JE (1986) Dental findings in chronic renal failure. Paper submitted to the British Dental Journal

Jones RWA, Dalton N, Start K, Bishti M and Chantler C (1980) Oral essential amino acid supplements in children with advanced chronic renal failure. *Am J Clin Nutr* **33**, 1966.

Jones RWA, Dalton N, Turner C, Haycock GB, Start K and Chantler C (1981) Oral essential amino acids and keto acid supplements in children with chronic renal failure. *Kidney Int* **24**, 95–103.

Kopple JD and Coburn JW (1973) Metabolic studies of low protein diets in uraemia I. *Medicine* **52**, 583.

Kopple JD (1978) Abnormal amino acid and protein metabolism in uraemia. *Kidney Int* **14**, 340.

Kopple JD and Blumenkrantz MJ (1983) Nutritional requirements for patients undergoing continuous ambulatory peritoneal dialysis. *Kidney Int* **S16**, [Suppl] 295–5302.

Lee HA (1978) *Nutrition in the clinical management of disease* p 230. Edward Arnold, London.

Lee HA (1980) Nutritional support in renal and hepatic failure In *Practical nutritional support* pp 275–82. Pitman Medical, London.

Lewis B (1976) *The hyperlipidaemias — clinical and laboratory practice* p 21 and p 314. Blackwell Scientific Publications, Oxford.

Lloyd JK (1984) Plasma lipid disorders. In *Chemical pathology and the sick child* Clayton B and Round J (Eds). Blackwell Scientific Publications, Oxford.

Manos J, Harrison A, Jones M, Adams PH and Mallick NP (1983) Protein/calorie balance in the nephrotic syndrome. *Kidney Int* **24**, (616) [Suppl] 347–8.

Maschio G, Oldrizzi R, Tessitore N D'Angelo A, Valvo E, Lupo A Loschiavo C, Fabris A, Gammaro L, Rugia C and Panzetta G (1982) Effects of dietary protein and phosphorus restriction on the progression of early renal failure. *Kidney Int* **22**, 371–6.

Mitch WE, Walser M, Buffington GA and Lemann J (1976) A simple method of estimating progression of chronic renal failure. *Lancet* **ii**, 1326–8.

Oreopolous DG (1979) Editorial. *Dialysis and Transplantation* **8**, 5.

Popovich RP, Moncrief JW, Decherd JB, Bomar JB and Pyle WK (1976) The definition of a novel portable/wearable equilibrium peritoneal dialysis. *Abstr Am Soc Art Intern Org* **5**, 64.

Pru C, Eaton J and Kjellstrand C (1985) Vitamin C intoxication and hyperoxalaemia in chronic haemodialysis patients. *Nephron* **39**, 112–6.

Rosman JB, Meijer S, Sluiler W, Terwee P M, Pires-Beckt TPM and Donker AJM (1984) Prospective randomized trial on early dietary protein restriction in chronic renal failure. *Lancet* **ii**, 1291–5.

Round JM (1973) Plasma calcium, magnesium, phosphorus and alkaline phosphatase levels in normal British school children. *Br Med J* **3**, 137–40.

Rubin J, Nolph K, Arfania D, Prowant B, Fruto L, Brown P and Moore H (1981) Protein losses in continuous ambulatory peritoneal dialysis. *Nephron* **28**, 218–21.

Sandoz P, Vallance D, Winder AF and Walls J (1984) Protein and amino acid losses from the peritoneum during CAPD and CCPD. *Proc III International Symposium on Peritoneal Dialysis* (in Press)

Shapiro FL et al (1974) Mortality, morbidity and rehabilitation results in regularly dialysed patients with diabetes mellitus. *Kidney Int* **6** [Suppl 1] S8—S14.

Shapiro FL (1983) Haemodialysis in diabetic patients. In *Prevention and treatment of diabetic nephropathy* Keen H and Legrain M (Eds) pp 247—59. MTP Press Ltd, Lancaster.

Start KM and Jones RWA (1983) Essential amino acids and keto acid analogues in children with chronic renal failure. *Proc Eur Dial Transplant Assoc* **12**, 147—52.

Start K, Rigden SPA and Master C (1985) Aluminium bone disease, a case report. *Council for Renal Nutrition* **March**

Tai-Ping Shyh, Beyer M and Freidman EA (1985) Treatment of the uraemic diabetic. *Nephron* **40**, 129—38.

Turgan C, Fehally J, Bennett SE, Davies TJ and Walls J (1981) Accelerated hypertriglyceridaemia in patients on continuous ambulatory peritoneal dialysis — a preventable abnormality. *Int J Art Org* **4**, (4), 158—60.

Van de Vyver FL, Vanheule AA, Majelyne WM, D'Haese P, Blockx PP, Bekaert AB, Buyssens N, Dekeersmaecker W and De Broe ME (1984) Serum ferritin as a guide for iron stores in chronic haemodialysis patients. *Kidney Int* **26**, 451—8.

Walser M (1975) Keto acids in the treatment of uraemia. *Clin Nephrol* **3**, 180.

Wauters JP (1983) Diabetic nephropathy: metabolic management of the patient with chronic renal failure. In *Prevention and treatment of diabetic nephropathy* Keen H and Legrain M (Eds) pp 197—211. MTP Press Ltd, Lancaster.

Williams AJ, Bennett SE, Russell GJ and Walls J (1984) Alteration in the course of chronic renal failure by dietary protein restriction. *Proc Eur Dial Transplant Assoc* **21**, 604—7.

Woods HF and Alberti KGMM (1972) Dangers of intravenous fructose. *Lancet* **ii** 1354.

4.17 Hyperuricaemia and Renal Stones

4.17.1 Hyperuricaemia

The role of purines in human disease has been of importance since the discovery that uric acid (to which they are metabolized) was a component of some renal stones and that serum uric acid levels were elevated in patients with gout. Hyperuricaemia may be primary or secondary, but whatever its aetiology it reflects either overproduction of purines, reduced renal clearance of uric acid or a combination of both.

The most common manifestation of hyperuricaemia is gout which appears to be a familial disease. Allopurinol inhibits the enzyme xanthine oxidase which is responsible for the conversion of xanthine and hypoxanthine to uric acid. This causes the serum uric acid to fall and the excretion of its precursors to be increased since they are more soluble and have a higher renal clearance rate than uric acid. Allopurinol is now used regularly in the treatment of gout, reducing the need for a strict low purine diet. Dietary purines are responsible for only a small part of the excess uric acid which accumulates in gout. However, it does no harm to reduce the intake of purines especially as the foods which are rich sources (such as fish roes, sardines, crab, anchovies, sprats and offal) are not difficult to avoid (see also p 176). Patients with chronic gout should be advised to attain ideal weight by gradual dieting. Fasting or strict dieting will increase serum uric acid levels. The diet should be reduced in fat, refined sugar and animal protein with emphasis on vegetable protein, fibre and unrefined carbohydrate. Over-indulgence in food or alcohol must be avoided. Fluid intake should be at least (1−2 l/day) to facilitate the passage of any small stones in the renal tract.

4.17.2 Renal stones

Waste products of metabolism and excess ions in a soluble form are disposed of by the kidney but certain combinations of ions, because they are only sparingly soluble in urine, may precipitate and become lodged in a narrow section of the urinary tract forming a nucleus around which a stone may grow.

Diagnosis is rarely difficult because the symptoms are so painful, ranging from dull loin pain if the stone is in the renal pelvis to agonising colic if it is lodged in the ureter.

In the UK the prevalence of urinary tract stone disease is relatively low about 1.5% (Currie and Turner 1979). The annual incidence of stone formation is around 7 per 10,000 of the population with a male/female ratio of about 2:1. The incidence of upper urinary tract stones containing calcium appears to be related to affluence (Robertson et al 1980; 1981a) and one dietary component implicated is animal protein. This is substantiated by the findings that the prevalence of stone disease in vegetarians is only about 50% of that in the general population (Robertson et al 1981b). A high intake of animal protein increases the urinary excretion of calcium and oxalate and the accompanying increase in purine intake increases uric acid excretion. These three products are all known risk factors for the formation of calcium-containing renal stones.

Stone formation is more common in hot climates. Low urine volume is the most likely cause but an increased exposure to ultra violet light which is known to increase the intestinal absorption of calcium from the diet may be a contributing factor and also account for the seasonal variation seen in this country (Robertson et al 1975).

Some workers have found that the concentration of inhibitors of crystallization of calcium salts in urine is lower in stone formers than the rest of the population (Robertson et al 1976). The inhibitors identified include glycoproteins, glycosaminoglycans and Tamm Horsfall glycoprotein. There may also be an inhibitor (not yet identified but certainly a macromolecule) which can reduce the rate of crystallization of urates and uric acid in urine (Sperling et al 1965; Porter 1966).

Environmental factors may be just as important as the concentration of inhibitors in determining stone formation but before aetiology and treatment can be specified the types of renal stones must be classified.

Classification of renal stones

Stones can be classified according to their chemical constituents. There are four main types: calcium, uric acid, magnesium ammonium phosphate together with calcium phosphate ('infection' stones), and cystine. In addition there are some rare forms but these account for less than 0.1% of all stone occurrence.

Calcium stones

In the UK, 70% of all stones contain calcium, about 50% contain pure calcium oxalate and the remainder are a mixture of calcium oxalate and calcium phosphate. In about 80% of cases there is no underlying cause and the stone can be described as idiopathic. In the remaining 20%, the stone is secondary to some other factor. The causes of secondary calcium stone disease are discussed on p 466.

Idiopathic calcium stone disease

Risk factors are listed below.

1 Sex. Men are particularly susceptible and account for 85% of cases.

2 Age. It occurs most commonly between the ages of 20 and 50 years but the incidence rises in the fourth decade.

3 Occupation. Cooks, below-deck sailors and heavy metal workers all have a greater than average incidence of calcium oxalate stones which may be linked with environmental factors. Hot working conditions may cause dehydration and heavy metal workers, for example, are often advised to consume a lot of milk and therefore have a high calcium intake.

4 Social class. The incidence is greater in social classes I and II and as previously suggested the higher protein intake in these groups may contribute to stone formation.

5 Diet. Dietary factors which may be involved in idiopathic hypercalcuria are calcium, vitamin D, fluids, fibre, protein and refined carbohydrate.

The role of excess calcium and vitamin D intake is obvious, as is that of a low fluid intake. Vegetable fibre contains phytic acid which binds dietary calcium and reduces its absorption. The role of protein is less clear. A high animal protein intake will lower urinary pH and, although urinary pH *per se* is not a major risk factor, calcium oxalate is less soluble in acid conditions. Dietary protein may have a more specific role; Tschope *et al* (1983) have reported that feeding certain amino acids increased urinary calcium and oxalate levels in normal subjects. Fellstrom *et al* (1983) have reported that a high protein diet fed to stone formers increased urinary saturation and decreased urinary citrate levels (an inhibitor to stone formation) and pH. Blacklock (1979) has also shown an epidemiological relationship between refined carbohydrate, especially sugar intake, and the incidence of renal stones.

6 Increased intestinal absorption of calcium. This can occur in people consuming a diet containing normal amounts of calcium and although it could be due to increased plasma levels of 1,25 dihydroxycholecalciferol or parathormone, both are usually normal in idiopathic hypercalcuria. Increased calcium absorption could also be a result of a decreased intake of dietary phosphate, fat, phytate or fibre.

7 Reduced tubular reabsorption of calcium. Some workers have reported a relatively high incidence of this [25% (Pak *et al* 1974) and 65% (Coe *et al* 1975)] but hypercalcuria alone does not cause calcium stone disease.

8 Increased urinary oxalate. Oxalate is absorbed by a passive process, with sodium oxalate being more readily absorbed than the insoluble calcium oxalate.

Finch *et al* (1981) found the amount of oxalate absorbed from different foods varied between 1.3% from strawberries to 22% from tea. The amount of fat and calcium in the diet will alter the percentage of oxalate which is absorbed. Fat will bind with calcium in preference to oxalate thus a high fat diet will result in more oxalate being available for absorption. In contrast, a high calcium intake will result in less free oxalate and hence less being absorbed.

The same authors have also shown that it is possible to increase the urinary oxalate excretion in normal subjects, from a mean of 0.17 mmol/24 hours by between 0.05 and 0.38 mmol/24 hours by adding various high oxalate foods (in normally consumed quantities) to a previously low oxalate diet. This indicates that dietary oxalate can be responsible for up to two-thirds of urinary oxalate. Oxalate crystals were found in the urine of the subjects when they ate the high oxalate foods and there is evidence that a raised urinary oxalate level is an important risk factor in the recurrence of calcium oxalate stones. Robertson and Peacock (1980) found that the rate of recurrence of idiopathic calcium oxalate stones was highly related to the urinary oxalate level, but only weakly related to the urinary calcium level.

Increased urinary oxalate levels may also be due to increased endogenous production of oxalate resulting from a high intake of animal protein.

9 Urinary uric acid. Total urinary uric acid output is usually normal in stone formers but the concentration is increased. This is thought to reduce the activity of the macromolecular inhibitors.

Diagnosis of idiopathic hypercalcuria

A range of tests and questions are needed to establish the cause and type of stone.

24-hour urine collection. An accurate 24-hour urine collection is needed to diagnose any type of stone. It is especially important in idiopathic hypercalcuria that this is done with the patient at home consuming their normal diet and carrying out their usual activities. In hospital a patient's diet and fluid intake can vary greatly from that at home. For example, a normal ward diet may contain 500–800 mg calcium, and if the patient usually consumes well over 1 g per day, any dietary hypercalcuria may disappear in hospital. Similarly, a patient at home may consume a large amount of one particular high oxalate food which is not present on the hospital menu, so dietary hyperoxaluria will disappear.

Dietary history. It is very important to determine the past and present intake of all relevant nutrients, especially calcium, to establish if hypercalcuria is of dietary origin or due to hyperabsorption. Hypercalcuria on a low or normal calcium diet indicates hyperabsorption. Vitamin D is present in many proprietary multivitamin preparations and fish liver oil capsules available over the counter in health food and chemists shops, so patients should be specifically asked about self-medication as they may not even realize they were taking vitamin D supplements.

Social history. Patient should be asked about past and present occupations to establish whether environment is likely to have caused long periods of dehydration. At risk jobs have been described previously and Caucasians who have worked abroad in a hot climate are at similar risk as a stone may have been formed during a period of dehydration many years previously, and has since been growing slowly. Alternatively, a period of bed rest sometime in the past may be responsible since this can lead to mobilization of calcium from the bones and thus to hypercalcuria. Furthermore, depending on the reason for bed rest, the patient may also have been encouraged to drink plenty of milk during his illness.

Early morning urine calcium/creatinine ratio. This is a useful diagnostic procedure because if after overnight starvation, the urine calcium/creatinine ratio is above 0.5 it probably indicates failure of tubular reabsorption of calcium.

Treatment of idiopathic hypercalcuria

Dietary. There are different schools of thought as to which dietary restrictions are necessary to treat idiopathic hypercalcuria and more importantly, prevent the recurence of stones. Modifying the intake of the following nutrients is currently considered to be important.

1 Calcium. It is common practice to recommend a reduction in calcium intake in idiopathic hypercalcuria, but the level of restriction imposed can vary. Only after a diet history has been taken can an appropriate diet be given. For instance, a patient with dietary hypercalcuria who is drinking two pints of milk a day may only need to be told to reduce this to half a pint in order to bring his calcium excretion within normal limits and will not need a strict low calcium diet. Conversely, a patient with hypercalcuria on a diet of under 1 g calcium daily will need to be restricted to approximately 300–500 mg calcium/day (see p 155).

2 Oxalate. A diet history will reveal which high oxalate foods the patient is consuming (see p 175). When calcium intake is reduced to below 500 mg daily, it is essential that the oxalate content of the diet is reduced because oxalate is usually bound to calcium in the gut. If there is less calcium present, the free oxalate will be absorbed leading to hyperoxaluria and the danger of further stone formation. It is usual to recommend that any patient being treated for hypercalcuria should avoid foods high in oxalate (see p 176).

3 Fibre. The phytic acid present in cereal fibre binds calcium in the gut and therefore a high fibre diet will help inhibit calcium absorption. In the UK all bread and flour except 100% wholemeal is fortified with calcium so changing to wholemeal bread also reduces the calcium content of the diet. For patients who dislike wholemeal bread, high fibre white bread is now available and wholemeal rice, pasta and breakfast cereals may be useful. Natural bran added to a low fibre diet is also effective in reducing calcium absorption.

4 Fluid. A high fluid intake helps to maintain a dilute urine and should be encouraged in all patients with stones. Except in very rare instances, it is not necessary for patients to purchase a water softener. Rose (1979a) demonstrated that when consuming 5 litres fluid per day, the difference in urinary calcium concentration was only 1 mmol/l when soft water was compared with London tap water. Extra care to drink plenty of fluids must be taken in hot weather, and especially when going on holiday to a hot climate.

5 Protein. Some workers (Rao *et al* 1982) recommend that all patients with renal stones be advised to consume a low animal protein diet, as well as reducing calcium and increasing fibre intake. There is evidence linking animal protein intake with stone formation but reducing the protein intake of stone formers results in a very restricted and complicated diet. Patients are expected to keep to these diets for many years and should therefore be given advice which is tolerable.

6 Sugar and refined carbohydrates. There is some evidence that a reduction in the intake of sugar and refined carbohydrate is beneficial (Rao *et al* 1983) but rather than eliminate them from the diet it is more conducive to compliance to advise a reduction in intake.

Thiazide diuretics. When dietary means alone cannot control hypercalcuria, thiazide diuretics such as bendrofluazide or chlorthalidone are often very effective. These act on the renal tubules causing greater reabsorption of calcium, putting the patient into positive calcium balance and reducing urinary calcium without increasing urinary oxalate. They are a cheap, easy and effective treatment, but occasionally have the unfortunate side effect of causing diabetes. The usual diabetic diet must then be given, and the present dietary guidelines fit in well with recommendations for stone formers apart from the major problem of whitening in tea and coffee. On a low calcium diet, a coffee whitener such as Coffeemate, can be used to replace milk but as these contain glucose they are not suitable for diabetics. A small amount of milk (150 ml) is permissible and, if this is insufficient, may be supplemented with 75 ml double cream diluted half and half with water. An unfortified soya milk could also be used.

Cellulose phosphate. This is another substance which is sometimes given to reduce hypercalcuria. It complexes with calcium in the gut, reducing its absorption and therefore its urinary excretion. However, it is more expensive than diuretics, has to be taken with all meals, causes an increase in urinary oxalate levels and may therefore even increase the risk of stones. In addition, it has some side effects, notably gastric discomfort and diarrhoea, and is not to be recommended.

Secondary calcium stone disease

Causation and treatment. Secondary calcium stone disease usually results from one of the following

1 Primary hyperparathyroidism. The treatment of primary hyperparathyroidism is a parathyroidectomy. However, if the parathyroidectomy is delayed or unsuccessful a low calcium diet can be prescribed to lower plasma and urine calcium levels (see p 465). In some cases surgical removal of the stone may be required.

2 Medullary sponge kidney. Because of the abnormal anatomy of the kidney, these patients make stones when the urinary calcium concentration is normal and should therefore reduce their calcium output below the level used for the treatment of idiopathic hypercalcuria (see p 465).

3 Renal tubular acidosis (RTA). This is a rare condition, caused by primary or secondary damage to the renal tubules. The patient cannot produce an acid urine, because of a failure of bicarbonate reabsorption and calcium phosphate stones are formed. Renal tubular acidosis can be treated by the use of alkalis and/or diet

a) Alkalis are given to form an acid urine (see p 467)

b) Diet. A diet rich in animal protein will cause a more acid urine, so patients should be advised to reduce their animal protein intake. Some patients may choose to make radical changes to their diet and become vegan since such a diet can have a dramatic effect in reducing symptoms. They should be given help to make sure their diet is nutritionally balanced.

4 Primary hyperoxaluria. This is caused by an inborn error of glyoxylic acid metabolism. Glyoxylic acid is normally transaminated to glycine or glycolic acid but if the necessary enzymes are absent, oxalic acid will be produced.

The full biochemistry of oxalic acid and glyoxylic acid metabolism is not known but in patients with primary hyperoxaluria the production and excretion of oxalic acid is vastly increased. Calcium oxalate is insoluble, so renal stones readily occur, and in addition, oxalosis (oxalate deposition in soft tissues) is common. When this happens the prognosis is very poor. Treatment of primary hyperoxaluria is outlined below

a) Pyridoxine. This is the only known effective treatment for primary hyperoxaluria. In doses of up to 1 g per day, pyridoxine has been shown to reduce urinary oxalate excretion from 1.4 mmol/24 hours to nearly normal (upper limit 0.5 mmol/24 hours; Rose 1979b). Not all patients respond to pyridoxine and work is in progress to see if other substances are effective in non-responders.

b) Fluid. The same regimen should be advised as for patients with uric acid stones and patients encouraged to drink enough to produce at least 3 litres urine/24 hours.

c) Diet. Patients should be advised to follow a low oxalate diet. A list of foods high in oxalate which should be avoided is given on p 176.

d) Increase solubility of calcium oxalate. Both magnesium hydroxide and disodium hydrogen phosphate can be given for this purpose.

5 Secondary hyperoxaluria. There are several causes of secondary hyperoxaluria

a) Treatment of hypercalcuria. (See idiopathic hypercalcuria.)

b) Intestinal bypass and bowel disease. In both these circumstances steatorrhoea may be present in which case the calcium in the gut will bind with fatty acids and be unavailable for binding with oxalate. Thus more oxalate is available for passive absorption. Gregory *et al* (1975) found that of 435 patients given an ileal bypass for obesity, 60% developed hyperoxaluria and 6% suffered from calcium oxalate stones.

Treatment revolves around reducing the steatorrhoea by prescribing a low fat diet. MCT oil has no effect on oxalate absorption and therefore can be used in patients with bowel disease to improve the palatability of the diet and increase the energy intake. A diet low in oxalate will also help to reduce the hyperoxaluria.

c) Excess vitamin C intake. This can lead to hyperoxaluria as ascorbic acid can be converted in the body to oxalic acid. However, it only happens when megadoses of vitamin C are taken, for instance as a 'cold cure', or as sometimes prescribed in cases of malabsorption, a procedure which must be avoided if hyperoxaluria occurs. A patient being investigated for hyperoxaluria should always be asked about any self-medication with vitamins or tonics.

6 Vitamin D overdose. This will cause increased intestinal absorption of calcium.

7 Immobilization. If prolonged, immobilization leads to bone resorption and consequent hypercalcaemia and hypercalcuria.

Uric acid stones

There is a high incidence of uric acid stones in industrialized societies which may indicate an environmental factor in their aetiology. However, only a small percentage of uric acid stone formers have a raised urinary uric acid attributable to a higher intake of purines from a diet rich in animal protein. More often, uric acid stone formers have a low urinary pH, and below pH 5.3, spontaneous precipitation of uric acid can occur.

Treatment of uric acid stones

Diet. If a patient with uric acid stones has hyperuricosuria, they should be advised to omit purine-rich foods (see Section 2.10.4, p 176) However, the necessity for such a diet has been superceded mainly by the use of allopurinol.

Fluid intake. As with all types of stones, a high fluid intake is beneficial. A daily urine output of at least 2 litres should be the target since precipitation will not occur when urine concentration is below the supersaturation level for uric acid.

Alkalis. Above pH 6, urine is unlikely to be supersaturated with uric acid, so treatment with alkalis to raise urine pH is useful. A combination of substances such as sodium or potassium bicarbonate or citrate can be used. The amount of alkali needed varies with the patient's diet, as a higher protein intake results in a more acid urine. A reduction in animal protein may therefore be a useful measure in some cases.

Allopurinol. This substance blocks the action of the enzyme xanthine oxidase in the pathway oxidizing hypoxanthine to urate and has few side effects. It appears to be very successful in preventing uric acid stone formation.

'Infection' stones (stones containing magnesium ammonium phosphate and calcium phosphate)

Chronic infection of the urinary tract with a urea-splitting organism is a very common cause of urinary stones. The organisms break down urea producing ammonia which causes an alkaline urine. Magnesium ammonium phosphate and calcium phosphate are extremely insoluble in alkali conditions and will crystallize spontaneously.

Treatment of infection stones

1 Surgery. Initially the stone must be surgically removed and any anatomical cause of the infection corrected.

2 Eradication of infection. Antibiotics must be used but results are often poor unless the stone is removed, as the source of infection is often within the stone itself.

3 Acidification of the urine. Ammonium chloride, ascorbic acid and methionine have all been used.

4 Urease inhibitor. It has been shown that it is possible to inhibit the action of the urea-splitting enzyme, urease, in the bacteria in the kidney, thus preventing ammonia release. The substance used is acetohydroxamic acid (1 g/day), but it is not as yet in general use in the UK.

Diet has little role in the treatment of these stones, but patients should be advised against an excessive calcium intake. On *very rare* occasions an acid ash diet may be indicated if it is not possible to acidify the urine by other methods. Generally this means a high intake of animal protein foods and minimal intake of fruit and vegetables, avoiding potatoes totally.

Cystine stones

This is a very rare type of kidney stone. It is caused by an autosomal recessive genetic disorder of renal tubular reabsorption of cystine, lysine, arginine and ornithine resulting in an increased concentration of cystine in the urine (see Table 4.43). The limit of solubility of cystine at pH range 5−7 at 37°C is 1250 µmol/l, so homozygous cystinurics readily precipitate cystine.

Table 4.43 Urinary concentration of cystine

Patient	Cystine concentration (µmol/l)
Normal	10−100
Heterozygous cystinurics	200−600
Homozygous cystinurics	1400−4200

Treatment of cystine stones

Dilution of urine. The patient should be instructed to drink enough fluid to pass at least 3 litres of urine each 24 hours, including getting up at night to pass urine. Approximately 600 ml of fluid should be drunk at bedtime and another 600 ml during the night. This treatment is simple, and, if complied with, will prevent the recurrence of stones.

Alkalinization of urine. Sodium bicarbonate can be given to increase the urinary pH to 7−7.4. The extra sodium may also help by making the patient thirsty thus encouraging them to drink.

D-penicillamine. This forms a more soluble complex with cystine and is an effective treatment for cystinuria. It is, however, toxic, causing rashes, fever, iron depletion and proteinuria. Sometimes nephrotic syndrome can develop. Another substance which forms an insoluble complex with cystine is Thiola (alpha-mercapto-propionylglycine). This has been shown to be effective and has fewer side effects than D-penicillamine but is not widely available in the UK.

Diet. Cystine is a non-essential amino acid and is synthesized in the body from methionine. A diet low in methionine will reduce urinary cystine. However, the diet is restrictive and difficult to follow. Animal protein is limited to 30 g/day from meat, fish, cheese and eggs, in addition to the protein contained in 300 ml milk. The remaining protein requirements are met by vegetable protein. The diet should only be used as a last resort when other treatments have failed.

Rare forms of stone disease

There are a number of uncommon forms of urinary stone disease which account for a very small percentage of all cases. These include xanthine, silica and 2,8 dihydroxyadenine stones but they are not amenable to dietary manipulation.

References

Blacklock NJ (1979) Epidemiology of renal lithiasis. In *Urinary calculus disease* Wickham JEA (Ed) pp 21−40. Churchill Livingstone, Edinburgh.

Coe FL, Lawton RL, Goldstein RB and Tembe V (1975) Sodium urate accelerates precipitation of calcium *in vitro*. *Proc Soc Exp Biol and Med* **149**, 926−9.

Currie WJC and Turner P (1979) The frequency of renal stones within Great Britain in a gouty and non-gouty population. *Br J Urol* **51**, 337−41.

Fellstrom BG, Danielson B, Karlstrom H, Lithell BJ, Ljunghall B and Vessby B (1983) The influence of a high dietary intake of purine-rich animal protein on urinary urate excretion and supersaturation in renal stone disease. *Clin Sci* **64**, (4), 399−405.

Finch AM, Kasieles GP and Rose GA (1981) Urine composition in normal subjects after oral ingestion of oxalate-rich foods. *Clin Sci* **60**, 411−8.

Gregory JG, Starkloff EB, Miyai K and Schoenberg HW (1975) Urological complications of ileal bypass operation for morbid obesity. *J Urol* **113**, 521−4.

Pak CYC, Ohata M, Lawrence EC and Snyder W (1974) The hypercalciurias. *J Clin Invest* **54**, 387−400.

Porter P (1966) Colloidal properties of urates in relation to calculus formation. *Res Vet Sci* **7**, 128−37.

Rao PN, Prendiville V, Buxton A, Moss DG and Blacklock NJ (1982) Dietary management of urinary risk factors in renal stone formers. *Br J Urol* **54**, 578−83.

Robertson WG and Peacock M (1980) The cause of idiopathic calcium stone disease: hypercalciuria or hyperoxaluria? *Nephron* **26**, 105−10.

Robertson WG, Peacock M, Marshall RW, Speed R and Nordin BEL (1975) Seasonal variations in the composition of urine in relation to calcium stone formation. *Clin Sci Mol Med* **49**, 597−602.

Robertson WG, Peacock M, Marshall RW, Marshall DH and Nordin BEL (1976) Saturation-inhibitor index as a measure of the risk of calcium oxalate stone formation in the urinary tract. *New Engl J Med* **294**, 249−52.

Robertson WG, Peacock M, Heyburn PJ and Hanes FA (1980) Epidemiological risk factors in calcium stone disease. *Scand J Urol Nephrol* [Suppl] **53**, 15−28.

Robertson WG, Peacock M, Heyburn PJ, Hanes FA and Swaminathan R (1981a) The risk of calcium stone formation in relation to affluence and dietary animal protein. In *Urinary calculus*

Brockis JG and Finlayson B (Eds) pp 3–12. PSG Publishing Co, Littleton, Massachusetts.

Robertson WG, Peacock M, Marshall DM and Speed R (1981b) The prevalence of urinary stone disease in practising vegetarians. *Fortschritte der Urologie and Nephrologie* **17**, 6–14.

Rose GA (1979a) *Urinary calculus disease* Wickham JEA (Ed) pp 131–2. Churchill Livingstone, Edinburgh.

Rose GA (1979b) *Urinary calculus disease* Wickham JEA (Ed) p 119. Churchill Livingstone, Edinburgh.

Sperling O, De Vries A and Keelem O (1965) Studies on the aetiology of uric acid lithiasis. Urinary non-dialysable substances in idiopathic uric acid lithiasis. *J Urol* **94**, 286–92.

Tschope E, Ritz E, Schmidt-Gayk H and Knebel L (1983) Different effects of oral glycine and methionine on urinary lithogenic substances. *Proc Eur Dial Transplant Assoc* **20**, 407–10. London.

E: Disorders of the Blood and Cardiovascular System

4.18 Diseases of the Blood

4.18.1 Anaemias

Anaemia can be defined as a reduction in the concentration of haemoglobin in blood below the normal for the age and sex of the patient. The WHO (1970) recommends that anaemia exists when in adults the haemoglobin levels are below 13 g/dl (males) or 12 g/dl (females). Children aged six months to six years are considered anaemic at levels below 11 g/dl and those aged six to twelve years below 12 g/dl.

Classification

Two main classifications are in use

1   The aetiological classification, based on the cause of the anaemia. (Table 4.44)

2   The morphological classification based on the characteristics of the red cells. Two main criteria are used, the mean cell volume (MCV) and the mean cell haemoglobin concentration (MCHC). Three main morphological types of anaemia are recognized

a)   Normocytic anaemias, in which the MCV is within the normal range (76−96 fl). Most are also normochromic, that is, the MCHC is within the normal range (30−35 g/dl).

b)   Hypochromic microcytic anaemias, in which both the MCV and MCHC are reduced.

c)   Macrocytic anaemias, in which the MCV is increased. Most are normochromic. Some macrocytic anaemias are also megaloblastic, this being a term to describe distinctive cytological changes in red cells and their precursors due to impaired DNA synthesis.

These two classifications are complementary. The investigation of a patient with anaemia involves first, a decision on the morphological type (which often gives a pointer to the cause) and secondly, the determination of the cause of the anaemia (necessary to institute appropriate treatment). Those forms of anaemias in which dietary treatment is relevant are described below.

Iron deficiency anaemia

Iron deficiency anaemia is by far the most common form of anaemia encountered in clinical practice. It can occur at all ages but is commonest in women of child bearing age, in whom it is an important cause of chronic ill health. Morphologically it is a hypochromic, microcytic anaemia.

There are three major factors in its pathogenesis 1. an increased physiological demand for iron, 2. loss of blood by haemorrhage and 3. inadequate iron intake. The relative importance of these three factors varies with age and sex but blood loss, often from an occult source such as the gastrointestinal tract, is by far the commonest cause in adults in industrialized societies. The body cannot control its iron content by excretion as, once iron has been absorbed, only traces of it are lost, mainly in epithelial cells desquamated from skin and mucous membrane; iron in the faeces consists almost entirely of iron unabsorbed from food.

An increased physiological demand for iron occurs in infants and children during the period of growth and in women during their reproductive period of life. The normal full-term infant is born with a reserve of iron sufficient for the first four to six months of life, derived partly from the mother *in utero*, and partly from iron released by breakdown of red cells shortly after birth. Iron stores from the mother are laid down mainly in the third trimester of pregnancy so that premature infants are born with inadequate iron stores. Infants of

Table 4.44 Classification of anaemia by aetiology

Blood loss	Acute or chronic
Impaired red cell production	1 Deficiency of substances essential for red cell formation (erythropoeisis) e.g. Iron deficiency anaemia. Megaloblastic macrocytic anaemia due to vitamin B12 or folate deficiency. Anaemia in scurvy. Anaemia associated with protein malnutrition.
	2 Disturbed bone marrow function not due to the deficiency of an essential substance. e.g. aplastic anaemia, anaemia associated with infection, renal failure, collagen diseases, liver disease and disseminated malignancy. Anaemia associated with bone marrow infiltration, e.g. in leukaemia, lymphoma and myelosclerosis. Anaemia in endocrine gland dysfunction, e.g. myxoedema and hypopituitarism. Sideroblastic anaemia. Congenital disorders of haemoglobin structure and synthesis, e.g. sickle cell anaemia and thalassaemia.
Increased red cell destruction	1 Haemolytic anaemia due to intrinsic red cell defect
	2 Haemolytic anaemia due to extrinsic factors

iron-deficient mothers may also have inadequate iron stores at birth.

During growth, which is maximal between six and twenty four months, there is a progressive increase in blood volume and a resultant increase in demand for iron by the bone marrow. It is during this period, when iron reserves are depleted and the infant becomes dependent on dietary iron, that most cases of iron deficiency in infancy and childhood occur as a result of inadequate intake from faulty feeding. An infant should start being weaned between four and six months so that the increasing iron requirement will be met by a mixed diet by the time the iron stores are exhausted.

In females of child bearing age, menstruation, pregnancy, parturition and lactation all increase the physiological requirements for iron. Between 15—30 mg are lost each month through menstruation whilst 500—600 mg are needed for each pregnancy to satisfy the foetal requirement and compensate for the blood loss at childbirth.

During the past 50 years, improved standards of living, reduction in family size, better antenatal care and the availability of infant welfare services have done much to reduce the incidence of iron deficiency in industrialized countries, especially in adults. Those most at risk are persons with a requirement above maintenance levels, such as young children and menstruating women, especially if they consume a vegetarian diet with a low citrus fruit content. Prevalence studies in women of child-bearing age in Western Europe have found a frequency of iron deficiency anaemia of between 15—20% (Dresch 1970; Vellar 1970). Another group at risk are the elderly living on a nutritionally deficient diet, in whom the incidence has been found to be as high as 6% in men and 9% in women (McLennan *et al* 1973). In tropical countries iron deficiency anaemia is a major problem: this subject is discussed in detail by Cowan and Bharucha (1973).

The major aetiological factors in iron deficiency anaemia are listed in Table 4.45

Table 4.45 Main aetiological factors in iron deficiency anaemia

Population group	Aetiological factor
Infants and children	Defective diet Diminished iron stores at birth
Females of child bearing age	Menstruation Pregnancy Pathological blood loss Defective diet
Adult males and post-menopausal females	Pathological blood loss

Dietary iron intake. The daily diet of a normal adult on a mixed western-type diet contains between 10—20 mg of iron. Only about 10%, about 1—2 mg (or sometimes even less) of this is absorbed so that a diet providing 10—15 mg of iron daily will barely meet the needs of adult men and post-menopausal women. The daily intakes of iron recommended by the WHO (1970) are listed in Table 4.46.

Iron is found in a wide variety of animal and plant foods, usually in low concentration, and occurs in two main forms: haem compounds and ferric iron complexes. Iron contained in haem, released from food by gastric digestion, appears to enter the intestinal epithelium unchanged. Most of the available iron in food is in the form of ferric iron: before this can be absorbed it has to be released from the ferric complexes by the action of gastric acid, both hydrochloric acid and organic acids, and then reduced to the ferrous form at an acid pH by reducing agents in the food,

Table 4.46 Recommended daily intake of iron (WHO 1970)

	Daily iron absorption required	Daily dietary intake required according to diet		
		Energy (kCal) derived from animal food (% of total energy intake)		
		10%	10—25%	25%
	(mg)	(mg)	(mg)	(mg)
Infants 0—4 months	0.5	—	—	—
Infants 5—12 months	1.0	10	7	5
Children 1—12 years	1.0	10	7	5
Boys 13—16 years	1.8	18	12	9
Girls 13—16 years	2.4	24	18	12
Menstruating women	2.8	28	19	14
Men and non-menstruating women	0.9	9	6	5

e.g. ascorbic acid and the sulphydryl groups of proteins. The free ferrous ions are then absorbed, mainly in the duodenum and proximal jejunum, passing across the mucosal cell by an active metabolic process.

The two main factors which influence the amount of iron absorbed are the size of the iron stores and the rate of red cell formation. A decrease in iron stores increases absorption and an increase lessens absorption. In iron-deficient humans, the amount of iron absorbed from food is increased from the usual 5–10% to a level up to three times as great (Callender 1981). Stimulation of red cell formation by blood loss or red cell breakdown increases the absorption of iron. The actual controlling mechanism which determines the amount of iron absorbed is, however, unknown.

Iron is better absorbed from some foods than others and, in addition, some dietary constituents may impair or facilitate absorption. The iron in meat and fish is well absorbed and that in cereals and vegetables, except soya beans, less well so. Animal protein, however, will enhance iron absorption from vegetable sources and from haemoglobin. A high phosphorus diet impairs absorption by forming insoluble ferric phosphate, while conversely, a low phosphorus diet may result in increased absorption. Bread, cereals and milk are rich in phosphate. Phytic acid, present in some cereals, converts ferrous and ferric salts into insoluble phytates and may impair absorption. Ascorbic acid, because of its powerful reducing action, increases the conversion of ferric to ferrous iron and so increases absorption. These factors to some extent account for the difficulty in calculating the percentage of dietary iron which is likely to be absorbed.

The role of ascorbic acid in reducing dietary iron to its more absorbable ferrous form is particularly important in vegetarian diets, where all the dietary iron is derived from non-haem sources and the intake of phosphates and phytates, known to reduce iron absorption, is high. Seshadri et al (1985) showed that, over a 60 day period, 100 mg of ascorbic acid, given twice a day with lunch and dinner, significantly improved both the haemoglobin level and the appearance of the red cells in anaemic pre-school children consuming a purely vegetarian diet deficient in ascorbic acid. It has been shown that 100 ml of orange juice or 100 g of raw green pepper (presumably because of their high ascorbic acid content), will enhance the relatively poor absorption of non-haem iron from eggs and bread, though eggs reduce iron absorption from other non-haem iron-containing foods taken simultaneously (Dister et al 1975).

Megaloblastic anaemias

The megaloblastic anaemias are particular forms of macrocytic anaemia distinguished by distinctive cytological changes in red cells and their precursors. They were first described by Ehrlich in 1880 and are now known to be due to impaired DNA synthesis. They are deficiency diseases nearly always caused by lack of either vitamin B12 or folate, both of which are necessary for the normal development of red cells. Though less common than iron deficiency anaemia, megaloblastic anaemia is a significant cause of ill health worldwide. In Britain and other temperate countries, pernicious anaemia (vitamin B12 deficiency, resulting from a failure of secretion of intrinsic factor by the stomach), and folate deficiency (due to dietary lack or malabsorption) are both common, but in tropical countries most cases are caused by folate deficiency from a combination of low intake and malabsorption, vitamin B12 deficiency being much less prevalent. The megaloblastic anaemias are of particular clinical importance because of their excellent response to treatment.

There are many similarities between the megaloblastic anaemias due to vitamin B12 and folate deficiency, especially in the clinical presentation and the morphological changes in the red cells. In addition to symptoms due to the anaemia, patients with both conditions often have a sore tongue and gastrointestinal upset, dyspepsia, anorexia, constipation or diarrhoea. Symptoms and signs due to degeneration of nerve tissue, in particular the spinal cord (subacute combined degeneration) and peripheral nerves, are, however, confined to those with vitamin B12 deficiency, in whom they may be the presenting feature.

The usual initial complaint is of parasthesiae, often numbness, tingling and pins and needles starting in the feet and spreading upwards. Weakness in the legs, unsteadiness of gait and clumsiness with fine movements are common. In severe cases impotence, loss of bladder and bowel control and even paraplegia are also present. It is important to make a firm diagnosis as to which deficiency is present because treating a patient with vitamin B12 deficiency with folate *per se* will often improve the anaemia but may cause a significant deterioration in the neurological state; serum assays of both substances are widely available. The main characteristics of vitamin B12 and folate are listed in Table 4.47.

Vitamin B12 deficiency anaemia. A mixed diet will provide about 30 μg vitamin B12/day but the vitamin is

Table 4.47 Characteristics of vitamin B12 and folate

	Vitamin B12	Folate
Parent form	Cyanocobalamin	Pteroylglutamic acid (folic acid)
Food source	Animal origin only (liver, meat, fish and dairy produce).	Yeast, liver, green vegetables, nuts, cereals and fruit.
Effect of cooking	10–30% loss	70–100% loss
Adult daily requirements	1–2 μg	100–200 μg
Adult daily intake	3–30 μg	400–700 μg
Site of absorption	Ileum	Duodenum and jejunum
Mechanism of absorption	Gastric intrinsic factor	Deconjugation, reduction and methylation.
Body stores	3–5 mg (2–4 years' supply)	6–20 mg (4 months' supply).

only present in foods of animal origin. The daily requirement for vitamin B12 is approximately 1–2 μg. It is a very stable vitamin, able to withstand heat and extremes of pH so little is lost in cooking. Dietary deficiency of vitamin B12 is therefore rare except in very strict vegetarians: the only B12 present in their diet will be by virtue of bacterial contamination. Many immigrants into Britain and other developed countries are strict vegetarians (Matthews and Wood 1984). The largest group of vegans are Hindus. Although more than 50% of vegans have low serum vitamin B12 levels (Wickramasinghe 1986), most vegans have normal haematological values and appear in good health. Some vegans do, however, develop a megaloblastic anaemia which responds to either oral or parenteral vitamin B12 therapy whilst breast fed infants of vegan mothers may develop vitamin B12 deficiency during the first year of life.

Most of the vitamin B12 in the diet is available for absorption. After release from foods by proteolytic enzymes it is bound to intrinsic factor, a glycoprotein secreted by the parietal cells of the gastric mucosa. The vitamin B12 – intrinsic factor complex, which is resistant to digestion, passes down to the terminal ileum where absorption takes place. The most common cause of vitamin B12 deficiency is a severe reduction or absence of intrinsic factor in the gastric secretion, secondary to atrophy of the gastric mucosa. Vitamin B12 present in the diet cannot therefore be absorbed and pernicious anaemia develops. The disease is most common in people of Northern European extraction, in whom the prevalence approaches 10% after the age of 60 years. It is relatively uncommon in Africans and

Asians. Treatment by regular subcutaneous injections of vitamin B12 is effective.

The great majority of other cases of acquired vitamin B12 deficiency are caused by disease of the gut. Surgical removal of part or whole of the stomach removes the source of intrinsic factor. However, the onset of megaloblastic anaemia following gastrectomy is often delayed for two years or more because of the high body stores of vitamin B12.

Disease or surgical resection of the ileum will also affect the absorption of the vitamin. In particular, megaloblastic anaemia is present in many patients with coeliac or Crohn's disease and in 60–90% of patients with tropical sprue. About 90% of patients with tropical sprue malabsorb vitamin B12 and many also malabsorb folate. The absorption of vitamin B12 frequently returns to normal after a course of broad-spectrum antibiotics and in the early stages of the disease may improve following therapy with folic acid (Wickramasinghe 1986).

Another important cause of vitamin B12 deficiency is infestation with the fish tapeworm (*Diphyllobothrium latum*), which still occurs in Finland and the Soviet Union. The tapeworm becomes attached to the lining of the small bowel and cause the deficiency by extracting vitamin B12 from the food as it passes down the bowel.

Malabsorption of vitamin B12 may also be drug-induced, e.g. by neomycin or paraminosalicylic acid (Jacobsen *et al* 1960; Heinivaara and Palva 1964) but in most cases the drug treatment is not continued for sufficiently long to produce clinical sequellae. The main causes of megaloblastic anaemia are listed in Table 4.48.

Folate deficiency anaemia. Folate compounds are present in all types of animal and vegetable foods. The richest sources are liver, yeast, green vegetables (especially spinach and Brussels sprouts), chocolate and nuts. In liver and other animal foods most of the folate is present as 5-methyltetrahydrofolate which is readily absorbed unaltered in the duodenum and jejunum. The folate content of an average mixed diet in Britain is about 680 μg/day (Wickramasinghe 1986). More than 75% of this is present as polyglutamates which have to be hydrolysed into monoglutamates prior to absorption. Hydrolysis is carried out by the enzyme folate conjugase, probably in the lumen of the gut. The larger the number of glutamate residues in the polyglutamate chain, the less well the compound is absorbed (Baugh *et al* 1971); probably only 100–200 μg folate/day is absorbed from a mixed diet in an adult. This is balanced by an equal loss of folate in sweat, desquamated epithelial cells and urine.

The relatively large daily requirement means that folate stores may become depleted and folate deficiency develop within three to four months of taking a folate-depleted diet. The daily requirement of folate is 50–100 μg during the first two years of life (Chanarin 1978) and 200–300 μg during pregnancy. Folates are rapidly destroyed by heat and 30–90% may be lost during cooking, especially by methods which involve keeping food warm. As this is a regular practice in some hospitals it is not surprising that many elderly people in some long stay geriatric wards have been found to be folate deficient.

The main causes of folate deficiency anaemia are listed in Table 4.48. Megaloblastic anaemia due to dietary deficiency tends to occur in developed countries in the poor, the neglected elderly, the mentally disturbed, chronic alcoholics and infants fed almost exclusively on goats' milk, which contains little folate. A macrocytic anaemia is common in chronic alcoholism; in about 70% of cases this is associated with normoblastic erythropoiesis and may be a result of impairment of cell proliferation in the bone marrow by a direct effect of alcohol on red cell precursors. Folate deficiency is common however, more so in spirit than beer drinkers because beer is a significant source of folate. Herbert et al (1963) found normal folate values in only 7% of patients with chronic alcoholism.

Table 4.48 Causes of megaloblastic anaemia due to vitamin B12 and folate deficiency

Vitamin B12 deficiency	
Inadequate intake	Veganism
Gastric lesions	Pernicious anaemia, total or partial gastrectomy, congenital intrinsic factor deficiency.
Intestinal lesions	Crohn's disease, ileal resection, stagnant loop syndrome, coeliac disease, tropical sprue and fish tapeworm infestation.
Folate deficiency	
Inadequate intake	Poverty, mental illness, alcoholism, infants fed on goat's milk, chronic illness, Kwashiorkor, etc.
Malabsorption	Coeliac disease, tropical sprue and jejunal resection.
Increased requirement	Pregnancy and lactation, prematurity and infancy, haemolytic anaemic (e.g. sickle cell disease and thalassaemia), malignancy (e.g. carcinoma, leukaemia and lymphoma), chronic inflammatory diseases (e.g. rheumatoid arthritis, malaria and tuberculosis).
Drugs	Anticonvulsants, oral contraceptives, treatment with dihydrofolate reductase inhibitors (methotrexate, trimethoprim, pyrimethamine and triamterene).

Diseases affecting the upper small bowel, in particular coeliac disease, tropical sprue and Crohn's disease, often cause anaemia due to malabsorption of folate.

Folate requirements are increased in the following conditions
1 In pregnancy due to the increase in maternal blood flow and the needs of the growing foetus.
2 In chronic haemolytic anaemias because of the increased red blood cell production.
3 In premature infants because of the rapid growth during the first two or three months.
4 In various malignant diseases, presumably in association with the increased production of tumour cells.

In all of these conditions this may result in megaloblastic anaemia, especially where the dietary intake is inadequate. In addition, folate deficiency in pregnancy can result in placental dysfunction and the premature birth of the infant. Before the use of folate supplements during pregnancy, megaloblastic red cells could be found in late pregnancy in up to 25% of women in the UK and up to 50% in southern India. However, the frequency of frank megaloblastic anaemia was then much lower, being 0.5–5.0% in the UK. It is still particularly common in twin pregnancies.

In patients with active chronic inflammation such as rheumatoid arthritis or tuberculosis; three different mechanisms of folate deficiency may apply, 1. inadequate intake, 2. increased urinary loss and 3. increased demand to support the continued formation of chronic inflammatory cells.

About 80% of a 200 μg dose of folic acid is absorbed so that oral treatment of the anaemia is effective. Even where there is malabsorption a dose of 1 mg/day is usually sufficient. In many countries, folic acid supplements are given to pregnant women. Where poor intake has been a factor, it is, of course, necessary to emphasize to the patient that their diet has been deficient and should be changed. Where alcohol has been a factor both folate supplementation and abstinence from alcohol are usually required to achieve a normal blood profile. It must also be remembered that deficiency of both folate and vitamin B12 often co-exist so attention should be paid to ensuring an adequate intake of both.

Other deficiency anaemias

Anaemia in scurvy. The role of ascorbic acid in red cell formation is unclear. Nevertheless, anaemia is present in about 80% of patients with scurvy and usually responds to treatment with small doses of vitamin C on its own, or in a minority of cases, in combination with other haematinics. The anaemia is usually normochromic but may be hypochromic if there is associated iron deficiency.

Anaemia of protein deficiency. Anaemia is a common complication of severe protein malnutrition or 'kwashiorkor' and protein-energy malnutrition or 'marasmus'. These conditions are most common in underdeveloped countries in the tropics, especially in young children and pregnant women, though they may occur at any age. Cases of protein malnutrition sometimes occur in industrialized societies in patients with gastrointestinal disease. The anaemia in uncomplicated cases is normocytic, of uncertain pathogenesis, and responds well to a high protein diet. Often, however, there are multiple associated deficiencies, especially of iron, folate, vitamin B12 and vitamin E and appropriate supplements to the diet are required.

4.18.2 Leukaemia

Leukaemia is a form of cancer of the blood-forming organs characterized by an uncontrolled, abnormal and widespread proliferation of leucocytes which infiltrate the bone marrow and body tissues, especially the liver, spleen and lymph nodes. This proliferation is usually accompanied by the appearance in the peripheral blood of immature leucocytes, many of which appear normal. In the past, leukaemia was invariably fatal. Now, with treatment, a significant number of patients with the acute form of the disease achieve remissions which may last for years and some are effectively cured. The aetiology is still uncertain but known precipitating factors are exposure to ionizing radiation, some toxic chemicals and cytotoxic drugs and certain viral infections. Leukaemia accounts for about 4% of all deaths from malignant disease.

Leukaemia occurs in a large number of forms, which differ in their clinical, pathological and haematological features. The two main criteria used in classification are the clinical course (acute or chronic) and the type and maturity of the dominant leukaemic cell. There are thus four main categories

1 Acute lymphoblastic leukaemia.
2 Acute myeloid leukaemia.
3 Chronic lymphocytic leukaemia.
4 Chronic granulocytic leukaemia.

However, as the leukaemias arise from clonal proliferations, i.e. the leukaemic cell population arises from a single cell, a comprehensive classification is difficult to undertake. For example, there are probably at least five morphologically separate forms of chronic granulocytic leukaemia and several specific subvarieties, such as hairy cell leukaemia, have been described.

Acute lymphoblastic leukaemia is more common in children and, untreated, runs a shorter course than the other categories which occur typically in adults and are more prevalent. It responds well to modern treatment so that many patients may, in effect, be cured, i.e. their survival is the same as that of unaffected persons. Significant, and often lengthy remissions may be produced by treatment of patients affected by the other categories.

Treatment of leukaemia, based on chemotherapy and/or radiotherapy, is variable depending on the type, but all regimens tend to result in side effects which affect the nutrition of the patient. The most common problems are nausea and vomiting caused by chemotherapy, throat and mouth infections provoked by radiation therapy and an altered immune state, and loss or impairment of the sense of taste. These are discussed further in Section 5.1.4. Patients who are unable to eat sufficiently well to meet their nutritional requirements may require tube feeding using a suitable proprietary product or even total parenteral nutrition (see Sections 1.12 and 1.13).

The immunosuppression which results from radiotherapy or chemotherapy may necessitate the use of a 'sterile' diet (see Section 5.2). This usually becomes necessary when the patient's neutrophil count is less than 50% of the total white cell count. All foods which may contain or convey pathogens must be avoided; essentially these are foods which are either uncooked or have been exposed to the air (e.g. salads, raw fruit, ice cream, unwrapped cakes, filled biscuits, bottled sauces). Instead, food must be freshly prepared and served to the patient as soon as it has been cooked (either in a diet kitchen or in a microwave oven on the ward). A daily supply of fresh milk should be kept refrigerated on the ward for each patient. Patients should be seen daily to ensure that they are receiving food which they enjoy and which meets their nutritional requirements.

The preparation of diets for immunosuppressed patients is discussed in detail in Section 5.2.

4.18.3 Haemorrhagic disease of the newborn

Haemorrhagic disease of the newborn is due to a deficiency of vitamin K which exacerbates the low activity of the vitamin K-dependent coagulation factors in the neonate. The fall in activity is greater in the premature infant.

THERAPEUTIC DIETETICS FOR DISEASE STATES

Bleeding, which can be severe, usually starts on the second or third day after birth and can be treated by injection of 0.5–1 mg of vitamin K (phylloquinone). It is routine practice in many hospitals however to give a single dose of vitamin K to infants immediately after birth. Thereafter the amount in human milk and modified milk feeds appears to be adequate (DHSS 1980).

References

Baugh CM, Krumdieck CL, Baker HJ and Butterworth CR Jr (1971) Studies on the absorption and metabolism of folic acid. *J Clin Invest* **50**, 2009–21.

Callender S (1981) Iron deficiency anaemia. In *Nutritional problems in modern society*. Howard AN (Ed). John Libbey and Co, London.

Chanarin I (1978) Anaemias and coagulation disorders of nutritional origin. In *Nutrition in the clinical management of disease*. Dickerson JWT and Lee HA (Eds). Edward Arnold, London.

Cowan B and Bharucha C (1973) Iron deficiency in the tropics. In *Clinics in haematology, Vol 2: Iron deficiency and iron overload*. Callender ST (Ed). WB Saunders, London.

Department of Health and Social Security (1980) *Artifical feeds for the young infant*. Report on Health and Social subjects No 18. HMSO, London.

Dister PB, Lynch SR, Charlton RW Torrance JD, Bothwell TH, Walker RB and Mayet F (1975) The effect of tea on iron absorption. *Gut* **16**, 193–200.

Dresch C (1970) Prevalence of iron deficiency in France. In *Iron deficiency*. Hallberg L, Harweth HG and Vannoth A (Eds). p 423. Academic Press, London.

Heinivaara O and Palva IP (1964) Malabsorption and deficiency of vitamin B12 caused by treatment with para aminosalicylic acid. *Acta Med Scand* **177**, 337–41.

Herbert V, Zalusky R and Davidson CS (1963) Correlation of folate deficiency with alcoholism and associated macrocytosis, anaemia and liver disease. *Ann Int Med* **58**, 977–88.

Jacobsen ED, Chodos RB and Faloon WW (1960) An experimental malabsorption syndrome induced by neomycin. *Am J Med* **28**, 524–33.

Matthews JH and Wood JK (1984) Megaloblastic anaemia in vegetarian Asians. *Clin Lab Haematol* **6**, 1–7.

McLennan WJ, Andrews GR, Macleod C and Caird FI (1973) Iron deficiency in the elderly. *Quart J Med* **42**, 1.

Seshadri S, Shah A and Bhade S (1985) Haematological response of anaemic pre-school children to ascorbic acid supplementation. *Hum Nutr: Appl Nutr* **39A**, 151–4.

Vellar (1970) Prevalence of iron deficiency in Norway. In *Iron deficiency*. Hallberg L, Harweth HG and Vannotti A (Eds). p 447. Academic Press, London.

Wickramasinghe SN (1986) *Systemic pathology: Vol 2: Blood and bone marrow*. Churchill Livingstone, Edinburgh.

World Health Organisation (1970) *Requirements of ascorbic acid, vitamin D, vitamin B12, folate and iron*. Technical Reports Series No 452, Geneva.

4.19   Hypertension

In young healthy adults the average systolic blood pressure is approximately 120 mm mercury (Hg) and average diastolic blood pressure 80 mm Hg. In Western societies blood pressure rises gradually with age so that the average blood pressure of a 65 year old is 160/90. This makes the definition of hypertension difficult, but it is usually accepted that essential hypertension (high blood pressure which is not secondary to a pre-existing medical condition) is present and classified as 'mild' when the diastolic pressure is between 90 and 105, 'moderate' between 105 and 120 and 'severe' when it exceeds 120 mm Hg (BNF 1981).

The advisability of treating mild or borderline hypertension and the feasibility of preventing its occurrence are controversial matters which are strongly debated (Brown *et al* 1984a, 1984b; de Wardener 1984, Rosenberg and Coleman 1984) and not clearly established.

However, the benefits of treating moderately severe hypertension are generally agreed and threshold values for the initiation of treatment have fallen steadily in most Western countries over the past two decades (Editorial 1984). As the number of people being treated increases so the use of non-pharmacological therapy becomes more attractive due to the cost and possible side effects of drug treatment.

Weight reduction and sodium restriction are the cornerstone of non-pharmacological therapy but more recently the dietary intakes of calcium and potassium have been implicated and may also have to be considered.

Weight reduction in hypertension

Weight loss by dietary restriction provides a cheap ethical means of treating hypertension and the association between obesity and hypertension is undisputed. It has been shown that hypertension is twice as prevalent in young overweight individuals and 50% more prevalent in older obese subjects than in control subjects within the normal weight range (Stamler *et al* 1978).

Patients who adhere to a diet are also more likely to follow a drug regimen and therefore have blood pressure which is easier to control (Hovell 1982) but none-theless studies investigating the effect of weight loss on hypertension strongly suggest it is effective and all hypertensive patients who are overweight should be encouraged to lose weight. Methods of weight reduction are described in Section 4.1

Sodium and potassium

One of the best known treatments in relation to sodium reduction for hypertension is the Kempner rice-fruit diet (Kempner 1948) which, although initially successful in over 50% of cases, is so rigid that few could adhere to it as out-patients and it is rarely used.

The effects of both drastic and moderate sodium restriction in patients who are clearly hypertensive are well established (Parijs *et al* 1973; Haddy 1980) but the effect in borderline hypertensives is less clear.

Some workers have claimed that blood pressure reduction caused by energy restriction is independent of sodium intake (Sowers *et al* 1982) but have failed to realize that the energy-reduced diet was also lower in sodium. Others have shown that either moderate weight reduction or a modest sodium restriction (70 mmol/day) produce substantial lowering of blood pressure in obese subjects with borderline hypertension (Gillum *et al* 1983) and the effect is greater if the two are combined. However, Fagerberg *et al* (1984) found that weight loss lowered blood pressure only when patients restricted both their energy and sodium intake.

There is considerable evidence from animal experiments that there is a genetic variation which determines individual sensitivity to sodium. This has been elegantly substantiated in human studies by Skrabai *et al* (1981) who showed that in 20 normotensive subjects (ten with a family history of hypertension) a reduction in salt intake from 200 to 50 mmol/day significantly reduced the rise in blood pressure induced by various doses of noradrenaline. Twelve subjects (eight with a family history of hypertension) responded to salt restriction with a fall of either diastolic or systolic blood pressure of at least 5 mmHg. A high potassium intake (200 mmol/day) reduced diastolic blood pressure by at least 5 mmHg in ten of the subjects, seven of whom had a family history of high blood pressure.

Studies in young adults with and without a family

history of hypertension have shown that whereas a high sodium intake causes an increased blood pressure in both groups, a high potassium intake only reduces blood pressure in those with a family history of hypertension (Parfrey *et al* 1981).

Calcium

There has been recent interest in the effect of calcium on blood pressure and Belizai *et al* (1983) showed that a daily supplement of 1 g calcium significantly reduced diastolic blood pressure in healthy individuals within a few weeks. Castenmiller *et al* (1985) have also found that in normotensive subjects, mean systolic and diastolic blood pressures were lower in subjects on a high calcium intake (4.1 mmol/MJ; 686 mg/1000 kcal) than those on a lower calcium intake (3.2 mmol/MJ; 535 mg/1000 kcal)

Dietary Recommendations

Although not all factors are fully established the following recommendations can be made for the non-pharmacological treatment of hypertension.

1 All overweight hypertensive individuals should adhere to a suitable weight reducing regimen.

2 The sodium intake of both the obese and non-obese hypertensive should be reduced. This should not be extreme and should require only that no salt be used either in cooking or at the table and that highly salted foods as described in Section 2.7, p 151 should be avoided.

3 A reduced sodium intake can be made more palatable by the liberal use of fresh fruit and vegetables. This will also increase the potassium intake and may be of additional benefit.

4 There is, as yet, insufficient evidence to make recommendations on the calcium content of the diet. However, care should be taken to ensure that all patients, especially post-menopausal women, are consuming at least the recommended daily intake of calcium.

References

Belizai JM, Vilar J and Peneda O (1983) Reduction of blood pressure with calcium supplementation in young adults. *J Am Med Assoc* **249**, 1161–5.

British Nutrition Foundation (1981) *Salt in the diet*. Briefing paper No 2.

Brown JJ, Lever AF, Robertson JIS, Semple PF, Bing RF, Heagerty AM, Swales JD, Thurston H, Leadingham JGG, Laragh JH, Hansson L, Nicholls MG and Espiner AE (1984a) Salt and hypertension. *Lancet* **ii**, 456.

Brown JJ, Lever AF, Robertson JIS, Semple PF, Bing RF, Heagerty AM, Swales JD, Thurston H, Ledingham JGG, Laragh JH, Hansson L, Nicholls MG and Espiner EA (1984b) Salt and hypertension. *Lancet* **ii**, 1333–4.

Castenmiller JJM, Mensink RP, van der Heyden L, Kouwenhoven T, Hautvast JGAJ, de Leeuw PW and Schaafsma G (1985) The effect of dietary sodium on urinary calcium and potassium excretion in normotensive men with different calcium intake. *Am J Clin Nutr* **41**, 52–60.

de Wardener HE (1984) Salt and hypertension. *Lancet* **ii**, 688.

Editorial (1984) Diet and hypertension. *Lancet* **ii**, 671–3.

Fagerberg B, Andersson OK, Isaksson B, Bjomtorp P (1984) Blood pressure control during weight reduction in obese hypertensive men: separate effects of sodium and energy restriction. *Br Med J* **288**, (i), 11–6.

Gillum RF, Elmer PJ and Prineas RJ (1981) Changing sodium intake in children. *Hypertension* **3**, 698–703.

Haddy FJ (1980) Mechanism, prevention and therapy of sodium-dependent hypertension. *Am J Med* **69**, 746–58.

Hovell MF (1982) The experimental evidence for weight loss treatment of essential hypertension: a critical review. *Am J Public Health* **72**, 359–68.

Kempner W (1948) Treatment of hypertensive vascular disease with rice diet. *Am J Med* **4**, 545–77.

Parfrey PS, Candon K, Wright P, Vandenburg MJ, Holly JMP, Goodwin FJ, Evans SJW and Ledinghain JM (1981) Blood pressure and hormonal changes following alteration in dietary sodium and potassium in young men with and without familial predisposition to hypertension. *Lancet* **i**, 113–7.

Parijs J, Joosens JV and Van de Linden (1973) Moderate sodium restriction and diuretics in the treatment of hypertension. *Am Heart J* **85**, 22–34.

Rosenberg E and Coleman BR (1984) Diet and hypertension. *Lancet* **ii**, 1334.

Skrabai F, Aubeck J and Hortnagi H (1981) Low sodium/high potassium diet for prevention of hypertension: probable mechanism of action. *Lancet* **ii**, 895–900.

Sowers JR, Nyby M and Stern N (1982) Blood pressure and hormone changes associated with weight reduction in the obese. *Hypertension* **4**, 686–91.

Stamler R, Stemler J, Reidlinger WF, Algera G and Roberts RH (1978) Weight and blood pressure. *J Am Med Assoc* **240**, 1607–10.

4.20 Atherosclerosis

Atherosclerosis is a disease of the medium and large arteries in which the intima layer of the artery wall becomes thickened with fibrous and fibro-fatty plaques. These plaques are composed of connective tissue, smooth muscle cells, cell debris and lipid deposits.

The consequences of atherosclerosis include coronary heart disease and cerebrovascular disease which are the cause of death in 40% of men and 38% of women in this country, greatly exceeding that due to any other group of diseases. Deaths from coronary heart disease out-number those from stroke by more than 2:1 (3.4:1 in men) (COMA 1984). Most deaths from cardiovascular disease occur in old age, the median age of death being 74 years. However, in England and Wales, deaths from coronary heart disease cause the annual loss of a quarter of a million years of working life with nearly 30,000 deaths in men under the age of 65.

In countries such as the USA, Canada and Australia deaths from coronary heart disease have declined considerably over the past decade. No similar decline has been observed in the UK and there are claims that this situation reflects the failure of successive Governments to take positive steps to prevent coronary heart disease (Salonen *et al* 1983).

A key point is whether there is sufficiently strong evidence of benefit in terms of reduced mortality from heart disease to be gained from dramatic changes in all aspects of lifestyle (diet, smoking and exercise) and it has been suggested that the mass approach is unnecessary and a screening programme to identify and treat high-risk individuals and their families would be more effective (Oliver 1984).

However, the National Advisory Committee on Nutrition Education (NACNE 1983) and more recently a Panel of the Government's Committee on Medical Aspects of Food Policy (COMA 1984) have examined the available evidence concerning the relationship between diet and the development of coronary heart disease and, while acknowledging that it is a multifactorial disease, were convinced that the evidence is strong enough to warrant dietary change for the whole population. The recommended changes have been summarized in Section 1.1.

The role of the dietitian is to inform people of these recommendations and show them how they can be carried out in everyday life. The COMA report called for clear labelling of food, especially in relation to the type and quantity of fat present. New legislation to enforce this is currently being prepared but labelling can only be of use to the public if they are aware of the significance and relevance of the information provided and can use it to plan a balanced diet. The majority of the population will require considerable health education in order to achieve this.

Further reading

American Heart Association, Nutrition Committee (1982) Rationale of the diet—heart statement of the American Heart Association. *Arteriosclerosis* **4**, 177—91.

Coronary heart disease prevention: plans for action (1984) A report based on an interdisciplinary workshop conference held at Canterbury, September 1983. Pitman Publishing Ltd, London.

Department of Health and Social Security (1974) *Diet and coronary heart disease.* Report of the Advisory Panel of the Committee on Medical Aspects of Food Policy (Nutrition) on diet in relation to cardiovascular and cerebrovascular disease. Report on Health and Social Subjects; No 7. HMSO, London.

Department of Health and Social Security (1981) *Report on avoiding heart attacks.* HMSO, London.

Shaper AG, Pocock SJ, Walker M, Cohen NM, Wale CJ and Thomson AG (1981) British Regional Heart Study: cardiovascular risk factors in middle aged men in 24 towns. *Br Med J* **283**, 179.

World Health Organisation (1982) *Prevention of coronary heart disease.* WHO, Geneva.

References

Committee on Medical Aspects of Food Policy (1984) *Diet and cardiovascular disease.* Report of the Panel on Diet in Relation to Cardiovascular disease. DHSS Report on Health and Social Subjects No 28. HMSO, London.

National Advisory Committee on Nutrition Education (1983) *Proposals for nutritional guidelines for health education in Britain.* Health Education Council, London.

Oliver MF (1984) Coronary heart disease: intervening in those at high risk. *Practitioner* **228**, 29—38.

Salonen JT, Puska P, Kottke TE, Fuomilheto J and Nissinen A (1983) Decline in mortality from coronary heart disease in Finland. *Br Med J* **286**, 1857—60.

4.21 Congestive heart failure

The clinical manifestations of congestive heart failure are related to fluid accumulation resulting from an inadequate renal flow. The weakened heart cannot pump sufficient blood to maintain renal blood pressure so sodium and water are reabsorbed by the kidney, increasing the volume of extracellular fluid and exacerbating the situation.

The failure usually starts as a result of disease (e.g. myocardial infarction) in the left ventricle which then is unable to pump efficiently. This creates a back pressure, initially in the left atrium which passes back through the pulmonary vessels to the right side of the heart. The right ventricle becomes stretched by accumulation of excessive blood and increases its force of contraction to push more blood into the pulmonary artery. This increases hydrostatic pressure causing loss of fluid into the interstitial spaces around the alveolar sacs. The pressure of fluid in the lungs may cause dyspnoea and orthopnea as diffusion of carbon dioxide and oxygen across the respiratory membrane becomes impaired.

When the right side of the heart fails there is a generalized fluid accumulation and oedema, particularly in the lower periphery.

Therapy

The primary symptom of congestive heart failure is oedema and thus diuretics are given to increase the excretion of fluids.

The principles of dietary management have been relaxed considerably since the days of the Karrell Diet (1886) when patients were prescribed 800 ml−1 litre of milk to be taken in small amounts throughout the day as the only source of nutrition! Even severe sodium restriction has become unnecessary with the improved efficiency of diuretic therapy. Nowadays patients with congestive heart failure should be advised to follow a no added salt diet (i.e. 80−100 mmol/day). (see p 151).

If they are overweight, appropriate advice on weight reduction should be given. While the patient remains oedematous, large meals should be avoided as stomach distension causes the diaphragm to elevate and displace the heart, further compromising cardiac function.

F: Disorders of the Brain and Nervous System

4.22 Stroke

The most important risk factor in the development of cerebrovascular disease and ischaemia leading to a stroke is hypertension (see Section 4.19). Smoking habits are also positively associated with the incidence of stroke. There is also an association between diabetes mellitus and mortality from stroke and the incidence appears to be related to blood glucose control (Fuller *et al* 1983).

Communicating with the stroke patient

The speech and language difficulties which often accompany stroke increase the patient's frustration and distress, and effective communication with the patient is essential in order to establish whether there are any feeding and swallowing difficulties as well as food preferences. Patients with communication problems may be divided into three groups

1 Group 1 dysphasia. Patients are clear in their own minds what they wish to say but cannot express themselves. Those severely affected may be able to say only one or two words which they repeat constantly.

2 Group 2 dysphasia. Patients who speak fluently but incoherently. They are unaware of their incoherence and often do not understand what is said to them, whilst appearing as if they do. These are the most difficult to communicate with.

3 Dysarthria. Patients can form speech in their mind and understand what is said to them. However, the muscles used to pronounce words are no longer properly co-ordinated and their speech is distorted. These patients are likely to also have swallowing, breathing and chewing difficulties.

Group 1 dysphasic patients and especially those with dysarthria can communicate their needs if their problems are approached intelligently and with compassion. The following guidelines should be observed when talking to the patient.

1 Never use baby talk; speak as you would to any other adult.

2 Do not raise your voice but speak at a normal pitch.

3 Do not allow frustration or impatience to edge your voice (or show in your face or manner).

4 Repeat your questions, quietly and slowly, as often as necessary.

5 Use different words to say the same thing to assist comprehension.

6 Give the patient plenty of time after you have asked a question to work out your meaning before trying again.

If the patient is mentally alert but unable to speak, answers may be written or an alphabet written in thick felt tip pen on cards can be used to make words.

The patient may be severely restricted in movement, in which case place both their hands on the bedclothes, palms upwards, and ask them to move a finger or half turn a hand over. If there is no movement, see whether a voluntary movement can be found elsewhere, for example a foot movement or tapping an object. Give a standard answering code and check the patient has understood. An example might be one move of an index finger means 'yes' and two 'no'. All questions should be simple and involve yes/no answers. This will all be tiring for the patient so do not continue without checking that he or she is alert and wishes to carry on.

Feeding the stroke patient

Following a stroke, a patient often has to relearn to eat. Some degree of dysphagia is likely and, in the initial stages, may be severe. Most patients will dribble due to loss of muscle tone on the affected side of the mouth.

Before any oral feeding is commenced, stroke patients should be tested (by a nurse or speech therapist) to see whether the gag reflex is present. If it is absent, the patient will be unable to swallow and tube feeding will be necessary. Where possible a fine bore nasogastric tube should be chosen.

While the patient is receiving total nasogastric feeding, the taste buds will require stimulation to prevent atrophy. Suitable stimulants which can be placed (in minute amounts) on the tongue are lemon juice (or a lemon slice), beef tea, yeast extract, blackcurrant cordial or similar bitter, salt, sweet or sour flavours. Mouth movement is also necessary for oral hygiene and the production of saliva.

When the gag reflex returns, tube feeding should gradually be replaced by an oral diet. Initially, overnight nasogastric feeding may be appropriate to supplement the food intake. Some guidelines for the reintroduction of oral diet are given below:

Assistance. The assistance of a speech therapist should be obtained. As a precaution, a suction machine should be nearby in case of emergency.

Position of the patient. The patients should be seated upright with their feet flat on the ground and the affected side supported. The patient's head should *not* be tipped back as this makes swallowing difficult.

Types of food. Suitable foods are those which are soft and tasty, e.g. thick custards, thick soup, yoghurt, mashed potatoes with eggs, ice cream or jellies. Cold foods are often better initially because they stimulate the gag reflex. Food preferences should be determined beforehand; the patient must not be offered something which is disliked.

Helping the patient to swallow. In order to facilitate swallowing, the patient should be given appropriate verbal instructions such as 'close the mouth' or 'chew the food well'. These actions may need to be illustrated. The cheeks may have to be manipulated and the instruction 'when you are ready, try to swallow' given. In order to help the larynx move upwards and assist swallowing, the neck area can be stroked upwards from the upper chest to the chin (patients may be able to do this for themselves).

Fluids. Fluids should only be introduced when swallowing has returned. Straws should *not* be given as their use requires considerable muscle co-ordination and cheek movements which will be difficult for some people. Feeding beakers may be necessary initially but the patient will find it more socially acceptable to take small sips from an ordinary cup or glass as soon as this is practicable.

As recovery progresses, patients will be able to try a wider range of foods and most will be able to feed themselves. Some patients with persisting physical disabilities may benefit from the use of specially developed cutlery. Care should be taken to ensure that the dietary intake is sufficient to meet nutritional needs and if necessary, appropriate supplements should be given.

When discharge from hospital is imminent, discussions should be held with members of the family and/ or those caring for the patient about the type and quantity of food which will be needed.

Support organisation

The Chest, Heart and Stroke Association, Tavistock House North, Tavistock Square, London WC1. (There are local support groups of this association in many areas.)

Further reading

Isaacs B (1985) *Understanding stroke illness.* Chest, Heart and Stroke Association, London.

References

Fuller JH, Shipley MJ, Rox G, Jarrett RJ and Keen H (1983) Mortality from coronary heart disease and stroke in relation to degree of glycaemia. The Whitehall Study. *Br Med J* **287**, 867–70.

4.23 Epilepsy

Epilepsy is a common disorder and one which has been recognized since biblical times. It is a symptom of cerebral dysfunction which may manifest itself in a number of ways. Epilepsy is classified according to the type of manifestations produced but these categories should not be regarded as separate disease entities.

A convulsion, or other epileptic manifestation, is thought to occur when there is a sudden disorganised discharge of electrical activity from a group of neurones, which spreads along existing anatomical pathways in such a manner as to produce symptoms ranging from sensory abnormalities to convulsive movements and unconsciousness. The grand mal (major or tonic clonic seizure) results from disturbances in the upper brain stem. Focal and temporal lobe epilepsy are other manifestations found in both children and adults. Myoclonic epilepsy occurs typically in children, presenting as massive violent muscular contractions; it can coexist with other types of fits and satisfactory drug therapy is difficult.

Diet and epilepsy

The ketogenic diet was first used as a treatment for childhood epilepsy in 1921 when Wilder documented his work showing that a high fat, restricted protein and carbohydrate diet could be of value in the management of children with intractable epilepsy.

This work was based on the clinical reports about the deliberate use of fasting to control epileptic seizures. Although the beneficial effects of fasting were clearly evident, deliberate starvation could only be used sporadically and was of limited value.

The ketogenic diet aims to mimic the effects of fasting and is effective for most forms of epilepsy, but particularly myoclonic, focal and temporal lobe epilepsy. However, the exact mode of action, if indeed it is a single action, still remains to be elucidated.

With the advent of modern anticonvulsants, the ketogenic diet went out of vogue until the late 1970s when interest in it as a treatment for childhood epilepsy was revived.

Ketogenic diets are usually, but not always, seen as the last line in treatment for the patient with intractable epilepsy. Anticonvulsants, even on a high dosage, do not always control seizures and the ketogenic diet can provide either an adjunct or an alternative to drug therapy. In cases where anticonvulsant therapy is refused, the ketogenic diet is the only other form of treatment. In addition, the possible long term side effects of anticonvulsant drugs are a further indication that a ketogenic diet may have a very positive role to play.

Selection of patients

The diet appears to be of most benefit to those patients (predominantly children) with myoclonic epilepsy, major motor epilepsy (grand mal) and minor motor epilepsy. Livingstone (1977) stated that children aged 3—5 years with grand mal and myoclonic seizures are most likely to respond to diet. Schwartz *et al* (1980) showed that the diet can be used in children between 6 months—16 years. Seizure improvement could occur when the diet was used with any form of epilepsy.

The ketogenic diet requires considerable commitment from patients, parents and the dietitian. Because it is restrictive and can affect social situations, it is only suitable for adults who are highly motivated.

Before a ketogenic diet is constructed, patients (or their parents) must have the full implications of the diet explained to them and must express willingness to co-operate. A diet history should then be taken to obtain meal patterns, food preferences and current energy intake.

Types of ketogenic diet

There are three types of ketogenic diet which can be used
1   The 4:1 classical ketogenic diet described by Livingstone.
2   The Medium Chain Triglyceride diet.
3   The John Radcliffe diet.
   The same principle is common to all in that they are high fat, low protein, low carbohydrate diets.

Classical ketogenic diet

The classical ketogenic diet contains 4 g fat:1 g (protein + carbohydrate). However, in children under 18 months, a ratio of 3:1 is more acceptable. The classical ketogenic diet is not recommended for adults because the quantities of food needed are unacceptable as a daily dietary regimen.

The calculation is based on the patient's actual body weight. The dietary energy content is calculated as 75 kcal g/kg body weight and the protein content as 1 g/kg body weight. If the patient is obese then adjustment taking account of ideal body weight may be necessary to prevent exacerbation of the obesity. The following formula can be used to calculate the dietary energy, fat, protein and carbohydrate content of a 4:1 ketogenic diet

If the patient's weight is W kg then

Energy content (kcal) $= 75 \times W$
Fat content (g) $= 7.5 \times W$
Protein content (g) $= W$
Carbohydrate content (g) $= \frac{7}{8} \times W$

The formula for calculating a 3:1 diet is

Fat content (g) $= 7.25* W$
Protein content (g) $= W$
Carbohydrate content (g) $= 1.44* W$

(W is the patient's weight in kg).

*rounded to two decimal places.

When the total protein, fat and carbohydrate for daily consumption have been calculated, each quantity is divided by three to give the amount available for each of three meals within a day (Table 4.49). Three meals are then devised which contain, as near as possible, the desired quantities of protein, fat and carbohydrate (Table 4.50).

Table 4.49 Example of a calculation of a 4:1 classical ketogenic diet for a patient of weight (W) 31.4 kg

Nutrient	Quantity per day	Quantity per meal (daily amount ÷ 3)
Energy	75 W kcal $= 75 \times 31.4$ $= 2355$ kcal	
Fat	7.5 W g $= 7.5 \times 31.4$ $= 235.5$ g	78.5 g
Protein	W g $= 31.4$ g	10.5 g
Carbohydrate	$\frac{7}{8} W$ g $= \frac{7 \times 31.4}{8}$ $= 27.5$ g	9.2 g

Table 4.50 Example of a classical ketogenic diet providing a total of 2355 kcal (Table 4.49) with a 4:1 ratio of fat to protein and carbohydrate

Meal	Fat (g)	Protein (g)	Carbohydrate (g)
Breakfast			
8 g Cornflakes	0.12	0.68	6.8
100 ml double cream	48.2	1.5	2.0
30 g fat	24.6	Tr	0.0
2 rye crispbread (Energen)	0.6	4.4	2.8
	73.52	6.58	11.6

6.58 g + 11.6 g = 18.18 g protein + carbohydrate
73.52 g fat ÷ 18.18 g = 4.

Meal	Fat (g)	Protein (g)	Carbohydrate (g)
Lunch			
30 g cod (raw weight)	Tr	5.22	0.0
30 g peas (cooked weight)	Tr	1.5	2.13
30 g fat	24.6	Tr	0.0
60 g stewed pear (no sugar)	Tr	Tr	5.58
100 ml double cream	48.2	1.5	2.0
	72.8	8.2	9.71

8.2 g + 9.71 g = 17.91 g protein + carbohydrate
72.8 g fat ÷ 17.91 g = 4

Meal	Fat (g)	Protein (g)	Carbohydrate (g)
Tea			
50 g egg	5.4	6.1	Tr
1 rye crispbread (Energen)	0.6	4.4	2.8
30 g fat	24.6	Tr	0.0
40 g stewed apple (no sugar)	Tr	Tr	3.28
100 ml double cream	48.2	1.5	2.0
	78.8	12.0	7.08

12.0 g + 7.08 g = 19.08 g protein + carbohydrate
78.8 g fat ÷ 19.08 g = 4

Table 4.51 Unrestricted foods on the classical ketogenic diet		
Salad vegetables	Celery, chicory, chinese cabbage, chives, cucumber, endive, lettuce, mint, mustard and cress, peppers, parsley and other herbs, radish, spring onion, tomatoes (not more than two a day) and watercress.
Green vegetables	Asparagus, bamboo shoots, beans (runner, French), bean sprouts, broccoli, cabbage, cauliflower, celeriac, courgettes, kale, leeks, mushroom, onions, spinach, spring greens and vegetable marrow,
Fruit	Rhubarb — stewed and sweetened with saccharine or aspartame (add sweetener to fruit after cooking)
Drinks	Black tea or coffee, diabetic and low calorie squash, diet and slimline fizzy drinks, PLJ, soda and mineral water.
Condiments	Salt, pepper, mustard, vinegar, Worcester sauce, herbs and spices, clear soup Bovril, Marmite, Oxo and soy sauce. Pickles (no added sugar), cauliflower, cucumber, gherkins, dill, red cabbage, onion, chillies and capers.
Miscellaneous	Essences, flavourings, vegetable colourings and gelatine. Artifical sweeteners — tablet and liquid saccharine, e.g. Hermesetas and the aspartame sweeteners Canderel and Nutrasweet.

These three meals form the basis of the classical ketogenic diet. To give variation, other meals can be calculated using the appropriate quantities of protein, carbohydrate and fat. One *whole* meal can then be exchanged for another *whole* meal. No other foods are allowed except those on the unrestricted food list (Table 4.51).

Practical guidelines

1 Double cream, Calogen (SHS), butter or margarine (not low fat spreads) are the source of fat in this diet. Any alternative to double cream/Calogen has to provide the same quantity of fat.
2 No sweet food or sugar is allowed.
3 No foods are allowed between meals other than unrestricted foods.
4 A full vitamin supplement must always be given, e.g. Ketovite vitamin supplement, tablets and liquid. (Paines and Byrne).
5 In very young children, supplements of minerals and calcium will be necessary. 8 g daily of metabolic mineral mixture (Allen and Hanburys) and Sandocal (Sandoz) calcium supplement is usually appropriate.
6 In very young children when a warm milky drink at bedtime is required, an extra 25 ml of double cream or substitute can be used, with water added to give the required volume.
7 Older children may require a snack mid-afternoon or at bedtime, in addition to the three main meals. This requirement usually arises after the children have been on the diet for 18 months — 2 years, or where circumstances suggest it would improve compliance. It should not be part of the suggested dietary regimen initially. Since including an extra snack will also in-

crease the overall energy intake it should be based on the same quantities as a whole meal exchange. It may contain less protein and more carbohydrate or vice versa, but the fat content should remain constant.
8 10 ml double cream or alternative can be exchanged for 5 g fat within any meal exchange.

General points

1 Due to the detailed calculations, the classical ketogenic diet is the most effective of all ketogenic diets. It is, however, very restrictive and requires a large amount of dietetic involvement in terms of calculations, monitoring, motivation of the family for adherence and patient support.
2 The possible long term risk of arterial disease from the high fat intake must be offset against the benefits from the diet in terms of a possible reduction in anticonvulsant dosage and drug-induced side effects. Furthermore, Schwartz et al (1980) have monitored the effects of the diet and have not found any increase in lipid levels.
3 Children on the classical ketogenic diet are likely to remain below the desired weight/height percentiles for age (Livingstone 1977). This is not necessarily a problem since there will be a compensatory growth spurt when the diet is discontinued (Schwartz et al 1980).
4 Patients must have a sufficient amount of unrestricted foods on the diet to provide bulk and alleviate hunger.

The medium chain triglyceride oil diet (MCT diet)

The MCT Diet is calculated on the desired energy

intake, usually taken as the RDA for energy for the patient's age. However, this must always be compared with the total energy intake derived from a diet history. If there is a significant difference, the MCT ketogenic diet should be based on an energy intake mid-way between the two figures. Weight of the patient must also be noted and adjustments made accordingly (the physically handicapped epileptic is often overweight due to drugs, excessive energy intake and/or inability to exercise).

The MCT diet energy can be apportioned in one of two ways

1 60:11:19:10 MCT oil: saturated fat: carbohydrate protein.

2 60:40 MCT oil: [saturated fat + carbohydrate + protein].

(MCT Oil contains 8.3 kcal/g.)

MCT diet 1

1 The nutrient content of the diet is calculated as

MCT oil (g)   = Total kcal × 0.60 ÷ 8.3
Saturated fat (g) = Total kcal × 0.11 ÷ 9
Carbohydrate (g) = Total kcal × 0.19 ÷ 4
Protein (g)   = Total kcal × 0.10 ÷ 4.

2 A system of exchanges is used to construct a diet containing the required quantities of macronutrients. Protein exchanges are based on

50 g (2 oz) meat exchange containing 12 g protein + 10 g fat
50 g (2 oz) egg exchange containing 6 g protein + 6 g fat

Carbohydrate is regulated by the 10 g carbohydrate exchange system used for diabetics (see p 131) but avoiding those foods which contain significant quantities of protein (e.g. fish fingers, beefburgers, all pulses (including baked beans), ice cream, yoghurt and tinned spaghetti).

Saturated fat is usually covered in the protein exchange. MCT oil is used for all cooking, but most of it is incorporated with skimmed milk to produce 'special milk'. Skimmed milk is calculated from the total quantities of protein, fat and carbohydrate in the initial calculation (Tables 4.52 a and b).

3 Patients are given a summary showing the quantity of MCT oil and skimmed milk to be taken daily and the total numbers of protein and carbohydrate exchanges to be incorporated as desired into the diet. The 'special milk' should be distributed throughout the day.

MCT diet 2. An alternative MCT-based diet can be calculated as follows

1 The required daily energy is divided into 60% kcal from MCT oil and 40% kcal from protein, fat and carbohydrate. The 40% kcal is incorporated into the diet using a 100 kcal exchange system.

2 MCT oil (or Liquigen, SHS) is given in the form of milk shakes as five or six drinks a day (Table 4.53).

To ensure that the patient consumes a minimum of 1 g protein/kg actual body weight/day, at least 2−3 of the 100 kcal exchanges should be protein exchanges. It is immaterial thereafter which 100 kcal exchanges are used, but they must be distributed throughout the day (Tables 4.54a,b).

Table 4.52a,b Example calculation of MCT diet 1

a) Calculation of nutrient content of diet. Desired energy intake = 1600 kcal.

60% energy as MCT oil =	954.5 kcal ÷ 8.3 = 115 ml MCT oil or 230 ml Liquigen.
11% energy as saturated fat =	170.1 kcal ÷ 9 = 18.9 g
19% energy as carbohydrate =	306.8 kcal ÷ 4 = 76.7 g
10% energy as protein =	159.2 kcal ÷ 4 = 39.8 g
	1591 kcal

b) The diet can then be made up as follows

	Fat (g)	Protein (g)	Carbohydrate (g)
60 g skimmed milk powder *	0.8	21.8	31.7
1 egg exchange	6.0	6.0	Tr
1 meat exchange	10.0	12.0	—
4½ carbohydrate exchanges	Tr	Tr	45.0
2.5 g fat (butter/margarine)	2.1	Tr	—
	18.9	39.8	76.7

* Made up to 600 ml with water. 600 ml skimmed milk + 230 ml Liquigen = 830 ml 'special' milk.

Table 4.53 Formula for MCT oil milk shake

30 ml diabetic squash or 1 teaspoon coffee powder or 1–2 drops
  vanilla essence.
20 ml MCT oil (or 40 ml Liquigen)
2 drops saccharine solution
Water to 100–200 ml

Table 4.54a,b MCT diet 2.

a) 2000 kcal diet based on kcal exchanges

60% kcal from MCT oil = 1200 kcal = 144 ml MCT oil*
40% kcal as 100 kcal exchanges = 800 kcal = 8 exchanges

* This can be given as 280 ml Liquigen, made into a milk shake, divided by six, and given with each meal and snack

b) Examples of 100 kcal exchanges

150 ml (6 fl.oz) milk
300 ml (12 fl.oz) skimmed milk
25 g (1 oz) cheddar cheese or cream cheese.
40 g (1½ oz) meat
50 g (2 oz) fish in batter, fried or fatty fish
40 g (1½ oz) bread
30 g (1¼ oz) cereals
150 g (6 oz), baked potato
40 g (1½ oz) chips
200 g (8 oz) peas
300 g (12 oz) eating apple or orange

Practical guidelines for MCT diets 1 and 2

1 It is preferable to use a MCT oil and water emulsion, i.e. Liquigen (SHS) rather than the oil itself, as this is easier to incorporate into the diet and, in particular, to mix with skimmed milk.

2 Skimmed milk may be calculated as either a liquid or a powder. The total volume must be one and a half times the total volume of Liquigen to be incorporated. An equal volume of skimmed milk + Liquigen is unpalatable.

3 The full amount of Liquigen *must never* be incorporated into the diet at the beginning of the treatment. It must always be added to the skimmed milk in increments, gradually increasing the amount until the desired level is reached. Treatment should commence with 10 ml Liquigen depending on tolerance and total volume, and increased by 10 ml daily. The increments can be increased to 15 ml and then 20 ml daily depending on tolerance. In very young children the increments should be 5 ml to begin with.

4 Some patients have a lower tolerance level than the amount calculated, in which case the amount should not be increased further.

5 MCT oil can produce side effects of abdominal pain, diarrhoea and vomiting. If any of these arise while introducing the Liquigen, patients should go back to the quantity previously tolerated and remain on this amount for 48 hours. The oil can then be increased to the maximum tolerated level in smaller increments.

6 The 'special milk' must be taken throughout the day.

7 Liquigen can be taken as a medicine or mixed with fruit juice.

8 MCT oil has a lower 'flash' point than ordinary cooking oil so care must be taken if it is used for frying.

9 Concentrated sugars (e.g. granulated, caster, icing sugar, sweets, jams, treacle, etc.) must be avoided.

General points for consideration with MCT oil diets 1 and 2

1 With the MCT diet 1, patients can become confused with protein exchanges.

2 Large volumes of 'special milk' cannot easily be incorporated into the diet throughout the day.

3 On the MCT diet 2, foods with a high sugar concentration may inadvertently be included and this may induce fits.

4 Some exchanges on each diet represent a large quantity of food and are impractical.

5 The MCT oil diet has greater flexibility than the classical ketogenic diet.

6 Foods which are favourites with children (such as fish fingers) are not allowed.

7 Vitamin and mineral supplementation may be necessary.

The John Radcliffe ketogenic diet

This has evolved as a result of the difficulties with the classical and MCT oil diets. The John Radcliffe diet has many similarities with the MCT diet but is now used more often.

The calculation of the diet is based on the recommended daily intake of energy as for the MCT diet but 30% of energy is provided by double cream and a slightly different system of exchanges is used.

1 Assess the desired daily energy intake (see MCT diet 1, p 492). Apportion the energy intake as follows

30% total kcal as MCT oil
30% total kcal as double cream
11% total kcal as saturated fat
19% total kcal as carbohydrate
10% total kcal as protein.

2 The protein exchange is based on 30 g (1 oz) meat providing 6 g fat and 6 g protein. The carbohydrate exchange follows the 10 g carbohydrate exchange system as used for diabetics (but avoiding foods with either a high sugar or significant protein content) (Table 4.55). Skimmed milk is used as the medium for incorporating the MCT oil.

Table 4.55 a–c Example calculation of John Radcliffe diet, based on a desired intake of 1500 kcal

a)

	Fat (g)	Protein (g)	Carbohydrate (g)
25 g skimmed milk powder	0.3	9.1	13.2
100 ml double cream	(48.0)	1.5	2.0
· 4 protein exchanges	24.0	24.0	0.0
5 carbohydrate exchanges	Tr	Tr	50.0
	24.3	34.6	65.2

b)

MCT Oil = 450 kcal = 50 ml MCT oil
From calculation:

MCT Oil	= 50 ml × 8.3	= 450 kcal	= 30%
Fat from double cream	= 48.0 g × 9 (1 g fat = 9 kcal)	= 433.8 kcal	= 29%
Saturated fat	= 24.3 g × 9 (1 g fat = 9 kcal)	= 218.7 kcal	= 14.5%
Protein	= 34.6 g × 4 (1 g Protein = 4 kcal)	= 138.4 kcal	= 9.2%
Carbohydrate	= 65.2 g × 4 (1 g CHO = 4 kcal)	= 260.8 kcal	= 17.3%
		1501.7 kcal	

This degree of variation in percentage energy from the formula given on p 493 is acceptable.

c) Total daily intake in 24 hours from calculation

4 protein exchanges
5 carbohydrate exchanges
25 g skimmed milk powder plus water to 250 ml
100 ml Liquigen
100 ml double cream presented as 50 ml double cream and
  25 g other fat (e.g. butter, margarine)

3 The patient is provided with a summary giving the quantities of double cream, MCT oil (usually in the form of Liquigen) and skimmed milk for daily use (Table 4.56) and the total number of protein and carbohydrate exchanges.

Practical guidelines for the John Radcliffe ketogenic diet

1 All guidelines given for the practical application for MCT diets 1 and 2 concerning the use of Liquigen and skimmed milk *must* be followed.
2 Fat used in cooking is not included in the dietary

Table 4.56 a–c John Radcliffe ketogenic diets
a) Examples of 30 g (1 oz) protein exchanges. (Each exchange contains 6 g protein and 6 g fat.)

30 g (1 oz) meat
40 g (1 oz) fish
50 g egg — 1 medium size
30 g (1 oz) cheddar cheese

b) Examples of 10 g carbohydrate exchanges

20 g wholemeal bread	1 small slice
10 g breakfast cereal	3 heaped tbs
15 g semi-sweet biscuit	2 plain
1 small bag crisps, plain	
50 g potato, plain boiled	1 size of an egg
25 g chips	4 large chips
230 fresh carrots	4 heaped tbs
100 g fresh apple or pear	1 medium fruit, raw with skin and core
50 g fresh banana	1 small without skin
100 ml natural orange juice	8 tbsp

c) Examples of protein and carbohydrate combined exchanges

100 g (4 level tbs) baked beans + 10 g fat	1 protein + 1 CHO exchange
50g (2 tbs) peas + 5 g fat	½ protein exchange
80 g (2 large or 4 chipolatas) beef sausage (cooked weight)	1 protein + 1 CHO exchange
60 g (2) fish fingers (cooked weight) + 5 g fat	1 protein + 1 CHO exchange
60 g (1 small) beefburger (cooked weight)	2 protein exchanges
80 g (1 heaped tbs) tinned spaghetti + 5 g fat	1 CHO exchange
40 g ice cream, vanilla plain	½ protein + 1 CHO exchange

calculations provided that it is not taken to extremes resulting in obesity.
3 If the number of carbohydrate exchanges consumed during the day are fewer than prescribed this does not matter provided that the patient is not losing weight. This problem usually only arises with the protein exchanges.
4 The amount of double cream calculated is usually divided into a specific amount of double cream and fat in the form of butter or margarine (but not low fat spreads). This is done on the basis of 10 ml double cream being equal to 5 g fat. For example, 50 ml double cream is equal to 30 ml double cream and 10 g fat.
5 Concentrated sugary foods must be avoided. Artificial sweeteners can be used but they must be of pure saccharine or aspartame derivative. Sorbitol should be avoided as a sweetener.
6 Oxo, Marmite, Bovril, gravy browning and Bisto can all be used for gravy. If cornflour and flour are used for thickening purposes they need not be counted as an exchange, provided they are not used to excess.
7 A combined protein and carbohydrate exchange can be given for foods not normally allowed, thus

giving greater flexibility to the diet. For example

a) 80 g beef sausage (cooked weight) = 1 protein and 1 carbohydrate exchange.

b) 40 g peanut butter = 1 protein exchange

c) 100 g baked beans plus 10 g extra fat = 1 protein exchange and 1 carbohydrate exchange.

General points for consideration with the
John Radcliffe ketogenic diet

1 The large volume of 'special milk' is reduced.
2 The diet can more easily be incorporated with the diet of the rest of the family.
3 There are only two basic exchange systems.
4 Vitamin and mineral supplementation may be necessary.

Monitoring dietary compliance

If a ketogenic diet has to be devised by a dietitian with little or no experience of this form of diet therapy, then hospital admission, of approximately five days, is advocated. This enables any adjustments to the regimen to be made and also enables the patient to become familiar with the diet in practice before it has to be attempted at home.

Once the most suitable diet for the patient has been implemented, the diet is monitored by regular testing of urinary ketone levels, the overall aim being to produce a ketone level in the region of 3.9–7.8 mmol/l.

Ideally the patient should be kept on clear fluids for the 24 hours preceding commencement of the diet to induce a state of ketosis. If the patient is a child, the parents often find this difficult to accept, so the diet may be started without this initial starvation period. If this is the case, then testing for ketones should not be carried out until the diet has been followed for at least ten days.

Testing for ketones should be done twice a day using Ketostix. Variations are usually seen with trace to small readings (1.5 mmol/l) in the morning specimens and moderate (3.9 mmol/l) to large (7.8–15.7 mmol/l) in the afternoon. In babies where a specimen cannot be collected, the Ketostix can be used on a wet nappy although the result is less accurate. A record of the Ketostix readings should be kept as they can often be correlated with seizure patterns. Many patients are sensitive to the levels of ketones; some are effectively controlled at a moderate ketone level, whereas others only improve if the reading is always high. Presence of urinary ketones reflects compliance with the diet. The ketone level depends on the type of

ketogenic diet used; higher levels occur on the classical ketogenic diet. A sudden fall in urinary ketones is often an indication of illness or the initial stages of an infection; ketones reappear with recovery.

If the ketone level remains low despite strict adherence to the diet and general good health, it may be due to one of the following reasons

1 The diet is being followed incorrectly. Check that all fat is consumed and that the protein and/or carbohydrate exchanges are not exceeded.
2 The last intake of fat may be consumed too early in the day. If the last meal is late afternoon, a specific medication of double cream or Liquigen should be taken at bedtime (20 ml double cream or 30 ml Liquigen is usually appropriate)
3 Concentrated carbohydrate foods such as sweets are being consumed.
4 The intake of total fluid may have been suddenly increased thus diluting ketones. If necessary, total fluid intake should be specified.

If none of these factors seem to apply, the diet itself may need adjustment and the carbohydrate intake should be reduced by half to one exchange.

Illness and ketogenic diet

If the patient is unable to tolerate the diet because of illness, in particular gastric upsets, the diet should be stopped and the following procedure carried out. In very young children and babies, medical help MUST be sought immediately.

1 Only clear fluids or sugar-free squash should be consumed for 24–48 hours.
2 When the symptoms subside, the diet should be reintroduced at a quarter of all daily allowances.
3 Food and fat should be increased gradually over a four day period until the normal regimen is reached.
4 If at any stage symptoms recur, there should be a return to the levels previously tolerated.
5 In any doubt, medical help should be sought immediately, especially if the symptoms have not resolved within 48 hours, or if the patient shows any sign of deterioration. If the patient requires hospital admission, sugary drinks and dextrose solutions should NOT be given (except for life-threatening conditions) as they can provoke seizures. Hypoglycaemia is not an immediate indication to give intravenous glucose as many children on the ketogenic diet have low blood glucose levels, especially those on the classical diet. If intravenous glucose has to be given, this must be done in conjunction with an enteral feed.

Ketogenic enteral feeds

When calculating enteral feeds, they should be based on the same total and percentage nutrient content as the oral diet.

For those patients following the MCT diet 1 or 2 and the John Radcliffe ketogenic diet, Liquigen and skimmed milk will form the basis of an enteral feed. For those following the classical ketogenic diet, double cream or Calogen (SHS) will form the basis of the enteral feed.

In all cases, other components, i.e. protein, carbohydrate, vitamins and minerals are added as necessary.

The ketogenic diet and special events

Parties, Christmas and Easter can cause particular problems due to the complex nature of the diet. The following are suggestions for these occasions and for situations where a 'reward' is required

1 Diabetic foods are generally not allowed because although sugar-free they can make a significant energy contribution to the diet. However, diabetic squash and all sugar-free low energy drinks are acceptable. Diabetic chocolate Christmas pennies and Easter eggs can be allowed as a special treat provided total consumption takes place over several weeks. Diabetic fruit gum-type sweets can be used occasionally as a reward.

2 Party suggestions include eclairs with no chocolate topping, sugar-free plain cake (ordinary sponge cake minus sugar) with a filling of whipped double cream, trifle using sugar-free cake, tinned fruit in natural juice and low energy jelly (made from sugar-free squash and gelatine) decorated with cream. Those patients using an exchange system can incorporate some of their exchanges into party foods such as crisps or sausages.

3 If the food taken on these occasions exceeds the dietary allowances, it must be counterbalanced by the addition of extra cream or other fat.

Duration and discontinuation of the ketogenic diet

In order to ascertain whether the diet is of benefit, it should be followed for a minimum of three months. If unsurmountable problems such as social crisis or complete intolerance arise during this period, then the diet may have to be stopped.

The ketogenic diet as a treatment for patients with intractable epilepsy is *not* a diet for life. The optimum duration of the diet is unknown, but the response, and

other related circumstances, have shown that the diet may be beneficial for a period of 18 months − 4 years. During this period anticonvulsant dosage will probably have been reduced and this, coupled with reduced seizure frequency, can produce an unwillingness to cease the diet.

When the decision has been made to discontinue the diet, it is imperative that dietary restrictions are released slowly, usually over a 1−2 week period. This is related to the length of time the patient has been on the diet. The ketones may well be acting as an anticonvulsant and a sudden increase in sugar consumption can easily precipitate seizures. The following steps are recommended

1 Reduce liquid fat intake by 10 ml/day and solid fat by 5 g daily until normal requirements are reached.

2 After seven days have elapsed following the initial discontinuation of the diet, introduce cows' milk.

3 Gradually increase the quantity of protein from the first day until the desired intake is reached.

4 From day seven, increase the quantity of carbohydrate foods but DO NOT introduce high sugar foods. This should remain a long term measure even after carbohydrate intake has returned to normal. If at any stage the seizures reappear or become more severe, the diet should be reinstated at the level where the patient was previously free of fits. Once stabilization has occurred, dietary discontinuation can be restarted but at a slower rate.

Summary

Ketogenic diets have a valuable therapeutic role in the treatment of intractable epilepsy. They can reduce, or sometimes completely eliminate, seizures and can be of particular benefit to children in terms of improving awareness, learning capacity and behaviour patterns. Ketogenic diets are, however, complex diets to administer and to follow and must never be instituted without close medical and dietetic supervision.

Further reading

Bower BD, Schwartz RH, Eaton J and Aynsley-Green A (1982) The use of ketogenic diets in the treatment of epilepsy In *Topics in perinatal medicine 2* pp 136−40. Pitman Publishing Ltd, London.

Clark B and House PM (1978) Medium chain triglyceride oil ketogenic diet in the treatment of childhood epilepsy. *J Hum Nutr* **32**, 111−6.

Coutts J (1978) Ketogenic diets. *J Hum Nutr* **32**, 214.

Dodson WE Prensky AL and Devivo DC (1976) Management of seizure disorders: selected aspects. *J Paediatr* **89**, 695−703.

Francis D (1978) Ketogenic diets. *J Hum Nutr* **32**, 212.

Gordon NS (1977) Medium chain triglycerides in a ketogenic diet. *Dev Med Child Neurol* **19**, 535–44.

Hamilton MB (1978) Ketogenic diets. *J Hum Nutr* **32**, 213.

Huttenlocher PR (1976) Ketonaemia and seizures: metabolic and anticonvulsant effects of two ketogenic diets in childhood epilepsy. *Paediatr Res* **10**, 536–40.

Stevenson JB (1977) Medium chain triglyceride in a ketogenic diet. *Develop Med Child Neurol* **19**, (5), 693–4.

Withrow CD (1980) Antiepileptic drugs: the ketogenic diet: mechanism of anticonvulsant action. *Adv Neurol* **27**, 643–54.

References

Livingston S (1977) Dietary treatment of epilepsy. In *Comprehensive management of epilepsy in infancy, childhood and adolescence*. Charles C. Thomas — Springfield, III pp 378–405

Schwartz R, Aynsley-Green A and Bower BD (1980) Clinical and metabolic aspects of ketogenic diets. *Res Clin Forums* **2**, (2), 63–74.

Wilder RM (1921) The effects of ketonuria on the course of epilepsy. *Mayo Clin Bull* **2**, 307.

4.24 Psychiatric Disorders

4.24.1 Depressive illness

Affective disorders (i.e. depressive illness, anxiety state, mania and hypomania) are a group of illnesses which fit into a continuum between sadness and excessive cheerfulness and in which the mood state (or affect) is the fundamental disturbance leading to the development of other symptoms.

Depression is an affect which may be defined as the subjective feeling of sadness, despondency, gloom, misery or unhappiness.

Types of depression

1 Normal reaction to common stress.
2 Depressive neurosis — relating to precipitating stress.
3 Endogenous depression — no precipitating cause.
a) Unipolar — mania or hypomania never occurs.
b) Bipolar — true manic depressive illness with swings between mania and depression.

Symptoms of depression

These may include psychomotor retardation, depressive ideas, depressive stupor, self reproach, mutism, paranoid ideas, agitation, restlessness and anxiety and suicidal thoughts.

Nutritional disturbances in depression

Anorexia

Loss of appetite is often severe and marked weight loss occurs. However, some depressed women may eat to excess.

Bowel disturbances

Constipation is common and may form the basis of hypochondriacal delusions. Anxious patients have increased bowel activity with frequent soft motions. Tricyclic antidepressant drug treatment will make constipation worse and this may greatly upset a patient.

Weight gain

Patients on tranquillisers (e.g. Benzodiazepines or lithium carbonate) may gain weight as a side effect of the drug. This is particularly common in female depressed patients who eat to excess as a symptom of their illness.

Low vitamin levels

Carney and co-workers (1979) reported a link between deficiencies of riboflavin and pyridoxine and affective illnesses. They have suggested that these deficciencies may have a primary role in the aetiology of affective disorders.

Dietary treatment in depressive illness

Dietary restriction due to medication

Depressed patients being treated by monoamine oxidase inhibitors (MAOI) must avoid taking food rich in tyramine (see p 175).

Weight reduction

Since many antidepressant drugs have the side effect of causing weight gain, and because an increase in weight in a depressed patient may make the mental condition worse, part of the treatment must be to control any potential weight problem. The use of an energy controlled diet works well and, once the mental state recovers, medication is reduced and the weight problem improves. Regular dietary counselling is important to encourage continuance of the diet.

Anorexia

To prevent weight loss becoming life threatening it is important to encourage eating in patients with severe anorexia. The use of oral supplements (see Section 2.12) to improve energy and protein intakes may be beneficial.

Constipation

Increasing the fibre and fluid content of the diet of

depressed patients will help to alleviate constipation. An increase in fluid intake will also to help relieve the dry mouth experienced by many patients using tricyclic antidepressants.

Low vitamin levels

Patients known to be at risk from deficiencies of B vitamins (e.g. alcoholics, patients using the contraceptive pill or those consuming a poor diet) should be given vitamin supplements as this measure may improve the mental condition.

Team approach

It is important that dietitians work in close co-operation with other members of the health care team so that patients are given dietary advice which is consistent and also appropriate for their needs.

4.24.2 Senile dementia

Diagnosis of senile dementia presents the clinician with considerable difficulty. The term 'senile dementia' is often taken to include Alzheimer's disease and senile dementia of Alzheimer type.

Dementia is the global disturbance of higher cortical functions — memory, the capacity to solve problems of daily living, the performance of perceptuomotor skills, the correct use of social skills and the control of emotional reactions.

Dementia occurs in 2.4% of persons aged 65–69 years but in 22% of those aged 80 years or more (Kay *et al* 1964, 1970). As the proportion of the population over the age of 65 years increases, what was once thought as an inevitable consequence of ageing has now become a major social problem.

To date no effective treatment is available. However, it is known that there is decreased activity of some of the neurotransmitters (such as homovanillic acid, 5 hydroxytryptamine and dopamine) in dementia and drug correction of these deficiencies may be possible in the future.

Nutrition and senile dementia

Some work has been carried out on nutritional status and dementia. Although a definite causative factor for dementia has not been found, deficiencies of some nutrients, in particular certain vitamins, have been shown to have an exacerbating effect on confusional states.

Folate

Reynolds *et al* (1971) suggested a causal relationship between folate deficiency and affective psychoses and dementia, and causes of dementia due to folate deficiency have been reported (Sneath *et al* 1973). The absence of any megaloblastic anaemia should not be taken as an indication of adequate folate status. Thomas *et al* (1985) have shown significant clinical improvement in a group of patients with early signs of dementia when supplemented with multivitamins including folic acid.

Ascorbic acid

Personality changes including 'hysteria' and depression have been produced by a clinical lack of vitamin C (Hughes 1982). Dopamine β hydroxylase is ascorbic acid-dependent and this enzyme converts dopamine to noradrenaline, a neurotransmitter likely to be implicated in depressed states. Biogenic amine pathways are known to be abnormal in dementia (Rosser *et al* 1984) and depressed symptoms are common in the condition, therefore these links with vitamin C make ascorbic acid of interest in this group of patients.

Patients in long stay hospitals and the elderly at home (especially the confused elderly) are very much at risk from vitamin C deficiency (Vir and Love 1979) and this could conceivably exacerbate the confusional state.

Thiamin

Many B vitamins, and especially thiamin, play important roles in brain metabolism and their deficiencies are associated with neurological or psychiatric diseases. Several workers (Older and Dickerson 1982; Katakity *et al* 1983) have shown an association between mental confusion and thiamin deficiency in elderly people. Shaw *et al* (1984) showed that 30% of a group of patients with senile dementia had increased levels of erythrocyte transketolase percentage activation, which is indicative of thiamin deficiency.

Tryptophan

This amino acid is a precursor of 5 hydroxytryptamine, a neurotransmitter in the central nervous system. Shaw *et al* (1981) found that patients with senile dementia had lower fasting levels of tryptophan than healthy community controls. When these patients' diets were supplemented with tryptophan, the patients showed signs of improvement. The authors suggested further investigation into the use of whole protein supplements in dementia.

Fluid

Patients with senile dementia may be unable to request extra drinks if thirsty and it is easy to forget that fluid intake may not be adequate. Dehydration can cause acute confusional states so fluid balance should be monitored.

Improving nutritional status

It should be remembered that patients with senile dementia are very confused and have poor short term memory, therefore nutritional intake is bound to be at risk. If specific nutrients do, as seem likely, have an influence on mental function, deficiencies could make the condition worse (Fig. 4.18). Ensuring that these patients have an adequate nutritional intake is therefore of paramount importance.

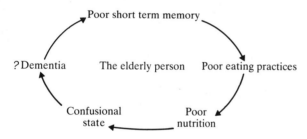

Fig. 4.18 The continuous circle of poor memory and failing nutrition.

Because distant memory tends to be better than that of the immediate past, it may be beneficial to reminisce about foods eaten when young and to talk about foods which they can prepare and eat now. These patients have often forgotten about various foods that they enjoy and may be unaware that modern convenience versions of some foods (such as fish) can be easy to cook and prepare. For those in hospital, menu cards with photographs of the menu items can help patients make a meal choice. Relatives and support groups should receive regular help and advice from dietetic personnel so that they realized the importance of good nutrition.

Interest in, and evidence of the value of, vitamin therapy in the treatment of confused states and senile dementia is growing and many centres routinely prescribe multivitamin therapy for these patients.

4.24.3 Schizophrenia

Schizophrenia is the name given to a group of mental disturbances which cause dramatic disturbance in the way a person's mind functions. The parts of the mind which control thinking and feeling are in conflict with one another. The person experiences the world around him in a different way and his behaviour changes strikingly.

The schizophrenic breakdown can happen at any time although people aged 18–33 years are especially at risk. The signs and symptoms vary from person to person; the most common are thought disturbance, hallucinations, delusions, disturbed feelings and withdrawal.

Nutrition and schizophrenia

The fundamental cause of schizophrenia is at present unknown. Whether nutrition is a factor in its aetiology is speculative but diet may be relevant to its treatment.

Gluten sensitivity

Dohan *et al* (1969) reported that patients with schizophrenia improved their mental state faster when put on a gluten and milk-free diet. This was substantiated by Singh and Kay (1976) in a double blind cross-over study. These studies suggested that the intestinal mucosa of some patients with schizophrenia is permeable to proteins or peptides which are not normally absorbed. In those patients whose mental function is associated with a sensitivity to wheat gluten, the adoption of a gluten-free diet may therefore help to keep them well. Unfortunately there is at present no simple test to determine gluten sensitivity and this is essential if this factor is to be considered in the treatment of schizophrenia.

Vitamin therapy

The use of megadoses of vitamins (notably niacin) may allow a reduction in drug dosage and has been reported to minimize the side effects of drugs in some patients (Osmond and Hoffer 1962). As with the effects of a gluten-free diet, there are no tests which can reliably help to distinguish those patients who may benefit from vitamin therapy.

Weight gain

Many schizophrenic patients will be treated with phenothiazines or benzodiazepines which have a tendency to cause an increase in weight. Weight gain can be very distressing to these patients and cause further anxiety states affecting their mental condition. Dietary treatment to treat or avert this may therefore be of benefit. However, the mental condition of these patients means that attention and concentration cannot be focused for long periods. Dietary interviews may take some time, with the patient's interest wandering from the topic. Advice therefore, is often more effective on a regular sessional basis in an attempt to introduce gradually any dietary changes which are necessary.

Special diets can present a problem for the schizophrenic patient. A meal that is different to the other members of the family or ward group may make the patient feel threatened and produce delusions of attempts to poison him.

For these reasons, plus the continued use of weight-enhancing medication, attempts at weight reduction are usually slow but can ultimately be successful (Knox 1980). Dietary counselling with these patients has the benefit of increasing their awareness of food and does help to curb weight gain.

4.24.4 Anorexia nervosa

Patients with anorexia nervosa (AN) are usually young and female. It most commonly occurs around the time of puberty but is becoming more apparent in older age groups and also in males. The AN patient is characterized by

1 An obsessional aim to achieve more and more weight loss. The desired weight goal is always decreased further when it has been reached.

2 An obsession with body size and fear of fatness. A distorted body image is common.

3 Lack of awareness, or refusal to admit, that there is a problem.

4 The wearing of loose bulky clothing (typically baggy shirts, jumpers and skirts and woolly socks or tights) to disguise size and for warmth. Food may be concealed in the pockets of garments.

5 Inability to sleep at night and over-activity during the day but with poor concentration. School or college work often starts to deteriorate.

The clinical features may include: emaciation, cessation of menstruation in most women, hypothermia of extremities, depression, hypertension, bradycardia and the appearance of lanugo hair (soft, downy fluff) on the back, arms, legs or face. Ultimately, death can, and often does, result.

Background

Social and family history

AN patients are usually, although not exclusively, from social classes I and II and often have a high IQ. They may have started dieting as a method of attention-seeking and they often have an immature personality — the typical 'Peter Pan Syndrome'. There may be fears of the adult world, of the pressure of work (despite being hard-working) or of their own sexuality.

The parents of an AN patient are often ambitious for the child — often pushing in a direction either not liked by the child and/or beyond his/her capabilities. There may be competition between siblings. Parents usually find the condition very difficult to understand and need to know 'where we have failed' and 'what has gone wrong'.

Previous dieting and attitude to foods

Fifty percent of AN patients have a pre-morbid history of obesity and most have lost at least 10% body weight in one or more bouts of dieting. They have a keen, often obsessional, interest in food and nutrition, an extensive knowledge of calorie values of food and will argue very forcefully with staff about diet.

Vegetarianism is often adopted after the start of the illness. If this is the case, a diet containing some animal products should be encouraged. It is very difficult to treat an AN patient with a vegan diet because the high energy level required results in a diet which is extremely bulky.

AN patients may spend hours in a kitchen creating meals and new recipes for family and friends to eat. They obtain great satisfaction from watching people consume the dishes they have prepared, but are always ready to find plausible excuses not to eat themselves, often claiming to have eaten while preparing food, or not to be hungry. In the early stages, the interest in food can make it more difficult for the family to recognize that a problem exists.

If they are observed eating, anorexics are very 'ritualistic'. They spend many minutes laying the table, collecting food, condiments, dishes and cutlery. They are very precise in placing food on to plates, always serving food in the same order. They often 'chant' or talk to themselves whilst this process is underway. When eating they take very small quantities and chew very slowly and deliberately. If food is left, it is often hidden under cutlery or other food in an attempt to make the quantity look less.

Like many starving people, AN patients are obsessed with the thought of food, both day and night, often dreaming of food or of eating or cooking it.

Treatment

In-patient treatment

Treatment in hospital is needed if weight drops below 75% ideal weight for height. Below 50% is life-threatening.

The aims of treatment are
1   To restore healthy weight with a more normal eating pattern.
2   To separate weight and eating control problems from wider personal issues.
3   To define and make progress on wider issues. Psychotherapy is often used. These personal problems may appear to be small and insignificant, but have become out of proportion to the patient.

Dietitians are mainly concerned with aim 1.

A *dietary history* is needed to establish intake prior to admission. If possible, a second opinion should be obtained from the parents as patients are likely to deny that a problem exists and may confine their descriptions of food consumption to phrases such as 'eating enough', 'eating regularly' or 'having a good appetite'. This interview may take place at an out-patient clinic and should be used as an opportunity to start gaining the patient's trust.

When planning the initial diet, the patient must be aware of what is expected of her. A limited list of dislikes should be allowed (a maximum of 3−5 is suggested) but these must be adhered to throughout so as to avoid any possibility of manipulation.

Dietary regimens

Refeeding an anorexic patient needs to be done with caution if the patient's intake has been very low.

If the patient has been fasting prior to admission, a fluid regimen is recommended until normal gastro-intestinal function returns. This may need to be administered via a nasogastric tube. As gut functions return and bowel movements occur, solid food can be introduced and the feed volume slowly decreased until the tube is removed.

A 500 kcal feed, increasing in approximately 200 kcal increments, can be used initially in very emaciated patients to prevent intolerance and possible obstruction.

Patients with low energy intakes, but actually eating on admission, can be given solid food. Initially, the energy intake should be similar to that taken prior to admission as judged by the dietary history. This should be increased in 200−500 kcal increments provided that normal gut function is maintained; vomiting and/or obstruction can occur in malnourished patients. 3000 kcal/day is the usual target to aim for, usually given as three meals with three snacks plus high energy drinks in between.

Adequate fluid intake is important to help normalize bowel function and should be specified on the diet plan.

Some patients require much higher levels, up to 5000 kcal/day, in order to overcome the starvation state, but this should still be given in a similar pattern to the 3000 kcal regimen. Some high fibre foods should be used and fluids encouraged, as laxative abuse prior to admission may lead to severe constipation.

Hiding sources of energy in foods should be avoided; if energy supplements are used the patient should be aware of the situation. This helps to keep the patient's confidence and trust in the dietitian and avoid any potential conflict situations should the patient accidentally find out.

Once food is tolerated and weight increases, energy supplements, if used, can be stopped and the number of high energy drinks reduced, leaving a more normal meal pattern. The aim is to establish the patient on three meals a day without snacks and supplements before discharge so that the patient experiences a normal eating pattern.

Detailed diet sheets must be distributed each time the diet is changed to everyone involved, i.e. the patient, dietetic, medical, nursing and catering staff. Amounts should be stated in an unambiguous form, in weights or acceptable measures, e.g. half-pint mug, one large slice, one tablespoon. Terms such as 'helping', 'small amount' and 'normal' should be avoided as they are too vague and leave room for argument between patient and staff. The patient may also have little concept of normal portion sizes. Once the regimen is decided, it must be adhered to. This allows everyone to become familiar with the routine and gives the patient a feeling of security.

The catering staff should never be asked to supply foods or supplements which are beyond their resources or to provide meals at unusual times. The catering department should also be aware that changes can only be made with agreement from all parties and, therefore, should only be accepted from some pre-determined source of authority, e.g. the dietitian or charge nurse. If this is to be enforced, both the ward and the catering staff must be informed of the accepted channel of communication.

The kitchen staff should also be asked to ensure that all food on the plate is edible, i.e. no fat, gristle, bones or poultry skin as this can cause conflict on the ward.

The time taken to eat a meal may need to be limited, e.g. to 20−30 min, as this gives the patient less time to ponder and worry over the meal. (It also discourages the time-wasting rituals previously mentioned).

The total team approach is very important for successful long term treatment.

Reward/contract system

These can be entered into from the beginning of treatment to encourage patient compliance. This system should try to operate positively by encouraging weight gain and good eating habits, and not negatively by punishing weight loss or bad behaviour. This is not always feasible as the patient will rarely increase weight steadily without any periods of weight loss. However, the positive side should always be stressed.

As the responsibility for decision-making about the diet is removed from the patient on admission, food cannot be used successfully as a reward. The reward system therefore tends to be linked with personal routines and freedoms.

These contracts are usually drawn-up by medical and nursing staff, but dietitians need to be aware of their content. Agreement about weight increments, target weights and nutritional points need to be agreed before the contract is 'signed'. Some restrictions which may be applied at the start of treatment and then relaxed as weight increases are

1 Restricted visitors. Visits from relatives (or friends) may be banned completely or limited to a specific number of occasions. This measure can also sometimes help distance the patient from any family conflict which may exist.

2 Limitation on recreations or hobbies. Basic school/college work may be allowed depending upon the physical and/or mental state of the patient.

3 Observation of the patient after mealtimes for a stated length of time.

4 A commode toilet and a sink with a disconnected waste pipe have to be used.

5 Hair washing and bathing/showering restricted.

6 Cigarettes limited.

7 Limited access to TV/radio.

8 Total bed rest, increasing in stages to periods in lounge with other patients, eventually allowing, firstly supervised, and then unsupervised trips off the ward.

9 Side room progressing to main ward.

10 Limited choice of meals.

11 Restrictions on preparation of own meals or drinks.

The contracts need to be designed individually as the extent of the restrictive measures will depend on the severity of the condition and the rewards will depend on the factors which matter most to each person.

Expected weight gain and target weight

The target weight set must be realistic and is not necessarily the ideal weight for height as set by Life Insurance Tables (see p 47). However, the target weight should not be so low that the patient has to remain on an energy restricted diet in order to maintain it; it must encourage normal eating. If the patient is female and in her late teens, the weight at which she first menstruated may be a good target. This is not as appropriate for older women. Growth charts are not always suitable for children as puberty may have been delayed or interrupted by the strict dieting and their heights may not, therefore, be appropriate for their ages. A compromise target must be found and the average weight for the population at the age the illness occurred may be more realistic. Once the initial crisis period is overcome new target weights may be negotiated.

These target weights should not be allowed to be exceeded. This will give the patient confidence and continue her trust in the team members. The expected weight gain should be in the region of 2 lbs (1 kg)/week once the full diet has been established. Too fast a weight gain will not help the patient adapt psychologically to their new size.

Failure to achieve expected weight gain. Patients not achieving the expected weight gain should be checked or observed for the following

1 Disposing of food and/or drinks by hiding it in lockers, carrying it to 'flush' toilets in toilet bags or clothes, throwing it out of windows (beware of flocks of birds outside her room), giving it to other patients (many patients may sympathize with the anorexic and

help out by eating unwanted food) or hiding it under the mattress.

2 Vomiting, and disposing of the products in similar ways to food. AN patients can vomit very quickly and quietly so close observation is necessary.

3 Laxative abuse, visitors may bring them in or patients may buy them on their trips away from the ward or have brought them into hospital.

4 Excessive exercise.

5 Wearing fewer clothes.

Patients may gain weight suddenly if they stop doing any of the above.

Patients may also try to give the impression they have gained weight by

1 Drinking vast amounts of fluid before being weighed.

2 Carrying weights hidden in underclothing.

3 Wearing hidden extra layers of clothes.

4 Being constipated.

These can cause unaccountable fluctuations in weight.

Because the weight is so important as a way of monitoring the patient's progress, it is better if the patient does not know when weighing will take place. The same procedures should always be followed. Patients should be weighed in the nude or in nightwear only, on the same set of scales and by the same staff. Care should be taken to ensure that the patient is standing, or sitting, squarely on the scales as this will eliminate weighing errors.

Follow-up and outcome

Psychotherapy and family therapy often have good long term results. These tend to be started once weight is back to acceptable levels. Younger patients generally have a better prognosis. Total cures are possible, but it can take many years and repeated admissions to hospital. Early treatment of symptoms gives better results and if long term treatment, i.e. four years or more, is needed this suggests that chronic AN is developing. This can be a form of bulimia (bulimia nervosa; see next section), where body weight is maintained, but, because of abnormal eating patterns and quantities of food eaten, self-induced vomiting is the only way that the patient can keep control.

Out-patient visits may be fortnightly initially, to check weight and dietary adequacy and to give patients the confidence to continue alone. It is usually found that these sessions will need to continue as long as the patient feels some benefit from them. Patients are weighed and changes discussed. They may be encour-

aged to keep a food diary and advised to spend 5–10 min each evening planning the next day's meals. This eliminates last minute decisions which often lead to the patient not eating. It also aims to reduce time spent thinking about food.

Bingeing is often a stage anorexics go through and the diaries can hopefully identify these problems in the early stages. Indicative signs include a large intake of sweets and drinks. The advice given to control eating must be flexible — banning foods is too authoritarian. The patient must be encouraged to control their own intake.

As weight and eating becomes less important the patient may gradually stop attending of their own accord. Relapses are not uncommon and should not be seen as a failure for either the patient or the therapist.

Patient support groups and suggestions for further reading are listed on p 506.

4.24.5 Bulimia

These patients often present as slightly obese and many are previous anorexia nervosa (AN) sufferers. Some centres categorize these chronic ANs as 'bulimia nervosa'. Bulimic patients tend to be slightly older than AN sufferers and have become trapped in a starving/bingeing/vomiting cycle (Fig. 4.19). Their eating pat-

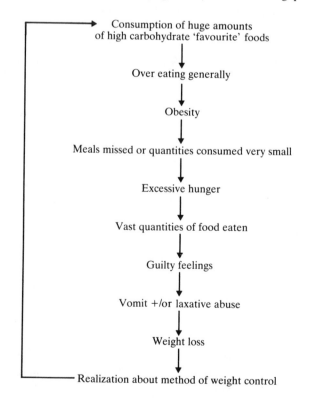

Fig. 4.19 Typical eating pattern of the bulimic patient.

tern is very erratic. Like AN patients, many overestimate their body size and this needs correction if a successful long term solution to their problems is to be achieved.

Vomiting and laxative abuse are the more commonly practised methods of weight control, but may also include excessive exercise (usually taken very secretively) or drug abuse. For example, slimming tablets may be taken in excess and some diabetics adjust their insulin to produce an adverse effect on their control and therefore, as a result of the glycosuria produced, their weight. Bulimics may consume excessive amounts of alcohol in order to forget their problems or to help eliminate hunger.

Because of the vast quantities of foods, laxatives, drugs or alcohol which are consumed, many bulimics develop financial problems. In some cases this has lead to petty crime to finance their habits, either by stealing food or by stealing goods to sell. It is often the financial problems which drive the patient or family to seek help.

Treatment of bulimia nervosa

The aims of treatment are
1 To gain patient's confidence and trust.
2 To reduce and eventually stop vomiting and any other forms of abusive behaviour.
3 To restore a normal eating pattern.
4 To restore a more normal body weight — which usually occurs when aim 3 is achieved.

Target weight

As with AN patients, the target weight should be negotiated between staff and patient and is not necessarily the weight for height obtained from the insurance tables. It should not be so low as to require continual dieting to maintain. The weight to which the body naturally settles once a good eating pattern has been established is the most desirable.

Dietary regimen

As in-patients, three regular meals without in-between snacks should be established, avoiding any foods on which the patient is known to binge. These are most commonly high carbohydrate foods which are easily eaten such as sweets, chocolate, biscuits, sweet desserts or lemonade. The energy content of the diet should be adjusted according to whether the patient presents at over, under-or normal body weight. Because many

bulimics abuse laxatives, high fibre foods should be included and careful monitoring of patient's bowel habits is needed to ensure obstruction does not occur. Patients will need great encouragement during this equilibrium phase as they may get a distended abdomen until normal gut movements are established and they may relate this normal bulk to obesity, panic and vomit. The patient should be made aware of the metabolic and medical effects of purging and vomiting so they can see the potential damage they are doing to themselves.

Time should be spent with the patient, discussing balanced healthy meals rather than letting the patient focus solely on 'calories'. Bulimics often believe that all carbohydrate is 'bad' and may also have distorted ideas about small quantities of food causing a disproportionately large increase in body weight. They need positive reinforcement that eating a complete meal is acceptable and is not gluttonish. Their previous quantities of food consumed may be a great source of embarrassment and guilt.

As their control over eating is regained, foods formerly 'binged' should be reintroduced in the form of snacks. The patient may have a great fear of these foods and will, at first, need close supervision both during and after the snack to ensure 'quantity control' is maintained and that vomiting does not occur. Eventually the patient should be encouraged to eat in various situations, e.g. the hospital snack bar or local cafe. The patient may be reluctant to spend time away from the 'safe' environment of the ward and initially returns speedily after eating to prevent loss of control.

The patient should be encouraged to plan shopping and cooking in order to make constructive use of the time allowed for thinking about food. This should be limited as in the treatment of AN. Many bulimics spread their purchasing over many shops so that no one sees the final quantity bought. Limiting the number of shops used may be a useful tactic, depending on the local stores available. Supermarkets are a great temptation and may be better avoided until later on. The increased cost of items in smaller shops will be offset by the reduced quantity being purchased. Storing food in cupboards out of sight rather than in open view may also help prevent impulses to binge.

Out-patient/follow-up

Out-patient treatment has to achieve the same aims, but, because of the lack of self control and the close supervision needed, it may not be as successful. Regular weekly visits will be required initially and the patient encouraged to complete small tasks in a stepwise regimen for recovery. Food diaries should be kept as this allows the therapist to discuss the nutritional content of the diet rather than relying solely on body weight as an indicator of progress. The patient may find that this procedure discourages binges if they have to be reported and discussed. If in-patients are allowed home for meals before their final discharge, food diaries should also be kept. Mood charts, to help the patient identify what triggers a binge session, may be useful. Ways of coping with potential trigger situations can then be discussed. The possibility that some patients may be allergic to the foods on which they binge should not be overlooked.

After discharge, regular follow-up visits to allow discussion about weight, eating habits and problems encountered will be needed. This can be in a group situation or on an individual basis.

Patient support groups

1 Anorexic Aid, Priory Centre, 11 Priory Road, High Wycombe, Bucks. Tel: 0494 21431.
2 Anorexic Family Aid, Sackville Place, 44/88 Magdalen Street, Norwich, Norfolk NR3 1JE.
3 Anorexic Counselling Service, 3 Woodbine Terrace, Leeds 6.
4 Anorexics Anonymous, 21 Kitson Road, Barnes, London SW13.
5 Society for the Advancement of Research into Anorexia (SARA), Stanthorpe, New Pound, Wisborough Green, Billinghurst, West Sussex.
6 Compulsive Eating Group, Mount Pleasant Community Centre, Sharrow Lane, Sheffield 11. Tel: 0533 53587.
7 Women's Therapy Centre, 6 Manor Gardens, London N7. Tel: 01 263 6200.
8 Overeaters Anonymous, St Philips Church Hall, London W8.

Further reading

Depression
Coppen A and Walk A (1968) Recent developments in affective disorders. *Br J Psychiat* Special publication No 2, Headley Brothers Ltd, Ashford.

Senile dementia
Kemm JR (Ed) (1985) *Vitamin deficiency in the elderly. Prevalence, clinical significance and effects on brain function.* Blackwell Scientific Publications, Oxford.
Roberts PJ (Ed) (1979) *Biochemistry of dementia.* John Wiley and Sons, Bristol.

Schizophrenia
Hemmings G and Hemmings WA (Eds) (1978) *The biological basis of schizophrenia.* MTP Press, Lancaster.

Anorexia nervosa/Bulimia nervosa
Bruch (1978) *Golden cage.* Harvard University Press, Cambridge.

Bruch (1974) *Eating disorders, obesity, anorexia nervosa and the person within.* Basic Books, New York.
Crisp AH (1980) *Anorexia nervosa — 'let me be'.* Academic Press, London.
Fairburn C (19) *Binge eating and bulimia nervosa.* Smith, Klyne & French, Welwyn Garden City.
MacLeod S (1981) *The art of starvation.* Virago Press Ltd, London.
Palmer RL (19) *Anorexia nervosa — a guide for sufferers and their families.* Pelican,
Wellbourne J and Piergold J (1984) *The eating sickness. Anorexia, bulimia and the myth of suicide by slimming.* Harvester Press Ltd, Brighton.

References

Carney MWD, Williams DG and Sheffield BF (1979) Thiamin and pyridoxine lack in newly admitted psychiatric patients. *Br J Psychiat* **135**, 249–54.
Dohan FC, Grasberger JC, Lowell FM, Johnston HT and Arbegas AW (1969) Relapsed schizophrenics: more rapid improvement on a milk and cereal-free diet. *Br J Psychiat* **115**, 595–6.
Hughes RE (1982) Recommended daily amounts and biochemical roles in the vitamin C, carnitine, fatigue relationship. In *Vitamin C.* Counsell JN and Horning DH (Eds) p 75. Applied Science Publishers Ltd, London.
Katakity M, Webb JF and Dickerson JWT (1983) Some effects of a food supplement in elderly hospitalized patients. *Hum Nutr: Appl Nutr* **37A**, 85–93.
Kay DWK, Beamish P and Roth M (1964) Old age mental disorders in Newcastle Upon Tyne. *Br J Psychiat* **110**, 146–58.
Kay DWK, Bergman K, Foster EM, McKechnie AA and Roth M (1970) Mental illness and hospitalization in the elderly: a random sample followed up. *Comprehensive Psychiatry* **11**, 26–35.
Knox JM (1980) A study of weight reducing diets in psychiatric in-patients. *Br J Psychiat* **136**, 287–9.
Older MWJ and Dickerson JWT (1982) Thiamin and the elderly orthopaedic patient. *Age and Ageing* **11**, 101–7.
Osmond H and Hoffer A (1962) Massive niacin treatment in schizophrenia: review of a nine year study. *Lancet* **i**, 316–9.
Reynolds EH, Preese J and Johnson AL (1971) Folate metabolism in epileptic and psychiatric patients. *J Neurol Neurosurg Psychiat* **34**, 726–32.
Rosser MN, Iverson LL, Reynolds GP, Mountjoy CW and Roth M (1984) Neurochemical characteristics of early and late onset types of Alzheimer's disease. *Br Med J* **288**, 961–4.
Shaw DM, Tidmarsh SF, Briscoe MH, Dickerson JWT, Chung a on KO (1984) Nutrition and patients with senile dementia. *Br Med J* **288**, 792–3.
Shaw DM, Tidmarsh SF, Sweeny EA, Williams S, Karajgi BM, Elameer M and Twining C (1981) Pilot study of amino acids in senile dementia. *Br J Psychiat* **139**, 580.
Singh MM and Kay SR (1976) Wheat gluten as a pathogenic factor in schizophrenia. *Science* **191**, 401–2.
Sneath P, Chanarin I, Hodkinson HM, McPherson CK and Reynolds EH (1973) Folate status in the geriatric population and its relation to dementia. *Age and Ageing* **2**, 177–82.
Thomas DE, Chung a on KO, Briscoe MH, Shaw DM and Dickerson JWT (1985) Vitamin supplementation in patients with early signs of dementia. Presentation at the British Dietetic Association Study Conference 1985, Keele University.
Vir D and Love AMG (1979) The nutritional status of the institutionalized and non-institutionalized aged in Belfast. *Am J Clin Nutr* **32**, 1934–47.

4.25   Multiple Sclerosis

Multiple Sclerosis (MS) is a degenerative disease of the central nervous system which is notoriously difficult to diagnose. It presents in two ways, the chronic progressive form and the more common remitting relapsing type. It can present at any age but usually starts in young adulthood. Symptoms include paraesthesia, episodes of blindness and weakness in various limbs. Remission can be long term but more typically is a course of attack, disability and partial recovery.

Very often no advice or medical treatment is offered, but drug therapy can be helpful for incontinence, frequency and for muscle spasm. Physiotherapy may also be beneficial. Most MS patients, and especially those recently diagnosed, are in need of considerable psychological support.

The role of diet in the mangement of MS

The role of diet in the treatment of MS is poorly documented and controversial.

Epidemiological studies have suggested that there may be a relationship between the amount and nature of dietary fat and the incidence of MS (Dean 1975). There is a higher prevalence of MS in Northern Europe in countries where the diet is commonly high in saturated fat than in countries such as Japan where the diet is based on fish and therefore high in polyunsaturated fat. The incidence of MS is also higher in the Shetlands than in the Faroes where the traditional fishing industry has been retained and fish consumption is higher (Bernsohn and Stephanides 1967).

60% of the solid matter of the brain and 70% of the myelin sheath is comprised of lipid, hence the interest in essential fatty acid nutrition and this disease of the central nervous system. Low levels of essential fatty acids (efa) have been found in the serum of MS patients (Swank 1950; Sinclair 1956) and this finding led to the double blind trial of linoleic acid supplementation in MS patients in Belfast and Newcastle (Millar *et al* 1973; Bates *et al* 1977). This indicated a decrease in frequency and duration of relapse in the supplemented group (87 patients) as against the control group (85 patients). During the study period of 28 months, 41 relapses occurred in the supplemented group, the majority being of short duration. 62 relapses occurred in the control group, most being for periods of 6−9

weeks or more than ten weeks. In addition, further reappraisal of this work (Dworkin *et al* 1984) has demonstrated that patients who had minimal or no disability and a shorter duration of illness benefited most from a diet high in linoleic acid. A fish oil trial is currently (1985) in progress at a London hospital.

A longitudinal study being conducted by the Action for Research into Multiple Sclerosis (ARMS) has been in progress for three years and has shown that a high percentage of patients maintained or decreased their disability level on the ARMS diet (see below) and exercise programme (Simpson *et al* 1985). Details of the subjects in this study and the preliminary findings are summarized in Tables 4.57 and 4.58.

Table 4.57 The ARMS diet and exercise programme study. General information on subjects

	Female	Male
Number of subjects	62	21
Mean (sd) age at entry to study (years)	40.2 (1.0)	39 (1.0)
Mean (sd) duration of disease (years)	10.8 (8.2)	6.8 (4.2)
Mean (sd) length on study (months)	34 (4.5)	33.8 (5.2)
Acute relapsing	49	13
Chronic progressive	13	8

Table 4.58   The ARMS diet and exercise programme study. Neurological data

	Acute relapsing	Chronic progressive
Mean (sd) Kurtzke disability status scale at entry to study	5.18 (0.98)	6.09 (0.8)
Mean (sd) Kurtzke disability status scale at end of study	5.20 (1.0)	6.07 (1.26)
No. Kurtzke scale decreased	10 (16%)	4 (19%)
No. Kurtzke scale maintained	32 (52%)	10 (45%)
No. Kurtzke scale increased	20 (32%)	7 (33%)
Mean no. of relapses during study	2.06 (2.17)	na
Mean no. of days of relapse during study	80 (114)	na
Mean % disability of activities of daily living (ADL) entry to study	3.7 (6)	19 (21)
Mean % disability of ADL end of study	5.4 (13)	16.8 (19)

Over 34 months disability would normally worsen.
Kurtzke disability scale 1−10 examples
Less than 5.0 — ambulatory without an aid.
       < 6.0 — in need of constant unilateral assistance.
       6.5 — in need of constant bilateral assistance.
       7.5 — wheelchair bound.

Swank (1970) has also suggested that a low animal fat diet started early in the course of the illness is beneficial. A diet containing less than 20 g saturated fat a day produced a marked improvement in life expectancy and disability over a 30 year period (Swank 1985). However it is debatable whether these benefits apply to patients who have had MS for a period of time or who have severe disability.

Dietary treatment of MS patients

It must be remembered that the relationships between diet and the progression or remission of MS are, at the present time, only suggestive rather than conclusive. Much more research in this area is needed, in particular prolonged trials of a double blind nature. However, such trials are especially difficult to conduct with MS patients who are often unwilling to commit themselves to one long term course of dietary treatment preferring, in their desperation to find a cure, to try a variety of dietary strategies.

Owing to the lack of conclusive proof of benefit, very few MS patients are prescribed a 'special' diet as part of their clinical care. Most clinicians feel that the only justifiable dietary measures are those which correct either an inappropriate energy intake or a diet of poor nutritional quality. Simple changes in diet may also help prevent constipation which, because of bowel spasticity, is a common problem.

However, for many MS patients these measures are not enough and large numbers of them will instigate their own dietary therapy in the hope of obtaining some remission from the disease. MS patients respond readily to any new suggestion, particularly from the media, that a particular diet may be of benefit and are inevitably very vulnerable to 'quack' diets.

At the present time, very few MS patients will receive any professional dietetic guidance. However, some MS patients may be referred to a dietitian at their own insistence and others will be referred either for general dietary assessment or for some disorder unconnected with the MS. In these instances, the dietitian can play a valuable role by answering queries about diet and MS, and putting the facts into perspective, and by ensuring that any self-imposed dietary regimen is at least nutritionally adequate. Dietitians should ensure that any changes in eating habits which are recommended should not cause the patient any more difficulty with regard to shopping or cooking than is already encountered; it is important that both stress and fatigue are avoided.

Some of the most common diets which the dietitian may either encounter or be asked about are outlined below. Support organisations (listed on p 509) may be able to help dietitians locate new research papers on the role of diet in the treatment of MS.

Diets commonly used by MS patients

Low fat diet This derives from the work of Swank (1983) who recommended a diet low in animal fat with elimination of hydrogenated margarines and oils.

The 'ARMS' diet. This diet was formulated by Professor Crawford (1979) and is a low saturated fat diet high in essential fatty acids (of the $\Omega6$ and $\omega3$ types). In addition, wholegrain cereals, vegetables and fruit are consumed in sufficient quantities to provide the necessary vitamins and minerals for conversion and utilization of the efa. For example, trace elements such as zinc, copper and iron are components of the desaturase and cyclo-oxygenase systems responsible for the synthesis of long chain derivatives and prostaglandins. The B vitamins are important for chain elongation reactions and vitamins C and E are vital as antioxidants (Crawford 1979; Hewson et al 1984). The diet has a P/S ratio greater than 1 and a vitamin E content of approximately 0.6 mg/g polyunsaturated fat.

Gluten-free (GF) diet (either with or without animal fat restriction). The Roger McDougall and Rita Greer diets are variations often followed by MS patients. There is no evidence to show they are beneficial; however many MS sufferers maintain they are helped by them.

Liversedge (1977) reported that in 37 (of 40) MS patients who completed a two year trial on a GF diet, the relapse rate was no better than average and disability scores worsened as would normally occur. A study of plasma samples of 36 MS patients showed only one with evidence of gluten antibodies and maintained that even this level did not justify a GF diet (Hunter et al 1984). Hewson (1984) studied 17 subjects on a GF diet and supported the view that there is no conclusive evidence that it is beneficial, but gives guidelines for dietitians dealing with MS patients who wish to follow such a diet.

'Allergy' diets. In desperation many MS patients undergo cytotoxic testing. This involves having a blood sample analysed for sensitivity to specific foods which

may then be eliminated from the diet. Many maintain that spasm is worsened by eating foods to which they are 'sensitive'. However, this type of dietary manipulation often results in a badly balanced diet.

Evening primrose oil (EPO). This is an efa (gamma linolenic acid) not directly obtainable from food, only by conversion of linoleic acid. It is expensive and not available on prescription. When taking EPO with the average British diet high in saturated fat, the non-essential fatty acids will compete with the efa and suppress their activity. It is probably only useful in conjunction with a low saturated fat diet and this may be scientifically demonstrated over the next few years.

Sunflower seed oil. This is rich in linoleic acid and often recommended. The dosage is usually six 0.5 ml sunflower seed oil capsules daily (a 23 ml supplement was used in a trial conducted by Millar *et al* (1973)) or 30 ml oil twice a day. Patients on the latter dosage who have a weight problem — as many disabled people do — must be advised how to reduce their energy intake without impairing dietary P/S ratio. As with evening primrose oil supplementation, a high intake of non-esterified fatty acids will diminish the effectiveness of any efa consumed.

Support organisations

1 Action for Research into Multiple Sclerosis (ARMS), 11 Dartmouth Street, London SW1. This organisation supports several research projects including a longitudinal management study which incorporates dietary assessment. ARMS provides information on physiothrapy, diet and on their therapy centres. They also run a counselling service.
2 The Multiple Sclerosis Society, 286 Munster Road, London SW6 6AP. The society also supports several research projects and has welfare officers throughout the country.

Both organisations produce regular news magazines.

Further reading

Graham J (1980) *MS A self help guide to management.* Thorsons, Wellingborough
Matthews B (19   ) *MS — the facts.* Oxford University Press, Oxford.

References

Bates D, Fawcett PR, Shaw DA and Weightman D (1977) Trial of polyunsaturated fatty acids in non-relapsing multiple sclerosis. *Br Med J* 2, 932−3.
Bernsohn J and Stephanides LM (1967) Aetiology of multiple sclerosis. *Nature (Lond)* 215, 821−3.
Crawford MA (1979) Dietary management in MS. *Proc Nutr Soc* 38, 373−89.
Dean C (1975) MRC Multiple Sclerosis research. In *Epidemiology: what is new and what remains to be done.* pp 39−42 Davison AN, Humphrey JH, Liversedge AL, McDonald WI and Porterfield JS (Eds). HMSO, London.
Dworkin RH, Bates D, Millar JH and Paty DW (1984) Linoleic acid and multiple sclerosis: a re-analysis of three double blind trials. *Neurology (Cleveland)* 34, 1441−5.
Liversedge LA (1977) Treatment and management of MS. *Br Med Bull* 33, 78−83.
Hewson DC, Phillips MA, Simpson KE, Drury P and Crawford MA (1984) Food intake in MS. *J Hum Nutr* 38A, 355−67.
Hewson DC (1984) Is there a role for GF diets in MS? *J Hum Nutr* 38A, 417−20.
Hunter L, Rees BWG and Jones LT (1984) Gluten antibodies in patients with MS. *J Hum Nutr* 38A, 142−3.
Millar JH, Zilkha KJ, Langman MJ, Payling Wright H, Smith AD, Belin J and Thompson RHS (1973) Double blind trial of linoleate supplementation of the diet in multiple sclerosis. *Br Med J* 1, 765−8.
Simpson KE, Fitzgerald GE and Harbige L (1985) Proceedings of the International Congress of Nutrition (August)
Sinclair HM (1956) Deficiency of essential fatty acids and atherosclerosis. *Lancet* i, 381.
Swank RL (1950) Multiple sclerosis: a correlation of its incidence with dietary fat. *Am J Med Sci* 220, 421−30.
Swank RL (1970) Multiple sclerosis: twenty years on low fat diets. *Arch Neurol* 23, 460−74.
Swank RL, Roth JG and Woody DC Jr (1983) Cerebral blood flow and red cell delivery in normal subjects and in multiple sclerosis. *Neurol Res* 5, 37−59
Swank RL (1985) International Fatty Acid Conference (London)

G: Disorders of the Skeletal System

4.26 Rickets and Osteomalacia

(See also Section 2.6, Vitamin D)

Rickets and osteomalacia are usually caused by either primary or secondary deficiency of vitamin D and the consequent failure to absorb calcium from the gastro-intestinal tract (Table 4.59).

Table 4.59 Causes of rickets and osteomalacia

Primary causes	Poor intake of dietary vitamin D relative to requirement (e.g. failure to meet an increased need due to growth/pregnancy).
	Inadequate synthesis of vitamin D due to insufficient exposure to sunlight.
	Poor absorption of calcium due to concomitant high fibre/phytate intakes.
Secondary causes	Malabsorption resulting from coeliac disease, gastric operations, bowel resection and bypass.
	Renal disease — chronic renal failure, renal tubular disorders and dialysis.
	Liver disease
	Primary disorder of parathyroid function — hypoparathyroidism or hyperparathyroidism.
	Familial vitamin D-resistant rickets.
	Prolonged use of drugs, e.g. anticonvulsants or glucocorticoids.

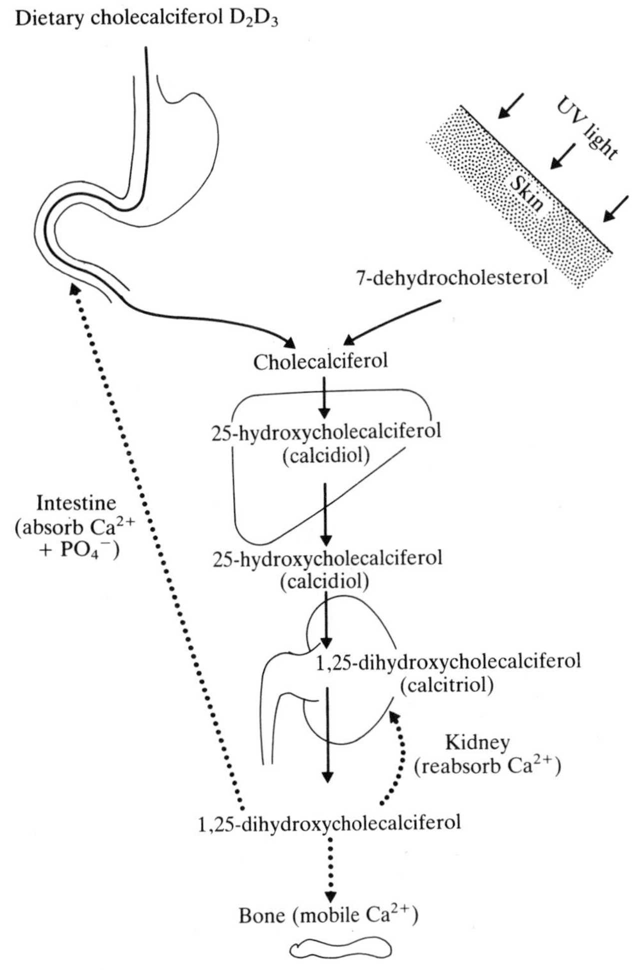

Vitamin D metabolism

Vitamin D status is dependent on both cutaneous production and dietary intake, so a deficiency is unlikely to occur unless the supply from both sources is defective or if there is an increased requirement for the vitamin. The vitamin D which is synthesized in the body is D^3 (cholecalciferol) but D^2 (ergocalciferol) is the form more commonly used therapeutically and for food fortification.

The metabolism of vitamin D has been clarified considerably in recent years (De Luca 1982). Although classed as a vitamin, the active metabolite (1,25 dihydroxycholecalciferol) may more properly be regarded as a hormone, and the dietary and endogenous precursors as prohormones (Fig. 4.20).

Contribution from diet and sunlight

Vitamin D provision from synthesis in the skin is efficient, minimizing the need for dietary forms of the vitamin in many populations. This is fortunate because the vitamin is not present in plentiful supply in food. The contribution to vitamin D status by sunlight is demonstrated by the seasonal variation in plasma 25

Fig. 4.20 Metabolism of vitamin D.

hydroxy vitamin D (25 (OH)D) levels (Dunnigan 1977; Poskitt et al 1979; Lawson et al 1979). From October to March no ultraviolet (UV) light reaches the earth's surface in Britain, so synthesis in the skin is restricted to the rest of the year. Where solar exposure is inadequate, the dietary intake of vitamin D has a more significant effect on vitamin D status, though debate about its importance continues (Lawson 1981).

Groups at risk of developing rickets and osteomalacia

1 Elderly and housebound people.
2 Immigrants from India, Pakistan and Turkey during infancy/early childhood, adolescence and pregnancy.

3 Children in poor socioeconomic circumstances.

4 Food faddists (particularly those on poorly constructed vegetarian or macrobiotic diets).

5 Patients with malabsorption, renal disease or on prolonged anticonvulsant therapy.

Aetiology

The relative importance of sunlight exposure and diet on vitamin D status is a complex and controversial issue.

Diet

Several dietary factors, singly or in combination, may contribute to the development of rickets and osteomalacia.

Vitamin D. Low dietary intakes of vitamin D have been suggested to be a cause of rickets and osteomalacia. Among Asians in Britain, some studies have shown dietary intakes to be lower than that of the indigenous population (Abraham 1983) but others (Dunnigan and Smith 1965) have found no difference and the tendency for Asian women to develop overt bone disease cannot be explained solely on a dietary basis. Among the elderly, low intake of vitamin D may well be relevant (Nayal *et al* 1978; Sheltawy *et al* 1984) (see Section 2.6, vitamin D).

Calcium. No differences in calcium intake have been found between rachitic and non-rachitic Asians though a poor Ca: P ratio may be an important factor (Dunnigan *et al* 1975). Among the elderly, low calcium intakes do not seem to be causative. Although extremely rare, rickets caused by low calcium intakes has been described in South African children (Marie *et al* 1982).

Fibre. The role of high extraction flours in the aetiology of nutritional rickets was first suggested by Mellanby (1949) and has been reconsidered as a result of the prevalence of rickets and osteomalacia among Asians in the UK (Robertson *et al* 1981). Supportive evidence has been derived from data from the Irish National Nutrition Survey (1943–8) (quoted by Robertson *et al* 1981), where a rise in the extraction rate of flour was believed to be responsible for the increased incidence of rickets in Dublin in 1942.

A possible mechanism may be the interruption of the entero-hepatic circulation of vitamin D metabolites by constituents of high extraction cereals and pulses (Batchelor and Compston 1983) or enhanced destruction of vitamin D in the liver (Clements and Fraser, in preparation). (See Section 2.6 vitamin D). In addition, unabsorbed fibre can bind calcium making it unavailable for absorption. The increasing use of wholemeal products in the population may precipitate deficiency in those groups already at risk.

Phytate. Phytic acid can bind calcium and the presence of phytates in chapatti flour has led to speculation that this may explain the increased incidence of rickets and osteomalacia in the Asian community. Healing of rickets has been reported following withdrawal of chapattis (Wills *et al* 1972), and Asian subjects have converted from negative to positive calcium balance on a chapatti-free diet (Ford *et al* 1972). However, O'Hara May and Widdowson (1976) felt that this hypothesis is unlikely because dietary calcium intakes exceed the amounts likely to be bound by phytic acid. Investigations are in progress to search for an alternative mechanism for the action of phytate.

Vegetarianism. Osteomalacia and rickets appeared in Austria and Germany at the end of the First World War during which people had reverted to a more vegetarian diet of bread and vegetables (Chick *et al* 1923).

Detailed analysis of the clinical findings, outdoor exposure and weighed dietary intakes of 84 Asian children in Glasgow showed that a lactovegetarian diet (as opposed to an omnivore diet) was rachitogenic independently of outdoor exposure (Robertson *et al* 1982). Dietary fibre, derived from high extraction rate wheat flour, fruit and pulses was the most important rachitogenic factor, while meat and fish (through their phosphorus content) were the most important protective foods. Dietary vitamin D intake *per se* was unimportant. It is thus not clear which component of the vegetarian diet makes it more rachitogenic than an omnivore diet. It is probably a combination of the low vitamin D, low phosphorus, high fibre and high phytic acid content.

Sunlight

Sunlight exposure. Seasonal variations in plasma levels of 25 hydroxyvitamin D (25 (OH)D) and differences in 25 (OH)D levels between indoor and outdoor workers (Neer *et al* 1977) emphasize the heavy dependence of vitamin D status on solar exposure. Calculations suggest that 1 cm² of exposed skin could provide up to 380 iu D³ per day in midsummer if there were no loss processes in the skin (Beadle 1977). Badges of polysulphone film, worn on the lapel can be used to monitor exposure to UV radiation (Challoner *et al* 1976).

The fact that 90% of circulating 25 hydroxyvitamin D is in the cholecalciferol (rather than ergocalciferol) form suggests that cutaneous synthesis is a quantitatively more important source than diet in the adult (Haddad and Hahn 1973). However, the fact that rickets and osteomalacia remain important health problems in parts of Asia, the Middle East and Africa, areas with abundant sunshine, while it has virtually disappeared from Europe and North America, shows that the relative contributions from diet and sunlight are not as clearly defined. However, many Asians avoid the sun and the mode of dress further reduces sunlight exposure, even on sunny days.

Measurements of sunlight exposure have not been shown to differ between Asian children with and without rickets and their European peers (Dunnigan 1977); however, these results must be interpreted with caution as valid measurements of total body UV exposure are extremely difficult to obtain. Among the elderly lack of sunlight exposure is likely to be an important risk factor (Hodkinson *et al* 1973).

Skin pigmentation. Hess and Unger (1917) noted that blacks in New York were more prone to develop osteomalacia than whites, but Stamp (1975) found no differences in the rise in serum 25 hydroxy vitamin D levels following UV radiation of White, Asian and West Indian subjects. If pigmentation is an important factor, rickets and osteomalacia would be expected to be much more common among West Indians and Africans in the UK but this is not the case.

Clinical features

Rickets and osteomalacia are most likely to occur at times when requirement for vitamin D is increased. These two deficiency states are differentiated solely on epiphyseal fusion. Rickets is a developmental disease of bone in children which manifests itself in defects in calcification which, if unchecked, can lead to skeletal deformities such as knock-knees, bow legs and curvature of the spine. The symptoms of rickets depend on the age at which vitamin D deficiency occurs.

Infantile rickets

At birth it presents as neonatal tetany and in infancy as craniotabes (unossified areas of the skull). Infants at risk include
1 Those born to vitamin D-deficient mothers.
2 Premature babies whose requirement is greater than that met by parenteral nutrition or breast milk.
3 Older babies given weaning foods with a low vitamin D content who are not given supplements or have little sunlight exposure.

Toddler rickets

Bow legs or knock-knees and 'rachitic rosary' (enlargement of the costochondral junction of the ribs) are classical signs. However, a milder form of rickets may be much more common and less easy to diagnose. This may be characterized by delays in mobility development (a child is slow to crawl, stand and walk), tooth eruption and closure of the anterior fontanelle.

Adolescent rickets

In older children, enlargement of the epiphysis at the lower end of the tibia, and later the femur and fibula, and chest deformities may be more apparent. Excessive head sweating and general irritability are also features of the disease. The growth spurt associated with puberty may precipitate this condition.

Osteomalacia

In the adult, the defective mineralization of the bone matrix (osteoid) is known as osteomalacia and can result in aching bone pain (often misdiagnosed as 'rheumatism', or even 'neurosis'). Muscular weakness caused by myopathy is common, and affects the proximal muscle groups. This may cause difficulty in rising from a chair, or climbing stairs. Spontaneous fractures, as distinct from the pseudofractures seen occasionally on X-ray, are uncommon. Blood tests may be normal, but the presence of a raised alkaline phosphatase of bone origin, or low plasma phosphate is suggestive. Plasma calcium concentrations are usually normal or only slightly reduced. In severe cases the presence of Looser's zones (pseudofractures) on X-ray, particularly of the long bones or pelvis, is diagnostic. In other patients the diagnosis can only be confirmed by bone biopsy. The essential histological criteria for osteomalacia are an increase in the volume and seam thickness of uncalcified bone (osteoid tissue), and reduction in calcification fronts at the surface of normal bone. These can be identified by the fluorescence caused by the antibiotic drug tetracycline, which is sometimes administered a day or two before bone biopsy for this purpose. In contrast to other bone diseases osteomalacia affects the whole skeleton, but the iliac crest is the most convenient site to biopsy.

Diagnosis

The classical clinical and radiological features of rickets and osteomalacia described above indicate an advanced state of vitamin D deficiency. Ideally the diagnosis should be made much earlier, but the early symptoms are often subtle and non-specific. However, the alert clinician should always consider the possibility in those groups now recognized as being at high risk of vitamin D deficiency. In such patients a history of muscle or bone aches, or proximal muscle weakness (easily tested by seeing if they are capable of rising from a squatting position) should indicate the need for appropriate blood tests. Plasma calcium is often normal, but in adults an elevated alkaline phosphatase (of bone origin), or low phosphate are strongly suggestive. The diagnosis can be confirmed by bone biopsy where radiology or biochemical testing is unhelpful.

Treatment

Primary deficiency

Simple nutritional rickets and osteomalacia usually respond rapidly to treatment with 2000–4000 i.u. of vitamin D daily. An oral supplement of calcium may help to restore the skeletal deficit more rapidly.

Secondary deficiency

Patients with osteomalacia caused by malabsorption syndromes may need large doses of vitamin D given by mouth. A gluten-free diet may restore 'sensitivity' to oral vitamin D in patients with coeliac disease, and vitamin D intoxication with hypercalcaemia may then occur. Alternatively, vitamin D may be administered by injection. This is usually recommended for patients with liver disease and chronic fat malabsorption due to prolonged obstructive jaundice.

Vitamin D-resistant osteomalacia, for example caused by chronic renal failure, requires very large doses of vitamin D (50,000–500,000 i.u. daily). Alternatively the active hormonal form of vitamin D (1,25 dihydroxy vitamin D), or synthetic analogues, may be used. In these patients the plasma calcium and alkaline phosphatase should be monitored carefully.

In all cases of secondary vitamin D deficiency, the underlying cause must be treated wherever possible.

Prevention

Effective prophylaxis may be achieved by the provision of vitamin D supplements to groups at risk of developing nutritional rickets or osteomalacia, in particular pregnant women (Brooke et al 1980). It may be helpful to encourage the use of foods rich in vitamin D such as margarine, butter, oily fish, milk, Ovaltine and fortified cereals. Emphasis on sunlight exposure is also important.

Health education measures should ensure that parents understand the importance of supplementation for children in at risk groups. Where anticonvulsant therapy is essential, concomitant vitamin D treatment should be considered.

References

Abraham R (1983) Ethnic and religious aspects of diet. In *Nutrition in pregnancy* pp 23–29. Royal College of Obstetricians and Gynaecologists, London.

Batchelor AJ and Compston JE (1983) Reduced plasma half life of radiolabelled 25 hydroxyvitamin D in subjects receiving a high fibre diet. *Br J Nutr* **49**, 213–6.

Beadle PC (1977) Sunlight, ozone and vitamin D. *Br J Dermatol* **97**, 585–91.

Brooke OG, Brown IRF, Bone CDM, Carter ND, Cleeve HJW, Maxwell JD, Robinson V and Winder SM (1980) Vitamin D supplements in pregnant Asian women: effects on calcium status and foetal growth. *Br Med J* **1**, 751–4.

Chick H, Dalyell EJ, Hume EM, Mackay HMM and Henderson Smith H (1923) Medical Research Council Special Report Series No 77 p 122. HMSO, London.

Challoner AVJ, Corless D, Davis A, Deane GHW, Diffey BL, Gupta SP and Magnus IA (1976) Personnel monitoring of exposure to ultraviolet radiation. *Clin Exp Dermatol* **1**, 175–9.

De Luca HF (1982) New developments in the vitamin D endocrine system. *J Am Diet Assoc* **80**, 231–6.

Dunnigan MG and Smith GM (1965) The aetiology of late rickets in Pakistani children in Glasgow. Report of a diet survey. *Scot Med J* **10**, 1–9.

Dunnigan MG, Childs WC, Smith CM (1975) The relative roles of ultraviolet deprivation and diet in the aetiology of Asian rickets. *Scott Med J* **20**, 217–8.

Dunnigan MG (1977) Asian rickets and osteomalacia in Britain. In *Child nutrition and its relation to mental and physical development* pp 43–70. Kellogg Company of Great Britain, Manchester.

Ford JA, Colhoun EM, McIntosh WB, Dunnigan MG (1972) Biochemical response of late rickets and osteomalacia to a chapatti-free diet. *Br Med J* **3**, 446–7.

Haddad JG and Hahn TJ (1973) Natural and synthetic sources of circulating 25 OHD in man. *Nature* **244**, 515–6.

Hess AF and Unger LJ (1917) Prophylactic therapy for rickets in a negro community. *J Am Med Assoc* **69**, 1583–6.

Hodkinson HM, Stanton BR, Round P and Morgan C (1973) Sunlight, vitamin D and osteomalacia in the elderly. *Lancet* **i**, 910–2.

Lawson DEM, Paul AA, Black AE, Cole TJ, Mande AR and Davie M (1979) Relative contributions of diet and sunlight to vitamin D state in the elderly. *Br Med J* **2**, 303–5.

Lawson DEM (1981) Dietary vitamin D: is it necessary? *J Hum Nutr* **35**, 61–3.

Marie PJ, Pettifor JM, Ross P and Glorieux FH (1982) Histological osteomalacia due to dietary calcium deficiency. *N Eng J Med* **307**, 584–8.

Mellanby E (1949) The rickets-producing and anti-calcifying action of phytate. *J Physiol Lond* **109**, 488–533.

Nayal AS, MacLennan WJ, Hamilton JC, Rose P and Kong M (1978) 25 hydroxy vitamin D and sunlight exposure in patients admitted to a geriatric unit. *Gerontology* **24**, 117–22.

Neer R, Clark M, Friedman V, Belsey R, Sweeney M, Buouchristiani J and Potts J (1977) Environmental and nutritional influences on plasma 25 hydroxy vitamin D concentration and calcium metabolism in man. In *Vitamin D: biochemical, chemical and clinical aspects related to calcium metabolism* Norman AW *et al* (Eds) p 595. Walter de Gruyter, Berlin.

O'Hara May J, Widdowson EM (1976) Diet and living conditions of Asian boys in Coventry with and without signs of rickets. *Br J Nutr* **36**, 23–36.

Poskitt EM, Cole T and Lawson DEM (1979) Diet, sunlight and 25 OHD in healthy children and adults. *Br Med J* **1**, 221–3.

Robertson I, Ford JA, McIntosh WB and Dunnigan MG (1981) The role of cereals in the aetiology of nutritional rickets: the lesson of the Irish National Nutrition Survey 1943–8. *Br J Nutr* **45**, 17–22.

Robertson I, Glekin BM, Henderson JB, McIntosh WB, Lakhani A and Dunnigan MG (1982) Nutritional deficiencies among ethnic minorities in the UK. *Proc Nutr Soc* **41**, (2), 243–56.

Sheltawy M, Newton H, Hay A, Morgan DB and Hullin RP (1984) The contribution of dietary vitamin D and sunlight to the plasma 25 OHD in the elderly. *Hum Nutr: Appl Nutr* **38C**, 191–4.

Stamp TCB (1975) Factors in human vitamin D nutrition and in the production and cure of classical rickets. *Proc Nutr Soc* **34**, 119–30.

Wills MR, Day RC, Phillips JB and Bateman EC (1972) Phytic acid and nutritional rickets in immigrants. *Lancet* **i**, 771–3.

4.27 Osteoporosis

Features and classification

In osteoporosis there is a decrease in bone mass; the bone is histologically normal, but each bone contains less osseous tissue. When the bone has become structurally weakened, fractures occur, frequently of the spinal vertebrae. Femoral neck fractures often occur about a decade later. Unless osteoporosis is secondary to some underlying disorder such as malabsorption or hyperthyroidism, a single aetiological factor is not found; the disorder is almost certainly multifactorial in origin (Heaney 1965). Osteoporosis may be classified by age

1 Juvenile. This can occur, rarely, in children aged about 8–15 years.
2 Young adult form. This is sometimes seen in pregnancy.
3 Postmenopausal (or Type I): This occurs predominantly in women who have passed normally through the menopause, or in oophorectomized women. It is characterized by accelerated and disproportionate loss of trabecular bone (Riggs and Melton 1983).
4 Senile (or Type II): This is characterized by a proportionate loss of both cortical and trabecular bone in the ageing process (Riggs and Melton 1983) and is commonly associated with fractures of the femoral neck and vertebrae in patients over the age of 75.

Juvenile osteoporosis

This is a very rare condition (Jowsey 1977). Where it is not secondary to leukaemia or Cushing's Syndrome, the disorder is of unknown origin and may remit spontaneously (Dent and Friedman 1965). There is no known effective form of treatment, but a restricted phosphorus intake or administration of small amounts of phosphate-binding agents have been recommended in cases which show no tendency to spontaneous remission (Jowsey and Johnson 1972). Sex hormones with dihydrotachysterol have been used with widely differing results (Dent and Friedman 1965).

Postmenopausal and senile osteoporosis

Most people lose bone steadily throughout adult life; peak bone mass is reached at around the age of 20–30 years. The rate of loss thereafter varies. In women the loss is accelerated for a few years after the menopause, thereafter probably slowing to the previous rate. Thus, since strength of the bones decreases in old age there is an increased tendency for fractures to occur, particularly of the spine, wrist and femur.

Dietary aetiology

There are several dietary factors which may be relevant to the development and progression of osteoporosis

Calcium intake. In Britain the recommended daily calcium intake for non-pregnant, non-lactating adults is 500 mg (DHSS 1979). In the USA the figure is 800 mg (NRC 1980). Recommendations are intended to be set at the level which is above the probable requirement of 90–95% of the population (Heaney *et al* 1982). Some recent work has questioned the adequacy of these levels. A review of published calcium balances of normal adults led Nordin *et al* (1979) to conclude that the recommended intake for adults should be nearer to 900 mg calcium. At a daily intake of 800 mg calcium a significant number of adults may be in negative calcium balance, and calcium balance may be significantly increased by the increase of calcium intake to 1200 mg (Spencer *et al* 1984). Calcium intakes greater than 1200 mg may not be beneficial as a plateau in balance is reached at this level. It has also been suggested that patients with osteoporosis are not able to absorb calcium from intakes greater than 1200 mg to the same extent as patients without osteoporosis (Spencer *et al* 1984).

At the time of the menopause or thereafter, calcium requirements may increase (Nordin *et al* 1979). Premenopausal and oestrogen-treated post-menopausal women may require an intake of around 1000 mg calcium daily to maintain zero calcium balance; in untreated post-menopausal women this requirement may be nearer 1500 mg (Heaney *et al* 1978). Perimenopausal women regularly consuming higher calcium intakes may be in more positive calcium balance than those on lower intakes (Heaney *et al* 1977).

Protein intake. There is some evidence that an increase of dietary protein as an isolated nutrient causes a proportional increase of urinary calcium. Since no change in calcium absorption or in endogenous faecal calcium excretion occurs, this may lead to a negative calcium balance (Licata *et al* 1981; Heaney *et al* 1982.) although this effect is disputed (Spencer *et al* 1978; Spencer *et al* 1983). However, phosphorus modifies the calciuric effect of high protein intakes, and foods which are high in protein are normally also high in phosphorus (Hegsted *et al* 1981). More work needs to be done on nutrient interactions which predispose to negative calcium balance. The evidence so far suggests that the net effect of protein intakes in excess of needs is reduced retention of absorbed calcium and therefore increased calcium requirement (Heaney and Recker 1982).

Sodium intake. It is known that the renal excretion of sodium and calcium are related. An infusion of calcium causes a temporary increase in urinary sodium excretion (Wills *et al* 1969). Similarly, sodium chloride loading causes an increase in urinary calcium excretion. This is accompanied by increased intestinal calcium absorption (Meyer *et al* 1976; Breslau *et al* 1982), through increased 1,25 dihydroxy vitamin D synthesis, probably mediated by parathyroid hormone (Breslau *et al* 1982). As a result of this adaptive process, net calcium balance does not change (Meyer *et al* 1976). However, Breslau *et al* hypothesize that on a high sodium diet, failure to adapt to increased renal calcium losses by increased intestinal calcium absorption may be a contributory factor to the bone disease of elderly osteoporotics and individuals with pseudohypoparathyroidism (Breslau *et al* 1982).

Fibre intake. A high dietary fibre intake may increase the faecal output of minerals, including calcium, and so tends to exacerbate negative calcium balance. However, whether this is significant in the long term is not yet known. Fibre intakes in Western diets are probably not as high as those in research studies, but some individuals may be at risk (Heaney *et al* 1982).

Lactase deficiency. In normal adults, lactose may enhance calcium absorption, but in subjects with intestinal lactase deficiency, calcium absorption is decreased in the presence of lactose (Condon *et al* 1970; Kocian *et al* 1973). Ingestion of lactose may therefore induce negative calcium balance in the long term, possibly predisposing individuals with alactasia to osteoporosis (Condon *et al* 1970). It has been suggested that post-menopausal women with osteoporosis have a high prevalence of lactose intolerance (Finkenstedt *et al* 1986). This, combined with a low consumption of milk and a subclinical disorder of glucose metabolism, is suggested to be a major factor in the development of idiopathic osteoporosis in women (Birge *et al* 1967). Other workers have failed to confirm a reduced calcium absorption from milk and yoghurt in lactase-deficient individuals. This may have been due to smaller, more physiological loads of lactose offered in the dairy products (Smith *et al* 1985). However, it seems prudent to ensure that lactose-intolerant individuals include plenty of low lactose, high calcium foods in the diet, or take calcium supplements.

Caffeine intake. Caffeine increases urinary calcium and sodium concentrations as well as urinary volume (Massey and Wise 1984). This may contribute to a more negative calcium balance, the significance of which is greater when combined with a low dietary calcium intake. The effect may be quite small at lower intakes of caffeine, but may be significant at extreme intakes (above 1g caffeine per day) (Heaney and Recker (1982). 1g caffeine would be obtained from about ten cups of percolated coffee or 15 cups of instant coffee daily, although this varies with brands and preparation methods (Bunker and McWilliams 1979).

Body weight and smoking. In women, Daniell (1976) noted a striking association between the early presence of osteoporosis and both cigarette smoking and lack of obesity in post-menopausal women. An association between low body weight and osteoporosis had already been noted, and it was suggested that fatty tissue may produce oestrogens in sufficient quantity to protect against the development of bone atrophy. Both smoking and low body weight tend to induce an earlier menopause which advances the development of osteoporosis by several years. However, more complex smoking-related phenomena other than an early menopause may be involved in this process.

Alcohol intake. Alcoholism accelerates bone loss, and in addition chronic alcoholics are likely to have a poor nutrient intake, adding to this risk factor. The likelihood of falls, predisposing to fractures, is also greater in alcoholics (WHO 1984).

In one study of post-menopausal women there was a three-fold increase in the incidence of alcoholism in women with fractures of the hip or distal radius compared with a control group without fractures (Hutchinson *et al* 1979).

Vitamin D intake. Vitamin D is essential for normal bone mineralization and metabolism, but there is little evidence that poor vitamin D status is causative in osteoporosis (WHO 1984).

Diet during immobilization. Prolonged bed rest leads to an increase in urinary and faecal calcium, with overall negative calcium balance and loss of bone mass. Reambulation will induce partial or complete remineralization of the skeleton (Donaldson *et al* 1970; Vogel and Whittle 1976). Supplementation with phosphate may ameliorate the negative calcium balance (Goldsmith *et al* 1969) although this effect may be only short term (Hulley *et al* 1971). Combined supplements of calcium and phosphate may also retard the development of disuse osteoporosis by making calcium balance less negative during immobilization (Hantman *et al* 1973).

Treatment of adult osteoporosis

Where osteoporosis is secondary to some other disorder such as malabsorption or hyperthyroidism, treatment is aimed at correction of the primary disorder, and the provision at the same time of an adequate calcium intake to enable the bones to heal. Where there is evidence of concomitant vitamin D deficiency, supplements should be given.

Adult osteoporosis is probably not a homogeneous disorder, and different sub-groups may respond to different treatments, but identification of these sub-groups is still in the research stage. In idiopathic, postmenopausal or senile osteoporosis it has been suggested that the first line of treatment should be the institution of a high calcium intake (Thalassinos *et al* 1982). Some short term reduction in bone loss has been reported with the administration of supplements of 1000 mg calcium daily (Horowitz *et al* 1984) and 800−1200 mg calcium daily (Nordin *et al* 1979). However, the evidence that sustained slowing of bone loss can be achieved in the long term by calcium supplementation alone is not conclusive (Heaney *et al* 1982).

Many of the current treatments for postmenopausal osteoporosis are still in the investigational or experimental stage. These proposed treatments have been reviewed by Chesnut (1981) and Milhaud *et al* (1983), and include

1 Non-hormonal
a) Sodium fluoride with or without calcium or vitamin D.
b) Diphosphonates.
2 Hormonal
a) Calcitonin.
b) Synthetic parathyroid hormone.
c) Oestrogen with or without gestagen.
d) Anabolic steroids.

Calcium balance studies may be used to monitor the progress of treatment (see metabolic balance diets, Section 5.6). The following factors should be noted when using this technique and interpreting the results

1 Level of activity. Immobilization leads to loss of calcium from the bones. During calcium balance studies patients should be encouraged to maintain their usual level of physical activity.
2 Weekly variations in calcium balance. There are week to week variations in calcium balance, both in normal subjects (Malm 1958) and in those with osteoporosis (Hesp *et al* 1979).
3 Annual variations in calcium balance. An annual cycle in calcium balance may occur in some subjects (Malm 1958).
4 Individual adaptation. Adaptation to the habitual diet may lead to a temporary negative balance if intake is reduced.

Prevention

Dietary aetiological risk factors for osteoporosis have been discussed above. The tendency for affluent Western societies to consume diets with a high protein and relatively low calcium content, combined with increasing fibre intakes, may predispose to negative calcium balance and to enhanced bone loss. Increased dietary calcium intake may help to balance this loss.

The preservation of mobility may also be an important factor in reducing the rate of bone loss.

Post-menopausally, calcium supplements may help to slow down the rate of bone loss, and if instituted early enough in subjects at risk, could slow down the advent of fractures. However, it is an important research objective to develop simple means to identify clearly those individuals at risk of developing clinical osteoporosis with eventual fractures. For these patients, combination therapy (an oestrogen with a sequential gestagen) may be the only effective preventive measure (Christiansen *et al* 1980).

Further reading

Exton-Smith AN (1976) The management of osteoporosis. *Proc Roy Soc Med* **69**, 931−4.

References

Birge SJ, Keutmann HT, Cuatrecasas P and Whedon G D (1967) Osteoporosis, intestinal lactase deficiency and low dietary calcium intake. *New Eng J Med* **276**, 445−8.

Breslau NA, McGuire J, Zerwekh JE and Pak CYC (1982) The role of dietary sodium on renal excretion and intestinal absorption of calcium and on vitamin D metabolism. *J Clin Endocrinol Metab* **55**, 369−73.

Bunker ML and McWilliams M (1979) Caffeine content of common beverages. *J Am Diet Assoc* **74**, 28−32.

Chesnut CH (1981) Treatment of post-menopausal osteoporosis: some current concepts. *Scot Med J* **26**, 72−80.

Christiansen C, Christiansen MS, McNair P, Hagen C, Stocklund K and Transbol IB (1980) Prevention of early post-menopausal bone loss: controlled two year study in 315 normal females. *Eur J Clin Invest* **10**, 273−9.

Condon JR, Nassium JR, Millard FJC, Hilbe A and Stainthorpe EM (1970) Calcium and phosphorus metabolism in relation to lactose intolerance. *Lancet* **i**, 1027−9.

Daniell HW (1976) Osteoporosis of the slender smoker. Vertebral compression fractures and loss of metacarpal cortex in relation to post-menopausal cigarette smoking and lack of obesity. *Arch Intern Med* **136**, 298−304.

Dent CE and Friedman M (1965) Idiopathic juvenile osteoporosis. *Quart J Med* **34**, 177−210.

Department of Health and Social Security (1979) *Recommended daily amounts of food energy and nutrients for groups of people in the United Kingdom.* Report on Public Health and Social Subjects No 15. HMSO, London.

Donaldson CL, Hulley SB, Vogel JM, Hattner RS, Bayers JH and McMillan DE (1970) Effect of prolonged bed rest on bone mineral. *Metabolism* **19**, 1071−84.

Finkenstedt G, Skrabal F, Gasser RW and Braunsteiner H (1986) Lactose absorption, milk consumption and fasting blood glucose concentrations in women with idiopathic osteoporosis. *Br Med J* **292**, 161−2.

Goldsmith RS, Killian P, Ingbar SH and Bass DE (1969) Effect of phosphate supplementation during immobilization of normal men. *Metabolism* **18**, 349−68.

Hantman DA, Vogel JM, Donaldson CL, Friedman R, Goldsmith RS and Hulley SB (1973) Attempts to prevent disuse osteoporosis by treatment with calcitonin, longitudinal compression and supplementary calcium and phosphate. *Clin Endocrinol Metab* **36**, 845−58.

Heaney RP (1965) A unified concept of osteoporosis. *Am J Med* **39**, 877−80.

Heaney RP, Recker RR and Saville PD (1977) Calcium balance and calcium requirements in middle aged women. *Am J Clin Nutr* **30**, 1603−11.

Heaney RP, Recker RR and Saville PD (1978) Menopausal changes in calcium balance performance. *J Lab Clin Med* **92**, 953−63.

Heaney RP, Gallagher JC, Johnston CC, Neer R, Parfitt AM, Chir B and Whedon GD (1982) Calcium nutrition and bone health in the elderly. *Am J Clin Nutr* **36**, 986−1013.

Heaney RP and Recker RR (1982) Effects of nitrogen, phosphorus and caffeine on calcium balance in women. *J Lab Clin Med* **99**, 46−55.

Hegsted M, Schuette SA, Zemel MB and Linkswiler HM (1981) Urinary calcium and calcium balance in young men as affected by level of protein and phosphorus intake. *J Nutr* **111**, 553−62.

Hesp R, Williams D, Rinsler M and Reeve J (1979) A comparison of chromium sesquioxide and [^{51}Cr] chromic chloride as inert markers in calcium balance studies. *Clin Sci* **57**, 89−92.

Horowitz M, Need AG, Philcox JC and Nordin BEC (1984) Effect of calcium supplementation on urinary hydroxyproline in osteoporotic post-menopausal women. *Am J Clin Nutr* **39**, 857−9.

Hulley SB, Vogel JM, Donaldson CL, Bayers JH, Friedman RJ and Rosen SN (1971) The effect of supplemental oral phosphate on the bone mineral changes during prolonged bed rest. *J Clin Invest* **50**, 2506−18.

Hutchinson TA, Polansky SM and Feinstein AL (1979) Post-menopausal oestrogens protect against fractures of hip and distal radius. A case-control study. *Lancet* **ii**, 705−9.

Jowsey J (1977) *Metabolic diseases of bone.* WB Saunders Company,

Jowsey J and Johnson KA (1972) Juvenile osteoporosis: bone findings in seven patients. *J Paediatr* **81**, 511−7.

Kocian J, Skala I and Bakos K (1973) Calcium absorption from milk and lactose-free milk in healthy subjects and patients with lactose intolerance. *Digestion* **9**, 317−24.

Licata AA, Bou E, Bartter FC and West F (1981) Acute effects of dietary protein on calcium metabolism in patients with osteoporosis. *J Gerontol* **36**, 14−9.

Malm OJ (1958) Calcium requirement and adaptation in adult man. *Scand J Clin Lab Invest* **10**, [Suppl 36], 1−290.

Massey LK and Wise KJ (1984) The effect of dietary caffeine on urinary excretion of calcium, magnesium, sodium and potassium in healthy young females. *Nutr Res* **4**, 43−50.

Meyer WJ III, Transbol I, Bartter FC and Delea C (1976) Control of calcium absorption: effect of sodium chloride loading and depletion. *Metabolism* **25**, 989−93.

Milhaud G, Christiansen C, Gallagher C, Reeve J, Seeman E, Chesnut C and Parfitt A (1983) Pathogenesis and treatment of post-menopausal osteoporosis. *Calcif Tissue Int* **35**, 708−11.

National Research Council (1980) *Recommended dietary allowances* 9e. Food and Nutrition Board, National Academy of Sciences NAS/NRC, Washington DC.

Nordin BEC, Horsman A, Marshall DH, Simpson M and Waterhouse GM (1979) Calcium requirement and calcium therapy. *Clin Orthop* **140**, 216−46.

Riggs BL and Melton LJ (1983) Evidence for two distinct syndromes of involutional osteoporosis. *Am J Med* **75**, 899−01.

Smith TM, Kolars JC, Savaiano DA and Levitt MD (1985) Absorption of calcium from milk and yoghurt. *Am J Clin Nutr* **42**, 1197−200.

Spencer H, Kramer L, Osis D and Norris C (1978) Effect of a high protein (meat) intake on calcium metabolism in man. *Am J Clin Nutr* **31**, 2167−80.

Spencer H, Kramer L, De Bartolo M, Norris C and Osis D (1983) Further studies on the effect of a high protein diet as meat on calcium metabolism. *Am J Clin Nutr* **37**, 924−9.

Spencer H, Kramer L, Lesniak M, DeBartolo M, Norris C and Osis D (1984) Calcium requirements in humans. *Clin Orthop* **184**, 270−80.

Thalassinos NC, Gutteridge DH, Joplin GF and Frazer TR (1982) Calcium balance in osteoporotic patients on long term oral calcium therapy with and without sex hormones. *Clin Sci* **62**, 221−6.

Vogel JM and Whittle MW (1976) Bone mineral content changes in the skylab astronauts. *Am J Roentgenology Radium Ther Nucl Med* **126**, 1296−7.

Wills MR, Gill JR and Bartter FC (1969) The interrelationships of calcium and sodium excretions. *Clin Sci* **37**, 621−30.

World Health Organisation (1984) *Prevention of osteoporosis.* A Nutrition/Public Health Concern Report on a WHO meeting Gothenberg, November 1984. WHO, Geneva.

4.28 Arthritis

4.28.1 Rheumatoid arthritis

Rheumatoid arthritis is the most common type of inflammatory arthritis. It affects 1:100 of the population and women more often than men.

Rheumatoid arthritis is usually a problem of middle or old age but can occur in children. The cause is not known. Conventional treatment is aimed at reducing pain, inflammation and stiffness and also attempts to prevent potential deformities. It includes physiotherapy, drug therapy (such as steroids, gold and aspirin) and surgery.

Diet therapy is an area of controversy. Dietary manipulation has been part of the folklore of rheumatoid management for decades and there is evidence that many patients alter their diets and claim relief from their symptoms by doing so (Darlington 1985). None of these dietary measures has been scientifically proved to be of benefit, although some warrant further investigation. In recent years there have been a number of claims, largely unsubstantiated, of an association between food 'allergy' and rheumatoid arthritis. There is some evidence that, in certain cases, some foods may exacerbate the symptoms of rheumatoid arthritis and that symptom relief can be obtained by their avoidance (Parke and Hughes 1981; Darlington 1985). The reason for such an association, if it exists, is not entirely clear. Although acute joint inflammation is a common feature of food intolerance, this is not necessarily relevant to the aetiology of the chronic forms of joint disease such as rheumatoid arthritis. It is perhaps more likely that any food intolerance is a *result of* the rheumatoid arthritis and the disordered immune system characteristic of the disease. Nevertheless, whether causal, consequential or even non-existent, it is an area which merits investigation and some rheumatologists may well refer patients with food-related symptoms to a dietitian for advice on exclusion diets.

However, dietitians are perhaps more likely to encounter patients with rheumatoid arthritis when they are referred for some other unrelated disorder. Dietitians should bear in mind that some of these patients may have put themselves on diets of dubious value and nutritional content. Tactful enquiries should therefore be made as to the nature of any self-imposed regimen so that any likely nutritional deficiencies (particularly in vulnerable groups such as the elderly) can be rectified.

Some of the diets commonly used to treat arthritis (not necessarily with any scientific support or medical approval) are outlined below.

Diets used in the treatment of arthritis

Elimination diets (see Section 5.9)

Where there is a convincing history of food-related symptoms a simple exclusion diet removing the food in question (e.g. citrus fruit) may be tried. If multiple food allergies are suspected, a stepwise elimination diet may be required.

Other diets

The Eskimo diet. This evolved from a study by Kremer *et al* (1985) where dietary fatty acids were manipulated. The diet was low in dairy produce (saturated fats) and high in polyunsaturated fats with an additional eicosapentaenoic acid supplement. Kremer reported clinical improvement on this diet.

Fish diet. The most commonly used diet for arthritis is that advocated by Dr Colin Dong. The diet is based on fish 'and the traditional Chinese diet', the rationale being that the Chinese have a very low incidence of rheumatoid arthritis. Although widely claimed to be beneficial, Panush *et al* (1983) failed to find evidence supporting clinical benefits of the diet.

Acid-reducing diets. These regimens are based on the idea that 'acids' produced in the body during digestion and metabolism, in particular oxalic and uric acids, cause arthritis. There is little evidence to support this hypothesis.

Health food and 'cleansing' diets. These have been developed on the basis that 'toxins' in the modern day diet cause arthritis. Typical advice is to eat wholegrain cereals and green leafy vegetables and avoid white sugar (but muscavado sugar can be used). The diet is often preceded by a 'cleansing' or 'purifying' regimen to get rid of the 'toxins' in the body. The only proof of benefit of these diets is anecdotal.

Supplements. Certain books on 'diets for arthritis' include advice on taking dietary supplement such as ascorbic acid or cod liver oil, sometimes in dangerously large doses.

Complications of rheumatoid arthritis

Steroid-induced diabetes and obesity

Steroids are commonly used in the treatment of rheumatoid arthritis and some people develop diabetes or obesity as a side effect. Conventional dietary advice should be given for these conditions.

Anaemia

This is a common complication of rheumatoid arthritis and may be aggravated by the avoidance of red meat (a common action) and the use of drugs, such as aspirin, which have a tendency to cause gastrointestinal bleeding.

4.28.2 Osteoarthritis

This is a degenerative joint disease also known as hypertrophic arthritis. It is a chronic disorder marked by degeneration of articular cartilage and hypertrophy of bone. It is accompanied by pain which appears with activity and subsides with rest. It tends to occur in middle age and the elderly.

Aetiology

The whole joint is normally involved, however the condition starts in the articular cartilage. Osteoarthritis takes years to become manifest and hence is more common after middle age. Biochemical changes in bone do occur with age, but the ageing process alone does not cause osteoarthritis. The essential factor is a discrepancy between the strength of the cartilage and the force to which it is subjected. Articular cartilage distributes the stress passing across a joint, thus spreading the load. If the load is too great, cartilage gives way; or if the load is normal, cartilage gives way if it has been weakened by damage or disease, or if it is unsupported by normal bone (Solomon 1976).

There are no known dietary factors involved in this condition but it is reasonable to regard all osteoarthritis as secondary to a cause which diligence will discover, such as a necrosis due to fracture and infection or other disorders such as Paget's disease (Apley 1984).

Rheumatoid arthritis is the most common inflammatory cause of weakened articular cartilage. There may be some congenital deformities as well as those which occur with repeated minor injuries in certain occupations or sports, for example, recurrent subluxation of the patella at the elbow with javelin throwing.

Treatment

There is as yet no form of treatment leading to a cure. Management is comprised chiefly of analgesics for pain or warmth from hot-water bottles, liniments, massage and radiant heat.

Obesity increases the load on the cartilage and should be treated and discouraged.

Activity may be modified and assisted by, for example, using a walking stick to reduce stress or a raised heel to permit walking without forcing the hip. Surgery is carried out as a last resort.

Occupational therapy and physiotherapy are usually recommended for rehabilitation.

Support organisation

British Rheumatism and Arthritis Association, 6 Grosvenor Crescent, London SW1X 7ER.

Further reading

Community Nutrition Group of the British Dietetic Association (1986) *Diet and arthritis.* Nutrition Group Information Sheet.
Swinson DR and Swinburn WR (1980) *Rheumatology.* Unibooks,
Wright V and Haslock I *Rheumatism for nurses and remedial therapist.* William Heinemann Medical Books Ltd, London.

References

Apley GA (1984) *System of orthopaedics and fractures.* Butterworth, London.
Darlington LG (1985) Does food intolerance have any role in the aetiology and management of rheumatoid disease? *Ann Rheum Dis* **44**, 801–4.
Dong C *New hope for the arthritic*
Kremer JM, Michalek AV, Lininger L, et al (1985) Effects of manipulation of dietary fatty acids on clinical manifestation of rheumatoid arthritis. *Lancet* i, 184–7.
Parke AL and Hughes GRV (1981) Rheumatoid arthritis and food: a case study. *Br Med J* **282**, 2027–9.
Panush RS, Carter RL, Katz P, Kowsari B, Kowsari B, Longley S, Finnie S (1983) Diet therapy for rheumatoid arthritis. *Arth Rheum* **26**, 462–71.
Solomon L (1976) Patterns of osteoarthritis of the hip. *J Bone Joint Surg* **58**, (2), 176–83.

4.29   Fractures

There are two types of fracture; they are either traumatic, caused by an accident, or pathological, caused by an underlying disease.

Traumatic fractures

Traumatic fractures are usually treated with mechanical support together with analgesics for pain relief. Early mobilization is normally recommended to prevent bone loss and muscle wastage. Pathological fractures require treatment of the underlying disease as well as of the fracture itself.

Pathological fractures

Aetiology

Osteoporosis (see also Section 4.27). Osteoporosis probably accounts for the majority of pathological fractures.

All individuals over a certain age have a degree of bone loss from the skeleton, involving both matrix and mineral. Formerly this was considered to be mainly a post-menopausal loss, largely confined to women over the age of 60 years. However, bone loss may start as early as the age of 21 (Trotter and Peterson 1955), and Gran (1970) has suggested that significant losses may have occurred by the age of 40. This resorption will continue and even increase during periods of diminished dietary nutrient intake, and this will inevitably lead to a reduction in bone mass (Newton-John and Morgan 1968) and an increase in the fracture rate. The changes which contribute to fracture occur over many years and to a varying extent in different bones.

The symptoms of a fracture will depend on the bone involved. Vertebral compression, common in osteoporosis, is associated with height loss with each compression and with localized severe pain. This may be periodic until the underlying pathology is treated.

Osteomalacia and rickets.   Osteomalacia and rickets may also result in fractures (Wootton *et al* 1979; Parfitt *et al* 1982). Fractures may occur through Looser's Zones, especially in tubular bones and the femoral neck (Gran 1975).

Other bone disorders.   Fractures may be an extension of microfractures as found in Paget's disease. In severe osteogenesis imperfecta, fractures may occur very easily with only slight pain.

Drugs.   Some drugs (e.g. anticonvulsants) may also make fractures more likely (Muckle 1976).

Treatment

The aim is to produce a positive calcium balance. This may be achieved by either one or a combination of the following preparations

1   Oral calcium, i.e. Ossopan or Sandocal, plus fluoride.
2   Vitamin D or its metabolites.
3   Calcitonin.
4   Anabolic steroids.
5   Biologically active fragments of parathyroid hormone.
6   Intermittent hypercalcaemic infusion.

Healing should start before surgery is attempted in cases of osteomalacia.

Further reading

Brereton PJ, Clark MB, Hesp R, Hodkinson HM, Klenerman L, Reeve J, Slavin G and Tellez-Yudilevich M Wootton R (1979) Fractured neck of femur in the elderly: an attempt to identify patients at risk. *Clin Sci* **57**, 93–101.
Vaughan J (1975) *Physiology of bone.* Clarendon Press, Oxford.

References

Gran SM (1970) *The earlier gain and the latter loss of cortical bone.* Thomas CC, Springfield, Illinois.
Gran SM (1975) Bone loss and ageing. In *The physiology and pathology of human ageing.* Academic Press, London.
Muckle DS (1976) Iatrogenic factors in femoral neck fractures. *Injury* **8**, 18–101.
Newton-John JF and Morgan DB (1970) The loss of bone with age, osteoporosis and fractures. *Clin Orthop* **71**, 229–52.
Parfitt AM, Gallagher JC, Heaney RP, Johnston CC, Neer R and Whedon GD (1982) Vitamin D and bone health in the elderly. *Am J Clin Nutr* **36**, 1014–31.
Trotter M and Peterson RR (1955) *Anat Rec* 123–341.

H: Disorders of the Skin

4.30   Atopic Eczema (Infantile Eczema, Dermatitis)

Eczema is one of several atopic diseases, including asthma, allergic rhinitis, allergic conjunctivitis and urticaria. Those affected commonly have a genetic predisposition to develop hypersensitivity to foreign proteins and other macromolecules.

Symptoms

Symptoms are a reddening of the skin (erythema), accompanied by itching, scratching and rubbing. Characteristic sites are the flexures, face, wrists, hands and legs, but lesions can occur anywhere. In most cases there is a varying degree of thickening of the skin and scaliness, described as either icthyosis or xeroderma. Many children with atopic eczema also have urticaria and eventually develop asthma and allergic rhinitis. Some have unexplained short stature.

Onset and course of the disease

The onset of atopic eczema can be at any time, but it is most common before the age of six months. The disease fluctuates in its severity and there is a general trend towards spontaneous improvement (Atherton 1982). However, the disease persists beyond early childhood in around 5% of cases, and for those who are severely affected, it can be a major handicap, physically and socially. Constant itching elicits scratching, which breaks the surface of the skin, causing bleeding and weeping of serous fluid. Infection is common, principally with streptococci, staphylococci, or the virus herpes simplex. Children acquire nicknames, most commonly 'scabby'. Passers-by in the street often mistake eczema for burns.

The itching and discomfort lead to countless nights without sleep for both the patient and parents, causing disruption to family life, tension and argument. Unsympathetic medical advice has been known to drive desperate parents to seek bizarre and scientifically unsound or dangerous treatment for their children (David 1985).

Treatment

Non-dietary measures which will improve symptoms and thus the quality of life for the patient, include the application of emollients and weak topical corticosteroids. The former are applied very liberally to the skin, as a means of keeping it moist, supple and unbroken. Infections are treated with topical antiseptics, or systemic antibiotics. Wool or man-made fibres in bedlinen and clothing often have to be avoided, being replaced by pure cotton. Biological washing powders are best avoided.

House-dust mite control measures, including removal of all fluffy toys, will help to improve symptoms for those who are sensitive to house-dust mite. Finger nails need to be kept short by filing in order to reduce damage from scratching.

Dietary exclusion is part of the treatment for a minority of difficult cases. For those in whom dietary exclusion is necessary, the treatment will be incomplete, unless accompanied by all the above-mentioned measures.

All exclusion diets are difficult to implement and are often highly restrictive. It is always necessary to consider whether the diet is worse than the disease.

Dietary treatment

A careful and detailed history is essential. It will help to pinpoint individual foods to which the patient reacts. There are no reliable investigations, skin tests or blood tests which will diagnose food allergy with any accuracy or predict allergy to single foods (David 1983; Cant 1985). The dietary treatment of atopic eczema ranges from simple exclusion of a single food, or a small number of foods, to the complete elimination of all foods, with nutritional intake maintained by an elemental formula, and followed by the reintroduction of foods one at a time. The prescription of a dietary regimen is a co-operative venture between clinician, dietitian, and patient or the patient's parents.

Simple exclusion. Dietary exclusion of cows' milk and eggs is advocated as a first step by some (Atherton *et al* 1978; Warner and Hathaway 1983), while others additionally exclude chicken, azo dyes and benzoate preservatives (Atherton 1985). (Details of exclusion diets are given in Section 5.9 and 2.11) The patient must be seen by a dietitian who will take a comprehensive and detailed diet history in order to ascertain how the current diet needs to be altered. A diet sheet should be provided detailing the exclusions and emphasizing those foods which are permitted. For infants and children up to five years of age, a properly formulated milk substitute is essential, as whole cows' milk normally provides a major part of a child's intake of energy and protein, as well as other nutrients, especially calcium (Francis 1980). If the clinician has not already prescribed a cows' milk substitute, the dietitian should contact him/her in order to ascertain whether there is a reason for this. It should be recognised that infants will, with persuasion, take more readily to a milk substitute than will an older child who is used to the taste of cows' milk. Parents should be encouraged to report a child's refusal to drink the milk substitute, so that a calcium and vitamin supplement can be prescribed.

Further exclusions.   If the simple elimination diet fails to produce an improvement in the patient's eczema during a trial period of not less than two weeks (Warner and Hathaway 1983) and, ideally, eight weeks (Atherton 1982), compliance with the prescribed exclusion should be checked by a dietitian, and maintenance of topical treatment and other measures should be reviewed by the clinician. If all appears to be in order, trial of a more rigorous diet may be attempted. Careful consideration should be given to whether the family of the affected patient or child will be able to cope with the disruption of routine caused by a major revision of the eating habits of one person. The food choice of the whole family may have to change to fit in more easily with the constraints of the diet. Families relying heavily on processed or convenience foods may find the diet more difficult than continuing to live with the eczema. If the diet history indicates that this is a possibility, the dietitian should bring it to the attention of the clinician.

Diets may be prescribed individually on the basis already described, or a patient may be assigned to a standard diet which eliminates a large number of common allergens or potentially provocative foods. Table 4.60 gives examples of such diets. Again, each patient should be seen by a dietitian who will explain how the diet may be best adhered to in the light of food preferences or meal pattern. A diet sheet must be provided for the patient. These multiple exclusion diets will probably include a milk substitute for the child under five years of age. After six weeks on such a diet a review will establish whether the diet has produced an improvement in the eczema and whether the improvement justifies the trouble taken over the diet. If the diet has not proved beneficial, then it may be abandoned, or eliminated foods may be reintroduced one

Table 4.60 Examples of multiple exclusion diets

Morgan (1980)	Warner and Hathaway (1983)	Graham et al (1984)	Price (1984)
To be avoided Milk, cheese and egg	*To be avoided* Dairy products (milk) and eggs	*To be avoided* Milk, cheese and egg	*To be avoided* Milk, milk products and eggs
Pork, bacon, liver, all offal, fish and shellfish	Pork, offal, fish and shellfish	Pork, bacon, offal, fish and shellfish	Chicken
Nuts and pips	Nuts	Nuts and pips	
Fruit	Fruit (except rhubarb and bananas)	Fruit	
Yeast Onions and garlic Honey Chewing gum	Vegetables Alcohol Herbs and spices	Yeasts Honey Sweets Gravy powder	Colouring in manufactured foods Coloured drinks, sweets, jellies and instant puddings. All foods with colouring added, e.g. sausages, tinned fish, soups, baked beans and flavoured crisps.
Allowed Carnation milk, tea, instant coffee, sugar, treacle, syrup, salt, butter, lard, beef, lamb, rabbit, green leafy vegetables, celery, lettuce, carrot, potatoes, mushrooms, bread, pastry, cakes and biscuits.			

Table 4.61 Examples of oligo allergenic diets

Morgan (1980)	Warner and Hathaway (1983)	Graham et al (1984)	Atherton (1985)
Food allowed	*Food allowed*	*Food allowed*	*Food allowed*
Lamb	Lamb or rabbit	Lamb	Turkey or rabbit
Sago	Sago	Sago flour	Sago or rice or potato
Fresh green leafy vegetables, carrots, celery and lettuce.	Cabbage, carrots, celery, lettuce and fresh rhubarb.	Fresh green vegetables, celery and rhubarb.	Cabbage or carrot or leek. Rhubarb or stewed apple.
Sugar, treacle and syrup.	Sugar, treacle and syrup.		
Water and tea	Water and tea (without milk)	Water and plain tea	
Salt	Tomor margarine	Kosher margarine	Tomor margarine, calcium, vitamins and sunflower seed oil.

at a time, or, a yet more rigorous diet may be attempted. If the diet is to continue, a diet survey should be conducted by the dietitian in order to monitor compliance and as a check on nutritional intake. Results should be forwarded to the clinician together with comments and recommendations for dietary modification or the prescription of vitamin and mineral supplements (David *et al* 1984). Although a diet may be theoretically adequate, individual food preference may well affect the nutritional intake.

An alternative course is to choose a diet consisting of a few rarely implicated or uncommon foods, a so-called oligo-allergenic diet (see also Section 5.9). Usually this consists of a meat protein food, a starchy food, a vegetable and a fat. For children under the age of five years, a milk substitute is again essential in the long term as they are unlikely to be able to eat sufficient bulk of the permitted foods to satisfy energy and other nutritional requirements. Examples of oligo-allergenic diets used in the treatment of eczema are shown in Table 4.61.

Complete withdrawal of food/elemental formula diets. For the most difficult cases, or when there is a long history of treatment as already outlined, with little or no improvement in the condition, as a last resort it may be worth considering complete withdrawal of all food. It is, of course, necessary to maintain an adequate nutritional intake and this may be attempted using an elemental formula such as those listed in Table 4.62

This procedure must only be undertaken during a hospital admission. It is hazardous, still experimental at present, and entails an eight to ten week residence in hospital for patient and parents.

Several authors give details of the use of Vivonex (Norwich-Eaton) as the elemental formula in the treatment of severe eczema (Hill and Lynch 1982; David

Table 4.62 Elemental formulae used in the treatment of eczema

Product	Manufacturer
Elemental feed 028A	Scientific Hospital Supplies
Flexical	Bristol-Myers
Nutranel	Casenne
Vivonex	Norwich Eaton
Vivonex HN	Norwich Eaton

Compositional data on these products can be found in Section 1.12 (Enteral feeding) p 77.

1983). There is no published description of the use of other elemental formulae although they may be suitable. Manufacturers' instructions regarding introduction, concentrations and quantities required should be followed.

As an example of an elemental formula, Vivonex is unsuitable for use in infants as it lacks the amino acid cystine. At full strength (32 g/100 ml water) it is hyperosmolar, 560 mosmol/kg, and teenagers and adults usually tolerate this concentration, provided that it is approached gradually over a number of days. However, experience shows that it is likely to cause osmotic diarrhoea in children under the age of five years, and it should be given at a lower concentration, 8 g/100 ml water, equivalent to 140 mosmol/kg, which is then increased over three days to 16 g/100 ml water, equivalent to 280 mosmol/kg. Children between the ages of five and ten years may tolerate concentrations greater than 16 g/100 ml, and a maximum concentration for each patient may be decided by trial and error.

The volume of formula given to the patient should be based on fluid requirement for age and weight. No flavouring should be added, and the initial use of low concentrations may help the patients become used to its unpleasant taste, but they may take up to a week to do so. Vivonex may be taken from a feeding bottle with a teat, from a covered feeding cup, or from a covered beaker with a straw, to suit the patient's age and preference. It may also be frozen and taken as 'ice lollies', or crushed and eaten with a spoon. The poor palatability of an unflavoured elemental formula may result in a child receiving less than the required amounts of energy and nutrients. However, no attempt should be made to force a particular volume on a patient with the aim of maximizing intake. Each child should be allowed to take as much or as little as they desire. No alternative drinks should be permitted, not even water, as it tastes better than an elemental formula and will be taken in preference. No toothpaste should be permitted, patients must use water to clean their teeth. All drugs should be taken as capsules or tablets. Capsules should be opened so that only their contents are administered, and any surface colour should be removed from tablets by washing under running water.

Although 5–20 days has been given as the limited period for trial of an elemental diet (Goldsborough and Francis 1983), 3–4 weeks or more is usually required for extensive resolution of eczema to occur (David 1983). Daily consumption charts should be used to check the intake of formula. Weight should be recorded on alternate days, and it is essential that serum electrolytes and protein are closely monitored. However, efforts must be made to draw the attention of parents away from their child's nutritional intake, which clinician and dietitian should realize may well be inadequate in the short term.

Experienced clinical judgement must decide the degree of improvement obtained from a trial of the elemental regimen. If the eczema has not improved significantly, the diet should be abandoned and a moderately restricted or normal diet resumed. If improvement has occurred single foods should be reintroduced following the pattern of an oligo-allergenic diet (see Table 4.61) The choice of food will depend not only on the previous history of foods known to exacerbate the eczema, but also on the patient's food preference. It is pointless, for example, to suggest the introduction of cabbage to the diet if the patient dislikes it. Foods should be introduced singly, and at intervals of 5–7 days, and if the eczema worsens during that period, the food is withdrawn, and then, when the skin has improved again, another food can be introduced.

If the first food to be introduced is a meat, for example lamb, it will need to be presented in large quantities. A child may have an apparently unlimited appetite for a food after several weeks on an elemental formula. There·should be close liaison between dietit-

ian and catering officer, who will need to understand the reason for the ordering of large quantities of meat for a single patient. However, in order to avoid boredom after a few days, it should also be presented in a variety of different ways to retain a child's interest. Lamb may be roasted and sliced, stewed, or served as chops. Minced, it may be turned into burgers, sausages or animal shapes. Lamb fat should be collected and retained for use in frying and roasting of foods to be added to the diet later. In order to achieve this and to avoid mistakes which can cause a setback to the treatment, it is essential to have a diet bay with a competent and co-operative diet cook who understands the reasoning behind the apparently bizarre meals being provided.

Once the patient is on a diet of four or five foods the Vivonex may be replaced by a casein hydrolysate formula, e.g. Pregestimil, prior to discharge. A programme should be devised of foods to be introduced and tried at home, singly and at weekly intervals. While the diet consists of only a small number of foods, diet surveys and estimates of nutritional intake are necessary from time to time, and serious inadequacies should be corrected (David et al 1984).

Support organisation

The National Eczema Society, Tavistock House North, Tavistock Square, London WC1H 9SR.

Further reading

Atherton DJ (1983) *Your child with eczema — a guide for parents.* Heinemann Medical Publishers Ltd, London.
MacKie R (1983) *Eczema and dermatitis — how to cope with inflamed skin.* Martin Dunitz Ltd, London.
Workman E, Hunter J and Jones VA (1984) *The allergy diet — how to overcome your food intolerance.* Martin Dunitz Ltd, London.

References

Atherton DJ, Sewell M, Soothill JF, Wells RS and Chilvers CED (1978) A double blind crossover trial of an antigen avoidance diet in atopic eczema. *Lancet* i, 401–3.
Atherton DJ (1982) Atopic eczema. In *Clinics in immunology and allergy 2, 1,* 77 Brostoff J and Challacombe SJ (Eds). W B Saunders Co Ltd, Eastbourne.
Atherton DJ (1985) Skin disorders and food allergy. In Food allergy in childhood. David TJ and Dinwiddie R (Eds). *J Roy Soc Med* [Suppl] (5), **78**, 7.
Cant AJ (1985) Food allergy in childhood. *Hum Nutr: Appl Nutr* **39A**, 277–93.
David TJ (1983) The investigation and treatment of severe childhood eczema. *Int Med* [Suppl] **6**, 19.
David TJ, Waddington Er and Stanton RHJ (1984) Nutritional hazards of elimination diets in children with atopic eczema. *Arch Dis Childh* **59**, (4), 323–5.

David TJ (1985) The overworked or fraudulent diagnosis of food allergy and food intolerance in children. In Food allergy in childhood David TJ and Dinwiddie R (Eds). *J Roy Soc Med* [Suppl] (5), **78**, 21.

Francis DEM (1980) Dietary management. In *Proceedings of the First Food Allergy Workshop* pp 85−93. MES Ltd, Oxford.

Goldsborough J and Francis DEM (1983) Dietary management. In *Proceedings of the Second Fisons Food Allergy Workshop*. MES Ltd, Oxford.

Graham P, Hall-Smith SP, Harris JR and Price ML (1984) A study of hypo allergenic diets and oral sodium cromoglycate in the management of atopic eczema. *Br. J Dermatol* **110**, 457−67.

Hill DJ and Lynch BC (1982) Elemental diet in the management of severe eczema in childhood. *Clin Allergy* **12**, 313−5.

Morgan JE (1980) In *Proceedings of the First Food Allergy Workshop* pp 93−4. MES Ltd, Oxford.

Price ML (1984) The role of diet in the management of atopic eczema. *Hum Nutr: Appl Nutr* **38A**, 409−15.

Warner JO and Hathaway MJ (1983) Dietary treatment of eczema due to food intolerance. In *Proceedings of the Second Fisons Food Allergy Workshop* pp 105−8. MES Ltd, Oxford.

4.31 Urticaria (Nettle Rash)

Symptoms

Urticaria is an eruption on the skin of erythematous (red) and oedematous patches which may appear on any part of the body. The affected skin usually itches, and the episode may last from minutes (acute urticaria) to years (chronic urticaria).

Aetiology

In a large proportion of cases, no cause can be found. The most common triggers are viral infections, and foodstuffs — azo dyes, benzoate preservatives, salicylates, foods naturally containing salicylates, various other foods, some containing high levels of histamine, yeasts or foods containing yeasts, have all been implicated in the provocation of urticaria, and are listed in Table 4.63.

Urticarial reactions may occur in children on contact with the food, in particular on the fingers, face or lips. Among adults, urticaria may be seen on the hands of those whose jobs involve the handling of foods.

Table 4.63 Foods and food constituents implicated in the causation of urticaria

Food additives	*Azo dyes* Tartrazine (E102) Amaranth (E123) Ponceau 4R/New Coccine (E124) Sunset Yellow (E110) *Preservatives* Benzoic Acid (E210) Sodium Benzoate (E211) Sodium Hydroxybenzoate 4-Hydroxy Benzoic Acid
Salicylate-containing foods	Apples, blueberries, beer, cider, grapes, liquorice, peas, plums, prunes (and jam), raspberries (and jam), red wine, sherry, rhubarb
Other foods and yeast products	Milk, egg, nuts, fruits, cheese, fish, shellfish, pork, mutton, aldehydes in fried foods, gluten/wheat, menthol, brewer's yeast, marmite (yeast extract), yeast tablets, bread, rice, wines, beer, sausages

Treatment

Many who have suffered an urticarial reaction to a food may never need to see a clinician in order to confirm the relationship between contact or ingestion and reaction. On taking a careful history the relationship may appear obvious, and no further advice is necessary other than to avoid the culprit food (Atherton 1985).

For chronic urticaria where no obvious relationship is manifest, a trial of an azo dye and preservative-free diet may be worthwhile (see Section 2.10; 2.15 and Section 5.9). If no improvement occurs, a diet diary may help to pinpoint the cause, relating the occurrence of symptoms to food ingestion. The suspect food or foods can then be eliminated. If a diet is prescribed involving the exclusion of more than one or two important foods, the patient should be seen by a dietitian. A detailed diet history will show when the implicated foods are taken and how they can be avoided. In cases of multiple exclusion, a diet sheet individually produced for each patient may be necessary (see Section 5.9).

Further reading

Denner WHB (1984) Colourings and preservatives in food. *Hum Nutr: Appl Nutr* **38A**, (6), 435–49.

Supramaniam G and Warner JO (1986) Artificial food additive intolerance in patients with angioedema and urticaria. *Lancet* **ii**, 907.

Suitable reading for patients

Hanssen M (1984) *E for additives*. Thorsons Publishers, Wellingborough.

Ministry of Agriculture, Fisheries and Food (1982) *Look at the label*. HMSO, London.

Workman E, Hunter J and Jones VA (1984) *The allergy diet: how to overcome your food intolerance*. Martin Dunitz, London.

References

Atherton DJ (1985) Skin disorders and food allergy. In Food allergy in childhood David TJ and Dinwiddie R (Eds). *J Roy Soc Med* [Suppl] (5) **78**, 7.

August PJ (1980) Urticaria. In *Proceedings of the First Food Allergy Workshop* pp 76–81. MES Ltd, Oxford.

4.32   Acrodermatitis Enteropathica

Symptoms

The symptoms result from a severe zinc deficiency (Bleehan 1979) and include a characteristic eruption around mouth and anus, bullous or verrucous eruptions on the extremities, hair loss and severe diarrhoea.

Onset

Onset is usually in early infancy, or may be delayed until after weaning in breastfed babies. The condition is sometimes familial and it is likely that there is an inherited defect in the absorption of zinc from the gut. Serum zinc levels are invariably low, and may be well below the normal level of $10-18$ μmol/l. (Halsted and Smith 1970; David *et al* 1984). The diagnosis is confirmed by a response to zinc supplements.

Treatment

There is no dietary treatment as such. Treatment is by zinc supplementation alone, and this is a life-long measure. The supplement is zinc sulphate 25 mg, twice daily with meals (Bleehan 1979). The optimum level of supplementation is 75 mg, twice daily (Moynahan 1979). Zinc sulphate is a potential gastrointestinal irritant, although it is well tolerated if given with food. Alternative zinc salts such as the oxide, carbonate or acetate may be preferred. There is no risk of zinc toxicity with doses in the ranges given, but very much higher doses may interfere with iron and copper absorption, causing anaemia (Hambidge 1977). Control of serum zinc levels is especially important in early pregnancy, as zinc deficiency may be teratogenic.

Further reading

Bleehan SS (1979) Acrodermatitis enteropathica. In *Textbook of dermatology* Vol II Rook A, Ebling FJG and Wilkinson DS (Eds). pp 2086. Blackwell Scientific Publications, Oxford.

References

David TJ, Wells FE, Sharpe TC and Gibbs ACC (1984) Low serum zinc in atopic eczema. *Br J Dermatol* **3**, 597−601.

Halsted JA and Smith JC (1970) Plasma zinc in health and disease. *Lancet* **i**, 322−4.

Moynahan EJ (1974) Acrodermatitis enteropathica — a lethal inherited human zinc deficiency disorder. *Lancet* **ii**, 399.

Hambidge KM (1977) The role of zinc and other trace metals in paediatric nutrition and health. *Paediatr Clin North Am* **24**, (1), 100.

4.33   Dermatitis Herpetiformis

This is a rare, chronic, recurrent skin disease.

Symptoms

The skin lesions, which itch intensely, are erythematous, urticarial and symmetrical. The associated jejunal villous atrophy is present in most cases, and appears to be indistinguishable from that of coeliac disease (see p 411).

Onset

Although the adult variety of the disease is seen occasionally in children, usually after the age of five years, the disease occurs mainly in adults between the ages of 20 and 55 years. The course of the disease is long term with many remissions and relapses. Relapse may be precipitated by acute infections and emotional disturbances (Sneddon 1979).

Treatment

Drug treatment is with dimethyl sulphone (Dapsone). Dietary treatment is with a gluten-free diet (see p 188). It has been reported (Fry et al 1973) that 80% of patients who adhered to a gluten-free diet for more than one year, were able to stop or significantly reduce the dose of Dapsone required to control symptoms. The time taken to stop the drug treatment completely, while remaining on a gluten-free diet varied between eight months and four years.

In a study of ten highly motivated patients, a gluten-free diet allowed a reduction of Dapsone in all but one of the patients, and in six of the patients Dapsone was stopped completely within a year of starting the gluten-free diet (Harrington and Read 1977). Another study of patients with dermatitis herpetiformis showed that they have an increased risk of developing malignant tumours. However, those treated with a gluten-free diet had a reduced risk of malignancy compared with those taking a normal diet (Leonard et al 1983). Jejunal biopsies show improvement in the associated jejunal villous atrophy of those patients maintaining a gluten-free diet (Marks and Whittle 1969; Fry et al 1968).

Reports suggesting no benefit from a gluten-free diet have been criticised (Fry et al 1973) as being based on a small number of patients with only a short follow-up period. As the time on a strictly maintained gluten-free diet may be considerable before the level of Dapsone can be reduced without a relapse, patients need a great deal of encouragement with the diet, and frequent checks to ensure that elimination of gluten is complete.

References

Fry L, McMinn, RMH, Cowan JD and Hoffbrand AV (1968) Effect of gluten-free diet on dermatological, intestinal and haematological manifestations of dermatitis herpetiformis. *Lancet* i, 557.

Fry L, Seah PP, Riches DJ and Hoffbrand AV (1973) Clearance of skin lesions in dermatitis herpetiforms after gluten withdrawal. *Lancet* i 288—91.

Harrington CI and Read NW (1977) Dermatitis herpetiformis: effect of gluten-free diet on skin IgA and jejunal structure and function. *Br Med J* **1**, 872.

Leonard JN, Tucker WF, Fry JS, Coulter CA, Boylston AW, McMinn RM, Haffenden GP, Swain AF and Fry L. (1983) Increased incidence of malignancy in dermatitis herpetiformis. *Br Med J* **286**, 16—18.

Marks R and Whittle HW (1969) Results of treatment of dermatitis herpetiformis with a gluten-free diet after one year. *Br Med J* **iv**, 772.

Sneddon IB (1979) Dermatitis herpetiformis: In *Textbook of dermatology* Vol II Rook A, Ebling FJG and Wilkinson DS (Eds) pp 1467—8. Blackwell Scientific Publications, Oxford.

Section 5 **Special Dietetic Procedures and Practice**

5.1 Catabolic States

5.1.1 Metabolic consequences of starvation and injury

Starvation, particularly for long periods, should not occur under medical supervision, but patients requiring complex examinations, particularly for investigation of gastrointestinal disease, often undergo repeated periods of starvation prior to medical or surgical treatment. Patients with a defective gastrointestinal tract may endure prolonged periods of undernutrition before seeking medical advice.

The changes in metabolism which occur during starvation aim to conserve body tissue, in particular body protein. This is achieved mainly by reducing metabolic rate and nitrogen losses.

The changes which occur following injury are different, being designed to mobilize tissues for defence and repair. The metabolic response to injury has three phases (Cuthbertson 1930, 1942)

1 The 'ebb' phase.
2 The catabolic or 'flow' phase.
3 The anabolic phase.

The *ebb phase* lasts only a few hours; there is a depression of metabolic function and a reduction of energy expenditure.

The *flow phase* soon follows; metabolic rate increases, energy reserves from fat are mobilized, and body protein reserves — mainly from muscle, are broken down to provide energy by gluconeogenesis. The negative nitrogen balance which occurs at this time may reflect reduced protein synthesis in addition to the increase in protein breakdown (O'Keefe *et al* 1974). Large nitrogen losses may be encountered and it is not always practical or necessary to replace the total amount of nitrogen lost per day. It is during this flow or catabolic phase that rapid weight losses occur. Nutritional therapy during this phase must be defensive. It should aim to reduce catabolism, minimize losses and the wasting of important tissues.

Eventually catabolism declines and the flow phase passes into the *anabolic phase*. This is usually coupled with an increase in appetite and ambulation. The nutritional therapy should now aim to restore muscle mass and increase protein synthesis.

The metabolic changes after injury are proportional to the severity of the injury and are most extreme following burn injuries (Wilmore 1978) (see Section 5.1.3).

The major effects of starvation and injury are summarized in Table 5.1. Seldom do patients simply fall into one category or the other. They may be injured after a period of undernutrition or underfed for some time after an injury.

Table 5.1 Comparision of the effects of starvation and injury (Woolfson 1978)

	Starvation	Injury
Metabolic rate	Decreased	Increased
Weight	Slow loss, almost all from fat stores	Rapid loss, 80% from fat stores. Remainder from body protein.
Nitrogen	Losses reduced	Losses increased
Hormones	Early small increases in catecholamines, cortisol, hGH. Then slow fall. Insulin decreased	Increases in catecholamines, glucagon, cortisol, hGH. Insulin increased but relative insulin deficiency.
Water and sodium	Initial loss Late retention	Retention

5.1.2 Surgery

Pre- and post-operative malnutrition

The term protein-energy malnutrition is usually associated with victims of starvation in underdeveloped countries and in particular, with malnourished children. However, it has been shown (Bistrain *et al* 1974; Hill *et al* 1977) that 40—50% of surgical patients in British and American hospitals have signs of protein-energy malnutrition after one week or more following surgery.

The following hypothetical example demonstrates how rapidly an energy deficit can build up in a patient who is not eating if the nutritional needs are ignored.

Female, weight 58 kg, maintained on 2 litres 5% dextrose daily for seven days after operation

Energy input	=	100 g dextrose × 3.75 kcal × 7 days	= 2625 kcal

Energy output	=	1315 kcal (Schofield BMR) × 1.2 activity factor × 1.4 injury factor	= 15,464 kcal

The deficit of nearly 14,000 kcal represents around 2 kg of adipose tissue or 14 kg of lean tissue.

The most fundamental nutritional requirement of the body is for energy. In surgical patients, energy requirement is usually above the normal range whereas their energy intake frequently falls below it.

The majority of surgical patients are anxious and unsure about the surgical procedure they are to undergo. Suddenly their surroundings have changed, friends and relatives are absent and the foods offered and methods of meal service are all very different. In addition, many patients need to be 'nil by mouth' for some periods of time due to peri-operative investigations. Physical difficulty with eating, pain, nausea and diarrhoea all affect a patient's ability to consume on adequate diet. Malnutrition can occur both pre- and post-operatively

Pre-operative malnutrition

This may be due to a number of causes, e.g. poor appetite, dysphagia, prolonged malabsorption, malignancy or inflammatory bowel disease.

Post-operative malnutrition

This is not a risk in all surgical patients and many patients can withstand a short stay in hospital for minor surgery with an inadequate intake of protein and calories and the consequent weight loss without becoming wasted. If major surgery is undertaken, malnutrition is more likely to occur if
1   Pre-operative malnutrition existed.
2   Oral intake is withheld or refused post-operatively for more than 5—7 days.
3   Post-operative complications occur, e.g. sepsis, wound breakdown, ileus.

From a nutritional point of view, malnourished surgical patients may be classified into four groups and their nutritional requirements must be assessed accordingly (Elwyn 1980)
1   Depleted
2   Hypercatabolic
3   Hypercatabolic and depleted
4   Chronic malabsorption

The significance of undernutrition in surgical patients

The objectives of nutritional support in surgical patients are
1   To enhance wound healing.
2   To reduce post-operative complications.

3   To reduce the period of convalescence.
4   To prevent further deterioration of the nutritional state.

Some controversy exists regarding the benefit of pre- and post-operative nutritional support and its effect on morbidity and mortality. However, protein-energy malnutrition in hospital patients has been associated with impaired cell-mediated immunity (Bistrian *et al* 1975) and prolonged post-operative recovery (Goode and Hawkins 1978). It may also reduce pulmonary function and increase the risk of the surgical procedure itself.

Peri-operative nutritional support has been shown to reduce significantly the incidence of wound infections (Williams *et al* 1977) and to improve the rate of wound healing (Moghissi *et al* 1977). Jeejeebhoy (1985) demonstrated that nutritional support improved muscle function and Bastow *et al* (1985) clearly showed that overnight nasogastric feeding of malnourished patients with a fractured femur improved their mobility and rehabilitation, increased their voluntary food intake and reduced their period of hospitalization.

Identification of patients at risk

Early identification of those patients with existing malnutrition and those likely to become malnourished is most important.

Routine pre-operative nutritional assessment and monitoring should be undertaken on all surgical patients by nursing and dietetic staff and include at least the following observations
1   Record of body weight — both on admission and regularly thereafter. Any recent marked loss of body weight should be noted.
2   Diet history — to include a brief account of any eating problems and loss of appetite.
3   Supervision of meal choice and assistance with eating if required.
4   Observation of food and fluids consumed — keeping an accurate record of nutritional intake if requested.

These simple measures, together with routine biochemical and haematological tests, and an understanding of the underlying medical conditional and surgical procedure can help to identify at an early stage those patients in need of nutritional support.

Methods of improving the nutritional status of surgical patients

If nutritional support is indicated, either pre- or post-operatively, it can be provided by one or more of the following methods:

The provision of appetising meals

Meals should be attractively served, the portion size being appropriate for the patient's appetite. Foods offered should be familiar to most patients and contain adequate amounts of energy and protein. The present national recommendations for high fibre, low fat dishes to be included in hospital menus is not necessarily appropriate for surgical patients. Such steps could result in a further reduction of their voluntary food intake.

Nutritional supplementation

Both protein and energy supplements (p. 74) should be used regularly on surgical wards. The nursing staff should be taught fully how and when to use them.

Total sip feeding

Patients with severe dysphagia and those with certain gastrointestinal conditions, e.g. inflammatory bowel disease, intestinal strictures or fistulae may require a liquid diet. The commercially produced nutritionally complete preparations are much more appropriate than liquidized hospital meals. It must be remembered that patients need to be well motivated and encouraged to take these drinks regularly in order to consume an adequate amount, and that the nursing staff should be given clear instructions regarding the sip feeding regimen. (see Section 1.12.2)

Naso-enteric tube feeding

If the oral diet is inadequate and the patient is already malnourished or likely to become so, total or supplementary overnight tube feeding should be instigated. A fine bore tube or jejunostomy feeding catheter can be inserted at the time of operation to provide post-operative nutrition. (see Section 1.12.3)

Total parenteral nutrition

If the gut is not functional and nutritional support is indicated, total parenteral nutrition (TPN) should be provided — preferably in consultation with the hospital nutrition team if one exists. Where possible, TPN should not be started unless a minimum of 7—10 days feeding is envisaged. Particular attention must be given to the patient's *total* nutritional needs remembering his requirements for vitamins, minerals, trace elements and fluid as well as energy and nitrogen. (See section 1.13)

Introduction of post-operative oral fluids and diet

After a general anaesthetic, gastric mobility and emptying is delayed. If gastrointestinal surgery has been undertaken, normal gut function may be slow to return. Oral fluids and food are usually withheld until the surgeon feels that gastric emptying and gut function are returning. Initially, the patient may only be offered sips of water. Small volumes, e.g. 15 ml and 30 ml may then be given hourly and if tolerated the volume is increased gradually over a few days. During this stage, fluid requirements but *not* nutritional requirements are met by intravenous infusion of saline and/or dextrose (2 litres of 5% dextrose provides a mere 400 kcal). Once the patient is taking fluids freely throughout the day, intravenous fluids can be reduced or discontinued and the patient can progress via soup and light sweet at lunch and supper to a light diet plus nutritional supplements if indicated. Throughout this time an accurate daily record of fluid balance should be kept.

Following other types of surgery, oral diet may well be given on the first post-operative day. However, Manners (1974) and Walesby *et al* (1979) reported very low energy and protein intakes in patients following cardiopulmonary bypass surgery, and post-operative anorexia is frequently seen on general surgical wards.

Monitoring

Regular monitoring of the patient's fluid intake and output, body weight, haematology, and serum and urinary biochemistry should be carried out throughout the hospital stay. This is discussed in detail in Section 1.10.

Most patients are discharged home before their natural appetite fully returns and dietetic advice and supervision should continue in the community and at follow-up clinics whenever possible.

Obesity and surgery

Gross obesity is associated with increased surgical risks. In the case of elective surgery, severe obesity should be remedied beforehand by planned weight reduction over a period of time, rather than by short term crash dieting.

Obesity can mask underlying malnutrition and should not be used as a reason for withholding nutritional support in surgical patients if post-operative complications exist or if anthropometric and biochemical nutritional indices show evidence of deficiencies and malnutrition. The obesity should be treated at a later stage when the patient has fully recovered.

5.1.3   Burn injury

Extensive thermal injury elicits the most pronounced response to stress that the human body is capable of generating. Resting metabolic expenditure (RME) increases as hormone-induced breakdown of body protein and fat occurs at greatly accelerated rates. Weight loss of 1.5 kg/day is possible. The patient is certain to die if weight loss approaches 30% of the pre-burn weight (Davenport 1979).

Nutritional therapy must provide sufficient nutrients to prevent weight loss, or in practice to restrict weight loss to less than 10%. The aim is to preserve lean body

mass, thereby ensuring that wound healing and the 'taking' of skin grafts proceed at maximal rates and immunocompetence is maintained. In order to maintain or restore lean body mass, Molnor et al (1983) recommend that aggressive nutritional therapy is undertaken in burn patients with the following features or complications.

1   >20% burn.
2   Pre-injury malnutrition.
3   Septic complications.
4   Associated injury including pulmonary.
5   Threat of >10% weight loss.

Fatal burn injuries

As a 'rule of thumb', a patient with a percentage body surface area burn and an age which when totalled together exceeds 100 is unlikely to survive, e.g. 86 year old with 30% burn = 116 — survival unlikely; 13 year

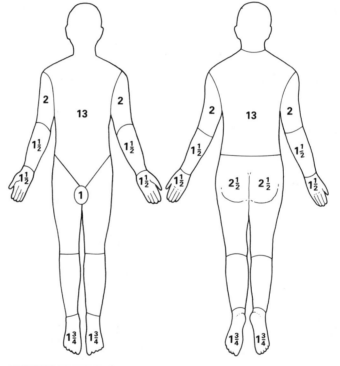

Area	Age (years)					
	0	1	5	10	15	Adult
Head and neck	21	19	15	13	11	9
Thigh	$5\frac{1}{2}$	$6\frac{1}{2}$	8	9	9	$9\frac{1}{2}$
Calf	5	5	$5\frac{1}{2}$	6	$6\frac{1}{2}$	7

Fig. 5.1 Percentage of different parts of the body at various ages (Kemble and Harvey 1984).

old with 55% burn = 68 — survival likely. This formula does not apply to children less than ten years old. More complicated formulae also exist for predicting mortality (Tobiasen *et al* 1982).

In cases of non-survivable injury, the patient should be kept well hydrated and given adequate pain-relief, but no nutritional therapy is attempted; the patient usually succumbs to the injury within a few days.

Minor burn injuries

Small percentage burn injuries (i.e. <15% in adults, <10% in children) do not require resuscitation with intravenous fluids. RME is not elevated to any great extent. Weight can usually be maintained on a high protein, high energy diet supplemented with *palatable* high energy and/or high protein drinks. (see p 74 and Section 2.12) Glucose polymers can be added to drinking water although the concentrated solutions designed for renal patients are best avoided because their high osmolarity can cause diarrhoea or dehydration. However, food intake may be low for various reasons. 'Nil by mouth' regimens for change of dressings or theatre procedures which require anaesthesia, lead to reduced intakes of food and fluids. Fear, pain or foul smelling dressings may reduce appetite. Patients cannot be made to eat to order, so flexibility in the catering arrangements is an advantage.

Major burn injuries

Ebb phase

The ebb phase (see Section 5.1.1.) from the time of burning up to 36—48 hours post-burn coincides with the resuscitation period. During this period, fluid moves from the circulation into the tissues and the patient becomes oedematous. Plasma and other fluids must be given intravenously to preserve blood volume and urine output. Oral fluids are restricted initially since, despite complaining of thirst, the patient frequently vomits after drinking.

No routine nutritional support is given in this period because the need to prevent hypovolaemia takes precedence. However, recently it has been claimed that early post-burn feeding has beneficial effects (McArdle *et al* 1983; Mochizuki *et al* 1984).

Flow phase

The flow phase begins some 48 hours post-burn and the depth of the burn determines its duration (Table 5.2). Increased production of catabolic hormones

Table 5.2 Burn wounds

	Superficial	Partial thickness	Full thickness
Depth of burn	Epidermis only	Some of dermis	All of dermis
Healing time	3—10 days	10—14 days	Many months or never
Scarring	No	Deep burns likely to produce scarring and contractures	Contractures unless grafted
Skin grafting	No	Deep burns may need grafting	Large areas need grafting

Pressure or infection may convert a partial thickness burn into a full thickness burn.

(adrenaline, noradrenaline, glucagon and the corticosteroids) leads to hypermetabolism, accelerated protein and fat breakdown, negative nitrogen balance and altered carbohydrate metabolism (Fig. 5.2).

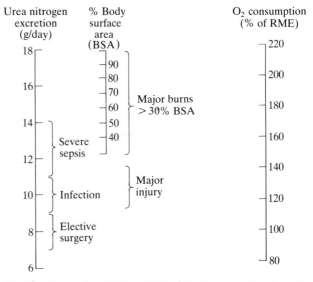

Fig. 5.2 Rates of hypermetabolism estimated from urinary urea nitrogen excretion (Blackburn *et al* 1977; Bistrian *et al* 1977).

The abnormalities of carbohydrate metabolism include elevated glucose levels, increased gluconeogenesis, altered insulin levels and profound insulin resistance. All are attributable to the hormonal imbalance which suppresses the influence of insulin on peripheral tissues (Richards 1977; Davies 1977; Wilmore and McDougal 1977).

Septicaemia will further accentuate post-injury glucose intolerance necessitating large doses of insulin (up to 600 units/day) but this requirement drops rapidly if treatment of sepsis is successful (Woolfson *et al* 1977). Insulin resistance often occurs in severe trauma or infection hence the name 'stress diabetes' or 'diabetes of trauma'. However, the patient seldom exhibits ketoacidosis so it is sometimes called 'pseudodiabetes'. More insulin, and not a reduction in nutrient intake, is required to treat the hyperglycaemia. Reduction of administered protein and energy will not prevent this stress response, and is detrimental to the patient.

The maximum catabolic response usually occurs 5—10 days post-burn. Thereafter healing of partial thickness burns and early excision and grafting of deep burns reduce wound size and thus the exogenous demand for nutrients.

Anabolic phase

Provided no weight loss has occurred, intakes can return to normal levels as healing progresses. Soroff *et al* (1961) showed that patients with major burn injuries were entering an 'anabolic' phase by 30 days post-burn. High protein high energy supplements (see p 74 and Section 2.12) will speed up convalescence.

Water and nutrient losses

Urine. Increased urinary urea is the principal route of nitrogen loss. Other non-urea nitrogen compounds are also increased in the urine.

Exudate. Fluid loss from a burn wound may be considerable and may contain 4—6 g protein/100 ml representing 25—50% of total nitrogen loss (Molnar *et al* 1983). Exudate losses vary in a patient from day to day. This loss cannot be measured routinely in burn units so it has to be estimated. Davies (1977) has reviewed the literature and suggests a figure of 0.2 g N/% burn /day for the first week post-burn. Subsequently the losses decrease as healing progresses. The exudate nitrogen loss from partial thickness burns rapidly decreases to 0.1 g N/% burn/day. When the burns are extensive and full thickness so that virtually no healing occurs, the exudate losses continue at 0.2 g N/% burn/day until the eschar (burned layer of skin) separates to reveal granulating tissue.

Evaporation. Burn patients lack the water impermeable barrier of the skin over large areas of their body. Evaporation losses are therefore high, despite attempts to reduce energy losses as heat by nursing in a warm, dry environment. Wilmore and McDougall (1977) estimate the evaporative water loss using the formula: (25 + % burn) × body surface area in m² = ml water lost/hour. This formula is in agreement with the finding of Michaels and Sorenson (1983) that a healthy non-burned volunteer on a Clinitron (air fluidized) bed lost 63.5 ml/hour/m². With burn injury the loss may be increased to 3 litres/day.

Faecal. Nitrogen losses via the faecal route are 1—3 g N/day (Davies 1977) and relatively small compared to urine and exudate losses. They will increase if the patient suffers from diarrhoea.

Vitamins and essential biological elements

With loss of skin tissue, increased muscle breakdown and increased fluid throughput, vitamin and mineral losses are likely to exceed the RDA for non-stressed individuals. However, there are no firm recommendations for replacement in burn patients (Molnar *et al* 1983). The following should be borne in mind

1 It may be advisable to give 500—1000 mg vitamin C/day because of its known role in collagen synthesis.
2 High intakes of carbohydrate, either enterally or parenterally, lead to an increased demand for thiamin.
3 Vitamin A may play a role in protection against stress ulceration.
3 Increased iron intake is needed to treat anaemia.
5 20% of the body's zinc is found in skin so burns inevitably cause zinc loss. Zinc losses in urine are also increased as a result of muscle breakdown. Zinc is a constituent of many metalloenzymes and important in DNA/RNA synthesis (Kay 1981) so adequate supplementation is important.

Estimating nutritional requirements

Many formulae have been devised to assess the energy and protein required to prevent weight loss in burns (Davies 1977). None take into account all the factors which affect requirements — weight, sex, age, height, % burn, % deep burn, respiratory involvement, activity level, infection and other injuries. Estimates of requirements must be regarded only as guidelines for intake which must be tailored for each individual patient.

The formula most often used in the UK for burned adults is that of Sutherland (1976)

Energy requirement = 20 kcal (84 kJ)/kg + 70 kcal (294 kJ)/% burn
Protein requirement = 1 g/kg + 3 g/% burn.

Example of calculation using the Sutherland formula

For a 65 kg patient with 30% burns
Energy requirement = (20 × 65) + (70 × 30)
= 3400 kcal

Protein requirement $= (1 \times 65) + (3 \times 30)$
$= 155$ g
Non-protein energy (NPE) $= 3400 - (155 \times 4)$
$= 2780$ kcal
Nitrogen $= 155/6.25 \quad = 24.8$ gN
NPE:N $= 112:1$

This emphasizes the parastic nature of the wound. If the requirement for nutrients is not met from exogenous sources it is met from endogenous sources with consequent weight loss. The formula gives a desirable non-protein energy to nitrogen (NPE:N) ratio for burn patients of between 100:1 and 120:1. This ratio is lower than most enteral/parenteral regimens and is imperative for weight maintenance. Regimens with a NPE:N of 150:1 may lead to weight losses of 10–15% (King, unpublished data).

However, with massive burns, it is rare for a patient's RME to exceed twice basal metabolic rate (BMR). Molnar et al (1983) suggest giving energy at BMR $\times$ 2 to minimize weight loss irrespective of burn size. This formula depends on knowing the patient's body surface area (see p. 68) and age, and uses a table (p. 69) to determine BMR. As no account is taken of burn size the formula overestimates the requirements for small burns, but in the main gives a lower, and more easily attainable, energy requirement than Sutherland's formula which seems to overestimate energy and protein requirements in burn patients.

Enteral feeding (see also Section 1.12)

Enteral feeding is always preferable to parenteral feeding in burn patients. Parenteral feeding is associated with a high incidence of septicaemia whether or not the parenteral feeding line goes through a burned area. Not only is enteral feeding unlikely to result in septicaemia, it is cheaper, more physiological since the liver is not bypassed, requires less biochemical monitoring, and may have a direct beneficial effect over parenteral feeding by preserving gut mucosal integrity which functions as a barrier against bacterial invasion (Mochizuki et al 1984).

Assuming that the patient does not have a compromized gut function prior to admission, a hyperosmolar polymeric tube feed can be started after 36–48 hours post-burn. The feed is given full strength but slowly (50 ml/hour) at first and over a period of hours. The osmolarity of the feed is not critical. Diluting the feed does not reduce the incidence of nausea and diarrhoea but does reduce the nutrient intake at a critical time. Diarrhoea is associated with the use of antibiotics during enteral feeding (Keohane et al 1984). Hopefully drugs causing the problem can be stopped or alternatives prescribed.

Up to 2 litres of feed is given in the first 24 hours; thereafter the full requirement can be given. Enteral pumps enable volumes exceeding 3 litres/24 hours to be given via a 1 mm internal diameter fine bore tube. Even patients with severe facial burns can be intubated with these tubes. If a fine bore tube cannot be kept in place, a Dobhoff tube can be used instead; its weighted end makes it difficult to cough or vomit up.

Enteral feeding should continue until either all the burns have healed with minimum weight loss or the burns have healed and biochemical parameters are within normal limits. If problems such as excessive weight loss, unhealed burns or graft rejection occur, enteral feeding should continue.

The enteral feed should contain: 1 kcal/ml (4.2 kJ/ml), 45 g protein/litre (NPE:N ratio 110–120:1). For example, (per litre)

Clinifeed 'Protein rich'	1 can
Clinifeed 'Favour'	1 can
Calogen	28 ml
Water	220 ml

Enteral feeds with an energy content of 1.5–2.0 kcal/ml (6.3–8.4 kJ/ml) can cause dehydration in patients not receiving additional fluid by other means. This is not such a problem with feed containing 1 kcal/ml.

Constipation may occur due to the side effects of pain killers or a lack of dietary fibre in a milk-based feed. Long term enteral tube feeding with no oral intake of dietary fibre can lead to diarrhoea, constipation or faecal impaction with 'overflow diarrhoea'. The use of a dietary fibre-containing feed 'Enrich' (Abbott), containing soy bran may alleviate these problems. If the patient is eating, a high fibre diet should be instituted.

Feeding gastrostomies have been described for burn patients (Kahn et al 1984).

There is no place for the routine use of elemental feeds in burn therapy (Wilmore and McDougal 1977).

Parenteral feeding (see Section 1.13)

Despite the risk of septicaemia, in the case of prolonged paralytic ileus there may be no choice other than to feed parenterally. The same nutritional principles should apply to total parental nutrition (TPN) as to enteral feeding. Total nitrogen input should, if possible, exceed total nitrogen output.

Fat-free regimens should be discouraged as the burns patient cannot oxidise glucose at as great a rate as healthy individuals. If glucose intake exceeds the maximal oxidation rate (Table 5.3), fat is synthesized. This is an energy-consuming process and large volumes of CO_2 are produced raising the respiratory quotient which may be dangerous to patients with pulmonary insufficiency. Overfeeding is known to increase metabolic rates in both normal and hypermetabolic humans. It is possible that extremely high energy intakes of 8−10,000 kcal (33−42 MJ)/day given to burns patients in the past may have contributed in part to the high measured metabolic rates (Molnar et al 1983). Synthesis of inappropriate quantities of fat from glucose can lead to fatty liver which in the past was thought to be caused by intravenously administered fat. In fact Intralipid has been used for many years in burns patients without apparent ill effect. Apart from supplying essential fatty acids (efa) one litre of Intralipid (20%) supplies 2000 kcal (8.4 MJ) and can be given peripherally (Davies 1977).

Many intravenous regimens have too high a NPE:N ratio for burns patients. Vitamin and mineral preparations often provide only basal requirements for healthy adults, not catabolic patients.

Table 5.3 Maximal glucose oxidation rate for 70 kg male

	Rate (mg/kg/minute)	Maximum amount of glucose which can be metabolized in 24 hours
Non-burned	7	706 g
Burned	5	504 g

Branched chain amino acids (BCAA)

BCAA are the only amino acids oxidised chiefly extra-hepatically. Insulin resistance in traumatic and septic states leads to poor utilization of fat and glucose by skeletal muscle, and consequently muscle protein is 'cannibalized' to provide BCAA (Richards 1977). The ketoacid of leucine partially suppresses proteolysis in post-operative patients (Sapir et al 1983). It has therefore been suggested that stressed patients require 0.5 g BCAA/kg/day (Cerra et al 1984; Echenique et al 1984). However, the use in burns patients of a BCAA-enriched solution which has an 'unbalanced' amino acid profile may not be appropriate to the altered metabolism found in these patients. The results of further studies may clarify the issue.

Monitoring progress

Morath et al (1983) reviewed the problems of monitoring nutritional therapy in burns patients and concluded that no single parameter indicates short term nutritional status but that regular repeated measurements can indicate trends (Table 5.4).

Table 5.4 Post-burn nutritional monitoring

Test	Frequency
24-hour urine collection	Daily
Maximum body temperature	Daily
Nutrient record	Daily
Body weight	When dressings are changed
Serum urea and electrolytes	Twice weekly
Serum transferrin	Twice weekly
Liver function tests	Twice monthly

Body weight. Oedema during the resuscitation period increases body weight by at least 10%. 'Dry weight' occurs some 14 days post-burn so weight measured before 14 days is distorted by oedema. Thereafter accurate repeated measurements of body weight help to assess nutritional therapy. Exudate soaked dressings invalidates daily weighing so the patient is weighed in dressings and before the dressings are changed. Discarded dressings are collected in a plastic bag and weighed to give an accurate body weight.

Nutrient intake. Food and drink consumed should be recorded by nursing staff. Total intake can be calculated from oral, enteral and parenteral records and compared to predicted requirements. Administered blood products are not usually included in nutrient totals.

Serum proteins. Serum albumin decreases very quickly post-burn and is slow to reflect improvement in nutritional status due to its long half life (20 days). Transferrin has a shorter half life (eight days) and may be a more sensitive short term indicator of nutritional status. Ogle and Alexander (1982) have found that transferrin levels of less than 2 g/litre are associated with an increased incidence of bacteraemia in burns.

Urinary urea. Urinary urea is the yardstick used to estimate stress. Twenty-four hour urinary urea nitrogen indicates internal nitrogen metabolism (Lee and Hartley 1975). However, nitrogen output depends on both nitrogen intake and nitrogen retention, and the latter is influenced by the magnitude of catabolic stress.

The catabolic index (Bistrian 1979) indicates the magnitude of this stress.

Catabolic index: urinary urea nitrogen $- (0.5 \times$ dietary nitrogen $+ 3$ g)

A value of < 0 indicates no stress

0.5 indicates moderate stress

> 5 indicates severe stress.

This assumes that 50% of ingested protein is catabolized via gluconeogenesis. The constant (3 g) added for non-urea nitrogen loss will almost always underestimate true losses in burns due to exudation, but nonetheless the catabolic index usefully indicates the change from stressed to non-stressed status.

Urinary creatinine. Urinary creatinine can be used to determine the creatinine/height index. This is so variable from day to day in burn patients that it is of no clinical use (Eve and Settle 1978).

Daily maximum body temperature. All the above tests give results retrospectively. A test is needed which is more immediately and freely available to all burn units. Body temperature indicates the extent of hypermetabolism at any given time. Each 1°C above normal produces a 10−12% rise in BMR.

Electrical burns

Care must be taken with the nutrition of patients with high voltage electrical injury. In addition to surface burn injury (entry and exit points) conduction through the body causes destruction of the underlying nerves, blood vessels, muscles, bones, tendons and visceral coverings. The more resistant the tissue, the more heat is generated as current flows through it (Diamond *et al* 1982) thus muscle close to bone may be necrosed. A high urinary urea output in these patients indicates that severe damage has occurred (Balogh and Bauer 1982). Burns feeding formulae based on % burn will understimate the amount of nutrients required by these patients.

Burn injuries in children

Davies (1977) reviewed burns feeding formulae and concluded that suggested inputs for burned adults, if scaled down in proportion to body weight, would be adequate for burned children. The formula of Sutherland and Batchelor (1968) has provided a useful guideline in the past for feeding burned children under ten years old

Energy = 60 kcal (252 kJ)/kg + 35 kcal (147kJ)/% burn

Protein = 3 g/kg + 1 g/% burn.

This formula illustrates the fact that children have a higher BMR than adults and a greater requirement for protein per kg body weight. Burn injury however, does not raise RME proportionally as much in children as in adults and when normally active children are confined to bed by burn injury, this saving in energy output partially offsets the increase in RME. If the average RDA for a non-burned child can be achieved, weight loss will be minimized.

Enteral feeding can often be avoided in burned children provided they will drink milky supplements. Milk can be fortified with dried milk powder (30 g to 500 ml). Alternatively Build Up reconstituted with milk can be given, provided it is diluted with an equal quantity of water to reduce the osmolarity. Both will boost protein intakes in burned children.

5.1.4 Cancer cachexia

Dietitians are often confronted with the cachectic cancer patient. The cachectic patient presents with

1 Anorexia.
2 Early satiety.
3 Weight loss.
4 Debilitation.
5 Depression.

Many patients with cancer are malnourished when admitted to hospital. Improving their nutritional status should be a vital part of their treatment as improved nutritional status leads to an increased tolerance to anti-cancer therapy and an improved quality of life. Nutritional support should continue beyond discharge throughout rehabilitation.

The side effects of anti-cancer therapy are not solely responsible for the cachectic state. The malignancy itself, as well as psychological, social and environmental factors, may play a large part in the patient's reluctance to eat.

Cancer treatments

Radiotherapy

On average, a course of radiotherapy consists of five treatments per week for six weeks. Nutritional problems may arise depending on the location and size of the treatment field. Radiation to the head and neck area, particularly to the tongue, palate and nasopharynx, causes many nutritional problems. Reactions include a burning sensation to the throat, loss of appetite, taste alterations and soreness of the mouth. Dry mouth is a common problem with patients receiving radiotherapy to the area including the salivary glands. This then causes problems with swallowing due to lack of saliva (see also p 386)

Decreased tolerance to foods can result from radiation to the upper abdomen which frequently causes cramping, malabsorption and diarrhoea.

Chemotherapy

The number of drugs used singly or in combination in the treatment of cancer is rapidly increasing. Most regimens involve several drugs given over a period of weeks. Nausea and vomiting are the common side effects affecting the patient's ability to eat. Depending on the dose and duration of treatment, other side effects can occur, such as taste changes (mouth blindness), stomatitis, mucositis, oesophagitis and malab-

sorption. These effects also severely affect the patient's food intake.

Surgery

As well as the general metabolic effects of surgery (see Section 5.1.2) patients undergoing surgery for treatment of cancer have further specific nutritional problems
1 Surgical removal of any tumour may frequently involve removal of considerable amounts of neighbouring tissue to reduce the likelihood of the malignancy spreading. Major surgery to any area of the gastrointestinal tract will lead to problems affecting the patient's ability to eat and possibly lead to malabsorption.
2 Surgical removal of head and neck tumours may involve long term enteral feeding and the possibility of soft and/or liquid feeds permanently.
3 An oesophagectomy, total or partial gastrectomy or colostomy can create its own specific problem (see Section 4.9; 4.10, 4.12).

The suggested dietary treatment of common nutritional problems related to cancer and its treatment are summarized in Table 5.5.

Table 5.5 Nutritional problems related to cancer and its treatment — suggested dietary treatment

Problem	Cause	Suggested Dietary Treatment
Anorexia	Disease state Radiotherapy Chemotherapy	Small attractive nourishing meals Snacks and/or nourishing drinks between meals. Use of energy and protein supplements, e.g. Maxijul/Caloreen, Fortical/Hycal, Maxipro/Casilan. Meals to be eaten slowly in a relaxed manner. Use of appetite stimulants, e.g. alcohol, prednisolone
Severe anorexia	As above	Tube feeding may be necessary
Inability to prepare meals due to tiredness or weakness	Disease state Treatment in general	Make use of store cupboard of convenience foods, tinned soups, tinned fruits and puddings, packet instant desserts, tinned meats, tinned snacks, etc. Arrange meals on wheels, home help if appropriate. Use meal replacements, e.g. Complan, Build Up
Sense of fullness	Disease state Radiotherapy to upper abdominal area	Small frequent meals. Reduction of fatty foods may help Avoidance of drinks with meals (to be taken ½ hour before or after) Use of nourishing drinks, e.g. milk shakes, egg nog (fortified if necessary with energy or protein supplements), Build-up, Complan, Ensure, Fortisip, Maxisorb, etc.
Nausea	Disease state Radiation to upper gastrointestinal tract Chemotherapy	Small frequent meals Keep patient away from cooking smells if possible. Suggest a short walk before meals to get some fresh air. For early morning nausea try unbuttered toast, cream crackers or plain biscuits Give dry meals with drinks before or after. Reduce very sweet or very greasy foods Try cold foods; these have less smell than cooked foods. Use of fizzy drinks, e.g. ginger ale may help
Severe nausea	As above	As above. Consult doctor regarding appropriate antiemetics
Severe vomiting	As above	Total parenteral nutrition may be necessary

Table 5.5 *contd*

Problem	Cause	Suggested Dietary Treatment	
Metallic taste in mouth	Certain types of chemotherapy	Elimination of foods accentuating this taste according to patient's individual tolerance	
Loss of taste (mouth blindness)	Certain types of chemotherapy Radiotherapy to mouth and throat	Emphasis on aroma of food. Marinate food to enhance flavour, use stronger seasonings and herbs. Avoid very hot foods, these often taste better at room temperature	
Dry mouth	Radiotherapy to mouth and throat	Frequent drinks. Give ice cubes to suck Give fruit drops, boiled sweets to suck. Regular mouthwashes. Lemon and glycerine mouth swabs. Avoidance of very dry foods. Artificial saliva — Salivex tablets are available on prescription. Hospital pharmacy may produce its own artificial saliva. Spray saliva, Glandosane (Fresenius), is also available.	
Sore mouth/throat (stomatitis, mucositis)	Certain types of chemotherapy Radiation to mouth and throat	Soft, moist foods. Use nourishing drinks. Avoidance of very salty or spicy foods. Cold foods are often soothing. Avoidance of very hot foods — allow to cool a little. Give drinks through a straw if necessary. Avoidance of rough or very dry foods	
General difficulties with chewing and swallowing	Radiotherapy to mouth and throat Oral surgery Oesophageal carcinoma, Insertion of palliative oesophageal tubes	Soft, semi-solid or liquid diet. Small frequent meals. Use of nourishing drinks. Use of fizzy drinks to clear oesophageal tubes	
Severe difficulties in chewing and swallowing	As above	Tube feeding	
Intestinal cramping, abdominal pain	Radiotherapy to lower abdomen Certain types of chemotherapy	Try low fibre diet	
Diarrhoea	As above	Low fibre diet with high fluid intake	
Severe diarrhoea	As above	Use of antidiarrhoeal agents	
Intermittent constipation	Certain types of chemotherapy	High fibre diet, plenty of fluids	
Severe constipation	As above	Possible use of laxatives	
Malabsorption	Radiotherapy to lower gastrointestinal tract Surgery to gastrointestinal tract	Low fat diet Low fibre diet Lactose-free diet Enteral feeds e.g. Ensure Isocal, etc. Total parenteral nutrition	As appropriate for the type of malabsorption problem

'Alternative diets'

The common 'alternative' dietary regimens publicized for the treatment of cancer are
1 The Bristol Diet.
2 The Macrobiotic Diet.
3 Gerson Therapy.

These are vegan style regimens claimed to be beneficial for cancer patients. In many patients, following such regimens leads to a further decrease in nutritional intake and further weight loss. There is no real scientific evidence to support any of these regimens or the megavitamin therapy which frequently accompanies

them. The important issue is the maintenance or improvement of nutritional status of the patient and conventional dietary advice from a qualified dietitian is more likely to achieve this.

Patients choosing to follow alternative regimens should be advised of the disadvantages (low energy, high bulk, possible high cost, etc.). The dietitian needs to be fully aware of the regimen in order to be able to advise the patient of likely problems and solutions to them. (see further reading and Section 2.16.2).

Continuous follow-up and monitoring of these patients is essential.

Further reading

Aihara H (1985) *Basic macrobiotics*. Japan Publications Inc.

DeWys WD and Hillenbrand Herbst S (1977) Oral feeding in the nutritional management of the cancer patient. *Cancer Research* **37**, 2429–31.

Dornan V (1985) Diet in terminal illness. *Nursing Mirror* **160**, (8), 39–41.

Forbes A (1984) *The Bristol diet*. Century Publishing, London.

Gerson M (1900) *A cancer therapy — results of 50 cases*. Wholefood Shop.

Hill GL (Ed) (1981) *Nutrition and the surgical patient*. Churchill Livingstone, Edinburgh.

Kushi M (1984) *The cancer prevention diet*. Thorsons, Wellingborough.

Kushi M (1985) *The macrobiotic way*. Avery,

Soukop M and Calman KC (1977) Nutrition support in patients with malignant disease. Nutrition and cancer 5. *J Hum Nutr* **33**, 179–88.

The Royal Marsden Hospital (1985) *Overcoming eating difficulties — a guide for cancer patients*. Patient Information Series No 9.

Roberts T (1980) *Oncology for nurses and health care professionals Vol I and II*. George, Allan and Unwin, London.

Tresillian M (1971) *Does diet cure cancer?* Thorsons, Wellingborough

Wesdorp RIC, Krause R and Von Meyenfeldt (1933) Cancer cachexia and its nutrition implications. *Br J Surg* **70**, 352–5.

References

Balogh D and Bauer M (1982) Determination of catabolism in the burn patient. *Chir Plastica* **7**, 67–74.

Bastow MD, Rawlings J and Allison SP (1985) Overnight nasogastric tube feeding. *Clin Nutr* **4**, 7–11.

Bistrian BR, Blackburn GL, Hallowell E and Heddle R (1974) Protein status of general surgical patients. *J Am Med Assoc* **230**, 858–60.

Bistrian BR, Blackburn GL, Scrimshaw NS and Flatt J (1975) Cellular immunity in semi-starved states in hospitalized adults. *Am J Clin Nutr* **28**, 1148–55.

Bistrian BR (1979) A simple technique to estimate the severity of stress. *Surg Gynaecol Obstet* **148**, 675–8.

Blackburn GL, Miller JDB, Bistrian BR, Flatt JP and Reinhoff HY (1977) Amino acids — key nutrients in the response to injury. In *Nutritional aspects of care in the critically ill*. Richard JR and Kinnery JM (Eds). Churchill Livingstone, Edinburgh.

Cerra FB, Mazuski JE, Chute E, Nuwer N, Teasley K, Lysne J, Shronts EP and Konstantinides FN (1984) Branch chain metabolic support. *Ann Surg* **199**, (3), 286–91.

Diamond TH, Twomey A and Myburgh DP (1982) High voltage electrical injury. *S Africa Med J* **27 Feb** 318–21.

Davies JWL (1977) The nutrition of patients with burns. In *Nutritional aspects of care in the critically ill*. Richards JR and Kinney JM (Eds). Churchill Livingstone, Edinburgh.

Davenport PJ (1979) Nutritional support in severe burns. *Res Clin Forums* **1**, (1). 79–82.

Echenique MM, Bistrian BR, Moldower LL, Palombo JD and Miller MM (1984) *Surg Gynaecol Obstet* **159**, 233–41.

Elwyn DH (1980) Nutritional requirements of adult surgical patients. *Crit Care Med* **8**, 9–20.

Eve MD and Settle JAD (1978) Elemental feeding in severe burns: monitoring a regime using Vivonex. *Burns* **5**, (1), 127–35.

Goode AW and Hawkins T (1978) In *Advances in parenteral nutrition*. Johnston IDA (Ed) p 557. MTP Press, Lancaster.

Hill GL, Blackett RL, Pickford I, Burkinshaw L, Young GA, Warren JV, Schorah CJ and Morgan DB (1977) Malnutrition in surgical patients: an unrecognized problem. *Lancet* **i**, 689–92.

Jeejeebhoy KN (1985) Changes in body composition and muscle function and effect of nutritional support. *Proceeding of the 4th World Congress on Intensive Critical Care Medicine* p 161.

Kahn AM, Kross ME and Goller FM (1984) Feeding gastrostomy for the severely burned patient. *Arch Surg* **119**, 1316–7.

Kay RG (1981) Zinc and copper in human nutrition. *J Hum Nutr* **35**, (1) 25–36.

Kemble JV and Harvey BE (1984) *Plastic surgical and burns nursing (current nursing practice)*. Balliere Tindall, Eastbourne.

Keohane PP, Attrill H, Love M, Frost P and Silk DBA (1984) Relation between osmolality of diet and gastronistestinal side effects in enteral nutrition. *Br Med J* **288**, 678–80.

Lee HA and Hartley TF (1975) A method of determining daily nitrogen requirements. *Postgrad Med J* **51**, 441–5.

Manners JM (1974) Nutrition after cardiac surgery. *Anaesthesia* **29**, 675–88.

McArdle AH, Palmason C, Brown RA, Brown HC and Williams HB (1983) Protection from catabolism in major burns; a new formula for the immediate enteral feeding of burn patients. *J Burn Care Rehab* **4**, (4), 245–50.

Michaels J and Sorensen B (1983) The physiology of a healthy normal person in the air-fluidized bed. *Burns* **9**, 158–68.

Mochizuki H, Trocki O, Dominioni L, Brackett KA, Joffe SN and Alexander JW (1984) Mechanism of prevention of postburn hypermetabolism and catabolism by early enteral feeding. *Ann Surg* **200**, (3), 297–308.

Moghissi K, Hornshaw J, Teasdale PR and Dawes EA (1977) Parenteral nutrition in carcinoma of the oesophagus treated by surgery: nitrogen balance and clinical studies. *Br J Surg* **64**, 125–8.

Molnar JA, Wolfe RR and Burke JF (1983) Burns: metabolism and nutritional therapy in thermal injury. In *Nutritional support of medical practice* 2e Schneider HA, Anderson CE and Coursin DB (Eds) pp 260–81. Harper and Row Publications, Philadelphia.

Morath MA, Miller SF, Finley RK and Jones LM (1983) Interpretation of nutritional parameters in burn patients. *J Burn Care Rehab* **4**, (5), 361–6.

Ogle CK and Alexander JW (1982) The relationship of bacteraemia to levels of transferrin, albumin and total serum proteins in burn patients. *Burns* **8**, 32–8.

Richards JR (1977) Metabolic responses to injury and starvation. An overview. In *Nutritional aspects of care in the critically ill* Richards JR and Kinney JM (Eds) pp 273–302. Churchill Livingstone, Edinburgh.

Sapir DG, Walser M, Moyer ED, Rosenshein NB, Steward PM, Moreadith C, Imbembo AL and Munoz S (1983) Effects of ketoisocaproate and of leucine on nitrogen metabolism in postoperative patients. *Lancet* **i**, 1010–4.

Soroff HS, Pearson E and Artz CP (1961) An estimation of the nitrogen requirements for equilibrium in burned patients. *Surg Gynaecol Obstet* **112**, 159–72.

Sutherland AB and Batchelor ADC (1968) Nitrogen balance in burned children. *Ann New York Acad Sci* **150**, 700.

Sutherland AB (1976) Nitrogen balance and nutritional requirements in the burn patient; a reappraisal. *Burns* **2**, 238–44.

Tobiasen J, Heibert JM and Edlich RF (1982) A practical burn severity index. *J Burn Care Rehab* **3**, (4), 229–32.

Walesby RK, Goode AW, Spinks TJ, Herring A, Ranicar AS and Bentall HH (1979) Nutritional status of patients requiring cardiac surgery. *J Thorac Cardiovasc Surg* **77**, 570–6.

Williams RHP, Heatley RV, Lewis MH and Hughes LE (1977) In *Clinical parenteral nutrition* Baxter DH and Jackson GM (Eds) p 52. Geistlich Education, Chester.

Wilmore DW and McDougal WS (1977) Nutrition in burns. In

Nutritional aspects of care in the critically ill Richards JR and Kinney JM (Eds) pp 583–94. Churchill Livingstone, Edinburgh.

Woolfson AMJ, Heatley RV and Allison SP (1977) Significance of insulin in the metabolic response to injury. In *Nutritional aspects of care in the critically ill* Richards JR and Kinney JM (Eds) pp 367–88. Churchill Livingstone, Edinburgh.

5.2   Diets for Immunosuppressed Patients ('Sterile' Diets)

Patients who have had their natural immunity to infection reduced by chemotherapy or radiation therapy may be at risk of microbiological contamination from the food eaten.

Many foods which we eat contain small and usually insignificant numbers of micro-organisms, but for patients who have undergone an immunosuppressive regimen, even minute amounts of these micro-organisms could prove to be harmful. It is therefore necessary to minimize microbiological contamination in the diet.

Complete sterilization of food is difficult and would result in an extremely unpalatable diet. However, in some specialist units 'commercially sterile' foods are prepared. This means that the food is not totally sterile but that it has an extremely low level of contamination. This level of 'sterility' is achieved by using gamma-irradiated and canned foods only. In some units the food is prepared in a Laminar Air-Flow cabinet. Canned foods, for example, are opened and warmed in the cabinet, then placed in special foil closed containers, double wrapped in sterile paper bags and taken straight to the patient.

For a patient not being treated in a specialist unit, the 'very clean food regimen' may be a practical alternative. This aims to provide a nutritionally adequate, palatable and practical diet with the minimum risk to the patient. There are four main aspects of the 'very clean food regimen'

1   Suitable foods.
2   Methods of cooking.
3   The shelf life of processed foods used.
4   Foods suitable after the period of isolation.

Suitable foods

Suitable food are summarized in Table 5.6.

Suitable methods of cooking

Cooking can be carried out in a
1   Conventional cooker, either gas or electric.
2   Pressure cooker or a hospital/industrial steamer.
3   Microwave oven.

Table 5.6 Foods suitable for a 'Very Clean Food Regimen'

Food	Comments
Water	Boiled, bottled sterile water, canned mineral water. Bottled mineral water is not suitable.
Milk	Sterilized or UHT; once opened keep refrigerated and use within 24 hours.
Drinks	Coffee and tea should be freshly made on an individual basis, water used must be boiling. Fruit juice — longlife cartons or small tetra packs of fruit juice or of diluted squashes. Once opened any remaining should be discarded after 24 hours. Canned and bottled fizzy drinks, e.g. lemonade, lucozade, etc. Fruit squash — bottles of squash may be used, but once opened any remaining should be discarded after 48 hours. Hycal may be useful if patient is on fluid restriction. Discard any remaining after 48 hours.
Bread	Use a wrapped loaf, fresh daily. This should be toasted to kill surface yeasts.
Butter	Individual portions, these should be kept refrigerated.
Meat and fish	Freshly cooked or high quality frozen entrees cooked by a suitable method. Canned meat or fish and vacuum packed meats can be used but, any remaining after 24 hours must be discarded.
Eggs	These must be well cooked, *not* lightly boiled or raw as in egg nog.
Cheese	Cheese may be used in cooked dishes. If used uncooked it must be vacuum packed and *well within* the 'sell by' date, and should be discarded 24 hours after opening.
Vegetables	Canned vegetables. Fresh and frozen vegetables may be used if they are suitably cooked. Avoid uncooked salad vegetables.
Fruit	Canned Fruit. Fresh or frozen fruit, cooked by a suitable method. Avoid raw fresh fruit.
Dried foodstuffs	Wherever possible breakfast cereals, biscuits, sugar and coffee should be individually packaged, and should preferably be opened and served in the cubicle. New large packets may be used, but discarded after three days. Dried foodstuffs which require cooking such as milk puddings, sponge puddings, cornflour, custard and packet soups can be used, but must be well cooked, preferably in a pressure cooker or industrial steamer.
Cold puddings	Cold uncooked puddings such as Angel Delight should be avoided. Ice cream and jelly should also be avoided.
Cake	Suitable if freshly baked and covered and cooled as quickly as possible after baking.

Table 5.6 contd.

Food	Comments
Pepper and other spices	These contain many bacterial spores; they may be used in cooked dishes, but should not be added to the meal after cooking.
Salt	Individual sachets are suitable.
Tube feeds	Wherever possible, commercially prepared 'sterile' tube feeds should be used in preference to 'home made' tube feeds
Infant feeding 1 Infant milks 2 Infant foods	'Ready to feed' milk formulae may be used Jars and canned baby foods are suitable. Dried baby foods must be made up with boiling water or boiling milk. The smallest possible packets should be used, and once opened should not be used for more than three days. The packet should be securely closed after each use.

Conventional gas or electric cooker

Oven. This method of cooking may be used, but certain precautions should be taken. The oven should always be preheated to mimimize the time when the food will be 'warm'. The aim is to ensure that the heat has thoroughly penetrated the food; the minimum acceptable core temperature of the food is 70°C. The core temperature of the food can be checked using a thermometer with a probe but this must *not* be used on the foods to be eaten by the patient.

Boiling on the hob. The food should always be put into rapidly boiling water, and brought back to boiling point as soon as possible. Once again the mimimum acceptable core temperature of the food is 70°C and can be checked (on duplicate food samples) with a probe thermometer.

Pressure cooking/steaming

Pressure cooking is an excellent way of preparing meals for the immunosuppressed patient, and is the method of choice in many hospitals. A domestic sized pressure cooker or large scale catering steamer may be used. It may then be possible for the patient to choose main meals from the general hospital menu and for these meals to be cooked under pressure. Care must be taken in transporting meals to the patient, as once the food has been cooked any subsequent contamination could put the immunosuppressed patient at risk.

Microwave oven

This may be a convenient way of reheating frozen or freshly cooked chilled foods for the immunosuppressed patient.

However, there is some evidence to suggest that the microwave oven may not be as efficient at killing micro-organisms as a conventional cooker. Fruin and Guthertz (1982) compared the destructive effect of

Table 5.7 Cooking foods for immunosuppressed patients — some examples

Food	Method of cooling	Cooking temperature	Cooking time	Core temperature of food after cooking
Lamb chops	Oven	200°C	35 min	80°C
Faggots in gravy	Oven	230°C	40 min	92°C
Fish fingers	Oven	200°C	10 min	90°C
Fish cakes	Oven	200°C	15 min	88°C
Minced beef/onion pie	Oven	220°C	35 min	99°C
Sausages	Oven	220°C	20 min	97°C
Oven chips	Oven	200°C	10 min	82°C
Chicken portion	Oven	200°C	25 min	87°C
Cod in batter	Oven	200°C	15 min	64°C
Chicken and mushroom casserole	Boil in the bag		15 min from water reboiling	90°C
Cod in parsley sauce	Boil in the bag		20 min from water reboiling	85°C
Roast beef in gravy	Boil in the bag		15 min from water reboiling	76°C

different cooking methods on certain bacteria. They found that the rapid increase in temperature which food underwent during cooking in a microwave oven did not kill the bacteria present as efficiently as a conventional oven in which the food is at a high temperature for a longer time. They also found that the microwave heating of non-fluid food items can be much less regular than in those cooked in a conventional oven.

Some examples of how specific foods may be cooked for the immunosuppressed patient are shown in Table 5.7.

Shelf life of processed foods

Canned foods can be stored for a very long time, (Table 5.8) Even after the times suggested, the food should be microbiologically safe for immunosuppressed patients but there may be a slight change in colour, texture or flavour.

Stored cans should be marked with the date they are received and used in rotation. They should always be stored in a cool dry place.

Table 5.8 Recommended storage times of canned foods for use by immunosuppressed patients

Canned food item	Recommended storage time
Milk products e.g.	
Cream Evaporated milk, Milk puddings	1 year
Rhubarb	9 months
Fruit juice	1 year
Prunes	1 year
Blackberries, blackcurrants, gooesberries, raspberries and strawberries	18 months
Other fruits	2 years
Vegetables (except new potatoes)	2 years
New potatoes	18 months
Baked beans	2 years
Pasta products, e.g. canned macaroni.	2 years
Soups	2 years
Fruit sauce	2 years
Solid pack cold meat products, e.g. ham, corned beef.	5 years
Fish in oil	5 years

All dried and frozen foods should be used well within the manufacturer's 'use by' date.

Foods after the period of isolation

When the previously immunosuppressed patient's white cell count has increased to a level where he or she can come out of isolation, a more normal diet can be followed. Patients can then choose their food from the hospital menu, provided that anything which is cooked is kept *hot* and served with *minimum* delay.

The following precautions should also be taken
1 Eggs should be well cooked, i.e. not soft boiled or lightly fried. Raw egg should be avoided.
2 Fresh fruit should be of a high quality, not overripe and should be peeled before being eaten.
3 Fresh vegetables. All cooked vegetables are suitable, but salad vegetables which cannot be skinned, (such as lettuce) should be avoided.

Patients should also be given advice on eating out. As far as possible, foods should be chosen which are freshly cooked and are still hot; cafeteria food which has been kept in a heated display cabinet should be avoided.

Further reading

Baldwin RE (1983) Microwave cooking: an overview. *J Food Protection* **46**, (3), 266–9.
Crespo FL *et al* (1977) Effect of conventional microwave heating on *Pseudomonas putrefaciens*, *Streptococcus faecalis* and *Lactobacillus plantorum* in meat tissue. *J Food Protection* **40**, (9), 588–91.
Cunningham FE (1980) Influence of microwave radiation on psychrotrophic bacteria. *J Food Protection* **43**, (8), 651–5.
Dahl CA *et al* (1980) Fate of *Staphylococcus aureus* in beef loaf, potatoes and frozen and canned green beans after microwave heating in a simulated cook/chill hospital food service system. *J Food Protection* **43**, (12), 916–23.
Dreyfuss MS and Chipley JR (1980) Comparison of effects of sublethal microwave radiation and conventional heating on the metabolic activity of *Staphylococcus aureus*. *Appl Environ Microbiol* **39**, (1), 13–6.
Page W and Martin WG (1978) Survival of microbial films in the microwave oven. *Can J Microbiol* **24**, (11), 1431–3.
Vela CR and Wu JF (1979) Mechanism of lethal action of 2450 MHz radiation on micro-organisms. *Appl Environ Microbiol* **37**, (3), 550–3.

Reference

Fruin J and Guthertz L (1982) Survival of bacteria in food cooked by microwave oven, conventional oven, and slow cookers. *J Food Protection* **45**, (8), 695–8.

5.3   Intensive Care Units

5.3.1   Intensive therapy units (ITUs)

Intensive therapy is not an alternative method of medical care but merely a concentration of existing techniques of diagnosis, measurement and treatment for the critically ill patient. Intensive therapy units (ITUs) have evolved over the past 30 years as a logical progression of patient care. In general wards those patients requiring most nursing care are usually sited nearest the nurses' station and progress out into the ward as their condition improves. The concentration of expertise and equipment required for critically ill patients into purpose-built units has advantages in terms of both patient care and economics.

Most ITUs in the UK are administered by an anaesthetist who shares the clinical care of the patient with the admitting consultant. The multiple problems associated with the care of the critically ill require a multi-disciplinary approach to intensive therapy. ITUs make a heavy demand on laboratory and para-medical services in the hospital — particularly biochemistry, haematology, bacteriology, radiology, pharmacy and physiotherapy. Experienced members of these departments are usually assigned to ITUs. Other specialists are called in to advise as required. Dietetic departments may not routinely designate a member of staff to cover ITUs. In fact, many dietitians may be apprehensive about visiting and advising the staff in ITU and feel that a visit is almost tantamount to territorial invasion! To overcome this, the dietitian should make frequent, regular visits to the ITU, not only when called but routinely to establish a rapport with the medical and nursing staff. The advent of nutritional care teams, which ought to include an experienced dietitian, should help to establish the dietitian as a member of the intensive therapy team.

Aims of intensive therapy

Selection of patients to ITU is usually based on clinical judgement and experience. Initial resuscitation should be followed by rapid and controlled transfer of the patient to ITU where the overall clinical status of the patient can be assessed more thoroughly. Measurement and monitoring techniques are established and priorities and therapy decided. Appropriate treatment is started and closely monitored. Where indicated, support systems such as mechanical ventilation are used. Therapy should aim to prevent malnutrition, sepsis and multiple organ failure.

The final aim of intensive care is the transfer and rehabilitation of successfully treated patients. The timing of the discharge is important as most patients are transferred to general medical or surgical wards where medical and nursing care is less concentrated.

Nutritional support in intensive care

An experienced dietitian should visit ITU regularly and be available to give dietary advice as required as part of a multi-disciplinary care team. However, such advice is not usually needed until the patient is established in the unit. One of the most fundamental points to remember is that patients in ITU seldom eat a normal diet and take only limited amounts of nutrients via the oral route. If patients are able to eat and if they require a therapeutic diet (e.g. diabetic or low fat, etc.), accurate control of each meal is not usually necessary as their intake of food is often self-limited and they are closely monitored to detect any biochemical changes. The nursing staff are generally well trained in recording the patient's fluid and food intake. Each 24-hour record can be analysed by the dietitian to calculate the nutrient intake if this information is required.

Most patients in ITUs require the use of artificial methods of feeding. The principles of tube feeding have been discussed in Section 1.12.3 and those of parenteral nutrition in Section 1.13. The choice of enteral or parenteral nutrition varies in different hospitals and may depend on available experience in the two techniques.

The critically ill patient is less likely to have a functioning gut and therefore more likely to require parenteral nutrition. However, if the gut is functional, enteral nutrition is the preferred method of feeding. Although the basic principles of enteral and parenteral nutrition apply, the metabolic changes which occur in intensive therapy patients necessitate particular consideration when planning the feeding regimens. Disorders of fluid and electrolyte balance occur and the calculation of accurate daily fluid balance is vital. The total fluid required for feeding regimens must be clearly understood — particularly when more than one route is being used for feeding at any one time. The use of indirect calorimetry has shown that the energy requirements of critically ill patients are often less than was previously thought. However, this technique for estimating energy requirements is not routinely available to all ITUs and nutritional requirements need to be estimated for each patient (see Section 1.11) including the appropriate additional allowance for pyrexia, sepsis, burns, fistula losses, etc. Over-feeding should be avoided, particularly in patients who are paralysed, heavily sedated or ventilated.

Enteral feeding considerations

Gastric Emptying. Many critically ill patients have delayed gastric emptying. It is important to ensure this function is adequate before commencing nasogastric feeding. A wide bore tube, e.g. Ryles or Salem should be passed and 60–100 ml of water infused over about 12 hours. If aspiration every four hours produces only a minimal return, nasogastric feeding may be started. The Ryles tube may be replaced by a fine bore tube once adequate gastric emptying has been well established. If there is any doubt regarding gastric emptying during feeding, intermittent feeding via a wider bore tube with aspiration before each feed may be more appropriate than a 24-hour continuous infusion. Such regimen will help reduce the likelihood of aspiration pneumonia occurring.

Introduction of enteral feed. In patients whose gastrointestinal function is gradually returning to normal, feeds introduced slowly and at half strength are usually well tolerated. The volume and then the density of the feed should be gradually increased; the rate of administration being controlled ideally by an infusion pump.

Hyperosmolar feeds may be more likely to cause gastrointestinal side effects and care should be taken if they are required (see fluid restriction below).

Fluid restriction. If total fluid intake has to be restricted it may be necessary to use a high energy, high nitrogen feed to achieve the required nutrient intake in a reduced volume. Such feeds are hyperosmolar and should be given slowly to reduce the risk of osmotic diarrhoea occurring.

Diarrhoea. Diarrhoea is often a result of antibiotic therapy and should be treated with an antidiarrhoeal agent such as codeine phosphate. Sterile proprietary feeds should be used and administered using an aseptic technique to reduce the risk of microbial contamination. It must be remembered that contamination of the feed can occur via the host pathogens.

Glucose intolerance. Enteral feeds have a fairly high carbohydrate content and patients may exhibit an intolerance to glucose with a resulting hyperglycaemia due to a resistance to the action of insulin (Allison et al 1968).

Parenteral feeding considerations

Fluid and electrolyte balance. Fluctuations in fluid and electrolyte balance may be more readily corrected using a multi-bottle regimen rather than a 3 litre big bag system. Some clinicians prefer to wait until the patient is more stable before changing to a 3 litre big bag method for administering parenteral solutions.

Glucose intolerance. Intravenous feeding regimens contain large amounts of glucose. Hyperglycaemia should be controlled by using insulin. Glucose tolerance may be improved by providing the patient's energy requirements from both glucose and fat rather than from glucose alone. The administration of concentrated glucose solutions to septic and critically ill patients causes an increase in O_2 consumption and CO_2 production. This imposes an additional burden for gas exchange in patients with respiratory insufficiency. The substitution of fat for some of the glucose energy lowers the production of CO_2 and the respiratory quotient (RQ) while maintaining O_2 consumption. (Jeejeebhoy et al 1976; Askanazi et al 1981).

Concurrent drug therapy and CVP monitoring. Ideally the feeding line should be used solely for feeding and not for taking blood, giving drugs or measuring central venous pressure (CVP). The use of the line for these purposes increases the risk of complications, particularly sepsis. In order to overcome this, two central lines may need to be inserted.

Modification of nutritional support for organ failure

The function of many organs is susceptible to metabolic changes induced by disease elsewhere in the body and to the effects of septic shock. Altered function of these organs may in turn result in additional changes in metabolism in general.

Post-traumatic respiratory insufficiency. Trauma patients often develop respiratory insufficiency because of direct or indirect pulmonary contusions, thoracic surgery, pneumonia, fat embolism or respiratory distress syndrome, and artificial ventilation is needed. Nutritional therapy should avoid overfeeding, overhydration and excessive carbohydrate loads.

Acute renal failure. The most common cause of oliguria is hypovolaemia. Anuria usually indicates renal damage. During severe shock, renal blood flow decreases and glomerular filtration rate and urine output are drastically reduced. Early frequent dialysis is beneficial as it allows adequate nutritional support by controlling fluid balance and uraemia. The management of renal failure is discussed in more detail in Section 4.16.

Hepatic failure. Failure of the liver has numerous effects on body function. The use of branched chain amino acids in the management of hepatic encephalopathy is currently being researched and both enteral and parenteral preparations enriched with branched chain amino acids are available but their value is uncertain. The management of hepatic failure is discussed in more detail in Section 4.13.

Abnormalities in liver function may be recorded during total parenteral nutrition and the possible reasons for this are explained in Section 1.13

Cardiac dysfunction. The restriction of fluid and sodium is often critical in patients with congestive cardiac failure. Energy-dense enteral feeds may be useful to provide adequate nutrition in a limited volume and concentrated glucose solutions together with lipid can be used to provide energy requirements intravenously. The use of salt-free albumin in hypoalbuminaemic patients may result in a diuresis. If diuretics are used, care should be taken to prevent hypokalaemia. Maintenance of phosphate balance is also important in patients with cardiac disease.

Pancreatic failure. Patients with acute pancreatitis or severe pancreatic injury (including pancreatic surgery) require nutritional support via the parenteral route. Intravenous feeding can suppress secretions of the upper gastrointestinal tract (Hamilton *et al* 1971). The infusion of elemental diets distal to the pylorus can also suppress pancreatic secretions (Voitk *et al* 1973; Ragins *et al* 1973, Blackburn *et al* 1976) and may be a suitable method of feeding enterally instead of parenterally.

Summary

The mortality rate of patients in ITUs is high; late mortality following trauma being due primarily to sepsis and multiple organ failure. The developments in clinical nutrition over recent years have been rapid and it is now possible to meet the nutritional requirements of the critically ill to reduce catabolism, minimize losses and improve survival, enabling the transfer and rehabilitation of successfully treated patients from ITU to the general wards.

5.3.2 Coronary care units

On admittance to a Coronary Care Unit (CCU) patients will normally require a light diet. Ideally this should be available from the normal hospital menu, with the emphasis being on small, regular meals offering appetising food.

Special diets, if necessary, should be requested by medical staff soon after admittance. Many patients in coronary care units will be recommended to lose some weight by medical staff, and the dietitian should start advising and re-educating the patient as soon as possible as incentive tends to be high in someone who has recently had a heart attack. The most appropriate time for giving this advice depends on the individual circumstances; patients may be in a stressful situation in the first few days and so may not remember advice given. Any dietary instructions given should be reiterated close to the time of discharge.

Those not requiring specific dietary advice may still require some general advice on diet, and it is important for dietitians to make medical and nursing staff aware of their role in this area. Patients are likely to be receptive to advice on changing and improving their normal dietary pattern, and may have many questions they wish to ask. The dietitian should therefore make herself available as an adviser on good nutrition for these patients and should also have the opportunity to talk to relatives. The discussion should include the following points

1 Energy balance – and the importance of achieving/ maintaining ideal body weight. Patients may become less active after a heart attack, their lifestyle may change if they are not working, or they may give up smoking, all of which could lead to an increase in weight, so even patients who are not overweight may benefit from advice on weight control after a heart attack.

2 Fat intake — the importance of reducing the total amount of fat in the diet to approximately 35% of the energy intake. Patients may have many questions about cholesterol and types of fat.

3 Fibre in the diet — a higher intake of fibre should be encouraged by promoting the use of wholemeal bread, wholegrain cereals and pasta and fruit and vegetables.

4 Sugar intake — particulary in relation to weight control. Identifying ways in which the individual can reduce sugar intake.

5 Alcohol consumption — advice given should be consistent with that given by medical staff.

6 Smoking and its effect on weight control.

7 General nutritional aspects — such as meal frequency (small regular meals are better than infrequent large ones) or how to choose wisely when eating out or for special occasions.

Literature outlining sensible healthy eating should be available for patients on cardiac wards. A dietary display in the patients' day room or giving talks to groups of patients are useful ways of reinforcing dietary education.

It is important that the hospital menu reflects the advice being given to patients and gives patients an example of a suitable diet to eat at home; patients should be encouraged to make a healthy choice of food while in hospital so that questions can be answered as they arise and any mistakes rectified.

Further reading

Abbott WC, Echenique MM, Bistrian BR, Williams S and Blackburn GL (1983) Nutritional care of the trauma patient. *Surg Gynaecol Obstet* **157**, 585—97.

Allison SP (1984) Clinical nutrition 4: Nutritional problems in intensive care. *Hosp Update* **10**, 1001—12.

Bain WH and Taylor KM (1983) *Handbook of intensive care*. Wright, Bristol.

Tweedle DEF (1982) *Metabolic care*. Churchill Livingstone, Edinburgh.

References

Allison SP, Hinton P and Chamberlain MJ (1968) Intravenous glucose tolerance, insulin and free fatty acid levels in burned patients. *Lancet* **ii**, 1113—6.

Askanazi J, Nordenstrom J, Rosenbaum SH *et al* (1981) Nutrition for the patient with respiratory failure: glucose vs fat. *Anesthesiology* **54**, 373—7.

Blackburn GL, Williams LF, Bistrian BR *et al* (1976) New approaches to the management of severe acute pancreatitis. *Ann Surg* **186**, 651—8.

Cuthbertson DP (1930) The disturbance of metabolism produced by bony and non-bony injury, with notes on certain abnormal conditions of bone. *Biochem J* **24**, 1244—63.

Cuthbertson DP (1942) Post shock metabolic response. *Lancet* **i**, 433—7.

Hamilton RF, Davis WC, Stephenson DV and McGee DF (1971) Effects of parenteral hyperalimentation on upper gastrointestinal tract secretion. *Arch Surg* **102**, 348—52.

Jeejeebhoy KN, Anderson GH, Nakhooda AF *et al* (1976) Metabolic studies in total parenteral nutrition with lipid in man. *J Clin Invest* **57**, 125—36.

O'Keefe SJD, Sender PM and James WPT (1974) 'Catabolic' loss of body nitrogen in response to surgery. *Lancet* **ii**, 1035—8.

Ragins H, Levenson SM, Signer R *et al* (1973) Intrajejunal administration of an elemental diet at neutral pH avoids pancreatic stimulation: studies in dog and man. *Am J Surg* **126**, 606—14.

Voitk A, Brown RH, Echave V *et al* (1973) Use of an elemental diet in the treatment of complicated pancreatitis. *Am J Surg* **125**, 223—7.

Wilmae DW and Aulick LH (1978) Metabolic changes in burned patients. *Surg Clin North Am* **58**, 1173—88.

Woolfson AMJ (1978) Metabolic considerations in nutritional support. In *Developments in clinical nutrition* Johnson IDA and Lee HA (Eds). Proceedings of a Symposium held at the Royal College of Physicians. London, October 1978. pp 35—47. MCS Consultants, Tunbridge Wells.

5.4 Low Birth Weight Infants and Special Care Baby Units

The low birth weight infant is defined as weighing less than 2500 g at birth. Very low birth weight (<1500 g) and extremely low birth weight (<1000 g) infants further categorize this group.

The prognosis for low birth weight infants has improved dramatically in recent years and over 50% of babies born weighing <1500 g now survive in special care baby units and develop normally.

There are two main reasons for low birth weight. The infant can either be *preterm* with a gestational age of 36 weeks or less or *small-for-gestational-age* (SFGA), defined as being below the 10th centile for weight at birth. The latter may have a more developed organ system, including the gastrointestinal tract, compared with preterm infants and so may be better able to digest and absorb feeds. SFGA infants should be fed to their expected 10th centile weight. Growth charts for infants preterm to 2 years are available from Castlemead Publications, Swain Mill, 4A Crane Mead, Ware, Herts SG12 9PY.

At present the aim when feeding the preterm low birth weight infant is to achieve a postnatal growth which mimics the intrauterine growth of a normal foetus of the same conceptual age. The American Academy of Pediatrics have recently reviewed their nutritional recommendations (AAP 1985).

5.4.1 Nutritional requirements of low birth weight infants

Energy

The energy requirement of low birth weight infants, taking into consideration their requirement for optimal weight gain, has been estimated to be 85–130 kcal/kg/day (Kerner 1983). Incubation will help reduce external heat loss and thus resting energy expenditure. Their actual needs are difficult to quantify because of the wide variation that exists between individual infants but intrauterine growth rates (20 g/day between 30–40 weeks gestational age) have been achieved in low birth weight infants receiving 120 kcal/kg/day (AAP 1985).

The percentage of energy provided by fat and carbohydrate is partially determined by tolerance but in commercial formulae specifically produced for the low birth weight infant they contribute 40–50% and 35–

40% respectively, which is similar to the ratio in mature human milk.

Protein

The normal term foetus lays down about 66% of its total body nitrogen during the last 8–9 weeks of gestation. It is therefore vital that the preterm infant receives adequate amounts of protein of suitable amino acid composition to achieve the rapid anabolism associated with brain development and general growth. An intake of 3.5–4.0 g/kg/day has been suggested (AAP 1985).

Amino acid pattern

The amino acid pattern of mature human milk is the reference standard against which the profile of formula feeds is compared. By adjusting the casein:whey ratio to 40:60, an amino acid pattern more closely resembling that of mature human milk is produced. This modification improves the digestibility and biological value of the feed. In addition the sulphur-containing amino acid content is increased, particularly cystine which is considered to be an essential amino acid for the immature infant. Taurine may also be an essential amino acid in low birth weight infants as they have a limited ability to synthesize it and human milk has a higher taurine content than cows' milk. Formula feeds for the low birth weight infant therefore provide at least the level of taurine found in human milk (5 mg/100 ml).

Fat

Fat contributes 50% of the energy of human milk and 40–50% in commercial formulae. Due to digestive tract immaturity the low birth weight infant has a reduced ability to absorb the saturated triglyceride found predominantly in cows' milk but absorbs unsaturated long chain triglycerides (LCT) from vegetable oils much more efficiently and medium chain triglycerides (MCT) even more so (AAP 1985). Thus low birth weight infant formulae now contain a mixture of LCT and MCT and more than adequately provide the essential fatty acid requirement.

The fat of human milk is well absorbed if it is not subjected to heat treatment which can denature the lipase naturally present in the milk (AAP 1985).

Carbohydrate

Low birth weight infants frequently have low intestinal lactase activity and therefore are relatively inefficient at digesting lactose. However, glucose polymers present no problem as glycosidase enzymes are active. On the basis of this, some low birth weight infant formulae provide 40–50% carbohydrate energy as lactose and 50–60% as glucose polymers (see Table 5.10).

Minerals and trace elements

Sodium and Potassium

The immature renal function of the low birth weight infant restricts the capacity to increase or decrease sodium excretion efficiently according to needs. Hyponatraemia and hypernatraemia are both potential problems for these infants (Aperia et al 1983). In relation to rapid growth, overall needs for sodium are generally higher in the low birth weight infant and hyponatraemia is a particular risk for very low birth weight infants during the first few weeks of life (Day et al 1975). Low birth weight infant formulae therefore have a higher sodium content than mature human milk (see Table 5.10). However, it should also be noted that some preparations are higher in sodium than others. Prematalac (Cow and Gate), for example, is especially suitable for infants with high sodium losses; Nenatal (Cow and Gate) is more suitable for those losing less sodium.

Potassium and chloride needs have not been well investigated but appear to be similar to those of term infants, that is, a minimum daily intake of 1.5 mmol potassium and 1.2 mmol chloride/kg body weight/day (Poole 1985).

Calcium and phosphorus

Since rickets is a high risk in the very low birth weight infant, formulae developed for these infants have a higher calcium and phosphorus content than mature human milk (Table 5.10). Studies have shown their use can lead to postnatal bone growth and mineralization comparable to foetal rates (Steichen et al 1980).

Zinc and manganese

There is evidence that zinc absorption in low birth weight infants is highly correlated with fat and nitrogen absorption and, providing that 40–50% of the fat is in the form of medium chain triglycerides, these nutrients can help produce a positive zinc balance (Voyer et al 1982). In the light of current knowledge the recommended levels for full term infant formulae (0.5 mg zinc/100 kcal and 5 μg manganese/100 kcal) are considered appropriate for low birth weight infant formulae (AAP 1985).

Iron

The low birth weight infant has a lower body content of iron than the full term infant and in addition frequent blood sampling may further deplete stores. However, the early anaemia of prematurity is not improved by oral iron supplementation and it should not usually be given before 1–2 months of age. If it is started earlier, vitamin E supplementation is essential as high intakes of iron interfere with its metabolism (Ziegler et al 1981).

Once a weight of 2000 g is achieved, or the infant is discharged, and is being fed wholly breast milk, iron supplementation (2–3 mg/kg/day) is essential. Low birth weight formulae on the other hand theoretically provide a sufficient iron intake.

Vitamins

Although the recommended oral intakes for the majority of vitamins do not differ between the low birth weight and full term infant (AAP 1985), some vitamins do require special consideration.

Vitamin D

The prevention of severe bone disease, including rickets, is dependent on an adequate intake of calcium and phosphorus (see Section 4.26) and at least 500 i.u. of vitamin D/day (AAP 1985). There is no evidence that any benefit can be obtained from giving the active metabolite of vitamin D.

Vitamin E

Low birth weight infants generally have a far lower body content of vitamin E at birth than full term infants (20 mg in a 3 kg infant compared with only 3 mg in 1000 g infant). The American Academy of Pediatrics (1985) recommend an intake of 0.7 i.u. vitamin E/100 kcal.

Energy density and fluid requirement

The use of an energy-dense feed allows the volume fed to the low birth weight infant to be smaller than would otherwise be the case. This can be advantageous when the gastric capacity is small. However, the use of such hyperosmolar feeds is associated with a high incidence of necrotising enterocolitis in the low birth weight infant (Book *et al* 1975).

Low birth weight formulae proving 80 kcal/100 ml fed at the rate of 120 kcal/kg/day have been estimated to provide sufficient water to permit adequate excretion of electrolytes and protein metabolites.

5.4.2 Feeding methods

Oral feeding

Breast milk

The advantages of breast feeding (Section 3.2.1) generally endorse its promotion in special care baby units whenever possible. Apart from the immunological benefits and the better absorption characteristics, the enhanced emotional bonding associated with breast feeding can be a particularly important reason for encouraging it.

It may initially be necessary to give the infant expressed breast milk, but if this is given via an enteral feed line, fat may adhere to the tube thus reducing the energy density of the feed.

Milk from mothers of preterm infants, especially during the first two weeks after delivery, has a higher concentration of energy, fat and protein than milk from mothers of full term infants (Table 5.9). This is unlikely to be an 'adaptive' effect but simply a consequence of low volume output by most mothers of preterm infants (Lucas and Hudson 1984). Nevertheless, it has been shown that pooled human milk from mothers of full term infants when given to low birth weight infants produces a slower rate of growth than the use of milk from mothers of preterm infants or low birth weight formulae (Fleischman and Finberg 1979).

Commercial milk formulae

Several formulations are available for feeding low birth weight infants (Table 5.10). Some have been specifically designed to meet the needs of those with particular problems such as high sodium losses (see previous section on nutritional requirements of low birth weight infants). Other differences in their nutrient profile reflect uncertainties about the most suitable form and amount of specific nutrients required. All formulae have been found to produce adequate growth and metabolic stability.

Longterm effects of different feeding methods in low birth weight infants

Research currently in progress will eventually elucidate the long term effects of feeding premature babies in the neonatal period (Lucas *et al* 1984a). A multicentre collaborative study in Cambridge, Sheffield, Norwich, Ipswich and Kings Lynn is following 950 infants of <1850 g birth weight in four randomized clinical trials comparing

1 Banked donor breast milk with a preterm formula (Osterprem) as sole diets.

2 A term formula (Osterfeed) with the preterm formula (Osterprem) as sole diets.

3 and **4** As in 1 and 2, but used as supplements to mothers own expressed breast milk.

These infants will be followed intermittently into adulthood.

Preliminary short term results have been published (Lucas *et al* 1984b). The main findings up to the 18 month post term follow-up will be published in 1987. Interim results from the follow-up of the first 400 infants have shown that the diet given to a premature baby whilst in hospital has major effects nearly two years later, and that these effects cannot be predicted from short term findings. For example, the preterm formula-fed group compared with the group fed donor

Table 5.9 Variations in energy and macronutrient content of breast milk/100 ml Adapted from Macy and Kelly (1961), DHSS (1977), and Anderson *et al* (1981)

Nutrient	Neonatal age				Mature breast milk		
	3−5 days		8−11 days		Range	Averages	
	Full term	Premature	Full term	Premature		Mothers	Banked donors
Protein (g)	1.9	2.1	1.7	1.9	0.7−2.0	1.3	1.1
Fat (g)	1.9	3.0*	2.9	4.1*	1.3−8.3	4.2	1.7
Carbohydrate (g) (lactose)	5.1	5.0	6.0	5.6	5.0−9.2	7.4	7.1
Energy (kcal)	48	58*	59	71*	45−119	70	46

*Significantly different in premature compared to full term.

Table 5.10 Composition of preterm infant formulae (All values are expressed per 200 ml prepared feed)

Nutrient	Mature breast milk (Range)[1,2]		Nenatal (Cow and Gate)	Prematalac (Cow and Gate)	Gold Cap SMA low birth weight (Wyeth)	Preaptamil (Milupa)	Osterprem (Farley)
Energy (kJ)	270	−315	320	330	334	308	334
(kcal)	65	−75	76	79	80	74	80
Protein (g)	1.2	−1.4	1.8	2.4	2.0	2.1	2.0
Casein (g)	0.5*		0.7	na	0.8	1.1	0.8
Whey (g)	0.8*		1.1	na	1.2	1.0	1.2
Fat (g)	3.7	−4.8	4.5	5.0	4.4	3.6	4.9
Carbohydrate (g)	7.1	−7.8	7.5	6.6	8.6	8.7	7.0
Calcium (mg)	32	−36	80	67	75	60	70
Phosphorus (mg)	14	−15	40	53	40	45	35
Ca:P ratio	2.3:1*		2:1	1.3:1	1.9:1	1.3:1	2:1
Sodium (mg)	11	−20	23	60	32	35	45
Potassium (mg)	57	−62	70	95	75	80	65
Chloride (mg)	35	−55	45	80	53	43	60
Magnesium (mg)	2.6	−3.0	8	11	7	7	5
Iron (μg)	62	−93	900	650	670	700	40
Zinc (μg)	260	−330	600	400	800	100	1000
Iodine (μg)	2	−12	6	4	8.3	na	7
Manganese (μg)	0.7	−1.5	11	10	20	10	3
Copper (μg)	37	−43	75	50	70	10	120
A retinol equiv (μg)	40	−76	80	80	96	150	100
D_3 cholecalciferol (μg)	na		3	1.1	1.3	1.1	8
E α−tocopherol (mg)	0.29−0.39		4	1.0	1.5	1.25	10
K_1 Phytomenadione (μg)	na		7	3.2	7	na	7
B_1 Thiamin (μg)	13	−21	100	70	80	100	95
B_2 Riboflavin (μg)	31		150	100	130	100	180
B_6 Pyridoxine (μg)	5.1	−7.2	70	80	50	100	100
B_{12} Cyanocobalamin (μg)	0.01		0.2	0.12	0.2	0.28	0.2
Nicotinic acid (μg)	210	−270	1000	850	630	1250	1000
Pantothenic acid (μg)	220	−330	500	250	360	na	500
Biotin (μg)	0.52−1.13		1.0	3.1	1.8	3.85	2
Folic acid (μg)	3.1	−6.2	13	3.5	10	12.5	50
C Ascorbic acid (mg)	3.1	−4.5	12	6.5	7	12.5	28
Choline (mg)	na		15	5.6	12.7	na	5.6
Inositol (mg)	na		23	na	na	na	3.2
Renal solute load (mosmol/l)	78*		113	169	173	132	133

[1] DHSS (1980)
[2] DHSS (1977)
*Average figure

breast milk became latently sensitized to cow's milk protein (Lucas *et al* 1984c) and left hospital with lower plasma IgG concentrations; however this had no detectable consequences in terms of clinical allergy or infection later in infancy. There are also indications that the type of feed given in hospital in the neonatal period can significantly influence development scores at follow-up. Dietitians should look out for publications from this major study.

Tube feeding (see also Section 1.12.3)

Infants born before 34 weeks gestation are likely to have poor co-ordination of sucking, swallowing and respiration and may therefore require to be tube fed. The preferred method is either continuous or bolus gastric feeds; intrajejunal tubes reduce the risk of pulmonary aspiration but at the expense of a slower weight gain (Whitefield 1982).

The volume of feed given should be advanced slowly over 10−14 days in infants weighing <1000 g and over 6−8 days in those of >1500 g. Progression often involves a transitional period of both oral and enteral feeding.

Parenteral feeding

Parenteral nutrition is a valuable means of providing

the nutritional requirements of the low birth weight infant, especially those weighing <1500 g. It may be used to supplement the enteral intake or as the sole means of nutritional support.

The non-protein energy sources used are glucose and lipid. The osmolality of a glucose solution and the relatively poor glucose tolerance of the low birth weight infant limit the amount of glucose which can be given and glucose infusion should start at a rate <6 mg/kg body weight/minute. Lipid provides a concentrated iso-osmotic source of energy but, to avoid hyperlipidaemia, should be infused at a rate <0.25 g/kg body weight/hour (AAP 1985). A positive nitrogen balance can be achieved with a non-protein energy intake of 60 kcal/kg body weight/day and 2.5−3.0 g/kg body weight/day (Rubecz et al 1981).

The commercially available parenteral amino acid solutions are not specifically designed for the low birth weight infant and indeed the ideal composition for such a solution is not known.

The parenteral trace element requirements for low birth weight infants have only been estimated from the requirements for full term infants or from animal studies. Further research is needed in this area.

Despite the gaps in knowledge of the parenteral needs of low birth weight infants this feeding method has undoubtedly helped to achieve a more optimistic outlook for some infants of particularly low birth weight.

Support organisations

National Information for Parents of Prematures, Education, Resources and Support (NIPPERS), St Mary's Hospjtal, Praed Street, London W2. Tel: 01−725−1487.

National Association for the Welfare of Children in Hospital (NAWCH), Argyle House, 29−31 Euston Road, London NW1.

Further reading

Alderson P (1983) *Special care for babies in hospital*. NAWCH Publication, London.

Dear PRF (1984) Nutritional problems in the newborn *Hosp Update*, 915.

Jonxis JHP (Ed) (1978) *Growth and development of the full term and premature infant*. Excerpta Medica.

McLaren DS and Burman D (Eds). (1982) *Textbook of paediatric nutrition* 2e Churchill Livingstone, Edinburgh.

References

American Academy of Paediatrics. Committee on Nutrition (1985) Nutritional needs of low birth weight infants. *Paediatrics* **75**, 976−86.

Anderson GH *et al* (1981) Energy and macronutrient content of human milk during early lactation from mothers giving birth prematurely and at term. *Am J Clin Nutr* **34**, 258−65.

Aperia A, Broberger O, Herin P, Thodenius K and Zetterstrom R (1983) *Acta Paediatr Scand* [Suppl] **305**, 61−5.

Book LS, Herbst JJ, Atherton SO and Jung AL (1975) Necrotizing enterocolitis in low birth weight infants fed an elemental formula. *J Paediatr* **87**, 602−5.

Day GM Chance GW and Raddle IC (1975) Growth and mineral metabolism in very low birth weight infants. *Paediatr Res* **9**, 568−75.

DHSS (1977) *The composition of mature human milk*. Report on Health and Social Subjects No 12. HMSO, London.

DHSS (1980) *Artificial feeds for the young infant*. Report on Health and Social Subjects No 18 HMSO, London.

Fleischman AR and Finberg L (1979) Breast milk for term and premature infants — optimal nutrition? *Semin Perinatol* **3**, 397−405.

Kerner JA (1983) *Manual of paediatric parenteral nutrition*. Kerner JA Jr (Ed) John Wiley and Sons, Chichester.

Lucas A and Hudson GJ (1984) Pre-term milk as a source of protein for low birth weight infants. *Arch Dis Childh* **59**, 831−6.

Lucas A, Cole TJ, Gore SM, Baker B, Bates CJ, Simpson P, Lucas PJ, Cork S, DiCarlo L, Brinkworth R, Bamford MF and Dossetor JFB (1984b) Multicentre clinical trial of diets for low birth weight infants: interim analysis of short term clinical and biochemical effects of diet. *Paediatr Res* **18**, 807 (Abstract).

Lucas A, Gore SM, Cole TJ, Bamford MF, Dosseter JFB, Barr I DiCarlo L, Cork S and Lucas PJ (1984a) Multicentre trial on feeding low birthweight infants: effects of diet on early growth. *Arch Dis Childh* **59**, 722−30.

Lucas A, McLaughlan P and Combs RRA (1984c) Latent anaphylactic sensitization of infants of low birth weight to cows' milk proteins. *Br Med J* **289**, 1254−6.

Macy IG and Kelly HJ (1961) *Milk, the mammary gland and its secretion*, Volume II. Academic Press, London.

Poole RL (1985) *Manual of paediatric parenteral nutrition* Kerner JA Jr (Ed). John Wiley and Sons, Chichester.

Rubecz I, Mestyan J and Varga P (1981) Energy metabolism substrate utilization and nitrogen balance in parenterally fed postoperative neonates and infants. *J Paediatr* **98**, 42−6.

Steichen JJ, Gratton TL and Tsang RC (1980) Osteopenia of prematurity: the cause and possible treatment. *J Paediatr* **96**, 528−34.

Voyer M, Darakis M, Antener I and Valleur D (1982) Zinc balance in preterm infants. *Biol Neonate* **42**, 87−92.

Whitefield MF (1982) Poor weight gain of the low birth weight infant fed nasojejunally. *Arch Dis Childh* **57**, 597−601.

Ziegler EE *et al* (1981) *Textbook of paediatric nutrition*. Suskind Rm (Ed) p 29. Raven Press, New York.

5.5 Milk Kitchens and Breast Milk Banks

5.5.1 Milk kitchens

A milk kitchen is an area used for the preparation of feeds for infants who are in hospital. Milk kitchens have traditionally been administered and run by nursing staff. However, the increasing use of 'ready-to-feed' baby milks in hospitals have resulted in many milk kitchens now being used only for the preparation of specialized feeds. This requires dietetic expertise and consequently many nursing administrations have passed their responsibility to the dietetic department. Dietitians who are requested to oversee the running of a milk kitchen should consider the probable difficulties if nursing staff are to be retained in the department. Conflicts can arise over administrative duties, for example, the organisation of duty rotas or the recruitment of staff.

If the milk kitchen is under the sole jurisdiction of the dietetic department, it can also be used for the preparation of nasogastric feeds and other liquid nutritional supplements. Some milk kitchens also take responsibility for providing a breast milk bank (see Section 5.5.2).

The following points need to be considered in the successful operation of a milk kitchen

1 Milk kitchen design.
2 Staffing.
3 Hygiene.
4 Bacteriological criteria.
5 Sterilization/pasteurization of prepared feeds.
6 Equipment required.
7 Refrigerator storage.

Milk kitchen design

The milk kitchen should be a self-contained department within the hospital. It should have two separate areas — one for feed preparation and the other for washing and cleaning the used feeding bottles and feed preparation equipment. All surfaces, particularly in the feed preparation area, should be smooth and able to be cleaned easily. There should be no inaccessible corners or cracks in walls, tiles or floors where bacteria can multiply. Adequate ventilation is essential to regulate the temperature and also an air filter system to eliminate undesirable particles from the outside air.

Staffing

Those employed in milk kitchens should be responsible and conscientious regarding matters of hygiene. They should be aware of the importance of careful and accurate measurements of ingredients. The grades of staff employed will vary from trained and auxiliary nurses, to cooks, assistant cooks and dietitians, depending on the hospital and the department supervising the milk kitchen. Domestic staff are usually employed to collect the used feeding bottles from the ward and to wash them.

Hygiene

Milk is an ideal medium for bacterial overgrowth. The staff employed in milk kitchens must be constantly reminded of this and taught to observe rigorous hygiene rules. Some milk kitchens have showering facilities and insist staff shower and change into sterile theatre gowns before entering the feed preparation area. If such facilities are not provided, strict personal hygiene must be practiced. All hair must be covered; clean dresses/gowns/uniforms must be worn and changed at least once daily; many hospitals insist on face masks. Hands and arms should be thoroughly scrubbed, all jewellery removed and nail varnish is forbidden. The consultant microbiologist's advice should be sought regarding the appropriate hand cleansing materials, disinfectant and detergents used in the milk kitchen. Staff should be frequently reminded to report any gastrointestinal upsets or respiratory and other infections they may have.

Microbiological criteria

Successful running of a milk kitchen depends on close liaison with the hospital microbiology department. The consultant microbiologist, in liaison with the paediatrician, will determine the bacteriological criteria for the feeds, i.e. whether they should be sterile or bacteriologically 'clean'. Milk kitchens should test feed samples for bacteriological contamination at predetermined regular times. If non-sterile feeds are acceptable, safe limits of bacteria will have been set by the microbiologist. Random swabs of staff and surfaces in the milk kitchen may be performed by the microbiology department, if considered necessary.

Sterilization/pasteurization of prepared feeds

Whether the prepared feeds are pasteurized or sterilized will depend on the paediatrician's and hospital microbiologist's criteria for the feeds.

Autoclaves will sterilize the prepared feed, bottles and utensils but they are expensive to install and can be unreliable so some 'back-up' method of sterilization may be necessary. Hypochlorite solution ('Milton') can be used to sterilize the bottles and mixing utensils, but not the prepared feed. However, if sterile water is used to mix the milk powders, the bacterial level in the feed can be kept to a mimium. For some hospitals this method may be perfectly acceptable but others use a pasteurization machine for the prepared feeds.

Equipment required

1 Autoclaves, or large tanks to immerse feeding bottles in hypochlorite solution or a pasteurizing machine will be required. The autoclaves and tanks are usually built into the milk kitchen department structure.

2 Two sets of scales accurate to +/− 1 g are essential.

3 A mixing machine or mixing utensils are required. The type and number of feeds prepared will determine whether the equipment should be electrically or hand-operated. Electrically operated machines should be capable of being dismantled for thorough cleaning. Simple hand mixing utensils are easier to clean but make feed preparation slow. However, if 'ready-to-use' feeds are available in the wards, the milk kitchen is probably only preparing individually calculated feeds and the use of mixing machines designed for bulk feeding preparation may be inappropriate.

4 If the prepared feeds are not to be autoclaved or pasteurized, a supply of sterile water at a suitable temperature must be available. A water heater with special filters can provide this.

5 Measuring jugs and cylinders for fluid volume measurement are necessary. Assorted sizes of syringes are also required for small accurate volumes of feeds or for the addition of small concentrated amounts of liquid additives.

6 Fine mesh metal sieves should be used wherever possible to strain feeds to ensure that powders and additives are thoroughly dissolved and that no lumps are present which may block teats.

7 An adequate supply of both small (100 −120 ml) sized and large (240 − 270 ml) sized feeding bottles with closely fitting tops must be available. The choice of plastic or glass feeding bottles and their tops, must be made depending on the sterilization method employed. Plastic bottles are unsuitable for autoclaving. If a pasteurizer is used, standard bottles designed to fit the machine must be used.

8 An electric bottle washing machine is necessary to ensure thorough cleansing of used feeding bottles. The machine should be capable of scrubbing the inside of the bottles with revolving brushes and also rinsing with clean water.

9 Containers or crates are useful in order to transport the prepared feeds to the wards and to enable each ward's feeds to be stored together, either in the milk kitchen itself or in the ward refrigerator, if possible.

Storage

Most milk kitchens will be preparing one day's supply of each infant's feed and some babies may require hourly feeds. Consequently there may be a large number of bottles containing prepared feeds to be stored in refrigerated conditions to avoid bacteriological overgrowth or contamination. It is unlikely that the ward refrigerators will be able to store their babies' 24-hour supply of feeds and therefore the milk kitchen should be able to do so. The refrigeration space must be large enough to accommodate the maximum expected number of prepared feeds and the shelving suited to the sizes of crates/containers being used. Additional refrigeration space may be considered necessary for the storage of certain solutions and ingredients used in the feed preparation.

5.5.2 Breast milk banks

A breast milk bank is where human milk is stored. The milk may also be treated to reduce the bacteriological contamination. Paediatricians have differing views as to the use of pasteurized versus raw breast milk for neonatal nutrition. There is a loss of some immunological factors and enzymes during pasteurization and some paediatricians will therefore elect to feed a mother's own raw milk to her own baby where this is possible. Other units, however, use pasteurized human milk which is less bacteriologically hazardous to a small, sick infant.

Many factors must be considered in the successful operation of a milk bank

1 Selection of donors.
2 Collection of milk.
3 Storage of untreated milk.
4 Transfer of milk to a milk bank.
5 Arrival of milk at a milk bank.

6 Pasteurization process.
7 Microbiological criteria.
8 Storage of pasteurized milk.

Selection of donors

This should ideally be done by a midwife who will obtain a medical history to determine if there are any contraindications to being a donor, for example, use of some drugs, disease, poor diet or poor hygiene.

Collection of milk

Donors are instructed to express their milk manually or to use a hand/machine operated pump*. Milk which drips from the non-feeding breast during a feed may also be collected (drip breast milk). Which ever method is used, the milk should be collected into a sterile container, preferably of plastic, as glass can shatter if it is deep-frozen. Strict hygiene must be practiced during the expressing and collection of milk. The container is labelled with the date, donor's name and address and details of any drugs taken.

Storage of untreated milk

Breast milk must be refrigerated immediately after it has been expressed and the total day's supply can then be delivered to the milk bank. Alternatively it can be deep-frozen in the donor's home freezer, and an arrangement made with the hospital for it to be delivered to the milk bank.

Transport of milk to the milk bank

This can be done in a variety of ways. Local geography will usually dictate each milk bank's preferred choice. Local midwives, health visitors, the donors themselves or their family may bring the milk to the hospital. Some hospitals may organise a collection service or use voluntary organisations. Insulated containers should be used for the transportation of the milk.

Arrival of milk at the milk bank

Records of all milk arriving at the milk bank are kept with details of the donor such as name, address, unit/hospital number, illnessess and medications being

*Small hand operated pumps are supplied by the hospital or may be purchased from organisations such as the National Childbirth Trust (NCT). Those who find hand pumps unsatisfactory can, if convenient, visit the hospital to use an electric pump or hire an electric pump from the NCT.

taken. Frozen milk is allowed to thaw overnight in a refrigerator or placed in a deep freeze if not being pasteurized within 24 hours. Refrigerated milk should be pasteurized within 24 hours or immediately deep frozen until it can be treated. Breast milk which has been frozen must be completely thawed before being pasteurized.

Pateurization process

The most common method of pasteurization is to heat the milk to 62.5°C and hold it at this temperature for 30 min. Other methods using higher temperatures for a shorter time have been tried. No method is regarded as better than another. Whichever method is used, a machine specifically designed for pasteurization should be employed. These machines rely on a thermostatically controlled water bath to regulate the temperature during the pasteurization process. Standard sized bottles containing the decanted raw breast milk are loaded into a crate which is fully immersed in the water bath. The bottles contain a maximum volume of 100 ml and some microbiologists may insist on the same amount of milk in each bottle to ensure each has received exactly the same treatment. If this is the case, agreement on a pre-determined volume should be sought from the paediatrician.

Microbiological criteria

Microbiological criteria will vary between hospitals but each milk bank should agree acceptable standards only after consultation with the microbiologist and paediatrician. These standards should determine whether

1 Raw untreated milk is safe to use.
2 Raw untreated milk is microbiologically safe for pasteurization.
3 Milk has been successfully pasteurized.

The following guidelines could be used as a basis for the microbiological testing of milk

1 A sample of raw milk from each donor should be tested. The microbiologist should indicate the appropriate amount required.
2 Either a sample of *pasteurized milk* from each donor or a sample of *pooled pasteurized* milk from a number of donors should be tested.

In this way each donor's milk has been subjected to a microbiological test before and after pasteurization. This procedure is summarized in Table 5.11. In order to identify each donor's milk after treatment, the pasteurization bottles should be marked with the name of the donor, date of pasteurization and other relevant data that the paediatrician or milk bank staff may

Table 5.11 Example of microbiological testing of milk

Assume the standard agreed amount of milk to be pasteurized is 50 ml from five donors — A, B, C, D and E.

Method 1		One sample of raw milk from each individual. The amount for testing to determined by microbiologist, e.g. 5 ml from each donor — A, B, C, D and E.
Method 2	a)	A sample of 50 ml pasteurized milk from each donor — A, B, C, D and E.
or	b)	A sample of 10 ml from each donor, giving a total of 50 ml pasteurized milk as a 'pooled' sample.

The advantage of using method 2b is less wastage of milk in microbiological testing.

require. The appropriate pasteurized samples for microbiological testing should also be clearly marked with any information which the microbiologist requires. Water-resistant marker pens are more suitable than labels which are likely to peel off in the water bath. Both the raw and pasteurized milk samples for testing should be taken to the microbiology department immediately to avoid bacterial overgrowth.

Storage of pasteurized milk

The pasteurized milk should be used within 24 hours if it has been agreed between the paediatrician and microbiologist that it is safe to do so. Some units freeze the pasteurized milk and do not use it until the microbiology results have shown it to be free of organisms. Frozen pasteurized milk should be used on a rotational basis using the oldest supply first. A double sided freezer is ideal — one side can be used for treated milk awaiting microbiological results and the other side for cleared milk. Pasteurized milk should not be stored deep-frozen for longer than three months.

Further reading

Those who are asked to be involved in the running of a milk bank are advised to read the DHSS (1981) Report No 22 *The collection and storage of human milk* HMSO, London.

Williams AF and Baum JD (Eds) (1984) *Human milk banking*. Nestle Nutrition Workshop Services Vol 5. Raven Press, New York.

5.6 Metabolic Balance Diets

The aim of a metabolic balance is to compare the amount of a nutrient or other chemical which enters the body with the amount which leaves it. An individual is said to be in positive balance when output is less than intake, or in negative balance when output exceeds intake.

Nutrients can enter the body both orally, via the diet and medications, and parenterally. The routes by which unwanted metabolites are excreted from the body are through faeces, urine, lungs, skin, and in special cases, by dialysis. Metabolites which control the balance are measured biochemically and isotopically in blood, lymph, bone and soft tissue. Accuracy of measurement of intake, excretion and tissue levels is crucial to the success of the investigation.

A *balance* diet, such as a calcium/phosphorous/magnesium balance, provides a constant daily intake of the specified nutrients, which is very carefully controlled and usually adhered to for a relatively lengthy period of time. Collections of both stools and urine are usually made.

A *constant* diet, such as a constant calcium diet, is less restricted in terms of the degree of accuracy, the number of nutrients and/or the time period involved. Collections are usually made of urine only, and not of stools.

Facilities

Because of the need for accuracy, the preparation of food for dietary balance studies should be undertaken by a trained diet cook or diet technician, in a specially equipped metabolic diet kitchen. A dietitian's office, diet store, food freezer and fridge should be located nearby. In addition to the usual ward facilities there should be dry toilets with refrigerated storage space for urine and faeces. Nursing staff must be trained in the accurate collection of urine, stools and any other metabolic products required. Phlebotomy and laboratory services must be available. Further details as to design of metabolic units may be found elsewhere (British Dietetic Association 1984).

Planning the study

The planning of the metabolic balance study is co-ordinated by a team of specialists consisting of physician, nursing staff, dietitian and laboratory staff. Figure 5.3 shows the involvement of these specialists during a typical calcium balance, and includes other departments whose help will be required. The specialist team plan the patient's protocol and at regular intervals monitor the progress of the study and resolve any problems. The protocol is the central source of information for all involved and will show

1 The type of balance study which is being undertaken, the nutrients being measured and any additional restriction in the diet, e.g. low protein for a patient with renal bone disease.

2 The timing of the 24-hour day for urine and stool collections, e.g. 8 am−8 am or 10 am−10 am. Note: it is useful to plan the collection period to commence in the working day and not at midnight.

3 The type of urine/stool/sweat, etc. collections which will be required, e.g. 24-hour urine collections for calcium measurement collected in boric acid preservative.

4 The length of the equilibration period, sometimes termed the 'run-in', and the length of the balance period.

5 All tests to be undertaken on the patient during the balance period which may require medical, dietetic, phlebotomy or clinical chemistry involvement.

Table 5.12 gives details of aspects to be considered when planning metabolic dietary studies.

Organisation of the metabolic diet

Foods used in balance diets and their preparation

Food included in the menus for metabolic balance studies should vary as little as possible in compositional analysis and should be kept simple in type and number to limit the variation inherent in foods. Regular availability, cost, storage properties, ease of preparation, palatability and acceptability of the foods must be considered. Foods should be bought in bulk for the period of the balance, including the stabilization period, and duplicate meals prepared for analysis (Reifenstein *et al* 1945; Isaksson and Sjorgen 1965). Foods such as meat can be prepared, cooked, weighed into portions, labelled and frozen before the balance commences. Likewise, dry goods can be weighed in

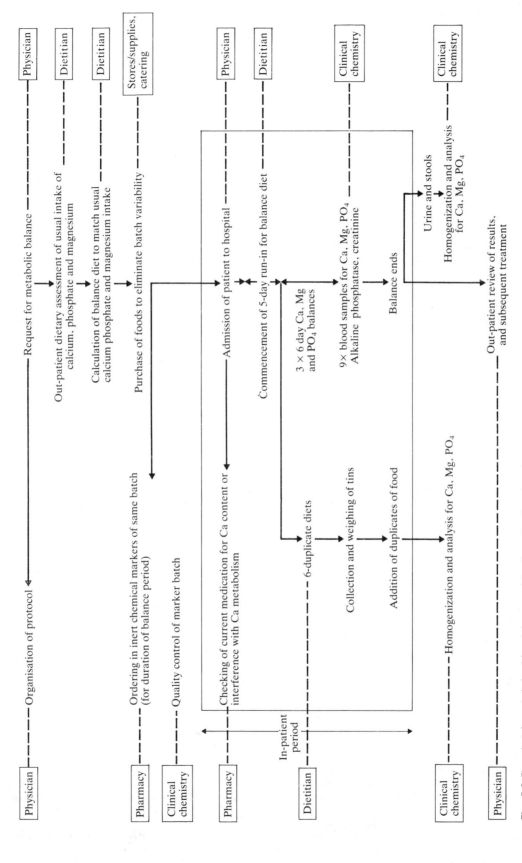

Fig. 5.3 Flow chart for a typical calcium balance — interaction with other departments.

Table 5.12 Aspects to be considered when planning metabolic balance studies

Type of study	Water	Food choice	Menu rotation	Length of run-in period	Length of balance periods	Types of Collection	Markers	Duplicate Diets	Toothpastes, medicaments and miscellaneous
Calcium, magnesium, phosphorus	Distilled or deionized for cooking and all beverages	Constant source, batched for entire study	1, 2 or 3 daily menus rotated. Matched for minerals being studied.	Balances 5–8 days. Constant diets 2–5 days.	may be 4 days × 4 5 days × 3 6 days × 3	*Balances* 24–hour urines in boric acid. Daily stool. Blood as necessary. *Constant diets* 24–hour urines in boric acid.	Continuous faecal markers	Essential for balance diets. 1 per balance period or 1 of each menu per balance period. Not required for constant diets.	Calcium-free toothpaste: use those with a silica abrasive.
Sodium potassium	Distilled or deionized for cooking and all beverages	Constant source, batched for entire study. Sodium — avoid high sodium foods. Potassium — avoid leaf tea and substitute instant tea.	1, 2 or 3 daily menus rotated	2–3 days. For large dietary changes allow longer run-in.	Variable	*Balances* 24-hour urines in boric acid. Daily stool. Blood as necessary. *Constant diets* 24-hour urines in boric acid.	Not usually required	Essential for balance diets	May require use of salt-free toothpaste
Nitrogen	Tap water for cooking and all beverages	Constant source; batched for entire study	1, 2 or 3 daily menus rotated	2–6 days	Variable	*Balances* 24-hour urines in boric acid Daily stool. Sometimes skin losses. *Constant diets* 24-hour urines in boric acid	Faecal or urinary	Essential for balance diets	Avoid use of all ointments, powder, purgatives and toothpaste unless authorised by clinician.
Purine-free	Tap water for cooking and all beverages	See Table 5.14. Not necessary to batch foods. Fresh foods may be used daily.	Single menu	5 days	3 days	24-hour urines in boric acid. Blood for uric acid creatinine.	Not required	Not required	Not restricted

advance. Tables 5.13 and 5.14 give details of foods suitable for metabolic dietary studies. Methods of cooking should be standardized and where possible foods should be served in the container in which they were cooked (Heaney *et al* 1977). Pressure cooking, casserole cooking and foil-wrap baking are all suitable cooking methods for preserving nutrient content.

Table 5.13 Description of foods used in metabolic studies, their preparation and storage

Food group	Comments
Cereals	
Breakfast cereals	From the same batch, weighed out into airtight containers before the study commences. Puffed Wheat, Shredded Wheat, Cornflakes, Rice Krispies, Weetabix, Special K and porridge are all commonly used.
·Bread	From the same batch. Wholemeal or white, weighed out before the study commences, crusts removed, trimmed to correct weight, packed appropriately and frozen. Alternatively, 'home made' bread may be baked to a standard recipe using ingredients of known, constant composition.

Table 5.13 contd.

Food group	Comments
Biscuits	From the same batch; only biscuits of uniform composition should be used, e.g. Rich Tea, Marie, digestives, cream crackers, Ryvita, scraped to correct weight and wrapped in cling film.
Puddings	Sago, rice, tapioca, semolina or custard, cooked in a pyrex dish in a microwave oven or bain-marie and served directly to the patient in this dish.
Dairy products, eggs and fats	
Milk	Fresh milk, homogenized to provide an even distribution of fat, Dried skimmed milk or whitener are alternatives.
Butter	Unsalted or salted can be used depending on whether or not constant sodium is required. Always obtain from the same batch and freeze beforehand if necessary.
Cheese	From the same batch, analysed by laboratory if necessary and frozen until required. Processed cheese may be more homogenous than hard cheeses. Avoid cheese in sodium-controlled studies.

Table 5.13 contd.

Food group	Comments
Eggs	Either homogenize eggs and use a constant quantity of homogenate or weigh eggs, e.g. 57 g egg provides 50 g whole egg and 7 g shell. Egg may be boiled, poached, scrambled or as omelette.
Margarine	Margarine may be used in preference to butter.
Vegetable oil	May be used in weighed quantities.
Meats	All meat used must be completely lean and be bone, skin and rind free. It must be cooked without salt before the balance commences, portioned, wrapped and frozen. It is advisable to use beef — topside or rump, lamb — leg; pork — loin and chicken breast. Ham may be included if the diet is not sodium-controlled.
Fish	Fish is not generally used in metabolic studies because of storage difficulties and variations in water lost. If used, care must be taken to ensure that the fish is free of bones.
Vegetables Salad vegetables	Fresh salad vegetables may be used, e.g. lettuce, tomato, cucumber, pepper, celery and cress. These must be very well washed in distilled water and dried before use.
Frozen vegetables	Frozen vegetables are preferable to fresh. Bought in batches before the balance commences. e.g. cauliflower, peas, runner beans, brussels sprouts and carrots. These are cooked in distilled water or deionized water, drained in a seive, then weighed.
Tinned vegetables	Should be avoided in sodium-controlled studies.
Potatoes	Instant potato flakes or powder reconstituted with distilled water are the most accurate. If fresh potatoes are used these should be steamed, or roasted in a weighed quantity of cooking oil.
Fruit Tinned fruit	From the same batch. Can be weighed into small containers with a measured quantity of fruit and syrup then frozen until required. Tinned grapefruit, mandarins, pears, pineapple and apricots are all suitable.
Fresh fruit	All fresh fruit must be peeled, cored and flesh weighed as required.
Fruit juice	From the same batch. May be weighed and frozen prior to the balance study.
Beverages Tea	A standard brew is made using tea bags or leaf tea. If potassium is being assessed instant tea should be used. In studies involving diuretic drugs use decaffeinated tea.
Coffee	Instant coffee is suitable. It can be weighed into small pots before the study commences. In studies involving diuretic drugs, decaffeinated should be used.
Bedtime drinks	Horlicks, drinking chocolate, cocoa and Ovaltine are all suitable.
Miscellaneous Ice cream	From the same batch
Jelly	From the same batch, made up to a standard recipe.
Fruit squash	Each portion of undiluted squash must be weighed.
Preserves	From the same batch. Marmalade, seedless jam and honey are all suitable.
Sugar	Weighed quantities in beverages if the patient requires it.
Boiled sweets, chocolate	Use, if required, in weighed quantities.
Salad cream	Use in weighed quantities.
Vinegar	Use in weighed quantities.

Table 5.14 List of food choices for purine-free constant diets

Foods to be avoided	Foods allowed
All meat, poultry, fish, offal, meat extracts, wholegrain cereals, potatoes peas, beans, lentils, spinach, asparagus, celery, onion, radishes, mushrooms, chocolate, drinking chocolate, Ovaltine, Bournvita, tea, coffee and alcohol.	Eggs, cheese (cheddar or processed cheese spread), Milk (homogenised), Cereals — white bread, plain biscuits, e.g. marie, rich tea, morning coffee. Cornflakes, custard powder, rice and semolina. Vegetables — cauliflower, carrots, lettuce, tomatoes and cucumber. Fruit (fresh) — apples and bananas. Fruit (tinned) — peaches, pears, pineapple, apricots, mandarins and grapefruit. Fruit (juice) — grapefruit, orange and pineapple. Fats — butter and oils. Beverages — fruit squashes. Miscellaneous — jams, marmalade, honey, sugar and boiled sweets.

The type of water (i.e. whether distilled, deionized or tap water) which should be used for cooking, drinking and in beverages in each type of study is indicated in Table 5.12.

The metabolic diet is prepared by a trained diet cook or diet technician using menu plans drawn up by the dietitian.

Planning the menu

The menu to be used during the balance period may be based on

1 A standard diet used by the metabolic unit.

2 A basic diet with selected increments to achieve the required intake.

3 Simulation of the patient's usual home intake of particular nutrient(s).

It may be necessary to keep patients in their current equilibrium, or steady state, for one or more nutrients. This steady state needs to be maintained where adaptation to different intakes of nutrients may take months, e.g. calcium (Isaksson and Sjorgen 1967; Lentner *et al* 1975). In this case a detailed dietary history of a typical week's food intake at home will be needed. With the help of the dietitian, the patient chooses the foods to be consumed during the balance period. The nutrient content of the chosen diet is calculated from standard food tables and adjusted to meet the required level of the nutrients to be investigated (see previous section on foods used in balance diets). Care should be taken to see that the choice provides a palatable, nutritious and attractive menu. The metabolic balance procedure is a demanding discipline for the patient, and the dietitian is responsible for providing a diet which is acceptable, while at the same time fulfilling the requirements of the dietary investigation.

Patient training

The dietitian is responsible for explaining to the patient
1 The purpose of the dietary procedure.
2 The necessity to consume all food and fluid provided.
3 How to clear all plates with either a small portion of bread included in the diet for this purpose or a flexible spatula (Reifenstein *et al* 1945).
4 How to rinse all drink containers with distilled water and to consume the rinsing water.
5 The importance of not taking any food or fluid other than those prescribed in the diet.
6 Where necessary, the restriction of toothpaste and talcum powder.

The physician should advise the patient regarding the desirable level of physical activity, for example, avoiding excessive sweating during sodium balances but keeping reasonable levels of physical activity during calcium balances.

Menu rotation

Constant or balance diets are planned on a one, two or three-day rotating menu. The single-day form has the advantage of ensuring greater constancy of nutrient intake. Two or three-day rotating menus calculated to provide an identical intake of nutrients are less monotonous but inevitably introduce greater daily variability of nutrient intake in practice. If rotating menus are used, each balance period must comprise the same number of each alternating menu. For constant nitrogen studies it is often useful to make exchanges of meals of similar nitrogen composition, with meats, cereals and vegetables grouped into separate exchange lists making three or four week menu cycles possible (see p 118). This is important for compliance in studies which continue for several weeks.

Drugs

Any drugs which the patient is taking must be checked for relevant mineral content or possible interference with the balance study. When preparing duplicate diets for analysis (see below), it may be desirable to include duplicate doses of any drugs taken which contain significant quantities of the mineral being measured.

If it is necessary to give a high sodium intake this may be achieved by giving weighed amounts of sodium chloride to be added to food and additional 'slow sodium' tablets if necessary. Similarly, an increase in potassium intake may be effected using 'slow potassium' tablets.

Toothpastes

For calcium studies a low calcium toothpaste should be used by patients who have their own teeth; suitable toothpastes are those with a silica abrasive (e.g. Signal, Close-Up, Pepsodent). Denture users should be taught to rinse their dentures thoroughly with distilled water after cleaning.

Sodium studies may require the use of salt-free toothpaste (made up by the pharmacy). A suitable formulation is given in Table 5.15.

The use of toothpaste may need to be restricted in nitrogen studies at the discretion of the physician in charge.

Table 5.15 Sodium-free toothpaste (Courtesy of the Glasgow Dental Hospital and School of Dentistry)

10 ml gum acacia
50 ml boiling water
10 ml glycerol
80 mg calcium carbonate
5 drops of carvone to flavour
5 drops of methylene blue to colour

This formulation contains no preservative so it should be kept refrigerated.

Ointments and powders

In nitrogen studies, ointments and powders should not used unless authorised by the physician in charge as they may directly or indirectly affect the nitrogen balance (for example, cortisol-based creams).

Stabilization or run-in period

Prior to commencing the balance study, the patient has a run-in period, which is a trial of the balance diet, and covers the period of time necessary for the patient's adaptation to the constant diet. This leads into the balance period. During the run-in period the patient becomes accustomed to the idea of being on a balance diet and learns the procedures required of him for the completion of the diet and for urine and stool collections (although no collections are made during this period). It is also a time when any problems over the diet are sorted out so that the final diet for the balance period can be tailored to suit the patient in both type and quantity of foods. The length of time of the run-in period will vary according to the type of balance and length of adaptation needed.

For calcium balances the run-in is 5−6 days and changes in the balance diet should not be made after about day 4. For gelatin-free diets for hydroxyproline excretion studies, 24 hours only are required (Gasser *et al* 1979).

For sodium and potassium balances the run-in may only be 2−3 days if the dietary change is not great, as adaptation to different intakes of these minerals is rapid. When significant increases or decreases of dietary nutrients are made, a run-in of five days may be required (for example, a 350 mmol sodium diet).

For purine-free diets, a five day run-in is necessary during which time dietary sources of uric acid are eliminated from the body.

During the run-in, the internal markers for the balance period will be given so that these have reached equilibrium in the gut by the time the balance starts (see below).

Balance periods

The length of balance will vary considerably according to the information required. Points to consider are

1 For minerals, longer studies give greater precision (Lentner *et al* 1975).

2 Where treatment changes are made during balance periods, a transitional period will occur before a new equilibrium is reached. Effectively another run-in period is required during this time before the balance can continue in the new equilibrium (for example in electrolyte studies).

3 There should be at least two metabolic periods for each regimen otherwise any trend creeping in due to unforeseen variables may be missed.

4 Balance periods longer than 6 days will involve volumes of faecal collections too large to be handled with ease (Reifenstein *et al* 1945).

Types of collection

Most balances require 24-hour urine and daily faecal collections. Daily faecal collections may be analysed individually or subsequently pooled for aliquot analysis. For constant diets (such as sodium and calcium) 24-hour urine collections are made without faecal collections.

Blood samples are often necessary, depending on the individual study, and sometimes measurements of skin losses are made during nitrogen, sodium or potassium balances (Isaksson and Sjorgen 1967). (See Table 5.12)

Markers — faecal and urinary

Faecal markers

For balance studies an inert faecal marker is necessary to correct for incomplete stool collections and variations in faecal output and transit time. There are two types of marker, intermittent and continuous.

Intermittent or visual markers. Intermittent markers are visible after transit through the gut, so that if markers are given at known times, stool collections can be made between the appearance of these markers. Examples of intermittent markers are Carmine markers (Rose 1964; Pak *et al* 1980) and Edicol Supra Blue.

Continuous markers. Continuous markers are given in known quantities throughout the run-in and balance periods. Since they remain totally unabsorbed during transit through the intestine, the quantitiy appearing in the stool can be used to correct for incomplete stool collections. Continuous markers are

1 Chromium sesquioxide (Cr_2O_3) (Rose 1964; Branch and Cummings 1978; Lentner *et al* 1975; Pak *et al* 1980). This marker can be a hazard during the analysis of faeces when chromium is oxidized to chromate with perchlorate; dry perchlorate salts may explode, and the material should be handled only in a fume cupboard with non-absorbent surfaces (Hesp *et al* 1979).

2 [^{51}Cr] chromic chloride (Hesp *et al* 1979).

3 Radio-opaque pellets (Branch and Cummings 1978).

4 Polyethylene glycol (4000−PEG) (Soergel 1968; Lentner *et al* 1975; Pak *et al* 1980).

Other substances sometimes used as markers in balance studies have disadvantages which limit their usefulness. For example, barium sulphate ($BaSO_4$) is time-consuming to analyse by the gravimetric method, and using flame photometry the method is insensitive and other elements interfere (Bacon 1980). Copper thiocyanate (CuSCN) may interfere with thyroid uptake of iodine. (Ingbar and Woeber 1968). However, the choice of marker is a matter of individual preference (Bacon 1980).

Intermittent and continuous markers may be used

concurrently (Pak *et al* 1980). The use of faecal markers may be invalid in gastrointestinal disease (Soergel 1968).

Urinary markers

Urine creatinine has been used as a measure of completeness of urine collections. Since creatinine excretion is related to lean body mass, it was assumed to be constant from day to day in any individual. However, urinary creatinine is also affected by diet, particularly meat consumption. Limited calorimetric studies have shown that even on a constant diet, day to day variations in urinary creatinine are quite large. It is advisable therefore to use a urine marker to check for completeness of urine collections.

Para-amino benzoic acid (in a dose of one 80 mg capsule three times daily) has a high percentage of recovery in urine. Collections containing less than 85% of the administered para-amino benzoic acid are probably incomplete (Bingham and Cummings 1983). These markers may be given combined with a faecal marker.

Duplicate diets

A duplicate diet consists of a 24-hour food intake, identical to the balance diet, which is submitted to the laboratory for analysis. This technique is employed as a measurement of the patient's actual food intake as opposed to the theoretical intake calculated from standard food tables.

A duplicate day's menu is prepared, cooked and sent to the laboratory for homogenization and analysis of an aliquot. Some food may be omitted, e.g. butter (because of its tendency to float to the top causing an unrepresentative aliquot to be taken), or tea infusions (where capacity of the homogenizing equipment is limited). The theoretical values for these omitted foods are added to the analysed values to give the true totals.

The total number of duplicates analysed varies with the number of menus and balance periods. If periods are short, with one menu, one duplicate should be prepared for each period; for alternating menus, one duplicate of each menu should be prepared for each balance period.

The precision of estimating true dietary intake increases with the number of duplicate diets analysed. For example, in the case of calcium, if one duplicate diet estimates the true dietary intake of calcium with a precision of 1.53 mmol (= 60 mg calcium), for six duplicate diets this figure is divided by $\sqrt{n}$, i.e.

$$\frac{1.53}{\sqrt{6}} = 25 \text{ mg.}$$

Duplicate diets are not usually required for constant diets.

Verification

The dietitian is responsible for checking all food which leaves the metabolic kitchen, for appearance, temperature and accuracy. Spot checks for weight error may at times be necessary. All trays from patients on metabolic balance diets should be returned to the metabolic kitchen to be checked for rejections.

Rejected food

This is kept to a minimum by patient co-operation. Where minor rejects occur, these should be analysed either individually or added to the stool pot for analysis with the faeces of the same date as the rejects. Rejections should be charted in a book kept in the metabolic kitchen. In some studies it may be necessary to make up the nutrient loss by replacing with alternative foods (for example, in fat balances). If it becomes apparent that rejections are so great as to invalidate the balance results, the possibility of terminating the balance study must be considered. In the event of a temporary illness it may be necessary to stop collections until the patient is well again, then allow a new run-in period before balance collections recommence.

Coding

In all metabolic wards a considerable amount of staff time is spent teaching the patient dietary and toilet regimens. In order to minimize possible errors, a system of coding (colour or letter) of equipment may be used. Each metabolic patient has his own colour or code and all equipment pertaining to his bedroom and toilet is labelled with his colour or code. All cooking dishes and crockery may be similarly coded.

Records

Throughout the study accurate records must be kept. These may include calculated dietary intakes of nutrients, fluid charts, prescription charts to show times that markers are given, and urine and stool charts.

Further reading

British Dietetic Association (1984) *Hankbook of metabolic dietetics.* Available from the British Dietetic Association.

References

Bacon S (1980) Faecal markers in metabolic balance studies. *J Hum Nutr* **34**, 445−9.

Bingham SA Cummings JH (1983) The use of 4-aminobenzoic acid as a marker to validate the completeness of 24-hour urine collections in man. *Clin Sci* **64**, 629−35.

Branch WJ and Cummings JH (1978) Comparison of radio-opaque pellets and chromium sesquioxide markers in studies requiring accurate faecal collections. *Gut* **19**, 371−6.

British Dietetic Association (1984) *Handbook of metabolic dietetics.* British Dietetic Association.

Gasser A, Celada A, Courvoisier B, Depierre D, Hulme PM, Rinsler M, Williams D and Wootton R (1979) The clinical measurement of urinary total hydroxyproline excretion. *Clin Chim Acta* **95**, 487−91.

Heaney RP, Recker RR and Saville PD (1977) Calcium balance and calcium requirements in middle-aged women. *Am J Clin Nutr* **30**, 1603−11.

Hesp R, Williams D, Rinsler M and Reeve J (1979) A comparison of chromium sesquioxide and [^{51}Cr]chromic chloride as inert markers in calcium balance studies. *Clin Sci* **57**, 89−92.

Ingbar SH and Woeber KA (1968) *Textbook of endocrinology.* Wiliams RH (Ed) p 105. WB Saunders, Philadelphia.

Isaksson B and Sjorgen B (1965) On the concept 'constant diet' in metabolic balance studies. *Nutritio Dieta* **7**, 175−85.

Isaksson B and Sjorgen B (1967) A critical evaluation of the mineral and nitrogen balances in man. *Proc Nutr Soc* **26**, 106−16.

Lentner C, Lauffenburger T, Guncaga J, Dambacher MA and Haas HG (1975) The metabolic balance technique: a critical reappraisal. *Metabolism* **24**, 461−71.

Pak CYC, Stewart A, Rasin P and Galosy RA (1980) A simple and reliable method for calcium balance using combined period and continuous faecal markers. *Metabolism* **29**, 793−6.

Reifenstein EC, Albright F and Wells SL (1945) The accumulation, interpretation and presentation of data pertaining to metabolic balances, notably those of calcium, phosphorus and nitrogen. *J Clin Endocrrinol* **5**,367−95.

Rose GA (1964) Experiences with the use of interrupted carmine red and continuous chromium sesquioxide marking of human faeces with reference to calcium, phosphorus and magnesium. *Gut* **5**, 274−9.

Soergel KH (1968) Inert markers. *Gastroenterology* **54**. 449−52.

5.7   Diagnostic Tests

5.7.1 Fat malabsorption — total faecal fat estimation

Dietary manipulation may be required to ensure that adequate fat (see below) is ingested for at least two days prior to the beginning of the test and for the duration of the test.

Many patients requiring this test have a poor fat tolerance and achieving an adequate fat intake can be a problem, causing further steatorrhoea and nausea.

An adequate fat intake is betwwen 50—150 g fat/day for adults; 100 g fat daily is commonly used. A minimum of 40 g fat daily is recommended for a child. In infants, the actual fat content of the current feeding regime is calculated and will be adequate unless steps have been taken to reduce the fat content. In hospital, the normal hospital diet plus a regimen of fat supplements can ensure a mimium daily fat intake of 100 g.
For example

5 butter/margarine portions (7 g each)	=	28 g fat
1 pint whole milk	=	21 g fat
50 g hard cheese	=	16 g fat
50 g chocolate (milk)	=	15 g fat
30 g peanuts	=	15 g fat
30 g double cream	=	15 g fat
		110 g fat

A record should be kept of food and fat supplements eaten during the two days prior to the test and for the duration of the test (three or five days) so that the validity of the test can be checked. The patient may be well enough to keep the record (Tietz 1983).

5.7.2 Gluten challenge

It is usual to confirm the diagnosis of coeliac disease by the reintroduction of gluten for a period of three months. This is followed by a jejunal biopsy to examine the villi of the intestinal mucosa. The challenge may be in a child or an adult. The method by which this is done varies from unit to unit but is based on (1) the use of gluten-containing foods or (2) the use of pure gluten powder.

Which ever method is used it is important to ensure that an adequate quantity of gluten is being ingested to constitute a challenge to the gut.

Gluten challenge using gluten-containing foods

An intake of at least 10 g wheat protein daily is recommended (Francis 1974) for children, and 15—20 g wheat protein daily for teenagers and adults.

This can be calculated using the protein content of foods whose protein source is wheat. For example, 10 g wheat protein can be provided by 4 large, thin slices of ordinary bread, brown of white *or* 4 Weetabix *or* 60 g raw spaghetti *or* 100 g digestive biscuits.

The introduction of foods which have previously been forbidden to the coeliac patient, especially if a child, may lead to problems of dietary compliance in the future if the challenge confirms the diagnosis of coeliac disease.

Gluten challenge using pure gluten powder

Gluten powder is added to foods which make up the gluten-free diet. The powder is very fine and has a strong taste. It does not mix with liquid but mixes well with thicker foods such as mashed potato, yoghurt or rice pudding. It can also be taken mixed with jam or other preserves as a 'medicine'. Children's dose is 20 g twice a day; teenage/adult dose is 20—40 g twice a day.

If during the challenge, unpleasant symptoms occur, the patient undergoes a jejunal biopsy before the three month period is completed. (Alderhay Children's Hospital, dietetic department, personal communication).

5.7.3 Glucose tolerance test

It is unlikely that the dietitian will be involved in the procedure for a glucose tolerance test. However, dietitians should be aware that the patient should not be placed on a diet which restricts carbohydrate intake prior to this diagnostic test being carried out, as this can impair the results.

The WHO (1980) have laid down diagnostic criteria and a classification of diagnosis, based on the results of an oral glucose tolerance test comprised of 75 g glucose in 250—300 ml of water for adults or 1.75 g glucose/kg body weight (to a maximum of 75 g glucose) for children.

5.7.4 Vanillylmandelic acid (VMA) test (for phaeochromocytoma)

Phaeochromocytoma is a rare syndrome caused by over-activity of the adrenal medulla, usually due to a benign adrenal medullary tumour. The disease is characterized by increased amounts of catecholamine metabolites such as vanillylmandelic acid (VMA) in the urine. Formerly, methods of measuring VMA also detected other phenolic acids so this test needed to be preceded by a diet free of: Tea, coffee, chocolate, nuts, bananas, vanilla essence, custard, blancmange, sponges, cakes, biscuits and sweets (except boiled).

However, the development of highly specific liquid chromatography estimation methods means that dietary restriction should no longer be necessary.

Further reading

Amery A and Conway J (1967) A critical review of diagnostic tests for phaeochromocytoma. *Am Heart J* **73**, 129.

References

Francis DEM (1986) *Diets for sick children* 4e. Blackwell Scientific Publications, Oxford.
Tietz NW (1983) *Clinical guide to laboratory tests* p 188. WB Saunders Co, Philadelphia.
World Health Organisation (1980) Second report of the Expert Committee on Diabetes Mellitus. WHO Technical Report Series 646. WHO, Geneva.

5.8 Preparation of the Bowel for Surgery, Barium Enema and Colonoscopy

Adequate preparation of the bowel is essential for double contrast examination of the large bowel (Dickie *et al* 1970) as it improves interpretation and the chances of a single diagnostic study. The preparation should result in a clean bowel with no residual faecal matter. Preparation of the bowel for surgery should also result in a clean, empty bowel, particularly if a bowel resection is to be performed. If a total colectomy is planned, e.g. for ulcerative colitis, it may not be necessary to thoroughly cleanse and empty the bowel.

A number of procedures have been advocated and the procedure of choice varies from one centre to another. Consideration should be given to the effects of the evacuant on the patient's mental, physical and metabolic state. Side effects should be minimal and the preparation be easily administered, preferably by the oral route.

Bowel preparation procedures

Whole gut irrigation

This is now seldom used. This procedure involved the administration of a large volume (10–15 litres) of normal saline into the gut by rapid, continuous drip via a nasogastric tube, until the anal effluent was clear. This would take a number of hours to complete and left the patient feeling weakened and exhausted.

Purgatives

The oral intake of 500 ml of 10% mannitol solution (flavoured with lemon or orange juice) and followed by 2 litres of clear fluids is a more acceptable, quicker and effective method of cleansing the bowel. Solutions of 25% magnesium sulphate are also used to purge and cleanse the bowel.

More recently, excellent results have been reported using a new preparation Picolax (sodium picosulphate/magnesium citrate) (De Lacey *et al* 1980, 1982). Picolax is presented in unit dose sachets containing 16.3 g of powder and administered orally. On the day prior to investigation two sachets of Picolax are taken: one before breakfast and one before the evening meal. A light, low residue diet may be taken during the day and patients are encouraged to drink as much clear

fluid as possible. A diet sheet is incorporated into the instructions (Table 5.16) although this may be modified to meet home or hospital catering arrangements (Table 5.17). The dietary instructions for patients taking Picolax prior to colonoscopy may be modified further (Table 5.17).

Table 5.16 Dietary advice for patients taking Picolax (Nordic). During this treatment carefully follow any instructions given by the hospital, the following *may* be allowed on the day before the examination. *Throughout the treatment drink as much water as desired*

Meal	Food allowed
Breakfast (8–9am) (After the first dose has been taken.)	1 boiled egg 1 slice white bread + honey (not jam or marmalade) 1 cup tea/coffee with sugar & milk if desired
Mid-morning (10.30am)	1 cup tea/coffee without milk. Sugar if liked. No food.
Lunch (12–1.30pm)	Small portion grilled/poached fish/chicken Cooked white rice Plain yoghurt, jelly or junket. No potatoes, fruit or vegetables 1 cup tea/coffee without milk.
Afternoon	No food but drink plenty of water
Supper (7–9pm)	Clear soup or meat extract drinks but no food.

No further food is allowed until after the examination but drink as much water as desired.

Rapid cleansing of the bowel with or without colonic lavage may result in a low blood sugar. Consideration of this must be given to patients with diabetes who require bowel preparation. Insulin dependent diabetics should undergo the procedure with hospital supervision and will require intravenous dextrose and regular blood glucose monitoring. Diabetic patients controlled by hypoglycaemic agents should also be carefully monitored to maintain acceptable blood glucose levels. It may be appropriate to omit their tablets on both the day of preparation and the day of investigation. In any event these diabetics should take glucose-containing clear fluids at regular intervals throughout the day.

Low residue diets in bowel preparation

Low residue diets may be used to prepare the bowel for surgery. Unless food is passing very rapidly through the gut it will take a number of days to prepare the

Table 5.17 Example of modified dietary instructions to prepare the bowel for barium enema and colonoscopy using Picolax

Investigation	Timing	Method	Precautions
Barium enema	Day before investigation	2 sachets Picolax: 1 before breakfast, 1 before evening meal. Diet — light, very low residue diet or high protein, high calorie fluids plus 3 litres clear fluids.	Careful blood glucose monitoring in paients with diabetes.
	Day of examination	Clear fluids only	
Colonoscopy		May use modified Picolax preparation.	Elderly patients may need preparation of bowel in hospital.
	Day 4 before investigation	Mild laxative at night.	Careful bood glucose monitoring in patients with diabetes, particularly on days 4 and 5.
	Days 2 and 3 before investigation	Low residue diet.	
	Day 1 before investigation	2 sachets Picolax: 1 early morning, 1 late afternoon. Diet — clear fluids, clear soups, plain jelly, very little milk in 1 or 2 cups of tea. 3 litres clear fluids.	
	Day of examination	Clear fluids only.	

bowel by this method. If patients are already established on a low residue diet as part of the management of inflammatory bowel disease, they may continue with the diet prior to surgery. Such patients are likely to have diarrhoea which obviously would result in regular emptying of the bowel and therefore the low residue diet may be quite adequate and no further dietary modification be required. Immediately prior to surgery or investigation, the bowel will need to be cleansed by bowel washout or disposable enema.

Proprietary enteral feeds — use in bowel preparation

Low residue enteral feeds alone are not an effective method of bowel preparation and bowel cleansing will also usually be necessary. However, deterioration of nutritional status in the pre-operative period may be prevented by sip feeding with enteral feeds. Elemental enteral feeds have been recommended for bowel preparation as they are absorbed mainly in the upper small bowel and leave a minimal residue in the large bowel, although clinicians disagree over the value of such products for this purpose (Keohane and Silk 1982). Elemental enteral feeds are hyperosmolar, unpleasant to take and more expensive than liquid whole protein foods. Provided that pancreatic, biliary and small intestinal absorption are not impaired, liquid whole protein enteral feeds result in a comparatively low residue in the large bowel (Jones *et al* 1983; Russell and Evans 1984) and may be equally as suitable as elemental enteral feeds.

In the preparation of the bowel for surgery or investigation it is probably more important to encourage the drinking of at least 3 litres of clear fluids per day rather than to assess the advantages or disadvantages of a pre-digested enteral feed over a whole protein enteral feed requiring normal digestion.

The preparation used to evacuate the bowel should result in a clean, residue-free bowel without causing undue distress to the patient or requiring unnecessary nursing time for lavage. The patient's metabolic state and general sense of well-being should be maintained and time spent in hospital ward and X-ray department kept to a minimum.

References

De Lacey G, Benson M, Wilkins R, Spencer J and Cramer B (1980) Colon preparation for double contrast enemas: a comparison of four regimens. Paper presented at Spring Meeting of British Society of Gastroenterologists and Association of Surgeons, Bournemouth, 1980.

De Lacey G, Benson M, Wilkins R, Spencer J and Cramer B (1982) Routine colonic lavage is unnecessary for double contrast barium enema in outpatients. *Br Med J* **284**, 1021–2.

Dickie J, James WB, Hume R and Robertson D (1970) A comparison of three substances used for bowel preparation prior to radiological examination. *Clin Radiol* **21**, 201–2.

Jones BJM, Lees R, Andrews J, Frost P and Silk DBA (1983) Comparison of an elemental and polymeric diet in patients with normal gastrointestinal function. *Gut* **24**, 78–84.

Keohane P and Silk DBA (1982) Low residue enteral diets and bowel preparation. *Nursing* **5**, 136–7.

Russell CA and Evans SJ (1984) A comparison of the absorption from 'chemically-defined elemental' and 'whole protein' enteral feeds by the human small bowel. *Proc Nutr Soc* **43**, 123A.

5.9   Food Allergy and Food Intolerance

In recent years, considerable publicity has been given to, and wild claims made about, the increasing problems caused by 'food allergies'. Much remains to be learnt about this complex and contentious subject. However, it is clear that only a minority of the unpleasant reactions to food are truly 'allergic' reactions, i.e. involving a specific immune reaction of the body, and the term 'food intolerance' should be the general term used to describe these conditions.

Food intolerance may be defined as a condition in which there are reproducible adverse effects after ingesting a specific food or food ingredient. Genuine food *intolerance* is quite distinct from psychologically based food *aversion* where a person merely believes that certain foods will provoke undesirable symptoms. The two can be distinguished by 'blind challenge' where the suspect item is given to the patient in a hidden form.

5.9.1   Causation of food intolerance

Food intolerance may be caused by a number of mechanisms.

Allergic reactions

It is important to realize that allergy is only one of a number of mechanisms provoking food intolerance and that it is the cause in only a minority of cases.

Allergy is defined as an altered or abnormal tissue reaction following exposure to a foreign antigen. Antigens are usually proteins (or items bound to proteins, e.g. food additives), but occasionally polysaccharides. An allergic reaction results from the combination of antigenic allergen with an antibody, Immunoglobulin E (IgE), within the tissues. The resulting cell damage releases histamine and other substances, which produce the clinical signs. Even a minute amount of the allergen can trigger the reaction.

Sensitization may occur; at the first time of consumption antigens may stimulate an immune response but no symptoms are produced due to rapid phagocytosis of the antigen. Later re-exposure to the antigen will result in a more rapid and more abundant antibody production and, therefore, an increased likelihood of interaction between antigen and IgE with consequent clinical manifestation.

Food allergies are probably due to one or more of the following reasons

1   An excessive absorption of food allergens due to gut mucosa defects.
2   An abnormal antibody response.
3   An inability to handle the immune complexes formed from absorbed food allergens and circulating antibodies.
4   Genetic factors.

True food allergy is characterized by raised blood levels of IgE and the presence of IgE antibodies to the food constituent, as assessed by radioallergosorbent tests (RAST) of the blood or by skin prick or intradermal testing. However, these methods are not infallible; false positive results can be produced in patients who no longer react clinically to the suspect food item and false negative results can be obtained in people who have delayed reactions. Other tests such as measurement of histamine release from basophil white blood cells may also be useful, but the search for the ideal diagnostic tool continues (Lessof *et al* 1980).

Non-allergic histamine release

Although histamine release is a feature of true allergic reaction, it may also be provoked by non-immunological mechanisms causing effects which are sometimes known as 'pseudo-allergy' (Moneret-Vautrin 1983). Foods which may cause this reaction include shellfish, strawberries and those rich in amines.

The clinical signs may be very similar to those of allergy and include headache, local oedema, urticaria and abdominal symptoms such as vomiting or diarrhoea.

However, unlike allergy, an abnormal immunological reaction cannot be demonstrated and the effects are usually only provoked by ingestion of relatively large quantities of the offending item.

Enzyme defects

A lack or deficiency of enzymes responsible for the digestion of food (e.g. lactase deficiency resulting in milk intolerance) or the metabolism of food (e.g.

phenylalanine hydroxylase deficiency causing phenyl-ketonuria) can cause many types of food intolerance. The treatment of these disorders is discussed in Section 4.12.1 and 4.7, respectively.

Pharmacological effects

Some food constituents can have a pharmacological effect, particularly if taken in large quantities.

The group of substances most likely to provoke pharmacological effects are the vasoactive amines which act as vasoconstrictors on blood vessels and affect the autonomous nervous system. The most familiar of these substances is caffeine, a methyl xanthine, consumed via coffee, tea and cola drinks. Large intakes of caffeine can induce a variety of toxic effects ranging from tremor to migraine or oesophageal reflux although unpleasant effects such as sweating and palpitations may be produced by as little as 200 mg (which can be obtained from 2−3 cups of coffee) (Turning 1978). Other vasoactive amines such as histamine, tryptamine, tyramine and serotonin may be consumed via foods such as red wine, cheese, yeast extracts and bananas. Other foods such as avocado, pears may also contain significant quantities. These foods can induce urticaria, facial flushing and headaches and may be an important trigger factor in migraine in susceptible people (Hannington 1983).

Irritant and toxic effects

Some foods (such as curry and strong coffee) can have a directly irritant effect on the gut mucosa, particularly if it is diseased. One or a number of foods may be responsible for some cases of the irritable bowel syndrome (Jones 1982). Management of the irritable bowel syndrome is discussed in Section 4.12.4.

Food intolerance of unknown origin

Some foods or food components may provoke reaction by mechanisms which at present remain unclear. There are a number of conditions, particularly skin disorders, such as eczema, which appear to be provoked by yeasts. Sensitivity to food additives, a topic which has attracted considerable media attention in recent years, may also fall into this category. Some food additives, in particular tartrazine and sodium benzoate, undoubtedly can provoke clinical reactions

such as urticaria, rhinitis and asthma in sensitive individuals (Freedman 1977). Some of these reactions can be identified as allergic responses but in other cases the aetiology is less clear. Behavioural changes (such as hyperkinesis) in children have also been reported to be linked with consumption of certain additives (Taylor 1985). Whilst care should be taken not to ascribe every instance of bad behaviour to dietary causes, the dramatic improvements achieved in some children following avoidance of some additives should not be ignored. Just because something cannot be as yet scientifically explained does not necessarily mean it does not exist. Dietitians should retain an open mind on this subject pending further investigation of the nature and incidence of such effects.

Foods which are most commonly associated with food intolerances and some effects of food intolerance are summarized in Tables 5.18 and 5.19.

Table 5.18 Foods commonly associated with food intolerances of varying aetiology

Cows' milk
Egg
Cereals, especially wheat
Fish, shellfish
Pork, bacon
Chocolate
Coffee, tea
Preservatives/colourings

5.9.2 Diagnosis of food intolerance

Non-dietary tests include sublingual testing (Breneman *et al* 1974), measurement of pulse rate after food ingestion (Coca 1942) and hair analysis. All have been used to discover 'sensitivity'; most are not reliable and have little place in clinical practice. Discovering which food or foods may provoke intolerance is not easy. Dietary investigations are currently the cornerstone of diagnosis. Dietary investigation is ideally conducted in 4 phases

1 Dietary enquiry or record-keeping.
2 Trial exclusion.
3 Reintroduction of foods.
4 Blind challenge (or other non-dietary confirmatory tests).

Dietary enquiry and record-keeping

In some cases of food intolerance the cause is obvious. Consumption of a certain item is immediately followed

Table 5.19 Some effects of food intolerance

	Mechanism and possible cause	Common precipitating foods or food components
Skin disorders		
Urticaria and rashes	1 Allergy 2 Pseudoallergy 3 Unknown	Almost any
Eczema	1 Allergy 2 Unknown	Dairy foods, fish, eggs, chocolate, citrus fruits, yeasts, nuts, Food colourings and preservatives beef, chicken.
Respiratory tract		
Rhinitis and nasal polyps	1 Allergy 2 Pseudoallergy	Wheat, eggs, salicylates, azo-dyes, sodium benzoate.
Asthma	1 Allergy 2 Unknown	Milk, azo dyes, sodium benzoate, monosodium glutamate, sulphur dixoide, sodium metabisulphite, e.g. white wine.
Nervous system		
Central nervous system	1 Allergy (rare) 2 Unknown	
Behavioural disturbances (e.g. hyperactivity)		Food additives
Mood changes (e.g. depression, anxiety)	1 Unknown if any	Debatable
Migraine	1 Pharmacological	Foods rich in vasoactive amines, e.g. cheese chocolate, yeasts, citrus fruits, yeast extract and red wine.
Gastrointestinal disorders		
Vomiting, abdominal pain, diarrhoea	1 Allergy 2 Pseudoallergy 3 Irritation	Almost any
Malabsorption	1 Primary or secondary enzyme deficiency	Lactose, sucrose, fructose, fat
Infantile colic	?	? Cows' milk
Coeliac disease	Gluten sensitivity	Wheat, rye, oats, barley
Crohn's disease	?	Wheat, dairy products, yeast, brassicas
Irritable bowel syndrome	1 Irritation 2 Allergy 3 Psychological cause	Wheat, corn, dairy products
Inflammatory disorders		
Arthritis	?	Cereals, milk, cheese, fruit with pips
Metabolic disorders		
Gout	Enzyme deficiency	Purines/pyrimidines
Inborn errors of metabolism	Enzyme deficiency	Various

by swelling of the lips, a tingling sensation in the mouth and sometimes difficulty in breathing. The remedy, avoidance of the item in question, is simple and the mechanism of the reaction, e.g. whether it is true or pseudo-allergy, is of little practical importance.

In most cases of suspected food intolerance, however, the cause is less apparent. Sometimes the patient will associate the consumption of certain foods with symptoms such as abdominal pain, vomiting or diarrhoea or with the exacerbation of disorders such as eczema, asthma or migraine. In such cases, dietary enquiry may produce sufficient evidence to justify a trial exclusion diet.

In other instances, any dietary link is even less obvious and in these patients a period of dietary and symptom record-keeping may yield useful clues. This is a time-consuming exercise from the patient's point of view but many patients will willingly comply, being only too pleased to try to discover the cause of their symptoms. Careful planning is needed beforehand on the part of the clinician and dietitian to determine

1 The dietary information required (e.g. if the suspected intolerance is to food additives, then brand names will need to be recorded).
2 Which symptoms should be recorded.
3 The duration of the record-keeping.
4 How frequently the record should be reviewed by the clinician and/or dietitian.

Some examples of suitable record-keeping formats are shown in Tables 5.20 and 5.21.

Other factors also may need to be recorded if it is considered that these may affect the symptoms, e.g. marital problems, difficulties with the children, menstrual-related effects or even the weather! The clinician also may advise cessation of smoking during the period of record-keeping as this can sometimes provoke the same symptoms as food intolerance (e.g. migraine). Medication also should be avoided or, if this is not possible, its composition (e.g. a lactose-base or a suspected colouring agent) taken into account, and possibly recorded, too.

It should be emphasized to the patient that meticulous record-keeping is essential if the procedure is to have any value. A definite willingness on the part of the patient to participate is essential if useful records are to be obtained.

Although undoubtedly a useful first step in the investigation of food intolerance, a period of dietary and symptom record-keeping may not be a realistic option in those with severe symptoms, e.g. a child with failure to thrive or life-threatening asthma.

Table 5.20 Suggested format of combined symptom record and food diary

Name	
Date	

*New Food**

Breakfast

Lunch

Evening

Symptoms

Vomiting

Headache

Diarrhoea

Constipation

Pain

Stress

   x when the symptoms are present
  xx when the symptoms are bad
 xxx when the symptoms are very bad

*The Brand name should be included if appropriate, also the cooking method and quantity.

Table 5.21 Suggested format of symptom record sheet for use in the investigation of food intolerance. Patients are asked to score twice daily how they feel

Date

General well-being	am	−5	0	5
	pm	−5	0	5
		Unwell		Well
Bowels	am	−5	0	5
	pm	−5	0	5
		Diarrhoea	Normal	Constipation
. . . .	am	−5	0	5
	pm	−5	0	5

Trial exclusion

Simple exclusion diets

When dietary enquiry or record-keeping suggests that a single (probably more) food(s) such as milk, egg or wheat may be the chief culprit(s), patients should be advised how to consume a diet free of this or these item(s).

Although simple in concept, such a diet is not necessarily simple in practice. Many manufactured products contain foods or food components in a non-obvious form. In children, exclusion of a food which normally makes a significant contribution to nutrient intake, e.g. milk, may require considerable dietetic expertise to ensure that dietary requirements are met.

The practicalities of dietary regimens free from milk, eggs, wheat, etc. are discussed in Section 2.11.

Multi-exclusion diets

If it is not clear from dietary enquiry or a simple exclusion diet which food or foods may be responsible, a more complex exclusion diet has to be tried on a trial-and-error basis. This can be achieved by one of two basic strategies

1 Initial exclusion ('decreasing' exclusion) diets. Initially a wide range of foods which may provoke intolerance is removed from the diet and, after a period of time, reintroduced singly into the diet so that the offending item(s) can be identified. There are various ways in which this can be done (see below).

2 Graduated or progressive exclusive ('increasing' exclusion) diets. The number of foods excluded from a diet is gradually increased in a step-wise programme until symptom relief is achieved (see p 584).

Initial ('decreasing') exclusion diets

Fasting. This is the most drastic method and one which is not recommended, the patient being asked to drink only bottled spring water for five days before gradually reintroducing foods. The symptoms of ketosis as well as withdrawal symptoms may magnify the food intolerance symptoms, making the patient feel wretched.

Oligo-antigenic of low allergen diet. All common food allergens and food items frequently causing intolerance are removed from the diet for a period of 2−3 weeks. If there is an improvement in symptoms during this time, foods are slowly and singly reintroduced into the diet so the offending foods can be identified. The foods which should be allowed in the basic elimination diets are a matter of some debate (Hathaway and Warner 1983), but one example of an oligo-antigenic diet is shown in Table 5.22.

The duration of this basic elimination diet should not exceed three weeks as more prolonged use may

Table 5.22 Example of foods allowed in an oligo-antigenic or low allergen diet

Foods excluded	Foods allowed
Milk, milk products, butter, cheese. Eggs.	Milk substitute (See Table 2.65)
Fish	
Ham, bacon, canned meats chicken, beef* and pork*	Lamb, rabbit
Butter margarine, lard and dripping*.	Olive or corn oil, Tomor margarine[†] Vitaquel margarine[§]
Fruits — tomatoes, oranges *, apples* and natural apple juice.	Pears, rhubarb Apricots* and peaches*
Vegetables — beans, peas, mushrooms, cucumber and potato powder.	Carrots, lettuce, fresh potatoes* and Other fresh vegetables*.
Nuts	
Drinks — fizzy drinks, squashes, vending machine drinks, Cola.	Bottled spring water, 7-Up Lemonade* Water, soda water, pure coffee* or tea* in small amounts.
Sweets, ice cream and chocolate.	Salt, sugar*, vinegar, honey* and golden syrup.
Cereals — oats*, wheat flour bread, biscuits, etc. rye. corn*.	Rice, cornflakes*, Rice Krispies*, Sago, barley and buckwheat.

*Varies from centre to centre and usually depends on the disorder being investigated.
[†]Tomor margarine is available from Jewish delicatessens.
[§]Vitaquel margarine is available from some Health Food shops.

result in poor compliance, inadequate energy intake and other nutritional deficiencies. If the symptoms have not improved within this time there are three possible reasons

1 The patient is not food intolerant.
2 The patient has failed to comply.
3 The diet still contains a food to which the patient is intolerant. If this is thought to be the case, a stricter hypo-allergenic diet should be tried — (see progressive exclusion diets Table 5.24).

If the symptoms improve, the patient is challenged with one food, usually every six days. It is important to introduce one food over a few days because delayed reactions can frequently occur. In children, only a small amount of the food is given on the first day in case of possible anaphylactic reactions. The order in which foods are reintroduced is flexible, and is usually influenced by a food preference and the degree of allergenicity of a food. It can take up to a year to reintroduce all the foods into a diet in both children and adults and regular contact is needed with a dietitian and clinician to check both the nutritional adequacy of the diet and, if relevant, growth. Appropriate vitamins and minerals should be given, if necessary.

There are many variations of the basic initial elimination diet. One such regimen is called the 'Stone-age diet', a limited regimen based on the exclusion of
1 All highly allergenic foods.
2 All processed food, including sugar.
3 All citrus fruits.
4 Tea and coffee.

Alternating oligo-antigenic diets. Another approach is to use two different alternating oligo-antigenic diets, each including a meat, a vegetable, a carbohydrate food and a fruit.
For example

	Diet 1	Diet 2
One meat	Lamb	Chicken
One vegetable	Carrots	Cabbage
One carbohydrate food	Rice	Potatoes
One fruit	Bananas	Apples
Plus a milk substitute, salt, sugar, tea and water.		

One of these diets is tried first for two weeks and if this does not produce any improvement in symptoms, the other is tried (Goldsborough and Francis 1983). Subsequently, foods are reintroduced.

The rotary diet. This is a modification of the oligo-antigenic diet which is widely favoured in the USA. A specific rotation of foods is consumed over a minimum of a five day period. Only three foods are allowed each day. Any one food is only allowed in one day in the rotation. There is no set rotation; foods are chosen and the rotation is planned by discussion with the patient. The following foods should be excluded
1 Foods known or suspected by the patient of causing symptoms.
2 Foods disliked by the patient.
3 Foods generally known to cause food intolerant reactions, e.g. oranges which may precipitate migraine, or cows' milk which may trigger eczema.

A plan should be made before starting the rotation and once the rotation is started, the order of foods in it must not be changed. It has been suggested that foods in the same biological families should not be used on consecutive days, e.g. pears should not be on a day following apples. A patient may eat as much as they like of any food allowed, but must only eat the foods allowed each day. In addition, sea salt may be used for seasoning, natural spring water for a beverage and herb teas if liked.

The rotation must be repeated twice. On the first rotation, results will not be significant because of the effects of previous foods. Patients must be warned about withdrawal symptoms possibly making them feel much worse. During the second rotation a record must be kept of the foods eaten and any symptoms. At the end of ten days it should be possible to assess whether or not a patient has a food intolerance. It may be necessary to repeat the rotation in some cases of eczema and possibly arthritis. If it is a case of food intolerance, then single foods are reintroduced in the same way as after an elimination diet. Provided the rotary diet is carefully planned, and provided the symptoms are severe enough, patients will manage this very limited diet.

Elemental diets. Sometimes, an elemental diet may be used as the initial exclusion diet. This often produces immediate symptom relief. However, such diets are unpalatable and monotonous and should only be used in those who are acutely ill or where it is important to maintain a good nutritional level before and whilst proceding with a formal exclusion diet (Workman *et al* 1984). Care must be taken with the use of any flavourings added to improve the taste of these preparations; additives such as tartrazine (E102) or sunset yellow (E110) found in, for example, milk shake syrups or fruit drink crystals, may provoke symptoms.

Elemental exclusion diets have been successfully used in children to produce relief from eczema (David 1983). However, not all the elemental products available are nutritionally adequate for children without modification (see Table 5.23).

Infants under 1 year with multiple food intolerances. Infants already receiving weaning foods who have severe food intolerant type symptoms (i.e. failing to thrive, vomiting, abdominal pain, diarrhoea and eczema), who do not respond to a simple milk-free diet may warrant a trial on a diet based on a milk-free baby rice and a casein hydrolysate milk, e.g. Nutramigen or Pregestimil. On this regimen, nutritional intake and growth require close monitoring. If the infant does improve on this diet, foods are not reintroduced until a catch-up weight gain is established. When this occurs, foods are introduced individually into the diet. Highly allergenic foods, e.g. milk, wheat and eggs, are avoided until after 8 months of age.

Diet for hyperactivity/The Feingold diet. Hyperactivity is a syndrome without very clear definitions or internationally agreed criteria for diagnosis. It is, therefore, difficult to diagnose, assess or compare treatments or

Table 5.23 Elemental preparations used in exclusion diets

Product and Manufacturer	Composition and analysis per 100 ml						Comments
	Protein	Fat	Carbohydrate	Energy		osmolality (mosm/kg)	
				(kcal)	(kJ)		
Elemental 028 (Scientific Hospital Supplies)	Crystalline L-amino acids 2.0 g	Arachis oil 1.32 g	Maltodextrin sucrose 15.6g	80	334	720. 1 to 5 dilution	Orange flavoured (tartrazine-free). Although a nutritionally complete adult feed, it should be used with caution in children 1–5 yrs, and appropriate supplements provided if necessary. Not suitable for children under 1 year. Unflavoured elemental 028 is available with separate flavoured sachets.
Neocate (Scientific Hospital Supplies)	Crystalline L-amino acids 1.87 g	Sunflower oil, MCT oil 3.5 g	Maltodextrin 8.4 g	71	298	360. 1 to 5 dilution	Unflavoured. Suitable for infants under 1 year.
Vivonex (Eaton Laboratories)	Pure L-amino acids 2.3 g	Safflower oil 0.15 g	Glucose solids 23 g	100	421	550. 1 sachet in 300 ml water.	Adult formula elemental feed. Cystine-free. Low in essential amino acids. Not suitable for children as a sole source of nutrition. Unsuitable for infants under 1 year. Vivonex HN also available. Both formulae contain vitamins and minerals.
Flexical (Mead Johnson)	Enzymatically hydrolysed casein plus L-tyrosine L-tryptophan L-methionine 2.3 g	Soya oil, MCT oil 3.4 g	Glucose syrup solids. Modified tapioca starch 15.2 g	100	421	550. 1 can in 2 litres water	Adult formula feed. Contains peptides and amino acids. Low in cystine. Contains vitamins and minerals. Not suitable for children as a sole source of nutrition. Unsuitable for infants under 1 year.

trials because a multiplicity of variables affect behaviour (Starr and Horder 1984). In recent years, the idea that chemicals added to food can cause children to exhibit a variety of behaviour patterns such as restlessness, irritability and short attention span has become popular (Pipes 1985). One of the most well-known proponents of this idea has been Benjamin Feingold (Taylor 1985). The basis of the Feingold diet is to eliminate the following groups of foods

1   All fruits and vegetables containing salicylates in a natural form.
2   All food and drink containing artificial colouring and flavouring.

As well as foods, items also excluded are aspirin, toothpaste, cough syrup, vitamins and most medications for children. If a child responds positively to the Feingold diet for approximately 4–6 weeks, then natural fruits and vegetables are reintroduced to the child's diet as tolerated. This is commonly referred to as the modified Feingold diet. Interestingly, currently available data on the salicylate contents of food are conflicting and there is no degree of parity in figures available in the USA, New Zealand and Australia (Starr and Horder 1984).

Although it is not clear how a Feingold diet works, a response rate of approximately 48% has been reported by Feingold (1974). However, other workers have failed to produce similar results and Feingold has been criticized because of the lack of control studies and the primarily subjective nature of the data (Leading article, *Lancet* 1979). Despite this, the diet has become popular with the general public.

The role of diet in hyperactivity in Britain has been pioneered by the lay organisation, the Hyperactive Children's Support Group (HACSG). In addition to Feingold's original diet, they exclude the following additives: monosodium glutamate, sodium glutamate, nitrate, nitrite, sodium benzoate, butylated hydroxytoluene, butylated hydroxyanisole and vanillin. The HACSG also recommend a supplement of 50 mg vitamin C daily due to the initial elimination of various fruits and vegetables.

It has been reported recently that many other foods such as milk, sugar and eggs in addition to the various additives are also implicated in causing hyperactivity (Egger *et al* 1985).

Graduated (or progressive) exclusion diets

This approach gradually increases the number of foods excluded from the diet. Initially, only the high aller-

Table 5.24 Outline of a graduated exclusion diet recommended by the National Society for Research into Allergy (NSRA). Reproduced by kind permission of Dr L McEwen

a) Diet 1

Category	Foods to avoid	Foods allowed
Milk	Ordinary milk, powdered and tinned milks	Carnation milk*
Eggs	Eggs, egg custard, salad cream, lemon curd	
Meat	Chicken and other poultry, pork, bacon, all offal and liver	Beef, salt beef, mince, lamb and mutton
Nuts, pips and chemical additives	Tomatoes, tomato sauce, Apples, pears, plums, cherries, apricots. Strawberries, raspberries, gooseberries, blackcurrants, etc. Marmalade and jam. Fruit juice, squash, fruit-flavoured drinks Grapes, sultanas and other dried fruit. Nuts, coconut, marzipan, peanuts, macaroons. All fizzy drinks (including cola), fruit sweets, peppermints, lollies, jellies, instant puddings, ice cream, chocolate. Fresh coffee, coffee whiteners, vending machine tea and coffee	Bananas (not more than one per day), rhubarb

Home made soda water (no flavourings)

Tea, instant coffee (powder not granules, not freeze dried |
Other vegetables	Peas, beans, lentils, soya. Melon, cucumber, marrow, cauliflower, broccoli, spinach Onions, garlic and leeks, Spices, pepper, mustard, curry, all herbs	Green leafy vegetables, celery, carrots, mushrooms (not more than 4 oz/week), fresh potatoes, home made crisps, small amounts of turnip, swede, parsnip and beetroot.
Oils and fats	Cooking oils	Tomor (kosher) margarine, pure corn oil for cooking
Yeast	Yeast, yeast and meat extracts, e.g. Marmite, Oxo, Bovril and gravy browning	
Fish	All fish and shellfish	
Cheese	All types	
Alcohol	All types	
Miscellaneous	Honey, chewing gum, vinegar	Sugar, treacle and syrup
Cereals	Bread, pastry, cakes or biscuits containing cream, egg, cherries, dried fruit, jam or fruit-flavoured cream or icing	Oats, rice, corn and rye Plain breakfast cereals

*Carnation brand milk is tolerated by 60% of people who are allergic to milk. Up to half a pint (undiluted quantity) may be included in Diet 1 in cases where the chances of milk allergy are not very high. Carnation milk should not be included in the diet of patients with eczema.

b) Diet 2

(Grain, fruit and chemical additive-free)

AVOID ALL FOODS *EXCEPT*

Sugar, treacle, syrup (unless testing for a psychological illness)
Salt
Pearl sago, sago flour
Lamb, mutton
Fresh green vegetables, celery, lettuce, carrots
Tomor (Kosher) margarine
Water
Home made soda water
Tea, without milk or lemon (unless testing for a psychological illness)
Rhubarb, fresh or frozen (avoid those brands containing dyes)

genic foods are avoided. If this is ineffective, a stricter hypoallergenic diet is consumed for a further two weeks. If no improvement occurs, the final stage involves a trial with an elemental diet. Once relief of symptoms is obtained, foods are reintroduced gradually so that the offending items can be identified. An example of a graduated exclusion diet is shown in Fig. 5.4.

The National Society for Research into Allergy (NSRA) recommends a modification of this strategy. Patients follow a moderately restricted Diet 1 for a period of three weeks and if relief of symptoms is not obtained they try a stricter Diet 2 for 1–2 weeks. Food are then gradually reintroduced. These diets are shown in Table 5.24.

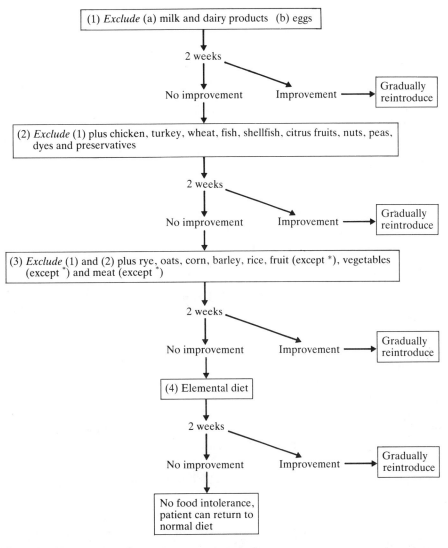

* *allow* lamb, cabbage, carrots, celery, lettuce, rhubarb, pears, treacle, syrup, sago, Vitaquel or Tomor margarine, water and tea.

Fig. 5.4 Example of a graduated (or progressive) exclusion diet.

Reintroduction of foods

In all the varying exclusion diet schemes, after a specified period of time excluded foods will need to be reintroduced. The order in which they are introduced will vary from patient to patient and the condition being treated. A list is given in Table 5.25 but it is not exhaustive. Foods not listed, such as convenience foods, are tested when the reintroduction of listed foods has been completed. All foods are either fresh or frozen. Foods which are rarely eaten or disliked should be left out.

Table 5.25 A suggested order of food reintroduction following an exclusion diet

Lamb	Apple	Lettuce	Oats
Pears	Chicken	Corn	Rhubarb
Rice	Port	Onion	Instant coffee
Broccoli	Yeast tablets	Parsnips	Honey
White fish	Potatoes	Cheddar cheese	Melon
Carrots	Butter	Mushrooms	Celery
Turkey	Eggs	White bread	Lemon
Tomatoes	Wheat	Spinach	Olive oil
Beef	Coffee beans	Grapefruit	Turnip/swede
Tap water	Leeks	Plain chocolate	Yoghurt
Banana	Cane sugar	Grapes	Rye bread
Milk	White wine	Courgettes or marrows	Monosodium glutamate
Peas	Oranges		
Tea	Brussel sprouts	Soya beans	Prawns/shrimps
Cabbage	Beet sugar	Cauliflower	Saccharin tablets

Rate of introduction

Where reactions are quickly demonstrated, e.g. swelling of lips and vomiting, it may be feasible to allow one new food daily, but where it is likely that there will be a delay, e.g. in Crohn's Disease, etc., it may be recommended that *either* one new food only is introduced weekly *or* that 3 foods are introduced three-weekly. This clearly will make patient compliance more difficult.

Quantity

The quantity of foods to be reintroduced should be discussed with the clinician. It may be desirable to introduce the suspect food gradually (this is often the best policy in children); in other cases it may be better to give larger quantities to ensure a realistic challenge.

The problems invariably come with reintroducting foods. Patients may rush along, introducing too many foods too quickly. A common mistake is that when a new food causes an adverse reaction, the patient does not allow these symptoms to subside completely before introducing another new food, and then it is difficult to establish which food is causing the symptoms.

If the patient has a reaction, however mild, he/she should be advised NOT to introduce any more new foods (as well as stopping the possible offending food) until the symptoms have completely disappeared.

Patient instruction

Some patients will quickly grasp what is required of them and will take great satisfaction from feeling better as well as trying to find the offending foods. Others will find it difficult to understand even what is meant by a 'simple' food such as a lamb chop and will want to include processed foods.

Blind food challenge

Once a suspect food (or foods) have been identified, it is important to confirm that a genuine food intolerance, rather than food aversion, exists. Exposing the patient to the suspect item(s) and observing the effect is termed 'challenge'. Immunological tests may be carried out at the same time if true allergy is suspected.

In order to distinguish between psychosomatic effects and genuine food intolerance, the challenge test should be 'blind', i.e. the suspect item is disguised and consumed without the patient's knowledge. This is not always easy to achieve but methods of doing this include:
1 Replacing a food free of a particular component (such as gluten-free bread or a colouring-free drink) with a similar item containing the suspect item (e.g. ordinary bread or a tartrazine-containing drink).
2 Incorporating a suspect food (e.g. egg) into an elemental diet.
3 Giving the suspect item in an encapsulated form. However, because of limitation in size, this test is only suitable if small quantities of the test food produce a reaction (Davies 1981).
4 Hiding the suspect item in soups, casseroles, puddings or cakes.
A realistic quantity should be given, a suggested guide for adults might be 2−3 times the usual portion size within 24 hours, e.g. 100 ml tartrazine-containing cordial in 24 hours. An adequate time period must be allowed for reactions to appear; these may occur within an hour but can take as long as a week, or even more, to become manifest. An objective assesment should be made.

Milk challenges in infants

Cows' milk (preferably using a modified infant formula milk) should be introduced slowly into the diet of infants with suspected milk intolerance. Five ml of cows' milk formula should be added to a feed of the usual milk substitute. If tolerated, the amount is gradually increased in subsequent feeds. Milk challenges in infants should be performed under medical supervision, in case of severe unpredictable reactions. Infants whose growth has been impaired should be allowed to catch up and achieve a steady growth rate before the challenge. If there is no growth disturbance, two months of the milk-free diet should be given before the challenge.

5.9.3 The role of the dietitian

Exclusion diets will stretch a dietitian's skills to the limits since immense practical expertise and patience is required.

Devising the scheme

As a member of the clinical team, the dietitian may be asked to draw up the dietary protocol to be followed. Before doing this, the dietitian must discuss fully with the clinician

1 The number of patients likely to be referred at any one time, since it will be a time-consuming commitment and the dietetic department has to consider whether the staffing resources are sufficient to undertake the work.

2 Where the patients are coming from. If the clinic or hospital is centrally placed, then patients will have no difficulty in attending frequently. In rural areas communication with patients might be a problem, unless they are on the telephone.

3 How often the clinician will be seeing them — whether this will be every time the patient attends the dietitian or only occasionally. Will the clinician be readily available if problems arise during the dietary programme?

4 Which method of recording symptoms and food consumption is the most appropriate.

5 What time-scale is required for the reintroduction of new foods, for example, one every six days, etc.

6 Whether the clinician envisages any of the patients being admitted to hospital; the diet-bay may not be able to manage exclusion diets without notice!

7 How the patients are going to be selected — are all patients with a certain disorder or only highly motivated patients in that group to be chosen? Will the clinician discuss fully with the patient what the test diets involve?

Practical problems in the diagnosis and management of food intolerance

There have been a number of books published recently for the general public on dietary topics so that it is not uncommon for patients or their relatives to question the possible link between their health and food. Whilst this possibility must not be ignored, it is important that the patient should always be advised to seek informed professionally qualified medical advice on the matter before being referred to the dietitian (British Dietetic Association, 1984).

As food intolerance is a fashionable subject, many patients will come with their own pre-conceived ideas of what they or their children are 'allergic' to, so that tactful handling will be required, especially if the intolerance is found to be psychologically based.

As far as possible, the type of exclusion diet should be chosen to suit the patient's clinical and practical needs. It is better to simplify a scheme in order to obtain patient compliance and improved health than to fail trying to follow a standard system.

Psychological support is often appreciated by the patient and family. Where possible, the same dietitian should maintain contact with the patient.

Some patients may find that their symptoms do not merit the effort of an exclusion diet! A trial period may be helpful so that the patient has the opportunity to start the diet and to report back after a short period. If the patient is feeling better then motivation and encouragement from the dietitian may help to continue the regimen.

Cheating may be a problem with this type of diet, especially in children, due to hunger or boredom. The social problems of adhering to an exclusion diet, e.g. school meals, works canteens, birthday parties, eating out in cafés, restaurants, visiting friends and relations must also be appreciated. It may be desirable to postpone starting a regimen until after a specific event, but once started, every encouragement should be given to follow the dietary instructions. If the diet is to be very restricted, either during the test or indefinitely in the maintenance period, the nutritional adequacy of the diet must be monitored. This is especially important in children and malnourished adults. Special supplements, including vitamins and minerals, may be necessary. It is important to give positive advice — emphasize which foods *can* be eaten, and include advice on how recipes can be adapted and how alternative foods can be used.

Dietitian's record cards

Where there are a number of patients on exclusion diets simultaneously, it may be helpful for the department to keep a file of cards (Table 5.26) or computerized records containing details of each patient, including the usual symptoms and the type of exclusion diet prescribed. When foods are reintroduced into the diet, the date should be recorded and the food underlined or encircled if reactions occur.

Patient support organisations

1 Asthma Society and Friends of the Asthma Research Council, St. Thomas' Hospital, Lambeth Palace Road, London SE1 7EH.

The aims of this society include sponsoring research into asthma. They produce useful leaflets for patients and a periodic newsletter.

2 Action Against Allergy, 43 The Downs, London SW20 8HS.

The aims of this association are 'to further the study of the role of modern foods, chemicals and biological materials in the causation of the allergic illnesses increasingly afflicting western man'. Membership is currently (1985) £5.00 per annum and services offered to members include a personal information service, postal book ordering services, reading list, the use of a lending library of Clinical Ecology books, film shows and lectures.

3 Coeliac Society, PO Box 220, High Wycombe, Bucks HP11 2HY.

This society aims to help coeliacs and patients with dermatitis herpetiformis with practical aspects of the gluten-free diet. Publications include a newsletter, recipe books, manufacturers' lists.

4 Migraine Trust, 45, Great Ormond Street, London WC1N 3HD.

Apart from supporting research, the trust funds a special clinic in London, produces a booklet for sufferers and a newsletter. Membership £5.00 annually (1985).

5 National Association for Colitis and Crohn's Disease, 98A London Road, St. Albans, Herts AL1 1NX.

This group supports research, produces a regular newsletter, as well as information literature for patients, Local groups also organise talks and social events for patients. Membership £3.00 annually (1985).

6 National Society for Research into Allergy, PO Box 45, Hinckley, Leicestershire.

This society aims to help the allergy sufferer and his/her family and to help people who think they may have an allergy. Services offered to members include a free 24 page elimination diet booklet, practical advice on the problems of allergy sufferers, periodic newsletters, advice on useful books and pamphlets and introductions to other members and allergy sufferers. The membership fee is currently (1985) £6.00 per annum (or £120.00 life membership).

7 Food and Chemical Allergy Association, 27, Ferringham Lane, Ferring, West Sussex.

Offers an advisory service by letter. They publish a booklet (1985) for £1 for patients on understanding allergies, based on Dr. Richard Mackarness' experience and others working in clinical ecology.

8 Food Watch, High Acre, East Stour, Gillingham, Dorset. Tel. 0747 85261.

Table 5.26 Example of dietitian's record of an exclusion diet and the reintroduction of foods

Patient's name	Referral doctor
Address	
Case-sheet number	
Telephone number	Diagnosis

Symptoms	
1.	5.
2.	6.
3.	7.
4.	8.
Any comments	

Diet record dates (Not necessarily in chronological order)
Low allergen diet . . . .   Elemental diet . . . .

Rice*		Eggs
Lamb*		Cabbage
Pears*		Cauliflower
Bread	If unwell	Yeast
		Wheat flour
Corn		Pork
Rye		Bananas
Oats		Mushrooms
Milk	If unwell try	Goats' milk
		Carnation milk
Cheese		Peas
Butter		Potato
Margarine		Tomato
Sugar		Apples
Tea		Chicken
Coffee		Fresh/frozen fish
Monosodium glutamate		Wine
Processed foods		Ham
Soya		
Citrus fruits		
Beef		

*Included on low allergen diet

A mail order service supplying many additive-free foods, special milks, etc. and a recipe book.

9 National Eczema Society, Tavistock House North, Tavistock Square, London WC1H 9SR.

This society supports research and produces literature for patients. Local groups. Annual membership £7.00 (1985).

10 British Goat Society, Rougham, Bury St. Edmunds, Suffolk.

11 British Sheep Dairying Association, Hon Sec Mrs Mills, Wield Wood Farm, Nr Alresford, Hants.

12 Hyperactive Children's Support Group, Sally Bunday (Secretary), 59 Meadowside, Angmering, West Sussex.

Further reading

Atherton DJ (1984) *Your child with eczema* Heinemann, London.

Bock SA (1983) Clinical aspects of food sensitivity. In *Proceedings of XI International Congress of Allergology and Clinical Immunology* Kerr JW and Ganderton MA (Eds) Macmillan, London.

Bower D and Jeffereys K (1984) *Cows' milk intolerance*. Community Nutrition Group. Information sheet No. 10, British Dietetic Association.

Brostoff J and Challacombe SJ (Eds) (1982) *Food allergy* WB Saunders Company, London.

Dodge JA (Ed) (1983) *Topics in paediatric nutrition* 1e. Pitman books, London.

Food Intolerance and Food Aversion A joint report of the Royal College of Physicians and the British Nutrition Foundation

Hanssen MH (Ed) (1983) *Clinical reactions to food* 1e. John Wiley and Sons, Chichester.

Hanssen M (1984) *E for additives*. Thorsons, Wellingborough.

Human Nutrition: Applied Nutrition, Volume 38A, No. 6 December 1984. *Contains a number of articles of interest.*

Lessof MH and Buisseret P (1981) Gastrointestinal reactions. In *Immunological and clinical aspects of allergy* Lessof MH (Ed). MTP Pres, Lancaster.

Ministry of Agriculture, Fisheries and and Food (1984) *Look at the Label*

MacKarness (1976) *Not all in the mind*. Pan Books, London.

Moore P (1983) *No milk, no eggs*. W Foulsham and Co, London.

McEwen LM and Morgan JE (1980) *Its something you ate: patients guide to elimination diets* 2e. Medical Education Services, Oxford.

Pepys J (1982) *Allergy*. Update Publications, London.

Proceedings from the First Food Allergy Workshop (1980) Medical Education Services, Oxford.

Proceedings from the Second Food Allergy Workshop (1983) Medical Education Services, Oxford.

Workman E, Hunter J and Jones VA (1984) *The Allergy Diet*. Positive Health Guide. Martin Dunitz, London.

References

Breneman JC, Hurst A, Heiner D, Leney FL, Morris D and Josephson BM (1974) Final report of the Food Allergy Committee of the American College of Allergists on the clinical evaluation of sublingual provocative testing method for diagnosis of food allergy. *Ann Allergy* **33**, 164–6.

British Dietetic Association (1984) Policy Statment on the Dietary Approach to Food Allergy and Food Intolerance. *Hum Nutr: Appl Nutr* **38A**, (6), 405.

Coca AF (1942) *Familial non-reaginic food allergy*. Oxford: Blackwell. Springfield, Illinois: Charles C. Thomas

David JJ (1983) The investigation and treatment of severe eczema in childhood. *Int Med Suppl.* **4**, 17–25.

Davies RJ (1981) *Immunological and clinical aspects of allergy*. Lessof MH (Ed) pp 67–8. MTP Press, Lancaster.

Egger J, Carter CM, Graham PJ, Gumley D and Soothill JF (1985) Controlled trial of oligo-antigenic treatment in the hyperkinetic syndrome. *Lancet* **i** (8428), 540–5.

Feingold BF (1974) *Why your child is hyperactive*. Random House Inc, New York.

Freedman BJ (1977) Asthma induced by sulphur dioxide, benzoate and tartrazine contained in orange drinks. *Clin Allergy* **7**, 407–15.

Goldsborough J and Francis DEM (1983) Dietary management. *The Second Fisons Food Allergy Workshop* pp 89–94.

Hannington E (1983) Migraine. In *Clinical reactions to food* Lessof M.H. (Ed). pp 155–80 John Wiley and Sons, Chichester.

Hathaway MJ and Warner JD (1983) Compliance problems in the dietary management of eczema. *Arch Dis Childh* **58**, 463–4.

Jones VA, McLaughlan P, Shorthouse M, Workman E and Hunter JO (1982) Food intolerance: a major factor in the pathogenesis of irritable bowel syndrome. *Lancet* **ii**, 1115-7.

Leading Article (1979) Feingold's regimen in hyperkinesis *Lancet* **ii**, 617–8.

Lessof MH, Wraith DG, Merrett TG, Merrett J and Buisseret PD (1980) Food Allergy and intolerance in 100 patients: local and systemic effects. *Quart J Med* **49**, 259–71.

Moneret-Vautrin DA (1983) False food allergies: Non-specific reactions to foodstuffs. In *clinical reactions to food* pp 135–53.

Pipes PL (1985) *Nutrition in infancy and childhood* 3e. Times Mirror/Mosby College Publishing, St Louis.

Starr J and Horder D (1984) Hyperactivity information sheet No 11. Community Nutrition Group. The British Dietetic Association.

Taylor E (1985) *The hyperactive child. A parent's guide*. Martin Dunitz, London.

Turnberg LA (1978) Coffee and the gastrointestinal tract. *Gastroenterology* **75**, 529–30.

Workman EM, Jones AV, Wilson AJ and Hunter OJ (1984) Diet in the management of Crohn's disease. *Hum Nutr: Appl Nutr* **38A**, 469–73.

5.10   Drug—Nutrient Interactions

The relationship between nutrition and drug metabolism is an important but poorly documented subject. Diet can affect drug action and metabolism in a number of ways and conversely, drugs themselves may affect nutrient intake and metabolism.

5.10.1   Effect of nutrition on drug action and metabolism

The metabolism of a drug usually involves the following stages
1   Absorption from the gastrointestinal tract (if the drug is orally administered).
2   Transport in the blood, usually bound to plasma proteins.
3   Deactivation by a two-stage metabolic process
a)   Oxidation by microsomal enzyme systems involving reduced nicotinamide adenine dinucleotide (NADPH) and cytochrome P450, predominantly in the liver but also in the lung and small intestine.
b)   Conjugation with glucuronic acid, sulphate or glycine.
4   Excretion of the conjugate in urine or bile.

Nutrient intake and drug absorption

The pharmacological response to a drug depends on the rate at which it is absorbed from the gastrointestinal tract.

The physical presence of food in the stomach and proximal intestine may delay the absorption of drugs from the gut (although it will not necessarily decrease the total amount absorbed). Food will modify gastric emptying and thus the rate of drug absorption. For this reason, some drugs (e.g. oral hypoglycaemics such as glipizide and glibenclamide, or antibiotics) must be taken on an empty stomach.

Cations in foods, e.g. Ca^{2+} can chelate with some drugs (e.g. tetracyclines and ferrous sulphate) and reduce their intestinal absorption; milk or milk products should therefore not be consumed within an hour or two of ingesting these drugs.

Other dietary constituents (e.g. fat) may impede the absorption of drugs which are hydrophilic. Foods which significantly alter the pH of the gut may also affect drug absorption. Absorption of drugs which are partly ionized (e.g. hexamethonium and amiloride) will be reduced by food. Some antihypertensives (atenolol and captopril) and antituberculous compounds (rifampicin and isoniazid) also have impaired absorption in the presence of food.

However, the absorption of some drugs (e.g. nitrofurantoin and hydrochlorthiazide) can be increased if taken with a meal and more recently it has been shown that the bioavailability of a number of drugs (including propanolol, metoprolol and hydralazine) is increased when given with food (Melander and McLean 1983).

Plasma protein binding

In severe malnutrition where energy intake is low, tissue protein is used as a source of energy, thus reducing the plasma protein available for transport of the drug from the gastrointestinal tract. Malnutrition therefore impairs the transport, and hence decreases the effectiveness, of drugs such as chloramphenicol, digoxin, phenylbutazone, salicylate and tetracycline.

Rate of deactivation and conjugation

Since the active constituent of a drug is very often one of its metabolic derivatives, abnormalities in the rate of deactivation and conjugation may considerably alter the pharmacological effects and/or toxicity of the drug.

Both short term starvation and prolonged periods of nutritional inadequacy can affect microsomal drug-metabolizing enzymes (Dickerson 1978; Cusack and Denham 1984). Either one of these features may occur in cases of severe illness where drug administration is also more likely.

5.10.2   Effects of drugs on nutrition

Absorption of nutrients

Laxatives can interfere with the biological availability of nutrients by decreasing intestinal absorption.

Chronic use of peristaltic stimulants (such as senna or phenolphthalein) and anticholinergic drugs can considerably reduce nutrient absorption while intestinal lubricants (such as liquid paraffin) impair the absorption of fat soluble vitamins.

Antibiotics are known to alter colonic flora and can cause diarrhoea which, if prolonged, can lead to a malnourished state. Other antibiotics such as neomycin can decrease carotene, glucose, fat and iron absorption. Drugs such as sulphasalazine cause folate malabsorption while cholestyramine impairs the absorption of fat soluble vitamins. The gut mucosa may be affected by cytotoxic drugs, producing villous atrophy leading to malabsorption.

Consumption of large doses of aspirin may cause malabsorption of vitamin C, and tetracycline increases its urinary excretion. This effect may be particularly important in the elderly, many of whom already have a low vitamin C intake.

Appetite

Appetite may be either increased or decreased by drug administration. Indomethacin and cytotoxic drugs have a directly anorectic effect while others such as theophylline, amphetamines and sulphonamides can cause nausea.

Conversely, drugs such as insulin, sulphonylureas, phenothiazines, benzodiazepines and alcohol can increase appetite. Drugs which can affect nutritional intake are shown in Table 5.27.

Increased nutrient requirement

Anticonvulsants, phenothiazines and tricyclics induce synthesis of cytochrome P-450 and increase the requirement for folic acid. Labadarios *et al* (1978) suggest that these drugs cause low blood levels of folate and deficiency will result if they are given for a sufficiently long period of time to patients with a low folate intake.

Penicillamine, used occasionally in the treatment of rheumatoid arthritis, chelates zinc and prolonged administration could lead to a deficiency of the mineral, especially when intake is also reduced.

Alterations in nutrient metabolism

Tyramine

Tyramine is an indirectly acting sympathomimetic amine which releases noradrenaline from adrenergic neurones causing a rise in blood pressure. Normally, tyramine is metabolized by the enzyme monoamine oxidase before any significant hypertension can occur. However, if the enzyme's activity is blocked by a monoamine oxidase inhibitor (MAOI) drug, a severe and possibly fatal rise in blood pressure can result from the ingestion of tyramine-rich foods. These foods (see p 175) must therefore be avoided by patients taking MAOI drugs.

Carbohydrate metabolism

Antidiabetic agents such as sulphonylureas are prescribed precisely because of their effect on carbohydrate metabolism. However, drugs such as oral contraceptives or corticosteroids can produce adverse effects on carbohydrate metabolism and provoke glucose intolerance.

Lipid metabolism

Similarly some drugs are used to correct lipid metabolism but others such as chlorpromazine and phenobarbitone induce hyperlipidaemia (Table 5.28)

Table 5.27 Effects of some drugs on nutritional intake

Drugs	Action affecting nutritional intake
Diethylpropion Mazindol Biguanides Fenfluramine Cytotoxic agents Neomycin sulphate Cyclophosphamide Digitalis Glucagon	Anorexia/decreased appetite
Amphetamines Indomethacin Digoxin Theophylline Clomipramine Diphenylhydrantoin Sulphonamides	Nausea
Androgens Sulphonylureas Corticosteroids Phenothiazines Benzodiazepines Antihistamines. Insulin Alcohol	Increased appetite

Table 5.28 Effect of drugs on carbohydrate and lipid metabolism

Drugs	Disturbance
Thiazides	Carbohydrate metabolism
Corticosteroids	
Oral contraceptives	
Diphenylhydantoin	
Sulphonylureas	
Aspirin	
Monoamine oxidase inhibitors	
Alcohol	
Asprin	Lipid metabolism
Chlortetracycline	
Colchicine	
Phenindione	
Indomethacin	
Oral contraceptives	
Ethanol	
Adrenal corticosteroids	
Growth hormone	
Chlorpromazine	
Phenobarbitone.	

Vitamin and mineral metabolism

Anticonvulsants such as phenytoin affect vitamin D metabolism resulting in impaired calcium absorption and, with prolonged treatment, osteomalacia or rickets.

Antimetabolite drugs such as methotrexate (used in the treatment of some cancers) directly antagonize folic acid metabolism by inhibiting the activity of the enzyme dehydrofolate reductase. Anticancer drugs can also affect thiamin status. Tables 5.29 and 5.30 show some other effects of some drugs on various vitamins and minerals.

Table 5.29 Effects of drugs on electrolytes and minerals

Drug	Effect
Thiazide diuretics	Depletion of body potassium
Purgatives	
Adrenal steroids	
Corticosteroids	Retention of water and salt
Phenylbutazone	
Oxyphenbutazone	
Carbenoxolone	
Oral contraceptives	
Phosphates	Decreased iron absorption
Antacids	
Tetracycline	
Sulphonylureas	Decreased iodine uptake by the thyroid gland
Phenylbutazone	
Cobalt	
Lithium	
Oral contraceptives	Reduction in plasma zinc
	Increase in plasma copper
Thiazide diuretics	Increased reabsorption of calcium from the kidney

Table 5.30 Effects of drugs on vitamin absorption and metabolism

Drug	Vitamin	Effect
Alcohol	Thiamin	Malabsorption
Antacids		
Isoniazid	Pyridoxine	Antagonists of the vitamin
Hydralazine		
Penicillamine		
Oral contraceptives		
Alcohol	Folate	Malabsorption
Aspirin		
Biguanides		
Metformin		
Oral contraceptives		
Sulphasalazine		
Anticonvulsants	Folate	Interaction between drugs and coenzymes
Phenothiazines		
Tricyclics		
Methotrexate		
Para amino salicylate	B_{12}	Malabsorption
Colchicine		
Metformin		
Phenformin		
Cholestyramine		
Oral contraceptives		
Trifluoperazine		
Tetracycline	C	Increase excretion and decrease storage levels
Aspirin		
Corticosteroids		
Barbiturates		
Oral contraceptives		
Anticonvulsants	D	Induce enzymes that convert the vitamin to its inactive form
Warfarin	K	Inhibit bacterial synthesis of the vitamin
Antibiotics		
Liquid paraffin	A, D, E, K	Malabsorption
Cholestyramine		

Further reading

Awad AG (1984) Diet and drug interactions in the treatment of mental illness — a review. *Can J Psychiat* **29**, 609–13.

Basu TK (1977) Interactions of drugs and nutrition. *J Hum Nutr* **31**, 449–58.

References

Cusack B and Denham MJ (1984) Nutritional status and drug disposition in the elderly. In *Drugs and nutrition in the geriatric patient* Roe DA (Ed) pp 71–91. Churchill Livingstone, Edinburgh.

Dickerson JWT (1978) The interrelationships of nutrition and drugs. In *Nutrition in the clinical management of disease*, Dickerson JWT and Lee HA (Eds) pp 308–31. Edward Arnold, London.

Labadarios D, Obuwa G, Lucas EG, Dickerson JWT and Parke DV (1978) The effects of chronic drug administration on hepatic enzyme induction and folate metabolism. *Br J Clin Pharmacol* **5**, 167–73.

Melander A and McLean A (1983) Influence of food intake on presystemic clearance of drugs. *Clin Pharmacokinet* **8**, 286–96.

5.11 Dietetic Research

Dietetic research can take many forms. It can evaluate the effectiveness of existing dietetic practices (e.g. in terms of patient compliance or response to treatment) or it may investigate the effects of a new type of treatment or a new way of administering an existing one. Studies can be based on individuals or different sized groups of people. They may take the form of case histories, direct measurements or controlled trials. They may require data reported by the participant, clinical measurements, biochemical measurements or measurements of food intakes. They may involve one-to-one interviews, questions or group interviews.

Whatever the type of research being undertaken the ultimate aim should be to improve dietetic practice and nutrition education (Table 5.31).

Table 5.31 The advantages of research

It improves the effectiveness of the dietitian's work
It widens the horizons of the work
It forces reading of relevant literature and other studies which have been undertaken
It enforces disciplined thinking and a more organised approach

Research does not have to be complex in order to be useful. Relatively simple studies conducted by one person can yield valuable information. However, all good research, whether large or small scale, does require careful planning in advance.

Research is also more likely to be successful and enjoyable if everyone concerned is happy about it and feels it to be important. Dietetic departments are not often involved in evaluating their own work so it is important to establish an interest in and support for the idea throughout the department. Regular discussions about each other's work and observations, formal allocation of time for all dietitians to read journals and published work, and interest and support from all members of staff, especially the most senior, are vital if an environment conducive to self-appraisal and advancement of knowledge is to be fostered.

5.11.1 General principles of research

There are a number of general principles which apply to all types of evaluative research. These are outlined below and described in detail by Calnan (1976). Table 5.32 summarizes the main steps.

Table 5.32 The main steps of a study

1   Make an observation about your work as accurately as possible
2   Try to repeat the observation. Be as objective and dispassionate as possible
3   Try to connect the conditions which explain your observations
4   Propose a hypothesis
5   Test the hypothesis
6   Think about the results — do they stand-up? Do they fit in with current knowledge? Do they contest current knowledge? Are they some completely new findings?
7   Draw your conclusions. Can a new hypothesis be formed?
8   Discuss the results with other people
9   Publish your work for the benefit of others

The hypothesis

In order to conduct any research there must be a hypothesis. The hypothesis should

1   Summarize the relevant known facts or close observations.
2   Be consistent with the known facts or observations.
3   Be as simple and straightforward as possible.
4   Explain what it is designed to do.
5   Be able to be verified or refuted, i.e. tested.

Literature search

Before any planning is undertaken it is very important and useful to look at previous research into similar hypotheses. Previous knowledge of faults, useful tips and tested methodologies can save a great deal of time and money. The first place to search is in the appropriate subject section of *Index Medicus* which is published monthly in the UK. A summary of the content of many nutritional papers can be found in *Nutrition Abstracts and Reviews*, also published monthly. The full text of any particularly relevant papers should then be read in detail.

Planning

All research must be well thought out and planned before it is begun. The aims and objectives must be absolutely clear in the researcher's mind. The primary objectives should be narrowed to two or three simple but important questions. Secondary objectives can answer other less important but, nevertheless, interesting questions.

Table 5.33 gives guidelines for drawing up a 'Project Planning Form' (Calnan 1976). No more than two sheets of A4 paper should be used and the plan should be as concise as possible.

Table 5.33 Project Planning Form

1. Name and date
2. Proposed work
3. Expected findings
4. Clinical significance or application of findings
5. Work previously done on the subject by others (two to four references)
6. Criticism of work done by others
7. Reasons for undertaking
8. Treatment/diet to be used
9. Methods of the experiment — Experimental design and experimental technique.
10. Duration of the experiment
11. Special technical assistance required
12. Other assistance required
13. Whether Ethical Committee permission is needed

The protocol

When the outline plan is clear, a full protocol can then be prepared. Writing a protocol helps the researcher to think all his/her ideas through clearly and discuss them with others in an organized way. It is a detailed written statement for everyone likely to be involved, e.g. the Ethical Committee and for those funding the project or giving other kinds of back-up and support. Table 5.34 outlines the basic structure of a useful protocol.

Ethics

Not all research is considered to be ethical, so it is essential to seek permission from the local Ethical Committee. Generally it is acceptable to undertake research if there is *no doubt* about the safety of the diet or treatment being tested. However, particularly strict rules apply to research with children. Also, if a research programme seems to be giving no useful results it may be judged more ethical to terminate it prematurely.

The sample

The number of participants involve in the study will depend primarily on the aims of the study. For studies hoping to show changes in behaviour or some other measurable factor, the sample size needed to show significant changes depends on the degree of change anticipated; the smaller the expected change the larger

Table 5.34 Protocol outline

Title	Title of project and names of all researchers (separate page).
Introduction	Outline why the study is being undertaken and any relevant previous research findings.
Aims	Give a short, clear statement of the hypothesis and how it is to be tested. (One of two sentences only.)
Outline of study	Give details of the hypothesis to be tested and describe the overall plan of the study.
Method	Give details of the exact methods to be used. For example: the sample to be tested, the treatment or diet, the measurement and assessment techniques to be used, the details of control populations, the duration of the study, etc.
Phases of the study	Give a simple step-by-step list of each phase and what it is hoped will be achieved at each stage.
Evaluation and interpretation	Give a detailed account of how all the data collected will be analysed and the statistical procedures to be used. Define the criteria for success or failure.
Applications of findings	Describe the expected benefits and uses of the findings.
Proposed time-scale	Give a timetable of the length of each phase of the study and when publication of results can be expected.
Facilities to be used	Give a brief description of what facilities are already available, what support and backing will be used and from whom.
Budget	If extra funds will be needed, draw up a budget for each phase of the study. This should include costs of extra staff, travel, equipment, computer analyses, extra stationery and postage.
Flow Chart	Give a simple diagrammatic summary of all the stages in the research.
Appendices	These should include questionnaires, coding methods, data processing methods and other information which is an integral part of the study.

the number of participants required in the study to give meaningful results. It is always best to ask a statistician's advice about sample size before embarking on any study since the required sample size is assessed by complicated mathematical formulae.

The type of participants to be studied should be clearly defined beforehand. There should be strict criteria about age, sex, social class, ethnic group, and type of patient (e.g. insulin dependent and/or non-insulin dependent diabetics).

If only a proportion of a group is being studied (e.g. one-fifth of the clinic population) selection of those people must be done on a random basis. This excludes the researcher's own preferences and bias and enables more balanced judgements to be made. Systematic or stratified sampling techniques can also be used. Simple statistics books explain these methods but the advice of a statistician is often a wise precaution.

The methodology

The methods of the study must be worked out in detail.

Criteria

The criteria to be measured must be clearly defined. For example, if the study is to measure dietary compliance, the exact definitions of 'compliance' and 'non-compliance' must be clarified.

Methods

It is important to work out in advance
1   Details of all the materials and equipment which will be required, e.g. questionnaires, diet history sheets, food diaries, scales and laboratory tests.
2   The exact procedures to be followed, e.g. questionnaire distribution, type of interview, presence of a control population, types of measurement to be made — indirect (e.g. interviews, impressions, or state of health of participant) or direct (e.g. blood tests, urine tests, weights or skinfold thickness).
3   How observations will be made and how they will be presented.
4   The calculations and statistics to be used.

Control groups

Not all studies will involve control groups but for those which do, the controls should be monitored at the same time as the treated group. They should also be matched for age, sex, social class, ethnic group and any other relevant factors.

Pilot studies

Pilot studies are designed to check the techniques to be used in the study — the data handling methods; whether there will be sufficient data from which to draw conclusions; whether the budget is realistic and whether completion of the project will be possible. They are carried out on a small number of people, similar to those who will be studied. The pilot study should identify any potential difficulties, enabling them to be eliminated before the main study. All questionnaires, survey methods and interview techniques *must* be piloted.

Communication

The language used must avoid jargon and be suitable for the population being studied. Attention should be paid to the needs of multi-ethnic populations and different literacy and language levels generally.

Questionnaires must be fully understood and stimulate replies. Before writing them, the questions they are designed to answer must be clear and they must be designed to find the answers to those questions. They should give the respondent the minimum amount of work but provide all the information needed (Bennett and Ritchie 1975).

Computers

Computers can relieve the researcher of many of the time-consuming and difficult aspects of statistical analysis. They are also useful for literature searches. Care must be taken to comply with the requirements of the Data Protection Act (1984) which places conditions on the storage of, for example, the names and addresses of individuals (see Section 1.7).

The results

The main stages in the analysis of results are outlined in Table 5.35 Results should be presented so they can be written up including tables, diagrams and simple statistics. Simple statistical techniques are described in many books (Swinscow 1978; Perry 1979; Greer 1980) but professional statistical guidance will help the inexperienced.

Table 5.35 Analysing results

Type of analysis	Purpose
Quantitative analysis	Sorting out material, editing, categorizing, coding and tabulating.
Qualitative analysis	People's views and impressions. (More difficult to analyse because bias can occur.)
Investigating bias	Bias may occur in the sample source, the questions asked or method used, or the analysis.
Testing for significance	Are any apparent effects, changes or differences found likely to be 'real' effects in statistical terms, or could they have arisen by chance?
Interpretation of facts	Bridging the gap between what has been discovered and what this means for the future.
Recommendations	These may support or refute the original hypothesis and may raise new questions to be answered.

The conclusions

Once the data has been analysed there are three possibilities. The conclusions may agree with and reinforce what is already known, or they may sustain ideas and views suspected to be true but as yet unsubstantiated, or they may be entirely new. If the third option is the case they may need to be confirmed and tested by others.

There is another possible, but less welcome, outcome which is that the results may be too inconclusive either to support or refute a hypothesis. This situation is highly undesirable since it means that the study has largely been a waste of time. It is precisely to avoid this outcome that careful planning in the early stages of a study is so important.

All conclusions must be justified by comparing them with theoretical knowledge and other people's results, by questioning the appropriateness of the methods used, by looking for the possibility of human error and any distorting environmental factors and by judging their relevance to the situation.

It is often possible for 'fallacies of logic' to occur. For example 'three men went into three pubs; at the first they drank whisky and water, at the second brandy and water, at the third vodka and water. Next morning they came to the conclusion that the cause of their hangover was from drinking water! Moreover, a modern hospital measuring the output of urine would have supported this hypothesis' (Calnan 1976). All results and conclusions should be widely discussed with colleagues and other intested people before anything is published. Dangers can occur in

1 Ambiguity of words.
2 Taking statements or events out of context.
3 Arguing from a position of power even if there is no evidence.

Table 5.36 Self-assessment fo the researcher

Methods	Were they reliable and accurate?
	Were they acceptable to the subjects?
	Were there any inherent errors?
	Were the methods up to date?
	Had the methods previously been tested and found to be competent?
	Would it have been possible to use any better methods?
Materials	Was the sample tested representative of the group under discussion?
	Was the control group matched?
	Were any comparisons justifiably made?
Conclusions	Are they supported by the evidence?
	Are they reliable?
	Are they feasible?
	Are they important?

Table 5.37 Guidelines for writing-up research findings

Title and Authors	The title of the project. The names of all the researchers. These may be in alphabetical order of surname or with the main workers first. The name of the department undertaking the research.
Summary	A brief description of the time of the reseach, the sample, the method and the main conclusions. (Usually not more than about 500 words.)
Introduction	Details of the background to the study, previous research and the need for the study.
Materials	Description of the subjects and any relevant advice they received.
Methods	Details of all the phases of the research including techniques for sampling, measuring, assessment and analysis.
Results	The main findings of the survey presented mainly in a textual format but with tables to illustrate points where necessary.
Discussion	Interpretation of the results in the light of current knowledge and the implications for the future.
Conclusion	Details of what exactly the study has shown or not shown.
Acknowledgements	Thanks to all people who have been involved with the research but are not included in the list of authors.
References	A list of all papers and publications referred to or used as background to the research. They should give enough detail to enable readers to find the articles from libraries with ease.
Appendices	In some instances further material which supports the body of the paper (e.g. diet sheets or questionnaires used) may be appended.

4 Constructing arguments based on feelings rather than facts.
5 Accepting lack of contradictory evidence as proof of the hypothesis.
6 Drawing conclusions on the basis of partial truths.
7 Misuse of statistics.
8 Forming irrelevant conclusions.

It is important to remember that in many aspects of nutrition or dietetic research absolute proof is not possible. Conclusions and recommendations have to be made on the basis of probabilities.

Reappraisal

At the end of the study it is important to assess how successful the study has been in order to pinpoint any weaknesses which could be avoided in future investigations. Table 5.36 suggests some of the ways in which this can be done.

Writing-up research

Publication of research findings is essential if dietitians are to improve the service offered throughout the country. Negative findings are just as interesting and useful as positive findings and all should be shared. Information gleaned in one department may save time and money for many departments but unless it is published few will know about it.

Table 5.37 gives guidelines for writing up research work. Authors must, however, check with specific journals for details of presentation as these differ.

5.11.2 Specific types of research

Controlled clinical trials

This type of major research project will probably be undertaken less frequently than other forms of research. Controlled clinical trials are likely to be larger studies involving considerable amounts of time and manpower and the implications will be very important. They may be used, for example, to test the efficacy of treatments which are new or already in use. The methodology can be complicated and controlled trials need to be carried out meticulously if useful results are to be achieved. There are a number of books available describing this type of research in detail (Schwartz et al 1980; Friedman et al 1981; Bulpitt 1983).

Controlled trials are prospective and are usually undertaken if

1 There is genuine doubt about the usefulness of a diet or treatment for a specific condition.
2 There is a new treatment which may be more effective than the one already in use.
3 There is a need to find out more about how the health problem responds to the dietary change.

Table 5.38 Principles of a controlled clinical trial

1 Aim to give a definitive answer to one or two precise questions.
2 Select the participants according to specific criteria.
3 Ensure the sample size is sufficient to show positive results if there are any to be found.
4 Randomly allocate participants to the control and intervention groups.
5 Ensure the control group will remain 'uncontaminated' by the advice given to the intervention group.
6 Make all observations in a systematic way.
7 Where relevant the study should be conducted 'blind', i.e. neither the dietitian nor the participant should know who is in the control group and who is in the intervention group (but make sure that somebody knows!).
8 If the control group becomes 'contaminated' accept that they are not a true control and that the results of the trial may not be conclusive.

Clinical trials need very careful planning and well thought out protocols. The problem being treated and the diet or treatment to be advised need to be very clearly defined. There must also be a properly matched control group. The main principles of a controlled clinical trial are outlined in Table 5.38.

Other methods

Research methods in general practice have been described by Howie (1979). The role of evaluation in nutrition education has been described by Wolf (1980) and Rodwell-Williams (1978). A course 'Learning about methods of research' has been offered in the past by the Open University (Jupp 1981). This course covered social surveys and sampling questionnaires, ethnography (putting emphasis on the collection of data in natural situations) and methodology (initial formulation of ideas, research design, data collection, analyses, presentation and reporting results).

Further reading

Burr ML and Fehily AM (1983) Epidemiology for nutritionists. *Hum Nutr: Appl Nutr* **37A**, (4), 37A (5) 339−347, 37A (6) 419−425

References

Bennett AE and Ritchie K (1975) *Questionnaires in medicine — a guide to their design and use*. Oxford University Press, London.
Bulpitt CJ (1983) *Randomized controlled clinical trials*. Martirnus Nijholf Publishers, The Hague.
Calnan J (1976) *One way to do research — the A−Z for those who must*. Heinemann Medical Books, London.
Friedman LM, Furberg CD and De Mets DL (1981) *Fundamentals of clinical trials*. John Wright and Sons, Bristol.
Greer A (1980) *A first course in statistics*. Stanley Thornes (Publishers), Cheltenham.
Howie JGR (1979) *Research in general practice* Croom Helm, London.
Jupp V (1981) Learning about methods of research with the Open University. *Nursing Times* 2nd Sept 1559.
Perry FE (1979) *Statistics revision cards* 4e. Michael Benn and Associates, Wetherby.
Rodwell-Williams S (1978) *Essentials of nutrition and diet therapy* 2e Chapter 11 p 143. The CV Mosby Company, St Louis.
Schwartz D, Flamant R and Lellouch J (1980) *Clinical trials*. Academic Press, London.
Swinscow TDV (1978) *Statistics at square one*. British Medical Association, London.
Wolf R (1980) The role of evaluation in nutrition education In *World nutrition and nutrition education* Sinclair HM and Howat GR (Eds) Chapter 13 p 109. Oxford University Press, Oxford.

Section 6 **Appendices**

6.1 Useful Conversion Factors and Formulae

6.1.1 General

Length/height

Table 6.1

1 inch	=	2.54 cm
1 foot	=	30.48 cm
1 yard	=	91.44 cm
1 cm	=	0.394 inch
1 m	=	39.37 inches

Height conversion tables

Table 6.2

Inches to centimetres		Centimetres to inches	
Inches	cm	cm	Inches
1	2.54	1	0.39
2	5.08	2	0.79
3	7.62	3	1.18
4	10.16	4	1.57
5	12.70	5	1.97
6	15.25	6	2.36
7	17.78	7	2.76
8	20.32	8	3.15
9	22.86	9	3.54
10	25.40	10	3.94
20	50.80	20	7.87
30	76.20	30	11.81
40	101.60	40	15.75
50	127.00	50	19.69
60	152.40	60	23.62
70	177.80	70	27.56
80	203.20	80	31.50
90	228.60	90	35.43
100	254.0	100	39.37
200	508.0	200	78.74
300	762.0	300	118.11
400	1016.0	400	157.48
500	1270.0	500	196.85
600	1524.0	600	236.22
700	1778.0	700	275.59
800	2032.0	800	314.96
900	2286.0	900	354.33
1000	2540.0	1000	393.70

Mass/weight

Table 6.3

1 ounce	=	28.35 cm
1 pound	=	454 g or 0.45 kg
1 g	=	0.0352 ounces
1 kg	=	2.203 pounds

Weight conversion tables

Table 6.4

Grams to ounces		Ounces to grams	
g	oz	oz	g
1	0.04	1	28.35
2	0.07	2	56.70
3	0.11	3	85.05
4	0.14	4	113.40
5	0.18	5	141.75
6	0.21	6	170.10
7	0.25	7	198.45
8	0.28	8	226.80
9	0.32	9	255.15
10	0.35	10	283.50
15	0.50	11	311.85
20	0.71	12	340.20
30	1.06	13	368.55
40	1.41	14	396.90
50	1.76	15	425.25
60	2.12	16	453.60
70	2.47		
80	2.82		
90	3.17		
100	3.53		

Table 6.5

Kilograms to pounds			Pounds to kilograms	
kg	lb	oz	lb	kg
0.2	0	7	1	0.453
0.3	0	11	2	0.907
0.4	0	14	3	1.361
0.5	1	2	4	1.814
0.6	1	5	5	2.268
0.7	1	9	6	2.272
0.8	1	13	7	3.175
0.9	2	0	8	3.629
1	2	3	9	4.082
2	4	7	10	4.536
3	6	10	20	9.072
4	8	13	30	13.608
5	11	0	40	18.144
6	13	3	50	22.680
7	15	7	60	27.215
8	17	10	70	31.752
9	19	13	80	36.287
10	22	1	90	40.823
20	44	1	100	45.359
30	66	2	200	90.718
40	88	3	300	136.077
50	110	4	400	181.436
60	132	4	500	226.795
70	154	5		
80	176	6		
90	198	7		
100	220	7		
200	440	15		

Table 6.6

Stones to pounds	
Stones	lb
1	14
2	28
3	42
4	56
5	70
6	84
7	98
8	122
9	126
10	140
11	154
12	168
13	182
14	196
15	210
16	224
17	238
18	252
19	266
20	280

Obesity

Table 6.7

Body Mass Index (BMI)	=	$\dfrac{Weight\ (kg)}{Height\ (m)^2}$
<20	=	Long term hazard to health
20–24.9	=	Desirable range
25–29.9	=	Moderate obesity
>30	=	Severe obesity

Volume

Table 6.8

1 pint	=	568 ml or 0.568 l
1 litre	=	1.76 pints

6.1.2 Dietary conversion factors

Dietary energy

Table 6.9 SI conversion factors*

Unit		Conversion factor
1 kilocalorie (kcal)	=	4.184 kilojoules (kJ)
	=	0.004184 megajoules (MJ)
1000 kilocalories (kcal)	=	4184 kilojoules (kJ)
	=	4.184 megajoules (MJ)
1 kilojoule (kJ)	=	0.239 kilocalories (kcal)
1 megajoule (MJ)	=	1000 kilojoules (kJ)
	=	239 kilocalories (kcal)

*For interconverting the total energy content of diets of normal composition, a conversion factor of 1 kcal = 4.2 kJ can be used.

To convert

1 kilocalories to kilojoules: $kJ = kcal \times 4.184$

2 kilojoules to kilocalories: $kcal = \dfrac{kJ}{4.184}$

3 kilocalories to megajoules: $MJ = kcal \times 0.0041$ (or $kcal \div 239$)

4 megajoules to kilocalories: $kcal = MJ \times 239$

Table 6.10 Nutrient energy yields

Nutrient	Energy yield	
1 g protein provides	4 kcal	(17 kJ)
1 g fat provides	9 kcal	(37 kJ)
1 g carbohydrate provides	3.75 kcal	(16 kJ)
1 g alcohol provides	7 kcal	(29 kJ)
1 g medium chain triglyceride (MCT) provides	8.4 kcal	(35 kJ)

Protein/nitrogen

Dietary protein/dietary nitrogen

Dietary protein* (g) = Dietary nitrogen (g) × 6.25

Dietary nitrogen (g) = Dietary protein* (g) ÷ 6.25

Nitrogen excretion from 24-hour urinary urea

$$\text{Nitrogen excretion (g)} = \begin{array}{c}\text{g urinary urea}\\ \text{excreted in}\\ \text{24 hours}\end{array} \times \frac{28^{\dagger}}{60} \times \frac{6^{\S}}{5}$$

For practical purposes, this formula can be condensed to

$$\text{Nitrogen excretion (g)} = \frac{\text{mmol urinary urea excreted in 24 hours}}{30}$$

Protein excretion from 24-hour urinary urea

Protein lost in 24 hours (g) = mmol urinary urea lost in 24 hours × 0.212

Correction factor for nitrogen excreted according to changes in plasma urea levels

$$(\text{Urea 2} - \text{Urea 1}) \times W \times 0.6 \times 0.028$$

where Urea 1 = plasma urea (mmol/l) at start of

*This conversion factor is only appropriate for a mixture of foods. For milk or cereals alone, the factors 6.4 or 5.7 respectively should be used.

†The molecular weight of urea is 60, of which 28 parts are nitrogen.

§Approximately 80% of the total urinary nitrogen is urea.

period; Urea 2 = plasma urea (mmol/l) at end of period; 0.6 = factor to estimate body water and W = body weight in kg.

In anuric patient or renal failure

$$[\text{Urea } 2 - \text{Urea } 1) \times W \times 0.6 + \\ (W \text{ gain} \times \text{Urea } 2)] \times 0.028$$

Calculation of nitrogen balance

1 Nitrogen input (g)   = g protein taken in 24 hours $\div$ 6.25

2 Nitrogen output (g) = g nitrogen lost in urine
   + 2−4 g (obligatory nitrogen losses in skin and faeces)
   + correction for rise in blood urea (subtracted if urea falls)*
   + nitrogen lost as protein in body fluids[†]

3 Nitrogen balance   = nitrogen input − nitrogen output

Vitamin A

The active vitamin A content of a diet is usually expressed in retinol equivalents.

1 µg retinol equivalent = 1 µg retinol or 6 µg β carotene

$\therefore$ µg retinol equivalents = µ retinol + $\dfrac{\text{µg β carotene}}{6}$

Occasionally, the vitamin A content of foods is still expressed in international units (i.u.).

1 i.u. vitamin A = 0.3 µg retinol or 0.6 µg β carotene.

To convert i.u. to µg retinol equivalents

µg retinol equivalents = i.u. vitamin A × 0.3 in animal foods (retinol)
   or i.u. vitamin A × 0.1 in plant foods (β carotene).

Vitamin D

1 µg vitamin D = 40 i.u.

To convert i.u. to µg

µg vitamin D = $\dfrac{\text{i.u.}}{40}$

*If applicable, e.g. in renal failure. For calculation of correction factor see calculation on previous page.
[†]If applicable, e.g. exudate losses from burns or fistulae.

Nicotinic acid/tryptophan

Tryptophan can be converted to nicotinic acid.

60 mg tryptophan are required to produce 1 mg nicotinic acid.

1 mg nicotinic acid equivalent = 1mg available nicotinic acid or 60 mg tryptophan.

Nicotinic acid content of a diet in mg equivalents = nicotinic acid (mg) + $\dfrac{\left(\text{tryptophan (mg)}\right)}{60}$

6.1.3 Biochemical conversion factors

Millimoles, milligrams and milliequivalents

1 1 millimole (mmol) = atomic weight in mg

To convert mg to mmol

mmol = mg $\div$ atomic weight.

To convert mmol to mg

mg = mmol × atomic weight.

2 1 milliequivalent (mEq) = atomic weight in mg divided by the valency.
   To convert mg to mEq

mEq = $\dfrac{\text{mg} \times \text{valency}}{\text{atomic weight}}$

To convert mEq to mg

mg = $\dfrac{\text{mEq} \times \text{atomic weight}}{\text{valency}}$.

For minerals with a valency of 1, mEq = mmol; for minerals with a valency of 2, mEq = mmol × 2. Table 6.11 lists the atomic weights and valencies of some minerals and trace elements.

Table 6.11 Atomic weights and valencies of some minerals and trace elements

Mineral	Atomic weight	Valency
Sodium	23.0	1
Potassium	39.0	1
Phosphorus	31.0	2
Calcium	40.0	2
Magnesium	24.3	2
Chlorine	35.4	1
Sulphur	32.0	2
Zinc	65.4	2

Table 6.12 Conversion tables

Mineral	mg/mmol		mg/mEq		mmol/mEq	
	mg =	mmol =	mg =	mEq =	mmol =	mEq =
Sodium	mmol × 23	mg ÷ 23	mEq × 23	mg ÷ 23	mEq	mmol
Potassium	mmol × 39	mg ÷ 39	mEq × 39	mg ÷ 39	mEq	mmol
Phosphorus	mmol × 31	mg ÷ 31	mEq × 15.5	mg ÷ 15.5	mEq ÷ 2	mmol × 2
Calcium	mmol × 40	mg ÷ 40	mEq × 20	mg ÷ 20	mEq ÷ 2	mmol × 2
Magnesium	mmol × 24.3	mg ÷ 24.3	mEq × 12.15	mg ÷ 12.15	mEq ÷ 2	mmol × 2
Chlorine	mmol × 35.4	mg ÷ 35.4	mEq × 35.4	mg ÷ 35.4	mEq	mmol
Sulphur	mmol × 32	mg ÷ 32	mEq × 16	mg ÷ 16	mEq ÷ 2	mmol × 2
Zinc	mmol × 65.4	mg ÷ 65.4	mEq × 32.7	mg ÷ 32.7	mEq ÷ 2	mmol × 2

Table 6.13 Mineral content of compounds and solutions

Solution/compound	Mineral content	
1 g sodium chloride	393 mg Na	(17.1 mmol Na^+)
1 g sodium bicarbonate	273 mg Na	(12 mmol Na^+)
1 g potassium bicarbonate	524 mg K	(13.4 mmol K^+)
1 g calcium chloride (hydrated)	273 mg Ca	(6.8 mmol Ca^{2+})
1 g calcium carbonate	400 mg Ca	(10 mmol Ca^{2+})
1 g calcium gluconate	93 mg Ca	(2.3 mmol Ca^{2+})
1 litre normal saline	3450 mg Na	(150 mmol Na^+)

SI units

The International System of Unit (Systeme International SI) was accepted in 1960 as a logical and coherent system for measurements. This system has been adopted by most laboratories in the UK. Table 6.14 contains the factor necessary to convert some clinical biochemistry constituents from SI units to traditional units and vice versa (Baron *et al* 1974).

Table 6.14 Conversion factors for SI units

Biochemical constituent	SI to traditional	Traditional to SI
Albumin	g/l × 0.1 = g/dl	g/dl × 10 = g/l
Bicarbonate	mmol/l = mEq/l	mEq/l = mmol/l
Bilirubin	μmol/l × 0.058 = mg/dl	mg/dl × 17 = μmol/l
pH	kPa × 7.5 = mm Hg	mm Hg × 0.133 = kPa
pCO_2	kPa × 7.5 = mm Hg	mm Hg × 0.133 = kPa
pO_2	kPa × 7.5 = mm Hg	mm Hg × 0.133 = kPa
Calcium	mmol/l × 4 = mg/dl	mg/dl × 0.25 = mmol/l
Chloride	mmol/l = mEq/l	mEq/l = mmol/l
Cholesterol	mmol/l × 39 = mg/dl	mg/dl × 0.0259 = mmol/l
Cortisol	mmol/l × 0.036 = μg/dl	μg/dl × 27.6 = mmol/l
Creatinine	μmol/l × 0.11 = mg/dl	mg/dl × 88.4 = μmol/l
Glucose	mmol/l × 18 = mg/dl	mg/dl × 0.055 = mmol/l
Iron	μmol/l × 5.6 = μg/dl	μg/dl × 0.179 = μmol/l
TIBC	μmol/l × 5.6 = μg/dl	μg/dl × 0.179 = μmol/l
Magnesium	mmol/l × 2.43 = mg/dl	mg/dl × 0.411 = mmol/l
Osmolality	mmol/kg = mosmol/kg	mosmol/kg = mmol/kg
Protein	g/l × 0.1 = g/dl	g/dl × 10 = g/l
Urate	mmol/l × 17 = mg/dl	mg/dl × 0.0595 = mmol/l
Urea	mmol/l × 6 = mg/dl	mg/dl × 0.166 = mmol/l
Potassium	mmol/l = mEq/l	mEq/l = mmol/l
Sodium	mmol/l = mEq/l	mEq/l = mmol/l
Triglyceride	mmol/l × 88.5 = mg/dl	mg/dl × 0.0113 = mmol/l
Calcium (urine)	mmol/24 h × 40 = mg/24 h	mg/24 h × 0.025 = mmol/24 h
Creatinine (urine)	mmol/24 h × 113 = mg/24 h	mg/24 h × 0.0088 = mmol/24 h
Phosphate (urine)	mmol/24 h × 31 = mg/24 h	mg/24 h × 0.032 = mmol/24 h
Urate (urine)	mmol/24 h × 168 = mg/24 h	mg/24 h × 0.0059 = mmol/24 h
Urea (urine)	mmol/24 h × 0.06 = g/24 h	g/24 h × 16.66 = mmol/24 h
Faecal fat	mmol/l × 0.3 = g/24 h	g/24 h × 3.33 = mmol/l

Correction of serum calcium for low albumin

$$\text{Corrected serum calcium level (mmol/)} = \text{Measured serum calcium (mmol/l)} + \left(\frac{40 - \text{measured albumin}}{40} \right)$$

An alternative (and possibly more accurate) formula is

$$\text{Corrected serum calcium level (mmol/l)} = \text{Measured serum calcium (mmol/l)} + \left[\left(40 - \text{measured albumin} \right) \times 0.02 \right]$$

To be even more accurate, the serum protein level should be considered as well

$$\text{Corrected serum calcium level (mmol/l)} = \text{Measured serum calcium (mmol/l)} + \left[\left(72 - \text{measured protein} \right) \times 0.02 \right]$$

This corrected calcium value should be added to that obtained from the correction for low albumin, and a mean of the 2 levels obtained, calculated to 2 decimal places.

Osmolality and osmolarity

Osmolality is the number of osmotically active particles (milliosmoles) in a *kilogram* of *solvent*. Osmolarity is the number of osmotically active particles in a *litre* of *solution* (i.e. solvent + solute).

In body fluids, there is only a small difference between the two. However, in commercially prepared feeds, osmolality is always much higher than osmolarity. Osmolality is therefore the preferred term for comparing the potential hypertonic effect of liquid diets (although in practice, it is often osmolarity which is stated).

The osmolality of a liquid feed is considerably influenced by the content of amino acids and electrolytes such as sodium and potassium. Carbohydrates with a small particle size (e.g. simple sugars) increase osmolality more than complex carbohydrates with a higher molecular weight. Fats do not increase the osmolality of solutions because of their insolubility in water.

The osmolality of blood plasma is normally in the range of 280–300 mosmol/kg and the body attempts to keep the osmolality of the contents of the stomach and intestine at an isotonic level. It does this by producing intestinal secretions which dilute a concentrated meal or drink. If enteral feeds with a high osmolality are administered, large quantities of intestinal secretions will be produced rapidly in order to reduce the osmolality. In order to avoid diarrhoea, it is therefore important to administer such feeds slowly; the number of mosmoles given per unit of time is more important than the number of mosmoles per unit of volume.

Reference

Baron DN, Broughton PMG, Cohen M, Lansley TS, Lewis SM and Shinton NK (1974) The use of SI units in reporting results obtained in hospital laboratories. *J Clin Path* **27**, 590–7.

6.2 Biochemical and Haematological Reference Ranges

The results of laboratory tests are interpreted by comparison to reference or normal ranges. These are usually defined as the mean ± 2 SD (standard deviation) this assumes a Gaussian or Normal (symmetrical) type distribution (Fig. 6.1). Unfortunately most biological data have a skewed rather than a symmetrical distribution and more complex statistical calculations are required to define the reference ranges.

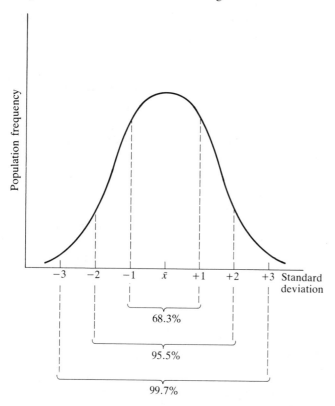

Fig. 6.1 Normal or Gaussian distribution curve.

The reference ranges as defined usually include approximately 95% of the normal 'healthy' population, consequently 5% of this population will have values outside the reference range but cannot be said to be abnormal. The use of reference ranges may be illustrated by taking the reference range for blood urea as 3.3 − 6.7 mmol/l. Approximately 95% of the normal 'healthy' population would come within these limits. However, it would be wrong to interpret a value of 6.4 mmol/l as normal while assuming a value of 7.0 mmol/l to be

abnormal. Nature 'abhors abrupt transitions', consequently there is no clear-cut division between 'normal' and 'abnormal', this applies equally well to body weight and height and also to measurements undertaken in the laboratory.

The majority of the normal 'healthy' population will have results close to the mean value for the population as a whole and all values will be distributed around that mean. Consequently the probability that a value is abnormal increases the further it is from the mean value (Fig. 6.2).

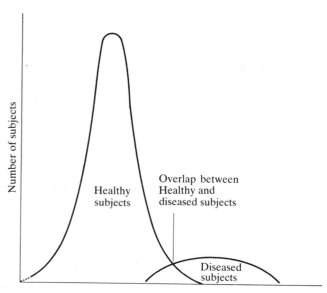

Fig. 6.2 Theoretical distribution of results from healthy and diseased subjects.

A variety of factors can cause variation in the biochemical and haematological constituents present within the blood. These can be conveniently divided into factors which cause variation within an individual and those causing variation between groups of individuals.

6.2.1 Variations within individuals

The following factors can cause significant variation in clinical biochemical and haematological data and should be considered when interpreting individual results.

Diet

Variation in diet can affect the levels of triglycerides, cholesterol, glucose, urea and other blood constituents.

Drugs

These can have significant effects on a number of biochemical determinations, often resulting from secondary effects on sensitive organs, e.g. liver, kidney and endocrine glands. Steroids, including oral contraceptives, can cause variations in a number of biochemical and haematological parameters including a reduction in albumin, increases in several carrier proteins, e.g. transcortin, thyroxine binding globulin, caeruloplasmin and transferrin, as well as increases in coagulation factors, e.g. fibrinogen, Factor VII and Factor X.

Menstrual cycle

Several biochemical constituents show marked variations with the phase of the cycle; these include the pituitary gonadotrophins, ovarian steroids and their metabolites. There is also a marked fall in plasma iron just prior to and during menstruation. This is probably produced by hormonal changes rather than blood loss.

Muscular exercise

Moderate exercise can cause increases in levels of potassium, together with a number of enzymes including aspartate transferase, lactate dehydrogenase, creatine kinase and hydroxybutyrate dehydrogenase.

Posture

Significant differences in the concentration of many blood constituents may be obtained by collecting blood samples from ambulant as compared to recumbent individuals. The red cell and white cell counts together with the concentration of proteins (albumin, immunoglobulins, etc.) and protein bound substances (e.g. calcium, cholesterol, T4, cortisol, etc.) may decrease by up to 15% following 30 min recumbency. This is probably due to fluid redistribution within the body. Hospitalized patients usually have their blood samples collected early in the morning following overnight recumbency and consequently have significantly lower values than the normal ambulant (out-patient) population.

Stress

Both emotional and physical stress can alter circulating biochemical constituents causing increases in the levels of pituitary hormones (ACTH, prolactin, growth hormone, etc.) and adrenal steroids (cortisol).

Time of day

Some substances exhibit a marked circadian (diurnal) variation which is independent of meals or other activities, e.g. serum cortisol, iron and the amino acids tyrosine, phenylalanine and tryptophan. Cortisol levels are at their highest in the morning (9 am) and at their lowest levels at midnight while iron concentration may decrease by 50% between the morning and evening. Plasma phenylalanine levels are at their lowest after midnight and reach their highest concentrations between 8.30−10.30 am.

6.2.2 Variation between groups of individuals

A number of factors influence the reference values quoted for individuals. These include age, sex and race.

Age

The blood levels of many biochemical and haematological constituents are age related, these include haemoglobin, total leucocyte count, creatinine, urea, inorganic phosphate and many enzymes, e.g. alkaline phosphatase, creatine kinase and γ-glutamyl transferase. Haemoglobin levels and total leucocyte counts are highest in the newborn and gradually decrease through childhood reaching the adult reference range at puberty. As creatinine is related to muscle mass, paediatric reference ranges are lower than those of adults. Urea levels rise slightly with age but this may well indicate impaired renal function. Alkaline phosphatase activity and inorganic phosphate levels are at their highest during childhood, reaching peak levels at puberty.

Sex

Many biochemical and haematological parameters show concentration differences which are sex dependant including creatinine, iron, urate, urea and of course the various sex hormones. Ferritin, haemoglobin and red cell counts are slightly higher in males than in females. Creatinine and urea levels are 15 – 20% lower in premenopausal females than in males. Premenopausal females also have lower serum iron levels than males, but after the menopause iron levels are similar in both sexes.

Race

Racial differences have been reported in some biochemical constituents, including cholesterol and protein. The reference ranges for cholesterol are higher in Europeans than in similar groups of Japanese. Similarly the Bantu Africans have higher serum globulins than corresponding Europeans. African and Middle-Eastern individuals have lower total leucocyte and neutrophil counts than other races. Some of these racial differences are probably genetic in origin, although the environment and diet may also be contributory.

6.2.3 Laboratory variations

Methods of analysis and standardizations vary considerably from laboratory to laboratory. These differences will influence the quoted reference ranges, and consequently readers are advised to use only those quoted by their local laboratory. Local reference ranges may be at variance with the levels quoted in the following sections.

6.2.4 Clinical biochemistry reference ranges

Table 6.15 Serum/plasma levels — general biochemistry

Blood constituent	Sex	Range	Units
Albumin		35–45	g/l
Bicarbonate		22–32	mmol/l
Bilirubin		<17	μmol/l
Calcium		2.25–2.65	mmol/l
Chloride		95–105	mmol/l
Cholesterol (desirable)		2.5–5.5	mmol/l
Creatinine		40–130	μmol/l
Glucose (fasting)		3.0–5.0	mmol/l
Inorganic phosphate		0.8–1.4	mmol/l
Magnesium		0.7–1.0	mmol/l
Osmolality		278–305	mosmol/kg
Potassium		3.5–5.0	mmol/l
Sodium		135–150	mmol/l
Total protein		60–80	g/l
Triglycerides		0.5–2.2	mmol/l
Urate	Male	0.25–0.45	mmol/l
	Female	0.15–0.35	mmol/l
Urea		3.3–6.7	mmol/l

Table 6.16 Serum/plasma lipid fractions

Lipid fraction	Sex	Range	Units
HDL cholesterol	Male	0.61–1.57	mmol/l
	Female	0.89–2.05	mmol/l
LDL cholesterol	Male	1.46–5.54	mmol/l
	Female	1.7–5.62	mmol/l
VLDL triglycerides	Male	0.3–2.32	mmol/l
	Female	0.1–0.76	mmol/l

Table 6.17 Serum/plasma enzyme levels

Enzyme	Sex	Range	Units
Acid phosphatase		<8	i.u./l
Alanine transaminase		<35	i.u./l
Alkaline phosphatase		90–300	i.u./l
Amylase		<300	i.u./l
Aspartate transaminase		10–40	i.u./l
Creatinine kinase	Male	<220	i.u./l
	Female	<150	i.u./l
Gamma glutamyl transferase	Male	<43	i.u./l
	Female	<28	i.u./l
Hydroxybutyrate dehydrogenase		<150	i.u./l

Table 6.18 Serum protein levels

Protein	Range	Units
α1–antitrypsin	1.8–3.0	g/l
Albumin	35–45	g/l
B2–microglobulin	1.1–2.4	mg/l
C Reactive protein	<10	mg/l
C3 complement	0.7–1.3	g/l
C4 complement	0.12–0.27	g/l
Caeruloplasmin	0.3–0.6	g/l
Fibrinogen (plasma)	2.0–4.0	g/l
Globulin	19–33	g/l
Haemoglobin A1c	5–8	%
Haptoglobin	0.3–2.0	g/l
Immunoglobulins IgA	0.9–3.4	g/l
Immunoglobulins IgG	5.4–16.1	g/l
Immunoglobulins IgM	0.5–2.0	g/l
Orosomucoid	0.5–1.0	g/l
Prealbumin	200–400	mg/l
Retinol binding protein (RBP)	30–65	mg/l
Thyroxine binding prealbumin (TBPA)	200–400	mg/l
Total protein	60–80	g/l
Transferrin	2.2–3.8	g/l

Table 6.19 Serum/plasma hormone levels

Hormone	Sex	Time	Range	Units
ACTH			<10-80	ng/l
Cortisol		am	280-700	nmol/l
		pm	140-280	nmol/l
Cortisol (urinary free)			<280	nmol/24 h
Follicle Stimulating Hormone (FSH)			2-8	U/l
Gastrin			<40	pmol/l
Growth Hormone			<20	mU/l
Insulin (fasting)			<15	mU/l
LH			2-8	U/l
17 β Oestradiol	Male		<150	pmol/l
	Female			
	follicular		80-250	pmol/l
	mid cycle		1000-1800	pmol/l
	luteal		400-900	pmol/l
	post-menopausal		<85	pmol/l
Parathormone			<0.73	μg/l
Progesterone	Male		<5	nmol/l
	Female		15-77	nmol/l
Prolactin	Male		<450	U/l
	Female		<600	U/l
TBG			7-17	mg/l
Testosterone	Male		10-30	nmol/l
	Female		0.8-2.8	nmol/l
Thyroxine (T4)			70-140	nmol/l
Tri-iodothyronine (T3)			1.2-3.0	nmol/l
Free Thyroxine			9-22	pmol/l
TSH			<6	mU/l

Table 6.20 Whole blood gases

Gas	Range	Units
pH	7.35-7.45	
Arterial carbon dioxide	4.7-6.0	kPa
Arterial oxygen	>10.6	kPa

Table 6.21 Serum/plasma vitamin levels

Vitamin	Range	Units
Ascorbate	34-68	μmol/l
β carotene	0.9-5.6	μmol/l
Folate	3.0-15.0	μg/l
Red cell folate	160-640	μg/l
Pyridoxine (B6)	>178	nmol/l
Riboflavin (B2)	Free <21.3	nmol/l
Riboflavin (B2)	Total <85.0	nmol/l
Thiamin (B1)	>40	nmol/l
Vitamin A	0.7-1.7	μmol/l
Vitamin B12	160-925	ng/l
Vitamin D	24-111	nmol/l

Table 6.22 Serum/plasma trace element and metal levels

Element	Sex	Range	Units
Cadmium (whole blood)		27-480	n mol/ι
Calcium		2.25-2.65	mmol/l
Chloride		95-105	mmol/l
Chromium		94-183	nmol/l
Cobalt		8.8-7.3	nmol/l
Copper		10-20	μmol/l
Gold		20-203	pmol/l
Iron	Male	14-31	μmol/l
	Female	11-30	μmol/l
Lead (whole blood)	Adult	<1.8	μmol/l
Magnesium		0.7-1.0	mmol/l
Manganese (whole blood)		100-200	nmol/l
Potassium		3.5-5.0	mmol/l
Sodium		135-150	mmol/l
Zinc		10-18	μmol/l

Table 6.23 Urine

Constituent	Range	Units
Calcium	<7.5	mmol/24 h
Creatinine	9–18	mmol/24 h
Inorganic phosphate	15–50	mmol/24 h
Osmolality	50–1500	mosmol/24 h
Potassium	40–120	mmol/24 h
Protein	<0.50	g/24 h
Sodium	100–250	mmol/24 h
Urate	<3.0	mmol/24 h
Urea	250–600	mmol/24 h

Table 6.24 Cerebrospinal fluid (CSF)

Constituent	Range	Units
Glucose	2.5–5.0	mmol/l
Protein	0.15–0.45	g/l

Table 6.25 Faeces

Constituent	Range	Units
Faecal fat	<18	mmol/24 h
Nitrogen	70–140	mmol/24 h

6.2.5 Haematological reference ranges

Table 6.26 Red cells

Parameter	Age/Sex	Range	Units
Haemoglobin	Male	13.5–17.5	g/dl
	Female	11.5–15.5	g/dl
	Newborn	15–21	g/dl
	3 Months	9.5–12.5	g/dl
Haematocrit (PCV)	Male	40–52	%
	Female	36–48	%
Red Cell Count	Male	4.5–6.3	10^{12}/l
	Female	4.2–5.4	10^{12}/l
Mean Cell Haemoglobin (MCH)		27–32	pg
Mean Cell Volume (MCV)		80–95	fl
Mean Cell Haemoglobin Concentration (MCHC)		32–36	g/dl

Table 6.27 White cells

Cells	Range	Units
White Blood Count (WBC)	4.0–11.0	10^9/l
Neutrophils	2.5–7.5	10^9/l
Eosinophils	0.04–0.4	10^9/l
Monocytes	0.2–0.8	10^9/l
Basophils	0.01–0.1	10^9/l
Lymphocytes	1.5–3.5	10^9/l
Platelets	150–350	10^9/l

Table 6.28 General

Parameter	Age/sex	Range	Units
Erythrocyte Sedimentation Rate (ESR)	Male	3–5	mm/h
	Female	4–7	mm/h
Ferritin	Male	40–340	µg/l
	Female	14–148	µg/l
	Children	7–142	µg/l
Serum B12		160–925	ngram/l
Serum folate		3.0–15.0	µg/l
Red cell folate		160–640	µg/l
Prothrombin time (PT)		10–14	seconds
Activated partial thromboplastin time (APTT)		30–40	seconds
Thrombin time (TT)		10–12	seconds

Sources

Giles AM and Ross BD (1983) Normal or reference values for biochemical data. In *Oxford textbook of medicine* Weatherall DJ, Ledingham JGC and Worrell DA (Eds) pp 27.3–27.8. Oxford University Press, Oxford.

Hoffbrand AV and Pettit JE (1980) *Essential haematology.* Blackwell Scientific Publications, Oxford.

Tietz NW (1976) *Fundamentals of clinical chemistry.* WB Saunders Co, Philadelphia.

Walmsey RN and White GH (1983) *A guide to diagnostic clinical chemistry.* Blackwell Scientific Publications, Oxford.

Whitby LG, Percy-Robb IW and Smith AF (1984) *Lecture notes on clinical chemistry.* Blackwell Scientific Publications, Oxford.

Wilding P and Bailey A (1978) The normal range. In *Scientific foundation of clinical biochemistry Vol 1. Analytical aspects.* Heinnemann Medical Books, London.

Williams DL, Nunn RF and Marks V (Eds).

Zilva JF and Pannall PR (1984) *Clinical chemistry in diagnosis and treatment.* Lloyd-Luke (Medical books) Ltd, London.

6.3 Abbreviations Used in Dietetic Practice

1, 25 (OH)$_2$D	1, 25 dihydroxy vitamin D
25(OH)D	25 hydroxy vitamin D
6-MP	6-mercaptopurine
AA	Amino acid
AAP	American Academy of Paediatrics
ACBS	Advisory Committee for Borderline Substances
ACTH	Arenocorticotrophic hormone
ADI	Acceptable Daily Intake
ADL	Activities of Daily Living
Al	Aluminium
Al (OH)$_3$	Aluminium hydroxide
AMA	American Medical Association
AN	Anorexia nervosa
ANF	Anti-nuclear factor
APTT	Activate Partial Thromboplastin time
ARF	Acute renal failure
ARMS	Action for Research into Multiple Sclerosis
ATN	Acute tubular neurosis
ATP	Adenosine triphosphate
AV	Arterio-venous
av	Audio-visual
BCAA	Branched chain amino acids
bd	Twice a day
BDA	British Dietetic Association
BEE	Basal energy expenditure (This is the same as the basal metabolic rate)
BHA	Butylated hydroxyanisole
BHT	Butylated hydroxytoluene
BIBRA	British Industrial Biological Research Association
BMA	British Medical Association
BMI	Body Mass Index (Weight (kg)/ Height (m)^2)
BMR	Basal metabolic rate
BNF	British Nutrition Foundation
BP	Blood pressure
BP	British Pharmacopoeia
C	Carbon
Ca	Calcium
Can	Canada
Ca:P	Calcium: phosphorus ratio

Cap	Capsule
CAPD	Continuous ambulatory peritoneal dialysis
CCPD	Continuous cyclic peritoneal dialysis
Cd	Cadmium
CF	Cystic fibrosis
CSF	Cerebrospinal fluid
CHI	Creatinine: Height index
CHO	Carbohydrate
Cl	Chlorine/chloride
cm	Centimetres
CNG	Community Nutrition Group
Co	Cobalt
CO$_2$	Carbon dioxide
COMA	Committee on Medical Aspects of Food Policy
COT	Committee on Toxicity of Chemicals in Food
CPAG	Child Poverty Action Group
CPSM	Council for the Professions Supplementary to Medicine
Cr	Chromium
CRF	Chronic renal failure
Cu	Copper
cv	Coefficient of variation
CVP	Central venous pressure
CyA	Cyclosporin A
D$_2$	Ergocalciferol
D$_3$	Cholecalciferol
DHSS	Department of Health and Social Security
dl	Decilitre (100 ml)
DNA	Deoxyribonucleic acid
dsp	Level dessertspoonful
E	European Economic Community Food additive number
E:T ratio	Ratio of essential amino acids (g) to total nitrogen (g)
eaa	Essential amino acids
edta	Ethylene diamine tetra-acetic acid
EDTA	European Dialysis and Transplant Association
EEC	European Economic Community

EEC SCF	European Economic Community Scientific Committee on Foods		IBS	Irritable bowel syndrome
EEG	Electroencephalogram		IBW	Ideal body weight
efa	Essential fatty acids		IDD	Insulin dependent diabetic
ENMH	Enrolled Nurse Mental Handicap		IDL	Intermediate density lipoproteins
EPO	Evening primrose oil		IgA	Immunoglobulin A
ERCP	Endoscopic retrograde cholangiopancreatography		IgG	Immunoglobulin G
			IgM	Immunoglobulin M
ESADI	Estimated safe and adequate daily intake		ILEA	Inner London Education Authority
			im	Intramuscular
ESN	Educationally sub-normal		IMHP	Intramuscular high potency
ESRF	End stage renal failure		IMM	Intramuscular maintenance
			IPD	Intermittent peritoneal dialysis
F	Fluorine		IQ	Intelligence quotient
FAC	Food Advisory Committee		ITU	Intensive therapy unit
FACC	Food Additives and Contaminants Committee		iu	International units
			iv	Intravenous
FAO	Food and Agriculture Organisation		IVHP	Intravenous high potency
Fe	Iron		JECFA	Joint Expert Committee on Food Additives
Fin	Finland			
fl oz	Fluid ounce		JVP	Jugular venous pressure
FP 10	Form used for the prescription of medicines in the UK		K	Potassium
			KI	Potassium iodide
FRG	West Germany		kJ	Kilojoules
FSH	Follicle stimulating hormone		kcal	Kilocalories
g	Grams		kg	Kilograms
GBM	Glomerular basement membrane		l	Litre
GF	Gluten-free		L-CAT	Lecithin-Cholesterol Acyl Transferase
GFR	Glomerular filtration rate		LACOTS	Local Authorities Co-ordinating Body on Trading Standards
GI	Gastrointestinal			
GLC	Greater London Council		lb	Pound
GN	Glomerulonephritis		LBV	Low biological value
GNU	Gerontology Nutrition Unit		LBW	Low birth weight
GP	General Practitioner		LCFA	Long chain fatty acids
GTF	Glucose tolerance factor		LCMG	Long chain monoglycerides
			LCT	Long chain triglycerides
HA	Healthy Authority		LDL	Low density lipoproteins
HbA$_1$	Haemoglobin Al		LFC	London Food Commission
HBV	High biological value		LH	Luteinizing hormone
HCO$_3$	Bicarbonate			
HCl	Hydrochloride or hydrochloric acid		m	Metres
HD	Haemodialysis		MAFF	Ministry of Agriculture, Fisheries and Food
HDL	High density lipoproteins			
HEA	Health Education Authority		MAMC	Mid arm muscle circumference
HF	Haemofiltration		MAOI	Monoamine oxidase inhibitors
Hg	Mercury		MCH	Mean cell haemoglobin
hGH	Human growth hormone		MCHC	Mean cell haemoglobin concentration
HLA	Human lymphocyte antigen		MCT	Medium chain triglycerides
HMSO	Her Majesty's Stationery Office		MCV	Mean cell volume
HSV	Highly selective vagotomy		mEq	Milliequivalents
I	Iodine		mg	Milligrams
IBD	Inflammatory bowel disease		Mg	Magnesium

Mg(OH)$_2$	Magnesium hydroxide	PDUO	Previous days urine output
MCHC	Mean cell haemoglobin concentration	PG	Prostaglandin
MIMS	Monthly Index of Medical Specialities	PGV	Proximal gastric vagotomy
MJ	Megajoules	Phe	Phenylalanine
ml	Millilitres	PKU	Phenylketonuria
mm	Millimetres	PN	Parenteral nutrition
mmol	Millimoles	PO$_4$	Phosphate
Mn	Manganese	PPF	Plasma protein fraction
Mo	Molybdenum	ppm	Parts per million
mosmol	Milliosmoles	pt (s)	Pint(s)
MRC	Medical Research Council	PT	Prothrombin time
MS	Multiple Sclerosis	PTH	Parathormone
MSG	Monosodium glutamate	PUFA	Polyunsaturated fatty acids
MSUD	Maple Syrup Urine Disease	PWS	Prader Willi Syndrome
MUAC	Mid upper arm circumference		
		RAST	Radioallergosorbent test
N	Nitrogen	RCP	Royal College of Physicians
Na	Sodium	RDA	Recommended Dietary Allowance (or Recommended Daily Amount)
NACNE	National Advisory Committee on Nutrition Education	RDI	Recommended Daily Intake (usually assumed to be the same as the Recommended Dietary Allowance)
NADPH	Reduced nicotinamide adenine dinucleotide phosphate		
NAMCW	National Association for Maternal and Child Welfare	RME	Resting metabolic expenditure
NAS	No added salt	RMR	Resting metabolic rate
NCHS	National Centre for Health Statistics	RNA	Ribonucleic acid
NCT	National Childbirth Trust	RNIB	Royal National Institute for the Blind
NFS	National Food Survey	RNMH	Registered Nurse Mental Handicap
NHANES	National Health and Nutrition Examination Survey	RQ	Respiratory quotient
		RTA	Renal tubular acidosis
NHS	National Health Service		
Ni	Nickel	sd	Standard deviation
NIDD	Non-insulin dependent diabetic	se	Standard error
NMCU	National Metrological Co-ordinating Unit	Se	Selenium
		SFGA	Small-for-gestational age
NPE:N	Non-protein energy: nitrogen ratio	SGOT	Serum glutamic-oxaloacetic transaminase activity
NRC	National Research Council		
NS	Nephrotic syndrome	SGPT	Serum glutamic-pyruvic transaminase activity
NSP	Non-starch polysaccharides		
NTD	Neural tube defect	SI	Systeme internationale
		SI	Statutory instrument
OTC	Over-the-counter	SLE	Systemic Lupus Erythematosis
Osmol	Osmoles	SRD	State Registered Dietitian
oz	Ounce	SRN	State Registered Nurse
		Swe	Sweden
P	Phosphorus		
P/S ratio	Ratio of polyunsaturated fatty acids to saturated fatty acids	T$_3$	Tri-iodothyronine
		T$_4$	Thyroxine
PABA	Para-amino benzoic acid	Tab	Tablet
Pb	Lead	TB	Tuberculosis
PCK	Polycystic disease of the kidney	TBPA	Thyroxine binding prealbumin
PCV	Packed cell volume	tbs	Level tablespoonful
PD	Peritoneal dialysis	TF	Transferrin
		TIBC	Total iron binding capacity

TLC	Total lymphocyte count	V	Vanadium
TPN	Total parenteral nutrition	VLCD	Very low calorie diet
TRP	Tubular reabsorption of filtered phosphate	VLDL	Very low density lipoproteins
		VMA	Vanillylmandelic acid
TSH	Thyroid stimulating hormone		
TSNS	Ten State Nutrition Survey	W/H^2	Weight (in kilograms) divided by Height (in metres) squared — the Quetelet Index or Body Mass Index
tsp	Level teaspoonful		
TST	Triceps skinfold thickness		
TT	Thrombin time	WBC	White blood cells
		WHO	World Health Organisation
UHT	Ultra-heat treatment	WRVS	Women's Royal Volunteer Service
UK	United Kingdom	wt	Weight
UN	United Nations		
USA	United States of America	Zn	Zinc
UTI	Urinary tract infections	µg	Micrograms
UV	Ultraviolet	µmol	Micromoles

6.4 Lists of Manufactured Food Products Free from Specified Ingredients

For the reasons given below, these lists are only available from a State Registered Dietitian as part of the dietary advice given to patients requiring a medically prescribed diet.

In 1965 the dietitian at the Hospital for Sick Children, Great Ormond Street, London, compiled a list of gluten-free foods to help coeliac patients. Over the years other dietitians collected information for their own patients on other types of products, e.g. lactose-free. In 1976 this was systematized when specific dietetic departments undertook responsibility for compiling specific food lists, e.g. lactose-free, wheat-free, etc., these were then made available to all from the British Dietetic Association (BDA). In 1984 the BDA took this a stage further when it centralized the collection of information and put it on computer.

However, in April 1984, a Joint Royal College of Physicians/British Nutrition Foundation (RCP-BNF) Report on Food Intolerance and Food Aversion recommended that food manufacturers consider the possibility of setting up a central databank where products free of ingredients known to be responsible for intolerance could be registered. As a result of this recommendation the Scientific and Technical Committee of the Food and Drink Federation set up a working party to examine the feasibility of setting up such a databank. The working party included representatives from the Food and Drink Federation, Leatherhead Food Research Association, the Food Research Institute, Norwich, the British Nutrition Foundation, the Royal College of Physicians and the British Dietetic Association.

Table 6.29 Definitions of 'free from' adopted by the Food Intolerance Working Party of the FDF in 1986

Food/food additive	Derivatives/additives covered	Notes
Milk and milk derivatives	Butter, caseinates, cheese, cream, lactose, margarine or shortening containing whey, whey, whey syrup sweetener, yoghurt	'Free from' is to be interpreted as contains no added milk or milk derivative
Egg and egg derivatives	Dried egg, egg albumen, egg lecithin, egg yolk, fresh egg	'Free from' is to be interpreted as contains no added egg or egg derivative
Wheat and wheat derivatives	Breadcrumbs, hydrolysed wheat protein, rusk, wheat bran, wheat binder, wheatflour, wheat germ, wheat germ oil, wheat gluten, raising agent containing wheat starch, wheat starch, wheat thickener, wholewheat	'Free from' is to be interpreted as contains no wheat or wheat derivative. NB the wheat-free list will be for actual wheat intolerance and not for gluten intolerance; gluten-free lists are already available from The Coeliac Society
Soya and soya derivatives	Flavouring (soya), hydrolysed vegetable protein (soya), lecithin (soya) (E322), soya protein products	'Free from' is to be interpreted as contains no added soya or soya derivative. NB a product declared as 'free from soya and soya derivatives' may contain soya oil and/or shortening. Such products will be separately identified in a manner similar to that undertaken in the current BDA list of soya-free manufactured foods, from products declared as free from soya and soya derivatives **and** free from soya oil and soya shortening
Cocoa	Cocoa powder, cocoa butter	
BHA and BHT		These are the permitted antioxidants butylated hydroxyanisole (E320 and butylated hydroxytoluene (E321) 'Free from' is to be interpreted as contains less than 1 mg/kg BHA and/or BHT calculated from the level of addition to the food but having due regard to the presence of these compounds in ingredients and thereby carried over into the food

Table 6.29 *contd.*

Food/food additive	Derivatives/additives covered	Notes
Sulphur dioxide	Sulphur dioxide (220), sodium sulphite (E221), sodium hydrogen sulphite (sodium bisulphite) (E222), sodium metabisulphite (E223), potassium metabisulphite (E224), calcium sulphite (E226), calcium hydrogen sulphite (calcium bisulphite) (E227)	'Free from' is to be interpreted as contains less than 1 mg/kg free sulphur dioxide as determined by the Tanner* method or an equivalent technique
Benzoate	Benzoic acid (E210), sodium benzoate (E211), potassium benzoate (E212), calcium benzoate (E213), ethyl 4−hydroxybenzoate (ethyl para-hydroxybenzoate) (E214), ethyl 4-hydroxybenzoate, Na Salt (sodium ethyl para-hydroxybenzoate) (E215), propyl 4−hydroxybenzoate (propyl para-hydroxybenzote) (E216), propyl 4−hydroxybenzoate, Na salt (sodium propyl para-hydroxybenzoate) (E217), methyl 4-hydroxybenzoate (methyl para-hydroxybenzoate) (E218), methyl 4-hydroxybenzoate, Na salt (sodium methyl para-hydroxybenzoate) (E219)	'Free from' is interpreted as contains less than 1 mg/kg benzoate as calculated from the level of addition to the food having due regard to the presence of these compounds in ingredients and thereby carried over into the final food
Glutamate	L-glutamic acid 620, sodium hydrogen L-glutamate (mono Sodium glutamate or MSG) (621), potassium hydrogen L-glutamate (mono Potassium glutamate) (622), calcium dihydrogen di-L-glutamate (calcium glutamate) (623)	'Free from' is to be interpreted as contains no added glutamate either in one of these forms or in the form of a protein hydrolysed before addition
Azo colour	Amaranth (E123), Black PH (E151), Brown FK (154), Brown HT (155), Carmoisine (122), Pigment Rubine (E180), Ponceau 4R (E124), Red 2G (128), Sunset Yellow (E110), Tartrazine (E102), Yellow 2G (107)	'Free from', is to be interpreted as contains no added azo colour

*Tanner H (1963) *Mitt Geb Lebensmitt u Hyg* **54**, 158. An English text is a suitable procedure based upon the Tanner method, included in the LFRA *Analytical Methods Manual*.

The databank was set up, and was in operation by the end of 1986. At the time of writing, lists of foods 'free' from any combination of wheat, milk, egg, soya, cocoa, sulphur dioxide, benzoate, glutamate, azo colour and the antioxidants BHA and BHT can be produced, and used in the diagnosis and management of food intolerances.

The definition of 'free from' caused the Working Party great problems, there being virtually no evidence in the medical literature on the levels of ingredients or additives in foods which can provoke reactions in a susceptible individual. The definitions finally adopted in September 1986 are given in Table 6.29.

The RCP/BNF Joint Report also concluded that 'The dietary approach to the management of food intolerance is particularly complex and may lead to nutritional difficulties and social disruption. There are considerable dangers in the unsupervised use of diets, especially for infants and young children'.

The working party accepted this conclusion. The information on the databank is therefore only available to State Registered Dietitians, and the lists can only be obtained from dietitians as part of a medically prescribed diet. They include a warning against the risks of self-diagnosis and self-treatment.

Reference

RCP/BNF (1984) Food intolerance and food aversion. A Joint Report of the Royal College of Physicians and the British Nutrition Foundation. *J Roy Coll Physicians London* **18**, No 2.

6.5 Useful Addresses

This list includes addresses of manufacturers/distributors of dietetic products professional associations and patient support organisations

Abbott Laboratories Ltd, Queensborough, Kent ME11 5 EL. Tel: Sheerness 663371

Action against Allergy, 43 The Downs, London SW20 8HS. Tel: 01 947 5082

Action for Research into Multiple Sclerosis (ARMS), 11 Dartmouth Street, London SW1.

ARMS Research Unit, Central Middlesex Hospital, Acton Lane, London NW10 7NS. Tel: 01 961 4911

Alembic Products Ltd, Oaklands House, Oaklands Drive, Sale, Manchester M33 1WS. Tel: 061 962 4423

The Alfawap Trust Fund Ltd, 4 Woodchurch Road, London NW6.

Allen and Hanbury Ltd, Horsenden House, Oldfield Lane North, Greenford, Middlesex UB6 OHB. Tel: 01 422 4225

Anorexic Aid, Priory Centre, 11 Priory Road, High Wycombe, Bucks.

Ashe Laboratories Ltd, Ashetree Works, Kingston Road, Leatherhead, Surrey KT22 7JZ. Tel: Leatherhead 376151

Association for Spina Bifida and Hydrocephalus, Tavistock House North, Tavistock Square, London WC1H 9HJ. Tel: 01 388 1382

Asthma Society and Friends of Asthma Research Council, St Thomas's Hospital, Lambeth Palace Road, London SE1 7EH. Tel: 01 261 0110

Bayer UK Ltd, Bayer House, Strawberry Hill, Newbury, Berks RG13 1JA. Tel: 0635 39000

Beecham Products, Beecham House, Great West Road, Brentford, Middlesex TW8 9BD. Tel: 01 560 5151

Bencard, Great West Road, Brentford, Middlesex TW8 9BD. Tel: 01 560 5151

Boots Company plc, 1 Thane Road West, Nottingham NG2 3AA. Tel: Nottingham 56111

Bow Produce Ltd, 15 Ashurst Close, Northwood Middlesex HA6 1 EL.

Braille Unit, Aylesbury Youth Custody Centre, HM Prison, Brereton Road, Aylesbury, Bucks.

Braille Unit, HM Prison Wakefield, 5 Live Lane, Wakefield WF2 9AG.

E Braun (Medical) Ltd, Evett Close, Stocklake, Aylesbury, Bucks HP 20 1DN. Tel: Aylesbury 32626

Bristol–Myers Pharmaceuticals, Swakeleys House, Milton Road, Ickenham, Uxbridge UB10 8NS.Tel: 0985 639911

British Diabetic Association, 10 Queen Anne Street, London W1M OBD. Tel: 01 323 1531

British Dietetic Association, Daimler House, Paradise Circus Queensway, Birmingham B1 2BJ. Tel: 021 643 5483

British Goat Society, Rougham, Bury St Edmunds, Suffolk.

British Institute of Mental Handicap, Wolverhampton Road Kidderminster, Worcs DY 10 3PP. Tel: 0562 850 251

British Kidney Patients Association, Bordon, Hants.

British Nutrition Foundation, 15 Belgrave Square, London SW1X 8PS Tel: 01 235 4904

British Rheumatism and Arthritis Association, 6 Grosvenor Crescent, London SW1X 7ER. Tel: 01 235 0902/5

British Sheep Dairying Association, Mrs Mills (Hon Sec), Wield Wood Farm, Nr Alresford, Hants.

Britannia Pharmaceuticals Ltd, Forum House, 41–75 Brighton Road, Redhill, Surrey RH1 6YS. Tel: 0737 73116

Butter Information Council Ltd, Tubs Hill House, London Road, Sevenoaks, Kent TN13 1BL. Tel: 0732 460060

Cantassium Company, Larkhall Laboratories, 225 Putney Bridge Road, London SW15 2PY. Tel: 01 870 0971

Carnation Foods Company Ltd, Danesfield House, Medmenham, Marlow, Bucks SL7 2ES.

Cassenne Ltd, Roussel House, Wembley, Middlesex HA9 ONF. Tel: 01 903 7881

Castle Priory College, Thames Street, Wallingford, Oxfordshire OX10 DHE.

Castlemead Publications, Swain Mill, 4A Crane Mead, Ware, Herts SG12 9PY.

Centre for Policy on Ageing, Nuffield Lodge, Regent's Park, London NW1 4RS. Tel: 01 722 8771

Chest, Heart and Stroke Association, Tavistock House North Tavistock Square, London WLIH 9JE. Tel: 01 387 3012/3/4

Child Poverty Action Group (CPAG), 1–5 Bath Street, London EC1V 9TY. Tel: 01 253 3406

CIBA Laboratories, Wimblehurst Road, Horsham, West Sussex RH12 4AB. Tel: Horsham 50101

Coeliac Society, PO Box 220, High Wycombe, Bucks HP11 2HY. Tel: 0494 37278

Coronary Prevention Group, Central Middlesex Hospital, Acton Lane, London NW10 7NS. Tel: 01 965 5733 ext 2330 or 01 961 6993

Cow and Gate Ltd, Cow and Gate House, Trowbridge, Wilts BA14 8YX. Tel: Trowbridge 68381

Crookes Products Ltd, PO Box 94, 1 Thane Road West, Nottingham NG2 3AA. Tel: Nottingham 57431

Cystic Fibrosis Research Trust, Alexandra House, 5 Blyth Road, Bromley, Kent BR1 3RS. Tel: 01 464 7211

Department of Agriculture and Fisheries in Scotland, Chesser House, 500 Gorgie Road, Edinburgh EH11 3AW.

Department of Health and Social Security, Hannibal House, Elephant and Castle, London SE1 6TE. Tel: 01 703 6380 (Dietetic officer: ext. 3470)

Disabled Living Foundation, 380–384 Harrow Road, London W9.

Down's Syndrone Association, 12/13 Clapham Common Southside, London SW4 7AA. Tel: 01 720 0008

Duncan, Flockhart and Company Ltd, 700 Oldfield Lane North, Greenford, Middlesex UB6 OHD. Tel: 01 422 2331

EEC Commission, 8 Storey's Gate, London SWIP 3AT.

Familial Hypercholesterolaemia Association, PO Box 133, High Wycombe, Bucks HP 13 6LF.,

Farley Health Products Ltd, Torr Lane, Plymouth PL3 5UA. Tel: 0752 24151

Farmitalia Carlo Erba Ltd Products distributed by Ultrapharm Ltd.

Food and Drink Federation, 6 Catherine Street, London WC2B 5JJ. 01 836 2460

Food Watch, High Acre, East Stour, Gillingham, Dorset. Tel: 0747 85261

Foresight, The Old Vicarage, Witley, Godalming, Surrey GU8 5PN. Tel: 042 879 4500

Foundation for Education and Research in Childbearing, 27 Walpole Street, London SW3.

Fresenius Ltd, 50 Brindley Road, Astmoor Industrial Estate, Runcorn, Cheshire WA7 1PG. Tel: 09285 65011

Geistlich Sons Ltd, Newton Bank, Long Lane, Chester CH2 3QZ. Tel: Chester 47534

General Designs Ltd, PO Box 38E, Worcester Park, Surrey KT4 7LX Tel: 01 337 9366

Gerontology Nutrition Unit, Royal Free Hospital School of Medicine, 21 Pond Street, London NW3 2PN.

GF Dietary Group of Companies Ltd, 494−496 Honeypot Lane, Stanmore, Middlesex HA7 1JH. Tel: 01 206 0522
01 951 5155
01 204 6968

Health Education Authority 78 New Oxford Street, London WC1A 1AH. Tel: 01 631 0930

Health Visitors Association, 50 Southwark Street, London SE1 1UN. Tel: 01 378 7255

Her Majesty's Stationery Office (HMSO), 49 High Holborn, London WC1V 6HB. Tel: 01 211 5656

Hospital Caterers Association, 43 Royston Road, Penge, London SE20 7QW.

Hyperactive Children's Support Group, Sally Bunday (Secretary), 59 Meadowside, Angmering, West Sussex BN14 4BW. Tel: 0706 725182

Hypoguard Ltd, Dock Lane, Melton, Woodbridge, Suffolk IP12 1PE.

Ileostomy Association of Great Britain and Ireland, Amblehurst House, Chobham, Woking, Surrey GU24 8PZ.

Kabi Vitrum Ltd, Kabi Vitrum House, Riverside Way, Uxbridge, Middlesex UB8 2YF. Tel: Uxbridge 51144

La Leche League. PO Box BM 3424, London WC1V 6XV. Tel: 01 404 5011

Local Authorities Co-ordinating Body on Trading Standards (LACOTS), PO Box 6, Fell Road, Croydon CR9 1LG.

London Food Commission, PO Box 291, London N5 1DU. Tel: 01 633 5782

Maternity Alliance, 59−61 Camden High Street, London NW1 7JL.

MCP Pharmaceuticals Ltd, Simpson Parkway, Kirkton Campus, Livingston, West Lothian EH54 7BH. Tel: Livingston 412512

Mead Johnson, Division of Bristol−Myers Co Ltd, Swakeleys House, Milton Road, Ickenham, Uxbridge UB10 8NS Tel: 0985 639911

MENCAP, 123 Golden Lane, London EC1Y ORT. Tel: 01 253 9433

E Merck Ltd, Winchester Road, Four Marks, Alton, Hants GU34 5HG. Tel: Alton 64011

Migraine Trust, 45 Great Ormond Street, London WC1N 3HD. Tel: 01 278 2676

Milk Marketing Board, Thames Ditton, Surrey KT7 OEL. Tel: 01 398 4101

Milupa Ltd, Rivermeade, Oxford Road, Denham, Uxbridge, Middlesex. Tel: 0895 72121

Ministry of Agriculture, Fisheries and Food, Horseferry Road, London SW1P 2AE.

Monastery of Poor Clares, Green Lane, Liverpool L18 2ES.

Multiple Sclerosis Society, 286 Munster Road, London SW6 6AP. Tel: 01 381 4022/5

Muscular Dystrophy Society, Natrass House, 35 Macauley Road, London SW4 OQP. Tel: 01 720 8055

National Association for Colitis and Crohn's Disease, 98A London Road, St Albans, Herts AL1 1NX. (Postal contact only)

National Association for Maternal and Child Wefare (NAMLW), 1 South Audley Street, London W1Y 6JS. Tel: 01 491 1315

National Association for the Welfare of Children in Hospital (NAWCH), Argyle House, 29−31 Euston Road, London NW1.

National Autistic Society, 276 Willesden Lane, London NW2 5RB.

National Childbirth Trust, 9 Queensborough Terrace, Bayswater, London W2 3TB Tel: 01 229 9319

National Coaching Foundation Information Service, 4 College Close, Beckett Park, Leeds LS6 3QH.

National Dairy Council, John Princes Street, London W1M OAP. Tel: 01 499 7822

National Eczema Society, Tavistock House North, Tavistock Square, London WC1H 9SR. Tel: 01 388 4097

National Extension College, 1 Brooklands Avenue, Cambridge CB2 2HN.

National Federation of Kidney Patients' Association (NFKPA), Mr B Pearmain (Chairman), Swan House, The Street, Wickham Skeith, Eye, Suffolk.

National Information for Parents of Prematures, Education, Resources and Support (NIPPERS), St Mary's Hospital, Praed Street, London W2.

National Metrological Co-ordination Unit (NMCU), PO Box 6, Fell Road, Croydon CR9 1LG.

National Society for Phenylketonuria and Allied Disorders, 26 Towngate Grove, Mirfield, West Yorkshire.

National Society for Research into Allergy, PO Box 45, Hinckley, Leicestershire LE10 1JY. (Postal contact only)

Nestlé Company Ltd, Health Care Division, St Georges House, Croydon, Surrey CR9 1NR. Tel: 01 686 3333

Newform Foods Ltd, 494−496 Honeypot Lane, Stanmore, Middlesex HA7 1JH. Tel: 01 206 0522
01 951 5155

Norwich Eaton Ltd, Hedley House, St Nicholas Avenue, Gosforth, Newcastle-upon-Tyne WC NE99 1EE. Tel: 091 279 2100

Novo Laboratories Ltd, Ringway House, Bell Road, Daneshill East, Basingstoke, Hampshire RG 24 0QN.

Nutrition Society, Grosvenor Gardens House, 35−37 Grosvenor Gardens, London SW1W OBS. Tel: 01 821 1243

Open University, PO Box 188, Milton Keynes MKJ 6DH.

Oxford Nutrition, PO Box 31, Oxford OX2 6HB.

Partially Sighted Society, 40 Wordsworth Street, Hove, Sussex BN3 5BH.

Patients' Association, Room 33, 18 Charing Cross Road, London WC2 OHR. Tel: 01 240 0671

Potato Marketing Board, 50 Hans Crescent, London SW1X ONB.

Prader Willi Syndrome Association, 30 Follett Drive, Abbot's Langley, Herts WD5 OLP.

Procea, Alexandra Road, Dublin 1, Eire. Tel: Dublin 741741

Roussel Laboratories Ltd, Roussel House, North End Road, Wembley Park Middlesex HA9 ONF. Tel: 01 903 1454

Royal College of Physicians, 11 St Andrews Place, Regents Park, London NW1 4LE. Tel: 01 935 1174

Royal National Institute for the Blind (RN1B), 224 Great Portland Street, London W1N 6AA. Tel: 01 388 1266

Rybar Laboratories Ltd, 25 Sycamore Road, Amersham, Bucks HP6 5PQ. Tel: Amersham 22741

Sandoz Products Ltd, Sandoz House, 98 The Centre, Feltham, Middlesex TW13 4EP. Tel: 01 890 1366

Schizophrenia Association of Great Britain, Tyr Twr, Llanfair Hall, Caernarvon, North Wales. Tel: 0248 670379

Scientific Hospital Supplies Ltd, 38 Queensland Street, Liverpool L7 3JG. Tel: 051 708 8008

Scottish Health Education Group, Woodburn House, Canaan Lane, Edinburgh EH10 4SG. Tel: 031 447 8044

Scottish Home and Health Department, St Andrew's House, Edinburgh EH1 3DE.

Searle Pharmaceuticals, PO Box 53, Lane End Road, High Wycombe, Bucks HP12 4HL. Tel: High Wycombe 21124

Spastics Society, 12 Park Crescent, London W1N 4EQ Tel: 01 636 5020

Travenol Laboratories Ltd, Caxton Way, Thetford, Norfolk IP24 3SE. Tel: Thetford 4581

Ultrapharm Ltd, PO Box 18, Henley on Thames, Oxon. RG9 Tel: 0491 578076

Unigreg Ltd, Spa House, 15–17 Worple Road, Wimbledon, London SW19 4JS. Tel:01 946 9871

Vegan Society, 47 Highlands Road, Leatherhead, Surrey.

Vegetarian Society, Parkdale, Denham Road, Altrincham, Cheshire.

Wander Ltd, Station Road, Kings Langley, Herts WD4 8LJ. Tel: 09277 66122

Welfare Foods (Stockport; Ltd, 63 London Road South, Poynton, Stockport, Cheshire SK12 ILA. Tel: 0625 877387

Wyeth Laboratories, Huntercombe Lane South, Taplow, Maidenhead, Berks SL6 OPH. Tel: Burnham 4377

Index

xanthine stones, 468
xylitol, 222
    dental caries and, 223
    diabetic use, 241
    gastrointestinal side effects, 223
    labelling, 241

yang foods, 303, 311
yeast sensitivity, 182, 176, 579
yin foods, 303, 311
Yom Kippur, 310

zen macrobiotic diets, 303
zinc
    absorption, 166
    alcohol and, 161, 167, 245, 246
    chelating agents and, 161, 167, 429
    in elderly, 284
    intake in tea and coffee, 165
    low birth weight infant formulae and,
       558
    in low income groups, 293
    oral contraceptives and, 246
    penicillamine interaction, 429
    pregnancy and, 248, 249, 250

zinc deficiency
    acrodermatitis enteropathica and, 435
    Crohn's disease and, 416, 418
    drugs and, 591
    end stage renal disease in children and,
      457
    small-for-dates babies and, 249
    sperm number and, 245
    thiazide diuretics and, 286
zinc supplements
    burn injury and, 542
    cystic fibrosis and, 404
    proprietary, 208